W9-BYG-311

BLACK'S
MEDICAL
DICTIONARY

BLACK'S
MEDICAL
DICTIONARY
41ST EDITION

Edited by
Dr Harvey Marcovitch

The Scarecrow Press, Inc.
Lanham, Maryland, and Oxford
2006

41st edition published in the United States of America in 2006
by Scarecrow Press, Inc.
A wholly owned subsidiary of
The Rowman & Littlefield Publishing Group, Inc.
4501 Forbes Boulevard, Suite 200, Lanham, Maryland 20706
www.scarecrowpress.com

ISBN 10: 0-8108-5713-8
ISBN 13: 978-0-8108-5713-1

This edition first published in Great Britain in 2005 by
A & C Black Publishers Limited
38 Soho Square, London W1D 3HB
www.acblack.com

Cataloging-in-Publication data is available from the Library of Congress

A & C Black uses paper produced with elemental chlorine-free pulp,
harvested from managed sustainable forests.

Typeset in Adobe Garamond by RefineCatch Limited, Bungay, Suffolk

Printed and bound in Great Britain by William Clowes Ltd, Beccles, Suffolk

CONTENTS

90,599

CONTENTS

PREFACE

Black's Medical Dictionary first appeared in 1906. That new century was to see health care in the United Kingdom evolve from a largely personal, paternalistic consultation between doctor and patient, based more on medical tradition than medical science, to a complex, science-based, team-oriented and managed service. Even so, the core of medical practice has survived: the face-to-face consultation between doctor and patient. But the nature of this core activity has been irreversibly altered by a shift in the 'balance of power' between the participants as patients became better informed about their health, illnesses and possible treatments. A significant catalyst in the emergence of the informed patient has been the media, including publications like this dictionary, the contents of which have during its 41 editions reflected these changes in medicine.

One modest constant in this sea of change, however, has been the objective of *Black's Medical Dictionary*. When launching the first edition, the editor, Edinburgh physician John D. Comrie, declared his aim as being to produce 'a work which would occupy a position somewhere between that of a Technical Dictionary of Medicine and one intended merely for the domestic treatment of common ailments . . . [giving] information in simple language upon medical subjects of importance and general interest'. That initial mission-statement underpins this first edition of the 21st century.

Entries in the 41st edition have undergone major revision where medical knowledge or research has resulted in greater understanding or changed practice. These include anaesthesia, breast screening and mammography, chronic fatigue syndrome, clinical guidelines, clinical trials, evidence-based medicine, Gulf War syndrome, hormone replacement therapy and post-traumatic stress disorder. Ironically the greatest changes in British medicine seem to be taking place in how doctors are required to work, rather than what they actually do. Many of the bodies which constitute the National Health Service have been replaced or merged, new ones have come into existence and functions changed. I predict that such reorganisation will continue throughout the life of this edition, so readers wishing to check on how the NHS works may need to refer to other sources to be absolutely sure of remaining up-to-date.

Black's Medical Dictionary is neither a textbook of medicine nor a formulary of therapeutic drugs. The many drugs that are included are given their generic title as used in the *British Pharmacopoeia.* Patients are individuals who react in varying ways to injuries, diseases and their treatments. Appendix 1 explains some basic first-aid procedures, but patients' own doctors are normally the appropriate source for personal medical advice. The dictionary should, however, help readers to decide when it would be wise to seek medical advice and subsequently help them to set such advice in context.

Although every effort has been made to ensure accuracy, neither the publishers nor the author can be held responsible for any consequences if readers use the book for the treatment of themselves or others.

Acknowledgements

I am grateful to colleagues who have updated or rewritten entries. They include: Dr Phil Alderson, Professor Michael Baum, Dr Karin Fuchs, Dr Pamela Laurie, Dr Richard Lehman, Mr John McGarry, Dr Klim McPherson, Mr Michael Paynton, Dr Rob Miller and Professor Simon Wessely.

HARVEY MARCOVITCH

Note: The use of small capitals – for instance – STOMACH, refers the reader to the entry of that name for additional information.

A & E Medicine

See ACCIDENT AND EMERGENCY MEDICINE.

Abdomen

The lower part of the trunk. Above, and separated from it by the diaphragm, lies the thorax or chest, and below lies the PELVIS, generally described as a separate cavity though continuous with that of the abdomen. Behind are the SPINAL COLUMN and lower ribs, which come within a few inches of the iliac bones. At the sides the contained organs are protected by the iliac bones and down-sloping ribs, but in front the whole extent is protected only by soft tissues. The latter consist of the skin, a varying amount of fat, three layers of broad, flat muscle, another layer of fat, and finally the smooth, thin PERITONEUM which lines the whole cavity. These soft tissues allow the necessary distension when food is taken into the STOMACH, and the various important movements of the organs associated with digestion. The shape of the abdomen varies; in children it may protrude considerably, though if this is too marked it may indicate disease. In healthy young adults it should be either slightly prominent or slightly indrawn, and should show the outline of the muscular layer, especially of the pair of muscles running vertically (recti), which are divided into four or five sections by transverse lines. In older people fat is usually deposited on and inside the abdomen. In pregnancy the abdomen enlarges from the 12th week after conception as the FETUS in the UTERUS grows (see PREGNANCY AND LABOUR; ANTENATAL CARE).

Contents The principal contents of the abdominal cavity are the digestive organs, i.e. the stomach and INTESTINE, and the associated glands, the LIVER and PANCREAS. The position

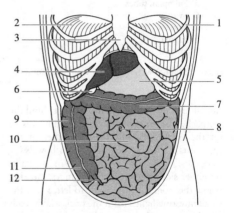

1	6th costal cartilage	7	transverse colon
2	diaphragm	8	position of umbilicus
3	xiphoid process	9	right flexure of colon
4	liver	10	small intestine
5	stomach	11	caecum
6	gall-bladder	12	appendix

Contents of the abdomen in position.

of the stomach is above and to the left when the individual is lying down, but may be much lower when standing. The liver lies above and to the right, largely under cover of the ribs, and occupying the hollow of the diaphragm. The two KIDNEYS lie against the back wall on either side, protected by the last two ribs. From the kidneys run the URETERS, or urinary ducts, down along the back wall to the URINARY BLADDER in the pelvis. The pancreas lies across the spine between the kidneys, and on the upper end of each kidney is a suprarenal gland

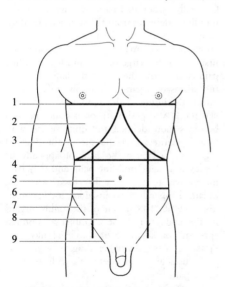

1	xiphisternal plane
2	hypochondriac region
3	epigastrium
4	right lumbar region
5	umbilical region
6	right iliac region
7	right anterior superior iliac spine
8	hypogastric region
9	inguinal region

Regions of the abdomen.

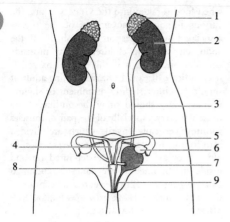

1 left adrenal gland
2 left kidney
3 left ureter
4 uterus
5 Fallopian tubes
6 ovary
7 bladder
8 vagina
9 urethra

Position of renal system on rear wall of abdomen.

(see ADRENAL GLANDS). The SPLEEN is positioned high up on the left and partly behind the stomach. The great blood vessels and nerves lie on the back wall, and the remainder of the space is taken up by the intestines or bowels (see INTESTINE). The large intestine lies in the flanks on either side in front of the kidneys, crossing below the stomach from right to left, while the small intestine hangs from the back wall in coils which fill up the spaces between the other organs. Hanging down from the stomach in front of the bowels is the OMENTUM, or apron, containing much fat and helping to protect the bowels. In pregnancy the UTERUS, or womb, rises up from the pelvis into the abdomen as it increases in size, lifting the coils of the small intestine above it.

The PELVIS is the part of the abdomen within the bony pelvis (see BONE), and contains the rectum or end part of the intestine, the bladder, and in the male the PROSTATE GLAND; in the female the uterus, OVARIES, and FALLOPIAN TUBES.

Abdomen, Acute

See ABDOMEN, DISEASES OF.

Abdomen, Diseases of

See under STOMACH, DISEASES OF; INTESTINE, DISEASES OF; DIARRHOEA; LIVER, DISEASES OF;

PANCREAS, DISEASES OF; GALL-BLADDER, DISEASES OF; KIDNEYS, DISEASES OF; URINARY BLADDER, DISEASES OF; HERNIA; PERITONITIS; APPENDICITIS; TUMOUR.

Various processes that can occur include inflammation, ulceration, infection or tumour. Abdominal disease may be of rapid onset, described as acute, or more long-term when it is termed chronic.

An 'acute abdomen' is most commonly caused by peritonitis – inflammation of the membrane that lines the abdomen. If any structure in the abdomen gets inflamed, peritonitis may result. Causes include injury, inflammation of the Fallopian tubes (SALPINGITIS), and intestinal disorders such as APPENDICITIS, CROHN'S DISEASE, DIVERTICULITIS or a perforated PEPTIC ULCER. Disorders of the GALL-BLADDER or URINARY TRACT may also result in acute abdominal pain.

General symptoms of abdominal disease include:

Pain This is usually ill-defined but can be very unpleasant, and is termed visceral pain. Pain is initially felt near the mid line of the abdomen. Generally, abdominal pain felt high up in the mid line originates from the stomach and duodenum. Pain that is felt around the umbilicus arises from the small intestine, appendix and first part of the large bowel, and low mid-line pain comes from the rest of the large bowel. If the diseased organ secondarily inflames or infects the lining of the abdominal wall – the PERITONEUM – peritonitis occurs and the pain becomes more defined and quite severe, with local tenderness over the site of the diseased organ itself. Hence the pain of appendicitis begins as a vague mid-line pain, and only later moves over to the right iliac fossa, when the inflamed appendix has caused localised peritonitis. PERFORATION of one of the hollow organs in the abdomen – for example, a ruptured appendix or a gastric or duodenal ulcer (see STOMACH, DISEASES OF) eroding the wall of the gut – usually causes peritonitis with resulting severe pain.

The character of the pain is also important. It may be constant, as occurs in inflammatory diseases and infections, or colicky (intermittent) as in intestinal obstruction.

Swelling The commonest cause of abdominal swelling in women is pregnancy. In disease, swelling may be due to the accumulation of trapped intestinal contents within the bowel, the presence of free fluid (ascites) within the abdomen, or enlargement of one or more of the abdominal organs due to benign causes or tumour.

Constipation is the infrequent or incomplete passage of FAECES; sometimes only flatus can be passed and, rarely, no bowel movements occur (see main entry for CONSTIPATION). It is often associated with abdominal swelling. In intestinal obstruction, the onset of symptoms is usually rapid with complete constipation and severe, colicky pain. In chronic constipation, the symptoms occur more gradually.

Nausea and vomiting may be due to irritation of the stomach, or to intestinal obstruction when it may be particularly foul and persistent. There are also important nonabdominal causes, such as in response to severe pain or motion sickness.

Diarrhoea is most commonly due to simple and self-limiting infection, such as food poisoning, but may also indicate serious disease, especially if it is persistent or contains blood (see main entry for DIARRHOEA).

Jaundice is a yellow discoloration of the skin and eyes, and may be due to disease in the liver or bile ducts (see main entry for JAUNDICE).

Diagnosis and treatment Abdominal diseases are often difficult to diagnose because of the multiplicity of the organs contained within the abdomen, their inconstant position and the vagueness of some of the symptoms. Correct diagnosis usually requires experience, often supplemented by specialised investigations such as ULTRASOUND. For this reason sufferers should obtain medical advice at an early stage, particularly if the symptoms are severe, persistent, recurrent, or resistant to simple remedies.

Abducent Nerve

This is the sixth nerve rising from the brain and controls the external rectus muscle of the EYE, which turns the eye outwards. It is particularly liable to be paralysed in diseases of the nervous system, thus leading to an inward squint.

Abduct

To abduct means to move a part of the body – for example, a limb – away from the mid line. (Opposite: ADDUCT.)

Ablation

Ablation means the removal of any part of the body by a surgical operation.

Abnormal

A structure or process that is not normal (typical, usual or conforming to the standard); differing from the usual condition of the body.

ABO Blood Groups

See BLOOD GROUPS.

Abortifacient

An abortifacient is a drug which causes artificial ABORTION.

Abortion

Abortion is defined as the expulsion of a FETUS before it is normally viable, usually before 24 weeks of pregnancy. (There are exceptional cases nowadays in which fetuses as young as 22 weeks' gestation have survived.) (See also PREGNANCY AND LABOUR.)

Spontaneous abortion Often called miscarriage, this may occur at any time before 28 weeks; 85 per cent occur in the first 12 weeks of pregnancy. Of all diagnosed pregnancies, 25 per cent end in spontaneous abortion.

Spontaneous abortions occurring in early pregnancy are almost always associated with chromosomal abnormalities of the fetus. Other causes are uterine shape, maternal disorders such as DIABETES MELLITUS, diseases of the thyroid gland (see under ENDOCRINE GLANDS), and problems with the immune system (see IMMUNITY). Recurrent spontaneous abortion (that is, three or more) seems to be a particular problem in women who have an abnormal response of their immune system to pregnancy. Other factors include being older, having had a lot of babies previously, cigarette smoking and spontaneous (but not therapeutic) abortions in the past.

Early ULTRASOUND scans have altered the management of spontaneous abortions. These make it possible to distinguish between threatened abortion, where a woman has had some vaginal bleeding but the fetus is alive; inevitable abortion, where the neck of the uterus has started to open up; incomplete abortion, where part of the fetus or placenta is lost but some remains inside the uterus; and complete abortion. There is no evidence that bed rest is effective in stopping a threatened abortion becoming inevitable.

Inevitable or incomplete abortion will usually require a gynaecologist to empty (evacuate) the uterus. (Complete miscarriage requires no treatment.) Evacuation of the uterus is carried out using local or general anaesthetic, usually gentle dilatation of the neck of the uterus (cervix), and curetting-out the remaining products of the pregnancy.

A few late abortions are associated with the cervix opening too early, abnormal structural abnormalities of the uterus, and possibly infection in the mother.

Drugs are often used to suppress uterine contractions, but evidence-based studies show that these do not generally improve fetal salvage. In proven cases of cervical incompetence, the cervix can be closed with a suture which is removed at 37 weeks' gestation. The evidence for the value of this procedure is uncertain.

Therapeutic abortion In the UK, before an abortion procedure is legally permitted, two doctors must agree and sign a form defined under the 1967 Abortion Act that the continuation of the pregnancy would involve risk – greater than if the pregnancy were terminated – of injury to the physical and/or mental health of the mother or any existing child(ren).

Legislation in 1990 modified the Act, which had previously stated that, at the time of the abortion, the pregnancy should not have exceeded the 24th week. Now, an abortion may legally be performed if continuing the pregnancy would risk the woman's life, or the mental health of the woman or her existing child(ren) is at risk, or if there is a substantial risk of serious handicap to the baby. In 95 per cent of therapeutic terminations in the UK the reason is 'risk of injury to the physical or mental health of the woman'.

There is no time limit on therapeutic abortion where the termination is done to save the mother's life, there is substantial risk of serious fetal handicap, or of grave permanent injury to the health of the mother.

About 190,000 terminations are carried out in the UK each year and only 1–1.5 per cent are over 20 weeks' gestation, with the vast majority of these late abortions being for severe, late-diagnosed, fetal abnormality.

The maternal mortality from therapeutic abortion is less than 1 per 100,000 women and, provided that the procedure is performed skilfully by experienced doctors before 12 weeks of pregnancy, it is very safe. There is no evidence that therapeutic abortion is associated with any reduction in future fertility, increased rates of spontaneous abortion or preterm birth in subsequent pregnancies.

Methods of abortion All abortions must be carried out in premises licensed for doing so or in NHS hospitals. The method used is either surgical or medical, with the latter being used more and the former less as time goes on. Proper consent must be obtained, signed for and witnessed. Women under 16 years of age can consent to termination provided that the doctors obtaining the consent are sure she clearly understands the procedure and its implications. Parental consent in the under-16s is not legally required, but counselling doctors have a duty to record that they have advised young people to inform their parents. However, many youngsters do not do so. The woman's partner has no legal say in the decision to terminate her pregnancy.

MEDICAL METHODS A combination of two drugs, mifepristone and a prostaglandin (or a prostaglandin-like drug, misoprostol – see PROSTAGLANDINS), may be used to terminate a pregnancy up to 63 days' gestation. A similar regime can be used between nine and 12 weeks but at this gestation there is a 5 per cent risk of post-treatment HAEMORRHAGE.

An ultrasound scan is first done to confirm pregnancy and gestation. The sac containing the developing placenta and fetus must be in the uterus; the woman must be under 35 years of age if she is a moderate smoker, but can be over 35 if she is a non-smoker. Reasons for not using this method include women with diseases of the ADRENAL GLANDS, on long-term CORTICOSTEROIDS, and those who have a haemorrhagic disorder or who are on ANTICOAGULANTS. The drugs cannot be used in women with severe liver or kidney disease, and caution is required in those with CHRONIC OBSTRUCTIVE PULMONARY DISEASE (COPD), disease of the cardiovascular system, or prosthetic heart valves (see PROSTHESIS), as well as with those who have had a CAESAREAN SECTION or an ECTOPIC PREGNANCY in the past or who are being treated for HYPERTENSION.

Some clinics use this drug combination for pregnancies older than 12 weeks. In pregnancies approaching viability (20 weeks), pre-treatment fetocide (killing of the fetus) with intrauterine drug therapy may be required.

SURGICAL METHODS Vacuum curettage is a method used up to 14–15 weeks. Some very experienced gynaecologists will perform abortions surgically by dilating the cervix and evacuating the uterine contents up to 22 weeks' gestation. The greater the size of the pregnancy, the higher the risk of haemorrhage and perforation of the uterus. In the UK, illegal abortion is rare but in other countries this is not the case. Where illegal abortions are done, the risks of infection and perforation are high and death a definite risk. Legal abortions are generally safe. In the USA, partial-birth abortions are spoken of but, in fact, there is no such procedure recorded in the UK medical journals.

Abrasion

Abrasion means the rubbing-off of the surface of the skin or of a mucous membrane due to some mechanical injury. Such injuries, though slight in themselves, are apt to allow the entrance of dirt-containing organisms, and so to lead to an ABSCESS or some more severe form of inflammation.

Treatment The most effective form of treatment consists in the thorough and immediate cleansing of the wound with soap and water. An antiseptic such as 1 per cent cetrimide can then be applied, and a sterile dry dressing.

Abreaction

An emotional release caused by the recall of past unpleasant experiences. This is normally the result of psychoanalytical treatment in which psychotherapy, certain drugs, or hypnosis (see HYPNOTISM) are used to effect the abreaction. The technique is used in the treatment of anxiety, hysteria, or other neurotic states.

Abruptio Placenta

Placental bleeding after the 24th week of pregnancy, which may result in complete or partial detachment of the placenta from the wall of the womb. The woman may go into shock. The condition is sometimes associated with raised blood pressure and PRE-ECLAMPSIA. (See also PREGNANCY AND LABOUR.)

Abscess

A localised collection of pus. A minute abscess is known as a PUSTULE; a diffused production of pus is known as CELLULITIS or ERYSIPELAS. An abscess may be acute or chronic. An acute abscess is one which develops rapidly within the course of a few days or hours. It is characterised by a definite set of symptoms.

Causes The direct cause is various BACTERIA. Sometimes the presence of foreign bodies, such as bullets or splinters, may produce an abscess, but these foreign bodies may remain buried in the tissues without causing any trouble provided that they are not contaminated by bacteria or other micro-organisms.

The micro-organisms most frequently found are staphylococci (see STAPHYLOCOCCUS), and, next to these, streptococci (see STREPTOCOC-

CUS) – though the latter cause more virulent abscesses. Other abscess-forming organisms are *Pseudomonas pyocyanea* and *Escherichia coli*, which live always in the bowels and under certain conditions wander into the surrounding tissues, producing abscesses.

The presence of micro-organisms is not sufficient in itself to produce suppuration (see IMMUNITY; INFECTION); streptococci can often be found on the skin and in the skin glands of perfectly healthy individuals. Whether they will produce abscesses or not depends upon the virulence of the organism and the individual's natural resistance.

When bacteria have gained access – for example, to a wound – they rapidly multiply, produce toxins, and cause local dilatation of the blood vessels, slowing of the bloodstream, and exudation of blood corpuscles and fluid. The LEUCOCYTES, or white corpuscles of the blood, collect around the invaded area and destroy the bacteria either by consuming them (see PHAGO-CYTOSIS) or by forming a toxin that kills them. If the body's local defence mechanisms fail to do this, the abscess will spread and may in severe cases cause generalised infection or SEPTICAEMIA.

Symptoms The classic symptoms of inflammation are redness, warmth, swelling, pain and fever. The neighbouring lymph nodes may be swollen and tender in an attempt to stop the bacteria spreading to other parts of the body. Infection also causes an increase in the number of leucocytes in the blood (see LEUCOCYTOSIS). Immediately the abscess is opened, or bursts, the pain disappears, the temperature falls rapidly to normal, and healing proceeds. If, however, the abscess discharges into an internal cavity such as the bowel or bladder, it may heal slowly or become chronic, resulting in the patient's ill-health.

Treatment Most local infections of the skin respond to ANTIBIOTICS. If pus forms, the abscess should be surgically opened and drained.

Abscesses can occur in any tissue in the body, but the principles of treatment are broadly the same: use of an antibiotic and, where appropriate, surgery.

Absorption

Uptake by the body tissues of fluids or other substances. For example, food is absorbed from the digestive tract into the blood and lymph systems. Food is absorbed mainly in the small INTESTINE (jejunum and ileum), which is lined by multiple villi that increase its surface area. (*See also* DIGESTION; ASSIMILATION.)

Abstract
(1) A dry powder produced by extracting the active principles from a crude drug. Abstracts are standardised so as to be twice the strength of the crude drug.
(2) Summary of scientific paper.

Acanthosis Nigricans
Acanthosis nigricans is a darkly pigmented verrucous skin change, usually occurring around the neck and axilla. It may be inherited but is most commonly acquired, and is associated with adenocarcinoma – usually of the stomach (see CANCER) – and certain hormonal disorders such as POLYCYSTIC OVARY SYNDROME, ADDISON'S DISEASE and CUSHING'S SYNDROME.

Acarina
The group of arthropod insects that include the parasitic MITES and TICKS.

Acarus
The group of animal parasites which includes *Sarcoptes scabiei*, the cause of the skin disease known as itch, or SCABIES. This parasite used to be known as *Acarus scabiei*.

Accidental Death
In 2000, more than 12,000 people died in or as a result of accidents in the UK, nearly half occurring at home and around a third in motor vehicle incidents. Many of these deaths would have been preventable, had appropriate safety measures been taken. A high proportion of deaths from accidents occur in males between five and 34 years of age; alcohol is a significant factor. Since the introduction of compulsory use of car seatbelts in the UK in the 1980s, the incidence of deaths from driving has fallen. With employers more aware of the risks of injury and death in the work place – with legislation reinforcing education – the number of such incidents has fallen over the past 50 years or more: this group now accounts for less than 2 per cent of all accidental deaths. Accidental deaths in the elderly are mainly caused by falls, mostly at home. In infants, choking is a significant cause of accidental death, with food and small objects presenting the main hazards. Poisoning (often from drug overdose) and drowning are notable causes between the mid-20s and mid-40s.

See www.rospa.com

Accident and Emergency Medicine
Accident and Emergency Medicine is the specialty responsible for assessing the immediate needs of acutely ill and injured people. Urgent treatment is provided where necessary; if required, the patient's admission to an appropriate hospital bed is organised. Every part of the UK has nominated key hospitals with the appropriately trained staff and necessary facilities to deal with acutely ill or injured patients. It is well-recognised that prompt treatment in the first hour or so after an accident or after the onset of an acute illness – the so-called 'golden hour' – can make the difference between the patient's recovery and serious disability or death.

A&E Medicine is a relatively new specialty in the UK and there are still inadequate numbers of consultants and trainees, despite an inexorable rise in the number of patients attending A&E departments. With a similar rise in hospital admissions there is often no bed available immediately for casualties, resulting in backlogs of patients waiting for treatment. A major debate in the specialty is about the likely need to centralise services by downgrading or closing smaller units, in order to make the most efficient use of staff.

See www.baem.org.uk

Accommodation
The process by which the refractive power of the lens of the EYE is increased by constriction of the ciliary muscle, producing an increased thickness and curvature of the lens. Rays of light from an object further than 6 metres away are parallel on reaching the eye. These rays are brought to a focus on the retina, mainly by the cornea. If the eye is now directed at an object

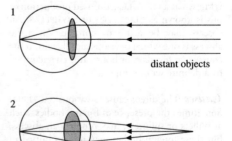

Diagram of eye in relaxed state (1), viewing a distant object; and in an accommodated state (2) with increased convexity of the lens for viewing a near object.

closer than 6 metres away, the rays of light from this near object will be diverging by the time they reach the eye. In order to focus these diverging beams of light, the refracting power of the lens must increase. In other words the lens must accommodate.

The lens loses its elasticity with age, and thus becomes less spherical when tension in the zonule relaxes. This results in an increased long-sightedness (presbyopia) requiring reading glasses for correction. (See AGEING.)

Accouchement

Archaic term for delivery of a baby (see PREG-NANCY AND LABOUR).

Accretion

Addition to an object of the substance of which it is comprised. An example is the growth of crystals in a fluid, or overgrowth of bone after injury. The term also describes foreign material collecting on the surface of a body structure: for example, PLAQUE on teeth.

Acebutolol

One of the BETA-ADRENOCEPTOR-BLOCKING DRUGS (beta blockers) used to treat HYPERTEN-SION and ANGINA. Like other beta blockers, it slows the heart rate and may precipitate heart failure, so should not be given to patients with incipient heart failure. Acebutolol can be used with caution in patients whose heart failure is satisfactorily controlled.

ACE Inhibitors

See ANGIOTENSIN-CONVERTING ENZYME (ACE) INHIBITORS.

Acetabulum

The cup-shaped socket on the pelvis in which rests the head of the femur or thigh-bone, the two forming the HIP-JOINT.

Acetazolamide

Acetazolamide is a sulphonamide drug which acts by inhibiting the ENZYME, carbonic anhy-drase. This enzyme is of great importance in the production of acid and alkaline secretions in the body. Acetazolamide is sometimes used as a second-line drug for partial seizures in EPILEPSY. It also has a diuretic action (see DIURETICS) and is used to treat GLAUCOMA. The drug has a range of side-effects. Related agents include dorzolamide and brinzolamide, used as eye-drops in patients resistant to beta blockers or who have contraindications to them.

Acetoacetic Acid

An organic acid produced by the LIVER when it is rapidly oxidising fatty acids – a metabolic process which occurs, for example, during star-vation. The acid produced is then converted to ACETONE, which is excreted.

Acetone

Acetone is a volatile, colourless organic com-pound of the KETONE group produced by the partial oxidation of fatty acids. In some abnormal conditions, such as starvation, uncontrolled diabetes (see DIABETES MELLITUS) or prolonged vomiting, acetone and other ketones can accumulate in the blood. Acetone may then appear in the urine, along with beta-hydroxybutyric and aceotacic acids, presaging developing COMA.

Acetylcholine

An acetic-acid ester of the organic base choline, acetylcholine is one of the substances which mediates the transmission of nerve impulses from one nerve to another, or from a nerve to the organ it acts on, such as muscles. It acts on both muscarinic receptors (blocked by ATRO-PINE and responsible for ganglionic and para-sympathetic transmission and also for sympa-thetic innervation of sweat glands – see under AUTONOMIC NERVOUS SYSTEM) and nicotinic receptors (responsible for the transmission of nerve impulses to muscles and blocked by cur-are, thus causing paralysis). Acetylcholine is rap-idly destroyed by cholinesterase, an ENZYME present in the blood. ANTICHOLINERGIC drugs such as PHYSOSTIGMINE prolong the action of acetylcholine.

Acetylcysteine

Acetylcysteine is a MUCOLYTIC drug that is used in the treatment of CYSTIC FIBROSIS and PARA-CETAMOL POISONING.

Acetylsalicyclic Acid

See ASPIRIN.

Achalasia

Achalasia is another term for SPASM, but indi-cates not so much an active spasm of muscle as a failure to relax.

Achalasia of the Cardia

A condition in which there is a failure to relax of the muscle fibres around the opening of the gullet, or oesophagus, into the stomach. (See OESOPHAGUS, DISEASES OF.)

A

Achilles Tendon

A thick tendon that joins the calf muscles to the heel bone (calcaneus) and pulls up that bone. The tendon is prone to rupture in middle-aged people playing vigorous sports such as squash or tennis. Named after the classical Greek hero Achilles, who was reputedly vulnerable to his enemies only in his heel.

Achlorhydria

Achlorhydria means an absence of HYDRO-CHLORIC ACID from the STOMACH's secretions. If the condition persists after the administration of HISTAMINE, the person probably has atrophy of the stomach lining. Achlorhydria occurs in about 4 per cent of healthy people and in several conditions, including PERNICIOUS ANAEMIA, carcinoma of the stomach and GASTRITIS.

Achondroplasia

The commonest form of inherited retarded growth. It is a dominant hereditary disorder of endochondral ossification, caused by mutations of fibroblast growth factor receptor 3 genes. The long bones of the arms and legs fail to grow properly, while the trunk and head develop normally. Achondroplasia affects both sexes and, while many infants are stillborn or die soon after birth, those who survive have normal intelligence, a normal expectation of life and good health.

Achromia

Loss of colour – for example, DEPIGMENTATION of the SKIN or of the iris of the EYE.

Aciclovir

Aciclovir is an antiviral drug that inhibits DNA synthesis in cells infected by HERPES VIRUSES, although it does not eradicate them. It is only effective if started at the onset of infection; uses include the systemic treatment of herpes simplex infections of the skin and mucous membranes (including genital herpes), as well as of varicella-zoster (chickenpox) pneumonia and encephalitis. It is also used topically in the eye. It is especially valuable for the treatment of herpes infections in those with IMMUNODEFICIENCY and may be required for the prevention of recurrence and for prophylaxis – indeed, it may be life-saving. Similar medications include famciclovir and valaciclovir.

Acid Base Balance

The balance between the acid and alkaline elements present in the blood and body fluids. The normal hydrogen ion concentration of the PLASMA is a constant pH 7·4, and the lungs and kidneys have a crucial function in maintaining this figure. Changes in pH value will cause ACIDOSIS or ALKALOSIS.

Acidosis

Acidosis is a condition in which there is either a production in the body of two abnormal acids – beta-hydroxybutyric and acetoacetic acids; or a diminution in the alkali reserve of the blood.

Causes The condition is usually due to faulty metabolism of fat, resulting in the production of beta-hydroxybutyric and acetoacetic acids. It occurs in DIABETES MELLITUS when this is either untreated or inadequately treated, as well as in starvation, persistent vomiting, and delayed anaesthetic vomiting. It also occurs in the terminal stages of glomerulonephritis (see KIDNEYS, DISEASES OF), when it is due to failure of the kidneys. A milder form of it may occur in severe fevers, particularly in children. (See also ACETONE.)

Symptoms General lassitude, vomiting, thirst, restlessness, and the presence of acetone in the urine form the earliest manifestations of the condition. In diabetes a state of COMA may ensue and the disease end fatally.

Treatment The underlying condition must always be treated: for example, if the acidosis is due to diabetes mellitus then insulin must be given. Sodium bicarbonate (see SODIUM) is rarely necessary for diabetic ketoacidosis; if it is used, it is invariably now given intravenously. Acidosis might be treated with oral sodium bicarbonate in cases of chronic renal failure. Anaesthetists dislike the administration of bicarbonate to acidotic patients, since there is some evidence that it can make intracellular acidosis worse. They almost always use HYPER-VENTILATION of the artificially ventilated patient to correct acidosis.

Aciduria

Excretion of an acid URINE.

Acinus

Acinus is the name applied to each of the minute sacs of which secreting glands are composed, and which usually cluster around the branches of the gland-duct like grapes on their stem. (See GLAND.)

Acne

A common skin condition starting after

puberty, and which may persist for many years. It involves plugged pores (blackheads and whiteheads), pimples and deeper nodules on the face, neck, trunk and even the upper arms. It arises from pilosebaceous glands (relating to hair follicles and associated SEBACEOUS GLANDS). SEBUM production is increased and bacterial proliferation causes inflammation with PAPULE and PUSTULE formation. Plugs of sebum and epidermal cells form blackheads (comedones); the colour is not due to dirt but to dried oil and shed skin cells in the hair-follicle openings.

Treatment Twice-daily washing with a salicylic-acid cleanser can help remove the pore-blocking debris, as can daily shampooing. Use only oil-free cosmetics and hide blackheads with a flesh-tinted acne lotion containing benzoyl peroxide, acid or sulphur. Never squeeze blackheads, however tempting; ask a skin specialist how to do this properly. Other treatments include microdermabrasion, and the antibiotic lotions erythromycin and clindamycin may be effective. Tretinoin and adapilene can be used on the skin but are not permitted in pregnancy and may cause problems such as hypersensitivity to sunlight, so medical advice is essential. In resistant cases, long-term suppressive oral therapy with one of the TETRA-CYCLINES or with ERYTHROMYCIN may be necessary. In females a combined oestrogen-antiandrogen 'pill' is an alternative. Severe resistant acne can be cleared by a 16- to 24-week course of oral isotretinoin, but this drug is teratogenic (see TERATOGENESIS) and can cause many side-effects including depression, so its use requires specialist supervision.

See www.skincarephysicians.com/acnenet/

Acne Rosacea

See ROSACEA.

Acoustic

Relating to hearing and the response to sound. For acoustic nerve, see VESTIBULOCOCHLEAR NERVE.

Acoustic Neuroma

A slow-growing, benign tumour in the auditory canal arising from the Schwann cells of the acoustic cranial nerve. The neuroma, which accounts for about 7 per cent of all tumours inside the CRANIUM, may cause facial numbness, hearing loss, unsteady balance, headache, and TINNITUS. It can usually be removed surgically, sometimes with microsurgical techniques that preserve the facial nerve.

Acriflavine

An aniline derivative, this is an orange-red crystalline powder, readily soluble in water, with strong antiseptic powers.

Acro-

Prefix meaning extremity or tip.

Acrocyanosis

A condition, occurring especially in young women, in which there is persistent blueness of hands, feet, nose and ears as a result of slow circulation of blood through the small vessels of the skin.

Acromegaly

A disorder caused by the increased secretion of growth hormone by an ADENOMA of the anterior PITUITARY GLAND. It results in excessive growth of both the skeletal and the soft tissues. If it occurs in adolescence before the bony epiphyses have fused, the result is gigantism; if it occurs in adult life the skeletal overgrowth is confined to the hands, feet, cranial sinuses and jaw. Most of the features are due to overgrowth of the cartilage of the nose and ear and of the soft tissues which increase the thickness of the skin and lips. Viscera such as the thyroid and liver are also affected. The overgrowth of the soft tissues is gradual.

The local effects of the tumour commonly cause headache and, less frequently, impairment of vision, particularly of the temporal field of vision, as a result of pressure on the nerves to the eye. The tumour may damage the other pituitary cells giving rise to gonadal, thyroid or adrenocortical insufficiency. The disease often becomes obvious in persons over about 45 years of age; they may also complain of excessive sweating, joint pains and lethargy. The diagnosis is confirmed by measuring the level of growth hormone in the serum and by an X-ray of the skull which usually shows enlargement of the pituitary fossa.

Treatment The most effective treatment is surgically to remove the pituitary adenoma. This can usually be done through the nose and the sphenoid sinus, but large adenomas may need a full CRANIOTOMY. Surgery cures about 80 per cent of patients with a microadenoma and 40 per cent of those with a large lesion; the rate of recurrence is 5–10 per cent. For recurrences, or for patients unfit for surgery or who refuse it, a combination of irradiation and drugs may be helpful. Deep X-ray therapy to the pituitary fossa is less effective than surgery but may also be helpful, and recently more sophisticated

X-ray techniques, such as gamma knife irradiation, have shown promise. Drugs – such as BROMOCRIPTINE, capergoline and quiangoline, which are dopamine agonists – lower growth-hormone levels in acromegaly and are particularly useful as an adjunct to radiotherapy. Drugs which inhibit growth-hormone release by competing for its receptors, octeotride and lanreotride, also have a place in treatment.

See www.niddk.nih.gov/health/endo/pubs/acro/acro.htm

www.umm.edu/endocrin/acromegaly.htm

Acromion
That part of the scapula, or shoulder blade, forming the tip of the shoulder and giving its squareness to the latter. It projects forwards from the scapula, and, with the CLAVICLE or collar-bone in front, forms a protective arch of bone over the shoulder-joint.

Acroparaesthesia
A disorder occurring predominantly in middle-aged women in which there is numbness and tingling of the fingers.

ACTH (Adrenocorticotrophic Hormone)
ACTH is the commonly used abbreviation for CORTICOTROPIN.

Actinomycin D
See DACTINOMYCIN.

Actinomycosis
A chronic infectious condition caused by an anaerobic micro-organism, *Actinomyces israelii*, that often occurs as a COMMENSAL on the gums, teeth and tonsils. Commonest in adult men, the sites most affected are the jaw, lungs and intestine, though the disease can occur anywhere. Suppurating granulomatous tumours develop which discharge an oily, thick pus containing yellowish ('sulphur') granules. A slowly progressive condition, actinomycosis usually responds to antibiotic drugs but improvement may be slow and surgery is sometimes needed to drain infected sites. Early diagnosis is important. Treatment is with antibiotics such as penicillin and tetracyclines. The disease occurs in cattle, where it is known as woody tongue.

Action on Smoking and Health
See ASH.

Acupuncture
A traditional Chinese method of healing by inserting thin needles into certain areas beneath the skin and rotating them. Its rationale is that disease is a manifestation of a disturbance of Yin and Yang energy in the body, and that acupuncture brings this energy back into balance by what is described as 'the judicious stimulation or depression of the flow of energy in the various meridians'. What is still unclear to western doctors is why needling, which is the essence of acupuncture, should have the effect it is claimed to have. One theory is that the technique stimulates deep sensory nerves, promoting the production of pain-relieving ENDORPHINS. Of its efficacy in skilled hands, however, there can be no question, and in China the technique is an alternative to anaesthesia for some operations. Acupuncture is increasingly used in the west, by medically qualified doctors as well as other practitioners of complementary medicine. As long as proper sterilisation procedures are followed, the treatment is safe: two recent and extensive UK studies detected no serious adverse effects.

Acute
A condition of short duration that starts quickly and has severe symptoms. It may also refer to a symptom, for example, severe pain. An 'acute' abdomen is a serious disorder of the abdomen requiring urgent treatment, usually surgery. Acute heart failure is the sudden stopping of or defect in the action of the heart. Acute LEUKAEMIA is a rapid growth in the number of white blood cells, which is fatal if untreated. (Opposite: chronic – see CHRONIC DISORDER.)

Acute Life-Threatening Event (ALTE)
See ALTE.

Acute Respiratory Distress Syndrome (ARDS)
Formerly known as adult respiratory distress syndrome. A form of acute respiratory failure in which a variety of different disorders give rise to lung injury by what is thought to be a common pathway. The condition has a high mortality rate (about 70 per cent); it is a complex clinical problem in which a disproportionate immuno-logical response plays a major role. (See IMMUNITY.)

The exact trigger is unknown, but it is thought that, whatever the stimulus, chemical mediators produced by cells of the immune system or elsewhere in the body spread and sustain an inflammatory reaction. Cascade mechanisms with multiple interactions are provoked. CYTO-TOXIC substances (which damage or kill cells) such as oxygen-free radicals and PROTEASE damage the alveolar capillary membranes (see ALVEOLUS). Once this happens, protein-rich fluid leaks into the alveoli and interstitial spaces. SURFACTANT is also lost. This impairs the exchange of oxygen and carbon dioxide in the lungs and gives rise to the clinical and pathological picture of acute respiratory failure.

The typical patient with ARDS has rapidly worsening hypoxaemia (lack of oxygen in the blood), often requiring mechanical ventilation. There are all the signs of respiratory failure (see TACHYPNOEA; TACHYCARDIA; CYANOSIS), although the chest may be clear apart from a few crackles. Radiographs show bilateral, patchy, peripheral shadowing. Blood gases will show a low PaO_2 (concentration of oxygen in arterial blood) and usually a high $PaCO_2$ (concentration of carbon dioxide in arterial blood). The lungs are 'stiff' – they are less effective because of the loss of surfactant and the PULMONARY OEDEMA.

Causes The causes of ARDS may be broadly divided into the following:

DIRECT INSULT
Viral, bacterial and fungal PNEUMONIA
Lung trauma or contusion
Inhalation of toxic gases or smoke
ASPIRATION of gastric contents
Near-drowning

INDIRECT INSULT
Septic, haemorrhagic and cardiogenic SHOCK
METABOLIC DISORDERS such as URAEMIA and pancreatitis (see PANCREAS, DISORDERS OF)
Bowel infarction
Drug ingestion
Massive blood transfusion, transfusion reaction (see TRANSFUSION OF BLOOD), CARDIO-PULMONARY BYPASS, disseminated intravascular coagulation

Treatment The principles of management are supportive, with treatment of the underlying condition if that is possible. Oxygenation is improved by increasing the concentration of oxygen breathed in by the patient, usually with mechanical ventilation of the lungs, often using continuous positive airways pressure (CPAP). Attempts are made to reduce the formation of pulmonary oedema by careful management of how much fluid is given to the patient (fluid balance). Infection is treated if it arises, as are the possible complications of prolonged ventilation with low lung compliance (e.g. PNEUMO-THORAX). There is some evidence that giving

surfactant through a nebuliser or aerosol may help to improve lung effectiveness and reduce oedema. Some experimental evidence supports the use of free-radical scavengers and ANTIOXI-DANTS, but these are not commonly used. Other techniques include the inhalation of NITRIC OXIDE (NO) to moderate vascular tone, and prone positioning to improve breathing. In severe cases, extracorporeal gas exchange has been advocated as a supportive measure until the lungs have healed enough for adequate gas exchange. (See also RESPIRATORY DISTRESS SYN-DROME; HYALINE MEMBRANE DISEASE; SARS.)

Acyclovir
See ACICLOVIR.

Adactyly
Absence of the digits.

Adaptation
A slowly diminishing reaction of a sense organ to persistent or repetitive stimulation. For example, a persistent smell may after a while result in the nose failing to signal its presence; the pressure-sensitive nerve endings in the skin may become accustomed to the presence of clothes on the body; regular background noise may be screened out by the cochlear nerve that links ear and brain.

Addiction
See DEPENDENCE.

Addison's Disease
The cause of Addison's disease (also called chronic adrenal insufficiency and hypocortiso-lism) is a deficiency of the adrenocortical hor-mones CORTISOL, ALDOSTERONE and andro-gens (see ANDROGEN) due to destruction of the adrenal cortex (see ADRENAL GLANDS). It occurs in about 1 in 25,000 of the population. In the past, destruction of the adrenal cortex was due to TUBERCULOSIS (TB), but nowadays fewer than 20 per cent of patients have TB while 70 per cent suffer from autoimmune damage. Rare causes of Addison's disease include metastases (see METASTASIS) from CARCINOMA, usually of the bronchus; granulomata (see GRANULOMA); and HAEMOCHROMATOSIS. It can also occur as a result of surgery for cancer of the PITUITARY GLAND destroying the cells which produce ACTH (ADRENOCORTICOTROPHIC HORMONE) – the hormone which provokes the adrenal cortex into action.

Symptoms The clinical symptoms appear slowly and depend upon the severity of the underlying disease process. The patient usually complains of appetite and weight loss, nausea, weakness and fatigue. The skin becomes pigmented due to the increased production of ACTH. Faintness, especially on standing, is due to postural HYPOTENSION secondary to aldosterone deficiency. Women lose their axillary hair and both sexes are liable to develop mental symptoms such as DEPRESSION. Acute episodes – Addisonian crises – may occur, brought on by infection, injury or other stressful events; they are caused by a fall in aldosterone levels, leading to abnormal loss of sodium and water via the kidneys, dehydration, low blood pressure and confusion. Patients may develop increased tanning of the skin from extra pigmentation, with black or blue discoloration of the skin, lips, mouth, rectum and vagina occurring. ANOREXIA, nausea and vomiting are common and the sufferer may feel cold.

Diagnosis This depends on demonstrating impaired serum levels of cortisol and inability of these levels to rise after an injection of ACTH.

Treatment consists in replacement of the deficient hormones. HYDROCORTISONE tablets are commonly used; some patients also require the salt-retaining hormone, fludrocortisone. Treatment enables them to lead a completely normal life and to enjoy a normal life expectancy. Before surgery, or if the patient is pregnant and unable to take tablets, injectable hydrocortisone may be needed. Rarely, treated patients may have a crisis, perhaps because they have not been taking their medication or have been vomiting it. Emergency resuscitation is needed with fluids, salt and sugar. Because of this, all patients should carry a card detailing their condition and necessary management. Treatment of any complicating infections such as tuberculosis is essential. Sometimes DIABETES MELLITUS coexists with Addison's disease and must be treated.

Secondary adrenal insufficiency may occur in panhypopituitarism (see PITUITARY GLAND), in patients treated with CORTICOSTEROIDS or after such patients have stopped treatment.

Adduct

To move a limb or any other part towards the midline of the body. (Opposite: ABDUCT.)

Adenitis

Adenitis means inflammation of a GLAND.

Adeno-

A prefix denoting relation to a GLAND or glands.

Adenocarcinoma

A malignant growth of glandular tissue. This tissue is widespread throughout the body's organs and the tumours may occur, for example, in the STOMACH, OVARIES and UTERUS. Adenocarcinomas may be subdivided into those that arise from mucous or serous secreting glandular tissue.

Adenoids

See NOSE, DISORDERS OF.

Adenolipoma

A non-malignant tumour arising from the EPITHELIUM and made up of ADIPOSE TISSUE and glandular tissues (see GLAND).

Adenoma

A growth or cyst arising from the EPITHELIUM, a lining layer of cells on the inside of organs. Although usually benign, adenomas can, as they enlarge, press on adjacent tissue such as nerves or, in the case of an adenoma of the PITUITARY GLAND, on brain tissue, causing symptoms. Where adenomas arise in ENDOCRINE GLANDS, such as the adrenals, pancreas, pituitary and thyroid, they can provoke excessive production of the hormone normally produced by the gland. If an adenoma is causing or is likely to cause symptoms it is usually surgically removed (see also TUMOUR).

Adenomatosis

A condition in which multiple glandular overgrowths occur.

Adenosine Triphosphate (ATP)

A compound comprising the chemical substances adenine, ribose and phosphates. The chemical bonds of the phosphates contain energy needed for cell METABOLISM that occurs when muscle cells contract. This energy is made available when ATP breaks up to form other chemical groupings – adenosine diphosphate (ADP) and adenosine monophosphate (AMP). The energy needed for recombining AMP and ADP to form ATP is produced by the breakdown of carbohydrates or other constituencies of food.

Adenoviruses

Viruses (see VIRUS) containing double-stranded DNA; these cause around 5 per cent of clinically recognised respiratory illnesses. Of the 40 or so known types, only a few have been properly studied to establish how they produce disease. Adenoviruses cause fever and inflammation of the respiratory tract and mucous membranes of the eyes – symptoms resembling those of the common cold. They also cause ENTERITIS, haemorrhagic CYSTITIS and life-threatening infections in newborn babies. Infections are generally benign and self-limiting, and treatment is symptomatic and supportive, although the elderly and people with chronic chest conditions may develop secondary infections which require antibiotic treatment.

ADHD
See ATTENTION DEFICIT DISORDER (HYPER-ACTIVITY SYNDROME).

Adhesion
The abnormal union of two normally separate tissues. Adhesion may occur after inflammation or surgery; the result is often a fibrous band between the adjacent tissues. Examples are adhesions between joint surfaces – which reduce mobility of a joint – or, after operation, between loops of intestine, where the fibrous band may cause obstruction. Movement of the heart may be restricted by adhesions between the organ and its membranous cover, the pericardial sac.

Adipose Tissue
Adipose tissue, or fat, is a loose variety of fibrous tissue in the meshes of which lie cells, each of which is distended by several small drops, or one large drop, of fat. This tissue replaces fibrous tissue when the amount of food taken is in excess of the bodily requirements. Adipose tissue occurs as a layer beneath the skin and also around several internal organs. (See DIET; FAT; OBESITY.)

Adiposis Dolorosa
Also known as Dercum's disease. A condition in which painful masses of fat develop under the skin – more common in women than in men.

Adiposity
See OBESITY.

Adjuvant
Any substance given in concert with another to boost its activity. For instance, a CYTOTOXIC drug used to reinforce radiotherapy or surgery in the treatment of cancer is described as adjuvant therapy.

The term is also used to describe an ingredient added to a VACCINE to boost the immune system's production of antibodies, thus enhancing the vaccine's effectiveness in promoting immunity.

Adler
Alfred Adler (1870–1937) was an Austrian psychiatrist who proposed psychoanalytical concepts based on individual psychology, his central thesis being that everyone is born with intrinsic feelings of inferiority. Thus life is a continuing struggle to overcome these feelings: failure results in neuroses.

Adolescence
See PUBERTY.

Adoption
See CHILD ADOPTION.

Adrenal Glands
Also known as suprarenal glands, these are two small triangular ENDOCRINE GLANDS situated one upon the upper end of each kidney. (See diagram of ABDOMEN.)

Structure Each suprarenal gland has an enveloping layer of fibrous tissue. Within this, the gland shows two distinct parts: an outer, firm, deep-yellow cortical (see CORTEX) layer, and a central, soft, dark-brown medullary (see MEDULLA) portion. The cortical part consists of columns of cells running from the surface inwards, whilst in the medullary portion the cells are arranged irregularly and separated from one another by large capillary blood vessels.

Functions Removal of the suprarenal glands in animals is speedily followed by great muscular prostration and death within a few days. In human beings, disease of the suprarenal glands usually causes ADDISON'S DISEASE, in which the chief symptoms are increasing weakness and bronzing of the skin. The medulla of the glands produces a substance – ADRENALINE – the effects of which closely resemble those brought about by activity of the SYMPATHETIC NERVOUS SYSTEM: dilated pupils, hair standing on end, quickening and strengthening of the heartbeat, immobilisation of the gut, increased output of sugar from the liver into the bloodstream. Several hormones (called CORTICOSTEROIDS) are produced in the cortex of the gland and play a vital role in the metabolism of the body. Some (such as aldosterone) control the electrolyte balance of the body and help to maintain the blood pressure and blood volume. Others are concerned in carbohydrate metabolism, whilst others again are concerned with sex physiology. HYDROCORTISONE is the most important hormone of the adrenal cortex, controlling as it does the body's use of carbohydrates, fats and proteins. It also helps to suppress inflammatory reactions and has an influence on the immune system.

Adrenaline

Adrenaline is the secretion of the adrenal medulla (see ADRENAL GLANDS). Its effect is similar to stimulation of the SYMPATHETIC NERVOUS SYSTEM as occurs when a person is excited, shocked or frightened. In the *United States Pharmacopoeia* it is known as epinephrine. It is also prepared synthetically. Among its important effects are raising of the blood pressure, increasing the amount of glucose in the blood, and constricting the smaller blood vessels.

Adrenaline has an important use when injected intramuscularly or intravenously in the treatment of ANAPHYLAXIS. Many patients prone to this condition are prescribed a pre-assembled adrenaline-containing syringe and needle (Min-i-Jet, Epipen) and are taught how to self-administer in an emergency. Adrenaline may be applied directly to wounds, on gauze or lint, to check haemorrhage; injected along with some local anaesthetic it permits painless, bloodless operations to be performed on the eye, nose, etc. Nowadays it is rarely, if ever, used hypodermically and is no longer given to treat ASTHMA. In severe cardiac arrest, adrenaline (1 in 10,000) by central intravenous injection is recommended. It can be given through an endotracheal tube as part of neonatal resuscitation.

Adrenergic Receptors

The sites in the body on which ADRENALINE and comparable stimulants of the SYMPATHETIC NERVOUS SYSTEM act. Drugs which have an adrenaline-like action are described as being adrenergic. There are five different types of adrenergic receptors, known as alpha$_1$, alpha$_2$, beta$_1$, beta$_2$ and beta$_3$ respectively. Stimulation of alpha receptors leads to constriction of the bronchi, constriction of the blood vessels with consequent rise in blood pressure, and dilatation of the pupils of the eyes. Stimulation of beta$_1$ receptors quickens the rate and output of the heart, while stimulation of beta$_2$ receptors dilates the bronchi. Beta$_3$ receptors are now known to mediate so-called non-shivering thermogenesis, a way of producing heat from specialised fat cells that is particularly relevant to the human infant.

For long it had been realised that in certain cases of ASTHMA, adrenaline had not the usual beneficial effect of dilating the bronchi during an attack; rather it made the asthma worse. This was due to its acting on both the alpha and beta adrenergic receptors. A derivative, isoprenaline, was therefore produced which acted only on the beta receptors. This had an excellent effect in dilating the bronchi, but unfortunately also affected the heart, speeding it up and increasing its output – an undesirable effect which meant that isoprenaline had to be used with great care. In due course drugs were produced, such as salbutamol, which act predominantly on the beta$_2$ adrenergic receptors in the bronchi and have relatively little effect on the heart.

The converse of this story was the search for what became known as BETA-ADRENOCEPTOR-BLOCKING DRUGS, or beta-adrenergic-blocking drugs. The theoretical argument was that if such drugs could be synthesised, they could be of value in taking the strain off the heart – for example: stress → stimulation of the output of adrenaline → stimulation of the heart → increased work for the heart. A drug that could prevent this train of events would be of value, for example in the treatment of ANGINA PECTORIS. Now there is a series of beta-adrenoceptor-blocking drugs of use not only in angina pectoris, but also in various other heart conditions such as disorders of rhythm, as well as high blood pressure. They are also proving valuable in the treatment of anxiety states by preventing disturbing features such as palpitations. Some are useful in the treatment of migraine.

Adrenocorticotrophic Hormone (ACTH)

See also CORTICOTROPIN. A hormone which is released into the body during stress. Made and stored in the anterior PITUITARY GLAND, ACTH regulates the production of corticosteroid hormones from the ADRENAL GLANDS, and is vital for the growth and maintenance of the adrenal cortical cells. Its production is in part controlled by the amount of HYDROCORTISONE in the blood and also by the HYPOTHALAMUS. ACTH participates in the FEEDBACK MECHANISM of hormone production and actions involving particularly the hypothalamus and pituitary gland. The hormone is used to test adrenal function and treat conditions such as ASTHMA. (See also CUSHING'S SYNDROME.)

Adrenogenital Syndrome

An inherited condition, the adrenogenital syndrome – also known as congenital adrenal hyperplasia – is an uncommon disorder affecting about 1 baby in 7,500. The condition is present from birth and causes various ENZYME defects as well as blocking the production of HYDROCORTISONE and ALDOSTERONE by the ADRENAL GLANDS. In girls the syndrome often produces VIRILISATION of the genital tract, often with gross enlargement of the clitoris and fusion of the labia so that the genitalia may be mistaken for a malformed penis. The metabolism of salt and water may be disturbed, causing dehydration, low blood pressure and weight loss; this can produce collapse at a few days or weeks of age. Enlargement of the adrenal glands occurs and the affected individual may also develop excessive pigmentation in the skin.

When virilisation is noted at birth, great care must be taken to determine genetic sex by karyotyping: parents should be reassured as to the baby's sex (never 'in between'). Blood levels of adrenal hormones are measured to obtain a precise diagnosis. Traditionally, doctors have advised parents to 'choose' their child's gender on the basis of discussing the likely condition of the genitalia after puberty. Thus, where the phallus is likely to be inadequate as a male organ, it may be preferred to rear the child as female. Surgery is usually advised in the first two years to deal with clitoromegaly but parent/patient pressure groups, especially in the US, have declared it wrong to consider surgery until the children are competent to make their own decision.

Other treatment requires replacement of the missing hormones which, if started early, may lead to normal sexual development. There is still controversy surrounding the ethics of gender reassignment.

See www.baps.org.uk

Advance Statements about Medical Treatment

See LIVING WILL.

Adverse Reactions to Drugs

When a new drug is introduced, it has usually been studied only in relatively few patients – typically 1,500. If n patients have been studied, and no serious effects observed, there is still a chance of a serious adverse effect occurring in the general population as frequently as $3/n$ (1:500).

Adverse effects can be divided into types. First, those which are closely related to the concentration of the drug and accord with what is known of its PHARMACOLOGY. These so-called type A (augmented pharmacological) effects are distinguished from type B (bizarre) effects which are unpredictable, usually rare, and often severe. ANAPHYLAXIS is the most obvious of these; other examples include bone-marrow suppression with CO-TRIMOXAZOLE; hepatic failure (see HEPATITIS) with SODIUM VALPROATE; and PULMONARY FIBROSIS with AMIODARONE. A more comprehensive classification includes reactions type C (chronic effects), D (delayed effects – such as teratogenesis or carcinogenesis) and E (end-of-dose effects – withdrawal effects). Examples of adverse reactions include nausea, skin eruptions, jaundice, sleepiness and headaches.

While most reported adverse reactions are minor and require no treatment, patients should remind their doctors of any drug allergy or adverse effect they have suffered in the past. Medical warning bracelets are easily obtained. Doctors should report adverse effects to the authorities – in the case of Britain, to the Committee on Safety of Medicines (CSM), using the yellow-card reporting machinery.

Aëdes Aegypti

The scientific name for the mosquito which conveys to humans (by biting) the viruses of YELLOW FEVER and of DENGUE or 'break-bone' fever.

Aegophony

The bleating or punchinello tone given to the voice as heard by AUSCULTATION with a stethoscope, when there is a small amount of fluid in the pleural cavity in the chest.

Aerobic Bacterium

A bacterium (see BACTERIA) that needs the presence of free oxygen for its life and multiplication.

Aerophagy

Swallowing abnormal quantities of air which can occur during rapid eating or drinking. Indigestion-sufferers sometimes do this to relieve their symptoms, and it is a common sign of anxiety.

Aerosol

See INHALANTS.

Aerotitis

See OTIC BARATRAUMA.

Aetiology
That part of medical science dealing with the causes of disease.

Afferent
An adjective to describe nerves, blood vessels or lymphatic vessels that conduct their electrical charge or contents inwards to the brain, spinal cord or relevant organ. (Opposite: EFFERENT.)

Afibrinogenaemia
A condition in which the blood will not clot because FIBRIN is absent. It is characterised by haemorrhage. There are two forms: (*a*) a congenital form, and (*b*) an acquired form. The latter may be associated with advanced liver disease, or may occur as a complication of labour. Treatment consists of the intravenous injection of fibrinogen, and blood transfusion. (See also COAGULATION.)

Afterbirth
See PLACENTA.

Afterpains
Pains similar to but feebler than those of labour, occurring in the two or three days following childbirth. (See PREGNANCY AND LABOUR.)

Causes are generally the presence of a blood clot or retained piece of PLACENTA which the womb (see UTERUS) is attempting to expel.

Agammaglobulinaemia
An inherited condition found in male infants, in which there is no GAMMA-GLOBULIN in the blood. These children are particularly susceptible to infections, as they are unable to form ANTIBODIES to any infecting micro-organism. Acquired agammaglobulinaemia is a rare disorder occurring in both sexes in their 20s and 40s, characterised by recurrent bacterial infections. The cause is a disturbance in the working of the immune system. (See IMMUNITY.)

Agar
Also known as agar-agar. A gelatinous substance made from seaweed, agar is used in preparing culture-media for use in bacteriological laboratories; it is also sometimes used to treat constipation.

Ageing
The result of a combination of natural, largely genetically programmed changes occurring in all body systems. Diseases or injuries may influence these changes, which impair the body's homeostatic mechanisms; environment and lifestyle also affect the ageing process.

The effects of ageing include: cessation of MENSTRUATION in females; wrinkling of the skin due to a loss of elastic tissue; failing memory (especially short term) and a reduced ability to learn new skills, along with slowed responses – changes caused by the loss of or less efficient working of nerve cells; the senses become less acute; the lungs become less efficient, as does heart muscle, both causing a fall in exercise tolerance; arteries harden, resulting in a rise in blood pressure and poor blood circulation; joints are less mobile, bones beome more brittle (OSTEOPOROSIS) and muscle bulk and strength are reduced; the lens of the EYE becomes less elastic, resulting in poorer sight, and it may also become opaque (CATARACT).

In developed countries people are living longer, in part because infant and child mortality rates have dropped dramatically over the past 100 years or so. Improved standards of living and more effective health care have also contributed to greater longevity: the proportion of people over 65 years of age has greatly increased, and that of the over-75s is still rising. The 2001 census found 336,000 people in the UK aged over 90 and there are 36,000 centenarians in the US. This extreme longevity is attributed to a particular gene (see GENES) slowing the ageing process. Interestingly, those living to 100 often retain the mental faculties of people in their 60s, and examination of centenarians' brains show that these are similar to those of 60-year-olds. (See MEDICINE OF AGEING; CLIMACTERIC.)

Help and advice can be obtained from Age Concern and Help the Aged.
See www.helpthaged.org.uk
www.ageconcern.org.uk

Agenesis
Agenesis means incomplete development, or the failure of any part or organ of the body to develop normally.

Agglutination
The adherence together of small bodies in a fluid. Thus, blood corpuscles agglutinate into heaps (rouleaux) when added to the serum of a person belonging to an incompatible blood group. Bacteria agglutinate into clumps and die when exposed to the presence of antibodies in the blood. This is important in regard to diagnosis of certain diseases due to bacteria. In typhoid fever (see ENTERIC FEVER), for example, the blood of an animal is immunised against typhoid bacilli by repeated injections of these.

The blood serum of the animal, known now as anti-typhoid serum, is issued to laboratories for use when bacilli are found in the excretions of a patient who is possibly suffering from typhoid fever. The bacilli are exposed to the action of a drop of the serum; if the serum shows the power of agglutinating these bacteria, this forms evidence that the bacteria in question are typhoid bacilli. The reaction may also be carried out in the contrary manner: that is to say, the serum from the blood of a patient who may be suffering from typhoid fever, but in whom the diagnosis is still doubtful, is added to a drop of fluid containing typhoid bacilli; if these are agglutinated into clumps by the patient's serum, the patient is then known to be suffering from typhoid fever. If they do not agglutinate, the symptoms are due to some other condition. This reaction for typhoid fever is known as the Widal reaction. Comparable agglutination reactions, using an appropriate serum, are used in the diagnosis of a number of diseases, including glandular fever (when it is known as the Paul-Bunnell reaction), typhus fever (when it is known as the Weil-Felix reaction), undulant fever, and Weil's disease. (For more information about these diseases, see under separate entries.)

Agglutinogen
An ANTIGEN that stimulates production of an agglutinin – an antibody that causes AGGLUTINATION or clumping of bacteria, blood cells or other antigenic particles. In the case of blood cells, this should not be confused with the clumping that happens in blood COAGULATION, which is a different process.

Aggression
A general term that covers a range of hostile behaviour, some of which may extend beyond normal social behaviour. Some physical diseases cause aggressive outbursts: temporal lobe EPILEPSY and hypoglycaemia (see DIABETES MELLITUS) are examples. Certain mental disorders – such as antisocial personality disorders, alcohol or drug abuse, and SCHIZOPHRENIA – may be associated with aggression.

Male sex hormones (see under ANDROGEN) appear to be linked to aggressive behaviour, and aggression is more common among adolescents and young adults than other sections of the population.

Agnosia
The condition in which, in certain diseases of the brain, the patient loses the ability to recognise the character of objects through the senses – touch, taste, sight, hearing.

Agonist
(1) A muscle which contracts and causes a movement. Contraction of an agonist is complemented by relaxation of its antagonist (see below).
(2) A drug that acts through receptors on the surface of the cell or within the cell and provokes a biological response. As the body contains natural agonists that combine with cell receptors, any 'occupation' of these cell receptors by drug molecules will have a pharmacological effect on the individual. The intensity of that pharmacological effect is believed to be directly proportional to the number of receptors on the cell that combine with the drug molecule. For example, the natural agonist noradrenaline contracts the smooth muscle of blood vessels; the drug agonist phenylnephrine has a similar effect.

Antagonists are drugs which will combine with the receptor site to prevent another agent from producing its greatest effect. If the drug has no efficacy of its own, but simply prevents the agonist from acting at the receptor site, it is called a full antagonist. A partial antagonist is a drug that provokes some activity at the receptor site. An example of an antagonist is prazosin, which acts against the natural agonist noradrenaline at the receptor site of the cells of blood-vessel muscle and prevents the vascular muscle from contracting.

Agoraphobia
A sense of fear experienced in large open spaces and public places, agoraphobia is a symptom of psychological disorder (see MENTAL ILLNESS). There are said to be 300,000 sufferers in the United Kingdom. Those who suffer from what can be a most distressing condition can obtain help and advice from the National Phobics Society.

Agranulocytosis
A condition in which the white cells or LEUCOCYTES in the blood of the polynuclear or granular variety become greatly lessened in numbers or disappear altogether. It is usually caused by taking such drugs as amidopyrine, thiourea, sulphonamides, chloramphenicol and the immunosuppressant drugs.

Agraphia
Loss of power to express ideas by writing. (See APHASIA.)

AI
See ARTIFICIAL INTELLIGENCE (AI).

AIDS/HIV

Acquired Immune Deficiency Syndrome (AIDS) is the clinical manifestation of infection with Human Immunodeficiency Virus (HIV). HIV belongs to the retroviruses, which in turn belong to the lentiviruses (characterised by slow onset of disease). There are two main HIV strains: HIV-1, by far the commonest; and HIV-2, which is prevalent in Western Africa (including Ivory Coast, Gambia, Mali, Nigeria and Sierra Leone). HIV attacks the human immune system (see IMMUNITY) so that the infected person becomes susceptible to opportunistic infections, such as TUBERCULOSIS, PNEUMONIA, DIARRHOEA, MENINGITIS and tumours such as KAPOSI'S SARCOMA. AIDS is thus the disease syndrome associated with advanced HIV infection.

Both HIV-1 and HIV-2 are predominantly sexually transmitted and both are associated with secondary opportunistic infections. However, HIV-2 seems to result in slower damage to the immune system. HIV-1 is known to mutate rapidly and has given rise to other subtypes.

HIV is thought to have occurred in humans in the 1950s, but whether or not it infected humans from another primate species is uncertain. It became widespread in the 1970s but its latency in causing symptoms meant that the epidemic was not noticed until the following decade. Although it is a sexually transmitted disease, it can also be transmitted by intravenous drug use (through sharing an infected needle), blood transfusions with infected blood (hence the importance of effective national blood-screening programmes), organ donation, and occupationally (see health-care workers, below). Babies born of HIV-positive mothers can be infected before or during birth, or through breast feeding.

Although HIV is most likely to occur in blood, semen or vaginal fluid, it has been found in saliva and tears (but not sweat); however, there is no evidence that the virus can be transmitted from these two body fluids. There is also no evidence that HIV can be transmitted by biting insects (such as mosquitoes). HIV does not survive well in the environment and is rapidly destroyed through drying.

Prevalence At the end of 2003 an estimated 42 million people globally were infected with HIV – up from 40 million two years earlier. About one-third of those with HIV/AIDS are aged 15–24 and most are unaware that they are carrying the virus. During 2003 it is estimated that 5 million adults and children worldwide were newly infected with HIV, and that 3 million adults and children died. In Africa in 2003, 3.4 million people were newly infected and 2.3 million died, with more than 28 million carrying the virus. HIV/AIDS was the leading cause of death in sub-Saharan Africa where over half of the infections were in women and 90 per cent of cases resulted from heterosexual sex. In some southern African countries, one in three pregnant women had HIV.

In Asia and the Pacific there were 1.2 million new infections and 435,000 deaths. The area with the fastest-growing epidemic is Eastern Europe, especially the Russian Federation where in 2002 around a million people had HIV and there were an estimated 250,000 new infections, with intravenous drug use a key contributor to this figure. Seventy-five per cent of cases occurred in men, with male-to-male sexual transmission an important cause of infection, though heterosexual activity is a rising cause of infection.

At the end of 2002 the UK had an estimated 55,900 HIV-infected adults aged between 15 and 59. More than 3,600 individuals were newly diagnosed with the infection in 2000, the highest annual figure since the epidemic started – in 1998 the figure was 2,817 and in 1999 just over 3,000 (Department of Health and Communicable Disease Surveillance Centre). The incidence of AIDS in the UK has declined sharply since the introduction of highly active antiretroviral therapy (HAART) and HIV-related deaths have also fallen: in 2002 there were 777 reported new AIDS cases and 395 deaths, compared with 1,769 and 1,719 respectively in 1995. (Sources: UNAIDS and WHO, *AIDS Epidemic Update*, December 2001; Public Health Laboratory Services AIDS and STD Centre Communicable Disease Surveillance and Scottish Centre for Infection and Environmental Health, *Quarterly Surveillance Tables*.)

Poverty is strongly linked to the spread of AIDS, for various reasons including lack of health education; lack of effective public-health awareness; women having little control over sexual behaviour and contraception; and, by comparison with the developed world, little or no access to antiretroviral drugs.

Pathogenesis The cellular target of HIV infection is a subset of white blood cells called T-lymphocytes (see LYMPHOCYTE) which carry the CD4 surface receptor. These so-called 'helper T-cells' are vital to the function of cell-mediated immunity. Infection of these cells leads to their destruction (HIV replicates at an enormous rate – 10^9) and over the course of several years the body is unable to generate sufficient new cells to keep pace. This leads to progressive destruction of the body's immune capabilities, evidenced clinically by the development of opportunistic infection and unusual tumours.

Monitoring of clinical progression It is possible to measure the number of viral particles present in the plasma. This gives an accurate guide to the likely progression rate, which will be slow in those individuals with fewer than 10,000 particles per ml of plasma but progressively more rapid above this figure. The main clinical monitoring of the immune system is through the numbers of CD4 lymphocytes in the blood. The normal count is around 850 cells per ml and, without treatment, eventual progression to AIDS is likely in those individuals whose CD4 count falls below 500 per ml. Opportunistic infections occur most frequently when the count falls below 200 per ml: most such infections are treatable, and death is only likely when the CD4 count falls below 50 cells per ml when infection is developed with organisms that are difficult to treat because of their low intrinsic virulence.

Simple, cheap and highly accurate tests are available to detect HIV antibodies in the serum. These normally occur within three months of infection and remain the cornerstone of the diagnosis.

Clinical features Most infected individuals have a viral illness some three weeks after contact with HIV. The clinical features are often non-specific and remain undiagnosed but include a fine red rash, large lymph nodes, an influenza-like illness, cerebral involvement and sometimes the development of opportunistic infections. The antibody test may be negative at this stage but there are usually high levels of virus particles in the blood. The antibody test is virtually always positive within three months of infection. HIV infection is often subsequently asymptomatic for a period of ten years or more, although in most patients progressive immune destruction is occurring during this time and a variety of minor opportunistic infections such as HERPES ZOSTER or oral thrush (see CANDIDA) do occur. In addition, generalised LYMPH-ADENOPATHY is present in a third of patients and some suffer from severe malaise, weight loss, night sweats, mild fever, ANAEMIA or easy bruising due to THROMBOCYTOPENIA.

The presentation of opportunistic infection is highly variable but usually involves either the CENTRAL NERVOUS SYSTEM, the gastrointestinal tract or the LUNGS. Patients may present with a sudden onset of a neurological deficit or EPILEPSY due to a sudden onset of a STROKE-like syndrome, or epilepsy due to a space-occupying lesion in the brain – most commonly TOXOPLASMOSIS. In late disease, HIV infection of the central nervous system itself may produce progressive memory loss, impaired concentration and mental slowness called AIDS DEMENTIA. A wide variety of opportunistic PROTOZOA or viruses produces DYSPHAGIA, DIARRHOEA and wasting. In the respiratory system the commonest opportunistic infection associated with AIDS, pneumonia, produces severe shortness of breath and sometimes CYANOSIS, usually with a striking lack of clinical signs in the chest.

In very late HIV infection, when the CD4 count has fallen below 50 cells per ml, infection with CYTOMEGALOVIRUS may produce progressive retinal necrosis (see EYE, DISORDERS OF) which will lead to blindness if untreated, as well as a variety of gastrointestinal symptoms. At this stage, infection with atypical mycobacteria is also common, producing severe anaemia, wasting and fevers. The commonest tumour associated with HIV is Kaposi's sarcoma which produces purplish skin lesions. This and non-Hodgkin's lymphoma (see LYMPHOMA), which is a hundred times more frequent among HIV-positive individuals than in the general population, are likely to be associated with or caused by opportunistic viral infections.

Prevention There is, as yet, no vaccine to prevent HIV infection. Vaccine development has been hampered
- by the large number of new HIV strains generated through frequent mutation and recombination.
- because HIV can be transmitted as free virus and in infected cells.
- because HIV infects helper T-cells – the very cells involved in the immune response.

There are, however, numerous research programmes underway to develop vaccines that are either prophylactic or therapeutic. Vaccine-development strategies have included: recombinant-vector vaccines, in which a live bacterium or virus is genetically modified to carry one or more of the HIV genes; subunit vaccines, consisting of small regions of the HIV genome designed to induce an immune response without infection; modified live HIV, which has had its disease-promoting genes removed; and DNA vaccines – small loops of DNA (plasmids) containing viral genes – that make the host cells produce non-infectious viral proteins which, in turn, trigger an immune response and prime the immune system against future infection with real virus.

In the absence of an effective vaccine, preventing exposure remains the chief strategy in reducing the spread of HIV. Used properly, condoms are an extremely effective method of preventing exposure to HIV during sexual intercourse and remain the most important public-health approach to countering the further acceleration of the AIDS epidemic. The spermicide nonoxynol-9, which is often included with condoms, is known to kill HIV *in vitro*; however, its effectiveness in preventing HIV infection during intercourse is not known.

Public-health strategies must be focused on avoiding high-risk behaviour and, particularly in developing countries, empowering women to have more control over their lives, both economically and socially. In many of the poorer regions of the world, women are economically dependent on men and refusing sex, or insisting on condom use, even when they know their partners are HIV positive, is not a straightforward option. Poverty also forces many women into the sex industry where they are at greater risk of infection.

Cultural problems in gaining acceptance for universal condom-use by men in some developing countries suggests that other preventive strategies should also be considered. Microbicides used as vaginal sprays or 'chemical condoms' have the potential to give women more direct control over their exposure risk, and research is underway to develop suitable products.

Epidemiological studies suggest that male circumcision may offer some protection against HIV infection, although more research is needed before this can be an established public-health strategy. Globally, about 70 per cent of infected men have acquired the virus through unprotected vaginal sex; in these men, infection is likely to have occurred through the penis with the mucosal epithelia of the inner surface of the foreskin and the frenulum considered the most likely sites for infection. It is suggested that in circumcised men, the glans may become keratinised and thus less likely to facilitate infection. Circumcision may also reduce the risk of lesions caused by other sexually transmitted disease.

Treatment AIDS/HIV treatment can be categorised as specific therapies for the individual opportunistic infections – which ultimately cause death – and highly active antiretroviral therapy (HAART) designed to reduce viral load

and replication. HAART is also the most effective way of preventing opportunistic infections, and has had a significant impact in delaying the onset of AIDS in HIV-positive individuals in developed countries.

Four classes of drugs are currently in use. Nucleoside analogues, including ZIDOVUDINE and DIDANOSINE, interfere with the activity of the unique enzyme of the retrovirus reverse transcriptase which is essential for replication. Nucleotide analogues, such as tenofovir, act in the same way but require no intracellular activation. Non-nucleoside reverse transcriptase inhibitors, such as nevirapine and EFAVIRENZ, act by a different mechanism on the same enzyme. The most potent single agents against HIV are the protease inhibitors, such as lopinavir, which render a unique viral enzyme ineffective. These drugs are used in a variety of combinations in an attempt to reduce the plasma HIV viral load to below detectable limits, which is achieved in approximately 90 per cent of patients who have not previously received therapy. This usually also produces a profound rise in CD4 count. It is likely, however, that such treatments need to be lifelong – and since they are associated with toxicities, long-term adherence is difficult. Thus the optimum time for treatment intervention remains controversial, with some clinicians believing that this should be governed by the viral load rising above 10,000 copies, and others that it should primarily be designed to prevent the development of opportunistic infections – thus, that initiation of therapy should be guided more by the CD4 count.

It should be noted that the drug regimens have been devised for infection with HIV-1; it is not known how effective they are at treating infection with HIV-2.

HIV and pregnancy An HIV-positive woman can transmit the virus to her fetus, with the risk of infection being particularly high during parturition; however, the risk of perinatal HIV transmission can be reduced by antiviral drug therapy. In the UK, HIV testing is available to all women as part of antenatal care. The benefits of antenatal HIV testing in countries where antiviral drugs are not available are questionable. An HIV-positive woman might be advised not to breast feed because of the risks of transmitting HIV via breastmilk, but there may be a greater risk associated with not breast feeding at all. Babies in many poor communities are thought to be at high risk of infectious diseases and malnutrition if they are not breast fed and may thus be at greater overall risk of death during infancy.

Counselling Confidential counselling is an essential part of AIDS management, both in terms of supporting the psychological well-being of the individual and in dealing with issues such as family relations, sexual partners and implications for employment (e.g. for health-care workers). Counsellors must be particularly sensitive to culture and lifestyle issues. Counselling is essential both before an HIV test is taken and when the results are revealed.

Health-care workers Health-care workers may be at risk of occupational exposure to HIV, either through undertaking invasive procedures or through accidental exposure to infected blood from a contaminated needle (needlestick injury). Needlestick injuries are frequent in health care – as many as 600,000 to 800,000 are thought to occur annually in the United States. Transmission is much more likely where the worker has been exposed to HIV through a needlestick injury or deep cut with a contaminated instrument than through exposure of mucous membranes to contaminated blood or body fluids. However, even where exposure occurs through a needlestick injury, the risk of seroconversion is much lower than with a similar exposure to hepatitis C or hepatitis B. A percutaneous exposure to HIV-infected blood in a health-care setting is thought to carry a risk of about one infection per 300 injuries (one in 1,000 for mucous-membrane exposure), compared with one in 30 for hepatitis C, and one in three for hepatitis B (when the source patient is e-antigen positive).

In the event of an injury, health-care workers are advised to report the incident immediately where, depending on a risk assessment, they may be offered post-exposure prophylaxis (PEP). They should also wash the contaminated area with soap and water (but without scrubbing) and, if appropriate, encourage bleeding at the site of injury. PEP, using a combination of antiretroviral drugs (in a similar regimen to HAART – see above), is thought to greatly reduce the chances of seroconversion; it should be commenced as soon as possible, preferably within one or two hours of the injury. Although PEP is available, safe systems of work are considered to offer the greatest protection. Double-gloving (latex gloves remove much of the blood from the surface of the needle during a needlestick), correct use of sharps containers (for used needles and instruments), avoiding the resheathing of used needles, reduction in the number of blood samples taken from a patient, safer-needle devices (such as needles that self-blunt after use) and needleless drug administration are all thought to reduce the risk of exposure to HIV and other blood-borne viruses. Although there have been numerous cases of health-care workers developing HIV through occupational exposure, there is little evidence of health-care workers passing HIV to their patients through normal medical procedures.

Air
The general constituents of air are:

	per cent
Oxygen	20·94
Nitrogen	78·09
Argon	0·94
Carbon dioxide	0·03

Besides these, there are always ozone, minerals and organic matter present in small and variable amounts, and more or less water vapour according to the weather. In the air of towns, sulphurous acid and sulphuretted hydrogen are important impurities derived from combustion. After air has been respired once, the oxygen falls by about 4 per cent and the carbonic acid rises to about 4 per cent, while organic matter and water vapour are greatly increased and the air rises in temperature. The cause of the discomfort felt in badly ventilated rooms and crowded halls is associated with the increase in the temperature and moisture of the air, but a high percentage of carbon dioxide may be present without causing any noticeable discomfort or appreciable quickening of the respiration. A combination of hot weather and emissions from vehicles and fossil-fuel combustion produces pollutants linked to a rise in the incidence of ASTHMA and other cardiorespiratory conditions. Falling levels of ozone in the upper atmosphere are also believed to contribute to global warming because ozone screens the earth from most of the sun's harmful ultraviolet radiation.

Air Embolism
A bubble of air in a blood vessel that affects the flow of blood from the heart. Air may enter the circulation after injury, infusions into the venous circulation, or surgery. The victim suffers breathlessness, chest discomfort, and acute heart failure.

Air Passages
These are the nose, pharynx or throat (the large cavity behind the nose and mouth), larynx,

A

trachea or windpipe, and bronchi or bronchial tubes. On entering the nose, the air passes through a high narrow passage on each side, the outer wall of which has three projections (the nasal conchae). It then passes down into the pharynx where the food and air passages meet and cross. The larynx lies in front of the lower part of the pharynx and is the organ where the voice is produced (see VOICE AND SPEECH) by aid of the vocal cords. The opening between the cords is called the glottis, and shortly after passing this the air reaches the trachea or windpipe.

The windpipe leads into the chest and divides above the heart into two bronchi, one of which goes to each lung, in which it splits into finer and finer tubes (see LUNGS). The larynx is enclosed in two strong cartilages: the thyroid (of which the most projecting part, the Adam's apple, is a prominent point on the front of the neck), and the cricoid (which can be felt as a hard ring about an inch below the thyroid). Beneath this, the trachea – which is stiffened by rings of cartilage so that it is never closed, no matter what position the body is in – can be traced down until it disappears behind the breastbone.

Air-Sickness
This condition is very similar to sea-sickness. (See MOTION (TRAVEL) SICKNESS.)

Akinesia
Loss or impairment of voluntary movement, or immobility. It is characteristically seen in PARKINSONISM.

Alastrim
Alastrim, or variola minor, is a form of SMALL-POX which differs from ordinary smallpox in being milder and having a low mortality.

Albendazole
A drug adjunct to surgery in the treatment of hydatid cysts (see under CYSTS) caused by *Taenia echinococcus*, a small tapeworm (see TAENIASIS). If surgery is not possible, albendazole can be used on its own. The drug is also used to treat STRONGYLOIDIASIS.

Albinism
A group of inherited disorders characterised by absence of or decrease in MELANIN in the skin, hair and eyes. The skin is pink, the hair white or pale yellow, and the iris of the eye translucent. Nystagmus (see under EYE, DISORDERS OF), PHOTOPHOBIA, SQUINT and poor eyesight are common. Photoprotection of both skin and eyes is essential. In the tropics, light-induced skin cancer may develop early.

Albumins
Albumins are water-soluble proteins which enter into the composition of all the tissues of the body. Albumins are generally divided according to their source of origin, as muscle-albumin, milk-albumin, blood- or serum-albumin, egg-albumin, vegetable-albumin, etc. These differ both in chemical reactions and also physiologically. Serum-albumin occurs in blood PLASMA where it is important in maintaining plasma volume.

When taken into the stomach, all albumins are converted into a soluble form by the process of DIGESTION and then absorbed into the blood, whence they go to build up the tissues. Albumin is synthesised in the liver, and in chronic liver disease this process is seriously affected. (See PROTEINURIA; KIDNEYS, DISEASES OF – Glomerulonephritis.)

Albuminuria
See PROTEINURIA.

Alcohol
A colourless liquid, also called ethanol or ethyl-alcohol, produced by the fermentation of carbohydrates by yeast. Medically, alcohol is used as a solvent and an antiseptic; recreationally it is a widely used drug, taken in alcoholic drinks to give a pleasant taste as well as to relax, reduce inhibitions, and increase sociability. Taken to excess, alcohol causes much mental and physical harm – not just to the individual imbibing it, but often to their family, friends, community and work colleagues.

Alcohol depresses the central nervous system and disturbs both mental and physical functioning. Even small doses of alcohol will slow a person's reflexes and concentration; potentially dangerous effects when, for example, driving or operating machinery. Drunkenness causes slurred speech, muddled thinking, amnesia (memory loss), drowsiness, erectile IMPOTENCE, poor coordination and dulled reactions – thereby making driving or operating machinery especially dangerous. Disinhibition may lead to extreme euphoria, irritability, misery or aggression, depending on the underlying mood at the start of drinking. Severe intoxication may lead to COMA and respiratory failure.

Persistent alcohol misuse leads to physical, mental, social and occupational problems, as well as to a risk of DEPENDENCE (see also ALCOHOL DEPENDENCE). Misuse may follow several patterns: regular but controlled heavy intake, 'binge' drinking, and dependence (alcoholism). The first pattern usually leads to mainly physical problems such as gastritis, peptic ulcer, liver disease, heart disease and impotence. The second is most common among young men and usually leads to mainly social and occupational problems – getting into fights, jeopardising personal relationships, overspending on alcohol at weekends, and missing days off work because of hangovers. The third pattern – alcohol dependence – is the most serious, and can severely disrupt health and social stability.

Many researchers consider alcohol dependence to be an illness that runs in families, with a genetic component which is probably passed on as a vulnerable personality. But it is hard to disentangle genetic, environmental and social factors in such families. In the UK there are estimated to be around a million people suffering from alcohol dependence and a similar number who have difficulty controlling their consumption (together about 1:30 of the population).

Alcohol causes tolerance and both physical and psychological dependence (see DEPENDENCE for definitions). Dependent drinkers classically drink early in the morning to relieve overnight withdrawal symptoms. These symptoms include anxiety, restlessness, nausea and vomiting, and tremor. Sudden withdrawal from regular heavy drinking can lead to life-threatening delirium tremens (DTs), with severe tremor, hallucinations (often visual – seeing spiders and monsters, rather than the pink elephants of romantic myth), and CONVULSIONS. This must be treated urgently with sedative drugs, preferably by intravenous drip. Similar symptoms, plus severe INCOORDINATION and double-vision, can occur in WERNICKE'S ENCEPHALOPATHY, a serious neurological condition due to lack of the B vitamin thiamine (whose absorption from the stomach is markedly reduced by alcohol). If not treated urgently with injections of thiamine and other vitamins, this can lead to an irreversible form of brain damage called Korsakoff's psychosis, with severe amnesia. Finally, prolonged alcohol misuse can cause a form of dementia.

In addition to these severe neurological disorders, the wide range of life-threatening problems caused by heavy drinking includes HEPATITIS, liver CIRRHOSIS, pancreatitis (see PANCREAS, DISEASES OF), gastrointestinal haemorrhage, suicide and FETAL ALCOHOL SYNDROME; pregnant women should not drink alcohol as this syndrome may occur with more than a glass of wine or half-pint of beer a day. The social effects of alcohol misuse – such as marital breakdown, family violence and severe debt – can be equally devastating.

Treatment of alcohol-related problems is only moderately successful. First, many of the physical problems are treated in the short term by doctors who fail to spot, or never ask about, heavy drinking. Second, attempts at treating alcohol dependence by detoxification or 'drying out' (substituting a tranquillising drug for alcohol and withdrawing it gradually over about a week) are not always followed-up by adequate support at home, so that drinking starts again. Home support by community alcohol teams comprising doctors, nurses, social workers and, when appropriate, probation officers is a recent development that may have better results. Many drinkers find the voluntary organisation Alcoholics Anonymous (AA) and its related groups for relatives (Al-Anon) and teenagers (Alateen) helpful because total abstinence from alcohol is encouraged by intensive psychological and social support from fellow ex-drinkers.

Useful contacts are: Alcoholics Anonymous; Al-Anon Family Groups UK and Eire (including Alateen); Alcohol Concern; Alcohol Focus Scotland; and Alcohol and Substance Misuse.

1 standard drink = 1 unit
      = ½ pint of beer
      = 1 measure of spirits
      = 1 glass of sherry or vermouth
      = 1 glass of wine

Limits within which alcohol is believed not to cause long-term health risks:

Women up to 2 units a day, 14 a week
(Pregnant women should avoid alcohol completely. If this is too difficult, 1 unit a day seems to be safe for the baby.) Women absorb alcohol more quickly than men.

Men up to 3 units a day, 21 a week

Alcohol Dependence

Alcohol dependence, or alcoholism, is described under ALCOHOL but a summary of the symptoms may be helpful in spotting the disorder. Behavioural symptoms vary but include furtiveness; aggression; inappropriately generous gestures; personality changes (selfishness, jealousy, irritability and outbursts of anger); empty promises to stop drinking; poor appetite; scruffy appearance; and long periods of drunkenness.

Alcuronium

Alcuronium is a drug which relaxes voluntary muscles. Given by injection during ANAESTHESIA to relax a patient undergoing surgery, the drug may delay the restart of spontaneous breathing.

Aldosterone

Aldosterone is a hormone secreted by the adrenal cortex (see ADRENAL GLANDS). It plays an important part in maintaining the electrolyte balance of the body by promoting the reabsorption of sodium and the secretion of potassium by the renal tubules. It is thus of primary importance in controlling the volume of the body fluids.

Alexia

Alexia is another name for WORD BLINDNESS. (See also APHASIA; DYSLEXIA.)

Alfacalcidol

Alfacalcidol is a synthetic form (or analogue) of vitamin D. (See APPENDIX 5: VITAMINS.)

Alglucerase

A drug used under specialist supervision for the rare hereditary disorder, GAUCHER'S DISEASE.

Algorithm

A set of instructions performed in a logical sequence to solve a problem. Algorithms are used increasingly in emergency situations, for example by ambulance controllers or by organisations such as NHS Direct. Each answer to a question leads on down a decision tree to the next question, eventually resulting in a recommended action or response.

Alimentary Canal

See GASTROINTESTINAL TRACT.

Alkali

A substance which neutralises an acid to form a salt, and turns litmus and other vegetable dyes blue. Alkalis are generally oxides or carbonates of metals.

Alkaloids

Substances found commonly in various plants. They are natural nitrogenous organic bases and combine with acids to form crystalline salts. Among alkaloids, morphine was discovered in 1805, strychnine in 1818, quinine and caffeine in 1820, nicotine in 1829, and atropine in 1833. Only a few alkaloids occur in the animal kingdom, the outstanding example being ADRENALINE, which is formed in the medulla of the suprarenal, or adrenal, gland. Alkaloids are often used for medicinal purposes. The name of an alkaloid ends in 'ine' (in Latin, 'ina').

Neutral principals are crystalline substances with actions similar to those of alkaloids but having a neutral reaction. The name of a neutral principal ends in 'in', e.g. digitalin, aloin.

The following are the more important alkaloids, with their source plants:

Aconite, *from Monkshood.*
Atropine, *from Belladonna* (juice of Deadly Nightshade).
Cocaine, *from Coca leaves.*
Hyoscine, *from Henbane.*
Morphine, Codeine, *from Opium* (juice of Poppy).
Thebaine, Nicotine, *from Tobacco.*
Physostigmine, *from Calabar beans.*
Pilocarpine, *from Jaborandi leaves.*
Quinidine, *from Cinchona or Peruvian bark.*
Strychnine, *from Nux Vomica seeds.*

Alkalosis

Alkalosis means an increase in the alkalinity (see ALKALI) of the blood, or, more accurately, a decrease in the concentration of hydrogen ions in the blood. It occurs, for example, in patients who have had large doses of alkalis for the treatment of gastric ulcer. (See ACID BASE BALANCE; ACIDOSIS.)

Alkaptonuria

See OCHRONOSIS.

Alkylating Agents

Alkylating agents are so named because they alkylate or chemically react with certain biochemical entities, particularly those concerned with the synthesis of NUCLEIC ACID. Alkylation is the substitution of an organic grouping in place of another grouping in a molecule.

Alkylating agents are important because they interfere with the growth and reproduction of cells, disrupting their replication. This CYTOTOXIC property is used to retard the division and growth of cancer cells, and alkylating drugs are widely used in the chemotherapy of malignant tumours – often in conjunction with surgery and sometimes with radiotherapy. Unfortunately, troublesome side-effects occur, such as: damage to veins when the drug is given intravenously, with resultant leakage into adjacent tissues; impaired kidney function due to the formation of URIC ACID crystals; nausea and vomiting; ALOPECIA (hair loss); suppression of BONE MARROW activity (production of blood cells); and adverse effects on reproductive function, including TERATOGENESIS. Indeed, cytotoxic drugs must not be given in pregnancy, especially during the first three months. Prolonged use of alkylating drugs, especially when accompanying radiotherapy, is also associated with a signficant rise in the incidence of acute non-lymphocytic LEUKAEMIA. Among the dozen or so alkylating drugs in use are CYCLOPHOSPHAMIDE, CHLORAMBUCIL, MELPHALAN, BUSULFAN and THIOTEPA. (See also CHEMOTHERAPY.)

Allantoin

Prepared synthetically, this powder, which occurs naturally in comfrey root, has been used as an ADJUVANT in the treatment of skin ulcers. It has been thought to stimulate the formation of the surface epithelial layer of skin, but its therapeutic value is now more dubious.

Allantois

A vascular structure which, very early in the life of an EMBRYO, grows out from its hind-gut. The end becomes attached to the wall of the womb (see UTERUS); it spreads out, becomes stalked, and later develops into the PLACENTA and umbilical cord, which forms the only connection between mother and embryo.

Allele

An allele, or allelomorph, is a gene (see GENES) which may exist in one or more forms, only one of which can occur in a given chromosome (see CHROMOSOMES). Two alleles of a given gene are at the same relative positions on a pair of homologous (similarly structured) chromosomes. If the two alleles are identical, the subject is homozygous for the gene – namely, the genes will exert a unanimous influence on a particular characteristic. If the alleles are different, with one having a dominant and the other a recessive influence, the subject is heterozygous.

Allergen

Any substance – usually a protein – which, taken into the body, makes the body hypersensitive or 'allergic' to it. Thus, in hay fever, the allergen is pollen. (See ALLERGY.)

Allergic Rhinitis

See HAY FEVER.

Allergy

A term generally used to describe an adverse reaction by the body to any substance ingested by the affected individual. Strictly, allergy refers to any reactions incited by an abnormal immunological response to an ALLERGEN, and susceptibility has a strong genetic component. Most allergic disorders are linked to ATOPY, the predisposition to generate the allergic antibody immunoglobulin E (IgE) to common environmental agents (see ANTIBODIES; IMMUNOGLOBULINS). Because IgE is able to sensitise MAST CELLS (which play a part in inflammatory and allergic reactions) anywhere in the body, atopic individuals often have disease in more than one organ. Since the allergic disorder HAY FEVER was first described in 1819, allergy has moved from being a rare condition to one afflicting almost one in two people in the developed world, with substances such as grass and tree pollen, house-dust mite, bee and wasp venom, egg and milk proteins, peanuts, antibiotics, and other airborne environmental pollutants among the triggering factors. Increasing prevalence of allergic reactions has been noticeable during the past two decades, especially in young people with western lifestyles.

A severe or life-threatening reaction is often termed ANAPHYLAXIS. Many immune mechanisms also contribute to allergic disorders; however, adverse reactions to drugs, diagnostic materials and other substances often do not involve recognised immunological mechanisms and the term 'hypersensitivity' is preferable. (See also IMMUNITY.)

Adverse reactions may manifest themselves as URTICARIA, wheezing or difficulty in breathing owing to spasm of the BRONCHIOLES, swollen joints, nausea, vomiting and headaches. Severe allergic reactions may cause a person to go into SHOCK. Although symptoms of an allergic reaction can usually be controlled, treatment of the underlying conditon is more problematic: hence, the best current approach is for susceptible individuals to find out what it is they are allergic to and avoid those agents. For some people, such as those sensitive to insect venom, IMMUNOTHERAPY or desensitisation is often effective. If avoidance measures are unsuccessful and desensitisation ineffective, the inflammatory reactions can be controlled with CORTICOSTEROIDS, while the troublesome symptoms can be treated with ANTIHISTAMINE DRUGS and SYMPATHOMIMETICS. All three types of drugs may be needed to treat severe allergic reactions.

One interesting hypothesis is that reduced exposure to infective agents, such as bacteria, in infancy may provoke the development of allergy in later life.

Predicted developments in tackling allergic disorders, according to Professor Stephen Holgate writing in the *British Medical Journal* (22 January 2000) include:

A

- Identification of the principal environmental factors underlying the increase in incidence, to enable preventive measures to be planned.
- Safe and effective immunotherapy to prevent and reverse allergic disease.
- Treatments that target the protein reactions activated by antigens.
- Identification of how IgE is produced in the body, and thus of possible ways to inhibit this process.
- Identification of genes affecting people's susceptibility to allergic disease.

Allocheiria
The name for a disorder of sensation in which sensations are referred to the wrong part of the body.

Allograft
A piece of tissue or an organ, such as the kidney, transplanted from one to another of the same species – from person to person, for example. Also known as a homograft.

Allopathy
A term applied sometimes by homeopaths (see HOMEOPATHY) to the methods used by regular practitioners of medicine and surgery. The term literally means curing by inducing a different kind of action in the body, and is an erroneous designation.

Allopurinol
A drug used to treat GOUT. It acts by suppressing the formation of uric acid. It is also being used in treatment of uric acid stone in the kidney.

Alopecia
Alopecia means hair loss. It may be localised or total in the scalp. The commonest type, which is hereditary, is male baldness (androgenic alopecia). Female balding spares the anterior hair line, develops later, and is less severe than the male variety. Diffuse hair loss is common after childbirth, severe illness or infection (telogen alopecia); it begins 8–12 weeks after the causative event and recovery is complete. Persistent diffuse hair loss may be caused by severe iron deficiency or HYPOTHYROIDISM, or may be drug-induced.

Patchy localised hair loss is commonly caused by fungal infections (tinea capitis – see RINGWORM), especially in the tropics. It may also be due to trauma, such as hair-pulling by children or disturbed adults, or hair-straightening by African or Afro-Caribbean women (traction alopecia). Rarely, diseases of the scalp-skin such as discoid lupus erythematosus (see under LUPUS) or lichen planus (see under LICHEN) may cause patchy alopecia with scarring which is irreversible. The long-term effects of radiotherapy may be similar.

Treatment depends on the cause. Specific antifungal drugs cure tinea capitis. Correction of thyroid or iron deficiency may be dramatic. Male baldness may be modified slightly by long-term use of minoxidil lotion, or improved permanently by various types of hair-follicle grafting of transplants from the occipital scalp. Female balding may be amenable to anti-androgen/oestrogen regimens, but severe forms require a wig.

Alopecia Areata
Alopecia areata is a common form of reversible hair loss which may be patchy, total on the scalp, eyebrows or eyelashes, or universal on the body. The onset is sudden at any age and the affected scalp-skin looks normal. The hair follicles remain intact but 'switched off' and usually hair growth recovers spontaneously. No consistently effective treatment is available but injections of CORTICOSTEROIDS, given with a spray gun into the scalp, may be useful. The regrown hair may be white at first but pigmentation recovers later.

Alpha Adrenergic Blockers
Also called adrenoceptor-blocking agents or alpha blockers, these drugs stop the stimulation of alpha-adrenergic receptors at the nerve endings of the SYMPATHETIC NERVOUS SYSTEM by HORMONES with ADRENALINE-like characteristics. The drugs dilate the arteries, causing a fall in blood pressure, so they are used to treat HYPERTENSION and also benign enlargement of the PROSTATE GLAND. Examples of this group of drugs are doxazosin, indoramin, phentolamine and prazosin. The drugs should be used with caution as some may cause a severe drop in blood pressure when first taken.

Alpha-Feto Protein
A protein produced in the gut and liver of the FETUS. Abnormality in the fetus, such as neural tube defect, may result in raised levels of alpha-feto protein in the maternal blood. In DOWN'S (DOWN) SYNDROME, levels may be abnormally low. In either case, screening of the pregnancy should be carried out, including AMNIOCENTESIS to check the amount of alpha-feto protein in the amniotic fluid. The protein may also be produced in some abnormal tissues in

the adult – in patients with liver cancer, for example.

ALTE

This is an abbreviation for 'acute life-threatening event'. It applies to infants, usually under one year of age, who suddenly and unexpectedly become pale or blue and appear to stop breathing. They generally recover spontaneously, although a parent or bystander often administers mouth-to-mouth resuscitation. By the time the baby reaches hospital he or she is usually well. Investigations show that the most common cause of ALTE is GASTRO-OESOPHAGEAL REFLUX, causing stomach acid to be regurgitated into the throat and provoking reflex closure of the GLOTTIS. Other causes may be brief epileptic seizures, identified by ELECTRO-ENCEPHALOGRAPHY (EEG); a heart ARRHYTHMIA; or a respiratory infection. In many cases the cause remains unknown, even though the events may be repeated, and the large majority of babies 'grow out' of the condition. Much controversy surrounds the suggestion – confirmed by hidden video-recording in hospitals – that a small minority of these babies have been subjected to repeated brief deliberate suffocation (see under MUNCHAUSEN'S SYNDROME).

Treatment is that of the underlying cause, if discovered. Parents may also be offered an APNOEA monitor, a device attached to the child – especially when asleep – which sounds an alarm if breathing stops for more than 20 seconds.

Alternative Medicine

See COMPLEMENTARY AND ALTERNATIVE MEDICINE (CAM).

Altitude Sickness

This condition, also known as mountain sickness, occurs in mountain climbers or hikers who have climbed too quickly to heights above 3,000 metres, thus failing to allow their bodies to acclimatise to altitude. The lower atmospheric pressure and shortage of oxygen result in hyperventilation – deep, quick breathing – and this reduces the amount of carbon dioxide in the blood. Nausea, anxiety and exhaustion are presenting symptoms, and seriously affected individuals may be acutely breathless because of pulmonary oedema (excess fluid in the lungs). Gradual climbing over two or three days should prevent mountain sickness. In serious cases the individual must be brought down to hospital urgently. Most attacks, however, are mild.

Aluminium

A light metallic element. It occurs in bauxite and other minerals and its compounds are found in low concentration in the body. Their function, if any, is unknown but they are believed to be harmful. Aluminium hydroxide is, however, a safe, slow-acting substance that is widely used in the treatment of indigestion, gastric ulcers (see STOMACH, DISEASES OF) and oesophagitis (see OESOPHAGUS, DISEASES OF), acting as an antacid (see ANTACIDS). Other ingested sources of aluminium include cooking utensils, kitchen foil and some cooking and food additives. Most aluminium is excreted; the rest is deposited in the brain, liver, lungs and thyroid gland. Prolonged use of aluminium-based antacids can cause loss of appetite, tiredness and weakness. It has been suggested that ALZHEIMER'S DISEASE is more common in areas with water which contains a high concentration of the element, but this issue is controversial.

Alveolitis

Inflammation of the alveoli (see ALVEOLUS) of the lungs caused by an allergic reaction. When the inflammation is caused by infection it is called PNEUMONIA, and when by a chemical or physical agent it is called pneumonitis. It may be associated with systemic sclerosis or RHEUMATOID ARTHRITIS.

Extrinsic allergic alveolitis is the condition induced by the lungs becoming allergic (see ALLERGY) to various factors or substances. It includes BAGASSOSIS, FARMER'S LUNG and BUDGERIGAR-FANCIER'S LUNG, and is characterised by the onset of shortness of breath, tightness of the chest, cough and fever. The onset may be sudden or gradual. Treatment consists of removal of the affected individual from the offending material to which he or she has become allergic. CORTICOSTEROIDS give temporary relief.

Fibrosing alveolitis In this disease there is diffuse FIBROSIS of the walls of the alveoli of the lungs. This causes loss of lung volume with both forced expiratory volume and vital capacity affected, but the ratio between them remaining normal. The patient complains of cough and progressive DYSPNOEA. Typically the patient will be cyanosed (blue – see CYANOSIS), clubbed (see CLUBBING), and have crackles in the mid- and lower-lung fields. Blood gases will reveal HYPOXIA and, in early disease, hypocapnia (deficiency of carbon dioxide in the blood due to hyperventilation). There is an association with RHEUMATOID ARTHRITIS (about one-eighth of cases), systemic lupus erythematosus (see under LUPUS), and systemic SCLEROSIS. Certain drugs – for example, bleomycin, busulphan and hexamethonium – may also cause this condition, as may high concentrations of oxygen, and inhalation of CADMIUM fumes.

Alveolus

(1) The minute divisions of glands and the air sacs of the lungs.
(2) The sockets of the teeth in the jawbone.

Alzheimer's Disease

Alzheimer's disease is a progressive degenerating process of neural tissue affecting mainly the frontal and temporal lobes of the BRAIN in middle and late life. There is probably a genetic component to Alzheimer's disease, but early-onset Alzheimer's is linked to certain mutations, or changes, in three particular GENES. Examination of affected brains shows 'senile plaques' containing an amyloid-like material distributed throughout an atrophied cortex (see AMYLOID PLAQUES). Many remaining neurons, or nerve cells, show changes in their NEUROFI-BRILS which thicken and twist into 'neurofibrillary tangles'. First symptoms are psychological with insidious impairment of recent memory and disorientation in time and space. This becomes increasingly associated with difficulties in judgement, comprehension and abstract reasoning. After very few years, progressive neurological deterioration produces poor gait, immobility and death. When assessment has found no other organic cause for an affected individual's symptoms, treatment is primarily palliative. The essential part of treatment is the provision of appropriate nursing and social care, with strong support being given to the relatives or other carers for whom looking after sufferers is a prolonged and onerous burden. Proper diet and exercise are helpful, as is keeping the individual occupied. If possible, sufferers should stay in familiar surroundings with day-care and short-stay institutional facilities a useful way of maintaining them at home for as long as possible.

TRANQUILLISERS can help control difficult behaviour and sleeplessness but should be used with care. Recently drugs such as DONEPEZIL and RIVASTIGMINE, which retard the breakdown of ACETYLCHOLINE, may check – but not cure – this distressing condition. About 40 per cent of those with DEMENTIA improve.

Research is in progress to transplant healthy nerve cells (developed from stem cells) into the brain tissue of patients with Alzheimer's disease with the aim of improving brain function.

The rising proportion of elderly people in the population is resulting in a rising incidence of Alzheimer's, which is rare before the age of 60 but increases steadily thereafter so that 30 per cent of people over the age of 84 are affected.

Amantadine

A drug used to treat certain virus infections which is also of value in the prevention of some forms of influenza. It is also used to treat PARKINSONISM.

Amaurosis Fugax

Sudden transitory impairment, or loss, of vision. It usually affects only one eye, and is commonly due to circulatory failure. In its simplest form it occurs in normal people on rising suddenly from the sitting or recumbent position, when it is due to the effects of gravity. It also occurs in migraine. A not uncommon cause, particularly in elderly people, is transient ocular ISCHAEMIA, resulting from blockage of the circulation to the retina (see EYE) by emboli (see EMBOLISM) from the common carotid artery or the heart. Treatment in this last group of cases consists of control of the blood pressure if this is raised, as it often is in such cases; and the administration of drugs that reduce the stickiness of blood platelets, such as aspirin. In some instances, removal of the part of the carotid artery from which the emboli are coming may be indicated.

Ambivalence

The psychological state in which a person concurrently hates and loves the same object or person.

Amblyopia

Defective vision for which no recognisable cause exists in any part of the eye. It may be due to such causes as defective development or excessive use of tobacco or alcohol. The most important form is that associated with SQUINT, or gross difference in refraction between the two eyes. It has been estimated that in Britain around 5 per cent of young adults have amblyopia due to this cause.

Amelia

This is absence of the limbs, usually a congenital defect.

Amenorrhoea

Absence of MENSTRUATION at the time of life at which it should normally occur. If menstruation has never occurred, the amenorrhoea is termed primary; secondary amenorrhoea is defined as menstruation ceasing after a normal cycle has been experienced for a number of years.

A few patients with primary amenorrhoea have an abnormality of their CHROMOSOMES or malformation of the genital tract such as absecence of the UTERUS (see TURNER'S SYNDROME). A gynaecological examination will rarely disclose an IMPERFORATE HYMEN in a young girl who may also complain of regular cycles of pain like period pains.

There are many causes of secondary amenorrhoea and management requires dealing with the primary cause. The commonest cause is pregnancy. Disorders of the HYPOTHALAMUS and related psychological factors such as anorexia nervosa (see EATING DISORDERS) also cause amenorrhoea, as can poor nutrition and loss of weight by extreme dieting. It is common in ballet dancers and athletes who exercise a great deal, but can also be triggered by serious illnesses such as tuberculosis or malaria. Excess secretion of prolactin, either due to a micro-adenoma (see ADENOMA) of the PITUITARY GLAND or to various prescription drugs will produce amenorrhoea, and sometimes GALACTORRHOEA as well. Malfunction of other parts of the pituitary gland will cause failure to produce GONADOTROPHINS, thus causing ovarian failure with consequent amenorrhea. In CUSHING'S SYNDROME, amenorrhoea is caused by excessive production of cortisol. Similarly, androgen-production abnormalities are found in the common POLYCYSTIC OVARY SYNDROME. These conditions also have abnormalities of the insulin/glucose control mechanisms. Taking the contraceptive pill is not now considered to provoke secondary amenorrhoea but OBESITY and HYPOTHYROIDISM are potential causes.

When the cause is weight loss, restoring body weight may alone restore menstruation. Otherwise, measuring gonadotrophic hormone levels will help show whether amenorrhoea is due to primary ovarian failure or secondary to pituitary disease. Women with raised concentrations of serum gonadotrophic hormones have primary ovarian failure. When amenorrhoea is due to limited pituitary failure, treatment with CLOMIPHENE may solve the problem.

Amentia

Amentia is the failure of the intellectual faculties to develop normally.

Amethocaine

An effective local anaesthetic for topical application. Rapidly absorbed from mucous membranes, it should never be applied to inflamed, traumatised or highly vascular surfaces – nor used when providing anaesthesia for bronchoscopy or cystoscopy. Amethocaine is used in ophthalmology and in skin preparations. It may sensitise the skin. (See ANAESTHESIA.)

Ametropia

See REFRACTION.

Amikacin

One of the AMINOGLYCOSIDES, amikacin is a semi-synthetic derivative of KANAMYCIN, which is used to treat infections caused by micro-organisms resistant to GENTAMICIN and TOBRAMYCIN.

Amiloride

A diuretic that acts without causing excessive loss of potassium (see DIURETICS).

Amines

Substances derived from ammonia or AMINO ACIDS which play an important part in the working of the body, including the brain and the circulatory system. They include ADRENALINE, NORADRENALINE and HISTAMINE. (See also MONOAMINE OXIDASE INHIBITORS (MAOIS).)

Amino Acids

Chemical compounds that are the basic building-blocks of all proteins. Each molecule consists of nitrogenous amino and acidic carboxyl groups of atoms joined to a group of carbon atoms. Polypeptides are formed by amino-acid molecules linking via peptide bonds. Many polypeptides link up in various configurations to form protein molecules. In humans, proteins are made up from 20 different amino acids: nine of these are labelled 'essential' (or, as is now preferred, 'indispensable') amino acids because the body cannot manufacture them and is dependent on the diet for their provision. (See also INDISPENSABLE AMINO ACIDS.)

Aminocaproic Acid

A drug used to treat hereditary angio-oedema (see under URTICARIA) – a serious anaphylactic (see ANAPHYLAXIS) reaction of the skin and respiratory tract resulting from a deficiency in the body's immunological defence mechanisms (see IMMUNITY).

Aminoglutethimide

A drug that inhibits the synthesis of adrenal CORTICOSTEROIDS. It is proving to be of value in the treatment of cancer of the breast in post-menopausal women.

Aminoglycosides

A group of antibiotics usually reserved for use in patients with severe infections. They are effective against a wide range of BACTERIA including some gram-positive and many gram-negative organisms (see GRAM'S STAIN). Aminoglycosides must be used cautiously because they can damage the inner ear – thus affecting hearing – and the kidneys. Examples of this group are AMIKACIN and GENTAMICIN (effective against *Pseudomonas aeuriginosa*), NEOMYCIN (used only for topical administration for skin infections), and STREPTOMYCIN (effective in combination with other drugs against *Mycobacterium tuberculosis*).

Aminophylline

A combination of theophylline and ethylenediamine. It is used intravenously in the treatment of acute severe ASTHMA, or as an oral preparation in the treatment of chronic asthma.

Amiodarone

(in the form of amiodarone hydrochloride) is a drug used to treat ARRHYTHMIA of the HEART and initiated only under supervision in hospital or by an appropriate specialist. Given by mouth or intravenous infusion, amiodarone can help to control paroxysmal supraventricular, nodal and ventricular TACHYCARDIA as well as FIBRILLATION of the auricles and ventricles of the heart. It may take some time to achieve control, and several weeks to be eliminated from the body when treatment is stopped. The drug has a range of potentially serious side-effects.

Amitriptyline

See ANTIDEPRESSANT DRUGS.

Ammonia

A compound of hydrogen and nitrogen that occurs naturally. The solution is colourless with a pungent smell; it is used in urine testing. In humans, certain inherited defects in the metabolism of ammonia can cause neurological symptoms including mental retardation. In vapour form it is a noxious gas.

Amnesia

Amnesia means loss of memory.

Amniocentesis

A diagnostic procedure for detecting abnormalities of the FETUS. Usually carried out between the 16th and 18th week of pregnancy, amniocentesis is performed by piercing the amniotic sac in the pregnant UTERUS with a hollow needle and withdrawing a sample of AMNIOTIC FLUID for laboratory analysis. As well as checking for the presence of abnormal fetal cells, the procedure can show the sex of the fetus. The risk of early rupture of the fetal membranes or of miscarriage is low (around 0.5 per cent).

Amnion

Amnion is the tough fibrous membrane which lines the cavity of the womb (UTERUS) during pregnancy, and contains between 0·5 and 1 litre (1–2 pints) of fluid in which the EMBRYO floats. It is formed from the ovum (egg) along with the embryo, and in labour the part of it at the mouth of the womb forms the 'bag of waters'. (See PREGNANCY AND LABOUR.) When a child is 'born with a CAUL', the caul is a piece of amnion.

Amnioscopy

The insertion of a viewing instrument (amnioscope) through the abdominal wall into the pregnant UTERUS to examine the inside of the amniotic sac (see AMNION). The growing FETUS can be viewed directly and its condition and sex assessed without disturbing the pregnancy. The amniotic sac may also be viewed late in pregnancy through the cervix or neck of the womb using an instrument called the fetoscope.

Amniotic Fluid

The clear fluid contained within the AMNION that surrounds the FETUS in the womb and protects it from external pressure. The fluid, comprising mainly water, is produced by the amnion and is regularly circulated, being swallowed by the fetus and excreted through the kidneys back into the amniotic sac. By the 35th week of pregnancy there is about 1 litre of fluid, but this falls to 0.5 litres at term. The amniotic sac normally ruptures in early labour, releasing the fluid or 'waters'.

Amniotic Sac

See AMNION.

Amoeba

A minute protozoan organism consisting of a single cell, in which a nucleus is surrounded by protoplasm that changes its shape as the protozoon progresses or absorbs nourishment. Several varieties are found under different conditions within the human body. One variety, *Entamoeba coli*, is found in the large intestine of humans without any associated disease; another, *Entamoeba gingivalis*, is found in the sockets of the teeth and associated with PYORRHOEA. *Entamoeba histolytica* is the causative organism of amoebic dysentery (see DYSENTERY); *Acanthamoeba* and *Naegleria fowleri* cause the infection of the brain known as MENINGOENCEPHALITIS. *Entamoeba histolytica* may also cause meningoencephalitis. Other forms are found in the genital organs.

Amoebiasis

See DYSENTERY.

Amoxicillin

See PENICILLIN; ANTIBIOTICS.

Amphetamines

A group of drugs closely related to ADRENALINE which act by stimulating the SYMPATHETIC NERVOUS SYSTEM. When taken by mouth they have a profound stimulating effect on the brain, producing a sense of well-being and confidence and seemingly increasing the capacity for mental work. They are, however, drugs of DEPENDENCE and their medical use is now strictly limited – for example, to the treatment of NARCOLEPSY.

Because amphetamines inhibit appetite, they rapidly achieved a reputation for slimming purposes. However, they should not be used for this purpose; their dangers far outweigh their advantages.

Amphoric

An adjective denoting the kind of breathing heard over a cavity in the lung. The sound is like that made by blowing over the mouth of a narrow-necked vase.

Amphotericin

A highly toxic, polygenic antifungal drug that must be given only under close medical supervision and for severe systemic fungal infections (see FUNGAL AND YEAST INFECTIONS). It is not absorbed from the gut so is normally given parenterally (see PARENTERAL). Oral and intestinal candidiasis (see CANDIDA) can, however, be treated with amphotericin tablets.

Ampicillin

See PENICILLIN; ANTIBIOTICS.

Ampoule

A small glass container having one end drawn out into a point capable of being sealed so as to preserve its contents sterile. It is used for containing solutions for hypodermic injection.

Ampulla of Vater

The dilated section of the common BILE DUCT when it is joined by the duct from the PANCREAS.

Amputation

Severance of a limb, or part of a limb, from the rest of the body. The leg is the most common site of amputation. It is usually performed as a controlled operation and may be required for a variety of reasons. In the young, severe injury is the most common cause, when damage to the limb is so extensive as to make it non-viable or functionally useless. In the elderly, amputation is more often the result of vascular insufficiency, resulting in gangrene or intractable pain.

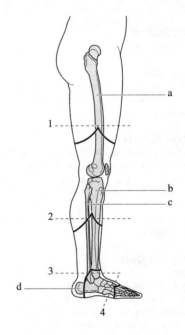

1   above knee (about 15 cm above joint)
2   below knee (about 8 cm below head of tibia bone)
3   Syme's heel flap
4   transmetatarsal
a   femur bone
b   tibia bone
c   fibula bone
d   calcaneus (heel bone)

Amputation sites of lower limb.

Sarcoma (see CANCER) of bone, muscle or connective tissues in a limb is another reason for amputation.

The aim is to restore the patient to full mobility with a prosthetic (artificial) limb, which requires both a well-fitting PROSTHESIS and a well-healed surgical wound. If this is not possible, the aim is to leave the patient with a limb stump that is still useful for balancing, sitting and transferring. Common types of lower-limb amputation are shown in the illustration. The Symes amputation can be walked upon without requiring a prosthesis. The below-knee amputation preserves normal flexion of the knee, and virtually normal walking can be achieved with a well-fitting artificial limb. Learning to walk is more difficult following an above-knee amputation, but some highly motivated patients can manage well. After any amputation it is not unusual for the patient to experience the sensation that the limb is still present: this is called a 'PHANTOM LIMB' and the sensation may persist for a long time.

Amsacrine
See under CYTOTOXIC.

Amylase
An ENZYME in pancreatic juice which facilitates the conversion of starch to maltose. (See PANCREAS.)

Amyl Nitrite
A volatile, oily liquid prepared by the action of nitric and nitrous acids on amyl alcohol. It was used for many years to treat angina but has been superseded by other nitrate drugs such as glyceril trinitrate. The substance is misused by drug abusers to produce a 'high' and is referred to as 'poppers'.

Amyloidosis
A rare condition in which deposits of complex protein, known as amyloid, are found in various parts of the body. It is a degenerative condition resulting from various causes such as chronic infection, including tuberculosis and rheumatoid arthritis.

Amyloid Plaques
Characteristic waxy deposits of amyloid found in primary AMYLOIDOSIS, the cause of which is unknown.

Amylose
The name applied to any carbohydrate of the starch group.

Amyotrophy
Loss of muscle bulk and strength caused by a disorder of the nerve that supplies the muscle. The loss is progressive and characterises chronic NEUROPATHY. Patients with DIABETES MELLITUS and MOTOR NEURONE DISEASE (MND) often suffer from amyotrophy as well as spasticity (see SPASTIC) of muscles.

Anabolic Steroids
The nitrogen-retaining effect of ANDROGEN, a steroid hormone, is responsible for the larger muscle mass of the male. This is called an anabolic effect. Attempts have been made to separate the anabolic effects of hormones from their virilising effects (see VIRILISATION), but these have been only partially successful. Thus, anabolic steroids have the property of protein-building so that when taken, they lead to an increase in muscle bulk and strength. All the anabolic steroids have some androgenic activity but they cause less virilisation than androgens in women. Androgenic side-effects may result from any of these anabolic compounds, especially if they are given for prolonged periods: for this reason they should all be used with caution in women, and are contraindicated in men with prostatic carcinoma. Jaundice due to stasis of bile in the intrahepatic canaliculi is a hazard, and the depression of pituitary gonadotrophin production is a possible complication.

Anabolic steroids have been used to stimulate protein anabolism in debilitating illness, and to promote growth in children with pituitary dwarfism and other disorders associated with interference of growth. Stimulation of protein anabolism may also be of value in acute renal failure, and the retention of nitrogen and calcium is of probable benefit to patients with OSTEOPOROSIS and to patients receiving corticosteroid therapy. Anabolic steroids may stimulate bone-marrow function in hypoplastic ANAEMIA.

They have been widely abused by athletes and body-builders aiming to improve their strength, stamina, speed or body size. However, there are considerable doubts over their efficacy, with little experimental evidence that they work. Dangerous adverse effects include precocious myocardial infarction (see HEART, DISEASES OF – Coronary thrombosis), DIABETES MELLITUS, liver disease, precocious carcinoma of the prostate, acne, and severe psychiatric disorders. Anabolic steroids should not be used by athletes, who face bans from official competitions if they take them.

The anabolic steroids in therapeutic use include nandrolone and stanozolol.

Anabolism

Production by the body of complex molecules like fat and proteins from simpler substances taken in the diet.

Anaemia

The condition characterised by inadequate red blood cells and/or HAEMOGLOBIN in the BLOOD. It is considered to exist if haemoglobin levels are below 13 grams per 100 ml in males and below 12 grams per 100 ml in adult non-pregnant women. No simple classification of anaemia can be wholly accurate, but the most useful method is to divide anaemias into: (*a*) microcytic hypochromic or iron deficiency anaemia; (*b*) megaloblastic hyperchromic anaemia; (*c*) aplastic anaemia; (*d*) haemolytic anaemia; (*e*) inherited anaemias (see below).

In Britain, anaemia is much more common among women than men. Thus, around 10 per cent of girls have anaemia at the age of 15, whilst in adult life the incidence is over 30 per cent between the ages of 30 and 40, around 20 per cent at 50, and around 30 per cent at 70. Among men the incidence is under 5 per cent until the age of 50; it then rises to 20 per cent at the age of 70. Ninety per cent of all cases of anaemia in Britain are microcytic, 7 per cent are macrocytic, and 3 per cent are haemolytic or aplastic. Inherited anaemias include sickle-cell anaemia and THALASSAEMIA.

Microcytic hypochromic anaemia

corresponds to a large extent with what used to be known as 'secondary anaemia'. It takes its name from the characteristic changes in the blood.

Causes

LOSS OF BLOOD

- As a result of trauma. This is perhaps the simplest example of all, when, as a result of an accident involving a large artery, there is severe haemorrhage.
- Menstruation. The regular monthly loss of blood which women sustain as a result of menstruation always puts a strain on the blood-forming organs. If this loss is excessive, then over a period of time it may lead to quite severe anaemia.
- Childbirth. A considerable amount of blood is always lost at childbirth; if this is severe, or if the woman was anaemic during pregnancy, a severe degree of anaemia may develop.

- Bleeding from the gastrointestinal tract. The best example here is anaemia due to 'bleeding piles' (see HAEMORRHOIDS). Such bleeding, even though slight, is a common cause of anaemia in both men and women if maintained over a long period of time. The haemorrhage may be more acute and occur from a DUODENAL ULCER or gastric ulcer (see STOMACH, DISEASES OF), when it is known as haematemesis.
- Certain blood diseases, such as PURPURA and HAEMOPHILIA, which are characterised by bleeding.

DEFECTIVE BLOOD FORMATION

- This is the main cause of anaemia in infections. The micro-organism responsible for the infection has a deleterious effect upon the blood-forming organs, just as it does upon other parts of the body.
- Toxins. In conditions such as chronic glomerulonephritis (see KIDNEYS, DISEASES OF) and URAEMIA there is a severe anaemia due to the effect of the disease upon blood formation.
- Drugs. Certain drugs, such as aspirin and the non-steroidal anti-inflammatory drugs, may cause occult gastrointestinal bleeding.

INADEQUATE ABSORPTION OF IRON

This may occur in diseases of intestinal malabsorption. A severe form of this anaemia in women, known as chlorosis, used to be common but is seldom seen nowadays.

INADEQUATE INTAKE OF IRON

The daily requirement of iron for an adult is 12 mg, and 15–20 mg for an adult woman during pregnancy. This is well covered by an ordinary diet, so that by itself it is not a common cause. But if there is a steady loss of blood, as a result of heavy menstrual loss or 'bleeding piles', the intake of iron in the diet may not be sufficient to maintain adequate formation of haemoglobin.

Symptoms These depend upon whether the anaemia is sudden in onset, as in severe haemorrhage, or gradual. In all cases, however, the striking sign is pallor, the depth of which depends upon the severity of the anaemia. The colour of the skin may be misleading, except in cases due to severe haemorrhage, as the skin of many Caucasian people is normally pale. The best guide is the colour of the internal lining of the eyelid. When the onset of the anaemia is sudden, the patient complains of weakness and

A

giddiness, and loses consciousness if he or she tries to stand or sit up. The breathing is rapid and distressed, the pulse is rapid and the blood pressure is low. In chronic cases the tongue is often sore (GLOSSITIS), and the nails of the fingers may be brittle and concave instead of convex (koilonychia). In some cases, particularly in women, the Plummer-Vinson syndrome is present: this consists of difficulty in swallowing and may be accompanied by huskiness; in these cases glossitis is also present. There may be slight enlargement of the SPLEEN, and there is usually some diminution in gastric acidity.

CHANGES IN THE BLOOD The characteristic change is a diminution in both the haemoglobin and the red cell content of the blood. There is a relatively greater fall in the haemoglobin than in the red cell count. If the blood is examined under a microscope, the red cells are seen to be paler and smaller than normal. These small red cells are known as microcytes.

Treatment consists primarily of giving sufficient iron by mouth to restore, and then maintain, a normal blood picture. The main iron preparation now used is ferrous sulphate, 200 mg, thrice daily after meals. When the blood picture has become normal, the dosage is gradually reduced. A preparation of iron is available which can be given intravenously, but this is only used in cases which do not respond to iron given by mouth, or in cases in which it is essential to obtain a quick response.

If, of course, there is haemorrhage, this must be arrested, and if the loss of blood has been severe it may be necessary to give a blood transfusion (see TRANSFUSION – Transfusion of blood). Care must be taken to ensure that the patient is having an adequate diet. If there is any underlying metabolic, oncological, toxic or infective condition, this, of course, must be adequately treated after appropriate investigations.

Megaloblastic hyperchromic anaemia There are various forms of anaemia of this type, such as those due to nutritional deficiencies, but the most important is that known as pernicious anaemia.

PERNICIOUS ANAEMIA An autoimmune disease in which sensitised lymphocytes (see LYMPHOCYTE) destroy the PARIETAL cells of the stomach. These cells normally produce INTRINSIC FACTOR, the carrier protein for vitamin B_{12} (see APPENDIX 5: VITAMINS) that permits its absorp-

tion in the terminal part of the ILEUM. Lack of the factor prevents vitamin B_{12} absorption and this causes macrocytic (or megaloblastic) anaemia. The disorder can affect men and women, usually those over the age of 40; onset is insidious so it may be well advanced before medical advice is sought. The skin and MUCOSA become pale, the tongue is smooth and atrophic and is accompanied by CHEILOSIS. Peripheral NEUROPATHY is often present, resulting in PARAESTHESIA and numbness and sometimes ATAXIA. A rare complication is subacute combined degeneration of the SPINAL CORD.

In 1926 two Americans, G R Minot and W P Murphy, discovered that pernicious anaemia, a previously fatal condition, responded to treatment with liver which provides the absent intrinsic factor. Normal development requires a substance known as extrinsic factor, and this depends on the presence of intrinsic factor for its absorption from the gut. The disease is characterised in the blood by abnormally large red cells (macrocytes) which vary in shape and size, while the number of white cells (LEUCOCYTES) diminishes. A key diagnostic find is the presence of cells in the BONE MARROW.

Treatment consists of injections of vitamin B_{12} in the form of hydroxocobalamin which must be continued for life.

Aplastic anaemia is a disease in which the red blood corpuscles are very greatly reduced, and in which no attempt appears to be made in the bone marrow towards their regeneration. It is more accurately called hypoplastic anaemia as the degree of impairment of bone-marrow function is rarely complete. The cause in many cases is not known, but in rather less than half the cases the condition is due to some toxic substance, such as benzol or certain drugs, or ionising radiations. The patient becomes very pale, with a tendency to haemorrhages under the skin and mucous membranes, and the temperature may at times be raised. The red blood corpuscles diminish steadily in numbers. Treatment consists primarily of regular blood transfusions. Although the disease is often fatal, the outlook has improved in recent years: around 25 per cent of patients recover when adequately treated, and others survive for several years. In severe cases promising results are being reported from the use of bone-marrow transplantation.

Haemolytic anaemia results from the excessive destruction, or HAEMOLYSIS, of the red blood cells. This may be the result of undue fragility of the red blood cells, when the condition is known as congenital haemolytic anaemia, or of acholuric JAUNDICE.

Sickle-cell anaemia A form of anaemia characteristically found in people of African descent, so-called because of the sickle shape of the red blood cells. It is caused by the presence of the abnormal HAEMOGLOBIN, haemoglobin S, due to AMINO ACID substitutions in their polypeptide chains, reflecting a genetic mutation. Deoxygenation of haemoglobin S leads to sickling, which increases the blood viscosity and tends to obstruct flow, thereby increasing the sickling of other cells. THROMBOSIS and areas of tissue INFARCTION may follow, causing severe pain, swelling and tenderness. The resulting sickle cells are more fragile than normal red blood cells, and have a shorter life span, hence the anaemia. Advice is obtainable from the Sickle Cell Society.

Anaerobe

The term applied to bacteria having the power to live without air. Such organisms are found growing freely, deep in the soil – as, for example, the tetanus bacillus.

Anaesthesia

The loss or absence of sensation or feeling. Commonly used to describe a reversible process which allows operations and painful or unpleasant procedures to be performed without distress to the patient.

The speciality of anaesthesia broadly covers its provision for SURGERY, intensive therapy (intensive care), chronic pain management, acute pain management and obstetric analgesia. Anaesthetists in Britain are trained specialists with a medical degree, but in many countries some anaesthetists may be nurse practitioners working under the supervision of a medical anaesthetist.

The anaesthetist will assess the patient's fitness for anaesthesia, choose and perform the appropriate type of anaesthetic while monitoring and caring for the patient's well-being, and, after the anaesthetic, supervise recovery and the provision of post-operative pain relief.

Anaesthesia may be broadly divided into general and local anaesthesia. Quite commonly the two are combined to allow continued relief of pain at the operation site after the patient awakens.

General anaesthesia is most often produced by using a combination of drugs to induce a state of reversible UNCONSCIOUSNESS. 'Balanced' anaesthesia uses a combination of drugs to provide unconsciousness, analgesia, and a greater or lesser degree of muscle relaxation.

A general anaesthetic comprises induction, maintenance and recovery. Historically, anaesthesia has been divided into four stages (see below), but these are only clearly seen during induction and maintenance of anaesthesia using inhalational agents alone.

(1) Onset of induction to unconsciousness
(2) Stage of excitement
(3) Surgical anaesthesia
(4) Overdosage

Induction involves the initial production of unconsciousness. Most often this is by INTRAVENOUS injection of a short-acting anaesthetic agent such as PROPOFOL, THIOPENTONE or ETOMIDATE, often accompanied by additional drugs such as ANALGESICS to smooth the process. Alternatively an inhalational technique may be used.

Maintenance of anaesthesia may be provided by continuous or intermittent use of intravenous drugs, but is commonly provided by administration of OXYGEN and NITROUS OXIDE or air containing a volatile anaesthetic agent. Anaesthetic machines are capable of providing a constant concentration of these, and have failsafe mechanisms and monitors which guard against the patient's receiving a gas mixture with inadequate oxygen (see HYPOXIC). The gases are adminstered to the patient via a breathing circuit either through a mask, a laryngeal mask or via ENDOTRACHEAL INTUBATION. In recent years, concerns about side-effects and pollution caused by volatile agents have led to increased popularity of total intravenous anaesthesia (TIVA).

For some types of surgery the patient is paralysed using muscle relaxants and then artificially ventilated by machine (see VENTILATOR). Patients are closely monitored during anaesthesia by the anaesthetist using a variety of devices. Minimal monitoring includes ELECTROCARDIOGRAM (ECG), blood pressure, PULSE OXIMETRY, inspired oxygen and end-tidal carbon-dioxide concentration – the amount of carbon dioxide breathed out when the lungs are at the 'empty' stage of the breathing cycle. Analgesic drugs (pain relievers) and local or regional anaesthetic blocks are often given to supplement general anaesthesia.

Volatile anaesthetics are either halogenated hydrocarbons (see HALOTHANE) or halogenated ethers (isoflurane, enflurane, desflurane and sevoflurane). The latter two are the most recently introduced agents, and produce the

A

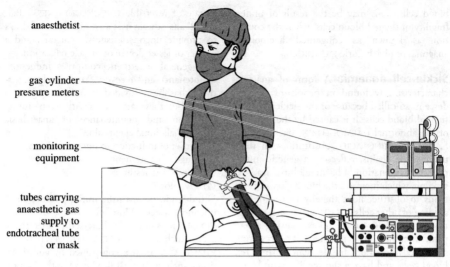

anaesthetist

gas cylinder pressure meters

monitoring equipment

tubes carrying anaesthetic gas supply to endotracheal tube or mask

equipment used for routine general anaesthesia with anaesthetic gases

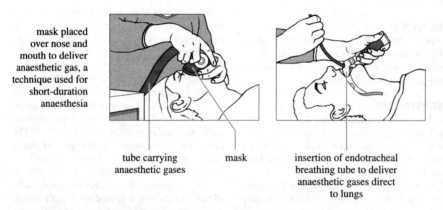

mask placed over nose and mouth to deliver anaesthetic gas, a technique used for short-duration anaesthesia

tube carrying anaesthetic gases

mask

insertion of endotracheal breathing tube to deliver anaesthetic gases direct to lungs

Patient under general anaesthesia (top). Use of a mask to deliver anaesthetic gases (bottom left). Delivering anaesthetic gases direct to the lungs (bottom right).

most rapid induction and recovery – though on a worldwide basis halothane, ether and chloroform are still widely used.

Despite several theories, the mode of action of these agents is not fully understood. Their efficacy is related to how well they dissolve into the LIPID substances in nerve cells, and it is thought that they act at more than one site within brain cells – probably at the cell membrane. By whatever method, they reversibly depress the conduction of impulses within the CENTRAL NERVOUS SYSTEM and thereby produce unconsciousness.

At the end of surgery any muscle relaxant still in the patient's body is reversed, the volatile agent is turned off and the patient breathes oxygen or oxygen-enriched air. This is the reversal or recovery phase of anaesthesia. Once the anaesthetist is satisfied with the degree of recovery, patients are transferred to a recovery area within the operating-theatre complex where they are cared for by specialist staff, under the supervision of an anaesthetist, until they are ready to return to the ward. (See also ARTIFICIAL VENTILATION OF THE LUNGS.)

Local anaesthetics are drugs which reversibly block the conduction of impulses in nerves. They therefore produce anaesthesia (and muscle relaxation) only in those areas of the body served by the nerve(s) affected by these drugs. Many drugs have some local anaesthetic action but the drugs used specifically for this purpose are all amide or ester derivatives of aromatic acids. Variations in the basic structure produce drugs with different speeds of onset, duration of action and preferential SENSORY rather than MOTOR blockade (stopping the activity in the sensory or motor nerves respectively).

The use of local rather than general anaesthesia will depend on the type of surgery and in some cases the unsuitability of the patient for general anaesthesia. It is also used to supplement general anaesthesia, relieve pain in labour (see under PREGNANCY AND LABOUR) and in the treatment of pain in persons not undergoing surgery. Several commonly used techniques are listed below:

LOCAL INFILTRATION An area of anaesthetised skin or tissue is produced by injecting local anaesthetic around it. This technique is used for removing small superficial lesions or anaesthetising surgical incisions.

NERVE BLOCKS Local anaesthetic is injected close to a nerve or nerve plexus, often using a peripheral nerve stimulator to identify the correct point. The anaesthetic diffuses into the nerve, blocking it and producing anaesthesia in the area supplied by it.

SPINAL ANAESTHESIA Small volumes of local anaesthetic are injected into the cerebrospinal fluid through a small-bore needle which has been inserted through the tissues of the back and the dura mater (the outer membrane surrounding the spinal cord). A dense motor and sensory blockade is produced in the lower half of the body. How high up in the body it reaches is dependent on the volume and dose of anaesthetic, the patient's position and individual variation. If the block is too high, then respiratory-muscle paralysis and therefore respiratory arrest may occur. HYPOTENSION (low blood pressure) may occur because of peripheral vasodilation caused by sympathetic-nerve blockade. Occasionally spinal anaesthesia is complicated by a headache, perhaps caused by continuing leakage of cerebrospinal fluid from the dural puncture point.

EPIDURAL ANAESTHESIA Spinal nerves are blocked in the epidural space with local anaesthetic injected through a fine plastic tube (catheter) which is introduced into the space using a special needle (Tuohy needle). It can be used as a continuous technique either by intermittent injections, an infusion or by patient-controlled pump. This makes it ideal for surgery in the lower part of the body, the relief of pain in labour and for post-operative analgesia. Complications include hypotension, spinal headache (less than 1:100), poor efficacy, nerve damage (1:12,000) and spinal-cord compression from CLOT or ABSCESS (extremely rare).

Analeptic

A restorative medicine, or one which acts as a stimulant of the central nervous system: for example, caffeine.

Analgesia

See ANALGESICS; PAIN.

Analgesics

Drugs which relieve or abolish PAIN. Unlike local anaesthetics, they are usually given systemically – affecting the whole body – and produce no SENSORY or MOTOR blockade stopping the activity in the sensory or motor nerves respectively that supply a part of the body. The many different types of analgesics have varying modes of action. The choice of drug and method of administration will depend upon the type and severity of pain being treated.

Non-opioid analgesics include ASPIRIN, PARACETAMOL and NON-STEROIDAL ANTI-INFLAMMATORY DRUGS (NSAIDS), which are used to treat mild or moderate pain such as headache (see also MIGRAINE), DYSMENOR-RHOEA, and transient musculoskeletal pain. Some analgesics – for example, aspirin and paracetamol – also reduce PYREXIA. A strong non-opioid analgesic is NEFOPAM HYDRO-CHLORIDE, which can be used for persistent pain or pain that fails to respond to other non-opioid analgesics, but does have troublesome side-effects. These non-opioid analgesics can be obtained without a doctor's prescription – over the counter (OTC) – but the sale of some has to be supervised by a qualified pharmacist. A wide range of compound analgesic preparations is available, combining, say, aspirin or paracetamol and CODEINE, while the weak stimulant CAFFEINE is sometimes included in the preparations. Most of these are OTC drugs. NSAIDs are especially effective in treating patients with chronic diseases accompanied by pain and inflammation. They, too, are sometimes combined with other analgesics.

Paracetamol acts within the central nervous system by inhibition of PROSTAGLANDINS. It is often combined with other analgesics – for example, aspirin or codeine; in proprietary compounds and in therapeutic doses it has few side-effects. Overdosage, however, can cause damage to the liver or kidneys (20–30 tablets are sufficient to do this). Paracetamol is often used by individuals attempting suicide. Even if there are no immediate symptoms, individuals suspected of having taken an overdose should be sent to hospital urgently for treatment.

The NSAIDs (including aspirin) inhibit prostaglandin synthesis. Prostaglandins are released by tissues that are inflamed, and may cause pain at peripheral pain sensors or sensitise nerve endings to painful stimuli: by inhibiting their production, pain and inflammation are reduced. NSAIDs are particularly effective for pain produced by inflammation – for example, ARTHRITIS. Side-effects include gastrointestinal bleeding (caused by mucosal erosions particularly in the stomach), inhibition of platelet aggregation (see PLATELETS), and potential for renal (kidney) damage.

Severe pain is often treated with opioid drugs. The original drugs were naturally occurring plant ALKALOIDS (e.g. MORPHINE), whilst newer drugs are man-made. They mimic the action of naturally occurring compounds (ENDORPHINS and ENCEPHALIN) which are found within the brain and spinal cord, and act on receptors to reduce the transmission of painful stimuli within the central nervous system (and possibly peripherally). They tend to produce side-effects of euphoria, respiratory depression, vomiting, constipation and itching. Chronic use or abuse of these drugs may give rise to addiction.

Analysis

Analysis means a separation into component parts by determination of the chemical constituents of a substance. The process of analysis is carried out by various means, for example: chromatographic analysis by means of the adsorption column; colorimetric analysis by means of various colour tests; densimetric analysis by estimation of the specific gravity; gasometric analysis by estimation of the different gases given off in some process; polariscope analysis by means of the polariscope; and volumetric analysis by measuring volumes of liquids. Analysis is also sometimes used as an abbreviation for PSYCHOANALYSIS.

Anaphylactoid Purpura

See HENOCH-SCHÖNLEIN PURPURA.

Anaphylaxis

An immediate (and potentially health- or life-threatening) hypersensitivity reaction produced by the body's immunoglobulin E (IgE) antibodies to a foreign substance (antigen); the affected tissues release histamine which causes local or systemic attack. An example is the pain, swelling, eruption, fever and sometimes collapse that may occur after a wasp sting or ingestion of peanut in a particularly sensitive person. Some people may suffer from anaphylaxis as a result of allergy to other foods or substances such as animal hair or plant leaves. On rare occasions a person may be so sensitive that anaphylaxis may lead to profound SHOCK and collapse which, unless the affected person receives urgent medical attention, including injection of ADRENALINE, may cause death. (See also ALLERGY; IMMUNITY.)

Anaplasia

The state in which a body cell loses its distinctive characters and takes on a more primitive form; it occurs, for example, in cancer, when cells proliferate rapidly.

Anastomosis

Direct intercommunication of the branches of two or more veins or arteries without any intervening network of capillary vessels. The term also describes the surgical joining of two hollow blood vessels, nerves or organs such as intestines to form an intercommunication.

Anatomy

The science which deals with the structure of the bodies of men and animals. Brief descriptions of the anatomy of each important organ are given under the headings of the various organs. It is studied by dissection of bodies bequeathed for the purpose, or of the bodies of those who die in hospitals and similar institutions, unclaimed by relatives.

Ancrod

An ENZYME present in the venom of the Malayan pit viper, which destroys the FIBRINOGEN in blood and thereby prevents the blood from clotting. In other words it is an anticoagulant (see ANTICOAGULANTS).

Ancylostomiasis

A parasitic infection caused by the nematodes *Ancylostoma duodenale* and *Necator americanus*, resulting in hookworm disease. These infections are exceedingly common in tropical and developing countries, millions of people being affected. Classically, *A. duodenale* occurred in the Far East, Mediterranean littoral, and Middle East, and *N. americanus* in tropical Africa, Central and South America, and the Far East; however, in recent years, geographical separation of the two human species is less distinct. In areas where standards of hygiene and sanitation are unsatisfactory, larvae (embryos) enter via intact skin, usually the feet. 'Ground itch' occasionally occurs as larvae enter the body. They then undergo a complex life-cycle, migrating through the lungs, trachea, and pharynx. Adult worms are 5–13 (mean 12) mm in length; their normal habitat is the small INTESTINE – especially the jejunum – where they adhere to the mucosa by hooks, thus causing seepage of blood into the lumen. A worm-pair produces large numbers of eggs, which are excreted in faeces; when deposited on moist soil they remain viable for many weeks or months. Clinical manifestations include microcytic hypochromic ANAEMIA, hypoalbuminaemia (low serum protein) and, in a severe case, OEDEMA. A chronic infection in childhood can give rise to physical, mental and sexual retardation. Treatment is with one of the benzimidazole compounds, usually mebendazole or albendazole; however, in developing countries, cheaper preparations are used, including tetrachloroethylene, bephenium hydroxynaphthoate, and pyrantel embonate. Anaemia usually responds to iron supplements; blood transfusion is rarely indicated.

Ancylostoma braziliensis A nematode infection of dogs, which in humans causes local disease (larva migrans) only, generally on the soles of the feet. It is usually acquired by walking on beaches contaminated with dog faeces in places such as the Caribbean.

Androgen
The general term for any one of a group of HORMONES which govern the development of the sexual organs and the secondary sexual characteristics of the male. TESTOSTERONE, the androgenic hormone formed in the interstitial cells of the testis (see TESTICLE), controls the development and maintenance of the male sex organs and secondary sex characteristics. In small doses it increases the number of spermatozoa (see SPERMATOZOON) produced, but in large doses it inhibits the gonadotrophic activity of the anterior PITUITARY GLAND and suppresses the formation of the spermatozoa. It is both androgenic and anabolic in action. The anabolic effect includes the ability to stimulate protein synthesis and to diminish the catabolism of amino acids, and this is associated with retention of nitrogen, potassium, phosphorus and calcium. Doses in excess of 10 mg daily to the female may produce VIRILISM.

Unconjugated testosterone is rarely used clinically because its derivatives have a more powerful and prolonged effect, and because testosterone itself requires implantation into the subcutaneous fat using a trocar and cannula for maximum therapeutic benefit. Testosterone propionate is prepared in an oily solution, as it is insoluble in water; it is effective for three days and is therefore administered intramuscularly twice weekly. Testosterone phenyl-propionate is a long-acting microcrystalline preparation which, when given by intramuscular or subcutaneous injection, is effective for four weeks. Testosterone enantate is another long-acting intramuscular preparation. Mesterolone is an effective oral androgen and is less hepatoxic: it does not inhibit pituitary gonadotrophic production and hence spermatogenesis is unimpaired. Testosterone undecanoate is also an effective oral form.

Anencephaly
The term given to the condition in which a child is born with a defect of the skull and absence of the brain. Anencephaly is the most common major malformation of the central nervous system. It has an incidence of 0·65 per 1,000 live births. There is complete absence of the cerebral hemispheres and overlying skull, and the brain stem and cerebellum are atrophic. If the pregnancy goes to term the infants rapidly die, but in 50 per cent of pregnancies associated with anencephaly, spontaneous abortion occurs. It is possible to detect the presence of anencephaly in the fetus by measuring the level of ALPHA-FETO PROTEIN in the mother's serum or in the amniotic fluid. (See also SPINA BIFIDA.)

Aneuploidy
The state in which there is an abnormal number of CHROMOSOMES: for example, DOWN'S (DOWN) SYNDROME and TURNER'S SYNDROME.

Aneurine
Aneurine is an alternative name for vitamin B_1. (See THIAMINE.)

Aneurysm
A localised swelling or dilatation of an artery (see ARTERIES) due to weakening of its wall. The most common sites are the AORTA, the arteries of the legs, the carotids and the subclavian arteries. The aorta is the largest artery in the body and an aneurysm may develop anywhere in it. A dissecting aneurysm usually occurs in the first part of the aorta: it is the result of degeneration in the vessel's muscular coat leading to a tear in the lining; blood then enters the wall and tracks along (dissects) the muscular coat. The aneurysm may rupture or compress

A

the blood vessels originating from the aorta: the outcome is an INFARCTION in the organs supplied by the affected vessel(s). Aneurysms may also form in the arteries at the base of the brain, usually due to an inherited defect of the arterial wall.

Aneurysms generally arise in the elderly, with men affected more commonly than women. The most common cause is degenerative atheromatous disease, but other rarer causes include trauma, inherited conditions such as MARFAN'S SYNDROME, or acquired conditions such as SYPHILIS or POLYARTERITIS NODOSA. Once formed, the pressure of the circulating blood within the aneurysm causes it to increase in size. At first, there may be no symptoms or signs, but as the aneurysm enlarges it becomes detectable as a swelling which pulsates with each heartbeat. It may also cause pain due to pressure on local nerves or bones. Rupture of the aneurysm may occur at any time, but is much more likely when the aneurysm is large. Rupture is usually a surgical emergency, because the bleeding is arterial and therefore considerable amounts of blood may be lost very rapidly, leading to collapse, shock and even death. Rupture of an aneurysm in the circle of Willis causes subarachnoid haemorrhage, a life-threatening event. Rupture of an aneurysm in the abdominal aorta is also life-threatening.

Treatment Treatment is usually surgical. Once an aneurysm has formed, the tendency is for it to enlarge progressively regardless of any medical therapy. The surgery is often demanding and is therefore usually undertaken only when the aneurysm is large and the risk of rupture is therefore increased. The patient's general fitness for surgery is also an important consideration. The surgery usually involves either bypassing or replacing the affected part of the artery using a conduit made either of vein or of a man-made fibre which has been woven or knitted into a tube. Routine X-ray scanning of the abdominal aorta is a valuable preventive procedure, enabling 'cold' surgery to be performed on identified aneurysms.

Angina
A feeling of constriction or suffocation often accompanied by pain (see ANGINA PECTORIS).

Angina Pectoris
Pain in the centre of the chest. Usually, exercise – sometimes acute anxiety – brings it on and pain may be severe and felt also in the arms and the jaw. The condition, which is aggravated by cold weather, is the result of the heart's demand for blood being greater than that which the coronary arteries can provide. This failure is most often due to narrowing of the coronary arteries by ATHEROMA; rarely, it may be caused by congenital defects in the arteries rendering them incapable of carrying sufficient blood to meet increased demands from the body.

Angina may be relieved or prevented by such drugs as glyceryl trinitrate and propranolol. If

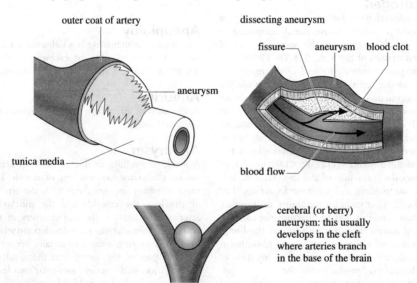

Aneurysm in wall of artery (top left). A dissecting aneurysm with the flow of blood splitting the arterial wall longitudinally (top right). A berry aneurysm in fork of the junction of two arteries (bottom).

drug treatment does not work, surgery on the coronary arteries such as angioplasty or bypass grafts may be necessary. People who suffer from angina pectoris need advice on their lifestyle, and in particular on diet, exercise and avoidance of smoking or excessive alcohol consumption. They may have high blood pressure, which will also require medical treatment (see HEART, DISEASES OF; HYPERTENSION).

Angiocardiography
Radiography of the heart after injection into it of a radio-opaque substance.

Angiography
Radiography of blood vessels made visible by injecting into them a radio-opaque substance. In the case of arteries this is known as arteriography; the corresponding term for veins being venography or phlebography. This procedure demonstrates whether there is any narrowing or ballooning of the lumen of the vessel, changes usually caused by disease or injury.

Angioma
A TUMOUR composed of blood vessels. (See NAEVUS.)

Angio-Oedema
Also called angioneurotic oedema; see under URTICARIA.

Angioplasty
A method of treating blockage or narrowing of a blood vessel by recanalising the vessel – that is, inserting a balloon into the constriction to reopen it. The technique is used to treat a narrowed artery in the heart or a limb. About 65 per cent of patients treated benefit, but when symptoms persist or recur the procedure may be repeated. There is a small risk of damage to the vessel or valve. New procedures under development include the use of lasers, cutting drills and suction to remove the deposits of ATHEROMA blocking the arteries.

Angiotensin
Angiotensin is a peptide that occurs in two forms: I and II. The former results from the action of the ENZYME, RENIN on alpha globulin (a protein) produced by the liver and passed into the blood. During passage of the blood through the lungs, angiotensin I is converted into an active form, angiotensin II, by an enzyme. This active form constricts the blood vessels and stimulates the release of two hormones – VASOPRESSIN and ALDOSTERONE – which raise the blood pressure. (See also ANGIOTENSIN-CONVERTING ENZYME (ACE) INHIBITORS.)

Angiotensin-Converting Enzyme (ACE) Inhibitors
The ENZYME that converts angiotensin I to angiotensin II (see ANGIOTENSIN) is called angiotensin-converting enzyme. Angiotensin II controls the blood pressure and is the most potent endogenous pressor substance produced in the body; angiotensin I has no such pressor activity. Inhibition of the enzyme that converts angiotensin I to angiotensin II will thus have marked effects on lowering the blood pressure, and ACE inhibitors have a valuable role in treating heart failure when thiazides and beta blockers cannot be used or fail to work, especially after myocardial infarction (see HEART, DISEASES OF). Captopril was the first ACE inhibitor to be synthesised: it reduces peripheral resistance by causing arteriolar dilatation and thus lowers blood pressure. Other drugs such as enalapril, lisinopril, cilazapril, quinapril and ramipril have since been developed. Some kidney disorders increase the production of angiotensin II and so cause HYPERTENSION.

Angitis
Angitis (or angiitis) means inflammation of a vessel such as a blood vessel, lymph vessel, or bile duct.

Ångström Unit
Called after the Swedish physicist, this is a measurement of length and equals 1/10,000 of a micrometre, or one-hundred-millionth of a centimetre. It is represented by the symbol Å and is used to give the length of electromagnetic waves.

Anhidrosis
Anhidrosis is an abnormal diminution in the secretion of sweat. This may be caused by disease or by a congenital defect.

Animal Starch
See GLYCOGEN.

Anisocytosis
This means inequality in the size of erythrocytes (red blood cells); it occurs in many forms but is prominent in megaloblastic ANAEMIA.

Ankle
The joint between the leg bones (TIBIA and FIBULA) above, and the TALUS (the Roman dice-bone) below. It is a very strong joint with powerful ligaments binding the bones together

at either side, and bony projections from the leg bones, which form large bosses on either side, called the outer and inner malleoli, extending about 12 mm (half an inch) below the actual joint. Two common injuries near the ankle are a sprain, on the inner side, consisting of tearing of the internal ligament; and fracture of the fibula (Pott's fracture) on the outer side. (See also JOINTS, DISEASES OF.)

Ankylosing Spondylitis
See SPINE AND SPINAL CORD, DISEASES AND INJURIES OF.

Ankylosis
The condition of a joint in which the movements are restricted by fibrous bands, or by malformation, or by actual union of the bones. (See JOINTS, DISEASES OF.)

Ankylostoma
See ANCYLOSTOMIASIS.

Anodynes
Any drug or treatment that eases pain. These may range from opium – the oldest and most powerful anodyne but a highly addictive substance – through ANALGESICS, to warmth and massage.

Anopheles
The generic name of a widely distributed group of mosquitoes, certain species of which transmit to humans the parasitic protozoa *Plasmodium*, the agent that causes MALARIA. *Anopheles maculipennis* and *A. bifurcatus* are both found in England and can both transmit the malaria parasite.

Anorexia
Loss of APPETITE.

Anorexia Nervosa
See under EATING DISORDERS.

Anorgasmia
An individual's inability to achieve ORGASM.

Anosmia
Loss of sense of smell. (See NOSE, DISORDERS OF.)

Anovular
Absence of OVULATION. Anovular menstruation occurs when a woman takes the contraceptive pill (see under CONTRACEPTION – Non-barrier methods).

Anoxaemia
Reduction of the oxygen content of the blood below normal limits.

Anoxia
That state in which the body tissues have an inadequate supply of OXYGEN. This may be because the blood in the lungs does not receive enough oxygen, or because there is not enough blood to receive the oxygen, or because the blood stagnates in the body.

Antabuse
See DISULFIRAM.

Antacids
Drugs traditionally used to treat gastrointestinal disorders, including peptic ulcer. They neutralise the hydrochloric acid secreted in the stomach's digestive juices and relieve pain and the discomfort of DYSPEPSIA (indigestion). A large number of proprietary preparations are on sale to the public and most contain compounds of aluminium or magnesium or a mixture of the two. Other agents include activated dimethicone – an antifoaming agent aimed at relieving flatulence; alginates, which protect against reflux oesophagitis; and surface anaesthetics. Antacids commonly prescribed by doctors include aluminium hydroxide, magnesium carbonate and magnesium trisilicate. Sodium bicarbonate and calcium and bismuth compounds are also used, although the latter is best avoided as it may cause neurological side-effects. (See DUODENAL ULCER; STOMACH, DISEASES OF.)

Antagonist
(1) A muscle the contraction of which opposes that of another muscle called the AGONIST. When the agonist contracts, the antagonist relaxes.
(2) The action of one drug in opposing the action of another.

Ante-
Prefix meaning before or forwards.

Anteflexion
The abnormal forward curvature of an organ in which the upper part is sharply bent forwards. The term is especially applied to forward displacement of the UTERUS.

Antenatal Care
The protocol which doctors and midwives follow to ensure that the pregnant mother and her FETUS are kept in good health, and that the pregnancy and birth have a satisfactory outcome. The pregnant mother is seen regularly at a clinic where, for example, her blood pressure is checked, the growth and development of her

child-to-be are carefully assessed, and any problem or potential problems dealt with. Most antenatal care deals with normal pregnancies and is supervised by general practitioners and midwives in primary-care clinics. If any serious problems are identified, the mother can be referred to specialists' clinics in hospitals. (See PREGNANCY AND LABOUR.)

Antepartum
An adjective describing an event before labour starts in pregnancy (see PREGNANCY AND LABOUR).

Anterior
An adjective that describes or relates to the front part of the body, limbs, or organs.

Anterior Tibial Syndrome
See under MUSCLES, DISORDERS OF – Compression syndrome.

Anteversion
The term applied to the forward tilting of an organ, especially of the UTERUS.

Anthelmintics
Substances which cause the death or expulsion of parasitic worms such as hook, tape and threadworms (see TAENIA; ENTEROBIASIS).

Anthracosis
The change which takes place in the lungs and bronchial glands of coal-miners, and others, who inhale coal-dust constantly. The lungs are amazingly efficient in coping with this problem; during a working lifetime a coal-miner may inhale around 5,000 grams of dust, but at POST-MORTEM EXAMINATION it is rare to find more than about 40 grams in the lungs. The affected tissues change in colour from greyish pink to jet black, owing to loading with minute carbon particles. (See PNEUMOCONIOSIS.)

Anthracyclines
ANTIBIOTICS that destroy tumour cells: examples include aclarubicin, daunorubicin, doxorubicin, epirubicin and idarubicin.

Anthrax
A serious disease occurring in sheep and cattle, and in those who tend them or handle the bones, skins and fleeces – even long after removal of the latter from the animals. It is sometimes referred to as malignant pustule, wool-sorters' disease, splenic fever of animals, or murrain. It is now a rare condition in the United Kingdom. The cause is a bacillus (*B. anthracis*) which grows in long chains and produces spores of great vitality. These spores retain their life for years, in dried skins and fleeces; they are not destroyed by boiling, freezing, 5 per cent carbolic lotion, or, like many bacilli, by the gastric juice. The disease is communicated from a diseased animal to a crack in the skin (e.g. of a farmer or butcher), or from contact with contaminated skins or fleeces. Nowadays skins are handled wet, but if they are allowed to dry so that dust laden with spores is inhaled by the workers, serious pneumonia may result. Instances have occurred of the disease being conveyed on shaving brushes made from bristles of diseased animals. A few countries are believed to have developed anthrax as a weapon of war to be delivered by shells or rockets, despite international agreements to ban such weapons.

In the wake of the devastating terrorist attacks on buildings in New York and Washington on 11 September 2001, modified anthrax spores were sent by mail from an unidentified source to some prominent Americans. Several people were infected and a few died. This was the first known use of anthrax as a terror weapon.

Prevention is most important by disinfecting all hides, wool and hair coming from areas of the world. An efficient vaccine is now available. Treatment consists of the administration of large doses of the broad-spectrum antibiotic, CIPROFLOXACIN. If bioterrorism is thought to be the likely source of anthrax infection, appropriate decontamination procedures must be organised promptly.

Symptoms

EXTERNAL FORM This is the 'malignant pustule'. After inoculation of some small wound, a few hours or days elapse, and then a red, inflamed swelling appears, which grows larger till it covers half the face or the breadth of the arm, as the case may be. Upon its summit appears a bleb of pus, which bursts and leaves a black scab, perhaps 12 mm (half an inch) wide. The patient is feverish and seriously ill. The inflammation may last ten days or so, when it slowly subsides and the patient recovers, if surviving the fever and prostration.

INTERNAL FORM This takes the form of pneumonia with haemorrhages, when the spores have been drawn into the lungs, or of ulcers of the stomach and intestines, with gangrene of the SPLEEN, when they have been swallowed.

It is usually fatal in two or three days. Victims may also develop GASTROENTERITIS or MENINGITIS.

Anti-
Prefix meaning against.

Antiarrhythmic Drugs
ARRHYTHMIA is a variation in the normal rhythm of the heartbeat. Management of the condition requires accurate diagnosis of the type, and ELECTROCARDIOGRAPHY is vital in this process (see HEART, DISEASES OF). Drug treatment is usually part of the management, and antiarrhythmic drugs can be divided clinically into those that act on supraventricular arrhythmias, those that act on both supraventricular and ventricular arrythmias, and those that act on ventricular arrythmias. Respective examples are VERAPAMIL, DISOPYRAMIDE and LIDOCAINE. This large group of drugs can also be classified according to their effects on the electrical reactions of active myocardial cells. The many drugs available are described in the *British National Formulary.*

Antibacterial Drugs
A group of drugs, which include ANTIBIOTICS, used to treat infections caused by BACTERIA. Drugs include CEPHALOSPORINS and cephamycins, TETRACYCLINES, AMINOGLYCOSIDES, MACROLIDES, and antituberculous compounds.

Antibiotics
Antibiotic is the term used to describe any antibacterial agent derived from micro-organisms, although most of them are now prepared synthetically. Such agents destroy or inhibit the growth of other micro-organisms: examples are penicillin, cephalosporin, amino-glycosides, streptomycin, and tetracycline.

Penicillin was the first antibiotic to be discovered and used in the 1940s. The discovery and isolation in 1958 of the penicillin nucleus, 6-amino penicillanic acid (6-PNA), allowed many new penicillins to be synthesised. These are now the largest single group of antibiotics used in clinical medicine. Most staphylococci (see STAPHYLOCOCCUS) have now developed resistance to benzylpenicillin, the early form of the drug, because they produce penicillinases – enzymes which break down the drug. Other types of penicillin such as cloxacillin and flucoxacillin are not affected and are used against penicillin-resistant staphylococci.

The cephalosporins are derived from the compound cephalosporin C, which is obtained by fermentation of the mould cephalosporium. The cephalosporin nucleus 7 amino cephalosporanic (7-ICA) acid has been the basis for the production of the semi-synthetic compounds of the cephalosporin nucleus. The first semi-synthetic cephalosporin, cephalothin, appeared in 1962; it was followed by cephaloridine in 1964. The original cephalosporins had to be given by injection, but more recent preparations can be given by mouth. The newer preparations are less readily destroyed by beta-lactamases and so they have a much broader spectrum of antibacterial activity. The newer cephalosporins include cephalexin, cefazolin, cephacetrile, cephapirin, cefamandole, cefuroxine, cephrodine, cefodroxil and cefotaxine. Inactivation of beta-lactamase is the basis of bacterial resistance both to the penicillins and to the cephalosporins, so that attempts to prepare these antibiotics with resistance to beta-lactamase is of great importance. A synthetic inhibitor of beta-lactamase called clavulanic acid has been synthesised; this is used in combination with the penicillins and cephalosporins to prevent resistance. The cephamycins are a new addition to the beta-lactam antibiotics. They are similar in structure to the cephalosporins but are produced, not by fungi, but by actinomycetes.

Overuse and misuse of antibiotics have resulted in many bacteria becoming resistant to them. Hospitals, in particular, have problems with METHICILLIN-RESISTANT STAPHYLOCOCCUS AUREUS (MRSA). Combinations of antibiotics are needed to combat resistant strains of bacteria, another example being *Mycobacterium tuberculosis.*

Antibodies
Antibodies are substances in the blood which destroy or neutralise various toxins or 'bodies' (e.g. bacteria), known generally as antigens (see ANTIGEN). The antibodies are formed, usually, as a result of the introduction into the body of the antigens to which they are antagonistic, as in all infectious diseases (see ALLERGY; IMMUNITY).

Anticholinergic
An action or drug that inhibits the activity of ACETYLCHOLINE.

Anticholinesterase
Any compound that inhibits the activity of CHOLINESTERASE, thus permitting ACETYLCHOLINE to continue its function of transmitting nerve impulses. Drugs with anticholinesterase properties include distigmine, NEOSTIGMINE and PHYSOSTIGMINE.

Anticoagulants

Anticoagulants are drugs which inhibit COAGU-LATION of the blood. They are used to prevent and treat abnormal clotting of the blood, to treat THROMBOSIS, and sometimes to prevent or treat STROKE or TRANSIENT ISCHAEMIC ATTACKS OR EPISODES (TIA, TIE). Anticoagulant drugs are also prescribed preventively in major surgery to stop abnormal clotting from occurring; HAEMODIALYSIS is another procedure during which these drugs are used. Anticoagulants are also prescribed to prevent thrombi (clots) forming on prosthetic heart valves after heart surgery.

The drugs are much more effective in the treatment and prevention of venous clotting – for example, deep vein thrombosis (DVT), see under VEINS, DISEASES OF – than in preventing thrombosis formation in arteries with their fast-flowing blood in which thrombi contain little fibrin (against which the anticoagulants work) and many PLATELETS.

The main anticoagulants now in use are the natural agent HEPARIN (a quick-acting variety and a low-molecular-weight long-acting type); synthetic oral anticoagulants such as WARFARIN and the less-often-used acenocoumarol and PHENINDIONE; and antiplatelet compounds such as ASPIRIN, clopidogrel dipyridamole and ticlopidines. Fondaparinux is an extract of heparin which can be given once daily by injection; ximelagatran, an inhibitor of thrombin, is being trialled as the first new oral anticoagulant since heparin.

Patients taking anticoagulants need careful medical monitoring and they should carry an Anticoagulant Card with instructions about the use of whatever drug they may be receiving – essential information should the individual require treatment for other medical conditions as well as for thrombosis.

Anticonvulsants

Drugs that reduce or prevent the severity of an epileptic convulsion or seizure (see EPILEPSY). The nature of the fit, and the patient's reaction to it, influences the type of anticonvulsant used. Anticonvulsants inhibit the high level of electrical activity in the brain that causes the fit. Among regularly used anticonvulsants are carbamazepine, sodium valproate, clonazopam, lamotrigine, gabapentin, vigabatrin, and topiramate. Older drugs such as phenytoin and primidone remain useful in some patients. Intravenous anticonvulsants, such as diazepam, are used for rapid control of epileptic status.

Antidepressant Drugs

These widely used drugs include a range of different preparations which relieve DEPRESSION. All the antidepressants available at the time of writing are more or less equally effective. In studies where patients agree to take either antidepressants or identical dummy PLACEBO pills (without knowing which), at least two-thirds of those who receive antidepressants feel much better within three months, while fewer than one-third of those on placebos recover naturally in the same period. In general these drugs are useful for severe and moderate depression including postnatal illness; they are not effective in milder forms of depression although they may be tried for a short time if other therapies have failed.

The most widely prescribed type of antidepressants are the tricyclics, so-called because their molecular structure includes three rings. The other commonly used types are named after the actions they have on chemicals in the brain: the SELECTIVE SEROTONIN-REUPTAKE INHIBITORS (SSRIS) and the MONOAMINE OXIDASE INHIBITORS (MAOIS) – see also below. All types of antidepressant work in similar ways. Tricyclic antidepressants have cured depression in millions of people, but they can cause unpleasant side-effects, particularly in the first couple of weeks. These include SEDATION, dry mouth, excessive sweating, CONSTIPATION, urinary problems, and impotence (inability to get an erection). Up to half of all people prescribed tricyclic drugs cannot tolerate the side-effects and stop treatment before their depression is properly treated. More seriously, tricyclics can upset the rhythm of the heart in susceptible people and should never be given in the presence of heart disease.

The SSRIs are newer, coming into wide use in the late 1980s. They increase the levels in the brain of the chemical messenger SEROTONIN, which is thought to be depleted in depression. Indeed, the SSRIs are as effective as tricyclics and, although they can cause nausea and excessive sweating at first, they generally have fewer side-effects. Their main disadvantage, however, is that they cost much more than the most commonly used tricyclic, amitriptyline. On the other hand, they are more acceptable to many patients and they cause fewer drop-outs from treatment – up to a quarter rather than a half. The money saved by completed, successful treatment may outweigh the prescribing costs. SSRIs have been reported as associated with an increased risk of suicide.

Another group of antidepressants, the MAOIs, have been in use since the late 1950s.

They are stimulants, rather than sedatives, and are particularly helpful for people who are physically and mentally slowed by depression. They work well but have one big disadvantage – a dangerous interaction with certain foods and other drugs, causing a sudden and very dangerous increase in blood pressure. People taking them must carry an information card explaining the risk and listing the things that they should avoid. Because of this risk, MAOIs are not used much now, except when other treatments have failed. A new MAOI, moclobemide, which is less likely to interact and so cause high blood pressure, is now available.

LITHIUM CARBONATE is a powerful antidepressant used for intractable depression. It should be used under specialist supervision as the gap between an effective dose and a toxic one is narrow.

St John's Wort is a popular herbal remedy which may be effective, but which is handicapped by differences of strength between different preparations or batches. It can interact with a number of conventional drugs and so needs to be used cautiously and with advice.

In general, antidepressants work by restoring the balance of chemicals in the brain. Improved sleep and reduced anxiety are usually the first signs of improvement, particularly among people taking the more sedative tricyclic drugs. Improvement in other symptoms follow, with the mood starting to lift after about two weeks of treatment. Most people feel well by three months, although a few residual symptoms, such as slowness in the mornings, may take longer to clear up. People taking antidepressants usually want to stop them as soon as they feel better; however, the risk of relapse is high for up to a year and most doctors recommend continuing the drugs for around 4–6 months after recovery, with gradual reduction of the dose after that.

Withdrawal reactions may occur including nausea, vomiting, headache, giddiness, panic or anxiety and restlessness. The drugs should be withdrawn gradually over about a month or longer (up to six months in those who have been on maintenance treatment).

A wide range of antidepressant drugs is described in the *British National Formulary*. Examples include:

● Tricyclics: amitryptyline, imipramine, doxepin.
● MAOIs: phenelzine, isocarboxazid.
● SSRIs: citalopram, fluoxetine, paraxtene.
(Antidepressant drugs not in these three groups include flupenthixol, mertazapine and venlafaxine.)

Antidiarrhoeal Treatments

Initial treatment of acute DIARRHOEA is to prevent or correct the loss of fluid and ELECTROLYTES from the body. This is a priority especially in infants and elderly people. Rehydration can be achieved orally or, in severe cases, by urgent admission to hospital for the replacement of fluid and electrolytes.

For adults with acute diarrhoea, short-term symptomatic treatment can be achieved with antimotility drugs such as codeine phosphate, co-phenotrope or loperamide hydrochloride. Adsorbent drugs, for example, KAOLIN, should not be used in acute diarrhoea, but bulk-forming drugs – ispaghula or methylcellulose – can help to control the consistency of faeces in patients with ileostomies and colostomies (see ILEOSTOMY; COLOSTOMY), or those with diarrhoea caused by DIVERTICULAR DISEASE.

Irritable bowel syndrome, malabsorption syndrom, ulcerative colitis, Crohn's disease and diverticular disease are often accompanied by diarrhoea; for more information on these conditions, see under separate entries.

ANTIBIOTICS may sometimes cause diarrhoea and this side-effect should be borne in mind when the cause of the condition is being investigated.

Antidiuretic Hormone (ADH)
See VASOPRESSIN.

Antidotes

An antidote is a therapeutic substance used to counteract the toxic action(s) of a specific substance. Very few substances have an antidote.

Antiemetic

A drug that counteracts nausea and sickness. Some antihistamines and anticholinergics have an antiemetic effect. They are used to combat motion sickness or nausea and vomiting brought on by other drugs – in particular, drugs used in ANAESTHESIA and anticancer agents – and by RADIOTHERAPY.

Antigen

Whenever the body identifies a substance entering it as foreign or potentially dangerous, the immune system (see IMMUNITY) produces an an antibody (see ANTIBODIES) to combat it. Antigens are normally proteins, but simple substances – for instance, metals – may become antigenic by combining with and changing the body's own proteins. Such a product is called a hapten.

Antihelminthic

See ANTHELMINTICS.

Antihistamine Drugs

Antihistamine drugs antagonise the action of HISTAMINE and are therefore of value in the treatment of certain allergic conditions (see ALLERGY). They may be divided into those with a central action (e.g. flupheniramine and cyclizine) and those such as loratidine and terfenadine with almost no central action. Antihistamines are also of some value in the treatment of vasomotor RHINITIS (see also under NOSE, DISORDERS OF); they reduce rhinorrhoea and sneezing but are usually less effective in relieving nasal congestion. All antihistamines are useful in the treatment of URTICARIA and certain allergic skin rashes, insect bites and stings, as well as in the treatment of drug allergies. Chlorpheniramine or promethazine injections are useful in the emergency treatment of angio-oedema (see under URTICARIA) and ANAPHYLAXIS.

There is little evidence that any one antihistamine is superior to another, and patients vary considerably in their response to them. The antihistamines differ in their duration of action and in the incidence of side-effects such as drowsiness. Most are short-acting, but some (such as promethazine) work for up to 12 hours. They all cause sedation but promethazine, trimeprazine and dimenhydrinate tend to be more sedating while chlorpheniramine and cyclizine are less so, as are astemizole, oxatomide and terfenadine. Patients should be warned that their ability to drive or operate machinery may be impaired when taking these drugs, and that the effects of ALCOHOL may be increased.

Antihypertensive Drugs

A group of drugs used to treat high blood pressure (HYPERTENSION). Untreated hypertension leads to STROKE, heart attacks and heart failure. The high incidence of hypertension in western countries has led to intensive research to discover antihypertensive drugs, and many have been marketed. The drugs may work by reducing the power of the heartbeat, by dilating the blood vessels or by increasing the excretion of salts and water in the urine (diuresis). Antihypertensive treatment has greatly improved the prognosis of patients with high blood pressure by cutting the frequency of heart and renal failure (see KIDNEYS, DISEASES OF), stroke, and

coronary thrombosis (see HEART, DISEASES OF). Drugs used for treatment can be classified as follows: diuretics; vasodilator antihypertensives; centrally acting antihypertensives; adrenergic neurone-blocking drugs; alpha-adrenoreceptor-blocking drugs; drugs affecting the renin-angiotensin system; ganglion-blocking drugs; and tyrosine hydroxylase inhibitors. The drugs prescribed depend on many factors, including the type of hypertension being treated. Treatment can be difficult because of the need to balance the effectiveness of a drug in reducing blood pressure against its side-effects.

Anti-Inflammatory Drugs

See ANALGESICS; NON-STEROIDAL ANTI-INFLAMMATORY DRUGS (NSAIDS).

Antimetabolites

A group of drugs used in the treatment of certain forms of malignant disease. Chemically, they closely resemble substances (or METABOLITES) which are essential for the life and growth of CELLS. Antimetabolites are incorporated into new nuclear material in the cell or combine irreversibly with essential cellular enzymes, thus disrupting normal cellular division (see MITOSIS and MEIOSIS) and causing death of the cell. There is now a range of antimetabolites including CYTARABINE, METHOTREXATE, FLUOROURACIL and MERCAPTOPURINE.

Antimuscarine

A pharmacological effect where the action of ACETYLCHOLINE, a chemical neurotransmitter released at the junctions (synapses) of parasympathetic and ganglionic nerves, is inhibited. The junctions between nerves and skeletal muscles have nicotinic receptors. A wide range of drugs with antimuscarinic effects are in use for various disorders including PSYCHOSIS, BRONCHOSPASM, disorders of the eye (see EYE, DISORDERS OF), PARKINSONISM, and problems of the GASTROINTESTINAL TRACT and URINARY TRACT. (See also ANTISPASMODICS.)

Antioxidant

A compound that can neutralise oxygen-free radicals in the body; these are atoms and chemical groups that can damage cells. Free radicals are the product of various disease processes as well as of such agents as poisons, radiation and smoking. Natural antioxidants also occur in the body.

Antiperistalsis

A movement in the bowels and stomach by which the food and other contents are passed upwards, instead of in the proper direction. (See PERISTALSIS.)

Antipsychotic Drugs

See NEUROLEPTICS.

Antipyretics

Measures used to reduce temperature in FEVER. Varieties include cold-sponging, wet-packs, baths and diaphoretic (sweat-reducing) drugs such as QUININE, salicylates and ASPIRIN.

Antiseptics

Antiseptics prevent the growth of disease-causing micro-organisms without damaging living tissues. Among chemicals used are boric acid, carbolic acid, hydrogen peroxide and products based on coal tar, such as cresol. Chlorhexidines, iodine, formaldehyde, flavines, alcohol and hexachlorophane are also used. Antiseptics are applied to prevent infection – for example, in preparing the skin before operation. They are also used externally to treat infected wounds.

Antispasmodics

These are antimuscarinic drugs (see ANTIMUS-CARINE) which have the property of relaxing smooth muscle. Along with other antimuscarinic drugs, antispasmodics may be helpful supportive treatment for patients with non-ulcer DYSPEPSIA, IRRITABLE BOWEL SYNDROME (IBS) and DIVERTICULAR DISEASE. Examples of antispasmodic drugs are ATROPINE sulphate, dicyclomine bromide and propantheline (a synthetic antimuscarinic drug used as a treatment adjunct in gastrointestinal disorders and also for controlling urinary frequency), bromide, alver-ine, mebervine and peppermint oil. With the arrival of more powerful and specific antisecre-tory drugs, such as the histamine H_2-receptor antagonists – examples are CIMETIDINE and RANITIDINE – the use of antispasmodics has declined.

Antitoxin

Any one of various preparations that contain ANTIBODIES which combine and neutralise the effects of a particular toxin (see TOXINS) released into the bloodstream by BACTERIA. Examples are the toxins produced by DIPH-THERIA and TETANUS. Antitoxins are produced from the blood of humans or animals that have been exposed to a particular toxin – whether by INFECTION or by INOCULATION – and thus have produced antibodies against it. They are usually given by intramuscular injection.

Antivenom

A therapeutic substance used to counteract the toxic action(s) of a specific animal toxin (see TOXINS) or venom. They are normally steril-ised, proteinaceous globulins (see GLOBULIN) extracted from the SERUM of animals, usually horses, immunised against the specific toxin/venom. Most are given by intravenous or intramuscular injection and are most effective when given shortly after the bite or sting has occurred. Some antivenoms may be effective against the venoms of several closely related animal species.

Antrostomy

Antrostomy is the operation in which an opening is made through the nose into the maxillary ANTRUM.

Antrum

Antrum means a natural hollow or cavity. The maxillary antrum is now known as the maxillary SINUS. The mastoid antrum is situated in the mastoid process, the mass of bone felt behind the ear. It may become the seat of an ABSCESS in cases of suppuration of the middle ear (see EAR, DISEASES OF). The pyloric antrum is the part of the stomach immediately preceding the PYLORUS.

Anuria

Anuria is a condition in which no URINE is voided. (See also KIDNEYS, DISEASES OF – Glomerulonephritis.)

Anus

The anus is the opening at the lower end of the bowel. It is kept closed by two muscles, the external and internal sphincters. The latter is a muscular ring which extends about 25 mm (1 inch) up the bowel, is nearly 6 mm (¼ inch) thick, and is kept constantly contracted by the action of a nerve centre in the spinal cord. In disease of the spinal cord the muscle may be paralysed, resulting in inability to retain the motions or stools.

Anus, Diseases of

See under RECTUM, DISEASES OF.

Anxiety State

See NEUROSIS.

Anxiolytics

Drugs for the relief of anxiety. They will induce sleep when given in large doses at night, and so are HYPNOTICS as well. Conversely, most hyp-notics will sedate when given in divided doses during the day. Prescription of these drugs is widespread but physical and psychological DEPENDENCE occurs as well as TOLERANCE to their effects, especially among those with personality disorders or who abuse drugs and alcohol. This is particularly true of the BARBITURATES which are now limited in their use, but also applies to the BENZODIAZEPINES, the most commonly used anxiolytics and hypnotics. Withdrawal syndromes may occur if drug treatment is stopped too abruptly; hypnotic sedatives and anxiolytics should therefore not be prescribed indiscriminately, but reserved for short courses. Among the anxiolytics are the widely used benzodiazepines, the rarely used barbiturates, and the occasionally prescribed drugs such as BUSPIRONE and beta blockers like OXPRENOLOL (see BETA-ADRENOCEPTOR-BLOCKING DRUGS).

Aorta

The large vessel which opens out of the left ventricle of the HEART and carries blood to all of the body. It is about 45 cm (1½ feet) long and 2·5 cm (1 inch) wide. Like other arteries it possesses three coats, of which the middle one is much the thickest. This consists partly of muscle fibre, but is mainly composed of an elastic substance called elastin. The aorta passes first to the right, and lies nearest the surface behind the end of the second right rib-cartilage; then it curves backwards and to the left, passes down behind the left lung close to the backbone, and through an opening in the diaphragm into the abdomen. There it divides, at the level of the navel, into the two common iliac arteries, which carry blood to the lower limbs.

Its branches, in order, are: two coronary arteries to the heart wall; the brachiocephalic, left common carotid, and left subclavian arteries to the head, neck and upper limbs; several small branches to the oesophagus, bronchi, and other organs of the chest; nine pairs of intercostal arteries which run around the body between the ribs; one pair of subcostal arteries which is in series with the intercostal arteries; four (or five) lumbar arteries to the muscles of the loins; coeliac trunk to the stomach, liver and pancreas; two mesenteric arteries to the bowels; and suprarenal, renal and testicular arteries to the suprarenal body, kidney, and testicle on each side. From the termination of the aorta rises a small branch, the median sacral artery, which runs down into the pelvis. In the female the ovarian arteries replace the testicular.

The chief diseases of the aorta are ATHEROMA

and ANEURYSM. (See ARTERIES, DISEASES OF; COARCTATION OF THE AORTA.)

Aortic Incompetence

See also REGURGITATION. This is the back flow of blood through the AORTIC VALVE of the HEART into the left ventricle, caused by an incompetent valve. The failure to close may be caused by a congenital defect or by damage from disease. The defect may be cured by surgical replacement of the damaged valve with an artificial valve. (See HEART, DISEASES OF.)

Aortic Stenosis

Narrowing of the AORTIC VALVE in the HEART which obstructs the flow of blood through it, with serious effects on the heart and the circulation. The muscle in the left ventricle works harder to compensate for the obstruction and thickens as a result. Stenosis is usually caused by the deposition of calcium on the valve and is commonly associated with ATHEROMA. Untreated, the condition leads to heart failure, but nowadays the stenosis can be treated surgically.

Aortic Valve

The valve that controls the flow of blood from the AORTA to the left ventricle of the HEART.

Aortitis

A rare degenerative condition of the lining of the AORTA. It may be the result of arteritis (inflammation of the arteries) or a consequence of untreated SYPHILIS. Aortitis may lead to thinning of the aorta's wall and development of an ANEURYSM.

Aortography

Aortography is the technique of rendering the AORTA visible in an X-ray film by injecting a radio-opaque substance into it. The procedure is used to detect the presence of an ANEURYSM. (See also ANGIOGRAPHY.)

Aperients

Medicines which produce a natural movement of the bowels. (See CONSTIPATION; PURGATIVES.)

Apex

The pointed portion of any organ which has a conical shape. The apex of each lung reaches about 3·5–5 cm (1½ or 2 inches) above the collar-bone into the neck. In health, the apex of the heart can be felt below the fifth rib immediately inside the nipple.

Apex Beat

This is the beat of the APEX of the HEART, which can be felt through the skin to the left of the breastbone between the fifth and sixth ribs.

Apgar Score

A method of assessing at birth whether or not a baby requires resuscitation. The newborn is routinely assessed at 1 minute of age and again at 5 minutes, and a value of 0, 1 or 2 given to each of five signs: colour, heart rate, muscle tone, respiratory (or breathing) effort, and the response to stimulation. A total score of 7 or more indicates that the newborn child is in excellent condition. An Apgar score of 5 or less at 15 or 20 minutes predicates an increased risk of subsequent CEREBRAL PALSY.

Aphakia

Absence of the lens of the EYE.

Aphasia

Inability to speak caused by disease in or injury to the cerebral cortex in the left half of the BRAIN (in a right-handed person), affecting the generation and content of speech as well as the understanding of language; often accompanied by problems with reading and writing (see DYSPHASIA). Comprehension and expression of language occur in two zones of the cerebral cortex (the outer layer of the main part of the brain). They are known as Wernicke's area (comprehension) and Broca's area (speech formulation).

Aphonia

Loss of voice, usually sudden. Commonly caused by emotional stress with no detectable physical abnormality in the LARYNX. Damage or disease of the larynx usually results in dysphonia (partial voice loss). Where no physical cause can be identified, reassurance and, if the voice does not quickly return, PSYCHOTHERAPY are the treatment.

Aphthous Ulcer

Single or multiple (and often recurrent) transiently painful ulcers in the oral mucous membrane that are usually self-limiting. The cause is unknown and treatment is symptomatic.

Apicectomy

Apicectomy is the minor operation carried out to try to save a tooth which has an ABSCESS on it or which does not respond to root treatment. In this, the abscess and the APEX of the tooth are removed.

Aplasia

The complete or partial failure of tissue or an organ to develop.

Apnoea

A general term meaning the cessation of breathing. Apnoea is a medical emergency: death soon follows if breathing is not quickly restored (see APPENDIX 1: BASIC FIRST AID). Apnoea may be caused by an obstruction to the airway, for example by the tongue during general ANAESTHESIA, or by a disturbance of the mechanisms that control breathing. Rapid heavy breathing reduces the blood levels of carbon dioxide and can lead to a brief period of apnoea.

Neonatal apnoeic attacks may represent a serious emergency, being caused by prematurity, milk aspiration, heart failure, infection, HYPOXIA, HYPOGLYCAEMIA or HYPOCALCAEMIA. If stimulation of the baby does not immediately restore breathing, then bag-and-mask ventilation should be used.

Apo-

Apo- is a prefix implying separation or derivation from.

Apodia

Absence of the foot.

Aponeurosis

Aponeurosis is the term applied to the white fibrous membrane which serves as an investment for the muscles and which covers the skull beneath the scalp.

Apoplexy

See STROKE.

Apoptosis

This is a genetically controlled type of cell death. There is an orchestrated collapse of a cell (see CELLS), typified by destruction of the cell's membrane; shrinkage of the cell with condensation of CHROMATIN; and fragmentation of DNA. The dead cell is then engulfed by adjacent cells. This process occurs without evidence of the inflammation normally associated with a cell's destruction by infection or disease.

Apoptosis, first identified in 1972, is involved in biological activities including embryonic development, ageing and many diseases. Its importance to the body's many physiological and pathological processes has only fairly recently been understood, and research into apoptosis is proceeding apace.

In adults, around 10 billion cells die each day – a figure which balances the number of cells arising from the body's stem-cell populations (see STEM CELL). Thus, the body's normal HOMEOSTASIS is regulated by apoptosis. As a person ages, apoptopic responses to cell DNA damage may be less effectively controlled and so result in more widespread cell destruction, which could be a factor in the onset of degenerative diseases. If, however, apoptopic responses become less sensitive, this might contribute to the uncontrolled multiplication of cells that is typical of cancers. Many diseases are now associated with changed cell survival: AIDS (see AIDS/HIV); ALZHEIMER'S DISEASE and PARKINSONISM; ischaemic damage after coronary thrombosis (see HEART, DISEASES OF) and STROKE; thyroid diseases (see THYROID GLAND, DISEASES OF); and AUTOIMMUNE DISORDERS. Some cancers, autoimmune disorders and viral infections are associated with reduced or inhibited apoptosis. Anticancer drugs, GAMMA RAYS and ULTRAVIOLET RAYS (UVR) initiate apoptosis. Other drugs – for example, NON-STEROIDAL ANTI-INFLAMMATORY DRUGS (NSAIDS) – alter the process of apoptosis. Research is in train to harness new knowledge about apoptosis for the development of new treatments and modifications of existing ones for serious disorders such as cancer and degenerative nervous diseases.

Appendicectomy

Appendicectomy, or appendectomy, is the operation for the removal of the vermiform appendix in the ABDOMEN (see APPENDICITIS).

Appendicitis

This is an inflammatory condition of the APPENDIX, and is a common surgical emergency, affecting mainly adolescents and young adults. It is usually due to a combination of obstruction and infection of the appendix, and has a variable clinical course ranging from episodes of mild self-limiting abdominal pain to life-threatening illness. Abdominal pain beginning in the centre of the abdomen but which later shifts position to the right iliac fossa is the classic symptom. The patient usually has accompanying fever and sometimes nausea, vomiting, loss of appetite, diarrhoea, or even constipation. The precise symptoms vary with the exact location of the appendix within the abdomen. In some individuals the appendix may 'grumble' with repeated mild attacks which resolve spontaneously. In an acute attack, the inflammatory process begins first in the wall of the appendix but, if the disease progresses, the appendix can become secondarily infected and pus may form within it. The blood supply

may become compromised and the wall become gangrenous. Eventually the appendix may rupture, giving rise to a localised abscess in the abdomen or, more rarely, free pus within the abdomen which causes generalised PERITONITIS. Rupture of the appendix is a serious complication and the patient may be severely unwell. Surgeons recognise that in order to make sure patients with appendicitis do not progress to peritonitis, a certain percentage of normal appendixes are removed when clinical signs are suspicious but not diagnostic of disease.

Treatment The best treatment is prompt surgical removal of the diseased appendix, usually with antibiotic cover. If performed early, before rupture occurs, APPENDICECTOMY is normally straightforward and recovery swift. If the appendix has already ruptured and there is abscess formation or free intra-abdominal pus, surgery is still the best treatment but postoperative complications are more likely, and full recovery may be slower.

Appendix

A term applied to the appendages of several hollow organs: for example, the larynx has two pouches called appendices, and the epiploic appendices are the tags of fat that hang from the exterior part of the large intestine. The commonest application, however, is to the vermiform appendix of the large intestine. This is a short, slim, blind-ended tube up to 10 cm long attached to the caecum (a pouch at the start of the large intestine). Its function is unknown, though it may once have had one in ancestral humans. It is, however, prone to inflammation and infection (see APPENDICITIS).

Appetite

Appetite is the craving for the food necessary to maintain the body and to supply it with sufficient energy to carry on its functions. The ultimate cause of appetite is a question of supply and demand in the muscles and various organs, but the proximate cause is doubtful. Unlike hunger, it is probably an acquired, rather than an inborn, sensation. Whatever other factors may be concerned, the tone of the STOMACH is of importance. Significant factors in stimulating appetite are anticipation and the sight and smell of well-cooked food. Individuals who eat unsuitable substances such as faeces are described as suffering from pica, which occurs sometimes during pregnancy, in children, and often in mental disorders. The two chief disorders, however, are excessive increase of appetite, and diminution or loss of appetite (see also EATING DISORDERS).

Excessive appetite may simply be a bad habit, due to habitual over-indulgence in good food and resulting in GOUT, OBESITY, etc. – according to the other habits and constitution of the person. It may also be a sign of DIABETES MELLITUS or thyrotoxicosis (see under THYROID GLAND, DISEASES OF).

Diminished appetite is a sign common to almost all diseases causing general weakness, because the activity of the stomach and the secretion of gastric juice fail early when vital power is low. It is the most common sign of DYSPEPSIA due to gastritis, and of cancer of the stomach. In some cases it is a manifestation of stress or strain such as domestic worry or difficulties at work. Indeed, appetite seems to be particularly susceptible to emotional disturbances, as is evidenced by the linked conditions of BULIMIA (pathological overeating) and anorexia nervosa (pathological dieting) – see also EATING DISORDERS.

Approved Names for Medicines

The term used for names devised or selected by the British Pharmacopoeia Commission for new drugs. European Union law (1992) requires the use of a Recommended International Non-proprietary Name (rINN) for medicinal substances. In most cases the British Approved Name (BAN) and rINN were the same when the legislation was introduced; where there were differences, the BAN was modified to meet the new requirements.

Pharmaceutical manufacturers usually give proprietary (brand) names to the drugs they develop, though doctors in the NHS are expected to prescribe using approved – nonproprietary or generic – titles. Most nonproprietary titles are those in the European Pharmacopoeia, British Pharmacopoeia Commission or the British Pharmaceutical Codex. The USA has its own legislation and arrangements covering the naming and prescribing of medicines. (See PROPRIETARY NAME; GENERIC DRUG; PATENT.)

Apraxia

Apraxia, or dyspraxia, is the loss of ability to make accurate skilled movements. The cause is a disorder of the cerebral cortex of the BRAIN: the patient is unable to coordinate his or her movements. Apraxia differs from clumsiness resulting from muscular weakness, loss of sensation or disease in the cerebellum (see BRAIN).

The condition is usually a consequence of disease in the brain's parietal lobes, though frontal-lobe disease may cause it. A person with gait apraxia has normal power in the legs and no abnormal signs suggesting cerebellar disease, but cannot perform the normal act of walking because of malfunction in the cerebrum.

Apyrexia

Absence of FEVER.

Arachnodactyly

Arachnodactyly, or MARFAN'S SYNDROME, is a congenital condition characterised by extreme length and slenderness of the fingers and toes – and, to a lesser extent, of the limbs and trunk; laxity of the ligaments; and dislocation of the lens of the eye. The antero-posterior diameter of the skull is abnormally long, and the jaw is prominent. There may also be abnormalities of the heart.

Arachnoid Membrane

One of the membranes covering the brain and spinal cord (see BRAIN). Arachnoiditis is the name applied to inflammation of this membrane.

Arboviruses

A heterogenous group of around 500 viruses, which are transmitted to humans by ARTHROPODS. Grouped in four families, they include the viruses of DENGUE and YELLOW FEVER which are transmitted by mosquitoes.

Arc Eye

Damage to the corneal surface of the EYE caused by ultraviolet light from arc welding. A painful condition, it usually heals if the eyes are covered with pads for a day or two. It can be prevented by the proper use of protective goggles. A similar condition occurs in snow-blindness or when someone fails to protect the eyes when using suntan lamps.

Arcus Senilis

See under EYE, DISORDERS OF.

Arenaviruses

A group of viruses, so-called because under the electron microscope they have a sand-sprinkled (Latin, *arenosus*) appearance. Among the diseases in humans for which they are responsible are LASSA FEVER in West Africa, Argentinian haemorrhagic fever (mortality rate 3–15 per cent), a similar disease in Bolivia (mortality rate 18 per cent), and lymphocytic choriomeningitis, in which deaths are uncommon.

Areola

Areola literally means a small space, and is the term applied to the red or dusky ring around the nipple, or around an inflamed part. Increase in the duskiness of the areola on the breast is an important early sign of pregnancy.

Argyll Robertson Pupil

A condition (described originally by Dr Argyll Robertson) in which the pupils contract when the eyes converge on a near object, but fail to contract when a bright light falls on the eye. It is found in several diseases, especially in locomotor ataxia and neurosyphilis, an advanced manifestation of SYPHILIS.

Argyria

Argyria, or argyriosis, means the effect produced by taking silver salts over a long period, and consists of a deep duskiness of the skin, especially of the exposed parts.

Aromatase Inhibitors

A group of drugs that stop the action of the ENZYME, aromatase. This enzyme converts androgens (see ANDROGEN) to OESTROGENS. If this conversion is inhibited, the concentrations of oestrogens in the body are reduced – so these drugs operate against tumours, such as breast cancer, that depend on oestrogen for their growth. Aromatase inhibitors include anastrazole and formestane, and they are usually prescribed as second-line treatment after TAMOXIFEN, the prime drug treatment for breast cancer.

Arrhythmia

Arrhythmia means any variation from the normal regular rhythm of the heartbeat. The condition is produced by some affection interfering with the mechanism which controls the beating of the heart, and includes the following disorders: sinus arrhythmia, atrial fibrillation, atrial flutter, heart block, extrasystoles, pulsus alternans, and paroxysmal atrial tachycardia, ventricular tachycardia and ventricular fibrillation. (See HEART, DISEASES OF; ELECTROCARDIOGRAM (ECG).)

Arsenic

A metalloid with industrial use in glass, wood preservative, herbicide, semiconductor manufacture, and as an alloy additive. It may be a component in alternative or traditional remedies both intentionally and as a contaminant. Common in the environment and in food, especially seafood, arsenic is odourless and tasteless and highly toxic by ingestion, inhalation and skin contact. It binds to sulphydryl groups inhibiting the action of many enzymes (see ENZYME) and also disrupts oxidative phosphorylation by substituting for PHOSPHORUS. Clinical effects of acute poisoning range from severe gastrointestinal effects to renal impairment or failure characterised by OLIGURIA, HAEMATURIA, PROTEINURIA and renal tubular necrosis. SHOCK, COMA and CONVULSIONS are reported, as are JAUNDICE and peripheral NEUROPATHY. Chronic exposures are harder to diagnose as effects are non-specific: they include gastrointestinal disturbances, hyperpigmentation and HYPERKERATOSIS of skin, localised OEDEMA, ALOPECIA, neuropathy, PARAESTHESIA, HEPATOMEGALY and jaundice. Management is largely supportive, particularly ensuring adequate renal function. Concentrations of arsenic in urine and blood can be measured and therapy instituted if needed. Several CHELATING AGENTS are effective: these include DMPS (2, 3-dimercapto-1-propanesulphonate), penicillamine and dimercaprol; DMPS is now agent of choice.

Artefact

See ARTIFACT.

Arteries

Arteries are vessels which convey oxygenated blood away from the heart to the tissues of the body, limbs and internal organs. In the case of most arteries the blood has been purified by passing through the lungs, and is consequently bright red in colour; but in the pulmonary arteries, which convey the blood to the lungs, it is deoxygenated, dark, and like the blood in veins.

The arterial system begins at the left ventricle of the heart with the AORTA, which gives off branches that subdivide into smaller and smaller vessels. The final divisions, called arterioles, are microscopic and end in a network of capillaries which perforate the tissues like the pores of a sponge and bathe them in blood that is collected and brought back to the heart by veins. (See CIRCULATORY SYSTEM OF THE BLOOD.)

The chief arteries after the aorta and its branches are:
(1) the common carotid, running up each side of the neck and dividing into the internal carotid to the brain, and external carotid to the neck and face;
(2) the subclavian to each arm, continued by the axillary in the armpit, and the brachial along the inner side of the arm, dividing at the elbow into the radial and the ulnar,

A

which unite across the palm of the hand in arches that give branches to the fingers;

(3) the two common iliacs, in which the aorta ends, each of which divides into the internal iliac to the organs in the pelvis, and the external iliac to the lower limb, continued by the femoral in the thigh, and the popliteal behind the knee, dividing into the anterior and posterior tibial arteries to the front and back of the leg. The latter passes behind the inner ankle to the sole of the foot, where it forms arches similar to those in the hand, and supplies the foot and toes by plantar branches.

Structure The arteries are highly elastic, dilating at each heartbeat as blood is driven into them, and forcing it on by their resiliency (see PULSE). Every artery has three coats: (*a*) the outer or adventitia, consisting of ordinary strong fibrous tissue; (*b*) the middle or media, consisting of muscular fibres supported by elastic fibres, which in some of the larger arteries form distinct membranes; and (*c*) the inner or intima, consisting of a layer of yellow elastic tissue on whose inner surface rests a layer of smooth plate-like endothelial cells, over which flows the blood. In the larger arteries the muscle of the middle coat is largely replaced by elastic fibres, which render the artery still more expansile and elastic. When an artery is cut across, the muscular coat instantly shrinks, drawing the cut end within the fibrous sheath that surrounds the artery, and bunching it up, so that a very small hole is left to be closed by blood-clot. (See HAEMORRHAGE.)

Arteries, Diseases of

ARTERIES are the blood vessels that convey blood away from the heart to the tissues. The commonest cause of arterial disease is a degenerative condition known as atherosclerosis. Less commonly, inflammation of the arteries occurs; this inflammation is known as arteritis and occurs in a variety of conditions.

Atherosclerosis is due to the deposition of CHOLESTEROL into the walls of arteries. The process starts in childhood with the development of fatty streaks lining the arteries. In adulthood these progress, scarring and calcifying to form irregular narrowings within the arteries and eventually leading to blockage of the vessel. The consequence of the narrowing or blockage depends on which vessels are involved – diseased cerebral vessels cause strokes; coronary vessels cause angina and heart attacks; renal vessels cause renal failure; and peripheral arteries cause limb ischaemia (localised bloodlessness).

Risk factors predisposing individuals to atherosclerosis include age, male gender, raised plasma cholesterol concentration, high blood pressure, smoking, a family history of atherosclerosis, diabetes and obesity.

Arteritis occurs in a variety of conditions that produce inflammation in the arteries. Examples include syphilis – now rare in Britain – which produces inflammation of the aorta with subsequent dilatation (aneurysm formation) and risk of rupture; giant cell arteritis (temporal arteritis), a condition usually affecting the elderly, which involves the cranial arteries and leads to headache, tenderness over the temporal arteries and the risk of sudden blindness; Takayasu's syndrome, predominantly affecting young females, which involves the aortic arch and its major branches, leading to the absence of pulse in affected vessels; and polyarteritis nodosa, a condition causing multiple small nodules to form on the smaller arteries. General symptoms such as fever, malaise, weakness, anorexia and weight loss are accompanied by local manifestations of ischaemia (bloodlessness) in different parts of the body.

Arteriography
See ANGIOGRAPHY.

Arteriole
A small artery (see ARTERIES).

Arterio-Venous Aneurysm
An abnormal communication between an artery and a vein. It is usually the result of an injury, such as a stab or a gunshot wound, which involves both a neighbouring artery and vein.

Arteritis
Arteritis means inflammation of an artery (see ARTERIES, DISEASES OF).

Arthralgia
Pain in a joint in which there is no swelling or other indication of ARTHRITIS.

Arthritis
Arthritis refers to any condition of joints of the limbs or spine associated with inflammatory or structural change. It is distinguished from ARTHRALGIA which simply implies joint pain with or without any inflammatory or structural change. The two main categories of arthritis are osteoarthritis, in which the primary change is

thought of as mechanical failure of articular cartilage; and rheumatoid arthritis, in which the primary problem is a chronic inflammation of the synovial lining of joints, tendon sheaths and bursae. Other, less common forms of inflammatory arthritis include psoriatic arthritis, Reiter's syndrome, colitic arthritis and Behçet's syndrome. Spondarthritis refers to an inflammatory arthritis with involvement of the spine and is often associated with the HLA B27 tissue type. (See OSTEOARTHRITIS;   RHEUMATOID ARTHRITIS; RHEUMATIC FEVER.)

Arthrodesis
An operation for fixating the bones in a diseased joint in a given position so that the joint cannot be moved. It is usually done if pain and deformity in a diseased joint – caused, for instance, by RHEUMATOID ARTHRITIS – are so bad that they cannot be relieved by drugs, PHYSIOTHERAPY, splinting or ARTHROPLASTY.

Arthropathy
A term applied to any form of joint disease.

Arthroplasty
The use of metal or plastic components to replace a joint or part of a joint. Arthroplasty was first used in the 1930s to replace diseased hip-joints and has been routinely used since the 1960s, enabling thousands of people, especially the older generation, to resume normal life free from pain and disability. Replacement of other joints – for instance, knees, fingers, shoulders and elbows – has now become routine. (See JOINTS, DISEASES OF and diagram.)

Arthropods
Arthropods are segmented invertebrates with jointed legs. They include a wide range of organisms, such as scorpions, mites, ticks, spiders and centipedes (see also ARBOVIRUSES).

Arthroscope
An endoscopic instrument (see ENDOSCOPE) that enables the operator to see inside a joint cavity and, if necessary, take a biopsy or carry out an operation.

Arthroscopy
Inspection of the interior of a joint (usually the knee) to diagnose any disorder there. The instrument used is a type of ENDOSCOPE called an ARTHROSCOPE. The knee is often affected by conditions that are not easy to diagnose and are not revealed by X-ray examination. Surgery can be performed using arthroscopy and this reduces the time a patient has to be in hospital.

Arthrotomy
Surgical exploration of a joint to examine the contents or to drain PUS in SEPTIC ARTHRITIS.

Articular
Articular means anything connected with a joint: for example, articular rheumatism.

Articulation
Articulation is a term employed in two senses in medicine, meaning either the enunciation of words and sentences, or the type of contact between the surfaces of joints – these surfaces are called articular surfaces.

Artifact (Artefact)
A foreign body found in living tissue viewed under a microscope. It is usually caused by faulty preparation of a specimen, with the result that disease or abnormality seems to be present.

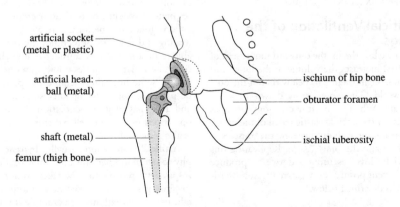

Arthroplasty of right hip (front view) showing how the artificial metal head fits into the metal socket set into the ischial part of the pelvis.

Artificial Insemination

In this method of fertilisation, SEMEN is collected either by the husband (AIH) or by a donor (AID) through masturbation and introduced into the cervix (neck of the womb) by means of an instrument around the time of OVULATION.

AIH is thought to be particularly useful for men with retrograde ejaculation or erectile IMPOTENCE. AID may be considered when the partner's sperm count is either very low or zero.

Insemination can be made with fresh or frozen semen. Donors should be tested for sexually transmitted diseases and their identity remain unknown to the infertile couple. The pregnancy rate over six months is 50–60 per cent. Artificial insemination is usually done at specially staffed centres with facilities to store semen and provide the individuals involved with appropriate counselling. Success rates are up to 70 per cent with fresh semen (used over a six-month period) and over 50 per cent with frozen semen.

Artificial Intelligence (AI)

The design and study of computer systems that have properties resembling human intelligence, such as natural language, problem-solving, and analysis of novel situations.

Artificial Joints

See ARTHROPLASTY.

Artificial Kidney

See DIALYSIS.

Artificial Limbs and Other Parts

See PROSTHESIS.

Artificial Respiration

See APPENDIX 1: BASIC FIRST AID.

Artificial Ventilation of the Lungs

When we breathe in, the outward movement of the chest increases the volume of the lungs and the pressure in them falls below that of the outside world. Therefore, air is drawn in automatically. When we breathe out, some air exits because of the normal elastic recoil of the lungs, but we also force air out by using the muscles of the chest and the DIAPHRAGM. Replicating this artificially involves using a device to produce intermittent positive or negative pressure ventilation as described below.

Intermittent positive pressure (IPP)

The simplest form of intermittent positive-pressure ventilation is mouth-to-mouth resuscitation (see APPENDIX 1: BASIC FIRST AID) where an individual blows his or her own expired gases into the lungs of a non-breathing person via the mouth or nose. Similarly gas may be blown into the lungs via a face mask (or down an endotracheal tube) and a self-inflating bag or an anaesthetic circuit containing a bag which is inflated by the flow of fresh gas from an anaesthetic machine, gas cylinder, or piped supply. In all these examples expiration is passive.

For more prolonged artificial ventilation it is usual to use a specially designed machine or ventilator to perform the task. The ventilators used in operating theatres when patients are anaesthetised and paralysed are relatively simple devices. They often consist of bellows which fill with fresh gas and which are then mechanically emptied (by means of a weight, piston, or compressed gas) via a circuit or tubes attached to an endotracheal tube into the patient's lungs. Adjustments can be made to the volume of fresh gas given with each breath and to the length of inspiration and expiration. Expiration is usually passive back to the atmosphere of the room via a scavenging system to avoid pollution.

In intensive-care units, where patients are not usually paralysed, the ventilators are more complex. They have electronic controls which allow the user to programme a variety of pressure waveforms for inspiration and expiration. There are also programmes that allow the patient to breathe between ventilated breaths or to trigger ventilated breaths, or inhibit ventilation when the patient is breathing.

Indications for artificial ventilation are when patients are unable to achieve adequate respiratory function even if they can still breathe on their own. This may be due to injury or disease of the central nervous, cardiovascular, or respiratory systems, or to drug overdose. Artificial ventilation is performed to allow time for healing and recovery. Sometimes the patient is able to breathe but it is considered advisable to control ventilation – for example, in severe head injury. Some operations require the patient to be paralysed for better or safer surgical access and this may require ventilation. With lung operations or very unwell patients, ventilation is also indicated.

Artificial ventilation usually bypasses the physiological mechanisms for humidification of inspired air, so care must be taken to humidify inspired gases. It is important to monitor the efficacy of ventilation – for example, by using blood gas measurement, pulse oximetry, and tidal carbon dioxide, and airways pressures.

Artificial ventilation is not without its hazards. The use of positive pressure raises the mean intrathoracic pressure. This can decrease venous return to the heart and cause a fall in CARDIAC OUTPUT and blood pressure. Positive-pressure ventilation may also cause PNEUMO-THORAX, but this is rare. While patients are ventilated, they are unable to breathe and so accidental disconnection from the ventilator may cause HYPOXIA and death.

Negative-pressure ventilation is seldom used nowadays. The chest or whole body, apart from the head, is placed inside an airtight box. A vacuum lowers the pressure within the box, causing the chest to expand. Air is drawn into the lungs through the mouth and nose. At the end of inspiration the vacuum is stopped, the pressure in the box returns to atmospheric, and the patient exhales passively. This is the principle of the 'iron lung' which saved many lives during the polio epidemics of the 1950s. These machines are cumbersome and make access to the patient difficult. In addition, complex manipulation of ventilation is impossible.

Jet ventilation is a relatively modern form of ventilation which utilises very small tidal volumes (see LUNGS) from a high-pressure source at high frequencies (20–200/min). First developed by physiologists to produce low stable intrathoracic pressures whilst studying CAROTID BODY reflexes, it is sometimes now used in intensive-therapy units for patients who do not achieve adequate gas exchange with conventional ventilation. Its advantages are lower intrathoracic pressures (and therefore less risk of pneumothorax and impaired venous return) and better gas mixing within the lungs.

Arytenoid
The name applied to two cartilages in the LARYNX.

Asbestosis
A form of PNEUMOCONIOSIS, in which widespread fine scarring occurs in the LUNGS, leading to severe breathing disability. The main hazard, however, is the risk of cancer (MES-OTHELIOMA) of the lung or PLEURA, or sometimes of the ovary (see OVARIES). It is caused by the inhalation of mainly blue or brown asbestos dust, either during mining or quarrying, or in one of the many industries in which it is used – for example, as an insulating material, in the making of paper, cardboard and brake linings. A person suffering from asbestosis is entitled to compensation, as the disease is legally pre-scribed. About 900 people a year in the UK claim compensation, and 600 of these for mesothelioma; most patients with asbestosis now being diagnosed have it as a consequence of industrial practices used before 1970. The use of asbestos is now strictly controlled and, when blue asbestos is found in old buildings, skilled workmen are employed to dispose of it.

Ascariasis
Ascariasis is the disease produced by infestation with the roundworm *Ascaris lumbricoides*, also known as the maw-worm. Superficially it resembles a large earthworm: the male measures about 17 cm (7 inches) and the female 23 cm (9 inches) in length. Ascariasis is a dirt disease, most prevalent where sanitation and cleanliness are lacking, particularly in the tropics and subtropics. Consumption of food contaminated by the ova (eggs), especially salad vegetables, is the commonest cause of infection. In children, infection is commonly acquired by crawling or playing on contaminated earth, and then sucking their fingers. After a complicated life-cycle in the body the adult worms end up in the intestines, whence they may be passed in the stools. A light infection may cause no symptoms. A heavy infection may lead to colic, or even obstruction of the gut. Occasionally a worm may wander into the stomach and be vomited up.

Treatment Mebendazole is the drug of choice in the UK, being given as a single dose. It should be combined with hygienic measures to break the cycle of autoinfection. All members of the family require treatment. Other ANTHELMINTICS include piperazine and pyrantel.

Ascaricides
Drugs used to treat ASCARIASIS, a disease caused by an infestation with the parasitic worm *Ascaris lumbricoides*. LEVAMISOLE, MEBENDA-ZOLE and PIPERAZINE are all effective against this parasite.

Ascaris
A worldwide genus of parasitic nematode worms (see ASCARIASIS).

Ascites
An accumulation of fluid in the abdomen. The causes include heart failure, CANCER, cirrhosis of the liver (see under LIVER, DISEASES OF), and infections. Treatment is directed at the underlying cause(s); if the amount of fluid is causing discomfort, it should be drained off.

Ascorbic Acid

Ascorbic acid, or vitamin C (see APPENDIX 5: VITAMINS), is a simple sugar found in living tissues – its highest concentrations being in the adrenal cortex (see ADRENAL GLANDS) and the eye. Stress and CORTICOTROPIN lead to a loss of ascorbic acid from the adrenal cortex. Fresh fruit and vegetables, particularly blackcurrants, citrus fruits, berries and green vegetables, are the richest dietary sources; it may also be synthetically prepared. Ascorbic acid is easily eliminated from the diet by traditional methods of cooking, being very soluble in water and easily destroyed by heat, alkalis, traces of copper or by an oxidase released by damage to plant tissues. Deficiency may lead to SCURVY, traditionally associated with sailors, among elderly people living alone or in poor communities living at subsistence level. It has been claimed that large doses (1–2 g daily) will prevent the common cold, but few large controlled trials have been carried out and it is inadvisable for people to dose themselves with large quantities of ascorbic acid, which may result in the formation of oxalate stones in the urinary tract. (See also VITAMIN.)

Asepsis

A technique to produce a germ-free environment to protect patients from infection. It is used for any procedure that might introduce infection into the body and is essential for all surgery – even minor procedures. Asepsis is achieved by ensuring that all people who come into contact with the patient scrub their hands and wear sterilised gowns with disposable masks and gloves. Operating-theatre air and equipment must also be clean. An aseptic technique is also necessary when caring for patients whose immune system (see IMMUNITY) is suppressed: one example is LEUKAEMIA, the treatment of which affects the immune system. Asepsis is aimed at preventing infection; antisepsis is the use of chemicals to destroy germs already on the body or in a wound (see ANTISEPTICS).

ASH

ASH, or Action on Smoking and Health, is a charity founded by the Royal College of Physicians in 1971 and supported by the Department of Health. It gathers information about the dangers of smoking, which it disseminates to the public. It also commissions surveys on public attitudes to smoking and helps people to give up the habit. ASH has contributed substantially to the cut in the number of smokers: six out of ten adults are now non-smokers, and an increasing number of public places are becoming smoke-free. The charity has a small headquarters in London from which further information may be obtained, with other national and regional branches in Scotland, Wales and Northern Ireland.

Asparaginase

Asparaginase is an ENZYME that breaks down the amino acid (see AMINO ACIDS), asparagine. This is of no significance to most cells in the body as they can make asparagine from simpler constituents. Certain tumours, however, are unable to do this; therefore, if they cannot receive ready-made supplies of the amino acid, they die. This property is utilised to treat acute lymphoblastic LEUKAEMIA.

Aspartame

Aspartame is an artificial sweetener, 200 times as sweet as sugar but without the bitter aftertaste of saccharine.

Asperger's Syndrome

A lifelong personality disorder, evident from childhood and regarded as a mild form of AUTISM. Persons with the syndrome tend to have great difficulty with personal relationships. They tend to take what is said to them as literal fact and have great difficulty in understanding irony, metaphors or even jokes. They appear shy with a distant and aloof character, emotional rigidity and inability to adapt to new situations. They are often mocked and ill-treated at school by their fellows because they appear unusual. Many people with Asperger's seem to take refuge in intense interests or hobbies, often conducted to an obsessional degree. Many become skilled in mathematics and particularly information technology. Frustration with the outside world which is so hard to comprehend may provoke aggressive outbursts when stressed.

Aspergillosis

A disease caused by invasion of the lung by the fungus, *Aspergillus fumigatus*. The infection is acquired by inhalation of air-borne spores of the fungus, which settle and grow in damaged parts of the lung such as healed tuberculous cavities, abscesses, or the dilated bronchi of BRONCHIECTASIS.

Aspergillus

A group of fungi including the common moulds. Several of these are capable of infecting the lungs and producing a disease resembling pulmonary TUBERCULOSIS.

Asphyxia

Asphyxia means literally absence of pulse, but is the name given to the whole series of symptoms which follow stoppage of breathing and of the heart's action. Drowning is one cause, but obstruction of the AIR PASSAGES may occur as the result of a foreign body or in some diseases, such as CROUP, DIPHTHERIA, swelling of the throat due to wounds or inflammation, ASTHMA (to a partial extent), tumours in the chest (causing slow asphyxia), and the external conditions of suffocation and strangling. Placing the head in a plastic bag results in asphyxia, and poisonous gases also cause asphyxia: for example, CARBON MONOXIDE (CO) gas, which may be given off by a stove or charcoal brazier in a badly ventilated room, can kill people during sleep. Several gases, such as sulphurous acid (from burning sulphur), ammonia, and chlorine (from bleaching-powder), cause involuntary closure of the entrance to the larynx, and thus prevent breathing. Other gases, such as nitrous oxide (or laughing-gas), chloroform, and ether, in poisonous quantity, stop the breathing by paralysing the respiration centre in the brain.

Symptoms In most cases, death from asphyxia is due to insufficiency of oxygen supplied to the blood. The first signs are rapid pulse and gasping for breath. Next comes a rise in the blood pressure, causing throbbing in the head, with lividity or blueness of the skin, due to failure of aeration of the blood, followed by still greater struggles for breath and by general CONVULSIONS. The heart becomes overdistended and gradually weaker, a paralytic stage sets in, and all struggling and breathing slowly cease. When asphyxia is due to charcoal fumes, coal-gas, and other narcotic influences, there is no convulsive stage, and death ensues gently and may occur in the course of sleep.

Treatment So long as the heart continues to beat, recovery may be looked for with prompt treatment. The one essential of treatment is to get the impure blood aerated by artificial respiration. Besides this, the feeble circulation can be helped by various methods. (See APPENDIX 1: BASIC FIRST AID – Choking; Cardiac/respiratory arrest.)

Aspiration

Aspiration means the withdrawal of fluid or gases from the natural cavities of the body or from cavities produced by disease. It may be performed for curative purposes; alternatively, a small amount of fluid may be drawn off for diagnosis of its nature or origin. An instrument called an aspirator is used to remove blood and fluid from a surgical-operation site – for example, the abdomen or the mouth (in dentistry).

PLEURISY with effusion is a condition requiring aspiration, and a litre or more of fluid may be drawn off by an aspirator or a large syringe and needle. Chronic abscesses and tuberculous joints may call for its use, the operation being done with a small syringe and hollow needle. PERICARDITIS with effusion is another condition in which aspiration is sometimes performed. The spinal canal is aspirated by the operation of LUMBAR PUNCTURE. In children the ventricles of the brain are sometimes similarly relieved from excess of fluid by piercing the fontanelle (soft spot) on the infant's head. (See HYDROCEPHALUS.)

Aspirin

Aspirin or acetylsalicylic acid is a white crystalline powder which is used like sodium salicylate as a remedy for reducing inflammation and fever. Taken orally, it has some action in relieving pain and producing sleep and is therefore often used for headache and slighter degrees of insomnia (sleeplessness). Daily doses are now used in the prevention of coronary thrombosis (see HEART, DISEASES OF); the dose is 75–300 mg. Aspirin should be used with caution in people with DYSPEPSIA or PEPTIC ULCER. (See also ANALGESICS.)

Aspirin Poisoning

ASPIRIN is a commonly available analgesic (see ANALGESICS) which is frequently taken in overdose. Clinical features of poisoning include nausea, vomiting, TINNITUS, flushing, sweating, HYPERVENTILATION, DEHYDRATION, deafness and acid-base and electrolyte disturbances (see ELECTROLYTES). In more severe cases individuals may be confused, drowsy and comatose. Rarely, renal failure (see KIDNEYS, DISEASES OF), PULMONARY OEDEMA or cardiovascular collapse occur. Severe toxicity may be delayed, as absorption of the drug may be prolonged due to the formation of drug concretions in the stomach. Treatment involves the repeated administration of activated CHARCOAL, monitoring of concentration of aspirin in the blood, and correction of acid-base and electrolyte imbalances. In more severely poisoned patients, enhanced excretion of the drug may be necessary by alkalinising the urine (by intravenous administration of sodium bicarbonate – see under SODIUM) or HAEMODIALYSIS.

Assisted Conception

(Further information about the subject and the terms used can be found at http://www.hfea.gov.uk/glossary)

This technique is used when normal methods of attempted CONCEPTION or ARTIFICIAL INSEMINATION with healthy SEMEN have failed. In the UK, assisted-conception procedures are governed by the Human Fertilisation & Embryology Act 1990, which set up the Human Fertilisation & Embryology Authority (HFEA).

Human Fertilisation & Embryology Act 1990 UK legislation was prompted by the report on *in vitro* fertilisation produced by a government-appointed committee chaired by Baroness Warnock. This followed the birth, in 1978, of the first 'test-tube' baby.

This Act allows regulation monitoring of all treatment centres to ensure that they carry out treatment and research responsibly. It covers any fertilisation that uses donated eggs or sperm (called gametes) – for example, donor insemination or embryos (see EMBRYO) grown outside the human body (known as licensed treatment). The Act also covers research on human embryos with especial emphasis on foolproof labelling and immaculate data collection.

Human Fertilisation & Embryology Authority (HFEA) Set up by the UK government following the Warnock report, the Authority's 221 members inspect and license centres carrying out fertilisation treatments using donated eggs and sperm. It publishes a code of practice advising centres on how to conduct their activities and maintains a register of information on donors, patients and all treatments. It also reviews routinely progress and research in fertility treatment and the attempted development of human CLONING. Cloning to produce viable embryos (reproductive cloning) is forbidden, but limited licensing of the technique is allowed in specialist centres to enable them to produce cells for medical treatment (therapeutic cloning).

In vitro **fertilisation (IVF)** In this technique, the female partner receives drugs to enhance OVULATION. Just before the eggs are released from the ovary (see OVARIES), several ripe eggs are collected under ULTRASOUND guidance or through a LAPAROSCOPE. The eggs are incubated with the prepared sperm. About 40 hours later, once the eggs are fertilised, two eggs (three in special circumstances) are transferred into the mother's UTERUS via the cervix (neck of the womb). Pregnancy should then proceed normally. About one in five IVF pregnancies results in the birth of a child. The success rate is lower in women over 40.

Indications In women with severely damaged FALLOPIAN TUBES, IVF offers the only chance of pregnancy. The method is also used in couples with unexplained infertility or male-factor infertility (where sperms are abnormal or their count low). Women who have had an early or surgically induced MENOPAUSE can become pregnant using donor eggs. A quarter of these pregnancies are multiple – that is, produce twins or more. Twins and triplets are more likely to be premature. The main danger of ovarian stimulation for IVF is hyperstimulation which can cause ovarian cysts. (See OVARIES, DISEASES OF.)

Gamete intrafallopian transfer (GIFT) Another method of helping infertile couples. In over half of women diagnosed as infertile, the Fallopian tubes are normal, and in many it is unknown why they cannot conceive – although some have ENDOMETRIOSIS.

Eggs are obtained and mixed with the partner's semen, then introduced into the woman's Fallopian tubes for fertilisation to take place. The fertilised egg travels to the uterus where IMPLANTATION occurs and pregnancy proceeds. A variation of GIFT is zygote intrafallopian transfer (ZIFT) in which early development of the fertilised eggs happens in the laboratory before the young embryo is transferred to the Fallopian tubes. GIFT is best used in couples with unexplained infertility or with minor degrees of male or female cervical factor infertility. The success rate is about 17 per cent. (See also ARTIFICIAL INSEMINATION.)

Association

In statistical terms, this represents two separate events apparently occurring together. Association does not necessarily mean cause and effect. For example, if a researcher finds that children wearing bicycle helmets have fewer injuries, this could imply that helmets protect them (cause and effect) or just that more careful children tend to be those who wear helmets (association).

Astereognosis

Astereognosis means the loss of the capacity to recognise the nature of an object by feeling it, and indicates a lesion (e.g. tumour) of the brain.

Asthenia
A traditional term meaning lack of strength.

Asthenopia
Asthenopia means a sense of weakness in the eyes, coming on when they are used. As a rule it is due to long-sightedness, slight inflammation, or weakness of the muscles that move the eyes. (See VISION.)

Asthma
Asthma is a common disorder of breathing characterised by widespread narrowing of smaller airways within the lung. In the UK the prevalence among children in the 5–12 age group is around 10 per cent, with up to twice the number of boys affected as girls. Among adults, however, the sex incidence becomes about equal. The main symptom is shortness of breath. A major feature of asthma is the reversibility of the airway-narrowing and, consequently, of the breathlessness. This variability in the obstruction may occur spontaneously or in response to treatment.

Cause Asthma runs in families, so that parents with asthma have a strong risk of having children with asthma, or with other atopic (see ATOPY) illnesses such as HAY FEVER or eczema (see DERMATITIS). There is therefore a great deal of interest in the genetic basis of the condition. Several GENES seem to be associated with the condition of atopy, in which subjects have a predisposition to form ANTIBODIES of the IgE class against allergens (see ALLERGEN) they encounter – especially inhaled allergens.

The allergic response in the lining of the airway leads to an inflammatory reaction. Many cells are involved in this inflammatory process, including lymphocytes, eosinophils, neutrophils and mast cells. The cells are attracted and controlled by a complex system of inflammatory mediators. The inflamed airway-wall produced in this process is then sensitive to further allergic stimuli or to non-specific challenges such as dust, smoke or drying from the increased respiration during exercise. Recognition of this inflammation has concentrated attention on anti-inflammatory aspects of treatment.

Continued inflammation with poor control of asthma can result in permanent damage to the airway-wall such that reversibility is reduced and airway-narrowing becomes permanent. Appropriate anti-inflammatory therapy may help to prevent this damage.

Many allergens can be important triggers of asthma. House-dust mite, grass pollen and animal dander are the commonest problems. Occupational factors such as grain dusts, hard-metals fumes and chemicals in the plastic and paint industry are important in some adults. Viral infections are another common trigger, especially in young children.

The prevalence of asthma appears to be on the increase in most countries. Several factors have been linked to this increase; most important may be the vulnerability of the immature immune system (see IMMUNITY) in infants. High exposure to allergens such as house-dust mite early in life may prime the immune system, while reduced exposure to common viral infections may delay the maturation of the immune system. In addition, maternal smoking in pregnancy and infancy increases the risk.

Clinical course The major symptoms of asthma are breathlessness and cough. Occasionally cough may be the only symptom, especially in children, where night-time cough may be mistaken for recurrent infection and treated inappropriately with antibiotics.

The onset of asthma is usually in childhood, but it may begin at any age. In childhood, boys are affected more often than girls but by adulthood the sex incidence is equal. Children who have mild asthma are more likely to grow out of the condition as they go through their teenaged years, although symptoms may recur later.

The degree of airway-narrowing, and its change with time and treatment, can be monitored by measuring the peak expiratory flow with a simple monitor at home – a peak-flow meter. The typical pattern shows the peak flow to be lowest in the early morning and this 'morning dipping' is often associated with disturbance of sleep.

Acute exacerbations of asthma may be provoked by infections or allergic stimuli. If they do not respond quickly and fully to medication, expert help should be sought urgently since oxygen and higher doses of drugs will be necessary to control the attack. In a severe attack the breathing rate and the pulse rate rise and the chest sounds wheezy. The peak-flow rate of air into the lungs falls. Patients may be unable to talk in full sentences without catching their breath, and the reduced oxygen in the blood in very severe attacks may produce the blue colour of CYANOSIS in the lips and tongue. Such acute attacks can be very frightening for the patient and family.

Some cases of chronic asthma are included in the internationally agreed description CHRONIC OBSTRUCTIVE PULMONARY DISEASE (COPD) – a chronic, slowly progressive disorder characterised by obstruction of the airflow persisting over several months.

Treatment The first important consideration in the treatment of asthma is avoidance of precipitating factors. When this is a specific animal or occupational exposure, this may be possible; it is however more difficult for house-dust mite or pollens. Exercise-induced asthma should be treated adequately rather than avoiding exercise.

Desensitisation injections using small quantities of specific allergens are used widely in some countries, but rarely in the UK as they are considered to have limited value since most asthma is precipitated by many stimuli and controlled adequately with simple treatment.

There are two groups of main drugs for the treatment of asthma. The first are the bronchodilators which relax the smooth muscle in the wall of the airways, increase their diameter and relieve breathlessness. The most useful agents are the beta adrenergic agonists (see ADRENERGIC RECEPTORS) such as salbutamol and terbutaline. They are best given by inhalation into the airways since this reduces the general side-effects from oral use. These drugs are usually given to reverse airway-narrowing or to prevent its onset on exercise. However, longer-acting inhaled beta agonists such as salmeterol and formoterol or the theophyllines given in tablet form can be used regularly as prevention. The beta agonists can cause TREMOR and PALPITATION in some patients.

The second group of drugs are the anti-inflammatory agents that act to reduce inflammation of the airway. The main agents in this group are the CORTICOSTEROIDS. They must be taken regularly, even when symptoms are absent. Given by inhalation they have few side-effects. In acute attacks, short courses of oral steroids are used; in very severe disease regular oral steroids may be needed. Other drugs have a role in suppressing inflammation: sodium cromoglycate has been available for some years and is generally less effective than inhaled steroids. Newer agents directed at specific steps in the inflammatory pathway, such as leukotriene receptor-antagonists, are alternative agents.

Treatment guidelines have been produced by various national and international bodies, such as the British Thoracic Society. Most have set out treatment in steps according to severity, with objectives for asthma control based on symptoms and peak flow. Patients should have a management plan that sets out their regular treatment and their appropriate response to changes in their condition.

Advice and support for research into asthma is provided by the National Asthma Campaign. See www.brit-thoracic.org.uk

Prognosis Asthma is diagnosed in 15–20 per cent of all pre-school children in the developed world. Yet by the age of 15 it is estimated that fewer than 5 per cent still have symptoms. A study in 2003 reported on a follow-up of persons born in 1972–3 who developed asthma and still had problems at the age of nine. By the time these persons were aged 26, 27 per cent were still having problems; around half of that number had never been free from the illness and the other half had apparently lost it for a few years but it had returned.

Astigmatism

An error of refraction in the EYE due to the cornea (the clear membrane in front of the eye) being unequally curved in different directions, so that rays of light in different meridians cannot be brought to a focus together on the retina. The curvature, instead of being globular, is egg-shaped, longer in one axis than the other. The condition causes objects to seem distorted and out of place, a ball for instance looking like an egg, a circle like an ellipse. The condition is remedied by suitable spectacles of which one surface forms part of a cylinder. A hard contact lens may be fitted to achieve an evenly curved surface. Astigmatism may be caused by any disease that affects the shape of the cornea – for example, a meibomian cyst (a swollen sebaceous gland in the eyelid) may press on the cornea and distort it.

Astroviruses

Small round viruses (see VIRUS) with no distinctive features, which have been isolated from the stools of infants with gastroenteritis (see DIARRHOEA). Most adults have antibodies against these viruses; this suggests that infection is common. There is no treatment.

Asymptomatic

The lack of any symptoms of disease, whether or not a disease is present.

Asynergia

The absence of harmonious and coordinated movements between muscles having opposite actions – for example, the flexors and extensors of a joint. Asynergia is a sign of disease of the nervous system.

Asystole

Arrest of the action of the heart.

Atavism

The principle of inheritance of disease or bodily characters from grandparents or remoter ancestors, the parents not having been affected by these.

Ataxia

Loss of coordination, though the power necessary to make the movements is still present. Thus an ataxic person may have a good grip in each hand but be unable to do any fine movements with the fingers; or, if the ataxia be in the legs, the person throws these about a great deal in walking while still being able to lift the legs and take steps quite well. This is due to a sensory defect or to disease of the cerebellum. (See FRIEDREICH'S ATAXIA; LOCOMOTOR ATAXIA.)

Atelectasis

Collapse of a part of the lung, or failure of the lung to expand at birth.

Atenolol

One of several BETA-ADRENOCEPTOR-BLOCKING DRUGS used in the treatment of high blood pressure, ANGINA and ARRHYTHMIA. One of its practical advantages is that only one dose a day need be taken. Atenolol, being a beta-blocking drug, may precipitate ASTHMA – an effect that may be dangerous. Among the side-effects are fatigue and disturbed sleep.

Atheroma

Degenerative changes in the inner and middle coats of arteries. (See ARTERIES, DISEASES OF.)

Atherosclerosis

A form of arteriosclerosis, in which there is fatty degeneration of the middle coat of the arterial wall. (See ARTERIES, DISEASES OF.)

Athetosis

Athetosis is the name for slow, involuntary writhing and repeated movements of the face, tongue, hands and feet, caused by disease of the brain. It is usually a manifestation of CEREBRAL PALSY. Drugs used to treat PARKINSONISM can also cause athetosis.

Athlete's Foot

A somewhat loose term applied to a skin eruption on the foot, usually between the toes. It is commonly due to RINGWORM, but may be due to other infections or merely excessive sweating of the feet. It usually responds to careful foot hygiene and the use of antifungal powder.

Athrombia

An inherited disorder in which there is a defect of blood-clotting caused by a deficiency in the formation of thrombin (see COAGULATION).

Atlas

The first cervical vertebra. (See SPINAL COLUMN.)

Atony

Absence of tone or vigour in muscles and other organs.

Atopy

Atopy, meaning out of place, is a form of hypersensitivity characterised – amongst other features – by a familial tendency. It is due to the propensity of the affected individual to produce large amounts of reagin ANTIBODIES which stick to MAST CELLS in the mucosa, so that when the ANTIGEN is inhaled, HISTAMINE is released from the mast cell. Atopy is the condition responsible for ASTHMA and HAY FEVER (see also ALLERGY). It is estimated that 10 per cent of the human race is subject to atopy. (See also DERMATITIS.)

Atresia

The absence of a natural opening, or closure of it by a membrane. Thus atresia may be found in newborn infants, preventing the bowels from moving. In young girls after puberty, absence of the menstrual flow may be due to such a malformation at the entrance to the VAGINA.

Atrial Natriuretic Peptide

The atria (see ATRIUM) of the heart contain peptides with potent diuretic and vasodilating properties. It has been known since 1980 that extracts of human atria have potent diuretic and natriuretic effects in animals (see DIURETICS). In 1984 three polypeptide species were isolated from human atria and were called alpha, beta and gamma human atrial natriuretic peptides. Plasma concentration of immunoreactive atrial natriuretic peptide can now be measured: the levels are low in healthy subjects and are increased in patients with congestive heart failure. Infusion of the peptides reduces blood pressure and causes a natriuresis and diuresis.

Atrial Septal Defect

See HEART, DISEASES OF – Congenital heart disease.

At-Risk Register

See RISK REGISTER.

Atrium

(Plural: atria.) Atrium is the name now given to the two upper cavities of the HEART. These used to be known as the auricles of the heart. The term is also applied to the part of the ear immediately internal to the drum of the ear.

Atrophy

Atrophy occurs when normal tissue, an organ or even the whole body wastes because the constituent cells die. Undernourishment, disease, injury, lack of use or AGEING may cause atrophy. Muscular atrophy occurs in certain neurological diseases such as POLIOMYELITIS or MUSCULAR DYSTROPHY. The ovary (see OVARIES) atrophies at the MENOPAUSE. (See also MUSCLES, DISORDERS OF.)

Atropine

Atropine is the active principle of belladonna, the juice of the deadly nightshade. Because of its action in dilating the pupils, it was at one time used as a cosmetic to give the eyes a full, lustrous appearance. Atropine acts by antagonising the action of the PARASYMPATHETIC NERVOUS SYSTEM. It temporarily impairs vision by paralysing accommodative power (see ACCOMMODATION). It inhibits the action of some of the nerves in the AUTONOMIC NERVOUS SYSTEM. The drug relaxes smooth muscle. It has the effect of checking the activity of almost all the glands of the body, including the sweat glands of the SKIN and the SALIVARY GLANDS in the mouth. It relieves spasm by paralysing nerves in the muscle of the intestine, bile ducts, bladder, stomach, etc. It has the power, in moderate doses, of markedly increasing the rate of the heartbeat, though by very large doses the heart, along with all other muscles, is paralysed and stopped.

Uses In eye troubles, atropine drops are used to dilate the pupil for more thorough examination of the interior of the eye, or to draw the iris away from wounds and ulcers on the centre of the eye. They also soothe the pain caused by light falling on an inflamed eye, and are further used to paralyse the ciliary muscle and so prevent accommodative changes in the eye while the eye is being examined with the OPHTHALMOSCOPE. Given by injection, atropine is used before general ANAESTHESIA to reduce secretions in the bronchial tree. The drug can also be used to accelerate the heart rate in BRADYCARDIA as a result of coronary thrombosis.

Atropine Poisoning

See ATROPINE; BELLADONNA POISONING.

Attention Deficit Disorder (Hyperactivity Syndrome)

A lifelong disorder characterised by overactive behaviour, short attention span and poor concentration. It is thought to be caused by a minor abnormality that affects the part of the brain that allows us to concentrate and focus on tasks. Some scientists have suggested that it may be caused by particular foods, particularly processed foods containing artificial additives, and recommend special diets. In some countries, attention deficit disorder is diagnosed in up to a tenth of all children; this may reflect differences in paediatric practice and diagnosis rather than a real variation in prevalence of the disorder. Behaviour therapy is the main treatment. Those children with very severe symptoms of restlessness, short attention span and disturbed behaviour may respond to additional treatment with methylphenidate (Ritalin®). This is an amphetamine-like drug that is thought to stimulate the part of the brain that is not working properly. Use of this drug has, however, been controversial.

Audiogram

A graph produced during hearing tests (with an audiometer) that shows the hearing threshold – the minimal audible loudness level – for a range of sound frequencies.

Audiometry

The testing of hearing.

Auditory Nerve

See VESTIBULOCOCHLEAR NERVE.

Aura

The peculiar feeling which persons who are subject to epileptic seizures (see EPILEPSY) experience just before the onset of an attack. It may be a sensation of a cold breeze, a peculiar smell, a vision of some animal or person, or an undefinable sense of disgust. An aura gives warning that a fit is coming and may enable a place of safety or seclusion to be reached. It may also occur as a precursor to a MIGRAINE headache.

Aural

Relating to the ear.

Auricle

A term applied both to the pinna or flap of the ear, and also to the ear-shaped tip of the atrium of the heart.

Auriscope

An instrument for examining the ear. The

source of illumination may be incorporated into the instrument, as in the electric auriscope, or it may be an independent light which is reflected into the ear by means of a forehead mirror. (See EAR, DISEASES OF.) .

Auscultation

The method used by physicians to determine, by listening, the condition of certain internal organs. The ancient physicians appear to have practised a kind of auscultation, by which they were able to detect the presence of air or fluids in the cavities of the chest and abdomen.

In 1819 the French physician, Laennec, introduced the method of auscultation by means of the STETHOSCOPE. Initially a wooden cylinder, the stethoscope has evolved into a binaural instrument consisting of a small expanded chest-piece and two flexible tubes, the ends of which fit into the ears of the observer. Various modifications of the binaural stethoscope have been introduced.

Conditions affecting the lungs can often be recognised by means of auscultation and the stethoscope. The same is true for the heart, in which disease can, by auscultation, often be identified with striking accuracy. But auscultation is also helpful in the investigation of aneurysms (see ANEURYSM) and certain diseases of the OESOPHAGUS and STOMACH. The stethoscope is also a valuable aid in the detection of some forms of uterine tumours, especially in the diagnosis of pregnancy.

Autism

A disorder, thought to be caused by a brain abnormality, that leads to a lifelong inability to relate in an ordinary way to people and situations. Autism is usually diagnosed before the age of three. It is rare, affecting around 20 people in every 10,000, and is three times more common in boys than in girls. The main features are a profound inability to form social relationships, delayed speech development, and a tendency to perform repeated compulsive actions or rituals. There is no cure at present, but behaviour therapy can help children to lead more normal lives.

Auto-

Prefix meaning self.

Autoantibody

An antibody (see ANTIBODIES) produced by a person's immune system (see IMMUNITY) that acts against the body's own tissues, resulting in AUTOIMMUNITY.

Autoclave

This is a very effective way of ensuring that material (e.g. surgical dressings) is completely sterilised, and that even the most resistant bacteria with which it may be contaminated are destroyed. Its use is based upon the fact that water boils when its vapour pressure is equal to the pressure of the surrounding atmosphere. This means that if the pressure inside a closed vessel is increased, the temperature at which water inside the vessel boils will rise above 100 degrees centigrade. By adjusting the pressure, almost any temperature for the boiling of the water will be obtained.

Autogenous

Autogenous means self-generated and is the term applied to products which arise within the body. It is applied to bacterial vaccines manufactured from the organisms found in discharges from the body and used for the treatment of the person from whom the bacteria were derived.

Autoimmune Disorders

A collection of conditions in which the body's immune system (see IMMUNITY) attacks its own tissues, identifying them as foreign substances. Genetic factors may play a part in this abnormal function, but the causes are not clear. The disorder may affect one organ (organ-specific) or type of cell, or several (non-organ-specific). Among the autoimmune disorders are ADDISON'S DISEASE; autoimmune haemolytic anaemia and pernicious anaemia (see under ANAEMIA); autoimmune chronic active HEPATITIS; DIABETES MELLITUS; MYASTHENIA GRAVIS; RHEUMATOID ARTHRITIS; and SYSTEMIC LUPUS ERYTHEMATOSUS (SLE).

Treatment Any major deficiencies, such as thyroxin or insulin lack, should be corrected. The activity of the immune system should then be reduced. CORTICOSTEROIDS and, in more severe cases, strong immunosuppressant drugs – AZATHIOPRINE, CYCLOPHOSPHAMIDE or METHOTREXATE – should be administered. Treatment is difficult because of the need to control the autoimmune condition without damaging the body's ability to combat other diseases.

Autoimmunity

Autoimmunity is a reaction to an individual's own tissues (self-antigens – see ANTIGEN) to which tolerance has been lost (see IMMUNITY). Autoantibodies are not necessarily harmful and are commonly encountered in healthy persons.

Autoimmune disease ensues when the immune system attacks the target cells of the autoimmune reaction.

Autointoxication

Literally means 'self-poisoning'. Any condition of poisoning brought about by substances formed in or by the body.

Autologous Blood Transfusion

See TRANSFUSION – Transfusion of blood.

Autolysis

The disintegration and softening of dead cells brought about by enzymes (see ENZYME) in the cells themselves.

Automatism

The performance of acts without conscious will, as, for example, after an attack of epilepsy or concussion of the brain. In such conditions the person may perform acts of which he or she is neither conscious at the time nor has any memory afterwards. It is especially liable to occur when persons suffering from epilepsy, mental subnormality, or concussion consume alcoholic liquors. It may also occur following the taking of barbiturates or PSYCHEDELIC DRUGS. There are, however, other cases in which there are no such precipitating factors. Thus it may occur following hypnosis, mental stress or strain, or conditions such as FUGUE or somnambulism (see SLEEP). The condition is of considerable importance from a legal point of view, because acts done in this state, and for which the person committing them is not responsible, may be of a criminal nature. According to English law, however, it entails complete loss of consciousness, and only then is it a defence to an action for negligence. A lesser impairment of consciousness is no defence.

Autonomic Nervous System

Part of the nervous system which regulates the bodily functions that are not under conscious control: these include the heartbeat, intestinal movements, salivation, sweating, etc. The autonomic nervous system consists of two main divisions – the SYMPATHETIC NERVOUS SYSTEM and the PARASYMPATHETIC NERVOUS SYSTEM. The smooth muscles, heart and most glands are connected to nerve fibres from both systems and their proper functioning depends on the balance between these two. (See also NERVES; NERVOUS SYSTEM.)

Autopsy

A POST-MORTEM EXAMINATION, or the examination of the internal organs of a dead body. (See NECROPSY.)

Autosomal Dominant Gene

See under GENETIC DISORDERS.

Auto-Suggestion

A self-induced receptive, hypnotic state which is believed to improve the body's ability to help itself. Doctors have long realised that if they suggested to a patient that a particular treatment would work, it often did – a type of placebo effect. Some techniques now make use of this idea. For instance, people can be taught muscular relaxation to control their anxiety states – the BIOFEEDBACK principle.

Avascular

Without a blood supply. Avascular necrosis is the death of a tissue because the blood supply has been cut off.

Aversion Therapy

A form of psychological treatment in which such an unpleasant response is induced to his or her psychological aberration that the patient decides to give it up. Thus the victim of alcoholism is given a drug that makes the subsequent drinking of alcoholic liquors so unpleasant, by inducing nausea and vomiting, that he or she decides to give up drinking. (See ALCOHOL; DISULFIRAM.) Aversion therapy may help in the treatment of alcoholism, drug addiction, sexual deviations such as transvestism, and compulsive gambling.

Avitaminosis

The condition of a human being or an animal deprived of one or more vitamins (see VITAMIN).

Avulsion

Forcible tearing away of one tissue from another. For example, a tendon may be avulsed from the bone to which it is attached, or a nerve may be injured and torn away – avulsed – from the tissue in which it runs.

Axilla

Anatomical name for the armpit.

Axis

The name applied to the second cervical vertebra. (See SPINAL COLUMN.)

Axon

Nerve fibre: an elongated projection of a nerve cell or NEURON(E) that carries an electrical impulse to the tissue at the end of the axon.

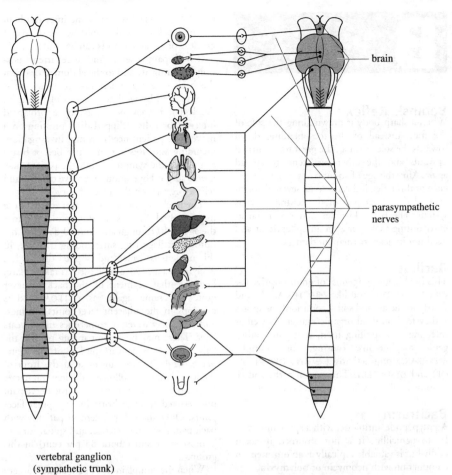

brain

parasympathetic
nerves

vertebral ganglion
(sympathetic trunk)

Schematic diagram of autonomic nervous system. (Left) Sympathetic nerves leaving middle section of spinal cord to connect via the vertebral ganglion (sympathetic trunk) to organs. (Right) Parasympathetic nerves leaving the brain and lower spinal cord to connect to organs.

Large axons are covered by a sheath of insulating myelin which is interrupted at intervals by nodes of Lanvier, where other axons branch out. An axon may be more than a metre long. It ends by branching into several filaments called telodendria, and these are in contact with muscle or gland membranes and other nerves (see NERVE).

Azathioprine

A CYTOTOXIC and an immunosuppressive drug (see IMMUNOSUPPRESSION). In the first of these capacities it is proving to be of value in the treatment of acute leukaemia. As an immunosuppressive agent it reduces the antibody response of the body (see ANTIBODIES), and is thereby helping to facilitate the success of transplant operations (see TRANSPLANTATION) by reducing the chances of the transplanted organ (e.g. the kidney) being rejected by the body. Azathioprine is also proving to be of value in the treatment of AUTOIMMUNE DISORDERS.

Azoospermia

The condition characterised by lack of spermatozoa (see SPERMATOZOON) in the SEMEN.

Azotaemia

Azotaemia means the presence of UREA and other nitrogenous bodies in greater concentration than normal in the blood. The condition is generally associated with advanced types of kidney disease (see KIDNEYS, DISEASES OF).

B

Babinski Reflex

When a sharp body is drawn along the sole of the foot, instead of the toes bending down towards the sole as usual, the great toe is turned upwards and the other toes tend to spread apart. After the age of about two years, the presence of this reflex indicates some severe disturbance in the upper part of the central nervous system. The Babinski reflex may occur transiently during COMA or after an epileptic fit and need not indicate permanent damage.

Bacillus

This is a big group (genus) of gram-positive (see GRAM'S STAIN) rod-like BACTERIA. Found widely in the air and soil – commonly as spores – they feed on dead organic matter. As well as infecting and spoiling food, some are pathogenic to humans, causing, for example, ANTHRAX, conjunctivitis (see EYE, DISORDERS OF) and DYSENTERY. They are also the source of some antibiotics (See under MICROBIOLOGY.)

Bacitracin

A polypeptide antibiotic, with a spectrum similar to penicillin. It is not absorbed if taken orally but is valuable topically as an ointment in conjunction with neomycin or polymyxin.

Backache

Most people suffer from backache at times during their lives, much of which has no identifiable cause – non-specific back pain. This diagnosis is one of the biggest single causes of sickness absence in the UK's working population. Certain occupations, such as those involving long periods of sedentary work, lifting, bending and awkward physical work, are especially likely to cause backache. Back pain is commonly the result of sporting activities.

Non-specific back pain is probably the result of mechanical disorders in the muscles, ligaments and joints of the back: torn muscles, sprained LIGAMENTS, and FIBROSITIS. These disorders are not always easy to diagnose, but mild muscular and ligamentous injuries are usually relieved with symptomatic treatment – warmth, gentle massage, analgesics, etc. Sometimes back pain is caused or worsened by muscle spasms, which may call for the use of antispasmodic drugs. STRESS and DEPRESSION (see MENTAL ILLNESS) can sometimes result in chronic backache and should be considered if no clear physical diagnosis can be made.

If back pain is severe and/or recurrent, possibly radiating around to the abdomen or down the back of a leg (sciatica – see below), or is accompanied by weakness or loss of feeling in the leg(s), it may be caused by a prolapsed intervertebral disc (slipped disc) pressing on a nerve. The patient needs prompt investigation, including MRI. Resting on a firm bed or board can relieve the symptoms, but the patient may need a surgical operation to remove the disc and relieve pressure on the affected nerve.

The nucleus pulposus – the soft centre of the intervertebral disc – is at risk of prolapse under the age of 40 through an acquired defect in the fibrous cartilage ring surrounding it. Over 40 this nucleus is firmer and 'slipped disc' is less likely to occur. Once prolapse has taken place, however, that segment of the back is never quite the same again, as OSTEOARTHRITIS develops in the adjacent facet joints. Stiffness and pain may develop, sometimes many years later. There may be accompanying pain in the legs: SCIATICA is pain in the line of the sciatic nerve, while its rarer analogue at the front of the leg is cruralgia, following the femoral nerve. Leg pain of this sort may not be true nerve pain but referred from arthritis in the spinal facet joints. Only about 5 per cent of patients with back pain have true sciatica, and spinal surgery is most successful (about 85 per cent) in this group.

When the complaint is of pain alone, surgery is much less successful. Manipulation by physiotherapists, doctors, osteopaths or chiropractors can relieve symptoms; it is important first to make sure that there is not a serious disorder such as a fracture or cancer.

Other local causes of back pain are osteoarthritis of the vertebral joints, ankylosing spondylitis (an inflammatory condition which can severely deform the spine), cancer (usually secondary cancer deposits spreading from a primary tumour elsewhere), osteomyelitis, osteoporosis, and PAGET'S DISEASE OF BONE. Fractures of the spine – compressed fracture of a vertebra or a break in one of its spinous processes – are painful and potentially dangerous. (See BONE, DISORDERS OF.)

Backache can also be caused by disease elsewhere, such as infection of the kidney or gall-bladder (see LIVER), inflammation of the PANCREAS, disorders in the UTERUS and PELVIS or osteoarthritis of the HIP. Treatment is effected by tackling the underlying cause. Among the many known causes of back pain are:

Mechanical and traumatic causes
Congenital anomalies.
Fractures of the spine.
Muscular tenderness and ligament strain.
Osteoarthritis.
Prolapsed intervertebral disc.
Spondylosis.

Inflammatory causes
Ankylosing spondylitis.
Brucellosis.
Osteomyelitis.
Paravertebral abscess.
Psoriatic arthropathy.
Reiter's syndrome.
Spondyloarthropathy.
Tuberculosis.

Neoplastic causes
Metastatic disease.
Primary benign tumours.
Primary malignant tumours.

Metabolic bone disease
Osteomalacia.
Osteoporosis.
Paget's disease.

Referred pain
Carcinoma of the pancreas.
Ovarian inflammation and tumours.
Pelvic disease.
Posterior duodenal ulcer.
Prolapse of the womb.

Psychogenic causes
Anxiety.
Depression.

People with backache can obtain advice from www.backcare.org.uk

Baclofen
A powerful muscle-relaxant used for patients with chronic severe spasticity – increased muscle rigidity – resulting from disorders such as CEREBRAL PALSY, MULTIPLE SCLEROSIS (MS) or traumatic partial section of the SPINAL CORD. Important adverse effects include SEDATION, HYPOTONIA and DELIRIUM.

Bacteraemia
Bacteraemia is the condition in which BACTERIA are present in the bloodstream.

Bacteria
(Singular: bacterium.) Simple, single-celled, primitive organisms which are widely distributed throughout the world in air, water, soil, plants and animals including humans. Many are beneficial to the environment and other living organisms, but some cause harm to their hosts and can be lethal.

Bacteria are classified according to their shape: BACILLUS (rod-like), coccus (spherical – see COCCI), SPIROCHAETE (corkscrew and spiral-shaped), VIBRIO (comma-shaped), and pleomorphic (variable shapes). Some are mobile, possessing slender hairs (flagellae) on the surfaces. As well as having characteristic shapes, the arrangement of the organisms is significant: some occur in chains (streptococci) and some in pairs (see DIPLOCOCCUS), while a few have a filamentous grouping. The size of bacteria ranges from around 0.2 to 5 μm and the smallest (MYCOPLASMA) are roughly the same size as the largest viruses (poxviruses – see VIRUS). They are the smallest organisms capable of existing outside their hosts. The longest, rod-shaped bacilli are slightly smaller than the human erythrocyte blood cell (7 μm).

Bacterial cells are surrounded by an outer capsule within which lie the cell wall and plasma membrane; cytoplasm fills much of the interior and this contains genetic nucleoid structures containing DNA, mesosomes (invaginations of the cell wall) and ribosomes, containing RNA and proteins. (See illustration.)

Reproduction is usually asexual, each cell dividing into two, these two into four, and so on. In favourable conditions reproduction can be very rapid, with one bacterium multiplying to 250,000 within six hours. This means that bacteria can change their characteristics by evolution relatively quickly, and many bacteria, including *Mycobacterium tuberculosis* and *Staphylococcus aureus*, have developed resistance to successive generations of antibiotics produced by man. (METHICILLIN-RESISTANT STAPHYLOCOCCUS AUREUS (MRSA)) is a serious hazard in some hospitals.

Bacteria may live as single organisms or congregate in colonies. In arduous conditions some bacteria can convert to an inert, cystic state, remaining in their resting form until the environment becomes more favourable. Bacteria have recently been discovered in an inert state in ice estimated to have been formed 250 million years ago.

Bacteria were first discovered by Antonj van Leewenhoek in the 17th century, but it was not until the middle of the 19th century that Louis Pasteur, the famous French scientist, identified bacteria as the cause of many diseases. Some act as harmful PATHOGENS as soon as they enter a host; others may have a neutral or benign effect on the host unless the host's natural immune defence system is damaged (see IMMUNOLOGY) so that it becomes vulnerable to any previously well-behaved parasites. Various benign bacteria that permanently reside in the human body are called normal flora and are found at certain sites, especially the SKIN, OROPHARYNX, COLON and VAGINA. The body's internal organs are usually sterile, as are the blood and cerebro-spinal fluid.

Bacteria are responsible for many human diseases ranging from the relatively minor – for example, a boil or infected finger – to the potentially lethal such as CHOLERA, PLAGUE or TUBERCULOSIS. Infectious bacteria enter the body through broken skin or by its orifices: by nose and mouth into the lungs or intestinal tract; by the URETHRA into the URINARY TRACT and KIDNEYS; by the vagina into the UTERUS and FALLOPIAN TUBES. Harmful bacteria then cause disease by producing poisonous endo-toxins or exotoxins, and by provoking INFLAMMATION in the tissues – for example, abscess or cellulitis. Many, but not all, bacterial infections are communicable – namely, spread from host to host. For example, tuberculosis is spread by airborne droplets, produced by coughing.

In scientific research and in hospital laboratories, bacteria are cultured in special nutrients. They are then killed, stained with appropriate chemicals and suitably prepared for examination under a MICROSCOPE. Among the staining procedures is one first developed in the late 19th century by Christian Gram, a Danish

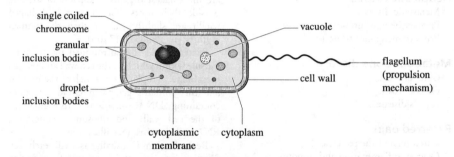

single coiled chromosome
granular inclusion bodies
droplet inclusion bodies
vacuole
flagellum (propulsion mechanism)
cell wall
cytoplasmic membrane   cytoplasm

Bacteria are micro-organisms that require special techniques such as electron microscopy to show details of their structures. They vary in their shape; examples are given below.

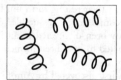

salmonella typhosa – a rod-like bacillus that causes typhoid fever

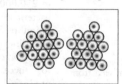

staphylococcus – groups of spherical-shaped (cocci) bacteria: cause infections such as boils

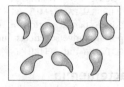

streptococcus – comprising a string of cocci: cause sore throats

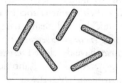

spirochaeta – a corkscrew-shaped bacterium that causes syphilis and leptospirosis

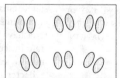

diplococci – pairs of motile cocci: among the diseases caused is pneumonia (pneumococcus)

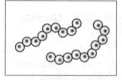

comma-shaped bacteria: an example is vibriocholerae which causes cholera

(Top) bacterial cell structure (enlarged to about 30,000 times its real size). (Centre and bottom) the varying shapes of different bacteria.

physician. His GRAM'S STAIN enabled bacteria to be divided into those that turned blue – gram positive – and those that turned red – gram negative. This straightforward test, still used today, helps to identify many bacteria and is a guide to which ANTIBIOTICS might be effective: for example, gram-positive bacteria are usually more susceptible to penicillin G than gram-negative organisms.

Infections caused by bacteria are commonly treated with antibiotics, which were widely introduced in the 1950s. However, the conflict between science and harmful bacteria remains unresolved, with the overuse and misuse of antibiotics in medicine, veterinary medicine and the animal food industry contributing to the evolution of bacteria that are resistant to antibiotics. (See also MICROBIOLOGY.)

Bacterial Meningitis
See MENINGITIS.

Bactericide
Anything which kills BACTERIA; the term is, however, usually applied to drugs and antiseptics which do this. Hence bactericidal.

Bacteriology
See MICROBIOLOGY.

Bacteriophage
A VIRUS which invades a bacterium (see BACTERIA). Containing either single-stranded or double-stranded DNA or RNA, a particular phage generally may infect one or a limited number of bacterial strains or species. After infection, once phage nucleic acid has entered the host cell, a cycle may result whereby the bacteria are programmed to produce viral components, which are assembled into virus particles and released on bacterial lysis (disintegration). Other (temperate) phages induce a non-lytic, or lysogenic, state, in which phage nucleic acid integrates stably into and replicates with the bacterial chromosome. The relationship can revert to a lytic cycle and production of new phages. In the process the phage may carry small amounts of donor bacterial DNA to a new host: the production of diphtheria toxin by *Corynebacterium diphtheriae* and of erythrogenic toxin by *Streptococcus pyogenes* are well-known examples of this effect.

Bacteriostatic
A term applied to substances that stop bacterial growth and cell division.

Bacterium
See BACTERIA.

Bacteriuria
The presence of unusual bacteria in the urine, usually a sign of infection in the kidneys, bladder or urethra. Normal urine usually contains some harmless bacteria; however, if bacterial numbers in a cleanly caught mid-stream specimen exceed 10,000 in each millilitre, that is abnormal. Investigation is necessary to find a cause and start treatment.

Patients found to have bacteriuria on SCREENING may never have consulted a doctor but nearly all have a few symptoms, such as frequency or urgency – so-called 'covert bacteriuria'.

Men have longer urethras and fewer urinary tract infections (UTIs) than women. Risk factors include diabetes mellitus, pregnancy, impaired voiding and genito-urinary malformations. Over 70 per cent of UTIs are due to *E. coli*, but of UTIs in hospital patients, only 40 per cent are caused by *E. coli*.

Treatment Patients should be encouraged to drink plenty of water, with frequent urination. Specific antibiotic therapy with trimethoprim or amoxicillin may be needed.

Bacteroides
A type of gram-negative (see GRAM'S STAIN), anaerobic, rod-like bacteria. They are generally non-motile and usually found in the alimentary and urogenital tracts of mammals. Often present in the mouth in association with periodontal disease (see TEETH, DISEASES OF).

Bacup
Bacup stands for the British Association of Cancer United Patients and their families and friends. It was founded by Dr Vicky Clement-Jones after she was treated for ovarian cancer, and it became fully operational on 31 October 1985. The aim of the Association is to provide an information service to cancer patients who want to know more about their illness or who need practical advice on how to cope with it. It does not seek to replace the traditional relationship between the doctor and patient, nor does it recommend specific treatment for particular patients; rather, its aim is to help patients to understand more about their illness so that they can communicate more effectively and freely with their medical advisers and their families and friends.

See www.cancerbacup.org.uk

Bagassosis
An industrial lung disease occurring in those who work with bagasse, which is the name

given to the broken sugar cane after sugar has been extracted from it. Bagasse, which contains 6 per cent silica, is used in board-making. The inhalation of dust causes an acute lung affection, and subsequently in some cases a chronic lung disease. (See ALVEOLITIS.)

BAL

BAL is the abbreviation for British Anti-Lewisite. (See DIMERCAPROL.)

Balance

The ability to balance is essential for a person to stand, walk and run. Maintaining this ability is a complex exercise of coordination dependent on the brain, sensory and motor nerves, and joints. There is a regular supply of information to the brain about the positions of various parts of the body and it responds with relevant instructions to the motor parts of the body. Eyes, the inner ear, skin and muscles all provide information. The cerebellum (part of the brain) collates all the information and initiates action. Balance may be affected by disorders in the balancing mechanism of the inner ear (semicircular canals) such as MENIERE'S DISEASE, and inflammation of the labyrinth (labyrinthitis). Infection of the middle ear, such as otitis media (see under EAR, DISEASES OF), can also disturb the ability to balance, sometimes accompanied by dizziness or VERTIGO. If the cerebellum is affected by disease – a tumour or a stroke, for example – the result will be faulty muscular coordination leading to clumsiness and the inability to walk properly.

Balanitis

Inflammation of the GLANS PENIS. Acute balanitis is associated with allergic DERMATITIS and HERPES GENITALIS. Diabetics are at increased risk of non-specific secondary infections; if recurrent balanitis occurs, circumcision is sometimes advised.

Balantidiasis

A form of dysentery caused by a protozoon known as *Balantidium coli* – a common parasite in pigs, which are usually the source of infection. It responds to metronidazole.

Baldness

See ALOPECIA.

Ballottement

The technique of examining a fluid-filled part of the body for the presence of a floating object. For example, a fetus can be pushed away by a finger inside the mother's vagina. The fetus floats away from the examining finger and then bounces back on to it.

Balsams

Substances which contain resins and benzoic acid. Balsam of Peru, balsam of tolu, and Friars' balsam (compound tincture of benzoin) are the chief. They are traditional remedies given internally for colds, and aid expectoration, while locally they are used to cover abrasions and stimulate ulcers.

BAN

See BRITISH APPROVED NAMES.

Bandages

Pieces of material used to support injured parts or to retain dressings in position. They come in various forms including elastic materials and plaster of Paris.

For more detailed information about bandaging, the reader is referred to *First Aid Manual*, the authorised manual of the St John's Ambulance Association, St Andrew's Ambulance Association and British Red Cross Society.

Barany's Test

A test for gauging the efficiency of the balancing mechanism (the vestibular apparatus) by applying hot or cold air or water to the external ear.

Barber's Itch

See SYCOSIS.

Barbiturates

A group of drugs which depress the CENTRAL NERVOUS SYSTEM by inhibiting the transmission of impulses between certain neurons. Thus they cause drowsiness or unconsciousness (depending on dose), reduce the cerebral metabolic rate for oxygen, and depress respiration. Their use as sedatives and hypnotics has largely been superseded by more modern drugs which are safer and more effective. Some members of this group of drugs – for instance, phenobarbitone – have selective anticonvulsant properties and are used in the treatment of GRAND MAL convulsions and status epilepticus (see EPILEPSY). The short-acting drugs thiopentone and methohexitone are widely used to induce general ANAESTHESIA. (See also DEPENDENCE.)

Barium Sulphate

A radio-opaque white powder used in X-ray examinations of the stomach and gastrointestinal tract. The barium sulphate may be swallowed to enable the oesophagus, stomach and small and large intestines to be assessed for disorders such as ulceration, tumours, DIVERTICULAR DISEASE and polyps. It may also be inserted into the RECTUM or descending COLON to investigate for possible disease. These procedures are usually done after endoscopy examinations have been carried out.

Baroreceptor
Specialised nerve ending which lines certain blood vessels and acts as a stretch receptor in the carotid sinus, aortic arch, atria, pulmonary veins and left ventricle. Increased pressure in these structures increases the rate of discharge of the baroreceptors. This information is relayed to the medulla and is important in the control of blood pressure.

Barrier Creams
Substances, usually silicone-based, applied to the skin before work to prevent damage by irritants. They are also used in medicine – for the prevention of bedsores and nappy rash, for example.

Barrier Nursing
The nursing of a patient suffering from an infectious disease in such a way that the risk of their passing on the disease to others is reduced. Thus, precautions are taken to ensure that all infective matter – such as stools, urine, sputum, discharge from wounds, and anything that may be contaminated by such infective matter (e.g. nurses' uniforms, bedding and towels) – is so treated that it will not convey the infection. (See NURSING.)

Bartholin's Glands
Two small glands opening either side of the external vaginal orifice. Their secretions help to lubricate the vulva, when a woman is sexually aroused. The glands may become infected and very painful; sometimes an abscess develops and local surgery is required. Otherwise antibiotics, analgesics and warm baths are usually effective.

Basal Cell Carcinoma
The most common form of skin cancer. Its main cause is cumulative exposure to ultraviolet light; most tumours develop on exposed sites, chiefly the face and neck. It grows very slowly, often enlarging with a raised, pearly edge, and the centre may ulcerate (rodent ulcer). It does not metastasise (see METASTASIS) and can be cured by surgical excision or RADIOTHERAPY. Small lesions can also be successfuly treated by curettage and cauterisation (see ELECTRO-

CAUTERY), LASER treatment or CRYOSURGERY. If the diagnosis is uncertain, a biopsy and histological examination should be done.

Basal Ganglion
Grey matter near the base of the cerebral hemispheres, consisting of the corpus striatum (caudate nucleus and lenticular nucleus [globus pallidus and putamen]), claustrum, and amygdaloid nucleus (see BRAIN). The basal ganglia are involved in the subconscious regulation of voluntary movement, and disorders in this region cause DYSKINESIA.

Basal Metabolism
See METABOLISM.

Basilic Vein
The prominent vein which runs from near the bend of the elbow upwards along the inner side of the upper arm.

Basophilia
The blueish appearance under the microscope of immature red blood corpuscles when stained by certain dyes. This appearance, with the blue areas collected in points, is seen in lead poisoning and the condition is called punctate basophilia. The term basophilia may also mean an increase in the numbers of basophil cells in the blood.

Bat Ears
The term commonly applied to prominent ears. The condition may be familial, but this is by no means the rule. Strapping the ears firmly back has no effect and is merely an embarrassment to the child. Where the patient wishes it, the condition can be rectified by plastic surgery.

Bather's Itch
Bather's itch, also called schistosome DERMATITIS, is the term given to a blotchy rash on the skin occurring in those bathing in water which is infested with the larvae of certain trematode worms known as schistosomes (see SCHISTOSOMIASIS). The worm is parasitic in snails. The skin rash is caused by penetration of the skin by the free-swimming larval cercaria. Bather's itch is common in many parts of the world.

BCG Vaccine
BCG (Bacillus Calmette-Guérin) vaccine, which was first introduced in France in 1908, is the only vaccine that has produced significant immunity against the tubercle bacillus (see TUBERCULOSIS) and at the same time has proved safe enough for use in human subjects. BCG

vaccination is usually considered for the following groups of people. (1) Schoolchildren: the routine programme in schools usually covers children aged between ten and 14. (2) Students, including those in teacher training colleges. (3) Immigrants from countries with a high prevalence of tuberculosis (TB). (4) Children and newborn infants born in the UK to parents from Group 3, or other newborns at parents' request. (5) Health workers, such as nurses, and others likely to be exposed to infection in their work. (6) Veterinary workers who handle animals susceptible to TB. (7) Staff of prisons, residential homes and hostels for refugees and the homeless. (8) Household contacts of people known to have active TB and newborn infants in households where there is a history of the disease. (9) Those staying for more than one month in high-risk countries.

A pre-vaccination tuberculin test is necessary in all age-groups except newborn infants, and only those with negative tuberculin reactions are vaccinated. Complications are few and far between. A local reaction at the site of vaccination usually occurs between two and six weeks after vaccination, beginning as a small papule that slowly increases in size. It may produce a small ulcer. This heals after around two months, leaving a small scar. (See IMMUNITY; TUBERCULIN.)

BDA
See BRITISH DENTAL ASSOCIATION.

Beclomethasone Dipropionate
One of the CORTICOSTEROIDS used as an aerosol inhalant. It must be used regularly for its best effect. Unlike systemic corticosteroids, inhaled forms are much less likely to suppress adrenal-gland activity and have fewer side-effects.

Bed Bath
A procedure for thoroughly washing a patient who is confined to bed. It helps to maintain a healthy skin, especially over pressure-points such as elbows, buttocks and heels. An invaluable preventive measure against the development of bed sores (see ULCER).

Bed-Blocking
The continued occupation of a hospital bed by a patient who is fit to be discharged but requires further care in a nursing home or in a community setting that cannot be arranged because of lack of suitable facilities and/or funding. Bed-blocking has become a common phenomenon in the NHS, particularly in the winter.

The result is that patients who need inpatient care cannot always be admitted. The term 'bed-blockers' is derogatory and should not be used.

Bed Bug
Bed bug, or *Cimex lectularius*, is a wingless, blood-sucking insect, parasitic on humans. It is a flat, rusty-brown insect, 5 mm long and 3 mm wide, which has an offensive, never-forgotten smell and cannot fly. The average life is 3–6 months, but it can live for a year without food. The bed bug remains hidden during the day in cracks in walls and floors, and in beds. It does not transmit any known disease. Eggs hatch out into larvae in 6–10 days, which become adult within about 12 weeks. A temperature of 44 °C kills the adult in an hour. Various agents have been used to disinfect premises, such as sulphur dioxide, ethylene oxide mixed with carbon dioxide, hydrogen cyanide and heavy naphtha, but insecticide is the most effective disinfecting agent.

Bedpan
A container made of metal, fibre or plastic into which a person confined to bed can defaecate and, in the case of a female, urinate. Men use a urinal – a flask-shaped container – to urinate. Hospitals have special cleaning and sterilising equipment for bedpans. They are much less used than in the past because patients are encouraged to be mobile as soon as possible, and also because bedside commodes are preferred where this is practical.

Bed Sores
See ULCER.

Bed-Wetting
See ENURESIS; NOCTURNAL ENURESIS.

Bee Stings
See BITES AND STINGS.

Behaviour Therapy
A form of psychiatric treatment based on learning theory. Symptoms are considered to be conditioned responses, and treatment is aimed at removing them, regardless of the underlying diagnosis. Desensitisation, operant conditioning, and aversion therapy are examples of behaviour therapy. (See MENTAL ILLNESS.)

Behçet's Syndrome
This is a syndrome characterised by oral and genital ulceration, UVEITIS and ARTHROPATHY. THROMBOPHLEBITIS is a common complication, and involvement of the central nervous system may occur.

Belching
See ERUCTATION.

Belladonna Poisoning
Atropa belladonna (deadly nightshade) is a relatively rare plant and severe poisoning is not common. The berries, which are black, ripen from August to October and are the most commonly ingested part of the plant. However, all parts of the plant are toxic. The berries contain ATROPINE and other unidentified ALKALOIDS, the leaves HYOSCINE and atropine, and the roots hyoscine. All these alkaloids have an ANTICHOLINERGIC effect which may cause a dry mouth, dilated pupils with blurred vision, TACHYCARDIA, HALLUCINATIONS and PYREXIA. There may also be ATAXIA, agitation, disorientation and confusion. In severe cases there may be CONVULSIONS, COMA, respiratory depression and ARRHYTHMIA. Clinical effects may be delayed in onset for up to 12 hours, and prolonged for several days. Treatment is supportive.

Bell's Palsy
Bell's palsy, or idiopathic facial nerve palsy, refers to the isolated paralysis of the facial muscles on one or both sides. It is of unclear cause, though damage to the seventh cranial, or FACIAL NERVE, possibly of viral origin, is thought likely. Occurring in both sexes at any age, it presents with a facial pain on the affected side, followed by an inability to close the eye or smile. The mouth appears to be drawn over to the opposite side, and fluids may escape from the angle of the mouth. Lines of expression are flattened and the patient is unable to wrinkle the brow. Rare causes include mastoiditis, LYME DISEASE, and hypertension.

Treatment Oral steroids, if started early, increase the rate of recovery, which occurs in over 90 per cent of patients, usually starting after two or three weeks and complete within three months. Permanent loss of function with facial contractures occurs in about 5 per cent of patients. Recurrence of Bell's palsy is unusual.

B Endorphin
A naturally occurring painkiller which is produced by the PITUITARY GLAND as part of a pro-hormone (pre-pro-opianomelanocortin). It is an agonist at opioid receptors, and its release is stimulated by pain and stress. (See ENDORPHINS.)

Bends
See COMPRESSED AIR ILLNESS.

Benign
Not harmful. Used especially to describe tumours that are not malignant.

Bennett's Fracture
Bennett's fracture – so-called after an Irish surgeon, Edward Hallaran Bennett (1837–1907) – is a longitudinal fracture of the first metacarpal bone in the wrist, which also involves the carpo-metacarpal joint.

Benzedrine
Proprietary name for amphetamine sulphate (see AMPHETAMINES).

Benzhexol
One of the antimuscarinic (see ANTIMUSCARINE) group of drugs used to treat PARKINSONISM. Acting by correcting the relative central cholinergic excess resulting from DOPAMINE deficiency, the drug has a moderate effect, reducing tremor and rigidity but with little action on BRADYKINESIA. It has a synergistic (see SYNERGIST) effect when used with LEVODOPA and is useful in reducing SIALORRHOEA. Valuable in treating cases of Parkinsonian side-effects occurring with neuroleptic drugs. Tardive DYSKINESIA is not improved and may be made worse.

There are few significant differences between the various antimuscarinic drugs available, but some patients may tolerate one drug better than another or find that they need to adjust their drug regimen in relation to food.

Benzocaine
Weak local anaesthetic found in some throat lozenges, creams and gels. It may cause allergic hypersensitivity.

Benzodiazepines
A large family of drugs used as HYPNOTICS, ANXIOLYTICS, TRANQUILLISERS, ANTICONVULSANTS, premedicants, and for intravenous sedation. Short-acting varieties are used as hypnotics; longer-acting ones as hypnotics and tranquillisers. Those with high lipid solubility act rapidly if given intravenously.

Benzodiazepines act at a specific central-nervous-system receptor or by potentiating the action of inhibitory neuro-transmitters. They have advantages over other sedatives by having some selectivity for anxiety rather than general sedation. They are safer in overdose. Unfortunately they may cause aggression, amnesia, excessive sedation, or confusion in the elderly. Those with long half-lives or with metabolites having long half-lives may produce

B

a hangover effect, and DEPENDENCE on these is now well recognised, so they should not be prescribed for more than a few weeks. Commonly used benzodiazepines include nitrazepam, flunitrazepam (a controlled drug), loprazolam, temazepam (a controlled drug) and chlormethiazole, normally confined to the elderly. All benzodiazepines should be used sparingly because of the risk of dependence.

Benzothiadiazines
See THIAZIDES.

Benzyl Benzoate
An emulson that was widely used as a treatment for SCABIES but is less effective and more irritant than newer scabicides. It is not advised for use in children.

Benzylpenicillin
See PENICILLIN.

Bereavement
The normal mental state associated with the death of a loved one, and the slow coming to terms with that death. The well-recognised stages of the bereavement reaction are: denial, bargaining, anger and acceptance. If bereavement symptoms are severe or prolonged, expert counselling may help. Bereavement-like symptoms may occur after divorce, retirement or other life-changing experiences.

Beriberi
(Singhalese: beri = extreme weakness.) Formerly a major health problem in many Asian countries, beriberi is a nutritional deficiency disease resulting from prolonged deficiency of the water-soluble vitamin, THIAMINE (vitamin B_1). It is often associated with deficiencies of other members of the the vitamin B complex (see APPENDIX 5: VITAMINS). A major public-health problem in countries where highly polished rice constitutes the staple diet, beriberi also occurs sporadically in alcoholics (see WERNICKE'S ENCEPHALOPATHY) and in people suffering from chronic malabsorptive states. Clinical symptoms include weakness, paralysis – involving especially the hands and feet (associated with sensory loss, particularly in the legs) – and 'burning sensations' in the feet (dry beriberi). Alternatively, it is accompanied by oedema, palpitations and a dilated heart (wet beriberi). Death usually results from cardiac failure. Thiamine deficiency can be confirmed by estimating erythrocyte transketolase concentration; blood and urine thiamine levels can be measured by high-pressure liquid chromatography.

Treatment consists of large doses of vitamin B_1 – orally or intramuscularly; a diet containing other vitamins of the B group; and rest.

Infantile beriberi This is the result of maternal thiamine deficiency; although the mother is not necessarily affected, the breast-fed baby may develop typical signs (see above). Optic and third cranial, and recurrent laryngeal nerves may be affected; encephalopathy can result in convulsions, coma and death.

Berylliosis
A disease of the lungs caused by the inhalation of particles of beryllium oxide.

Beta Adrenoceptor
See ADRENERGIC RECEPTORS.

Beta-Adrenoceptor-Blocking Drugs
Also called beta blockers, these drugs interrupt the transmission of neuronal messages via the body's adrenergic receptor sites. In the HEART these are called $beta_1$ (cardioselective) receptors. Another type – $beta_2$ (non-cardioselective) receptors – is sited in the airways, blood vessels, and organs such as the eye, liver and pancreas. Cardioselective beta blockers act primarily on $beta_1$ receptors, whereas non-cardioselective drugs act on both varieties, $beta_1$ and $beta_2$. (The neurotransmissions interrupted at the beta-receptor sites through the body by the beta blockers are initiated in the ADRENAL GLANDS: this is why these drugs are sometimes described as beta-adrenergic-blocking agents.)

They work by blocking the stimulation of beta adrenergic receptors by the neurotransmitters adrenaline and noradrenaline, which are produced at the nerve endings of that part of the SYMPATHETIC NERVOUS SYSTEM – the autonomous (involuntary) network – which facilitates the body's reaction to anxiety, stress and exercise – the 'fear and flight' response.

$Beta_1$ blockers reduce the frequency and force of the heartbeat; $beta_2$ blockers prevent vasodilation (increase in the diameter of blood vessels), thus influencing the patient's blood pressure. $Beta_1$ blockers also affect blood pressure, but the mechanism of their action is unclear. They can reduce to normal an abnormally fast heart rate so the power of the heart can be concomitantly controlled: this reduces the oxygen requirements of the heart with an advantageous knock-on effect on the respiratory system. These are valuable therapeutic effects in patients with ANGINA or who have had a myocardial infarction (heart attack – see HEART, DISEASES OF), or who suffer from HYPERTENSION. Beta$_2$ blockers reduce tremors in muscles elsewhere in the body which are a feature of anxiety or the result of thyrotoxicosis (an overactive thyroid gland – see under THYROID GLAND, DISEASES OF). Non-cardioselective blockers also reduce the abnormal pressure caused by the increase in the fluid in the eyeball that characterises GLAUCOMA.

Many beta-blocking drugs are now available; minor therapeutic differences between them may influence the choice of a drug for a particular patient. Among the common drugs are:

Primarily cardioselective	*Non-cardioselective*
Acebutolol	Labetalol
Atenolol	Nadolol
Betaxolol	Oxprenolol
Celiprolol	Propanolol
Metoprolol	Timolol

These powerful drugs have various side-effects and should be prescribed and monitored with care. In particular, people who suffer from asthma, bronchitis or other respiratory problems may develop breathing difficulties. Long-term treatment with beta blockers should not be suddenly stopped, as this may precipitate a severe recurrence of the patient's symptoms – including, possibly, a sharp rise in blood pressure. Gradual withdrawal of medication should mitigate untoward effects.

Beta Blockers
See BETA-ADRENOCEPTOR-BLOCKING DRUGS.

Betamethasone
One of the CORTICOSTEROIDS which has an action comparable to that of PREDNISOLONE, but in much lower dosage. In the form of betamethasone valerate it is used as an application to the skin as an ointment or cream.

Betatron
See RADIOTHERAPY.

Bezoar
A mass of ingested foreign material found in the stomach, usually in children or people with psychiatric illnesses. It may cause gastric obstruction and require surgical removal. The commonest type consists of hair and is known as a trichobezoar.

Bias
A statistical term describing a systematic influence which leads to consistent over- or under-estimation of the true value. For example, if a researcher is studying the effects of two different drugs on the same disease and personally favours one, unless they have been blinded to which patient is receiving which treatment, they may unwittingly cause bias in the results by regarding those treated with their preferred drug as being healthier.

Bicarbonate of Soda
Also known as baking soda. Bicarbonate of soda is an alkali, sometimes used as a home remedy for indigestion or for soothing insect bites.

Biceps
A term used for a muscle that has two heads. The biceps femoris flexes the knee and extends the hip, and the biceps brachii supinates the forearm and flexes the elbow and shoulder.

Bicuspid
Having two cusps. The premolars are bicuspid teeth, and the mitral valve of the HEART is a bicuspid valve.

Bifid
Split into two parts.

Bifocal Lens
A spectacle lens in which the upper part is shaped to assist distant vision and the lower part is for close work such as reading.

Bifurcation
The point at which a structure (for example, a blood vessel) divides into two branches.

Biguanides
Biguanides are a group of oral drugs, of which METFORMIN is the only one available for treatment, used to treat non-insulin-dependent diabetics when strict dieting and treatment with SULPHONYLUREAS have failed. Metformin acts mainly by reducing GLUCONEOGENESIS and by increasing the rate at which the body uses up glucose. Hypoglycaemia is unusual, unless taken in overdose. Gastrointestinal side-effects such as anorexia, nausea, vomiting and transient diarrhoea are common initially and may persist, particularly if large doses are taken. Metformin should not be given to patients with renal failure, in whom there is a danger of inducing lactic acidosis. (See also DIABETES MELLITUS.)

Bilateral
Occurring on both sides of the body.

B

Bile

A thick, bitter, greenish-brown fluid, secreted by the liver and stored in the gall-bladder (see LIVER). Consisting of water, mucus, bile pigments including BILIRUBIN, and various salts, it is discharged through the bile ducts into the intestine a few centimetres below the stomach. This discharge is increased shortly after eating, and again a few hours later. It helps in the digestion and absorption of food, particularly fats, and is itself reabsorbed, passing back through the blood of the liver. In JAUNDICE, obstruction of the bile ducts prevents discharge, leading to a build-up of bile in the blood and deposition in the tissues. The skin becomes greenish-yellow, while the stools become grey or white and the urine dark. Vomiting of bile is a sign of intestinal obstruction, but may occur in any case of persistent retching or vomiting, and should be fully investigated.

Bile Duct

The channel running from the gall-bladder (see LIVER) to the DUODENUM; carries BILE.

Bilharziasis

Bilharziasis is another name for SCHISTOSOMIASIS.

Biliary Colic

Severe pain caused by the attempted (and sometimes successful) expulsion of a gall-stone from the gall-bladder via the BILE DUCT. The pain, which is felt in the upper right corner of the abdomen, may last for an hour or more. Strong ANALGESICS are required to subdue the pain and the patient may need hospital admission for examination and eventual surgery. Attacks may recur, and the pain is sometimes mistakenly diagnosed as signalling a heart attack.

Bilirubin

The chief pigment in human BILE. It is derived from HAEMOGLOBIN which is the red pigment of the red blood corpuscles. The site of manufacture of bilirubin is the RETICULO-ENDOTHELIAL SYSTEM. When bile is passed into the intestine from the gall-bladder (see LIVER), part of the bilirubin is converted into stercobilin and excreted in the FAECES. The remainder is reabsorbed into the bloodstream, and of this portion the bulk goes back to the liver to be re-excreted into the bile, whilst a small proportion is excreted in the urine as urobilinogen.

Binaural

Relating to both ears.

Binocular

Relating to both eyes. Binocular vision involves focusing on an object with both eyes simultaneously and is important in judging distance.

Binovular Twins

Twins who result from the fertilisation of two separate ova. (See MULTIPLE BIRTHS.)

Bio-Availability

Bio-availability refers to the proportion of a drug reaching the systemic circulation after a particular route of administration. The most important factor is first-pass metabolism – that is, pre-systemic metabolism in either the intestine or the liver. Many lipid-soluble drugs such as beta blockers (see BETA-ADRENOCEPTOR-BLOCKING DRUGS), some tricyclic ANTIDEPRESSANT DRUGS, and various opiate ANALGESICS are severely affected. Food may affect bio-availability by modifying gastric emptying, thus slowing drug absorption. Ingested calcium may combine with drugs such as tetracyclines, further reducing their absorption.

Biofeedback

A technique whereby an auditory or visual stimulus follows on from a physiological response. Thus, a subject's ELECTROCARDIO-GRAM (ECG) may be monitored, and a signal passed back to the subject indicating his or her heart rate: for example, a red light if the rate is between 50 and 60 beats a minute; a green light if it is between 60 and 70 a minute. Once the subject has learned to discriminate between these two rates, he or she can then learn to control the heart rate. How this is learned is not clear, but by utilising biofeedback some subjects can control heart rate and blood pressure, relax spastic muscles, bring migraine under control and even help constipation.

Biological Warfare

The use of living organisms – or infectious agents derived from them – to disable or kill men, animals or plants in the pursuit of war. Such warfare, along with chemical warfare, was condemned in 1925 by the Geneva Convention, and the United Nations has endorsed this policy. Even so, some countries have experimented with possible biological agents, including those causing ANTHRAX and BOTULISM, with the intention of delivering them by land, sea or water-based missiles. These developments have prompted other countries to search for ways of annulling the lethal consequences of biological warfare.

Biomechanical Engineering

The joint utilisation of engineering and biological knowledge to illuminate normal and abnormal functions of the human body. Blood flow, the reaction of bones and joints to stress, the design of kidney dialysis machines, and the development of artificial body parts are among the practical results of this collaboration.

Biopsy

Biopsy means the removal and examination of tissue from the living body for diagnostic purposes. For example, a piece of a tumour may be cut out and examined to determine whether it is cancerous.

Bioremediation

The use of the natural properties of living things to remove hazards that threaten human and animal health. When a pollutant first appears in a local environment, existing microorganisms such as bacteria attempt to make use of the potential source of energy and as a side-effect detoxify the polluting substance. This is an evolutionary process that normally would take years.

Scientists have engineered appropriate genes from other organisms into BACTERIA, or sometimes plants, to accelerate this natural evolutionary process. For effective 'digestion of waste', a micro-organism must quickly and completely digest organic waste without producing unpleasant smells or noxious gases, be non-pathogenic and be able to reproduce in hostile conditions. For example, American researchers have discovered an anaerobic bacterium that neutralises dangerous chlorinated chemical compounds such as trichlorethane, which can pollute soil, into a harmless molecule called ethens. But the bacteria do not thrive in soil. So the dechlorinating genes in this bacterium are transferred to bacteria that are acclimatised to living in toxic areas and can more efficiently carry out the required detoxification. Other research has been aimed at detoxifying the byproducts of DDT, a troublesome and resistant pollutant. Bioremediation should prove to be an environmentally friendly and cost-effective alternative to waste incineration or chemically based processes for washing contaminated soils.

Bioterrorism

Terror attacks on civilian communities using biological agents such as ANTHRAX and SMALL-POX. Particular problems in detecting and handling attacks are the time lags between exposure of a population to dangerous agents and the onset of victims' symptoms, and the fact that early symptoms might initially be taken as the result of a naturally occurring disease. Management of any biological attack must depend on systems already in place for managing new diseases, new epidemics or traditional diseases. The effectiveness of public-health surveillance varies widely from country to country, and even advanced economies may not have the staff and facilities to investigate anything other than a recognised epidemic. As attacks might well occur without warning, tackling them could be a daunting task. Intelligence warnings about proposed attacks might, however, allow for some preventive and curative measures to be set up. Medical experts in the US believe that deployment of existing community disaster teams working to pre-prepared plans, and the development of specially trained strike teams, should cut the numbers of casualties and deaths from a bioterrorist attack. Nevertheless, bioterrorism is an alarming prospect.

Biotin

One of the dozen or so vitamins included in the vitamin B complex. It is found in liver, eggs and meat, and also synthesised by bacteria in the gut. Absorption from the gut is prevented by avidin, a constituent of egg-white. The daily requirement is small: a fraction of a milligram daily. Gross deficiency results in disturbances of the skin, a smooth tongue and lassitude. (See APPENDIX 5: VITAMINS.)

Bipolar Disorder

A type of mental illness typified by mood swings between elation (mania) and depression (see MENTAL ILLNESS).

Bird Fancier's Lung

Also known as pigeon breeder's lung, this is a form of extrinsic allergic ALVEOLITIS resulting from sensitisation to birds. In bird fanciers, skin tests sometimes show sensitisation to birds' droppings, eggs, protein and serum, even through there has been no evidence of any illness.

Birth Canal

The passage that extends from the neck of the womb (UTERUS), known as the CERVIX UTERI, to the opening of the VAGINA. The baby passes along this passage during childbirth.

Birth Control
See CONTRACEPTION.

Birth Defects
See CONGENITAL.

Birth Marks
Birth marks are of various kinds; the most common are port-wine marks (see NAEVUS). Pigment spots are found, very often raised above the skin surface and more or less hairy, being then called moles (see MOLE).

Birth Pool
A pool of warm water in which a woman can give birth to her baby. The infant is delivered into the water. The method was introduced during the 1980s and is claimed to make delivery less painful and upsetting.

Birth Rate
In 2003, 695,500 live births were registered in the United Kingdom; 38 per cent occurred outside marriage. Overall, total fertility is falling slowly. The number of births per 1,000 women aged over 40 years has been rising, and in 1999 was 8.9 per cent. In Great Britain in 2003, 193,817 legal abortions were performed under the Abortion Act 1967.

Bisacodyl
Bisacodyl is a laxative which acts by stimulation of the nerve endings in the colon by direct contact with the mucous lining.

Bisexual
Having the qualities of both sexes. The term is used to describe people who are sexually attracted to both men and women.

Bismuth
Various bismuth chelates and complexes, such as sucralfate, effective in healing gastric and duodenal ulcers are available. They may act by a direct toxic effect on gastric HELICOBACTER PYLORI, or by stimulating mucosal prostaglandin (see PROSTAGLANDINS) or bicarbonate secretion. Healing tends to be longer than with H_2-RECEPTOR ANTAGONISTS and relapse still occurs. New regimens are being developed involving co-administration with antibiotics. ENCEPHALOPATHY, described with older high-dose bismuth preparations, has not been reported.

Bisphosphonates
Bisphosphonates, of which disodium etidronate is one, are a group of drugs used mainly in the treatment of PAGET'S DISEASE OF BONE and in established vertebral osteoporosis (see BONE, DISORDERS OF). Their advantage over CALCITONIN (which has to be given by subcutaneous or intramuscular injection) is that they can be taken orally. They act by reducing the increased rate of bone turnover associated with the disease. Disodium etidronate is used with calcium carbonate in a 90-day cycle (duration of therapy up to three years) in the treatment of osteoporosis.

Bites and Stings
Animal bites are best treated as puncture wounds and simply washed and dressed. In some cases ANTIBIOTICS may be given to minimise the risk of infection, together with TETANUS toxoid if appropriate. Should RABIES be a possibility, then further treatment must be considered. Bites and stings of venomous reptiles, amphibians, scorpions, snakes, spiders, insects and fish may result in clinical effects characteristic of that particular poisoning. In some cases specific ANTIVENOM may be administered to reduce morbidity and mortality.

Many snakes are non-venomous (e.g. pythons, garter snakes, king snakes, boa constrictors) but may still inflict painful bites and cause local swelling. Most venomous snakes belong to the viper and cobra families and are common in Asia, Africa, Australia and South America. Victims of bites may experience various effects including swelling, PARALYSIS of the bitten area, blood-clotting defects, PALPITATION, respiratory difficulty, CONVULSIONS and other neurotoxic and cardiac effects. Victims should be treated as for SHOCK – that is, kept at rest, kept warm, and given oxygen if required but nothing by mouth. The bite site should be immobilised but a TOURNIQUET must not be used. All victims require prompt transfer to a medical facility. When appropriate and available, antivenoms should be administered as soon as possible.

Similar management is appropriate for bites and stings by spiders, scorpions, sea-snakes, venomous fish and other marine animals and insects.

Bites and stings in the UK The adder (*Vipera berus*) is the only venomous snake native to Britain; it is a timid animal that bites only when provoked. Fatal cases are rare, with only 14 deaths recorded in the UK since 1876, the last of these in 1975. Adder bites may result in marked swelling, weakness, collapse, shock, and in severe cases HYPOTENSION, non-specific changes in the electrocardiogram and peripheral leucocytosis. Victims of adder bites should be transferred to hospital even if asymptomatic, with the affected limb being immobilised and the bite site left alone. Local incisions, suction, tourniquets, ice packs or permanganate must not be used. Hospital management may include use of a specific antivenom, Zagreb®.

The weever fish is found in the coastal waters of the British Isles, Europe, the eastern Atlantic, and the Mediterranean Sea. It possesses venomous spines in its dorsal fin. Stings and envenomation commonly occur when an individual treads on the fish. The victim may experience a localised but increasing pain over two hours. As the venom is heat-labile, immersion of the affected area in water at approximately 40 °C or as hot as can be tolerated for 30 minutes should ease the pain. Cold applications will worsen the discomfort. Simple ANALGESICS and ANTIHISTAMINE DRUGS may be given.

Bees, wasps and hornets are insects of the order *Hymenoptera* and the females possess stinging apparatus at the end of the abdomen. Stings may cause local pain and swelling but rarely cause severe toxicity. Anaphylactic (see ANAPHYLAXIS) reactions can occur in sensitive individuals; these may be fatal. Deaths caused by upper-airway blockage as a result of stings in the mouth or neck regions are reported. In victims of stings, the stinger should be removed as quickly as possible by flicking, scraping or pulling. The site should be cleaned. Antihistamines and cold applications may bring relief. For anaphylactic reactions ADRENALINE, by intramuscular injection, may be required.

Black Death
An old name for PLAGUE.

Blackheads
See ACNE.

Blackwater Fever
This is caused by rapid breakdown of red blood cells (acute intravascular haemolysis), with resulting kidney failure as the breakdown products block the vessels serving the kidney filtration units (see KIDNEYS). It is associated with severe *Plasmodium falciparum* infection.

The complication is frequently fatal, being associated with HAEMOGLOBINURIA, JAUNDICE, fever, vomiting and severe ANAEMIA. In an extreme case the patient's urine appears black. Tender enlarged liver and spleen are usually present. The disease is triggered by quinine usage at subtherapeutic dosage in the presence of *P. falciparum* infection, especially in the nonimmune individual. Now that quinine is rarely used for prevention of this infection (it is reserved for treatment), blackwater fever has become very unusual. Treatment is as for severe complicated *P. falciparum* infection with renal impairment; dialysis and blood transfusion are usually indicated. When inadequately treated, the mortality rate may be over 40 per cent but, with satisfactory intensive therapy, this should be reduced substantially.

Bladder, Diseases of
See URINARY BLADDER, DISEASES OF and GALLBLADDER, DISEASES OF; see also URINE.

Bladders
Sacs formed of muscular and fibrous tissue and lined by a mucous membrane, which is united loosely to the muscular coat so as freely to allow increase and decrease in the contained cavity. Bladders are designed to contain some secretion or excretion, and communicate with the exterior by a narrow opening through which their contents can be discharged. In humans there are two: the gall-bladder and the urinary bladder.

Gall-bladder This is situated under the liver in the upper part of the abdomen, and its function is to store the BILE, which it discharges into the intestine by the BILE DUCT. For further details, see LIVER.

Urinary bladder This is situated in the pelvis, in front of the last part of the bowel. In the full state, the bladder rises up into the abdomen and holds about 570 ml (a pint) of urine. Two fine tubes, called the ureters, lead into the bladder, one from each kidney; and the urethra, a tube as wide as a lead pencil when distended, leads from it to the exterior – a distance of 4 cm (1½ inches) in the female and 20 cm (8 inches) in the male. The exit from the bladder to the urethra is kept closed by a muscular ring which is relaxed every time urine is passed.

Bleeding
See HAEMORRHAGE; VENESECTION.

Blenorrhoea
An excessive discharge of mucus or slimy material from a surface, such as that of the eye, nose, bowel, etc. The word 'catarrh' is used with the same meaning, but also includes the idea of inflammation as the cause of such discharge.

Bleomycin

A CYTOTOXIC antibiotic, obtained from *Streptomyces verticillus*, used to treat solid cancerous tumours of the upper part of the gut and genital tract, and lymphomas. Like other cytotoxic drugs it can have serious side-effects, and bleomycin may cause pulmonary fibrosis and skin pigmentation.

Blepharitis

Inflammation of the eyelids. (See EYE, DISORDERS OF.)

Blepharospasm

See EYE, DISORDERS OF.

Blind Loop Syndrome

A disorder in which abnormal FAECES occur as a result of a redundant loop in the small INTESTINE. The loop obstructs the normal flow of the contents of the bowel, causing stagnation. The syndrome is characterised by light-yellow, smelly, fatty, bulky faeces. The patient suffers from tiredness, malaise and loss of weight. Previous abdominal surgery is sometimes the cause, but the condition can be inherited. Blockage of intestinal contents upsets the bowel's normal bacterial balance and hinders the normal absorption of nutrients. Treatment is either with antibiotics or, if that fails, surgery.

Blindness

The statutory definition – for the purposes of registration as a blind person under the National Assistance Act 1948 – is that the person is 'so blind as to be unable to perform any work for which eyesight is essential'. Generally this is vision worse than 6/60 in the better eye, or with better acuity than this but where 'the field of vision is markedly contracted in the greater part of its extent'. Partial sight has no statutory definition, but there are official guidelines for registering a person as partially sighted: generally these are a corrected visual acuity of 3/60 or less in the better eye with some contraction of the peripheral field, or better with gross field defects. In the UK more than 100,000 people are registered as legally blind and some 50,000 as partially sighted. The World Health Organisation has estimated that there are over 40 million binocularly blind people in the world. The causes of blindness vary with age and degree of development of the country. In western society the commonest causes are glaucoma, diabetic retinopathy, other retinal diseases and senile cataract. (See also VISION.)

Any blind person, or his or her relatives, can obtain help and advice from the Royal National Institute for the Blind (www.rnib.org.uk).

Night blindness An inability to see in the dark. It can be associated with retinitis pigmentosa or vitamin A deficiency (see EYE, DISORDERS OF).

Blood

Blood consists of cellular components suspended in plasma. It circulates through the blood vessels, carrying oxygen and nutrients to the organs and removing carbon dioxide and other waste products for excretion. In addition, it is the vehicle by which hormones and other humoral transmitters reach their sites of action.

Composition The cellular components are red cells or corpuscles (ERYTHROCYTES), white cells (LEUCOCYTES and lymphocytes – see LYMPHOCYTE), and platelets.

The red cells are biconcave discs with a diameter of 7.5μm. They contain haemoglobin – an iron-containing porphyrin compound, which takes up oxygen in the lungs and releases it to the tissue.

The white cells are of various types, named according to their appearance. They can leave the circulation to wander through the tissues. They are involved in combating infection, wound healing, and rejection of foreign bodies. Pus consists of the bodies of dead white cells.

Platelets are the smallest cellular components and play an important role in blood clotting (see COAGULATION).

Erythrocytes are produced by the bone marrow in adults and have a life span of about 120 days. White cells are produced by the bone

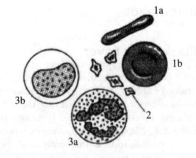

1 red blood cell (erythrocyte): (a) side view
(b) plan view
2 platelets
3 white blood cells (leucocytes): (a) neutrophil or granular leucocyte; (b) lymphocyte

Red and white blood cells and platelets.

marrow and lymphoid tissue. Plasma consists of water, ELECTROLYTES and plasma proteins; it comprises 48–58 per cent of blood volume. Plasma proteins are produced mainly by the liver and by certain types of white cells. Blood volume and electrolyte composition are closely regulated by complex mechanisms involving the KIDNEYS, ADRENAL GLANDS and HYPOTHALAMUS.

Blood Bank

A department in which blood products are prepared, stored, and tested prior to transfusion into patients.

Blood Brain Barrier

A functional, semi-permeable membrane separating the brain and cerebrospinal fluid from the blood. It allows small and lipid-soluble molecules to pass freely but is impermeable to large or ionised molecules and cells.

Blood Clot

A blood clot arises when blood comes into contact with a foreign surface – for example, damaged blood vessels – or when tissue factors are released from damaged tissue. An initial plug of PLATELETS is converted to a definitive clot by the deposition of FIBRIN, which is formed by the clotting cascade and erythrocytes. (See COAGULATION.)

Blood Corpuscle

See ERYTHROCYTES and LEUCOCYTES.

Blood Count

The number of each of the cellular components per litre of blood. It may be calculated using a microscope or by an automated process.

Blood, Diseases of

See ANAEMIA; LEUKAEMIA; LYMPHOMA; MYELO-MATOSIS; THROMBOSIS.

Blood Donor

An individual who donates his or her own blood for use in patients of compatible blood group who require transfusion.

Blood Gases

Specifically, this describes the measurement of the tensions of oxygen and carbon dioxide in blood. However, it is commonly used to describe the analysis of a sample of heparinised arterial blood for measurement of oxygen, carbon dioxide, oxygen saturation, pH, bicarbonate, and base excess (the amount of acid

required to return a unit volume of the blood to normal pH). These values are vital in monitoring the severity of illness in patients receiving intensive care or who have severe respiratory illness, as they provide a guide to the effectiveness of oxygen transport between the outside air and the body tissues. Thus they are both a guide to whether the patient is being optimally ventilated, and also a general guide to the severity of their illness.

Blood Groups

People are divided into four main groups in respect of a certain reaction of the blood. This depends upon the capacity of the serum of one person's blood to cause the red cells of another's to stick together (agglutinate). The reaction depends on antigens (see ANTIGEN), known as agglutinogens, in the erythrocytes and on ANTIBODIES, known as agglutinins, in the serum. There are two of each, the agglutinogens being known as A and B. A person's erythrocytes may have (1) no agglutinogens, (2) agglutinogen A, (3) agglutinogen B, (4) agglutinogens A and B: these are the four groups. Since the identification of the ABO and Rhesus factors (see below), around 400 other antigens have been discovered, but they cause few problems over transfusions.

In blood transfusion, the person giving and the person receiving the blood must belong to the same blood group, or a dangerous reaction will take place from the agglutination that occurs when blood of a different group is present. One exception is that group O Rhesus-negative blood can be used in an emergency for anybody.

Group	Agglutinogens in the erythrocytes	Agglutinins in the plasma	Frequency in Great Britain
AB	A and B	None	2 per cent
A	A	Anti-B	46 per cent
B	B	Anti-A	8 per cent
O	Neither A nor B	Anti-A and Anti-B	44 per cent

Rhesus factor In addition to the A and B agglutinogens (or antigens), there is another one known as the Rhesus (or Rh) factor – so named because there is a similar antigen in the red blood corpuscles of the Rhesus monkey. About 84 per cent of the population have this Rh factor in their blood and are therefore known as 'Rh-positive'. The remaining 16 per cent who do not possess the factor are known as 'Rh-negative'.

The practical importance of the Rh factor is that, unlike the A and B agglutinogens, there are no naturally occurring Rh antibodies. However, such antibodies may develop in a Rh-negative person if the Rh antigen is introduced into his or her circulation. This can occur (*a*) if a Rh-negative person is given a transfusion of Rh-positive blood, and (*b*) if a Rh-negative mother married to a Rh-positive husband becomes pregnant and the fetus is Rh-positive. If the latter happens, the mother develops Rh antibodies which can pass into the fetal circulation, where they react with the baby's Rh antigen and cause HAEMOLYTIC DISEASE of the fetus and newborn. This means that, untreated, the child may be stillborn or become jaundiced shortly after birth.

As about one in six expectant mothers is Rh-negative, a blood-group examination is now considered an essential part of the antenatal examination of a pregnant woman. All such Rh-negative expectant mothers are now given a 'Rhesus card' showing that they belong to the rhesus-negative blood group. This card should always be carried with them. Rh-positive blood should never be transfused to a Rh-negative girl or woman.

Blood-Letting
See VENESECTION.

Blood-Poisoning
See SEPTICAEMIA.

Blood Pressure
Blood pressure is that pressure which must be applied to an artery in order to stop the pulse beyond the point of pressure. It may be roughly estimated by feeling the pulse at the wrist, or accurately measured using a SPHYGMO-MANOMETER. It is dependent on the pumping force of the heart, together with the volume of blood, and on the elasticity of the blood vessels.

The blood pressure is biphasic, being greatest (systolic pressure) at each heartbeat and falling (diastolic pressure) between beats. The average systolic pressure is around 100 mm Hg in children and 120 mm Hg in young adults, generally rising with age as the arteries get thicker and harder. Diastolic pressure in a healthy young adult is about 80 mm Hg, and a rise in diastolic pressure is often a surer indicator of HYPERTENSION than is a rise in systolic pressure; the latter is more sensitive to changes of body position and emotional mood. Hypertension has various causes, the most important of which are kidney disease (see KIDNEYS, DISEASES OF), genetic predisposition and, to some extent, mental stress. Systolic pressure may well be over 200 mm Hg. Abnormal hypertension is often

accompanied by arterial disease (see ARTERIES, DISEASES OF) with an increased risk of STROKE, heart attack and heart failure (see HEART, DISEASES OF). Various ANTIHYPERTENSIVE DRUGS are available; these should be carefully evaluated, considering the patient's full clinical history, before use.

HYPOTENSION may result from superficial vasodilation (for example, after a bath, in fevers or as a side-effect of medication, particularly that prescribed for high blood pressure) and occur in weakening diseases or heart failure. The blood pressure generally falls on standing, leading to temporary postural hypotension – a particular danger in elderly people.

Blood Test
Removal of venous, capillary or arterial blood for haematological, microbiological or biochemical laboratory investigations.

Blood Transfusion
See TRANSFUSION – Transfusion of blood.

Blood Vessel
Tube through which blood is conducted from or to the heart. Blood from the heart is conducted via arteries and arterioles through capillaries and back to the heart via venules and then veins. (See ARTERIES and VEINS.)

BMA
See BRITISH MEDICAL ASSOCIATION (BMA).

BMI
See BODY MASS INDEX.

Body Mass Index
Body Mass Index (BMI) provides objective criteria of size to enable an estimation to be made of an individual's level or risk of morbidity and mortality. The BMI, which is derived from the extensive data held by life-insurance companies, is calculated by dividing a person's weight by the square of his or her height (kilograms/metres^2). Acceptable BMIs range from 20 to 25 and any degree above 30 characterises obesity. The Index may be used (with some modification) to assess children and adolescents. (See OBESITY.)

Boils (Furunculosis)
A skin infection caused by *Staphylococcus aureus*, beginning in adjacent hair follicles (see FOLLICLE). As the folliculitis becomes confluent, a tender red lump develops which becomes necrotic (see NECROSIS) centrally with pus formation. A cluster of boils becoming confluent is

called a carbuncle. Release of the pus and an oral antibiotic lead to rapid healing.

Recurrent boils are usually due to a reservoir of staphylococcal bacteria (see STAPHYLOCOCCUS) in a nostril or elsewhere, so an intranasal antibiotic cream may be prescribed. Underlying DIABETES MELLITUS should always be excluded.

Bolam Test

A medico-legal defence for a clinician accused of failing to provide an acceptable standard of care for one of his or her qualification and experience. The defence is that a responsible body of medical practitioners would have taken the same action, even though others would have acted differently. The precise size of a 'responsible body' has not been defined. The test has been modified following a case referred to as Bolitho, in which it was held that the Bolam defence failed if it could be shown that the actions relied upon, although shown to be carried out by some responsible doctors, were nonetheless illogical.

Bolus

A lump of food prepared for swallowing by chewing and mixing with saliva. The term is also used to describe the rapid intravenous injection of fluid or a drug, as opposed to a slower infusion.

Bonding

The formation of a close, selective attachment between two individuals, as in the relationship between a mother and her baby.

Bone

The framework upon which the rest of the body is built up. The bones are generally called the skeleton, though this term also includes the cartilages which join the ribs to the breastbone, protect the larynx, etc.

Structure of bone Bone is composed partly of fibrous tissue, partly of bone matrix comprising phosphate and carbonate of lime, intimately mixed together. The bones of a child are about two-thirds fibrous tissue, whilst those of the aged contain one-third; the toughness of the former and the brittleness of the latter are therefore evident.

The shafts of the limb bones are composed of dense bone, the bone being a hard tube surrounded by a membrane (the periosteum) and enclosing a fatty substance (the BONE MARROW); and of cancellous bone, which forms the short bones and the ends of long bones, in which a fine lace-work of bone fills up the whole interior, enclosing marrow in its meshes. The marrow of the smaller bones is of great importance. It is red in colour, and in it red blood corpuscles are formed. Even the densest bone is tunnelled by fine canals (Haversian canals) in which run small blood vessels, nerves and lymphatics, for the maintenance and repair of the bone. Around these Haversian canals the bone is arranged in circular plates called lamellae, the lamellae being separated from one another by clefts, known as lacunae, in which single bone-cells are contained. Even the lamellae are pierced by fine tubes known as canaliculi lodging processes of these cells. Each lamella is composed of very fine interlacing fibres.

GROWTH OF BONES Bones grow in thickness from the fibrous tissue and lime salts laid down by cells in their substance. The long bones grow in length from a plate of cartilage (epiphyseal cartilage) which runs across the bone about 1·5 cm or more from its ends, and which on one surface is also constantly forming bone until the bone ceases to lengthen at about the age of 16 or 18. Epiphyseal injury in children may lead to diminished growth of the limb.

REPAIR OF BONE is effected by cells of microscopic size, some called osteoblasts, elaborating the materials brought by the blood and laying down strands of fibrous tissue, between which bone earth is later deposited; while other cells, known as osteoclasts, dissolve and break up dead or damaged bone. When a fracture has occurred, and the broken ends have been brought into contact, these are surrounded by a mass of blood at first; this is partly absorbed and partly organised by these cells, first into fibrous tissue and later into bone. The mass surrounding the fractured ends is called the callus, and for some months it forms a distinct thickening which is gradually smoothed away, leaving the bone as before the fracture. If the ends have not been brought accurately into contact, a permanent thickening results.

VARIETIES OF BONES Apart from the structural varieties, bones fall into four classes: (*a*) long bones like those of the limbs; (*b*) short bones composed of cancellous tissue, like those of the wrist and the ankle; (*c*) flat bones like those of the skull; (*d*) irregular bones like those of the face or the vertebrae of the spinal column (backbone).

The skeleton consists of more than 200 bones. It is divided into an axial part, comprising the skull, the vertebral column, the ribs with their cartilages, and the breastbone; and an appendicular portion comprising the four limbs. The hyoid bone in the neck, together with the cartilages protecting the larynx and windpipe, may be described as the visceral skeleton.

AXIAL SKELETON The skull consists of the cranium, which has eight bones, viz. occipital, two parietal, two temporal, one frontal, ethmoid, and sphenoid; and of the face, which has 14 bones, viz. two maxillae or upper jaw-bones, one mandible or lower jaw-bone, two malar or cheek bones, two nasal, two lacrimal, two turbinal, two palate bones, and one vomer bone. (For further details, see SKULL.) The vertebral column consists of seven vertebrae in the cervical or neck region, 12 dorsal vertebrae, five vertebrae in the lumbar or loin region, the sacrum or sacral bone (a mass formed of five vertebrae fused together and forming the back part of the pelvis, which is closed at the sides by the haunch-bones), and finally the coccyx (four small vertebrae representing the tail of lower animals). The vertebral column has four curves: the first forwards in the neck, the second backwards in the dorsal region, the third forwards in the loins, and the lowest, involving the sacrum and coccyx, backwards. These are associated with the erect attitude, develop after a child learns to walk, and have the effect of diminishing jars and shocks before these reach internal organs. This is aided still further by discs of cartilage placed between each pair of vertebrae. Each vertebra has a solid part, the body in front, and behind this a ring of bone, the series of rings one above another forming a bony canal up which runs the spinal cord to pass through an opening in the skull at the upper end of the canal and there join the brain. (For further details, see SPINAL COLUMN.) The ribs – 12 in number, on each side – are attached behind to the 12 dorsal vertebrae, while in front they end a few inches away from the breastbone, but are continued forwards by cartilages. Of these the upper seven reach the breastbone, these ribs being called true ribs; the next three are joined each to the cartilage above it, while the last two have their ends free and are called floating ribs. The breastbone, or sternum, is shaped something like a short sword, about 15 cm (6 inches) long, and rather over 2·5 cm (1 inch) wide.

APPENDICULAR SKELETON The upper limb consists of the shoulder region and three segments – the upper arm, the forearm, and the wrist with the hand, separated from each other

by joints. In the shoulder lie the clavicle or collar-bone (which is immediately beneath the skin, and forms a prominent object on the front of the neck), and the scapula or shoulder-blade behind the chest. In the upper arm is a single bone, the humerus. In the forearm are two bones, the radius and ulna; the radius, in the movements of alternately turning the hand palm up and back up (called supination and pronation respectively), rotating around the ulna, which remains fixed. In the carpus or wrist are eight small bones: the scaphoid, lunate, triquetral, pisiform, trapezium, trapezoid, capitate and hamate. In the hand proper are five bones called metacarpals, upon which are set the four fingers, each containing the three bones known as phalanges, and the thumb with two phalanges.

The lower limb consists similarly of the region of the hip-bone and three segments – the thigh, the leg and the foot. The hip-bone is a large flat bone made up of three – the ilium, the ischium and the pubis – fused together, and forms the side of the pelvis or basin which encloses some of the abdominal organs. The thigh contains the femur, and the leg contains two bones – the tibia and fibula. In the tarsus are seven bones: the talus (which forms part of the ankle joint); the calcaneus or heel-bone; the navicular; the lateral, intermediate and medial cuneiforms; and the cuboid. These bones are so shaped as to form a distinct arch in the foot both from before back and from side to side. Finally, as in the hand, there are five metatarsals and 14 phalanges, of which the great toe has two, the other toes three each.

Besides these named bones there are others sometimes found in sinews, called sesamoid bones, while the numbers of the regular bones may be increased by extra ribs or diminished by the fusion together of two or more bones.

Bone, Disorders of

Bone is not an inert scaffolding for the human body. It is a living, dynamic organ, being continuously remodelled in response to external mechanical and chemical influences and acting as a large reservoir for calcium and phosphate. It is as susceptible to disease as any other organ, but responds in a way rather different from the rest of the body.

Bone fractures These occur when there is a break in the continuity of the bone. This happens either as a result of violence or because the bone is unhealthy and unable to withstand normal stresses.

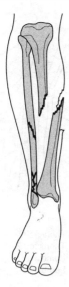

Examples of fractures: the fibula (thin bone) has a simple fracture of its shaft and a comminuted fracture at its lower end; the tibia has a compound fracture of its shaft.

SIMPLE FRACTURES Fractures where the skin remains intact or merely grazed.

COMPOUND FRACTURES have at least one wound which is in communication with the fracture, meaning that bacteria can enter the fracture site and cause infection. A compound fracture is also more serious than a simple fracture because there is greater potential for blood loss. Compound fractures usually need hospital admission, antibiotics and careful reduction of the fracture. Debridement (cleaning and excising dead tissue) in a sterile theatre may also be necessary.

The type of fracture depends on the force which has caused it. Direct violence occurs when an object hits the bone, often causing a transverse break – which means the break runs horizontally across the bone. Indirect violence occurs when a twisting injury to the ankle, for example, breaks the calf-bone (the tibia) higher up. The break may be more oblique. A fall on the outstretched hand may cause a break at the wrist, in the humerus or at the collar-bone depending on the force of impact and age of the person.

FATIGUE FRACTURES These occur after the bone has been under recurrent stress. A typical example is the march fracture of the second toe, from which army recruits suffer after long marches.

PATHOLOGICAL FRACTURES These occur in bone which is already diseased – for example,

by osteoporosis (see below) in post-menopausal women. Such fractures are typically crush fractures of the vertebrae, fractures of the neck of the femur, and COLLES' FRACTURE (of the wrist). Pathological fractures also occur in bone which has secondary-tumour deposits.

GREENSTICK FRACTURES These occur in young children whose bones are soft and bend, rather than break, in response to stress. The bone tends to buckle on the side opposite to the force. Greenstick fractures heal quickly but still need any deformity corrected and plaster of Paris to maintain the correction.

COMPLICATED FRACTURES These involve damage to important soft tissue such as nerves, blood vessels or internal organs. In these cases the soft-tissue damage needs as much attention as the fracture site.

COMMINUTED FRACTURES A fracture with more than two fragments. It usually means that the injury was more violent and that there is more risk of damage to vessels and nerves. These fractures are unstable and take longer to unite. Rehabilitation tends to be protracted.

DEPRESSED FRACTURES Most commonly found in skull fractures. A fragment of bone is forced inwards so that it lies lower than the level of the bone surrounding it. It may damage the brain beneath it.

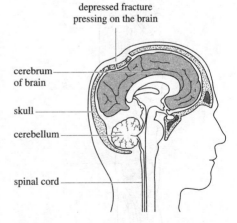

Depressed fracture of the skull (sagittal view).

HAIR-LINE FRACTURES These occur when the bone is broken but the force has not been severe enough to cause visible displacement. These fractures may be easily missed.

Symptoms and signs The fracture site is usually painful, swollen and deformed. There is asymmetry of contour between limbs. The limb is held uselessly. If the fracture is in the upper

B

limb, the arm is usually supported by the patient; if it is in the lower limb then the patient is not able to bear weight on it. The limb may appear short because of muscle spasm.

Examination may reveal crepitus – a bony grating – at the fracture site. The diagnosis is confirmed by radiography.

Treatment Healing of fractures (union) begins with the bruise around the fracture being resorbed and new bone-producing cells and blood vessels migrating into the area. Within a couple of days they form a bridge of primitive bone across the fracture. This is called callus.

The callus is replaced by woven bone which gradually matures as the new bone remodels itself. Treatment of fractures is designed to ensure that this process occurs with minimal residual deformity to the bone involved.

Treatment is initially to relieve pain and may involve temporary splinting of the fracture site. Reducing the fracture means restoring the bones to their normal position; this is particularly important at the site of joints where any small displacement may limit movement considerably.

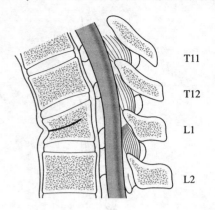

T11   Thoracic 11
T12   Thoracic 12
L1   Lumbar 1
L2   Lumbar 2

Injury to the spine: compression fracture of 1st lumbar vertebra with no damage to spinal cord.

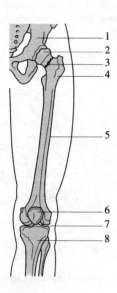

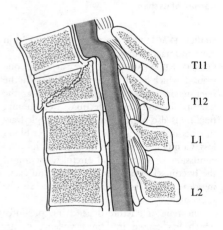

T11   Thoracic 11
T12   Thoracic 12
L1   Lumbar 1
L2   Lumbar 2

Injury to the spine: fracture/dislocation of 12th thoracic vertebra with damage to spinal cord.

1   pubic bone
2   head of femur (ball and socket joint)
3   fracture of neck of femur
4   greater trochanter of femur
5   shaft of femur
6   patella (knee cap)
7   knee joint (hinge)
8   tibia

Impacted fracture of neck of left femur.

Reduction may be done under a general anaesthetic which relaxes muscles and makes manipulation easier. Traction, which means sustained but controlled pulling on the bone, then restores the fragments of the fracture into their normal position: these are kept in position with plaster of Paris. If closed traction does not work, then open reduction of the fracture may be needed. This may involve fixing the fracture with internal-fixation methods, using metal plates, wires or screws to hold the fracture site in a rigid position with the two ends closely opposed. This allows early mobilisation after fractures and speeds return to normal use.

External fixators are usually metal devices applied to the outside of the limb to support the fracture site. They are useful in compound fractures where internal fixators are at risk of becoming infected.

Consolidation of a fracture means that repair is complete. The time taken for this depends on the age of the patient, the bone and the type of fracture. A wrist fracture may take six weeks, a femoral fracture three to six months in an adult.

Complications of fractures are fairly common. In non-union, the fracture does not unite – usually because there has been too much mobility around the fracture site. Treatment may involve internal fixation (see above). Malunion means that the bone has healed with a persistent deformity and the adjacent joint may then develop early osteoarthritis.

Myositis ossificans may occur at the elbow after a fracture. A big mass of calcified material develops around the fracture site which restricts elbow movements. Late surgical removal (after 6–12 months) is recommended.

Fractured neck of FEMUR typically affects elderly women after a trivial injury. The bone is usually osteoporotic. The leg appears short and is rotated outwards. Usually the patient is unable to put any weight on the affected leg and is in extreme pain. The fractures are classified according to where they occur:

● subcapital where the neck joins the head of the femur.
● intertrochanteric through the trochanter.
● subtrochanteric transversely through the upper end of the femur (rare).

Most of these fractures of the neck of femur need fixing by metal plates or hip replacements, as immobility in this age group has a mortality of nearly 100 per cent. Fractures of the femur shaft are usually the result of severe trauma such as a road accident. Treatment may be conservative or operative.

In fractures of the SPINAL COLUMN, mere damage to the bone – as in the case of the so-called compression fracture, in which there is no damage to the spinal cord – is not necessarily serious. If, however, the spinal cord is damaged, as in the so-called fracture dislocation, the accident may be a very serious one, the usual result being paralysis of the parts of the body below the level of the injury. Therefore the higher up the spine is fractured, the more serious the consequences. The injured person should not be moved until skilled assistance is at hand; or, if he or she must be removed, this should be done on a rigid shutter or door, not on a canvas stretcher or rug, and there should be no lifting which necessitates bending of the back. In such an injury an operation designed to remove a displaced piece of bone and free the spinal cord from pressure is often necessary and successful in relieving the paralysis. DISLOCATIONS or SUB-LUXATION of the spine are not uncommon in certain sports, particularly rugby. Anyone who has had such an injury in the cervical spine (i.e. in the neck) should be strongly advised not to return to any form of body-contact or vehicular sport.

Simple fissured fractures and depressed fractures of the skull often follow blows or falls on the head, and may not be serious, though there is always a risk of damage which is potentially serious to the brain at the same time.

Compound fractures may result in infection within the skull, and if the skull is extensively broken and depressed, surgery is usually required to check any intercranial bleeding or to relieve pressure on the brain.

The lower jaw is often fractured by a blow on the face. There is generally bleeding from the mouth, the gum being torn. Also there are pain and grating sensations on chewing, and unevenness in the line of the teeth. The treatment is simple, the line of teeth in the upper jaw forming a splint against which the lower jaw is bound, with the mouth closed.

Congenital diseases These are rare but may produce certain types of dwarfism or a susceptibility to fractures (osteogenesis imperfecta).

Infection of bone (osteomyelitis) may occur after an open fracture, or in newborn babies with SEPTICAEMIA. Once established it is very difficult to eradicate. The bacteria appear capable of lying dormant in the bone and are not easily destroyed with antibiotics so that prolonged treatment is required, as might be surgical drainage, exploration or removal of dead bone. The infection may become chronic or recur.

Osteomalacia (rickets) is the loss of mineralisation of the bone rather than simple loss of bone mass. It is caused by vitamin D deficiency and is probably the most important bone disease in the developing world. In sunlight the skin can synthesise vitamin D (see APPENDIX 5:

B

VITAMINS), but normally rickets is caused by a poor diet, or by a failure to absorb food normally (malabsorbtion). In rare cases vitamin D cannot be converted to its active state due to the congenital lack of the specific enzymes and the rickets will fail to respond to treatment with vitamin D. Malfunction of the parathyroid gland or of the kidneys can disturb the dynamic equilibrium of calcium and phosphate in the body and severely deplete the bone of its stores of both calcium and phosphate.

Osteoporosis A metabolic bone disease resulting from low bone mass (osteopenia) due to excessive bone resorption. Sufferers are prone to bone fractures from relatively minor trauma. With bone densitometry it is now possible to determine individuals' risk of osteoporosis and monitor their response to treatment.

By the age of 90 one in two women and one in six men are likely to sustain an osteoporosis-related fracture. The incidence of fractures is increasing more than would be expected from the ageing of the population, which may reflect changing patterns of exercise or diet.

Osteoporosis may be classified as primary or secondary. Primary consists of type 1 osteoporosis, due to accelerated trabecular bone loss, probably as a result of OESTROGENS deficiency. This typically leads to crush fractures of vertebral bodies and fractures of the distal forearm in women in their 60s and 70s. Type 2 osteoporosis, by contrast, results from the slower age-related cortical and travecular bone loss that occurs in both sexes. It typically leads to fractures of the proximal femur in elderly people.

Secondary osteoporosis accounts for about 20 per cent of cases in women and 40 per cent of cases in men. Subgroups include endocrine (thyrotoxicosis – see under THYROID GLAND, DISEASES OF, primary HYPERPARATHYROIDISM, CUSHING'S SYNDROME and HYPOGONADISM); gastrointestinal (malabsorption syndrome, e.g. COELIAC DISEASE, or liver disease, e.g. primary biliary CIRRHOSIS); rheumatological (RHEUMATOID ARTHRITIS or ANKYLOSING SPONDYLITIS); malignancy (multiple MYELOMA or metastatic CARCINOMA); and drugs (CORTICOSTEROIDS, HEPARIN). Additional risk factors for osteoporosis include smoking, high alcohol intake, physical inactivity, thin body-type and heredity.

Individuals at risk of osteopenia, or with an osteoporosis-related fracture, need investigation with spinal radiography and bone densitometry. A small fall in bone density results in a large increase in the risk of fracture, which has important implications for preventing and treating osteoporosis.

Treatment Antiresorptive drugs: hormone replacement therapy – also valuable in treating menopausal symptoms; treatment for at least five years is necessary, and prolonged use may increase risk of breast cancer. Cyclical oral administration of disodium etidronate – one of the bisphosphonate group of drugs – with calcium carbonate is also used (poor absorption means the etidronate must be taken on an empty stomach). Calcitonin – currently available as a subcutaneous injection; a nasal preparation with better tolerance is being developed. Calcium (1,000 mg daily) seems useful in older patients, although probably ineffective in perimenopausal women, and it is a safe preparation. Vitamin D and calcium – recent evidence suggests value for elderly patients. Anabolic steroids, though androgenic side-effects (masculinisation) make these unacceptable for most women.

With established osteoporosis, the aim of treatment is to relieve pain (with analgesics and physical measures, e.g. lumbar support) and reduce the risk of further fractures: improvement of bone mass, the prevention of falls, and general physiotherapy, encouraging a healthier lifestyle with more daily exercise.

Further information is available from the National Osteoporosis Society.

Paget's disease (see also separate entry) is a common disease of bone in the elderly, caused by overactivity of the osteoclasts (cells concerned with removal of old bone, before new bone is laid down by osteoblasts). The bone affected thickens and bows and may become painful. Treatment with calcitonin and bisphosphonates may slow down the osteoclasts, and so hinder the course of the disease, but there is no cure.

If bone loses its blood supply (avascular necrosis) it eventually fractures or collapses. If the blood supply does not return, bone's normal capacity for healing is severely impaired.

For the following diseases see separate articles: RICKETS; ACROMEGALY; OSTEOMALACIA; OSTEOGENESIS IMPERFECTA.

Tumours of bone These can be benign (non-cancerous) or malignant (cancerous). Primary bone tumours are rare, but secondaries from carcinoma of the breast, prostate and kidneys are relatively common. They may form cavities in a bone, weakening it until it breaks under normal load (a pathological fracture). The bone eroded away by the tumour may also cause problems by causing high levels of calcium in the plasma.

EWING'S TUMOUR is a malignant growth affecting long bones, particularly the tibia (calf-bone). The presenting symptoms are a throbbing pain in the limb and a high temperature. Treatment is combined surgery, radiotherapy and chemotherapy.

MYELOMA is a generalised malignant disease of blood cells which produces tumours in bones which have red bone marrow, such as the skull and trunk bones. These tumours can cause pathological fractures.

OSTEOID OSTEOMA is a harmless small growth which can occur in any bone. Its pain is typically removed by aspirin.

OSTEOSARCOMA is a malignant tumour of bone with a peak incidence between the ages of ten and 20. It typically involves the knees, causing a warm tender swelling. Removal of the growth with bone conservation techniques can often replace amputation as the definitive treatment. Chemotherapy can improve long-term survival.

Bone Graft
See BONE TRANSPLANT.

Bone Marrow
Bone marrow is the soft substance occupying the interior of bones. It is the site of formation of ERYTHROCYTES, granular LEUCOCYTES and PLATELETS.

Bone Marrow Transplant
The procedure by which malignant or defective bone marrow in a patient is replaced with normal bone marrow. Sometimes the patient's own marrow is used (when the disease is in remission); after storage using tissue-freezing technique (cryopreservation) it is reinfused into the patient once the diseased marrow has been treated (autologous transplant). More commonly, a transplant uses marrow from a donor whose tissue has been matched for compatibility. The recipient's marrow is destroyed with CYTOTOXIC drugs before transfusion. The recipient is initially nursed in an isolated environment to reduce the risk of infection.

Disorders that can be helped or even cured include certain types of LEUKAEMIA and many inherited disorders of the immune system (see IMMUNITY).

Bone Transplant
The insertion of a piece of bone from another site or from another person to fill a defect, provide supporting tissue, or encourage the growth of new bone.

Borborygmus
Flatulence in the bowels ('tummy rumbling').

Bornholm Disease
Bornholm disease, also known as devil's grip, and epidemic myalgia, is an acute infective disease due to COXSACKIE VIRUSES. It is characterised by the abrupt onset of pain around the lower margin of the ribs, headache, and fever; it occurs in epidemics, usually during warm weather, and is more common in young people than in old. The illness usually lasts seven to ten days. It is practically never fatal. The disease is named after the island of Bornholm in the Baltic, where several epidemics have been described.

Botulinum Toxin
The toxin of the anaerobic bacterium CLOSTRIDIUM botulinum is now routinely used to treat focal DYSTONIA in adults. This includes blepharospasm (see EYE, DISORDERS OF), SPASMODIC TORTICOLLIS, muscular spasms of the face, squint and some types of tremor. Injected close to where the nerve enters the affected muscles, the toxin blocks nerve transmissions for up to four months, so relieving symptoms. The toxin is also used in cerebral palsy. Although very effective, there are many possible unwanted effects, especially if too high a dose is used or the injection is misplaced.

Botulism
A rare type of food poisoning with a mortality greater than 50 per cent, caused by the presence of the exotoxin of the anaerobic bacterium *Clostridium botulinum*, usually in contaminated tinned or bottled food. Symptoms develop a few hours after ingestion.

The toxin has two components, one having haemagglutinin activity and the other neurotoxic activity which produces most of the symptoms. It has a lethal dose of as little as 1 mg/kg and is highly selective for cholinergic nerves. Thus the symptoms are those of autonomic parasympathetic blockade (dry mouth, constipation, urinary retention, mydriasis, blurred vision) and progress to blockade of somatic cholinergic transmission (muscle weakness). Death results from respiratory muscle paralysis. Treatment consists of supportive measures and

4 aminopyridine and 3, 4 di-aminopyridine, which may antagonise the effect of the toxin.

Bougies

Solid instruments for introduction into natural passages in the body – in order either to apply medicaments which they contain or with which they are coated, or, more usually, to dilate a narrow part or stricture of the passage. Thus we have, for example, urethral bougies, oesophageal bougies and rectal bougies, made usually of flexible rubber or, in the case of the urethra, of steel.

Bovine Spongiform Encephalopathy (BSE)

Known colloquially as 'mad cow disease', this is a fatal and untreatable disease. Along with scrapie in sheep and CREUTZFELDT-JACOB DISEASE (CJD) in humans, BSE belongs to a class of unusual degenerative diseases of the brain known as transmissible spongiform encephalopathies. The disease is caused by abnormal PRION proteins, which are resistant to cellular degradation. These abnormal prion proteins accumulate in and eventually cause the death of nerve cells, both in the spinal cord and the brain. The rare human disease CJD occurs throughout the world and is of three types: sporadic, iatrogenic (see IATROGENIC DISEASE) and inherited.

Since the BSE epidemic in cattle developed in the UK in the 1980s, however, a new variant of CJD has been identified and is believed to be the result of consumption of the meat of BSE-infected cattle. Studies in transgenic mice have confirmed that BSE caused variant CJD. The new variant has affected younger people and may have a shorter incubation period. If this incubation period turns out to be the same as for the other types of CJD, however, it could be 2005–2010 before the peak of this outbreak is reached. Over 148 people had died, or were dying, from variant CJD in the UK by the year 2005.

The appearance of BSE in cattle is believed to have been caused by a gene mutation (see GENETIC DISORDERS), although whether this mutation first occurred in cattle or in some other animal remains uncertain. Although the first case of BSE was officially reported in 1985, the first cattle are thought to have been infected in the 1970s. BSE spread to epidemic proportions because cattle were fed meat and bone meal, made from the offal of cattle suffering from or incubating the disease. Mother-to-calf transfer is another likely route of transmission, although meat and bone meal in cattle feed were the main cause of the epidemic. The epidemic reached its peak in 1992 when the incidence of newly diagnosed cases in cattle was 37,545.

A two-year UK government inquiry into the BSE epidemic concluded that BSE had caused a 'harrowing fatal disease in humans', and criticised officials for misleading the public over the risk to humans from BSE. Consequently, a compensation package for patients and relatives was made available. Meanwhile, a ban on the export of UK beef and restrictions on the type of meat and products made from beef that can be sold to the public were put in place. Although initially thought to be a problem primarily confined to the UK, several other countries – notably France, Germany, Spain, Switzerland and the United States – have also discovered BSE in their cattle.

Bowels

See INTESTINE.

Bowen's Disease

An uncommon chronic localised skin disease, presenting as a solitary chronic fixed irregular plaque mimicking eczema or psoriasis. It is a fairly benign form of CARCINOMA *in situ* in the EPIDERMIS but can occasionally become invasive. It is curable by CRYOTHERAPY or surgical excision.

Bow Leg

Also known as genu varum: a deformity of the legs which comprises outward curvature between knee and ankle. It may be normal in infancy, and occurs in osteoarthritis, RICKETS and other metabolic bone diseases. In early childhood it may correct with growth, but in other cases surgical correction by osteotomy or ephiphyseal stapling is possible.

Boxing Injuries

Boxing injuries rank eighth in frequency among sports injuries. According to the *Report on the Medical Aspects of Boxing* issued by the Committee on Boxing of the Royal College of Physicians of London in 1969, of 224 ex-professional boxers examined, 37 showed evidence of brain damage and this was disabling in 13.

The first type of damage occurs as an acute episode in which one or more severe blows leads to loss of consciousness and occasionally to death. Death in the acute phase is usually due to intracranial haemorrhage and this carries a mortality of 45 per cent even with the sophisticated surgical techniques currently available. The second type of damage develops over a much longer period and is cumulative, leading to the atrophy of the cerebral cortex and brain stem. The repair processes of the brain are very limited and even after mild concussion it may suffer a small amount of permanent structural damage. Brain-scanning techniques now enable brain damage to be detected during life, and brain damage of the type previously associated with the punch-drunk syndrome is now being detected before obvious clinical signs have developed. Evidence of cerebral atrophy has been found in relatively young boxers including amateurs and those whose careers have been considered successful. The tragedy is that brain damage can only be detected after it has occurred. Many doctors are opposed to boxing, even with the present, more stringent medical precautions taken by those responsible for running the sport. Since the Royal College's survey in 1969, the British Medical Association and other UK medical organisations have declared their opposition to boxing on medical grounds, as have medical organisations in several other countries.

In 1998, the Dutch Health Council recommended that professional boxing should be banned unless the rules are tightened. It claimed that chronic brain damage is seen in 40–80 per cent of boxers and that one in eight amateur bouts end with a concussed participant.

There is currently no legal basis on which to ban boxing in the UK, although it has been suggested that an injured boxer might one day sue a promoter. One correspondent to the *British Medical Journal* in 1998 suggested that since medical cover is a legal requirement at boxing promotions, the profession should consider if its members should withdraw participation.

Brachial

Brachial means 'belonging to the upper arm'. There are, for example, a brachial artery, and a brachial plexus of nerves through which run all the nerves to the arm. The brachial plexus lies along the outer side of the armpit, and is liable to be damaged in dislocation at the shoulder.

Brachycephalic

Brachycephalic means short-headed and is a term applied to skulls the breadth of which is at least four-fifths of the length.

Brachydactyly

The conditions in which the fingers or toes are abnormally short.

Bradycardia

Slowness of the beating of the heart with corresponding slowness of the pulse (below 60 per minute). (See HEART, DISEASES OF.)

Bradykinesia

Bradykinesia refers to the slow, writhing movements of the body and limbs that may occur in various brain disorders (see ATHETOSIS).

Bradykinin

Bradykinin is a substance derived from plasma proteins; it plays an important role in many of the reactions of the body, including INFLAMMATION. Its prime action is in producing dilatation of arteries and veins. It has also been described as 'the most powerful pain-producing agent known'.

Braille

A system of printing or writing devised for blind people. Developed by the Frenchman Louis Braille, the system is based on six raised dots which can be organised in different combinations within two grades. Each system in Grade I represents an individual letter or punctuation mark. Grade II's symbols represent common combinations of letters or individual words. Braille is accepted for all written languages, mathematics, science and music, with Grade II the more popular type.

Brain

The brain and spinal cord together form the central nervous sytem (CNS). Twelve cranial nerves leave each side of the brain (see NERVES, below) and 31 spinal nerves from each side of the cord: together these nerves form the peripheral nervous system. Complex chains of nerves lying within the chest and abdomen, and acting largely independently of the peripheral system, though linked with it, comprise the AUTONOMIC NERVOUS SYSTEM and govern the activities of the VISCERA.

The control centre of the whole nervous system is the brain, which is located in the skull or cranium. As well as controlling the nervous system it is the organ of thought, speech and emotion. The central nervous system controls the body's essential functions such as breathing, body temperature (see HOMEOSTASIS) and the heartbeat. The body's various sensations, including sight, hearing, touch, pain, positioning and taste, are communicated to the CNS by nerves distributed throughout the relevant tissues. The information is then sorted and interpreted by specialised areas in the brain. In response these initiate and coordinate the motor output, triggering such 'voluntary' activities as movement, speech, eating and swallowing. Other activities – for example, breathing, digestion, heart contractions, maintenance of BLOOD PRESSURE, and filtration of waste products from blood passing through the kidneys – are subject to involuntary control via the autonomic system. There is, however, some overlap between voluntary and involuntary controls.

Divisions

CEREBRUM This forms nearly 70 per cent of the brain and consists of two cerebral hemispheres which occupy the entire vault of the cranium and are incompletely separated from one another by a deep mid-line cleft, the longitudinal cerebral fissure. At the bottom of this cleft the two hemispheres are united by a thick band of some 200 million crossing nerve fibres – the corpus callosum. Other clefts or fissures (sulci) make deep impressions, dividing the cerebrum into lobes. The lobes of the cerebrum are the frontal lobe in the forehead region, the parietal lobe on the side and upper part of the brain, the occipital lobe to the back, and the temporal lobe lying just above the region of the ear. The outer 3 mm of the cerebrum is called the cortex, which consists of grey matter with the nerve cells arranged in six layers. This region is concerned with conscious thought, sensation and movement, operating in a similar manner to the more primitive areas of the brain except that incoming information is subject to much greater analysis.

Numbers of shallower infoldings of the surface, called furrows or sulci, separate raised areas called convolutions or gyri. In the deeper part, the white matter consists of nerve fibres connecting different parts of the surface and passing down to the lower parts of the brain. Among the white matter lie several rounded masses of grey matter, the lentiform and caudate nuclei. In the centre of each cerebral hemisphere is an irregular cavity, the lateral ventricle, each of which communicates with that on the other side and behind with the third ventricle through a small opening, the inter-ventricular foramen, or foramen of Monro.

BASAL NUCLEI Two large masses of grey matter embedded in the base of the cerebral hemispheres in humans, but forming the chief part of the brain in many animals. Between these masses lies the third ventricle, from which the infundibulum, a funnel-shaped process, projects downwards into the pituitary body, and

above lies the PINEAL GLAND. This region includes the important HYPOTHALAMUS.

MID-BRAIN or mesencephalon: a stalk about 20 mm long connecting the cerebrum with the hind-brain. Down its centre lies a tube, the cerebral aqueduct, or aqueduct of Sylvius, connecting the third and fourth ventricles. Above this aqueduct lie the corpora quadrigemina, and beneath it are the crura cerebri, strong bands of white matter in which important nerve fibres pass downwards from the cerebrum. The pineal gland is sited on the upper part of the mid-brain.

PONS A mass of nerve fibres, some of which run crosswise and others are the continuation of the crura cerebri downwards.

CEREBELLUM This lies towards the back, underneath the occipital lobes of the cerebrum.

MEDULLA OBLONGATA The lowest part of the brain, in structure resembling the spinal cord, with white matter on the surface and grey matter in its interior. This is continuous through the large opening in the skull, the foramen magnum, with the spinal cord. Between the medulla, pons, and cerebellum lies the fourth ventricle of the brain.

Structure   The grey matter consists mainly of billions of neurones (see NEURON(E)) in which all the activities of the brain begin. These cells vary considerably in size and shape in different parts of the brain, though all give off a number of processes, some of which form nerve fibres. The cells in the cortex of the cerebral hemispheres, for example, are very numerous, being set in layers five or six deep. In shape these cells are pyramidal, giving off processes from the apex, from the centre of the base, and from various projections elsewhere on the cell. The grey matter is everywhere penetrated by a rich supply of blood vessels, and the nerve cells and blood vessels are supported in a fine network of fibres known as neuroglia.

The white matter consists of nerve fibres, each of which is attached, at one end, to a cell in the grey matter, while at the other end it splits up into a tree-like structure around another cell in another part of the grey matter in the brain or spinal cord. The fibres have insulating sheaths of a fatty material which, in the mass, gives the white matter its colour; they convey messages from one part of the brain to the other (association fibres), or, grouped into bundles, leave the brain as nerves, or pass down into the spinal cord where they end near, and exert a control upon, cells from which in turn spring the nerves to the body.

Both grey and white matter are bound together by a network of cells called GLIA which make up 60 per cent of the brain's weight. These have traditionally been seen as simple structures whose main function was to glue the constituents of the brain together. Recent research, however, suggests that glia are vital for growing synapses between the neurons as they trigger these cells to communicate with each other. So they probably participate in the task of laying down memories, for which synapses are an essential key. The research points to the likelihood that glial cells are as complex as neurons, functioning biochemically in a similar way. Glial cells also absorb potassium pumped out by active neurons and prevent levels of GLUTAMATE – the most common chemical messenger in the brain – from becoming too high.

The general arrangement of fibres can be best understood by describing the course of a motor nerve-fibre. Arising in a cell on the surface in front of the central sulcus, such a fibre passes inwards towards the centre of the cerebral hemisphere, the collected mass of fibres as they lie between the lentiform nucleus and optic thalamus being known as the internal capsule. Hence the fibre passes down through the crus cerebri, giving off various small connecting fibres as it passes downwards. After passing through the pons it reaches the medulla, and at this point crosses to the opposite side (decussation of the pyramids). Entering the spinal cord, it passes downwards to end finally in a series of branches (arborisation) which meet and touch (synapse) similar branches from one or more of the cells in the grey matter of the cord (see SPINAL CORD).

BLOOD VESSELS Four vessels carry blood to the brain: two internal carotid arteries in front, and two vertebral arteries behind. These communicate to form a circle (circle of Willis) inside the skull, so that if one is blocked, the others, by dilating, take its place. The chief branch of the internal carotid artery on each side is the middle cerebral, and this gives off a small but very important branch which pierces the base of the brain and supplies the region of the internal capsule with blood. The chief importance of this vessel lies in the fact that the blood in it is under especially high pressure, owing to its close connection with the carotid artery, so that haemorrhage from it is liable to occur and thus give rise to stroke. Two veins, the internal cere-bral veins, bring the blood away from the interior of the brain, but most of the small veins come to the surface and open into large venous sinuses, which run in grooves in the skull, and finally pass their blood into the internal jugular vein that accompanies the carotid artery on each side of the neck.

MEMBRANES The brain is separated from the skull by three membranes: the dura mater, a thick fibrous membrane; the arachnoid mater, a more delicate structure; and the pia mater, adhering to the surface of the brain and containing the blood vessels which nourish it. Between each pair is a space containing fluid on which the brain floats as on a water-bed. The fluid beneath the arachnoid membrane mixes with that inside the ventricles through a small opening in the fourth ventricle, called the median aperture, or foramen of Magendie.

These fluid arrangements have a great influence in preserving the brain from injury.

NERVES Twelve nerves come off the brain:
I.   Olfactory, to the nose (smell).
II.   Optic, to the eye (sight).
III. Oculomotor
IV.   Trochlear, to eye-muscles.
V.   Abducent
VI.   Trigeminal, to skin of face.
VII. Facial, to muscles of face.
VIII. Vestibulocochlear, to ear (hearing and balancing).
IX.   Glossopharyngeal, to tongue (taste).
X.   Vagus, to heart, larynx, lungs, and stomach.
XI.   Spinal accessory, to muscles in neck.
XII. Hypoglossal, to muscles of tongue.

Brain, Diseases of

These consist either of expanding masses (lumps or tumours), or of areas of shrinkage (atrophy) due to degeneration, or to loss of blood supply, usually from blockage of an artery.

Tumours

All masses cause varying combinations of headache and vomiting – symptoms of raised pressure within the inexpansible bony box formed by the skull; general or localised epileptic fits; weakness of limbs or disordered speech; and varied mental changes. Tumours may be primary, arising in the brain, or secondary deposits from tumours arising in the lung, breast or other organs. Some brain tumours are benign and curable by surgery: examples include meningiomas and pituitary tumours. The symptoms depend on the size and situation of the mass. Abscesses or blood clots (see HAEMATOMA) on the surface or within the brain may resemble tumours; some are removable. Gliomas (see GLIOMA) are primary malignant tumours arising in the glial tissue (see GLIA) which despite surgery, chemotherapy and radiotherapy usually have a bad prognosis, though some astrocytomas and oligodendronogliomas are of low-grade malignancy. A promising line of research in the US (in the animal-testing stage in 2000) suggests that the ability of stem cells from normal brain tissue to 'home in' on gliomal cells can be turned to advantage. The stem cells were chemically manipulated to carry a poisonous compound (5-fluorouracil) to the gliomal cells and kill them, without damaging normal cells. Around 80 per cent of the cancerous cells in the experiments were destroyed in this way.

Clinical examination and brain scanning (CT, or COMPUTED TOMOGRAPHY; magnetic resonance imaging (MRI) and functional MRI) are safe, accurate methods of demonstrating the tumour, its size, position and treatability.

Strokes When a blood vessel, usually an artery, is blocked by a clot, thrombus or embolism, the local area of the brain fed by that artery is damaged (see STROKE). The resulting infarct (softening) causes a stroke. The cells die and a patch of brain tissue shrinks. The obstruction in the blood vessel may be in a small artery in the brain, or in a larger artery in the neck. Aspirin and other anti-clotting drugs reduce recurrent attacks, and a small number of people benefit if a narrowed neck artery is cleaned out by an operation – endarterectomy. Similar symptoms develop abruptly if a blood vessel bursts, causing a cerebral haemorrhage. The symptoms of a stroke are sudden weakness or paralysis of the arm and leg of the opposite side to the damaged area of brain (HEMIPARESIS), and sometimes loss of half of the field of vision to one side (HEMIANOPIA). The speech area is in the left side of the brain controlling language in right-handed people. In 60 per cent of left-handers the speech area is on the left side, and in 40 per cent on the right side. If the speech area is damaged, difficulties both in understanding words, and in saying them, develops (see DYSPHASIA).

Degenerations (atrophy) For reasons often unknown, various groups of nerve cells degenerate prematurely. The illness resulting is determined by which groups of nerve cells are affected. If those in the deep basal ganglia are affected, a movement disorder occurs, such as Parkinson's disease, hereditary Huntington's chorea, or, in children with birth defects of the brain, athetosis and dystonias. Modern drugs, such as DOPAMINE drugs in PARKINSONISM, and other treatments can improve the symptoms and reduce the disabilities of some of these diseases.

Drugs and injury Alcohol in excess, the abuse of many sedative drugs and artificial brain stimulants – such as cocaine, LSD and heroin (see DEPENDENCE) – can damage the brain; the effects can be reversible in early cases. Severe head injury can cause localised or diffuse brain damage (see HEAD INJURY).

Cerebral palsy Damage to the brain in children can occur in the uterus during pregnancy, or can result from rare hereditary and genetic diseases, or can occur during labour and delivery. Severe neurological illness in the early months of life can also cause this condition in which stiff spastic limbs, movement disorders and speech defects are common. Some of these children are learning-disabled.

Dementias In older people a diffuse loss of cells, mainly at the front of the brain, causes ALZHEIMER'S DISEASE – the main feature being loss of memory, attention and reasoned judgement (dementia). This affects about 5 per cent of the over-80s, but is not simply due to ageing processes. Most patients require routine tests and brain scanning to indicate other, treatable causes of dementia.

Response to current treatments is poor, but promising lines of treatment are under development. Like Parkinsonism, Alzheimer's disease progresses slowly over many years. It is uncommon for these diseases to run in families. Multiple strokes can cause dementia, as can some organic disorders such as cirrhosis of the liver.

Infections in the brain are uncommon. Viruses such as measles, mumps, herpes, human immunodeficiency virus and enteroviruses may cause ENCEPHALITIS – a diffuse inflammation (see also AIDS/HIV).

Bacteria or viruses may infect the membrane covering the brain, causing MENINGITIS. Viral meningitis is normally a mild, self-limiting infection lasting only a few days; however, bacterial meningitis – caused by meningococcal groups B and C, pneumococcus, and (now rarely) haemophilus – is a life-threatening condition. Antibiotics have allowed a cure or good control of symptoms in most cases of meningitis, but early diagnosis is essential. Severe headaches, fever, vomiting and increasing sleepiness are the principal symptoms which demand urgent advice from the doctor, and usually admission to hospital. Group B meningococcus is the commonest of the bacterial infections, but Group C causes more deaths. A vaccine against the latter has been developed and has reduced the incidence of cases by 75 per cent.

If infection spreads from an unusually serious sinusitis or from a chronically infected middle ear, or from a penetrating injury of the skull, an abscess may slowly develop. Brain abscesses cause insidious drowsiness, headaches, and at a late stage, weakness of the limbs or loss of speech; a high temperature is seldom present. Early diagnosis, confirmed by brain scanning, is followed by antibiotics and surgery in hospital, but the outcome is good in only half of affected patients.

Cerebral oedema Swelling of the brain can occur after injury, due to engorgement of blood vessels or an increase in the volume of the extravascular brain tissue due to abnormal uptake of water by the damaged grey (neurons) matter and white (nerve fibres) matter. This latter phenomenon is called cerebral oedema and can seriously affect the functioning of the brain. It is a particularly dangerous complication following injury because sometimes an unconscious person whose brain is damaged may seem to be recovering after a few hours, only to have a major relapse. This may be the result of a slow haemorrhage from damaged blood vessels raising intracranial pressure, or because of oedema of the brain tissue in the area surrounding the injury. Such a development is potentially lethal and requires urgent specialist treatment to alleviate the rising intracranial pressure: osmotic agents (see OSMOSIS) such as mannitol or frusemide are given intravenously to remove the excess water from the brain and to lower intracranial pressure, buying time for definitive investigation of the cranial damage.

Brain Injuries
Most blows to the head cause no loss of consciousness and no brain injury. If someone is knocked out for a minute or two, there has been a brief disturbance of the brain cells (concussion); usually there are no after-effects. Most patients so affected leave hospital within 1–3 days, have no organic signs, and recover and return quickly to work without further complaints.

Severe head injuries cause unconsciousness for hours or many days, followed by loss of memory before and after that period of unconsciousness. The skull may be fractured; there may be fits in the first week; and there may develop a blood clot in the brain (intracerebral haematoma) or within the membranes covering the brain (extradural and subdural haematomata). These clots compress the brain, and the pressure inside the skull – intracranial pressure – rises with urgent, life-threatening consequences. They are identified by neurologists and neurosurgeons, confirmed by brain scans (see COMPUTED TOMOGRAPHY; MRI), and require urgent surgical removal. Recovery may be complete, or in very severe cases can be marred by physical disabilities, EPILEPSY, and by changes in intelligence, rational judgement and behaviour. Symptoms generally improve in the first two years.

A minority of those with minor head injuries have complaints and disabilities which seem disproportionate to the injury sustained. Referred to as the post-traumatic syndrome, this is not a diagnostic entity. The complaints are headaches, forgetfulness, irritability, slowness, poor concentration, fatigue, dizziness (usually not vertigo), intolerance of alcohol, light and noise, loss of interests and initiative, DEPRESSION, anxiety, and impaired LIBIDO. Reassurance and return to light work help these symptoms to disappear, in most cases within three months. Psychological illness and unresolved compensation-claims feature in many with implacable complaints.

People who have had brain injuries, and their relatives, can obtain help and advice from Headwat and from www.neuro.pmr.vcu.edu and www.biausa.org

Brain-Stem Death
Brain damage, resulting in the irreversible loss of brain function, renders the individual incapable of life without the aid of a VENTILATOR. Criteria have been developed to recognise that 'death' has occurred and to allow ventilation to be stopped: in the UK, these criteria require the patient to be irreversibly unconscious and unable to regain the capacity to breathe spontaneously. (See also GLASGOW COMA SCALE and PERSISTENT VEGETATIVE STATE (PVS).)

All reversible pharmacological, metabolic, endocrine and physiological causes must be excluded, and there should be no doubt that irreversible brain damage has occurred. Two senior doctors carry out diagnostic tests to confirm that brain-stem reflexes are absent. These tests must be repeated after a suitable interval before death can be declared. Imaging techniques are not required for death to be diagnosed. The test for brain-stem death are:

- Fixed dilated pupils of the eyes
- Absent CORNEAL REFLEX
- Absent VESTIBULO-OCULAR REFLEX
- No cranial motor response to somatic (physical) stimulation
- Absent gag and cough reflexes
- No respiratory effort in response to APNOEA despite adequate concentrations of CARBON DIOXIDE in the arterial blood.

Bran

The meal derived from the outer covering of a cereal grain. It contains little or no carbohydrate, and is mainly used to provide ROUGHAGE in the control of bowel function and the prevention of constipation.

Branchial Cyst

A cyst arising in the neck from remnants of the embryological branchial clefts. They are usually fluid-filled and will therefore transilluminate.

Breasts

Breasts, or mammary glands, occur only in mammals and provide milk for feeding the young. These paired organs are usually fully developed only in adult females, but are present in rudimentary form in juveniles and males. In women, the two breasts over-lie the second to sixth ribs on the front of the chest. On the surface of each breast is a central pink disc called the areola, which surrounds the nipple. Inside, the breast consists of fat, supporting tissue and glandular tissue, which is the part that produces milk following childbirth. Each breast consists of 12–20 compartments arranged radially around the nipple: each compartment opens on to the tip of the nipple via its own duct through which the milk flows. The breast enlargement that occurs in pregnancy is due to development of the glandular part in preparation for lactation. In women beyond childbearing age, the glandular part of the breasts reduces (called involution) and the breasts become less firm and contain relatively more fat.

Breasts, Diseases of

The female breasts may be expected to undergo hormone-controlled enlargement at puberty, and later in pregnancy, and the glandular part of the breast undergoes evolution (shrinkage) after the menopause. The breast can also be affected by many different diseases, with common symptoms being pain, nipple discharge or retraction, and the formation of a lump within the breast.

Benign disease is much more common than cancer, particularly in young women, and includes acute inflammation of the breast (mastitis); abscess formation; and benign breast lumps, which may be fibroadenosis – diffuse lumpiness also called chronic mastitis or fibrocystic disease – in which one or more fluid-filled sacs (cysts) develop.

Women who are breast feeding are particularly prone to mastitis, as infection may enter the breast via the nipple. The process may be arrested before a breast abscess forms by prompt treatment with antibiotics. Non-bacterial inflammation may result from mammary duct ectasia (dilatation), in which abnormal or

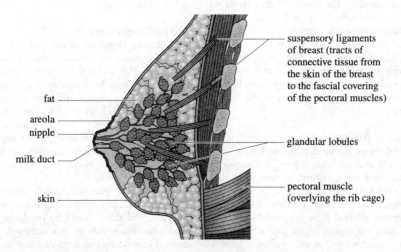

fat
areola
nipple
milk duct
skin

suspensory ligaments of breast (tracts of connective tissue from the skin of the breast to the fascial covering of the pectoral muscles)

glandular lobules

pectoral muscle (overlying the rib cage)

Lateral view of female breast showing internal structure and chest wall.

blocked ducts may overflow. Initial treatments should be with antibiotics, but if an abscess does form it should be surgically drained.

Duct ectasia, with or without local mastitis, is the usual benign cause of various nipple complaints, with common symptoms being nipple retraction, discharge and skin change.

Breast lumps form the chief potential danger and may be either solid or cystic. Simple examination may fail to distinguish the two types, but aspiration of a benign cyst usually results in its disappearance. If the fluid is bloodstained, or if a lump still remains, malignancy is possible, and all solid lumps need histological (tissue examination) or cytological (cell examination) assessment. As well as having their medical and family history taken, any women with a breast lump should undergo triple assessment: a combination of clinical examination, imaging – mammography for the over-35s and ultrasonagraphy for the under-35s – and fine-needle aspiration. The medical history should include details of any previous lumps, family history (up to 10 per cent of breast cancer in western countries is due to genetic disposition), pain, nipple discharge, change in size related to menstrual cycle and parous state, and any drugs being taken by the patient. Breasts should be inspected with the arms up and down, noting position, size, consistency, mobility, fixity, and local lymphadenopathy (glandular swelling). Nipples should be examined for the presence of inversion or discharge. Skin involvement (*peau d'orange*) should be noted, and, in particular, how long changes have been present. Fine-needle aspiration and cytological examination of the fluid are essential with ULTRASOUND, MAMMOGRAPHY and possible BIOPSY being considered, depending on the patient's age and the extent of clinical suspicion that cancer may be present.

The commonest solid benign lump is a fibroadenoma, particularly in women of childbearing age, and is a painless, mobile lump. If small, it is usually safe to leave it alone, provided that the patient is warned to seek medical advice if its size or character changes or if the lump becomes painful. Fibroadenosis (diffuse lumpiness often in the upper, outer quadrant) is a common (benign) lump. Others include periductal mastitis, fat NECROSIS, GALACTOCELE, ABSCESS, and non-breast-tissue lumps – for example, a LIPOMA (fatty tissue) or SEBACEOUS CYST. A woman with breast discharge should have a mammograph, ductograph, or total duct excision until the cause of any underlying duct ectasia is known. Appropriate treatment should then be given.

Malignant disease

most commonly – but not exclusively – occurs in post-menopausal women, classically presenting as a slowly growing, painless, firm lump. A bloodstained nipple discharge or eczematous skin change may also be suggestive of cancer.

The most commonly used classification of invasive cancers has split them into two types, ductal and lobular, but this is no longer suitable. There are also weaknesses in the tumour node metastases (TNM) system and the International Union Against Cancer (UICC) classification.

The TNM system – which classifies the lump by size, fixity and presence of affected axillary glands and wider metastatic spread – is best combined with a pathological classification, when assessing the seriousness of a possibly cancerous lump. Risk factors for cancer include nulliparity (see NULLIPARA), first pregnancy over the age of 30 years, early MENARCHE, late MENOPAUSE and positive family history. The danger should be considered in women who are not breast feeding or with previous breast cancer, and must be carefully excluded if the woman is taking any contraceptive steroids or is on hormone-replacement therapy (see under MENOPAUSE).

Screening programmes involving mammography are well established, the aim being to detect more tumours at an early and curable stage. Pick-up rate is five per 1,000 healthy women over 50 years. Yearly two-view mammograms could reduce mortality by 40 per cent but may cause alarm because there are ten false positive mammograms for each true positive result. In premenopausal women, breasts are denser, making mammograms harder to interpret, and screening appears not to save lives. About a quarter of women with a palpable breast lump turn out to have cancer.

Treatment This remains controversial, and all options should be carefully discussed with the patient and, where appropriate, with her partner. Locally contained disease may be treated by local excision of the lump, but sampling of the glands of the armpit of the same side should be performed to check for additional spread of the disease, and hence the need for CHEMOTHERAPY or RADIOTHERAPY. Depending on the extent of spread, simple mastectomy or modified radical mastectomy (which removes the lymph nodes draining the breast) may be required. Follow-up chemotherapy, for example, with TAMOXIFEN (an oestrogen antagonist), much improves survival (it saves 12 lives over 100 women treated), though it may occasionally cause endometrial carcinoma. Analysis in the mid-1990s of large-scale international studies of breast-cancer treatments showed wide variations in their effectiveness. As a result the NHS has encouraged hospitals to set up breast-treatment teams containing all the relevant health professional experts and to use those treatments shown to be most effective.

As well as the physical treatments provided, women with suspected or proven breast cancer should be offered psychological support because up to 30 per cent of affected women develop an anxiety state or depressive illness within a year of diagnosis. Problems over body image and sexual difficulties occur in and around one-quarter of patients. Breast conservation and reconstructive surgery can improve the physical effects of mastectomy, and women should be advised on the prostheses and specially designed brassieres that are available. Specialist nurses and self-help groups are invaluable in supporting affected women and their partners with the problems caused by breast cancer and its treatment. Breast Cancer Care, British Association of Cancer United Patients (BACUP), Cancerlink, and Cancer Relief Macmillan Fund are among voluntary organisations providing support.

Breastbone
See STERNUM.

Breast Feeding
This is the natural way to feed a baby from birth to WEANING. Human milk is an ideal food, containing a proper balance of nutrients as well as an essential supply of antibodies to protect the infant against infections. Breast feeding also strengthens the physical bond between mother and child. For the first few weeks, feeding should be on demand. Difficulties over breast feeding, discouragement from health-care providers and the pressures of modern life, especially for working mothers, can make it hard to continue breast feeding for more than a few weeks, or even to breast feed at all. Sometimes infections occur, producing soreness and even an abscess. Mothers should seek advice from their health visitor about breast feeding, especially if problems arise.

Breast Reconstruction
See MAMMOPLASTY.

Breast Reduction
See MAMMOPLASTY.

Breast Screening
A set of investigations aimed at the early detection of breast cancer. It includes self-screening by monthly examination of the breasts, and formal programmes of screening by palpation and mammography in special clinics. In the UK the NHS offers regular mammography examinations to all women between 50 and 64 years of age; in 1995–6, 1.1 million women were screened – 76 per cent of those invited. More than 5,500 cancers were detected – 5.3 per 1,000 women screened.

Breath-Holding
Breath-holding attacks are not uncommon in infants and toddlers. They are characterised by the child suddenly stopping breathing in the midst of a bout of crying evoked by pain, some emotional upset, or loss of temper. The breath may be held so long that the child goes blue in the face. The attack is never fatal and the condition disappears spontaneously after the age of 3–5 years, but once a child has acquired the habit it may recur quite often.

It is important for a paediatrician to determine that such events are not epileptic (see EPILEPSY). Generally they require no treatment other than reassurance, as recovery is spontaneous and rapid – although a small number of severely affected children have been helped by a PACEMAKER. Parents should avoid dramatising the attacks.

Breathing
See RESPIRATION.

Breathlessness
Breathlessness, or dyspnoea, may be due to any condition which renders the blood deficient in oxygen, and which therefore produces excessive involuntary efforts to gain more air. Exercise is a natural cause, and acute anxiety may provoke breathlessness in otherwise healthy people. Deprivation of oxygen – for example, in a building fire – will also cause the victim to raise his or her breathing rate. Disorders of the lung may diminish the area available for breathing – for example, ASTHMA, PNEUMONIA, TUBERCULOSIS, EMPHYSEMA, BRONCHITIS, collections of fluid in the pleural cavities, and pressure caused by a TUMOUR or ANEURYSM.

● Pleurisy causes short, rapid breathing to avoid the pain of deep inspiration.

● Narrowing of the air passages may produce sudden and alarming attacks of difficult breathing, especially among children – for example, in CROUP, asthma and DIPHTHERIA.

● Most cardiac disorders (see HEART, DISEASES OF) cause breathlessness, especially when the person undergoes any special exertion.
● Anaemia is a frequent cause.
● Obesity is often associated with shortness of breath.

Mountain climbing may cause breathlessness because, as altitude increases, the amount of oxygen in the air falls (see ALTITUDE SICKNESS). (See also LUNGS and RESPIRATION.)

Breath Sounds
The transmitted sounds of breathing, heard when a stethoscope is applied to the chest. Normal breath sounds are described as vesicular. Abnormal sounds may be heard when there is increased fluid in the lungs or fibrosis (crepitation or crackles), when there is bronchospasm (rhonchi or wheezes), or when the lung is airless (consolidated – bronchial breathing). Breath sounds are absent in people with pleural effusion, pneumothorax, or after pneumonectomy.

Breech Delivery
See BREECH PRESENTATION.

Breech Presentation
By the 32nd week of pregnancy most babies are in a head-down position in the womb. Up to 4 per cent of them, however, have their buttocks (breech) presenting at the neck of the womb. If the baby is still a breech presentation at the 34th to 35th week the obstetrician may, by external manipulation, try to turn it to the head-down position. If this is not successful, the fetus is left in the breech position. Breech deliveries are more difficult for mother and baby because the buttocks are less efficient than the head at dilating the cervix and vagina. An EPISIOTOMY is usually necessary to assist delivery, and obstetric FORCEPS may also have to be applied to the baby's head. If the infant and/or the mother become unduly distressed, the obstetrician may decide to deliver the baby by CAESAREAN SECTION; some obstetricians prefer to deliver most breech-presentation babies using this method. (See PREGNANCY AND LABOUR.)

Bright's Disease
See KIDNEYS, DISEASES OF – Glomerulonephritis.

British Approved Names (BAN)
The officially approved name for a medicinal substance used in the UK. A 1992 European Union directive required the use of a Recommended International Non-proprietary Name (rINN) for these substances. Usually the BAN and rINN were identical; where there was a difference, the rINN nomenclature is now used. An exception is adrenaline, which remains the official name in Europe with the rINN – epinephrine – being a synonym.

British Dental Association
See APPENDIX 8: PROFESSIONAL ORGANISATIONS.

British Medical Association (BMA)
See APPENDIX 8: PROFESSIONAL ORGANISATIONS.

British National Formulary (BNF)
A pocket-book for those concerned with the prescribing, dispensing and administration of medicines in Britain. It is produced jointly by the Royal Pharmaceutical Society and the British Medical Association, is revised twice yearly and is distributed to NHS doctors by the Health Departments. The *BNF* is also available in electronic form.

British Pharmacopoeia
See PHARMACOPOEIA.

British Thermal Unit (BTU)
An officially recognised measurement of heat: a unit is equal to the quantity of heat needed to raise the temperature of one pound of water by 1°Fahrenheit. One BTU is equivalent to 1,055 joules (see JOULE).

Brittle Bone Disease
Brittle Bone Disease is another name for OSTEOGENESIS IMPERFECTA.

Bromocriptine
A drug that stimulates DOPAMINE receptors in the brain. It inhibits production of the hormone PROLACTIN and is used to treat GALACTORRHOEA (excessive milk secretion) and also to suppress normal LACTATION. The drug is helpful in treating premenstrual breast engorgement and also ACROMEGALY.

Bronchial Tubes
See AIR PASSAGES; BRONCHUS; LUNGS.

Bronchiectasis
A condition characterised by dilatation of the bronchi (see BRONCHUS). As a rule, this is the result of infection of the bronchial tree leading to obstruction of the bronchi. Due to the obstruction, the affected individual cannot get rid of the secretions in the bronchi beyond the obstruction; these accumulate and become

infected. The initial infection may be due to bacterial or viral pneumonia or to the infection of the lungs complicating measles or whooping-cough. Once a common disease, immunisation of infants against infectious diseases and the use of antibiotics have greatly reduced the incidence of bronchiectasis. (See CHRONIC OBSTRUCTIVE PULMONARY DISEASE (COPD).)

Treatment consists of postural drainage of excessive lung secretions, and antibiotics.

Bronchioles
The term applied to the finest divisions of the bronchial tubes of the LUNGS.

Bronchiolitis
The name sometimes applied to bronchitis affecting the finest bronchial tubes, also known as capillary bronchitis. Major epidemics occur every winter in Northern Europe in babies under 18 months due to respiratory syncytial virus (RSV). Many are admitted to hospital; some need artificial ventilation for a time and a very small number die.

Bronchiolitis Obliterans
A rare disorder involving gradually increasing FIBROSIS and destruction of lung tissue following an attack of BRONCHIOLITIS.

Bronchitis
Inflammation of the bronchial tubes (see AIR PASSAGES; BRONCHUS; LUNGS). This may occur as an acute transient illness or as a chronic condition.

Acute bronchitis is due to an acute infection – viral or bacterial – of the bronchi. This is distinguished from PNEUMONIA by the anatomical site involved: bronchitis affects the bronchi whilst pneumonia affects the lung tissue. The infection causes a productive cough, and fever. Secretions within airways sometimes lead to wheezing. Sometimes the specific causative organism may be identified from the sputum. The illness is normally self-limiting but, if treatments are required, bacterial infections respond to a course of antibiotics.

Chronic bronchitis is a clinical diagnosis applied to patients with chronic cough and sputum production. For epidemiological studies it is defined as 'cough productive of sputum on most days during at least three consecutive months for not less than two consecutive years'. Chronic bronchitis is classified as a CHRONIC PULMONARY OBSTRUCTIVE DISEASE (COPD);

chronic ASTHMA and EMPHYSEMA are the others.

In the past, industrial workers regularly exposed to heavily polluted air commonly developed bronchitis. The main aetiological factor is smoking; this leads to an increase in size and number of bronchial mucous glands. These are responsible for the excessive mucus production within the bronchial tree, causing a persistent productive cough. The increased number of mucous glands along with the influx of inflammatory cells may lead to airway-narrowing: when airway-narrowing occurs, it slows the passage of air, producing breathlessness. Other less important causative factors include exposure to pollutants and dusts. Infections do not cause the disease but frequently produce exacerbations with worsening of symptoms.

Treatments involve the use of antibiotics to treat the infections that produce exacerbations of symptoms. Bronchodilators (drugs that open up the airways) help to reverse the airway-narrowing that causes the breathlessness. PHYSIOTHERAPY is of value in keeping the airways clear of MUCUS. Cessation of smoking reduces the speed of progression.

Bronchodilator
This type of drug reduces the tone of smooth muscle in the lungs' BRONCHIOLES and therefore increases their diameter. Such drugs are used in the treatment of diseases that cause bronchoconstriction, such as ASTHMA and BRONCHITIS. As bronchiolar tone is a balance between sympathetic and parasympathetic activity, most bronchodilators are either B_2 receptor agonists or cholinergic receptor antagonists – although theophyllines are also useful.

Bronchography
A radiographic procedure using a radio-opaque substance injected into the bronchial tree to show its outline. This is a simple procedure carried out under general anaesthesia and allows the accurate location of, for example, a lung ABSCESS, BRONCHIECTASIS, or a TUMOUR in the lung.

Bronchopleural Fistula
An abnormal communication between the tracheo-bronchial tree and the pleural cavity (see LUNGS). Most commonly occurring from breakdown of the bronchial stump following pneumonectomy, it may also be caused by trauma, neoplasia or inflammation.

Broncho-Pneumonia

See PNEUMONIA.

Bronchoscope

An instrument constructed on the principle of the telescope, which on introduction into the mouth is passed down through the LARYNX and TRACHEA and enables the observer to see the interior of the larger bronchial tubes. The bronchoscope has largely been superseded by fibreoptic bronchoscopy. (See ENDOSCOPE.)

Bronchoscopy

The use of a bronchoscope to visualise the interior of the bronchial tubes.

Bronchospasm

Muscular contraction of the bronchi (air passages) in the LUNGS, causing narrowing. The cause is usually a stimulus, as in BRONCHITIS and ASTHMA. The result is that the patient can inhale air into the lungs but breathing out becomes difficult and requires muscular effort of the chest. Exhalation is accompanied by audible noises in the airways which can be detected with a STETHOSCOPE. Reversible obstructive airways disease can be relieved with a BRON-CHODILATOR drug; if the bronchospasm cannot be relieved by drugs it is called irreversible. (See CHRONIC OBSTRUCTIVE PULMONARY DISEASE (COPD).)

Bronchus

Bronchus, or bronchial tube, is the name applied to tubes into which the TRACHEA divides, one going to either lung. The name is also applied to the divisions of these tubes distributed throughout the lungs, the smallest being called bronchioles.

Brucellosis

Also known as undulant fever, or Malta fever.

Causes In Malta and the Mediterranean littoral, the causative organism is the bacterium *Brucella melitensis* which is conveyed in goat's milk. In Great Britain, the US and South Africa, the causative organism is the *Brucella abortus*, which is conveyed in cow's milk: this is the organism which is responsible for contagious abortion in cattle. In Great Britain brucellosis is largely an occupational disease and is now prescribed as an industrial disease (see OCCUPATIONAL DISEASES), and insured persons who contract the disease at work can claim industrial injuries benefit. The incidence of brucellosis in the UK has fallen from more than 300 cases a year in 1970 to single figures.

Symptoms The characteristic features of the disease are undulating fever, drenching sweats, pains in the joints and back, and headache. The liver and spleen may be enlarged. The diagnosis is confirmed by the finding of *Br. abortus*, or antibodies to it, in the blood. Recovery and convalescence tend to be slow.

Treatment The condition responds well to one of the tetracycline antibiotics, and also to gentamicin and co-trimoxazole, but relapse is common. In chronic cases a combination of streptomycin and one of the tetracyclines is often more effective.

Prevention It can be prevented by boiling or pasteurising all milk used for human consumption. In Scandinavia, the Netherlands, Switzerland and Canada the disease has disappeared following its eradication in animals. Brucellosis has been eradicated from farm animals in the United Kingdom.

Bruises

Bruises, or contusions, result from injuries to the deeper layers of the skin or underlying tissues, with variable bleeding but without open wounds. Bruises range from a slight bluish discoloration, due to minimal trauma and haemorrhage, to a large black swelling in more severe cases. Diseases such as HAEMOPHILIA and SCURVY, which reduce COAGULATION, should be suspected when extensive bruises are produced by minor injuries. Bruises change colour from blue-black to brown to yellow, gradually fading as the blood pigment is broken down and absorbed. Bruising in the abdomen or in the back in the area of the kidneys should prompt the examining doctor to assess whether there has been any damage to internal tissues or organs. Bruising in children, especially repeated bruising, may be caused by physical abuse (see CHILD ABUSE and NON-ACCIDENTAL INJURY (NAI)). Adults, too, may be subjected to regular physical abuse.

Bruit and Murmur

Abnormal sounds heard in connection with the heart, arteries and veins on AUSCULTATION.

Bruxism

Bruxism, or teeth-grinding, refers to a habit of grinding the teeth, usually while asleep and without being aware of it. The teeth may feel uncomfortable on wakening. It is common in children and is usually of no significance. In adults it may be associated with stress or a malpositioned or overfilled tooth. The underlying cause should be treated but, if unsuccessful, a plastic splint can be fitted over the teeth.

Bubo

(Plural: buboes.) A swelling of a lymphatic gland in the groin in venereal disease (see SEXUALLY TRANSMITTED DISEASES (STDS)) or in PLAGUE.

Buccal

Relating to the mouth or inside of the cheek.

Budgerigar-Fancier's Lung

Budgerigar-fancier's lung is a form of extrinsic allergic ALVEOLITIS, resulting from sensitisation to budgerigars, or parakeets as they are known in North America. Skin tests have revealed sensitisation to the birds' droppings and/or serum. As it is estimated that budgerigars are kept in 5–6 million homes in Britain, current figures suggest that anything up to 900 per 100,000 of the population are exposed to the risk of developing this condition.

Buerger's Disease

See THROMBOANGIITIS OBLITERANS.

Bulbar Paralysis

See PARALYSIS; MOTOR NEURONE DISEASE (MND).

Bulimia

Bulimia means insatiable appetite of psychological origin. This eating-disorder symptom may be of psychological origin or the result of neurological disease – for example, a lesion of the HYPOTHALAMUS. Bulimia nervosa is linked to anorexia nervosa and is sometimes called the binge and purge syndrome. Bulimia nervosa is characterised by overpowering urges to eat large amounts of food, followed by induced vomiting or abuse of laxatives to avoid any gain in weight. Most of the victims are prone to being overweight and all have a morbid fear of obesity. They indulge in bouts of gross overeating, or 'binge rounds' as they describe them, to 'fill the empty space inside'. By their bizarre behaviour, most of them manage to maintain a normal weight. The condition is most common in women in their 20s; it is accompanied by irregular menstruation, often amounting to amenorrhoea (see MENSTRUATION). Although there are many similarities to anorexia nervosa, bulimia nervosa differs in that there is no attempt at deceit; sufferers freely admit to an eating disorder and feel distress about the symptoms that it produces. In spite of this, the response to treatment is, as in anorexia nervosa, far from satisfactory. (See EATING DISORDERS.)

Bulla

An air- or fluid-filled bubble occurring in the skin or lungs. The latter may be congenital or the result (in adults) of EMPHYSEMA. Skin bullae are really blisters.

Bumetanide

Bumetanide is a strong loop diuretic which is active when taken by mouth. It acts quickly – within a half-hour – and its action is over in a few hours. (See THIAZIDES; DIURETICS.)

Bundle Branch Block ·

An abnormality of the conduction of electrical impulses through the ventricles of the HEART, resulting in delayed depolarisation of the ventricular muscle. The electrocardiograph (see ELECTROCARDIOGRAM (ECG)) shows characteristic widening of the QRS complexes. Abnormalities of the right and left bundle branches cause delayed contraction of the right and left ventricles respectively.

Bundle of His

Bundle of His, or atrioventricular bundle, is a bundle of special muscle fibres which pass from the atria to the ventricles of the HEART and which form the pathway for the impulse which makes the ventricles contract, the impulse originating in the part of the atria known as the sinuatrial node.

Bunions

See CORNS AND BUNIONS.

Bupivacaine

A local anaesthetic, about four times as potent as LIDOCAINE. It has a slow onset of action (up to 30 minutes for full effect), but its effect lasts up to eight hours, making it particularly suitable for continuous epidural analgesia in labour (see PREGNANCY AND LABOUR). It is commonly used for spinal anaesthesia, particularly lumbar epidural blockade (see ANAESTHESIA). It is contraindicated in intravenous regional anaesthesia.

Burkitt's Lymphoma

Malignant LYMPHOMA in children previously infected with EPSTEIN BARR VIRUS. It occurs mainly in the jaw and abdominal organs. It is common in parts of Africa where MALARIA is endemic.

Burning Feet

A SYNDROME characterised by a burning sensation in the soles of the feet. It is rare in temperate climes but widespread in India and the Far

East. The precise cause is not known, but it is associated with malnutrition; lack of one or more components of the vitamin B complex is the likeliest cause (see APPENDIX 5: VITAMINS).

Burnout

A mental state of physical and emotional exhaustion; an anxiety disorder that is a stress reaction to a person's reduced capability to cope with the demands of his or her occupations. Symptoms of burnout include tiredness, poor sleeping pattern, irritability and reduced performance at work; increased susceptibility to physical illness and abuse of alcohol and addictive drugs can also occur. Treatment can be difficult and may require a change to a less stressful lifestyle, counselling and, in severe cases, psychotherapy and carefully supervised use of ANXIOLYTICS or ANTIDEPRESSANT DRUGS.

Burns and Scalds

Burns are injuries caused by dry heat, scalds by moist heat, but the two are similar in symptoms and treatment. Severe burns are also caused by contact with electric wires, and by the action of acids and other chemicals. The burn caused by chemicals differs from a burn by fire only in the fact that the outcome is more favourable, because the chemical destroys the bacteria on the affected part(s) so that less suppuration follows.

Severe and extensive burns are most frequently produced by the clothes – for example, of a child – catching fire. This applies especially to cotton garments, which blaze up quickly. It should be remembered that such a flame can immediately be extinguished by making the individual lie on the floor so that the flames are uppermost, and wrapping him or her in a rug, mat or blanket. As prevention is always better than cure, particular care should always be exercised with electric fires and kettles or pots of boiling water in houses where there are young children or old people. Children's clothes, and especially night-clothes, should be made of non-inflammable material: pyjamas are also much safer than nightdresses.

Severe scalds are usually produced by escape of steam in boiler explosions. Cigarettes are a common cause of fires and therefore of burns; people who have fallen asleep in bed or in a chair while smoking may set fire to the bed or chair. Discarded, unextinguished cigarettes are another cause.

Degrees of burns Burns are referred to as either superficial (or partial-thickness) burns, when there is sufficient skin tissue left to ensure regrowth of skin over the burned site; and deep (or full-thickness) burns, when the skin is totally destroyed and grafting will be necessary.

Symptoms Whilst many domestic burns are minor and insignificant, more severe burns and scalds can prove to be very dangerous to life. The main danger is due to SHOCK, which arises as a result of loss of fluid from the circulating blood at the site of a serious burn. This loss of fluid leads to a fall in the volume of the circulating blood. As the maintenance of an adequate blood volume is essential to life, the body attempts to compensate for this loss by withdrawing fluid from the uninjured areas of the body into the circulation. If carried too far, however, this in turn begins to affect the viability of the body cells. As a sequel, essential body cells, such as those of the liver and kidneys, begin to suffer, and the liver and kidneys cease to function properly. This will show itself by the development of JAUNDICE and the appearance of albumin in the urine (see PROTEINURIA). In addition, the circulation begins to fail with a resultant lack of oxygen (see ANOXIA) in the tissues, and the victim becomes cyanosed (see CYANOSIS), restless and collapsed: in some cases, death ensues. In addition, there is a strong risk of infection occurring. This is the case with severe burns in particular, which leave a large raw surface exposed and very vulnerable to any micro-organisms. The combination of shock and infection can all too often be life-threatening unless expert treatment is immediately available.

The immediate outcome of a burn is largely determined by its extent. This is of more significance than the depth of the burn. To assess the extent of a burn in relation to the surface of the body, what is known as the Rule of Nine has been evolved. The head and each arm cover 9 per cent of the body surface, whilst the front of the body, the back of the body, and each leg each cover 18 per cent, with the perineum (or crutch) accounting for the remaining 1 per cent. The greater the extent of the burn, the more seriously ill will the victim become from loss of fluid from his or her circulation, and therefore the more prompt should be his or her removal to hospital for expert treatment. The depth of the burn, unless this is very great, is mainly of import when the question arises as to how much surgical treatment, including skin grafting, will be required.

Treatment This depends upon the severity of the burn. In the case of quite minor burns or scalds, all that may be necessary if they are seen

B

immediately is to hold the part under cold running water until the pain is relieved. Cooling is one of the most effective ways of relieving the pain of a burn. If the burn involves the distal part of a limb – for example, the hand and forearm – one of the most effective ways of relieving pain is to immerse the burned part in lukewarm water and add cold water until the pain disappears. As the water warms and pain returns, more cold water is added. After some three to four hours, pain will not reappear on warming, and the burn may be dressed in the usual way. Thereafter a simple dressing (e.g. a piece of sterile gauze covered by cotton-wool, and on top of this a bandage or adhesive dressing) should be applied. The part should be kept at rest and the dressing kept quite dry until healing takes place. Blisters should be pierced with a sterile needle, but the skin should not be cut away. No ointment or oil should be applied, and an antiseptic is not usually necessary.

In slightly more severe burns or scalds, it is probably advisable to use some antiseptic dressing. These are the cases which should be taken to a doctor – whether a general practitioner, a factory doctor, or to a hospital Accident & Emergency department. There is still no general consensus of expert opinion as to the best 'antiseptic' to use. Among those recommended are CHLORHEXIDINE, and antibiotics such as BACITRACIN, NEOMYCIN and polymixin. An alternative is to use a Tulle Gras dressing which has been impregnated with a suitable antibiotic.

In the case of severe burns and scalds, the only sound rule is immediate removal to hospital. Unless there is any need for immediate resuscitation, such as artificial respiration, or attention to other injuries there may be, such as fractures or haemorrhage, nothing should be done on the spot to the patient except to make sure that s/he is as comfortable as possible and to keep them warm, and to cover the burn with a sterile (or clean) cloth such as a sheet, pillowcases, or towels wrung out in cold water. If pain is severe, morphine should be given – usually intravenously. Once the victim is in hospital, the primary decision is as to the extent of the burn, and whether or not a transfusion is necessary. If the burn is more than 9 per cent of the body surface in extent, a transfusion is called for. The precise treatment of the burn varies, but the essential is to prevent infection if this has not already occurred, or, if it has, to bring it under control as quickly as possible. The treatment of severe burns has made great advances, with quick transport to specialised burns units, modern resuscitative measures, the use of skin grafting and other artificial covering techniques

and active rehabilitation programmes, offering victims a good chance of returning to normal life.

CHEMICAL BURNS Phenol or lysol can be washed off promptly before they do much damage. Acid or alkali burns should be neutralised by washing them repeatedly with sodium bicarbonate or 1 per cent acetic acid, respectively. Alternatively, the following buffer solution may be used for either acid or alkali burns: monobasic potassium phosphate (70 grams), dibasic sodium phosphate (70 grams) in 850 millilitres of water. (See also PHOSPHORUS BURNS.)

Burr (Bur) Hole

A circular hole made in the SKULL using a special surgical drill with a rounded tip, called the burr. The operation is done to relieve pressure on the BRAIN. This pressure – raised intracranial tension – is commonly the result of blood collecting between the skull and the brain after a head injury. The presence of PUS or an increase in the amount of CEREBROSPINAL FLUID as a result of infection or tumours in the brain can also cause a potentially fatal rise in intracranial pressure which can be relieved by drilling a burr hole. A neurosurgeon may make several burr holes when doing a CRANIOTOMY, a procedure in which a section of the skull is removed to provide access to the brain and surrounding tissues. Archaeological evidence suggests that modern man's ancestors used burr holes probably to treat physical ailments and mental illness.

Bursae

Natural hollows in the fibrous tissues, lined by smooth cells and containing a little fluid. They are situated at points where there is much pressure or friction, and their purpose is to allow free movement without stretching or straining the tissues: for example, on the knee-cap or the point of the elbow, and, generally speaking, where one muscle rubs against another or against a bone. They develop also beneath corns and bunions, or where a bone presses on the skin.

Bursitis

Inflammation within a bursa (see BURSAE). Acute bursitis is usually the result of injury, especially on the knee or elbow, when the prominent part of the joint becomes swollen, hot, painful and red.

Chronic bursitis is due to too much movement of, or pressure on, a bursa, with fluid building up therein. Fluid may need to be drained and the affected area rested. Excision of a chronically inflamed bursa is sometimes necessary. For example, the condition of housemaid's knee is a chronic inflammation of the patellar bursa in front of the knee, due to too much kneeling.

Chronic bursitis affecting ligaments round the wrist and ankle is generally called a GANGLION.

Buspirone

A non-benzodiazepine drug used to treat anxiety. It is believed to act at specific serotonin receptors of NEURON(E) cells. The patient may take as long as two weeks to respond to treatment.

Busulfan

A drug used almost exclusively to treat chronic myeloid LEUKAEMIA; it is given by mouth. Excessive suppression of myelocytes may lead to irreversible damage to BONE MARROW and therefore to the manufacture of blood cells, so frequent blood counts are necessary to check on the numbers of red and white cells.

Butyrophenones

Butyrophenones are a group of drugs, including haloperidol, used to treat psychotic illness (see MENTAL ILLNESS).

Bypass Operation

A technique by which narrowing or blockage of an artery (see ARTERIES), vein (see VEINS) or a section of the gastrointestinal tract is bypassed using surgery. Arterial blockages – usually caused by ATHEROSCLEROSIS – in the carotid, coronary or iliofemoral arteries are bypassed utilising sections of artery or vein taken from elsewhere in the patient. Tumour growths in the intestines are sometimes too large to remove and can be bypassed by linking up those parts of the intestines on each side of the growth.

Byssinosis

Chronic inflammatory thickening of the lung tissue, due to the inhalation of dust in textile factories. It is found chiefly among cotton and flax workers and, to a lesser extent, among workers in soft hemp. It is rare or absent in workers in jute and the hard fibres of hemp and sisal. With much-improved working conditions in the UK, where byssinosis is one of the PRESCRIBED DISEASES, the disease is rare, but it is still common in some Asian countries where textiles are manufactured.

Byte

Computer terminology describing a group of neighbouring bits, usually four, six or eight, working as a unit for the storage and manipulation of data in a computer.

C

Cachet
An oval capsule that encloses a dose of unpleasant medicine.

Cachexia
Severe weight loss and listlessness produced by serious disease such as cancer or tuberculosis, or by prolonged starvation.

Cadaver
A dead body.

Cadmium
A metallic element which, when molten, gives off fumes that can cause serious irritation of the lungs if inhaled.

Cadmium Poisoning
Cadmium poisoning is a recognised hazard in certain industrial processes, such as the manufacture of alloys, cadmium plating and glass blowing. Sewage sludge, which is used as fertiliser, may be contaminated by cadmium from industrial sources; such cadmium could be taken up into vegetable crops and cadmium levels in sewage are carefully monitored.

A tin-like metal, cadmium accumulates in the body. Long-term exposure can lead to EMPHYSEMA, renal failure (see KIDNEYS, DISEASES OF) and urinary-tract CALCULI. Acute exposure causes GASTROENTERITIS and PNEUMONITIS. Cadmium contamination of food is the most likely source of poisoning. The EU Directive on the Quality of Water for Human Consumption lays down 5 milligrams per litre as the upper safe level.

Caecum
The dilated first part of the large intestine lying in the right lower corner of the abdomen. The small intestine and the appendix open into it, and it is continued upwards through the right flank as the ascending colon.

Caesarean Section
The operation used to deliver a baby through its mother's abdominal wall. It is performed when the risks to mother or child of vaginal delivery are thought to outweigh the problems associated with operative delivery. One of the most common reasons for Caesarean section is 'disproportion' between the size of the fetal head and the maternal pelvis. The need for a Caesarean should be assessed anew in each pregnancy; a woman who has had a Caesarean section in the past will not automatically need to have one for subsequent deliveries. Caesarean-section rates vary dramatically from hospital to hospital, and especially between countries, emphasising that the criteria for operative delivery are not universally agreed. The current rate in the UK is about 23 per cent, and in the USA, about 28 per cent. The rate has shown a steady rise in all countries over the last decade. Fear of litigation by patients is one reason for this rise, as is the uncertainty that can arise from abnormalities seen on fetal monitoring during labour. Recent research suggesting that vaginal delivery is becoming more hazardous as the age of motherhood rises may increase the pressure from women to have a Caesarean section – as well as pressure from obstetricians.

The operation is usually performed through a low, horizontal 'bikini line' incision. A general anaesthetic in a heavily pregnant woman carries increased risks, so the operation is often performed under regional – epidural or spinal – ANAESTHESIA. This also allows the mother to see her baby as soon as it is born, and the baby is not exposed to agents used for general anaesthesia. If a general anaesthetic is needed (usually in an emergency), exposure to these agents may make the baby drowsy for some time afterwards.

Another problem with delivery by Caesarean section is, of course, that the mother must recover from the operation whilst coping with the demands of a small baby. (See PREGNANCY AND LABOUR.)

Caesium-137
An artificially produced radioactive element that is used in RADIOTHERAPY treatment.

Caffeine
A white crystalline substance obtained from coffee, of which it is the active principle. Its main actions are as a cerebral stimulant, a cardiac stimulant, and a diuretic. It is a constituent of many tablets for the relief of headache, usually combined with aspirin and paracetamol, but its pain-killing properties are controversial. One unusual use is in treating apnoeic attacks in premature babies (see APNOEA).

Caisson Disease
See COMPRESSED AIR ILLNESS.

Calamine
A mild astringent used, as calamine lotion, to

soothe and protect the skin in many conditions such as eczema and urticaria.

Calcaneus
The heel-bone or os calcis, and the largest bone in the foot.

Calcicosis
Calcicosis is a traditional term applied to disease of the lung caused by the inhalation of marble dust by marble-cutters.

Calciferol
This is an outdated term for ergocalciferol or vitamin D$_2$ (see APPENDIX 5: VITAMINS).

Calcification
The deposition of CALCIUM salts in body tissues, normally BONE and TEETH, though abnormal deposits can occur in damaged muscles or the walls of arteries.

Calcinosis
Abnormal deposition of CALCIUM in the body tissue.

Calcitonin
A hormone, produced by the THYROID GLAND, which is involved in the metabolism of bone. Acting to lower concentrations of CALCIUM and PHOSPHATES in the blood, calcitonin is given by injection in the treatment of some patients with HYPERCALCAEMIA (especially when associated with malignant disease). In severe cases of PAGET'S DISEASE OF BONE it is used mainly for pain relief, but also relieves some of the neurological complications such as deafness.

Calcium
The metallic element present in chalk and other forms of lime. The chief preparations used in medicine are calcium carbonate (chalk), calcium chloride, calcium gluconate, calcium hydroxide (slaked lime), liquor of calcium hydroxide (lime-water), calcium lactate, and calcium phosphate. Calcium gluconate is freely soluble in water and is used in conditions in which calcium should be given by injection.

Calcium is a most important element in diet; the chief sources of it are milk and cheese. Calcium is especially needed by the growing child and the pregnant and nursing mother. The uptake of calcium by the baby is helped by vitamin D (see APPENDIX 5: VITAMINS). A deficiency of calcium may cause TETANY, and an excess may result in the development of

CALCULI (stones) in the KIDNEYS or gall-bladder (see LIVER).

The recommended daily intakes of calcium are: 500 mg for children, 700 mg for adolescents, 500–900 mg for adults and 1,200 mg for pregnant or nursing mothers.

Calcium-Channel Blockers
Calcium-channel blockers inhibit the inward flow of calcium through the specialised slow channels of cardiac and arterial smooth-muscle cells. By thus relaxing the smooth muscle, they have important applications in the treatment of HYPERTENSION and ANGINA PECTORIS. Various types of calcium-channel blockers are available in the United Kingdom; these differ in their sites of action, leading to notable differences in their therapeutic effects. All the drugs are rapidly and completely absorbed, but extensive first-pass metabolism in the liver reduces bioavailability to around one-fifth. Their hypotensive effect is additive with that of beta blockers (see BETA-ADRENOCEPTOR-BLOCKING DRUGS); the two should, therefore, be used together with great caution – if at all. Calcium-channel blockers are particularly useful when beta blockers are contraindicated, for example in asthmatics. However, they should be prescribed for hypertension only when THIAZIDES and beta blockers have failed, are contraindicated or not tolerated.

Verapamil, the longest-available, is used to treat angina and hypertension. It is the only calcium-channel blocker effective against cardiac ARRHYTHMIA and it is the drug of choice in terminating supraventricular tachycardia. It may precipitate heart failure, and cause HYPOTENSION at high doses. Nifedipine and diltiazem act more on the vessels and less on the myocardium than verapamil; they have no antiarrhythmic activity. They are used in the prophylaxis and treatment of angina, and in hypertension. Nicardipine and similar drugs act mainly on the vessels, but are valuable in the treatment of hypertension and angina. Important differences exist between different calcium-channel blockers so their use must be carefully assessed. They should not be stopped suddenly, as this may precipitate angina. (See also HEART, DISEASES OF.)

Calcium Gluconate
A salt of the element CALCIUM used to treat deficiency of the mineral or to prevent osteoporosis (see BONE, DISORDERS OF). Tablets can be obtained without a doctor's prescription. It is used intravenously to treat low calcium levels causing symptoms in newborn babies.

Calculi

The general name given to concretions in, for example, the URINARY BLADDER, KIDNEYS or gall-bladder (see LIVER).

Caldicott Guardian

A senior health professional in all NHS trusts, whose responsibility it is to preserve the confidentiality of patient information.

Calibre

A talking-book service which is available to all blind and handicapped people who can supply a doctor's certificate confirming that they are unable to read printed books in the normal way. Its catalogue contains more than 370 books for adults and more than 250 for children, and additions are being made at the rate of around three a week. Full details can be obtained from Calibre.

www.calibre.org.uk

Calliper

A two-pronged instrument with pointed ends, for the measurement of diameters, such as that of the pelvis in obstetrics.

Calliper Splint

This is applied to a broken leg in such a way that in walking, the weight of the body is taken by the hip-bone and not by the foot.

Callosities

Areas of gross thickening of the epidermis in response to trauma. They usually occur on a foot due to bony deformity or ill-fitting footwear. (See CORNS AND BUNIONS.)

Callus

The new tissue formed around the ends of a broken bone. (See BONE, DISORDERS OF.)

Caloric Test

A test for vestibular function (see EAR). It is performed by irrigating the external auditory meatus of the ear with alternate cold and hot water. This usually stimulates the vestibular apparatus, causing nystagmus (see DIABETES MELLITUS – Diabetic eye disease). If the vestibular apparatus is affected by disease, the response may be absent or reduced.

Calorie

A unit of energy. Two units are called by this name. The small calorie, or gram calorie, is the amount of heat required to raise one gram of water one degree centigrade in temperature. The large Calorie or kilocalorie, which is used in the study of dietetics and physiological processes, is the amount of heat required to raise one kilogram of water one degree centigrade in temperature. The number of Calories required to carry on the processes necessary for life and body warmth – such as the beating of the heart, the movements of the chest in breathing, and the chemical activities of the secreting glands – is, for an adult person of ordinary weight, somewhere in the neighbourhood of 1,600. For ordinary sedentary occupations an individual requires about 2,500 Calories; for light muscular work slightly over 3,000 Calories; and for hard continuous labour around 4,000 Calories daily.

Under the International System of Units (SI UNITS – see APPENDIX 6: MEASUREMENTS IN MEDICINE) the kilocalorie has been replaced by the joule, the abbreviation for which is J (1 kilocalorie=4,186·8 J). The term Calorie, however, is so well established that it has been retained in this edition. Conversion from Calories (or kilocalories) to joules is made by multiplying by 4·2 .

Calyx

Calyx means a cup-shaped cavity, the term being especially applied to the recesses of the pelvis of the kidney.

CAM

See COMPLEMENTARY AND ALTERNATIVE MEDICINE (CAM).

Campylobacter

A species of bacterium found in farm and pet animals, from which it can be transmitted to humans, in whom it is a major cause of bacterial FOOD POISONING: outbreaks of infection have followed drinking unpasteurised milk from infected cows and eating undercooked meat and poultry. It causes diarrhoea.

In the United Kingdom, the number of cases of food poisoning (by all types of infection) has risen from 102.9 to 162.9 per 100,000 population over the last 15 years. In 2003, more then 70,000 cases of food poisoning were notified. The use of preventive methods throughout the food production process, marketing and consumption of food is most important in controlling infection, as is taking hygienic precautions, such as hand-washing, after handling animals – including domestic pets.

Mild cases can be treated at home with no solid food but plenty of liquids and some salt. Serious cases require hospital care.

Canaliculus

Canaliculus means a small channel, and is applied to (*a*) the minute passage leading from the lacrimal pore on each eyelid to the lacrimal sac on the side of the nose; (*b*) any one of the minute canals in bone.

Cancellous

A term applied to loose bony tissues as found in the ends of the long bones.

Cancer

The general term used to refer to a malignant TUMOUR, irrespective of the tissue of origin. 'Malignancy' indicates that (i) the tumour is capable of progressive growth, unrestrained by the capsule of the parent organ, and/or (ii) that it is capable of distant spread via lymphatics or the bloodstream, resulting in development of secondary deposits of tumour known as 'metastases'. Microscopically, cancer cells appear different from the equivalent normal cells in the affected tissue. In particular they may show a lesser degree of differentiation (i.e. they are more 'primitive'), features indicative of a faster proliferative rate and disorganised alignment in relationship to other cells or blood vessels. The diagnosis of cancer usually depends upon the observation of these microscopic features in biopsies, i.e. tissue removed surgically for such examination.

Cancers are classified according to the type of cell from which they are derived as well as the organ of origin. Hence cancers arising within the bronchi, often collectively referred to as 'lung cancer', include both adenocarcinomas, derived from epithelium (surface tissue), and carcinomas from glandular tissue. Sarcomas are cancers of connective tissue, including bone and cartilage. The behaviour of cancers and their response to therapy vary widely depending on this classification as well as on numerous other factors such as how large the cancer is, how fast the cells grow and how well defined they are. It is entirely wrong to see cancer as a single disease entity with a universally poor prognosis. For example, fewer than one-half of women in whom breast cancer (see BREASTS, DISEASES OF) is discovered will die from the disease, and 75 per cent of children with lymphoblastic LEUKAEMIA can be cured.

Incidence In most western countries, cancer is the second most important cause of death after heart disease and accounts for 20–25 per cent of all deaths. In the United Kingdom in 2003, more than 154,000 people died of

malignant disease. There is wide international variation in the most frequently encountered types of cancer, reflecting the importance of environmental factors in the development of cancer. In the UK as well as the US, carcinoma of the BRONCHUS is the most common. Since it is usually inoperable at the time of diagnosis, it is even more strikingly the leading cause of cancer deaths. In women, breast cancer was for a long time the most common malignant disease, accounting for a quarter of all cancers, but figures for the late 1990s show that lung cancer now heads the incidence list – presumably the consequence of a rising incidence of smoking among young women. Other common sites are as follows: males – colon and rectum, prostate and bladder; females – colon and rectum, uterus, ovary and pancreas.

In 2003, of the more than 154,000 people in the UK who died of cancer, over 33,000 had the disease in their respiratory system, nearly 13,000 in the breast, over 5,800 in the stomach and more than 2,000 in the uterus or cervix, while over 4,000 people had leukaemia. The incidence of cancer varies with age; the older a person is, the more likely it is that he or she will develop the disease. The over-85s have an incidence about nine times greater than those in the 25–44 age group. There are also differences in incidence between sexes: for example, more men than women develop lung cancer, though the incidence in women is rising as the effects of smoking work through. The death rate from cancer is falling in people under 75 in the UK, a trend largely determined by the cancers which cause the most deaths: lung, breast, colorectal, stomach and prostate.

Causes In most cases the causes of cancer remain unknown, though a family history of cancer may be relevant. Rapid advances have, however, been made in the past two decades in understanding the differences between cancer cells and normal cells at the genetic level. It is now widely accepted that cancer results from acquired changes in the genetic make-up of a particular cell or group of cells which ultimately lead to a failure of the normal mechanisms regulating their growth. It appears that in most cases a cascade of changes is required for cells to behave in a truly malignant fashion; the critical changes affect specific key GENES, known as oncogenes, which are involved in growth regulation. (See APOPTOSIS.)

Since small genetic errors occur within cells at all times – most but not all of which are repaired – it follows that some cancers may develop as a result of an accumulation of random changes which cannot be attributed to environmental or other causes. The environmental factors known to cause cancer, such as radiation and chemicals (including tar from tobacco, asbestos, etc.), do so by increasing the overall rate of acquired genetic damage. Certain viral infections can induce specific cancers (e.g. HEPATITIS B VIRUS and HEPATOMA, EPSTEIN BARR VIRUS and LYMPHOMA) probably by inducing alterations in specific genes. HORMONES may also be a factor in the development of certain cancers such as those of the prostate and breast. Where there is a particular family tendency to certain types of cancer, it now appears that one or more of the critical genetic abnormalities required for development of that cancer may have been inherited. Where environmental factors such as tobacco smoking or asbestos are known to cause cancer, then health education and preventive measures can reduce the incidence of the relevant cancer. Cancer can also affect the white cells in the blood and is called LEUKAEMIA.

Treatment Many cancers can be cured by surgical removal if they are detected early, before there has been spread of significant numbers of tumour cells to distant sites. Important within this group are breast, colon and skin cancer (melanoma). The probability of early detection of certain cancers can be increased by screening programmes in which (ideally) all people at particular risk of development of such cancers are examined at regular intervals. Routine screening for CERVICAL CANCER and breast cancer (see BREASTS, DISEASES OF) is currently practised in the UK. The effectiveness of screening people for cancer is, however, controversial. Apart from questions surrounding the reliability of screening tests, they undoubtedly create anxieties among the subjects being screened.

If complete surgical removal of the tumour is not possible because of its location or because spread from the primary site has occurred, an operation may nevertheless be helpful to relieve symptoms (e.g. pain) and to reduce the bulk of the tumour remaining to be dealt with by alternative means such as RADIOTHERAPY or CHEMOTHERAPY. In some cases radiotherapy is preferable to surgery and may be curative, for example, in the management of tumours of the larynx or of the uterine cervix. Certain tumours are highly sensitive to chemotherapy and may be cured by the use of chemotherapeutic drugs alone. These include testicular tumours, LEUKAEMIA, LYMPHOMA and a variety of tumours occurring in childhood. These tend to be rapidly growing tumours composed of primitive cells which are much more vulnerable to the toxic effects of the chemotherapeutic agents than the normal cells within the body.

Unfortunately neither radiotherapy nor currently available chemotherapy provides a curative option for the majority of common cancers if surgical excision is not feasible. New effective treatments in these conditions are urgently needed. Nevertheless the rapidly increasing knowledge of cancer biology will almost certainly lead to novel therapeutic approaches – including probably genetic techniques utilising the recent discoveries of oncogenes (genes that can cause cancer). Where cure is not possible, there often remains much that can be done for the cancer-sufferer in terms of control of unpleasant symptoms such as pain. Many of the most important recent advances in cancer care relate to such 'palliative' treatment, and include the establishment in the UK of palliative care hospices.

Families and patients can obtain valuable help and advice from Marie Curie Cancer Care, Cancer Relief Macmillan Fund, or the British Association of Cancer United Patients.

www.cancerbacup.org.uk
www.mariecurie.org.uk

Cancrum Oris

Cancrum oris, also called noma, is a gangrenous ulcer about the mouth which affects sickly children, especially after some severe disease such as measles. It is due to the growth of bacteria in the tissues.

Candida

Candidosis (moniliasis) is an infection with the yeast, *Candida albicans*. It is encouraged by pregnancy, DIABETES MELLITUS, prolonged wide-spectrum ANTIBIOTICS or CORTICOSTEROIDS therapy, and is also seen in debilitated infants, the elderly and immunocompromised patients, e.g. those with AIDS/HIV. It may cause white patches in the mouth or vulvovaginal area (thrush) and a red vesicular and scaly rash in the finger clefts, beneath the breasts or in the groin or anogenital folds. Fingernail-fold infection causes chronic PARONYCHIA with secondary nail DYSTROPHY and may complicate RAYNAUD'S DISEASE. CLOTRIMAZOLE and similar 'azoles' as creams, oral gels or vaginal pessaries are rapidly effective, but severe systemic infections require oral itraconazole or even intravenous AMPHOTERICIN B.

Canine Teeth

Or eye-teeth – see TEETH.

Cannabis

Psychoactive substances obtained from *Cannabis sativa* or Indian hemp, they are the oldest euphoriants. Also called marijuana, these substances do not usually result in physical DEPENDENCE but chronic abuse leads to passivity, apathy and inertia. Acute adverse effects include transient panic reactions and toxic psychoses. The panic reactions are characterised by anxiety, helplessness and loss of control and may be accompanied by florid paranoid thoughts and hallucinations. The toxic psychoses are characterised by the sudden onset of confusion and visual hallucinations. Even at lower doses, cannabis products can precipitate functional psychoses in vulnerable individuals. The acute physical manifestations of short-term cannabis abuse are conjunctival suffusion and tachycardia.

The chopped leaves are usually smoked but can be eaten in food or taken as tea. The active ingredient is tetrahydrocannibol. There is much public debate in western countries over the social use of cannabis: it is illegal to possess or supply the substance in the United Kingdom, but nevertheless cannabis is quite widely used. Cannabis is classified as a Schedule 1 drug under the Misuse of Drugs Act 1971 and has not officially been used medicinally – despite some claims that it is helpful in ameliorating painful symptoms in certain serious chronic diseases such as multiple sclerosis. A related agent, NABILONE, is a synthetic cannabinoid licenced for use in treating nausea and vomiting caused by CYTOTOXIC drugs.

Cannula

A tube for insertion into the body, designed to fit tightly round a trocar – a sharp, pointed instrument which is withdrawn from the cannula after insertion, so that fluid may run out through the latter.

Canthus

The name applied to the angle at either end of the aperture between the eyelids.

CAPD

Chronic ambulatory peritoneal dialysis – an outpatient technique for treating failure of the KIDNEYS. (See HAEMODIALYSIS.)

Capillaries

The minute vessels which join the ends of the arteries to venules, the tiny commencement of veins. Their walls consist of a single layer of fine, flat, transparent cells, bound together at the edges, and the vessels form a meshwork all through the tissues of the body, bathing the latter in blood with only the thin capillary wall interposed, through which gases and fluids readily pass. These vessels are less than 0·025 mm in width.

Capillary Return

A test for the adequacy of blood circulation by pressing on the skin and seeing how long it takes for the colour to return. (See PERFUSION.)

Capsule

A term used in several senses in medicine. It is applied to a soluble case, usually of gelatine, for enclosing small doses of unpleasant medicine.

Enteric-coated capsules, which have been largely superseded by enteric-coated tablets, are capsules treated in such a manner that the ingredients do not come in contact with the acid stomach contents but are only released when the capsule disintegrates in the alkaline contents of the intestine.

The term is also applied to the fibrous or membranous envelope of various organs, as of the spleen, liver or kidney. Additionally, it is applied to the ligamentous bag surrounding various joints and attached by its edge to the bones on either side.

Captopril

An ACE-inhibitor drug introduced for the treatment of patients with severe HYPERTENSION. It acts by lowering the concentration in the blood of angiotensin II which is one of the factors responsible for high blood pressure. (See ANGIOTENSIN; RENIN.)

Caput Medusae (Medusa's Head)

The term describing the abnormally dilated veins that form around the umbilicus in CIRRHOSIS of the liver.

Caput Succedaneum

Usually shortened by obstetricians to 'caput', this is the temporary swelling which is sometimes found on the head of the newborn infant. It is due to OEDEMA in and around the scalp, caused by pressure on the head as the child is born. It is of no significance and quickly disappears spontaneously.

Carbachol

A drug which stimulates the parasympathetic nervous system, for example, for relieving GLAUCOMA and retention of urine due to ATONY.

Carbamazepine

An anticonvulsant drug used to treat most types of EPILEPSY, including simple and complex partial seizures and tonic-clonic seizures secondary to a focal discharge. Monitoring of concentrations in the blood may be of help in finding the most effective dose. Carbamazepine has generally fewer side-effects than other antiepileptic drugs; even so, it should be started at a low dose and increased incrementally. The drug is also used to treat TRIGEMINAL NEURALGIA and other types of nerve pain, as well as pain from a PHANTOM LIMB. DEPRESSION resistant to LITHIUM CARBONATE may also benefit from carbamazepine.

Carbaryl

A pesticide used to kill head and crab lice (see PEDICULOSIS). Available as a lotion, some of which contains alcohol (not recommended for use on crab lice), the substance may irritate skin and should not be used near damaged skin, eyes or ears.

Carbimazole

One of the most widely used drugs in the treatment of HYPERTHYROIDISM. It acts by interferring with the synthesis of thyroid hormone in the thyroid gland.

Carbohydrate

The term applied to an organic substance in which the hydrogen and oxygen are usually in the proportion to form water. Carbohydrates are all, chemically considered, derivatives of simple forms of sugar and are classified as monosaccharides (e.g. glucose), disaccharides (e.g. cane sugar), polysaccharides (e.g. starch). Many of the cheaper and most important foods are included in this group, which comprises sugars, starches, celluloses and gums. When one of these foods is digested, it is converted into a simple kind of sugar and absorbed in this form. Excess carbohydrates, not immediately needed by the body, are stored as glycogen in the liver and muscles. In DIABETES MELLITUS, the most marked feature consists of an inability on the part of the tissues to assimilate and utilise the carbohydrate material. Each gram of carbohydrate is capable of furnishing slightly over 4 Calories of energy. (See CALORIE; DIET.)

Carbolic Acid

Carbolic acid, or phenol, was the precursor of all ANTISEPTICS. It paralyses and then destroys most forms of life, particularly organisms such as bacteria. It has been superseded by less penetrative and harmful antiseptics.

Carbon

A non-metallic element, the compounds of which are found in all living tissues and which is a constituent (as carbon dioxide) of air exhaled from the LUNGS. Two isotopes of carbon, ^{11}C and ^{14}C, are used in medicine. Carbon-11 is used in positron-emission tomography (see PET SCANNING); carbon-14 is used as a tracer element in studying various aspects of METABOLISM.

Carbon Dioxide (CO$_2$)

Formed by the body during metabolism and exhaled by the lungs. Seen in sparkling waters and wines, it is also used in baths as a stimulant to the skin. Combined with oxygen in cylinders, it is used to control breathing in ANAESTHESIA and in the treatment of victims of CARBON MONOXIDE (CO) poisoning.

Measuring the partial pressure of the gas by taking blood for blood gas estimation provides information on the adequacy of breathing. A high partial pressure may indicate impending or actual respiratory failure.

Carbonic Anhydrase Inhibitor

A drug that curbs the action of an ENZYME in the blood controlling the production of carbonic acid or bicarbonate from CARBON DIOXIDE (CO$_2$). Called carbonic anhydrase, the enzyme is present in ERYTHROCYTES and it has a key part in maintaining the acid-base balance in the blood. Inhibiting drugs include ACETAZOLAMIDE and DORZOLAMIDE, and these are used as weak DIURETICS to reduce the increased intraocular pressure in ocular hypertension or open-angle GLAUCOMA (see EYE, DISORDERS OF).

Carbon Monoxide (CO)

This is a colourless, odourless, tasteless, non-irritating gas formed on incomplete combustion of organic fuels. Exposure to CO is frequently due to defective gas, oil or solid-fuel heating appliances. CO is a component of car exhaust fumes and deliberate exposure to these is a common method of suicide. Victims of fires often suffer from CO poisoning. CO combines reversibly with oxygen-carrying sites of HAEMOGLOBIN (Hb) molecules with an affinity 200 to 300 times greater than oxygen itself. The carboxyhaemoglobin (COHb) formed becomes unavailable for oxygen transportation. In addition the partial saturation of the Hb molecule results in tighter oxygen binding, impairing delivery to the tissues. CO also binds to MYOGLOBIN and respiratory cytochrome enzymes. Exposure to CO at levels of 500 parts per million (ppm) would be expected to cause mild symptoms only and exposure to levels of 4,000 ppm would be rapidly fatal.

Each year around 50 people in the United Kingdom are reported as dying from carbon monoxide poisoning, and experts have suggested that as many as 25,000 people a year are exposed to its effects within the home, but most cases are unrecognised, unreported and untreated, even though victims may suffer from long-term effects. This is regrettable, given that Napoleon's surgeon, Larrey, recognised in the 18th century that soldiers were being poisoned by carbon monoxide when billeted in huts heated by woodburning stoves. In the USA it is estimated that 40,000 people a year attend emergency departments suffering from carbon monoxide poisoning. So prevention is clearly an important element in dealing with what is sometimes termed the 'silent killer'. Safer designs of houses and heating systems, as well as wider public education on the dangers of carbon monoxide and its sources, are important.

Clinical effects of acute exposure resemble those of atmospheric HYPOXIA. Tissues and organs with high oxygen consumption are affected to a great extent. Common effects include headaches, weakness, fatigue, flushing, nausea, vomiting, irritability, dizziness, drowsiness, disorientation, incoordination, visual disturbances, TACHYCARDIA and HYPERVENTILATION. In severe cases drowsiness may progress rapidly to COMA. There may also be metabolic ACIDOSIS, HYPOKALAEMIA, CONVULSIONS, HYPOTENSION, respiratory depression, ECG changes and cardiovascular collapse. Cerebral OEDEMA is common and will lead to severe brain damage and focal neurological signs. Significant abnormalities on physical examination include impaired short-term memory, abnormal Rhomberg's test (standing unsupported with eyes closed) and unsteadiness of gait including heel-toe walking. Any one of these signs would classify the episode as severe. Victims' skin may be coloured pink, though this is very rarely seen even in severe incidents. The venous blood may look 'arterial'. Patients recovering from acute CO poisoning may suffer neurological sequelae including TREMOR, personality changes, memory impairment, visual loss, inability to concentrate and PARKINSONISM. Chronic low-level exposures may result in nausea, fatigue, headache, confusion, VOMITING, DIARRHOEA, abdominal pain and general malaise. They are often misdiagnosed as influenza or food poisoning.

First-aid treatment is to remove the victim from the source of exposure, ensure an effective airway and give 100-per-cent oxygen by tight-fitting mask. In hospital, management is largely suppportive, with oxygen administration. A blood sample for COHb level determination should be taken as soon as practicable and, if possible, before oxygen is given. Ideally, oxygen therapy should continue until the COHb level falls below 5 per cent. Patients with any history of unconsciousness, a COHb level greater than 20 per cent on arrival, any neurological signs, any cardiac arrhythmias or anyone who is pregnant should be referred for an expert opinion about possible treatment with hyperbaric oxygen, though this remains a controversial therapy. Hyperbaric oxygen therapy shortens the half-life of COHb, increases plasma oxygen transport and reverses the clinical effects resulting from acute exposures. Carbon monoxide is also an environmental poison and a component of cigarette smoke. Normal body COHb levels due to ENDOGENOUS CO production are 0.4 to 0.7 per cent. Non-smokers in urban areas may have level of 1–2 per cent as a result of environmental exposure. Smokers may have a COHb level of 5 to 6 per cent.

Carboxyhaemoglobinaemia
The term applied to the state of the blood in carbon monoxide poisoning, in which this gas combines with the haemoglobin, displacing oxygen from it. (See CARBON MONOXIDE (CO).)

Carbuncle
See BOILS (FURUNCULOSIS).

Carcinogenesis
Carcinogenesis is the means or method whereby the changes responsible for the induction of CANCER are brought about.

Carcinogens
Agents, such as tobacco smoke, certain chemicals, asbestos fibres and high-dose radiation, that have the property of causing CANCER.

Carcinoma
A type of CANCER developing from cells found in the surface layer of an organ in the body.

Carcinoma in Situ
The first stage of CARCINOMA in which the malignant tumour is present only in the EPITHELIUM, and when surgical excision of the local growth, with its pathological status confirmed in the laboratory, should ensure a cure.

Carcinomatosis
The spread of cancer cells from their original

site of growth to other tissues in the body. Such a spread of cancer, which takes place mainly via blood and lymph vessels, is usually fatal. CHEMOTHERAPY and RADIOTHERAPY may, however, check the spread or sometimes destroy the cancerous growth.

Cardia

Cardia is a term applied to the upper opening of the stomach into which the oesophagus empties. The cardia lies immediately behind the heart.

Cardiac Arrest

Cardiac arrest occurs when the pumping action of the heart stops. This may be because the heart stops beating (see ASYSTOLE) or because the heart muscle starts contracting too fast to pump effectively (ventricular systole, the period when the heart contracts). Coronary thrombosis is the most frequent cause of arrest. Irreversible brain damage and death result without prompt treatment. Heart massage, defibrillation and artificial respiration are customary treatment. Other causes of cardiac arrest are respiratory arrest, anaphylactic shock and electrocution. Up to one-third of patients treated in hospital whose heart rhythm is restored recover to an extent that enables them to return home. (See APPENDIX 1: BASIC FIRST AID – Cardiac/respiratory arrest.)

Cardiac Arrhythmia

Abnormal rhythm of the heartbeat. Most commonly seen after someone has had a myo-cardial infarction, but also present in some normal individuals – especially if they have taken a lot of coffee or other stimulant – and in those with a congenital abnormality of the heart-muscle conducting system. The cause is interference in the generation or transmission of electrical impulses through the heart's conducting system. Occasional isolated irregular beats (ectopic beats) do not necessarily mean that conduction is faulty. Arrhythmias can be classified as tachycardias (more than 100 beats a minute) or bradycardias (slower than 60 beats a minute). Heartbeats may be regular or irregular. (See HEART, DISEASES OF.)

Cardiac Catheterisation

A diagnostic procedure in which a tube is inserted into a blood vessel under local anaesthetic and threaded through to the chambers of the heart to monitor blood flow, blood pressure, blood chemistry and the output of the heart, and to take a sample of heart tissue. The technique is used to diagnose congenital heart disease and coronary artery disease. Another application is in the diagnosis and treatment of valvular disease in the heart.

Cardiac Cycle

The various sequential movements of the heart that comprise the rhythmic relaxation and expansion of the heart muscles as first the atria contract and force the blood into the ventricles (diastole), which then contract (systole) to pump the blood round the body. (See ELECTROCARDIOGRAM (ECG).)

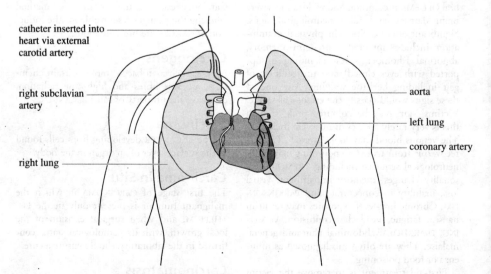

catheter inserted into heart via external carotid artery

right subclavian artery

right lung

aorta

left lung

coronary artery

Catheterisation of coronary artery, a diagnostic procedure to determine patency of the artery.

Cardiac Disease
See HEART, DISEASES OF.

Cardiac Glycosides

Drugs whose main actions are to increase the force of myocardial contraction and reduce the conductivity of the nerve fibres in the atrioventricular node of the heart. They are useful in treating supraventricular tachycardias (rapid heart rhythm) and some forms of heart failure. Glycosides are a traditional group of cardiac drugs, originally derived from the leaves of foxglove plants and used as digitalis. The active principle has long been synthesised and used as DIGOXIN. They are potentaially toxic and their use, especially during initial treatment, should be monitored. Side-effects include ANOREXIA, nausea, vomiting, diarrhoea and abdominal pain; drowsiness, confusion and DEPRESSION may occur. An abnormally slow heart rate may develop. The glycosides should be used with special care in the elderly who are sometimes particularly susceptible to their toxic effects.

Cardiac Massage

The procedure used to restart the action of the heart if it is suddenly arrested. In many cases the arrested heart can be made to start beating again by rhythmic compression of the chest wall. This is done by placing the patient on a hard surface – a table or the floor – and then placing the heel of the hand over the lower part of the sternum and compressing the chest wall firmly, but not too forcibly, at the rate of 60–80 times a minute. At the same time artificial respiration must be started by the mouth-to-mouth method. (See APPENDIX 1: BASIC FIRST AID.) Open heart massage is sometimes undertaken if an arrest occurs during a chest operation – the heart being directly handled by the resuscitator.

Cardiac Muscle

The muscle, unique to the heart, which comprises the walls of the atria and ventricles. It consists of long broadening cells (fibres) with special physiological characteristics which enable them to keep contracting and expanding indefinitely.

Cardiac Neurosis

Obsessional fear about the state of the heart. It tends to occur after a heart attack and may result in the patient's experiencing the symptoms of another attack.

Cardiac Output

The volume of blood pumped out per minute by the ventricles of the heart. It is one measure of the heart's efficiency. At rest, the heart of a healthy adult will pump between 2.5 and 4.5 litres of blood every minute. Exercise will raise this to as much as 30 litres a minute but, if this figure is low, it suggests that the heart muscle may be diseased or that the person has suffered severe blood loss.

Cardiac Pacemaker

The natural pacemaker is the sinuatrial node, found at the base of the heart. The heart normally controls its rate and rhythm; heart block occurs when impulses cannot reach all parts of the heart. This may lead to ARRHYTHMIA, or even cause the heart to stop (see HEART, DISEASES OF). Artificial pacemakers may then be used; in the United Kingdom these are required for around one person in every 2,000 of the population. Usually powered by mercury or lithium batteries, and lasting up to 15 years, they are either fixed to the outside of the chest or implanted in the armpit, and connected by a wire passing through a vein in the neck to the heart. Normally adjusted to deliver 65–75 impulses a minute, they also ensure a regular cardiac rhythm. Patients with pacemakers may be given a driving licence provided that their vehicle is not likely to be a source of danger to the public, and that they are receiving adequate and regular medical supervision from a cardiologist.

Although there are numerous possible sources of electrical interference with pacemakers, the overall risks are slight. Potential sources include anti-theft devices, airport weapon detectors, surgical diathermy, ultrasound, and short-wave heat treatment. Nevertheless, many pacemaker patients lead active and fulfilling lives.

Cardiac Pump
See HEART, ARTIFICIAL.

Cardiac Tamponade

Compression of the heart due to abnormal accumulation of fluid within the fibrous covering of the heart (PERICARDIUM). The result is irregular rhythm and death if the fluid is not removed.

Cardioangiography

Rendering the outline of the heart visible on an X-ray film by injecting a radio-opaque substance into it.

Cardiology

That branch of medical science devoted to the study of the diseases of the heart.

Cardiomegaly

Enlargement of the heart (see HEART, DISEASES OF).

Cardiomyopathy

A general term covering primary disease of the heart muscle. (See HEART, DISEASES OF.)

Cardioplegia

A procedure whereby the heart is stopped by reducing its temperature (hypothermia), by injecting the muscle with a solution of salts or by electrostimulation. This enables surgeons to operate safely on the heart.

Cardiopulmonary Bypass

A procedure in which the body's circulation of blood is kept going when the heart is intentionally stopped to enable heart surgery to be carried out. A HEART-LUNG MACHINE substitutes for the heart's pumping action and the blood is oxygenated at the same time.

Cardiopulmonary Resuscitation (CPR)

The use of life-saving measures of mouth-to-mouth resuscitation and external cardiac compression massage in a person who has collapsed with CARDIAC ARREST. Speedy restoration of the circulation of oxygenated blood to the brain is essential to prevent damage to brain tissues from oxygen starvation. The brain is irreversibly damaged if it is starved of oxygen for more than 4–5 minutes. Someone whose heart has stopped will be very pale or blue-grey (in particular, round the lips) and unresponsive; he or she will not be breathing and will have no pulse. It is important to determine that the collapsed person has not simply fainted before starting CPR. The procedure is described under cardiac/respiratory arrest in APPENDIX 1: BASIC FIRST AID. In hospital, or when paramedical staff are attending an emergency, CPR may include the use of a DEFIBRILLATOR to apply a controlled electric shock to the heart via the chest wall.

Cardiospasm

The spasmodic contraction of the muscle surrounding the opening of the oesophagus into the stomach: also termed achalasia of the cardia. (See OESOPHAGUS, DISEASES OF.)

Cardiovascular System

This refers to the whole circulatory system: the heart, the systemic circulation (the arteries and veins of the body) and the pulmonary circulation (the arteries and veins of the lungs). Blood circulates throughout the cardiovascular system bringing oxygen and nutrients to the tissues and removing carbon dioxide and other waste products.

Cardioversion

Cardioversion, or DEFIBRILLATION, is indicated in patients with ventricular fibrillation or tachycardia, fast or irregular heartbeat, if other treatments have failed. A general anaesthetic is given if the patient is conscious, following which a carefully timed direct-current shock is applied to the patient's chest wall using a DEFIBRILLATOR. The patient's ECG rhythm should then be monitored and anticoagulants considered, as the risk of EMBOLISM is increased.

Care in Community

See COMMUNITY CARE.

Care Standards Act

Legislation (approved by the UK parliament in 2001) that sets up a new, independent regulatory body for social care and private and voluntary health-care services. The new body is called the National Care Standards Commission and covers England and Wales, but in the latter the National Assembly is the regulatory body. Independent councils register social-care workers, set social-care work standards and regulate the education and training of social workers in England and Wales. The Act also gives the Secretary of State for Health the authority to keep a list of individuals considered unsuitable to work with vulnerable adults. In addition, the legislation reforms the regulation of childminders and day-care provision for young children, responsibility for overseeing these services having been transferred from local authorities to the Chief Inspector of Schools. Services covered by the Act range from residential care homes and nursing homes, children's homes, domiciliary-care agencies, fostering agencies and voluntary adoption agencies through to private and voluntary health-care services. This includes private hospitals and clinics and private primary-care premises. For the first time, local authorities will have to meet the same standards as independent-sector providers.

Caries

See TEETH, DISORDERS OF.

Carminatives

Preparations to relieve FLATULENCE, and any resulting griping, by the bringing up of wind, or ERUCTATION. Their essential constituent is an aromatic volatile oil, usually of vegetable extraction.

Carneous Mole
An ovum which has died in the early months of pregnancy. It usually requires no treatment and evacuates itself.

Carotene
A colouring matter of carrots, other plants, butter and yolk of egg, carotene is the precursor of vitamin A, which is formed from carotene in the liver. (See VITAMIN and APPENDIX 5: VITAMINS.)

Carotid Body
A small reddish-brown structure measuring 5–7 × 2·5–4 millimetres, situated one on each side of the neck, where the carotid artery divides into the internal and external carotid arteries. Its main function is in controlling breathing so that an adequate supply of oxygen is maintained to the tissues of the body. Oxygen levels are controlled by a reflex operating between the carotid body and the respiratory centre in the brain.

Carpal Tunnel Syndrome
A condition characterised by attacks of pain and tingling in the first three or four fingers of one or both hands. The attacks usually occur at night. Carpal tunnel syndrome is caused by pressure on the median nerve as it passes under the strong ligament that lies across the front of the wrist. The condition may respond to use of a night splint on the hand; otherwise a corticosteroid injection under the ligament may help. If not, pressure is relieved by surgical division of the compressing ligament.

Carpus
The Latin term for the WRIST, composed of eight small bones firmly joined together with ligaments, but capable of a certain amount of sliding movement over one another.

Carriers of Disease
See INFECTION.

Cartilage
A hard but pliant substance forming parts of the skeleton – for example, the cartilages of the ribs, of the larynx and of the ears. Microscopically, cartilage is found to consist of cells arranged in twos or in rows, and embedded in a ground-glass-like material devoid of blood vessels and nerves. The end of every long bone has a smooth layer of hyaline cartilage on it where it forms a joint with other bones (articular cartilage), and in young persons up to about the age of 16 there is a plate of cartilage (epiphyseal cartilage) running right across the bone about 12 mm (half an inch) from each end. The latter, by constantly thickening and changing into bone, causes the increase in length of the bone. (See also BONE.) In some situations there is found a combination of cartilage and fibrous tissue, as in the discs between the vertebrae of the spine. This fibro-cartilage, as it is known, combines the pliability of fibrous tissue with the elasticity of cartilage. (For cartilages of the knee, see KNEE.)

Caruncle
Any small fleshy eminence, whether normal or abnormal.

Caseation
A process which takes place in the tissues in TUBERCULOSIS and some other chronic diseases. The central part of a diseased area, instead of changing into pus and so forming an ABSCESS, changes to a firm cheese-like mass which may next be absorbed or may be converted into a calcareous deposit and fibrous tissue, and so healing results in the formation of a scar.

Case-Control Study
Research in which 'cases' – that is, persons with a particular condition or receiving a particular medication – are compared with a group similar in age, sex distribution and social class, etc. who do not have the condition or who are not receiving the drug.

Casein
That part of milk which forms cheese or curds. It is produced by the union of a substance, caseinogen, dissolved in the milk, with lime salts also dissolved in the milk – the union being produced by the action of rennin, a ferment from the stomach of the calf. The same change occurs in the human stomach as the first step in the digestion of milk, and therefore when milk is vomited curdled it merely shows that digestion has begun.

Castration
This is literally defined as 'deprivation of the power of generation'. In practical terms this involves surgical removal of both OVARIES, or both testicles (see TESTICLE). Such an operation is most commonly associated with the treatment of malignant lesions. In women who have reached the menopause, bilateral oophorectomy

is routinely performed during HYSTERECTOMY, especially in cases of uterine carcinoma, and is usually performed when removing an ovarian tumour or malignant cyst. It is essential that the surgeon discusses with a woman before an operation when it might prove beneficial to remove her ovaries in addition to carrying out the main procedure. In men, orchidectomy is routine for testicular tumours, and is sometimes carried out when treating prostatic cancer.

Casts

Casts of hollow organs are found in various diseases. Membraneous casts of the air passages are found in diphtheria and in one form of bronchitis, and are sometimes coughed up entire. Casts of the interior of the bowels are passed in cases of mucous colitis associated with constipation, and casts of the microscopic tubules in the kidneys passed in the urine form one of the surest signs of glomerulonephritis. (See KIDNEYS, DISEASES OF.)

Catabolism

The breakdown by the body of complex substances to form simpler ones, a process that is accompanied by the release of energy. Among the substances catabolised are nutrients, such as CARBOHYDRATE and PROTEIN in food, and in storage in the body – for example, GLYCOGEN.

Catalepsy

A physical condition in which part or all of the body becomes rigid. It is characterised by the adoption of strange – often statue-like – poses (CATATONIA), which may pass off within a few minutes or may last for several hours (rarely, days). Typically brought on by a sudden mental trauma, catalepsy may occur with prolonged depression or some other serious MENTAL ILLNESS, and occasionally with EPILEPSY. Successful treatment must depend upon due recognition of all precipitating factors and circumstances.

Cataplexy

Cataplexy is a condition in which the patient has a sudden attack of muscular weakness affecting the whole body. (See also NARCOLEPSY.)

Cataract

An opacity of the lens sufficient to cause visual impairment (see EYE, DISORDERS OF).

Catarrh

Inflammation of the mucous membranes, particularly those of the air passages, associated with a copious secretion of mucus. Commonly the result of infection or local allergy, catarrh can affect the nose, middle ear and sinuses.

Catatonia

A condition in which an individual takes up odd postures, often accompanied by muteness or semi-coma. The arms and legs may be moved passively by someone else into positions that the sufferer then holds for many hours. Catatonia occurs in SCHIZOPHRENIA. It may also be associated with organic brain disease such as encephalitis lethargica (see ENCEPHA-LITIS), tumours and carbon monoxide intoxication.

Catecholamines

Substances produced in the body from the dietary AMINO ACIDS, PHENYLALANINE and TYRO-SINE. They include ADRENALINE, NORADREN-ALINE and DOPAMINE which have varying functions, usually as NEUROTRANSMITTERS, in the sympathetic and central nervous systems (see under NERVOUS SYSTEM). Their chemical structure is based on a benzene ring with hydroxyl and amine side-chains.

Catgut

A traditional absorbable SUTURE used in surgery for tying cut arteries and stitching wounds. Consisting of twisted COLLAGEN (from sheep or cattle intestines), catgut is absorbed by phagocytes (see under PHAGOCYTE) over a variable period. There are two types: plain, and chromatised or chromic. Synthetic absorbable sutures cause less reaction, have a predictable absorption period and are more effective.

Cathartics

Substances which produce an evacuation of the bowels (see LAXATIVES). The term 'cathartic' also means possessing the power to cleanse.

Catherisation

Use of a catheter (see CATHETERS).

Catheters

Hollow tubes, usually made of rubber or plastic, used for passing into various organs of the body, either for investigational purposes or to give some form of treatment. They are used under strict sterile conditions.

Cardiac catheters are introduced through a vein in the arm and passed into the heart in order to diagnose some of the more obscure forms of congenital heart disease, and often as a preliminary to operating on the heart.

Endotracheal catheters are used to pass

down the TRACHEA into the lungs, usually in the course of administering anaesthetics (see under ANAESTHESIA).

Eustachian catheters are small catheters that are passed along the floor of the nose into the Eustachian tube in order to inflate the ear.

Nasal catheters are tubes passed through the nose into the stomach to feed a patient who cannot swallow – so-called nasal feeding.

Rectal catheters are passed into the REC-TUM in order to introduce fluid into the rectum.

Suprapubic catheters are passed into the bladder through an incision in the lower abdominal wall just above the pubis, either to allow urine to drain away from the bladder, or to wash out an infected bladder.

Ureteric catheters are small catheters that are passed up the ureter into the pelvis of the kidney, usually to determine the state of the kidney, either by obtaining a sample of urine direct from the kidney or to inject a radio-opaque substance preliminary to X-raying the kidney. (See PYELOGRAPHY.)

Urethral catheters are catheters that are passed along the urethra into the bladder, either to draw off urine or to wash out the bladder.

It is these last three types of catheters that are most extensively used.

'Cat Scanner'

See CT SCANNER.

Cat-Scratch Fever

An infection in humans caused by a small gram-negative BACILLUS (*Bartonella henselae*). The domestic cat is a reservoir for the bacteria, and up to 50 per cent of the cat population may be affected. The disorder manifests itself as a skin lesion 3–10 days after a minor scratch; within two weeks the victim's lymph glands enlarge and may produce pus. Fever, headache and malaise occur in some patients. Antibiotics do not seem to be effective. The skin lesion and lymph-gland enlargement subside spontaneously within 2–5 months.

Cauda

A tail or a tail-like structure. For example, the cauda equina ('horse's tail') is a collection of nerve roots arising from the lumbar, sacral and coccygeal spinal nerves. The resulting bundle, fancifully resembling a horse's tail, runs down inside the spinal column until the individual fibres leave through their respective openings.

Caul

The piece of AMNION which sometimes covers a child when he or she is born.

Cauliflower Ear

The term applied to the distortion of the external ear produced by repeated injury in sport. Initially it is due to a HAEMATOMA in the auricle (see EAR). To prevent deformity the blood should be drawn off from this haematoma as soon as possible, and a firm pressure bandage then applied. Subsequent protection can be given to the ear by covering it with a few layers of two-way-stretch strapping wound around the head.

Causalgia

A severe burning pain in a limb in which the sympathetic and somatic nerves have been damaged.

Caustics and Cauteries

Caustics and cauteries are used to destroy tissues – the former by chemical action, the latter by their high temperature. (See ELECTROCAUTERY.)

Cavernous Breathing

A peculiar quality of the respiratory sounds heard on AUSCULTATION over a cavity in the lung.

Cavernous Sinus

A channel for venous blood placed either side of the sphenoid bone at the base of the SKULL behind the eye sockets. Blood drains into it from the eye, the nose, the brain and part of the cheek, and leaves via the internal jugular and facial veins. Sometimes the sinus becomes blocked by a blood clot (thrombus), usually a complication of a nearby bacterial infection. A potentially serious condition, it should be treated with thrombolysis and antibiotics.

CD4/CD8 Count

An immunological assessment used to monitor for signs of organ rejection after transplantation; it is also used to check the progress of treatment in patients with HIV (see AIDS/ HIV). The count measures the ratio of helper-induced T-lymphocytes to cytotoxic-suppressor lymphocytes. (See LYMPHOCYTE; IMMUNOLOGY.)

Cefoxitin

Cefoxitin is a semi-synthetic antibiotic, given by injection, which is used in the treatment of infections due to gram-negative micro-organisms such as *Proteus* which are resistant to many other antibiotics.

Cell Salvage Transfusion

See TRANSFUSION.

Cells

The basic structural unit of body tissues. There are around 10 billion cells in the human body and they are structurally and functionally linked to carry out the body's many complex activities.

Every cell consists essentially of a cell-body of soft albuminous material called cytoplasm, in which lies a kernel or nucleus which seems to direct all the activities of the cell. Within the nucleus may be seen a minute body, the nucleolus; and there may or may not be a cell-envelope around all. (See also MITOCHONDRIA.) Each cell nucleus carries a set of identical CHROMOSOMES, the body's genetic instructions.

Cells vary much in size, ranging in the human body from 0·0025 mm to about 0·025 mm.

All animals and plants consist at first of a single cell (the egg-cell, or ovum), which begins to develop when fertilised by the sperm-cell derived from the opposite sex. Development begins by a division into two new cells, then into four, and so on till a large mass is formed. These cells – among them stem cells (see STEM CELL) which have the potential to develop into a variety of specialised cells – then arrange themselves into layers, and form various tubes, rods, and masses which represent in the embryo the organs of the fully developed animal. (See FETUS.)

When the individual organs have been laid down on a scaffolding of cells, these gradually change in shape and in chemical composition. The cells in the nervous system send out long processes to form the nerves; those in the muscles become long and striped in appearance; and those which form fat become filled with fat droplets which distend the cells. Further, they begin to produce, between one another, the substances which give the various tissues their special character. Thus, in the future bones, some cells deposit lime salts and others form cartilage, while in tendons they produce long white fibres of a gelatinous substance. In some organs the cells change little: thus the liver consists of columns of large cells packed together, while many cells, like the white blood corpuscles, retain their primitive characters almost entire.

Thus cells are the active agents in forming the body, and they have a similar function in repairing its wear and tear. Tumours, and especially malignant tumours, have a highly cellular structure, the cells being of an embryonic type, or, at best, forming poor imitations of the tissues in which they grow (see TUMOUR).

Cellulitis

Inflammation taking place in cellular tissue, and usually referring to infection in the sub-cutaneous tissue. A related word, cellulite, which has no medical meaning, is used in the slimming business to refer to excess fatty tissue in the arms, buttocks and thighs. (See ABSCESS; ERYSIPELAS.)

Cellulose

A carbohydrate substance forming the skeleton of most plant structures. It is colourless, transparent, insoluble in water and is practically unaffected by digestion. In vegetable foods it therefore adds to the bulk, but it is of no value as a food-stuff. It is found in practically a pure state in cotton-wool.

Cement

See TEETH.

Central Nervous System

This comprises the nervous tissue of the brain and spinal cord, but does not include the cranial and spinal nerves and the autonomic nervous system. This latter group makes up the peripheral nervous system. (See BRAIN and SPINAL CORD; NERVOUS SYSTEM.)

Central Venous Pressure

The pressure of blood within the right atrium of the HEART as measured by a catheter and manometer.

Cephalosporins

These are broad-spectrum antibiotics. Most are semi-synthetic derivatives of cephalosporin C, an antibiotic originally derived from a sewage outfall in Sardinia.

First-generation examples still in use include cephalexin and cefadroxil. They are orally active and, along with second-generation cefaclor, have a similar antimicrobial spectrum. They are used for 'resistant' urinary infections and urinary infections in pregnancy. Cephalosporins have a similar pharmacology to that of penicillin, and about 10 per cent of patients allergic to penicillin will also be hypersensitive to cephalosporins. They are effective in treating SEPTICAEMIA, PNEUMONIA, MENINGITIS, biliary-tract infections and PERITONITIS.

Second-generation cefuroxime and cefamandole are less vulnerable to penicillinases and are useful for treating 'resistant' bacteria and *Haemophilus influenzae* and *Neisseria gonorrhoea*. Third-generation cephalosporins include cefotaxime, ceftazidime and others; these are more effective than the second-generation in treating some gram-negative infections, especially those causing septicaemia.

Cereal

Any grass-like plant bearing an edible seed. The important cereals are wheat, oats, barley, maize, rice and millet. Along with these are usually included tapioca (derived from the cassava plant), sago (derived from the pith of the sago palm) and arrowroot (derived from the root of a West Indian plant), all of which consist almost entirely of starch. Semolina, farola and macaroni are preparations of wheat.

	per cent
Water	10–12
Protein	10–12
Carbohydrate	65–75
Fat	0·5–8
Mineral matter	2

Composition of cereals

Cereals consist predominantly of carbohydrate. They are therefore an excellent source of energy. On the other hand, their deficiency in protein and fat means that to provide a balanced diet, they should be supplemented by other foods rich in protein and fat.

per cent

	Water	Protein	Fat	Carbo-hydrate	Cellu-lose	Ash
Wheat	12·0	11·0	1·7	71·2	2·2	1·9
Oatmeal	7·2	14·2	7·3	65·9	3·5	1·9
Barley	12·3	10·1	1·9	69·5	3·8	2·4
Rye	11·0	10·2	2·3	72·3	2·1	2·1
Maize	12·5	9·7	5·4	68·9	2·0	1·5
Rice (polished)	12·4	6·9	0·4	79·4	0·4	0·5
Millet	12·3	10·4	3·9	68·3	2·9	2·2
Buck wheat	13·0	10·2	2·2	61·3	11·1	2·2

Composition of certain cereals

Cerebellar Ataxia

Uncoordinated movements, including an unsteady gait, caused by damage to or disease of the cerebellum (see BRAIN). Brain tumours, MULTIPLE SCLEROSIS (MS) and stroke can result in ataxia – as can excessive consumption of alcohol, and degeneration of the cerebellum as a result of an inherited disease. Affected victims may have slurred speech, hand tremors and nystagmus (see under EYE, DISORDERS OF).

Cerebellum and Cerebrum
See BRAIN.

Cerebral Palsy

The term used to describe a group of conditions characterised by varying degrees of paralysis and originating in infancy or early childhood. In some 80 per cent of cases this takes the form of spastic paralysis (muscle stiffness), hence the now obsolete lay description of sufferers as 'spastics'. The incidence is believed to be around 2 or 2·5 per 1,000 of the childhood community. In the majority of cases the abnormality dates from well before birth: among the factors are some genetic malformation of the brain, a congenital defect of the brain, or some adverse effect on the fetal brain as by infection during pregnancy. Among the factors during birth that may be responsible is prolonged lack of oxygen such as can occur during a difficult labour; this may be the cause in up to 15 per cent of cases. In some 10–15 per cent of cases the condition is acquired after birth, when it may be due to KERNICTERUS, infection of the brain, cerebral thrombosis or embolism, or trauma. Acute illness in infancy, such as meningitis, may result in cerebral palsy.

The disease manifests itself in many ways. It may not be finally diagnosed and characterised until the infant is two years old, but may be apparent much earlier – even soon after birth. The child may be spastic or flaccid, or the slow, writhing involuntary movements known as athetosis may be the predominant feature. These involuntary movements often disappear during sleep and may be controlled, or even abolished, in some cases by training the child to relax. The paralysis varies tremendously. It may involve the limbs on one side of the body (hemiplegia), both lower limbs (paraplegia), or all four limbs (DIPLEGIA and QUADRIPLEGIA). Learning disability (with an IQ under 70) is present in around 75 per cent of all children but children with diplegia or athetoid symptoms may have normal or even high intelligence. Associated problems may include hearing or visual disability, behavioural problems and epilepsy.

The outlook for life is good, only the more severely affected cases dying in infancy. Although there is no cure, much can be done to help these disabled children, particularly if the condition is detected at an early stage. Assistance is available from NHS developmental and assessment clinics, supervised by community paediatricians and involving a team approach from experts in education, physiotherapy, occupational therapy and speech training. In this way many of these handicapped children reach adulthood able to lead near-normal lives. Much help in dealing with these children can be obtained from SCOPE (formerly the Spastics Society), and Advice Service Capability Scotland (ASCS).

Cerebrospinal Fluid

The fluid within the ventricles of the brain and bathing its surface and that of the spinal cord. Normally a clear, colourless fluid, its pressure when an individual is lying on one side is 50 to 150 mm water. A LUMBAR PUNCTURE should not be done if the intracranial pressure is raised (see HYDROCEPHALUS).

The cerebrospinal fluid (CSF) provides useful information in various conditions and is invaluable in the diagnosis of acute and chronic inflammatory diseases of the nervous system. Bacterial MENINGITIS results in a large increase in the number of polymorphonuclear LEUCO-CYTES, while a marked lymphocytosis is seen in viral meningitis and ENCEPHALITIS, tuberculous meningitis and neurosyphilis. The total protein content is raised in many neurological diseases, being particularly high with neurofibromatosis (see VON RECKLINGHAUSEN'S DISEASE) and Guillan-Barré syndrome, while the immunoglobulin G fraction is raised in MULTIPLE SCLEROSIS (MS), neurosyphilis, and connective-tissue disorders. The glucose content is raised in diabetes (see DIABETES MELLITUS), but may be very low in bacterial meningitis, when appropriately stained smears or cultures often define the infecting organism. The CSF can also be used to measure immune proteins produced in response to infection, helping diagnosis in cases where the organism is not grown in the laboratory culture.

Cerebrovascular Accident

See STROKE.

Cerumen

The name for the wax-like secretion found in the external ear.

Cervical

Cervical means anything pertaining to the neck, or to the neck of the womb.

Cervical Cancer

Cancer of the cervix – the neck of the womb – is one of the most common cancers affecting women throughout the world. In some areas its incidence is increasing. This cancer has clearly identifiable precancerous stages with abnormal changes occurring in the cells on the surface of the cervix: these changes can be detected by a CERVICAL SMEAR test. Early cancer can be cured by diathermy, laser treatment, electrocoagulation or cryosurgery. If the disease has spread into the body of the cervix or beyond, more extensive surgery and possibly radiotherapy may be needed. The cure rate is 95 per cent if treated in the early stages but may fall as low as 10 per cent in some severe cases. Around 3,000 patients are diagnosed as having cervical cancer every year in the United Kingdom, and around 1,500 die from it. Latest figures in England show that the incidence rates have fallen to under 11 per 100,000 women, while death rates fell by more than 40 per cent during the 1990s. The sexual behaviour of a woman and her male partners influences the chances of getting this cancer; the earlier a woman has sexual intercourse, and the more partners she has, the greater is the risk of developing the disease.

Cervical Smear

This screening test detects abnormal changes in the cells of the cervix (see CERVIX UTERI), enabling an affected woman to have early treatment. The National Health Service has arrangements to check women regularly. A woman's first test should be within six months of her first experience of intercourse and thereafter at three-yearly intervals for the rest of her life. The test is simple, with some cells being scraped off the cervix with a spatula and the tissue then being examined microscopically.

Cervical Vertebrae

The seven bones of the top end of the backbone that form the neck. The first cervical vertebra is the atlas and this articulates with the base of the skull. The axis is the second vertebra, which contains a shaft of bone that allows the atlas to rotate on it, thus permitting the head to turn. (See SPINAL COLUMN.)

Cervicitis

Inflammation of the cervix uteri or neck of the womb.

Cervix Uteri

The neck of the womb or uterus, placed partly above and partly within the vagina. (See UTERUS.)

Cetavlon
See CETRIMIDE.

Cetrimide
Also known as cetavlon, cetrimide is the official name for a mixture of alkyl ammonium bromides. It is a potent antiseptic, and as a 1 per cent solution is used for cleaning and disinfecting wounds, and in the first-aid treatment of burns. As it is also a detergent, it is particularly useful for cleaning the skin, and also for cleansing and disinfecting greasy and infected bowls and baths.

Chagas' Disease
Chagas' disease, or American trypanosomiasis, is a disease widespread in Central and South America, and caused by the *Trypanosoma cruzi*. The disease is transmitted by the biting bugs, *Panstrongylus megistus* and *Triatoma infestans*. It occurs in an acute and a chronic form. The former, which is most common in children, practically always affects the heart, and the prognosis is poor. The chronic form is commonest in adolescents and young adults and the outcome depends upon the extent to which the heart is involved. There is no effective drug treatment. (See also SLEEPING SICKNESS.)

Chalazion
See EYE, DISORDERS OF.

Chalicosis
A disorder of the lungs found among stonecutters, and due to the inhalation of fine particles of stone.

Chalk-Stones
See GOUT.

Chancre
The primary lesion of SYPHILIS.

Chancroid
A soft or non-syphilitic venereal sore, caused by a micro-organism known as *Haemophilus ducreyi*. It is usually acquired by sexual contact, and responds well to treatment with antibiotics. The disease is rare in the UK.

Change of Life
See CLIMACTERIC; MENOPAUSE.

Chapped Hands
Chapped hands occur in cold weather, when reduced sweat and sebaceous activity leads to decreased natural protection of the skin. Prolonged immersion in soapy water, followed by exposure to cold air, results in cracking of the skin.

Prevention consists of minimising exposure to detergents and soapy water, and wearing rubber gloves for all routine household duties.

Chapped Lips
See LIPS.

Charcoal
Activated charcoal is a finely powdered material with a huge surface area ($1,000$ m^2/g) prepared from vegetable matter by carbonisation. It is capable of binding a variety of drugs and chemicals and is used in the treatment of poisoning as a method of gastric decontamination. It is not systemically absorbed. It is also used occasionally for flatulence and as a deodorant for skin ulcers.

Charcot's Joint
Named after a 19th-century French physician, this condition presents as a painless swelling and disorganisation of the joints resulting from damage to the pain fibres that occurs in diabetic neuropathy (see DIABETES MELLITUS – Complications), LEPROSY, SYRINGOMYELIA and syphilitic infection of the spinal cord (see SYPHILIS).

Cheilosis
Inflammation of the lips. It is common at the angles of the lips (angular stomatitis), usually as a consequence of sagging facial muscles or ill-fitting dentures producing folds at the corners of the mouth which retain food debris and allow proliferation of bacteria and candida. Atopic eczema (see SKIN, DISEASES OF) is a common cause of cheilosis of the whole of the lips.

Cheiropompholyx
Pompholyx is an old name for vesicular eczema (see DERMATITIS) on the palms and fingers (cheiropompholyx) or soles of the feet (podopompholyx).

Chelating Agents
Chelating agents are compounds that will render an ion (usually a metal) biologically inactive by incorporating it into an inner ring structure in the molecule. (Hence the name, from the Greek *chele* = claw.) When the complex formed in this way is harmless to the body and is excreted in the urine, such an agent is an effective way of ridding the body of toxic metals such

as mercury. The main chelating agents are DIMERCAPROL, PENICILLAMINE, desferrioxamine and sodium calciumedetate, used for example, in iron poisoning.

Chemosis
Swelling of the conjunctiva of the EYE, usually caused by inflammation from injury or infection.

Chemotaxis
The ability of certain cells to attract or repel others.

Chemotherapy
The prevention or treatment of disease by chemical substances. The term is generally used in two senses: the use of antibacterial and other drugs to treat infections; and the administration of ANTIMETABOLITES and other drugs to treat cancer. The discovery by Paul Ehrlich in 1910 of the action of Salvarsan in treating syphilis led to the introduction of sulphonamides in 1935, followed by PENICILLIN during World War II, which revolutionised the treatment of common infections. Many ANTIBACTERIAL DRUGS have been developed since then: these include CEPHALOSPORINS, cephamycins, TETRACYCLINES, AMINOGLYCOSIDES, MACROLIDES and CLINDAMYCIN as well as antituberculous drugs such as STREPTOMYCIN and METRONIDAZOLE. Unfortunately, overuse of chemotherapeutic drugs in medicine and in animal husbandry has stimulated widespread resistance among previously susceptible pathogenic microorganisms. Chemotherapy also plays an important role in treating tropical diseases, especially MALARIA, SLEEPING SICKNESS and LEPROSY.

Recently chemotherapy has become increasingly effective in the treatment of cancer. Numerous drugs, generally CYTOTOXIC, are available; great care is required in their selection and to minimise side-effects. Certain tumours are highly sensitive to chemotherapy – especially testicular tumours, LEUKAEMIA, LYMPHOMA and various tumours occurring in childhood (e.g. Wilm's tumour – see NEPHROBLASTOMA) – and may even be cured.

Chenodeoxycholic Acid
One of the bile acids (see BILE), used in the treatment of cholesterol gall-stones for patients with mild symptoms when other modern techniques are unsuitable. (See GALL-BLADDER, DISEASES OF.)

Chest
The chest, or THORAX, is the upper part of the trunk. It is enclosed by the breastbone (sternum) and the 12 ribs which join the sternum by way of cartilages and are attached to the spine behind. At the top of the thorax, the opening in between the first ribs admits the windpipe (TRACHEA), the gullet (OESOPHAGUS) and the large blood vessels. The bottom of the thorax is separated from the abdomen below by the muscular DIAPHRAGM which is the main muscle of breathing. Other muscles of respiration, the intercostal muscles, lie in between the ribs. Overlying the ribs are layers of muscle and soft tissue including the breast tissue.

Contents The trachea divides into right and left main bronchi which go to the two LUNGS. The left lung is slightly smaller than the right. The right has three lobes (upper, middle and lower) and the left lung has two lobes (upper and lower). Each lung is covered by two thin membranes lubricated by a thin layer of fluid. These are the pleura; similar structures cover the heart (pericardium). The heart lies in the middle, displaced slightly to the left. The oesophagus passes right through the chest to enter the stomach just below the diaphragm. Various nerves, blood vessels and lymph channels run through the thorax. The thoracic duct is the main lymphatic drainage channel emptying into a vein on the left side of the root of the neck. (For diseases affecting the chest and its contents, see HEART, DISEASES OF; LUNGS, DISEASES OF; CHEST, DEFORMITIES OF.)

Chest, Deformities of
The healthy chest is gently rounded all over, its contour being more rounded in women by the breast tissue. In cross-section it is oval-shaped with a longer dimension from side to side than from back to front.

Barrel chest is found in long-standing ASTHMA or chronic BRONCHITIS and EMPHYSEMA, when the lungs are chronically enlarged. The anterio-posterior dimension of the chest is increased and the ribs are near horizontal. In this position they can produce little further expansion of the chest, and breathing often relies on accessory muscles in the neck lifting up the whole thoracic cage on inspiration.

Pigeon chest is one in which the cross-section of the chest becomes triangular with the sternum forming a sort of keel in front. It may be related to breathing problems in early life.

Rickety chest is uncommon now and is caused by RICKETS in early life. There is a hollow down each side caused by the pull of muscles on the softer ribs in childhood. The line of knobs produced on each side where the ribs join their costal cartilages is known as the rickety rosary.

Pectus excavatum, or funnel chest, is quite a common abnormality where the central tendon of the diaphragm seems to be too short so that the lower part of the sternum is displaced inwards and the lower ribs are prominent. When severe, it may displace the heart further to the left side.

Local abnormalities in the shape of the chest occur when there is a deformity in the spine such as scoliosis which alters the angles of the ribs. The chest wall may be locally flattened when the underlying lung is reduced in size locally over a prolonged period. (See SPINE AND SPINAL CORD, DISEASES AND INJURIES OF.) This may be seen over a scarred area of lung such as that observed in pulmonary TUBERCULOSIS.

Cheyne-Stokes Breathing
A type of breathing which gets very faint for a short time, then gradually deepens until full inspirations are taken for a few seconds, and then gradually dies away to another quiet period, again increasing in depth after a few seconds and so on in cycles. It is seen in some serious neurological disorders, such as brain tumours and stroke, and also in the case of persons with advanced disease of the heart or kidneys. When well marked it is a sign that death is impending, though milder degrees of it do not carry such a serious implication in elderly patients.

Chiasma
This is an X-shaped crossing. The optic chiasma is where the nerve fibres from the nasal half of each retina cross over the mid line to join the optic tract from the other side.

Chickenpox
Also known as varicella. An acute, contagious disease predominantly of children – although it may occur at any age – characterised by fever and an eruption on the skin. The name, chickenpox, is said to be derived from the resemblance of the eruption to boiled chickpeas.

Causes The disease occurs in epidemics affecting especially children under the age of ten years. It is due to the varicella zoster virus, and the condition is an extremely infectious one from child to child. Although an attack confers life-long immunity, the virus may lie dormant and manifest itself in adult life as HERPES ZOSTER or shingles.

Symptoms There is an incubation period of 14–21 days after infection, and then the child becomes feverish or has a slight shivering, or may feel more severely ill with vomiting and pains in the back and legs. Almost at the same time, an eruption consisting of red pimples which quickly change into vesicles filled with clear fluid appears on the back and chest, sometimes about the forehead, and less frequently on the limbs. These vesicles appear over several days and during the second day may show a change of their contents to turbid, purulent fluid. Within a day or two they burst, or, at all events, shrivel up and become covered with brownish crusts. The small crusts have all dried up and fallen off in little more than a week and recovery is almost always complete.

Treatment The fever can be reduced with paracetamol and the itching soothed with CALAMINE lotion. If the child has an immune disorder, is suffering from a major complication such as pneumonia, or is very unwell, an antiviral drug (aciclovir) can be used. It is likely to be effective only at an early stage. A vaccine is available in many parts of the world but is not used in the UK; the argument against its use is that it may delay chickenpox until adult life when the disease tends to be much more severe.

Chigger
Another name for *Trombicula autumnalis*, popularly known as the harvest mite (see BITES AND STINGS).

Chilblain
Chilblain, or erythema pernio (see under ERYTHEMA), is an inflamed condition of the hands or feet, or occasionally of the ears, and should not be confused with cracked or CHAPPED HANDS. Most commonly found in childhood and old age, it may be associated with generally poor health, though there may also be a genetic predisposition. Prevention with good food, warm clothing, a warm environment, and

regular exercise to maintain the circulation, is the best treatment.

Child Abuse

This traditional term covers the neglect, physical injury, emotional trauma and sexual abuse of a child. Professional staff responsible for the care and well-being of children now refer to physical injury as 'non-accidental injury'. Child abuse may be caused by parents, relatives or carers. In England around 35,000 children are on local-authority social-service department child-protection registers – that is, are regarded as having been abused or at risk of abuse. Physical abuse or non-accidental injury is the most easily recognised form; victims of sexual abuse may not reveal their experiences until adulthood, and often not at all. Where child abuse is suspected, health, social-care and educational professionals have a duty to report the case to the local authority under the terms of the Children Act. The authority has a duty to investigate and this may mean admitting a child to hospital or to local-authority care. Abuse may be the result of impulsive action by adults or it may be premeditated: for example, the continued sexual exploitation of a child over several years. Premeditated physical assault is rare but is liable to cause serious injury to a child and requires urgent action when identified. Adults will go to some lengths to cover up persistent abuse. The child's interests are paramount but the parents may well be under severe stress and also require sympathetic handling.

In recent years persistent child abuse in some children's homes has come to light, with widespread publicity following offenders' appearances in court. Local communities have also protested about convicted paedophiles, released from prison, coming to live in their communities.

In England and Wales, local-government social-services departments are central in the prevention, investigation and management of cases of child abuse. They have four important protection duties laid down in the Children Act 1989. They are charged (1) to prevent children from suffering ill treatment and neglect; (2) to safeguard and promote the welfare of children in need; (3) when requested by a court, to investigate a child's circumstances; (4) to investigate information – in concert with the NSPCC (National Society for the Prevention of Cruelty to Children) – that a child is suffering or is likely to suffer significant harm, and to decide whether action is necessary to safeguard and promote the child's welfare. Similar provisions exist in the other parts of the United Kingdom.

When anyone suspects that child abuse is occurring, contact should be made with the relevant social-services department or, in Scotland, with the children's reporter. (See NON-ACCIDENTAL INJURY (NAI); PAEDOPHILIA.)

Child Adoption

Adoption was relatively uncommon until World War II, with only 6,000 adoption orders annually in the UK. This peaked at nearly 25,000 in 1968 as adoption became more socially acceptable and the numbers of babies born to lone mothers rose in a climate hostile to single parenthood.

Adoption declined as the availability of babies fell with the introduction of the Abortion Act 1968, improving contraceptive services and increasing acceptability of single parenthood.

However, with 10 per cent of couples suffering infertility, the demand continued, leading to the adoption of those previously perceived as difficult to place – i.e. physically, intellectually and/or emotionally disabled children and adolescents, those with terminal illness, and children of ethnic-minority groups.

Recent controversies regarding homosexual couples as adoptive parents, adoption of children with or at high risk of HIV/AIDS, transcultural adoption, and the increasing use of intercountry adoption to fulfil the needs of childless couples have provoked urgent consideration of the ethical dilemmas of adoption and its consequences for the children, their adoptive and birth families and society generally.

Detailed statistics have been unavailable since 1984 but in general there has been a downward trend with relatively more older children being placed. Detailed reasons for adoption (i.e. interfamily, step-parent, intercountry, etc.) are not available but approximately one-third are adopted from local-authority care.

In the UK all adoptions (including interfamily and step-parent adoption) must take place through a registered adoption agency which may be local-authority-based or provided by a registered voluntary agency. All local authorities must act as agencies, the voluntary agencies often providing specialist services to promote and support the adoption of more difficult-to-place children. Occasionally an adoption allowance will be awarded.

Adoption orders cannot be granted until a child has resided with its proposed adopters for 13 weeks. In the case of newborn infants the mother cannot give formal consent to placement until the baby is six weeks old, although informal arrangements can be made before this time.

In the UK the concept of responsibility of birth parents to their children and their rights to continued involvement after adoption are acknowledged by the Children Act 1989. However, in all discussions the child's interests remain paramount. The Act also recognises adopted children's need to have information regarding their origins.

BAAF – British Agencies for Adoption and Fostering – is the national organisation of adoptive agencies, both local authority and voluntary sector. The organisation promotes and provides training service, development and research; has several specialist professional subgroups (i.e. medical, legal, etc.); and produces a quarterly journal.

Adoption UK is an effective national support network of adoptive parents who offer free information, a 'listening ear' and, to members, a quarterly newsletter.

National Organisation for Counselling Adoptees and their Parents (NORCAP) is concerned with adopted children and birth parents who wish to make contact.

The Registrar General operates an Adoption Contact Register for adopted persons and anyone related to that person by blood, half-blood or marriage. Information can be obtained from the Office of Population Censuses and Surveys. For the addresses of these organisations, see Appendix 2.

Childbirth
See PREGNANCY AND LABOUR.

Child Health
Paediatrics is the branch of medicine which deals with diseases of children, but many paediatricians have a wider role, being employed largely outside acute hospitals and dealing with child health in general.

History Child health services were originally designed, before the NHS came into being, to find or prevent physical illness by regular inspections. In the UK these were carried out by clinical medical officers (CMOs) working in infant welfare clinics (later, child health clinics) set up to fill the gap between general practice and hospital care. The services expanded greatly from the mid 1970s; 'inspections' have evolved into a regular screening and surveillance system by general practitioners and health visitors, while CMOs have mostly been replaced by consultant paediatricians in community child health (CPCCH).

Screening Screening begins at birth, when every baby is examined for congenital conditions such as dislocated hips, heart malformations, cataract and undescended testicles. Blood is taken to find those babies with potentially brain-damaging conditions such as HYPO-THYROIDISM and PHENYLKETONURIA. Some NHS trusts screen for the life-threatening disease CYSTIC FIBROSIS, although in future it is more likely that finding this disease will be part of prenatal screening, along with DOWN'S (DOWN) SYNDROME and SPINA BIFIDA. A programme to detect hearing impairment in newborn babies has been piloted from 2001 in selected districts to find out whether it would be a useful addition to the national screening programme. Children from ethnic groups at risk of inherited abnormalities of HAEMO-GLOBIN (sickle cell disease; thalassaemia – see under ANAEMIA) have blood tested at some time between birth and six months of age.

Illness prevention At two months, GPs screen babies again for these abnormalities and start the process of primary IMMUNISATION. The routine immunisation programme has been dramatically successful in preventing illness, handicap and deaths: as such it is the cornerstone of the public health aspect of child health, with more potential vaccines being made available every year. Currently, infants are immunised against pertussis (see WHOOPING COUGH), DIPHTHERIA, TETANUS, POLIOMYEL-ITIS, haemophilus (a cause of MENINGITIS, SEPTICAEMIA, ARTHRITIS and epiglottitis) and meningococcus C (SEPTICAEMIA and meningitis – see NEISSERIACEAE) at two, three and four months. Selected children from high-risk groups are offered BCG VACCINE against tuberculosis and hepatitis vaccine. At about 13 months all are offered MMR VACCINE (measles, mumps and rubella) and there are pre-school entry 'boosters' of diphtheria, tetanus, polio, meningococcus C and MMR. Pneumococcal vaccine is available for particular cases but is not yet part of the routine schedule.

Health promotion and education Throughout the UK, parents are given their child's personal health record to keep with them. It contains advice on health promotion, including immunisation, developmental milestones (when did he or she first smile, sit up, walk and so on), and graphs – called centile charts – on which to record height, weight and head circumference. There is space for midwives, doctors, practice nurses, health visitors and parents to make notes about the child.

Throughout at least the first year of life, both parents and health-care providers set great store by regular weighing, designed to pick up children who are 'failing to thrive'. Measuring length is not quite so easy, but height measurements are recommended from about two or three years of age in order to detect children with disorders such as growth-hormone deficiency, malabsorption (e.g. COELIAC DISEASE) and psychosocial dwarfism (see below).

All babies have their head circumference measured at birth, and again at the eight-week check. A too rapidly growing head implies that the infant might have HYDROCEPHALUS – excess fluid in the hollow spaces within the brain. A too slowly growing head may mean failure of brain growth, which may go hand in hand with physically or intellectually delayed development.

At about eight months, babies receive a surveillance examination, usually by a health visitor. Parents are asked if they have any concerns about their child's hearing, vision or physical ability. The examiner conducts a screening test for hearing impairment – the so-called distraction test; he or she stands behind the infant, who is on the mother's lap, and activates a standardised sound at a set distance from each ear, noting whether or not the child turns his or her head or eyes towards the sound. If the child shows no reaction, the test is repeated a few weeks later; if still negative then referral is made to an audiologist for more formal testing.

The doctor or health visitor will also go through the child's developmental progress (see above) noting any significant deviation from normal which merits more detailed examination. Doctors are also recommended to examine infants developmentally at some time between 18 and 24 months. At this time they will be looking particularly for late walking or failure to develop appropriate language skills.

Child development teams (CDTs)

Screening and surveillance uncover problems which then need careful attention. Most NHS districts have a CDT to carry out this task – working from child development centres – usually separate from hospitals. Various therapists, as well as consultant paediatricians in community child health, contribute to the work of the team. They include physiotherapists, occupational therapists, speech therapists, psychologists, health visitors and, in some centres, pre-school teachers or educational advisers and social workers. Their aims are to diagnose the child's problems, identify his or her therapy needs and make recommendations to the local health and educational authorities on how these should be met. A member of the team will usually be appointed as the family's 'key worker', who liaises with other members of the team and coordinates the child's management. Regular review meetings are held, generally with parents sharing in the decisions made. Mostly children seen by CDTs are under five years old, the school health service and educational authorities assuming responsibility thereafter.

Special needs The Children Act 1989, Education Acts 1981, 1986 and 1993, and the Chronically Sick and Disabled Persons Legislation 1979 impose various statutory duties to identify and provide assistance for children with special needs. They include the chronically ill as well as those with impaired development or disabilities such as CEREBRAL PALSY, or hearing, vision or intellectual impairment. Many CDTs keep a register of such children so that services can be efficiently planned and evaluated. Parents of disabled children often feel isolated and neglected by society in general; they are frequently frustrated by the lack of resources available to help them cope with the sheer hard work involved. The CDT, through its key workers, does its best to absorb anger and divert frustration into constructive actions.

There are other groups of children who come to the attention of child health services. Community paediatricians act as advisers to adoption and fostering agencies, vital since many children needing alternative homes have special medical or educational needs or have behavioural or psychiatric problems. Many see a role in acting as advocates, not just for those with impairments but also for socially disadvantaged children, including those 'looked after' in children's homes and those of travellers, asylum seekers, refugees and the homeless.

Child protection Regrettably, some children come to the attention of child health specialists because they have been beaten, neglected, emotionally or nutritionally starved or sexually assaulted by their parents or carers. Responsibility for the investigation of these children is that of local-authority social-services departments. However, child health professionals have a vital role in diagnosis, obtaining forensic evidence, advising courts, supervising the medical aspects of follow-up and teaching doctors, therapists and other professionals in training. (See CHILD ABUSE.)

School health services Once children have reached school age, the emphasis changes. The prime need becomes identifying those with problems that may interfere with learning – including those with special needs as defined above, but also those with behavioural problems. Teachers and parents are advised on how to manage these problems, while health promotion and health education are directed at children. Special problems, especially as children reach secondary school (aged 11–18) include accidents, substance abuse, psychosexual adjustment, antisocial behaviour, eating disorders and physical conditions which loom large in the minds of adolescents in particular, such as ACNE, short stature and delayed puberty.

There is no longer, in the UK, a universal school health service as many of its functions have been taken over by general practitioners and hospital and community paediatricians. However, most areas still have school nurses, some have school doctors, while others do not employ specific individuals for these tasks but share out aspects of the work between GPs, health visitors, community nurses and consultant paediatricians in child health.

Complementing their work is the community dental service whose role is to monitor the whole child population's dental health, provide preventive programmes for all, and dental treatment for those who have difficulty using general dental services – for example, children with complex disability. All children in state-funded schools are dentally screened at ages five and 15.

Successes and failures Since the inception of the NHS, hospital services for children have had enormous success: neonatal and infant mortality rates have fallen by two-thirds; deaths from PNEUMONIA have fallen from 600 per million children to a handful; and deaths from MENINGITIS have fallen to one-fifth of the previous level. Much of this has been due to the revolution in the management of pregnancy and labour, the invention of neonatal resuscitation and neonatal intensive care, and the provision of powerful antibiotics.

At the same time, some children acquire HIV infection and AIDS from their affected mothers (see AIDS/HIV); the prevalence of atopic (see ATOPY) diseases (ASTHMA, eczema – see DERMATITIS, HAY FEVER) is rising; more children attend hos-pital clinics with chronic CONSTIPATION; and little can be done for most viral diseases.

Community child health services can also boast of successes. The routine immunisation programme has wiped out SMALLPOX, DIPHTHERIA and POLIOMYELITIS and almost wiped out haemophilus and meningococcal C meningitis, measles and congenital RUBELLA syndrome. WHOOPING COUGH outbreaks continue but the death and chronic disability rates have been greatly reduced. Despite these huge health gains, continuing public scepticism about the safety of immunisation means that there can be no relaxation in the educational and health-promotion programme.

Services for severely and multiply disabled children have improved beyond all recognition with the closure of long-stay institutions, many of which were distinctly child-unfriendly. Nonetheless, scarce resources mean that families still carry heavy burdens. The incidence of SUDDEN INFANT DEATH SYNDROME (SIDS) has more than halved as a result of an educational programme based on firm scientific evidence that the risk can be reduced by putting babies to sleep on their backs, avoidance of parental smoking, not overheating, breast feeding and seeking medical attention early for illness.

Children have fewer accidents and better teeth but new problems have arisen: in the 1990s children throughout the developed world became fatter. A UK survey in 2004 found that one in five children are overweight and one in 20 obese. Lack of exercise, the easy availability of food at all times and in all places, together with the rise of 'snacking', are likely to provoke significant health problems as these children grow into adult life. Adolescents are at greater risk than ever of ill-health through substance abuse and unplanned pregnancy. Child health services are facing new challenges in the 21st century.

Children Act

The Children Act 1989 (Children Act) introduced major reforms of child-care law. It encourages negotiation and cooperation between parents, children and professionals to resolve problems affecting children. The aim is to enable children to stay within their own families with appropriate back-up from local-authority and professional resources. The emphasis is on empowering families rather than paternalistic control. The Act set up a court made up of three tiers – the High Court, county court and magistrates' court – each with concurrent jurisdiction. The Act has been broadened, clarified and interpreted by subsidiary legislation, rules, case law and official guidance. An equivalent act is in force in Scotland.

Chills
See COLD, COMMON.

Chimera
Chimera is an organism, whether plant, animal or human being, in which there are at least two kinds of tissue differing in their genetic constitution.

Chinese Avian Influenza
A variety of influenza in chickens occurring in southern China that in 1997 appeared to jump the species barrier and infect humans. Some cases of the human version of the infection occurred in Hong Kong. There were fears of a serious epidemic which, because of a lack of natural resistance among humans, might have led to its worldwide spread. This has not so far occurred.

Chiropody
Chiropody (also termed podiatry) is that part of medical science which is concerned with the health of the feet. Its practitioners are specialists capable of providing a fully comprehensive foot-health service. This includes the palliation of established deformities and dysfunction, both as short-term treatment for immediate relief of painful symptoms and as long-term management to secure optimum results. This requires the backing of effective appliances and footwear services. It also involves curative foot-care, including the use of various therapeutic techniques, including minor surgery and the prescription and provision of specialised and individual appliances.

Among conditions routinely treated are walking disorders in children, injuries to the feet of joggers and athletes, corns, bunions and hammer toes, ulcers and foot infections. Chiropody also has a preventative role which includes inspection of children's feet and the detection of foot conditions requiring treatment and advice and also foot-health education. The chiropodist is trained to recognise medical conditions which manifest themselves in the feet, such as circulatory disorders, DIABETES MELLITUS and diseases causing ulceration.

The only course of training in the United Kingdom recognised for the purpose of state registration by the Health Professionals Council is the Society of Chiropodists' three-year full-time course. The course includes instruction and examination in the relevant aspects of anatomy and physiology, local analgesia, medicine and surgery, as well as in podology and therapeutics. The Council holds the register of podiatrists. (See APPENDIX 2: ADDRESSES: SOURCES OF INFORMATION, ADVICE, SUPPORT AND SELF-HELP.)

Chiropractor
A person who practises chiropractic – mainly a system of physical manipulations of minor displacements of the spinal column. These minor displacements (see SUBLUXATION) of the spine are believed to affect the associated or neighbouring nerves and so cause malfunctions of the muscles throughout the body. By manipulating the affected part of the spinal column the patient's complaint, whatever it may be – for example, backache – is relieved.

Chlamydia
A genus of micro-organisms which include those responsible for NON-SPECIFIC URETHRITIS (NSU), ORNITHOSIS, PSITTACOSIS and TRACHOMA. *Chlamydia trachomitis* can be sexually transmitted by both men and women and in developed countries is the most significant cause of NSU. Chlamydia and *Neisseria gonorrhoea* (see GONORRHOEA) are the major cause of PELVIC INFLAMMATORY DISEASE (PID) which affects around 100,000 women a year in the UK, most of whom are under 25 years of age. Chlamydia does not usually cause symptoms unless it spreads to the upper genital tract; such spread, however, may cause miscarriage (see PREGNANCY AND LABOUR) or ECTOPIC PREGNANCY. The number of diagnoses of chlamydia has doubled in the past five years and the incidence of ectopic pregnancies has also been rising. The infection may well be the main preventable cause of ectopic pregnancy, one estimate being that no fewer than half of such pregnancies are linked to chlamydia infection – a figure that is probably much higher in young women. A preventive campaign in Sweden found that over 15 years, the incidence of ectopic pregnancies fell at the same rate as that of chlamydia diagnoses. Chlamydia infection responds well to antibiotic treatment, but education of the public about this often 'silent' infection, coupled with screening programmes, would go a long way to reducing the incidence.

Chloasma
This is an increase in the melanin pigment of the skin as a result of hormonal stimulation. It is commonly seen in pregnancy and sometimes

in women on the contraceptive pill. It mainly affects the face.

Chloral Hydrate
This drug is now rarely used but chloral betaine (Welldorm) is occasionally used in the elderly and in newborns with fits or cerebral irritation after a difficult delivery.

Chlorambucil
One of several ALKYLATING AGENTS widely used in cancer chemotherapy, chlorambucil is an oral drug commonly used to treat chronic lymphocytic LEUKEMIA, non-Hodgkin's lymphomas, Hodgkin's disease (see LYMPHOMA) and ovarian cancer (see OVARIES, DISEASES OF). Apart from suppression of bone-marrow activity, side-effects are few.

Chloramphenicol
An antibiotic derived from a soil organism, *Streptomyces venezuelae*. It is also prepared synthetically. A potent broad-spectrum antibiotic, chloramphenicol may, however, cause serious side-effects such as aplastic ANAEMIA, peripheral NEURITIS, optic neuritis and, in neonates, abdominal distension and circulatory collapse. The drug should therefore be reserved for the treatment of life-threatening infections such as *Haemophilus influenzae*, SEPTICAEMIA or MENINGITIS, typhoid fever (see ENTERIC FEVER) and TYPHUS FEVER, when the causative organism proves resistant to other drugs. However, because it is inexpensive, it is used widely in developing countries. This antibiotic is available as drops for use in eye and ear infection, where safety is not a problem.

Chlordane
An insecticide which has been used sucessfully against flies and mosquitoes resistant to DDT (see DICHLORODIPHENYL TRICHLOROETHANE), and for the control of ticks and mites. It requires special handling as it is toxic to humans when applied to the skin.

Chlordiazepoxide
A widely used anti-anxiety drug. (See TRANQUILLISERS; BENZODIAZEPINES.)

Chlorhexidine
An antiseptic which has a bacteriostatic action against many bacteria.

Chlorine
See SODIUM HYPOCHLORITE.

Chloroma
Chloroma, or green cancer, is the name of a disease in which greenish growths appear under the skin, and in which a change takes place in the blood resembling that in leukaemia.

Chlorophyll
The green colouring matter of plants. Its main use is as a colouring agent, principally for soaps, oils and fats. It is also being found of value as a deodorant dressing to remove, or diminish, the unpleasant odour of heavily infected sores and wounds.

Chloroquine
Chloroquine, which is a 4-aminoquinoline, was introduced during World War II for the treatment of MALARIA. The drug is also used for PROPHYLAXIS against malaria where the risk of chloroquine-resistant falciparum is still low. It has also been found of value in the treatment of the skin condition known as chronic discoid lupus erythematosus, and of rheumatoid arthritis.

Chlorpromazine
Chlorpromazine is chemically related to the antihistamine drug, PROMETHAZINE HYDROCHLORIDE. One of the first antipsychotic drugs to be marketed, it is used extensively in psychiatry on account of its action in calming psychotic activity without producing undue general depression or clouding of consciousness. The drug is used particularly in SCHIZOPHRENIA and mania. It carries a risk of contact sensitisation, so should be handled with care, and the drug has a wide range of side-effects.

Chlorpropamide
An oral hypoglycaemic agent, chlorpropamide was for many years used to treat diabetes (see DIABETES MELLITUS). It has been largely superseded by more effective oral agents with fewer side-effects, such as gliclazide.

Chlortetracycline
See TETRACYCLINES.

Choking
Choking is the process which results from an obstruction to breathing situated in the larynx (see AIR PASSAGES). It may occur as the result of disease causing swelling round the glottis (the entrance to the larynx), or of some nervous disorders that interfere with the regulation of the muscles which open and shut the larynx. Generally, however, it is due to the irritation of a piece of food or other substance introduced by the mouth, which provokes coughing but only

partly interferes with breathing. As the mucous membrane lining the upper part of the latter is especially sensitive, coughing results in order to expel the cause of irritation. At the same time, if the foreign body is of any size, lividity of the face appears, due to partial suffocation (see ASPHYXIA).

Treatment The choking person should take slow, deep inspirations, which do not force the particle further in (as sudden catchings of the breath between the coughs do), and which produce more powerful coughs. If the coughing is weak, one or two strong blows with the palm of the hand over either shoulder blade, timed to coincide with coughs, aid the effect of the coughing. If this is ineffective, the Heimlich manoeuvre may be used. This involves hugging the person from behind with one's hands just under the diaphragm. A sudden upward compressive movement is made which serves to dislodge any foreign body. In the case of a baby, sit down with left forearm resting on thigh. Place the baby chest-down along the forearm, holding its head and jaw with the fingers and thumb. The infant's head should be lower than its trunk. Gently deliver three or four blows between the shoulder blades with the free hand. The resuscitator should not attempt blind finger-sweeps at the back of the mouth; these can impact a foreign body in the larynx.

If normal breathing (in adult or child) cannot be quickly restored, seek urgent medical help. Sometimes an emergency TRACHEOSTOMY is necessary to restore the air supply to the lungs. (See APPENDIX 1: BASIC FIRST AID.)

Cholagogues
Substances which increase the flow of BILE by stimulating evacuation of the gall-bladder (see LIVER). The great majority of these act only by increasing the activity of the digestive organs, and so producing a flow of bile already stored up in the gall-bladder. Substances which stimulate the liver to secrete more bile are known as CHOLERETIC.

Cholangiography
The process whereby the bile ducts (see BILE DUCT) and the gall-bladder (see LIVER) are rendered radio-opaque and therefore visible on an X-ray film.

Cholangitis
Inflammation of the bile ducts (see BILE DUCT; GALL-BLADDER, DISEASES OF).

Cholecystectomy
Removal of the gall-bladder (see LIVER) by operation.

Cholecystitis
Inflammation of the gall-bladder (see GALL-BLADDER, DISEASES OF).

Cholecystography
The process whereby the gall-bladder (see LIVER) is rendered radio-opaque and therefore visisble on an X-ray film.

Cholecystokinin
The hormone (see HORMONES) released from the lining membrane of the DUODENUM when food is taken, and which initiates emptying of the gall-bladder (see LIVER).

Cholelithiasis
The presence of gall-stones in the bile ducts and/or in the gall-bladder. (See GALL-BLADDER, DISEASES OF.)

Cholelithotomy
The removal of gall-stones from the gall-bladder or bile ducts (see GALL-BLADDER, DISEASES OF), when CHOLECYSTECTOMY or LITHOTRIPSY are inappropriate or not possible. It involves a cholecystomy, an operation to open the gall-bladder.

Cholera
Bacterial infection caused by *Vibrio cholerae*. The patient suffers profuse watery DIARRHOEA, and resultant dehydration and electrolyte imbalance. Formerly known as the Asiatic cholera, the disease has occurred in epidemics and pandemics for many centuries. When it entered Europe in 1853, Dr John Snow, a London anaesthetist, carried out seminal epidemiological work in Soho, London, which established that the source of infection was contaminated drinking water derived from the Broad Street pump. Several smaller epidemics involved Europe in the latter years of the 19th century, but none has arisen in Britain or the United States for many years. In 1971, the El Tor biotype of *V. cholerae* emerged, replacing much of the classical infection in Asia and, to a much lesser extent, Europe; parts of Africa were seriously affected. Recently a non-01 strain has arisen and is causing much disease in Asia. Cholera remains a major health problem (this is technically the seventh pandemic) in many countries of Asia, Africa and South America. It is one of three quarantinable infections.

Incubation period varies from a few hours to

five days. Watery diarrhoea may be torrential and the resultant dehydration and electrolyte imbalance, complicated by cardiac failure, commonly causes death. The victim's skin elasticity is lost, the eyes are sunken, and the radial pulse may be barely perceptible. Urine production may be completely suppressed. Diagnosis is by detection of *V. cholerae* in a faecal sample. Treatment consists of rapid rehydration. Whereas the intravenous route may be required in a severe case, in the vast majority of patients oral rehydration (using an appropriate solution containing sodium chloride, glucose, sodium bicarbonate, and potassium) gives satisfactory results. Proprietary rehydration fluids do not always contain adequate sodium for rehydration in a severe case. ANTIBIOTICS, for example, tetracycline and doxycycline, reduce the period during which *V. cholerae* is excreted (in children and pregnant women, furazolidone is safer); in an epidemic, rapid resistance to these, and other antibiotics, has been clearly demonstrated. Prevention consists of improving public health infrastructure – in particular, the quality of drinking water. When supplies of the latter are satisfactory, the infection fails to thrive. Though there have recently been large epidemics of cholera in much of South America and parts of central Africa and the Indian subcontinent, the risk of tourists and travellers contracting the disease is low if they take simple precautions. These include eating safe food (avoid raw or undercooked seafood, and wash vegetables in clean water) and drinking clean water. There is no cholera vaccine at present available in the UK as it provides little protection and cannot control spread of the disease. Those travelling to countries where it exists should pay scrupulous attention to food and water cleanliness and to personal hygiene.

Choleretic

The term applied to a drug that stimulates the flow of BILE.

Cholestasis

A reduction or stoppage in the flow of BILE into the intestine caused either by a blockage such as a stone in the BILE DUCT or by liver disease disturbing the production of bile. The first type is called extrahepatic biliary obstruction and the second, intrahepatic cholestasis. The patient develops jaundice and itching and passes dark urine and pale faeces. Cholestasis may occasionally occur during pregnancy.

Cholesterol

A LIPID that is an important constituent of body cells and so widely distributed throughout the body. It is especially abundant in the brain, nervous tissue, adrenal glands and skin. It is also found in egg yolk and gall-stones (see GALL-BLADDER, DISEASES OF). Cholesterol plays an important role in the body, being essential for the production of the sex hormones as well as for the repair of membranes. It is also the source from which BILE acids are manufactured. The total amount in the body of a man weighing 70 kilograms (10 stones) is around 140 grams, and the amount present in the blood is 3·6–7·8 mmol per litre or 150–250 milligrams per 100 millilitres.

A high blood-cholesterol level – that is, one over 6 mmol per litre or 238 mg per 100 ml – is undesirable as there appears to be a correlation between a high blood cholesterol and ATHEROMA, the form of arterial degenerative disease associated with coronary thrombosis and high blood pressure. This is well exemplified in DIABETES MELLITUS and HYPOTHYROIDISM, two diseases in which there is a high blood cholesterol, sometimes going as high as 20 mmol per litre; patients with these diseases are known to be particularly prone to arterial disease. There is also a familial disease known as hypercholesterolaemia, in which members of affected families have a blood cholesterol of around 18 mmol per litre or more, and are particularly liable to premature degenerative disease of the arteries. Many experts believe that there is no 'safe level' and that everybody should attempt to keep their cholesterol level as low as possible.

Cholesterol exists in three forms in the blood: high-density lipoproteins (HDLs) which are believed to protect against arterial disease, and a low-density version (LDLs) and very low-density type (VLDLs), these latter two being risk factors.

The rising incidence of arterial disease in western countries in recent years has drawn attention to this relationship between high levels of cholesterol in the blood and arterial disease. The available evidence indicates that there is a relationship between blood-cholesterol levels and the amount of fat consumed; however, the blood-cholesterol level bears little relationship to the amount of cholesterol consumed, most of the cholesterol in the body being produced by the body itself.

On the other hand, diets high in saturated fatty acids – chiefly animal fats such as red meat, butter and dripping – tend to raise the blood-cholesterol level; while foods high in unsaturated fatty acids – chiefly vegetable products such as olive and sunflower oils, and oily fish such as mackerel and herring – tend to lower it. There is a tendency in western society to eat too much animal fat, and current health recommendations are for everyone to decrease saturated-fat intake, increase unsaturated-fat intake, increase daily exercise, and avoid obesity. This advice is particulary important for people with high blood-cholesterol levels, with diabetes mellitus, or with a history of coronary thrombosis (see HEART, DISEASES OF). As well as a low-cholesterol diet, people with high cholesterol values or arterial disease may be given cholesterol-reducing drugs such as STATINS, but this treatment requires full clinical assessment and ongoing medical monitoring. Recent research involving the world's largest trial into the effects of treatment to lower concentrations of cholesterol in the blood showed that routine use of drugs such as statins reduced the incidence of heart attacks and strokes by one-third, even in people with normal levels of cholesterol. The research also showed that statins benefited women and the over-70s.

Choline

One of the many constituents of the vitamin B complex. Lack of it in the experimental animal produces a fatty liver. It is found in egg-yolk, liver, and meat. The probable daily human requirement is 500 mg, an amount amply covered by the ordinary diet. Choline can be synthesised by the body (see APPENDIX 5: VITAMINS).

Cholinergic

A description of nerve fibres that release ACETYLCHOLINE as a NEUROTRANSMITTER.

Cholinesterase

An ENZYME that helps to break down the neurotransmitter compound ACETYLCHOLINE.

Chondroma

A TUMOUR composed in part of cartilage.

Chorda

A nerve-fibre, tendon or cord.

Chorea

Chorea, or St Vitus's dance, is the occurrence of short, purposeless involuntary movements of the face, head, hands and feet. Movements are sudden, but the affected person may hold the new posture for several seconds. Chorea is often accompanied by ATHETOSIS, when it is termed choreoathetosis. Choreic symptoms are often due to disease of the basal ganglion in the brain. The withdrawal of phenothiazines may cause the symptoms, as can the drugs used to treat PARKINSONISM. Types of chorea include HUNTINGTON'S CHOREA, an inherited disease, and SYDENHAM'S CHOREA, which is autoimmune. There is also a degenerative form – senile chorea.

Choriocarcinoma

A form of cancer affecting the CHORION, in the treatment of which particularly impressive results are being obtained from the use of methotrexate.

Chorion

This is the more external of the two fetal membranes. (See PLACENTA.)

Chorionic Gonadotrophic Hormone

A hormone produced by the PLACENTA during pregnancy. It is similar to the pituitary GONADOTROPHINS, which are blocked during pregnancy. Large amounts appear in a woman's urine when she is pregnant and are used as the basis for pregnancy tests. Human gonadotrophins are used to treat delayed puberty and premenstrual tension.

Choroid

See EYE.

Choroiditis

See UVEITIS.

Choroid Plexus

An extensive web of blood vessels occurring in the ventricles of the BRAIN and producing the CEREBROSPINAL FLUID.

Christmas Disease

A hereditary disorder of blood coagulation which can only be distinguished from HAEMOPHILIA by laboratory tests. It is so-called after the surname of the first case reported in this country. About one in every ten patients clinically diagnosed as haemophiliac has in fact Christmas disease. It is due to lack in the blood of Factor IX (see COAGULATION).

Chromaffin

A term applied to certain cells and organs in the body, such as part of the adrenal glands, which have a peculiar affinity for chrome salts. These cells and tissues generally are supposed to secrete substances which have an important action in maintaining the tone and elasticity of the blood vessels and muscles.

Chromatin

The genetic material found in the nucleus of a cell. It consists of PROTEIN and deoxyribonucleic acid (DNA). During mitotic division of the cell, chromatin condenses into CHROMOSOMES.

Chromic Acid

Chromic acid is used in several industries, particularly in chromium plating. Unless precautions are taken it may lead to dermatitis of the hands, arms, chest and face. It may also cause deep ulcers, especially of the nasal septum and knuckles.

Chromosomes

The rod-shaped bodies to be found in the nucleus of every cell in the body. They contain the GENES, or hereditary elements, which establish the characteristics of an individual. Composed of a long double-coiled filament of DNA, they occur in pairs – one from the maternal, the other from the paternal – and human beings possess 46, made up of 23 pairs. The number of chromosomes is specific for each species of animal. Each chromosone can duplicate an exact copy of itself between each cell division. (See GENETIC CODE; GENETICS; HEREDITY; MEIOSIS; SEX CHROMOSOMES.)

Chronic Disorder

A persistent or recurring condition or group of symptoms. Chronic disorders are customarily contrasted with acute diseases which start suddenly and last a short time. The symptoms of acute disease often include breathlessness, fever, severe pain and malaise, with the patient's condition changing from day to day or even hour to hour. Those suffering from chronic conditions – for example, severe arthritis, protracted lung disease, ASTHMA or SILICOSIS – should be distinguished from those with a 'static disability' following a stroke or injury. Chronic disorders steadily deteriorate, often despite treatment and the patient is increasingly unable to carry out his or her daily activities.

Chronic Fatigue Syndrome (CFS)

See also MYALGIC ENCEPHALOMYELITIS (ME). A condition characterised by severe, disabling mental and physical fatigue brought on by mental or physical activity and associated with a range of symptoms including muscle pain, headaches, poor sleep, disturbed moods and impaired concentration. The prevalence of the condition is between 0.2 and 2.6 per cent of the population (depending on how investigators define CFS/ME). Despite the stereotype of 'yuppie flu', epidemiological research has shown that the condition occurs in all socio-economic and ethnic groups. It is commoner in women and can also occur in children.

In the 19th century CFS was called neurasthenia. In the UK, myalgic encephalomyelitis (ME) is often used, a term originally introduced to describe a specific outbreak such as the one at the Royal Free Hospital, London in 1955. The term is inaccurate as there is no evidence of inflammation of the brain and spinal cord (the meaning of encephalomyelitis). Doctors prefer the term CFS, but many patients see this as derogatory, perceiving it to imply that they are merely 'tired all the time' rather than having a disabling illness.

The cause (or causes) are unknown, so the condition is classified alongside other 'medically unexplained syndromes' such as IRRITABLE BOWEL SYNDROME (IBS) and multiple chemical sensitivity – all of which overlap with CFS. In many patients the illness seems to start immediately after a documented infection, such as that caused by EPSTEIN BARR VIRUS, or after viral MENINGITIS, Q FEVER and TOXOPLASMOSIS. These infections seem to be a trigger rather than a cause: mild immune activation is found in patients, but it is not known if this is cause or effect. The body's endocrine system is disturbed, particularly the hypothalamo-pituitary-adrenal axis, and levels of cortisol are often a little lower than normal – the opposite of what is found in severe depression. Psychiatric disorder, usually depression and/or anxiety, is associated with CFS, with rates too high to be explained solely as a reaction to the disability experienced.

Because we do not know the cause, the underlying problem cannot be dealt with effectively and treatments are directed at the factors leading to symptoms persisting. For example, a slow increase in physical activity can help many, as can COGNITIVE BEHAVIOUR THERAPY. Too much rest can be harmful, as muscles are rapidly weakened, but aggressive attempts at coercing patients into exercising can be counter-productive as their symptoms may worsen. Outcome is influenced by the presence of any pre-existing psychiatric disorder and the sufferer's beliefs about its causes and treatment. Research continues.

Chronic Obstructive Pulmonary Disease (COPD)

This is a term encompassing chronic BRONCHITIS, EMPHYSEMA, and chronic ASTHMA where the airflow into the lungs is obstructed.

Chronic bronchitis is typified by chronic productive cough for at least three months in two successive years (provided other causes such as TUBERCULOSIS, lung cancer and chronic heart failure have been excluded). The characteristics of emphysema are abnormal and permanent enlargement of the airspaces (alveoli) at the furthermost parts of the lung tissue. Rupture of alveoli occurs, resulting in the creation of air spaces with a gradual breakdown in the lung's ability to oxygenate the blood and remove carbon dioxide from it (see LUNGS). Asthma results in inflammation of the airways with the lining of the BRONCHIOLES becoming hypersensitive, causing them to constrict. The obstruction may spontaneously improve or do so in response to bronchodilator drugs. If an asthmatic patient's airway-obstruction is characterised by incomplete reversibility, he or she is deemed to have a form of COPD called asthmatic bronchitis; sufferers from this disorder cannot always be readily distinguished from those people who have chronic bronchitis and/ or emphysema. Symptoms and signs of emphysema, chronic bronchitis and asthmatic bronchitis overlap, making it difficult sometimes to make a precise diagnosis. Patients with completely reversible airflow obstruction without the features of chronic bronchitis or emphysema, however, are considered to be suffering from asthma but not from COPD.

The incidence of COPD has been increasing, as has the death rate. In the UK around 30,000 people with COPD die annually and the disorder makes up 10 per cent of all admissions to hospital medical wards, making it a serious cause of illness and disability. The prevalence, incidence and mortality rates increase with age, and more men than women have the disorder, which is also more common in those who are socially disadvantaged.

Causes The most important cause of COPD is cigarette smoking, though only 15 per cent of smokers are likely to develop clinically significant symptoms of the disorder. Smoking is believed to cause persistent airway inflammation and upset the normal metabolic activity in the lung. Exposure to chemical impurities and dust in the atmosphere may also cause COPD.

Signs and symptoms Most patients develop inflammation of the airways, excessive growth of mucus-secreting glands in the airways, and changes to other cells in the airways. The result is that mucus is transported less effectively along the airways to eventual evacuation as sputum. Small airways become obstructed and the alveoli lose their elasticity. COPD usually starts with repeated attacks of productive cough, commonly following winter colds; these attacks progressively worsen and eventually the patient develops a permanent cough. Recurrent respiratory infections, breathlessness on exertion, wheezing and tightness of the chest follow. Bloodstained and/or infected sputum are also indicative of established disease. Among the symptoms and signs of patients with advanced obstruction of airflow in the lungs are:

- RHONCHI (abnormal musical sounds heard through a STETHOSCOPE when the patient breathes out).
- marked indrawing of the muscles between the ribs and development of a barrel-shaped chest.
- loss of weight.
- CYANOSIS in which the skin develops a blue tinge because of reduced oxygenation of blood in the blood vessels in the skin.
- bounding pulse with changes in heart rhythm.
- OEDEMA of the legs and arms.
- decreasing mobility.

Some patients with COPD have increased ventilation of the alveoli in their lungs, but the levels of oxygen and carbon dioxide are normal so their skin colour is normal. They are, however, breathless so are dubbed 'pink puffers'. Other patients have reduced alveolar ventilation which lowers their oxygen levels causing cyanosis; they also develop COR PULMONALE, a form of heart failure, and become oedematous, so are called 'blue bloaters'.

Investigations include various tests of lung function, including the patient's response to bronchodilator drugs. Exercise tests may help, but radiological assessment is not usually of great diagnostic value in the early stages of the disorder.

Treatment depends on how far COPD has progressed. Smoking must be stopped – also an essential preventive step in healthy individuals. Early stages are treated with bronchodilator drugs to relieve breathing symptoms. The next stage is to introduce steroids (given by inhalation). If symptoms worsen, physiotherapy – breathing exercises and postural drainage – is valuable and annual vaccination against INFLUENZA is strongly advised. If the patient develops breathlessness on mild exertion, has cyanosis, wheezing and permanent cough and tends to HYPERVENTILATION, then oxygen therapy should be considered. Antibiotic treatment is necessary if overt infection of the lungs develops.

Complications Sometimes rupture of the pulmonary bullae (thin-walled airspaces produced by the breakdown of the walls of the alveoli) may cause PNEUMOTHORAX and also exert pressure on functioning lung tissue. Respiratory failure and failure of the right side of the heart (which controls blood supply to the lungs), known as cor pulmonale, are late complications in patients whose primary problem is emphysema.

Prognosis This is related to age and to the extent of the patient's response to bronchodilator drugs. Patients with COPD who develop raised pressure in the heart/lung circulation and subsequent heart failure (cor pulmonale) have a bad prognosis.

Chronic Sick and Disabled Act 1970

UK legislation that provides for the identification and care of individuals who have an incurable chronic or degenerative disorder. The patients are usually distinguished from elderly people with chronic disorders. Local authorities identify relevant individuals and arrange for appropriate services. The legislation does not, however, compel doctors and nurses in the community to inform local authorities of potential beneficiaries. This may be because the individuals concerned dislike being on a register of disabled, or because questions of confidentiality prevent health staff from reporting the person's condition.

Chyle

The milky fluid which is absorbed by the lymphatic vessels of the intestine. The absorbed portion consists of fats in very fine emulsion, like milk, so that these vessels receive the name of lacteals (L. *lac*, milk). This absorbed chyle mixes with the lymph and is discharged into the thoracic duct, a vessel, which passes up through the chest to open into the jugular vein on the left side of the neck, where the chyle mixes with the blood.

Chyluria

The passage of CHYLE in the urine. This results in the passing of a milky-looking urine. It is one of the manifestations of FILARIASIS, where it is due to obstruction of the LYMPHATICS by the causative parasite.

Chyme

Partly digested food as it issues from the stomach into the intestine. It is very acid and grey in colour, containing salts and sugars in solution, and the animal food softened into a semi-liquid mass. It is next converted into CHYLE.

Chymopapain

An ENZYME obtained from the paw-paw, which is being used in the treatment of prolapsed INTERVERTEBRAL DISC. When injected into the disc it dissolves the cartilage tissue.

Chymotrypsin

An ENZYME produced by the PANCREAS which digests protein. It is used as an aid in operations for removal of a cataract (see ZONULOLYSIS), and also by inhalation to loosen and liquefy secretions in the windpipe and bronchi.

Cicatrix

Another word for scar.

Ciclosporin A

A drug used to prevent the rejection of transplanted organs such as the heart and kidneys. (See TRANSPLANTATION.)

Cilia

A term applied to minute, lash-like processes which are seen with the aid of the microscope upon the cells covering certain mucous membranes – for example, the TRACHEA (or windpipe) and nose – and which maintain movement in the fluid passing over these membranes. They are also found on certain bacteria which have the power of rapid movement.

Ciliary Body

That part of the EYE that connects the iris and the choroid. The ciliary ring is next to the choroid; the ciliary processes comprise many ridges behind the iris, to which the lens's suspensory ligament is attached; and the ciliary muscle contracts to change the curvature of the lens and so adjust the accommodation of the eye.

Cimetidine

Cimetidine is a drug (known as an H_2 receptor antagonist) that is widely used in the treatment of PEPTIC ULCER. It acts by reducing the hyperacidity of the gastric juice by antagonising histamine receptors in the stomach.

Cimex Lectularius

See BED BUG.

Cinchona

The general name for several trees in the bark of which QUININE is found. This bark is also known as Jesuit's bark, having been first brought to notice by Spanish priests in South America, and first brought to Europe by the Countess of Cinchon, wife of the Viceroy of Peru, in 1640. The red cinchona bark contains the most quinine; quinine is usually prepared from this. Various extracts and tinctures are made direct from cinchona bark, and used in place of quinine.

Ciprofloxacin

A quinolone antibiotic (see QUINOLONES) used to treat typhoid and paratyphoid infections (see ENTERIC FEVER).

Circle of Willis

A circle of arteries at the base of the brain, formed by the junction of the basilar, posterior cerebral, internal carotid and anterior cerebral arteries. Congenital defects may occur in these arteries and lead to the formation of aneurysm (see ANEURYSM).

Circulatory System of the Blood

The course of the circulation is as follows: the veins pour their blood, coming from the head, trunk, limbs and abdominal organs, into the right atrium of the HEART. This contracts and drives the blood into the right ventricle, which then forces the blood into the LUNGS by way of the pulmonary artery. Here it is contained in thin-walled capillaries, over which the air plays freely, and through which gases pass readily out and in. The blood gives off carbon dioxide (CO_2) and takes up oxygen (see RESPIRATION), and passes on by the pulmonary veins to the left atrium of the heart. The left atrium expels it into the left ventricle, which forces it on into the aorta, by which it is distributed all over the body. Passing through capillaries in the various tissues, it enters venules, then veins, which ultimately unite into two great veins, the superior and the inferior vena cava, these emptying into the right atrium. This complete circle is accomplished by any particular drop of blood in about half a minute.

In one part of the body there is a further complication. The veins coming from the bowels, charged with food material and other products, split up, and their blood undergoes a second capillary circulation through the liver. Here it is relieved of some food material and purified, and then passes into the inferior vena cava, and so to the right atrium. This is known as the portal circulation.

The circle is maintained always in one direction by four valves, situated one at the outlet from each cavity of the heart.

The blood in the arteries going to the body generally is bright red, that in the veins dull red in colour, owing to the former being charged with oxygen and the latter with carbon dioxide (see RESPIRATION). For the same reason the blood in the pulmonary artery is dark, that in the pulmonary veins is bright. There is no direct communication between the right and left sides of the heart, the blood passing from the right ventricle to the left atrium through the lungs.

In the embryo, before birth, the course of circulation is somewhat different, owing to the fact that no nourishment comes from the bowels nor air into the lungs. Accordingly, two large arteries pass out of the navel, and convey blood to be changed by contact with maternal blood (see PLACENTA), while a large vein brings this blood back again. There are also communications between the right and left atria, and between pulmonary artery and aorta. The latter is known as the ductus arteriosus. At birth all these extra vessels and connections close and rapidly shrivel up.

Circumcision

A surgical procedure to remove the prepuce of the PENIS in males and a part or all of the external genitalia in females (see below). Circumcision is mainly done for religious or ethnic reasons; there is virtually no medical or surgical reason for the procedure. (The PREPUCE is not normally retractable in infancy, so this is not an indication for the operation – by the age of four the prepuce is retractable in most boys.) Americans are more enthusiastic about circumcision, and the reason offered is that cancer of the penis occurs only when a foreskin is present. This is however a rare disease. In the uncircumcised adult there is an increased transmission of herpes and cytomegaloviruses during the reproductive years, but this can be reduced by adequate cleansing. PHIMOSIS (restricted opening of the foreskin) is sometimes an indication for circumcision but can also be dealt with by division of adhesions between the foreskin and glans under local anesthetic. Haemorrhage, infection and meatal stenosis are rare complications of circumcision.

Circumcision in women is a damaging procedure, involving the removal of all or parts of the CLITORIS, LABIA majora and labia minora, sometimes combined with narowing of the entrance to the VAGINA. Total removal of the external female genitalia, including the clitoris, is called INFIBULATION. The result may be psychological and sexual problems and complications in childbirth, with no known benefit to the woman's health, though cultural pressures have resulted in its continuation in some Muslim and African countries, despite widespread condemnation of the practice and campaigns to stop it. It has been estimated that more than 80 million women in 30 countries have been circumcised.

Cirrhosis

Cirrhosis, or FIBROSIS, is a diseased condition, in which the proper tissue is replaced by fibrous tissue similar to scar tissue. The name cirrhosis was originally given by Laennec to the disease as occurring in the liver, because of its yellow colour. (See LIVER, DISEASES OF.)

Cirsoid Aneurysm

The condition in which a group of arteries become abnormally dilated and tortuous.

Cisplatin

A toxic drug with an alkylating action that gives it useful anti-tumour properties, especially against solid tumours such as ovarian and testicular cancers (see CYTOTOXIC).

Citric Acid

This is responsible for the sharp taste associated with citrus fruits, such as lemons and limes, and other fruits such as currants and raspberries. Although chemically different from, it is similar in action and appearance to tartaric acid, obtained from grapes and other fruits, and similar to malic acid, found in apples and pears.

CJD

See CREUTZFELDT-JAKOB DISEASE (CJD).

Claudication

A cramp-like pain that occurs in the legs on walking. It may cause the sufferer to limp or, if severe, stop him or her from walking. The usual cause is narrowing or blockage of the arteries in the legs due to ATHEROSCLEROSIS: smoking is a contributory factor. Intermittent claudication occurs when a person has to stop every so often to let the pain – caused by the build-up of waste products in the muscles – to subside. The condition may be improved by exercise, for example, for an hour a day (resting when the pain starts). Pentoxifylline, a vasodilator, may help, as may CALCIUM-CHANNEL BLOCKERS. Patients must avoid all tobacco products.

Claustrophobia

Morbid fear of being in a confined space, or the fear experienced while in it. Claustrophobia may develop because of a previous unpleasant experience in a confined space. COGNITIVE BEHAVIOUR THERAPY may help patients whose daily lives are seriously affected by this disorder.

Clavicle

The bone which runs from the upper end of the breastbone towards the tip of the shoulder across the root of the neck. It supports the upper limb, keeps it out from the side, and gives breadth to the shoulders. The bone is shaped like an 'f' with two curves, which give it increased strength. It is, however, liable to be broken by falls on the hand or on the shoulder, and is the most frequently fractured bone in the body. (See BONE, DISORDERS OF.)

Claw-Foot

Claw-foot, or PES CAVUS, is a familial deformity of the foot characterised by an abnormally high arch of the foot accompanied by shortening of the foot, clawing of the toes, and inversion, or turning inwards, of the foot and heel. Its main effect is to impair the resilience of the foot resulting in a stiff gait and aching pain. Milder cases are treated with special shoes fitted with a sponge rubber insole. More severe cases may require surgical treatment.

Claw-Hand

A (contraction) deformity of the hand and fingers, especially of the ring and little fingers. The condition is generally due to paralysis of the ULNAR NERVE. A somewhat similar condition is produced by contraction of the fibrous tissues in the palm of the hand, partly due to rheumatic changes and partly to injury caused by the constant pressure of a tool against the palm of the hand. (See DUPUYTREN'S CONTRACTURE.)

Claw-Toes

See CLAW-FOOT.

Cleft Foot

A rare congenital abnormality characterised by the absence of one or more toes and a deep central cleft that divides the foot into two. It is sometimes known as lobster foot, or lobster claw. It may be accompanied by other congenital defects, such as CLEFT HAND, absent permanent teeth, CLEFT PALATE (and/or lip), absence of the nails, and defects of the eye.

Cleft Hand

A rare congenital abnormality characterised by the absence of one or more fingers and a deep central cleft that divides the hand into two. It is sometimes known as lobster hand. It may be accompanied by other congenital defects, such as CLEFT FOOT, absent permanent teeth, CLEFT PALATE (and/or lip), absence of the nails and defects of the eye.

Cleft Palate

A fissure in the roof of the mouth (palate) and/or the lip which is present at birth. It is found in varying degrees of severity in about one in 700 children. Modern plastic surgery can greatly improve the functioning of lips and palate and the appearance of the baby. Further cosmetic surgery later may not be necessary. The parent of the child who has cleft lip and/or palate will be given detailed advice specific to his or her case. In general the team of specialists involved are the paediatrician, plastic surgeon, dentist or orthodontic specialist, and speech therapist. (See PALATE, MALFORMATIONS OF.)

Clicking Finger

A condition usually occurring in middle-aged people in which the victim finds on wakening in the morning that he or she cannot straighten the ring or middle finger spontaneously, but only by a special effort, when it suddenly straightens with a painful click. Hence the name. In due course the finger remains bent at all times unless a special effort is made to straighten it with the other hand. The condition is due to a swelling developing in one of the tendons of the affected finger. If the tendon sheath is slit open surgically, the condition is relieved. Many cases recover spontaneously if the patient is prepared to wait.

Climacteric

This was a word originally applied to the end of certain epochs or stages in the life of an individual, at which some great change was supposed to take place. (See also MENOPAUSE.)

Clindamycin

An antibiotic used in the treatment of serious infections. It is active against gram-positive cocci, including penicillin-resistant staphylococci (see STAPHYLOCOCCUS) and also many anaerobes (see ANAEROBE), especially *Bacteroides fragilis*. It is recommended for staphylococcal bone and joint infections such as OSTEOMYELITIS and intra-abdominal sepsis, as well as ENDOCARDITIS prophylaxis. Clindamycin has only limited use because of its adverse effects; patients should discontinue immediately if diarrhoea or colitis develops.

Clinical

Clinical means literally 'belonging to a bed', but the word is used to denote anything associated with the practical study or observation of sick people – as in clinical medicine, clinical thermometers.

Clinical Audit

A MEDICAL AUDIT carried out by health professionals.

Clinical Governance

A concept, introduced in a UK government White Paper in 1997, aimed at 'ensuring that all NHS organisations have in place proper processes for continuously monitoring and improving clinical audit'. All clinicians and managers are now expected to understand their individual and collective responsibilities for assuring accountability for the quality of patient care. Clinical governance is now included in the NHS legislation based on the 1997 White Paper. (See also MEDICAL AUDIT; HEALTH CARE COMMISSION; NATIONAL INSTITUTE FOR CLINICAL EXCELLENCE (NICE).)

Clinical Guidelines

Systematically developed statements which assist clinicians and patients to decide on appropriate treatments for specific conditions. The guidelines are attractive to health managers and patients because they are potentially able to reduce variation in clinical practice. This helps to ensure that patients receive the right treatment of an acceptable standard. In England and Wales, the NATIONAL INSTITUTE FOR CLINICAL EXCELLENCE (NICE) is developing national guidelines with advice from health-care professionals and patients to improve clinical effectiveness of NHS care. Some doctors have reservations about guidelines because (1) health-care managers might use them primarily to contain costs; (2) inflexibility would discourage clinical innovations; (3) they could encourage litigation by patients. (See also HEALTH CARE COMMISSION; MEDICAL LITIGATION.)

Clinical Psychology

Psychology is the scientific study of behaviour. It may be applied in various settings including education, industry and health care. Clinical psychology is concerned with the practical application of research findings in the fields of physical and mental health. Training in clinical psychology involves a degree in psychology followed by postgraduate training. Clinical psychologists are specifically skilled in applying theoretical models and objective methods of observation and measurement, and in therapeutic interventions aimed at changing patients' dysfunctional behaviour, including thoughts and feelings as well as actions. Dysfunctional behaviour is explained in terms of normal processes and modified by applying principles of normal learning, adaption and social interaction.

Clinical psychologists are involved in health care in the following ways: (1) Assessment of thoughts, emotions and behaviour using standardised methods. (2) Treatment based on theoretical models and scientific evidence about behaviour change. Behaviour change is considered when it contributes to physical, psychological or social functioning. (3) Consultation with other health-care professionals about problems concerning emotions, thinking and behaviour. (4) Research on a wide variety of topics including the relationship between stress, psychological functioning and disease; the aetiology of problem behaviours; methods and theories of behaviour change. (5) Teaching other professionals about normal and dysfunctional behaviour, emotions and functioning.

Clinical psychologists may specialise in work in particular branches of patient care, including surgery, psychiatry, geriatrics, paediatrics, mental handicap, obstetrics and gynaecology, cardiology, neurology, general practice and physical rehabilitation. Whilst the focus of their work is frequently the patient, at times it may encompass the behaviour of the health-care professionals.

Clinical Risk Management

Initially driven by anxiety about the possibility of medical negligence cases, clinical risk management has evolved into the study of IATROGENIC DISEASE. The first priority of risk managers is to ensure that all therapies in medicine are as safe as possible. Allied to this is a recognition that errors may occur even when error-prevention strategies are in place. Lastly, any accidents that occur are analysed, allowing a broader understanding of their cause. Risk management is generally centred on single adverse events. The threat of litigation is taken as an opportunity to expose unsafe conditions of practice and to put pressure on those with the authority to implement change. These might include senior clinicians, hospital management, the purchasing authorities, and even the Secretary of State for Health. Attention is focused on organisational factors rather than on the individuals involved in a specific case.

Clinical Signs

The physical manifestations of an illness elicited by a doctor when examining a patient – for example, a rash, lump, swelling, fever or altered physical function such as reflexes.

Clinical Symptoms

The experiences of a patient as communicated to a doctor, for example, pain, weakness, cough. They may or may not be accompanied by confirmatory CLINICAL SIGNS.

Clinical Trials

(See EVIDENCE-BASED MEDICINE.) Clinical trials aim to evaluate the relative effects of different health-care interventions. They are based on the idea that there must a fair comparison of the alternatives in order to know which is better. Threats to a fair comparison include the play of chance and bias, both of which can cause people to draw the wrong conclusions about how effective a treatment or procedure is.

An appreciation of the need to account for chance and bias has led to development of methods where new treatments are compared to either a PLACEBO or to the standard treatment (or both) in a controlled, randomised clinical trial. 'Controlled' means that there is a comparison group of patients not receiving the test intervention, and 'randomised' implies that patients have been assigned to one or other treatment group entirely by chance and not because of their doctor's preference. If possible, trials are 'double-blind' – that is, neither the patient nor the investigator knows who is receiving which intervention until after the trial is over. All such trials must follow proper ethical standards with the procedure fully explained to patients and their consent obtained.

The conduct, effectiveness and duplication of clinical trials have long been subjects of debate. Apart from occasional discoveries of deliberately fraudulent research (see RESEARCH FRAUD AND MISCONDUCT), the structure of some trials are unsatisfactory, statistical analyses are sometimes disputed and major problems have been the – usually unwitting – duplication of trials and non-publication of some trials, restricting access to their findings. Duplication occurs because no formal international mechanism exists to enable research workers to discover whether a clinical trial they are planning is already underway elsewhere or has been completed but never published, perhaps because the results were negative, or no journal was willing to publish it, or the authors or funding authorities decided not to submit it for publication.

In the mid 1980s a proposal was made for an international register of clinical trials. In 1991 the NHS launched a research and development initiative and, liaising with the COCHRANE COLLABORATION, set out to collect systematically data from published randomised clinical trials. In 1994 the NHS set up a Centre for Reviews and Dissemination which, among other responsibilities, maintains a database of research reviews to provide NHS staff with relevant information.

These efforts are hampered by availability of information about trials in progress and unpublished completed trials. With a view to improving accessibility of relevant information, the publishers of *Current Science*, in 1998, launched an online metaregister of ongoing randomised controlled trials.

Subsequently, in October 1999, the editors of the *British Medical Journal* and the *Lancet* argued that the case for an international register of all clinical trials prior to their launch was unanswerable. 'The public', they said, 'has the right to know what research is being funded. Researchers and research funders don't want to waste resources repeating trials already underway.' Given the widening recognition of the importance to patients and doctors of the practice of EVIDENCE-BASED MEDICINE, the easy availability of information on planned, ongoing and completed clinical trials is vital. The register was finally set up in 2005.

Clitoris
A small, sensitive organ comprising erectile tissue at the top of the female genitalia where the labial folds meet below the pubic bone. Clitoral tissue extends into the anterior roof of the vagina. During sexual excitement the clitoris enlarges and hardens and may be the focus of orgasm. (See CIRCUMCISION.)

Clofazimine
A drug used in the treatment of LEPROSY.

Clofibrate
See HYPERLIPIDAEMIA.

Clomiphene
An anti-oestrogen drug that stimulates ovulation, or the production of ova, through the medium of the PITUITARY GLAND. When used in the treatment of female infertility, one of its hazards is that, if given in too-big doses, it may produce multiple births.

Clomipramine
One of the tricyclic ANTIDEPRESSANT DRUGS.)

Clonazepam
A drug to treat EPILEPSY, including STATUS EPILEPTICUS, and MYOCLONUS. (See also TRANQUILLISERS.)

Clone
A group of cells genetically identical to each other that have arisen from one cell by asexual reproduction (see CLONING).

Clonic
A word applied to short spasmodic movements.

Clonidine
A drug used for HYPERTENSION, MIGRAINE, GILLES DE LA TOURETTE'S SYNDROME, and menopausal flushing. It can cause drowsiness so caution is needed when driving or using machinery.

Cloning
Cloning – from the Greek *klon*, meaning a cutting such as is used to propagate plants – is essentially a form of asexual reproduction. The initial stages were first successfully achieved in rabbits. In essence the technique consists of destroying the nucleus of the egg and replacing it with the nucleus from a body cell of the same species – either a male or a female. This provides the egg with a full complement of CHROMOSOMES and it starts to divide and grow just as it would if it had retained its nucleus and been fertilised with a spermatozoon. The vital difference is that the embryo resulting from this cloning process owes nothing genetically to the female egg. It is identical in every respect with the animal from which the introduced nucleus was obtained.

In 1997 the first mammal to be cloned from the tissue of an adult animal was born. A technique that scientists have been trying to perfect for decades, the success of the Roslin Institute, near Edinburgh, in producing 'Dolly', a cloned sheep, has profound implications. Already some scientists are talking of cloning humans, although this has great medical, legal and ethical consequences. The key to the scientists' success in producing Dolly was the ability to coordinate the fusion of a donor cell (from an adult) containing all its DNA with a recipient egg from which DNA had been removed. The difficulty of the technique is shown by the fact that, out of 277 fused pairs of cells where the donor cell was from adult tissue, Dolly was the only survivor and she has developed premature arthritis. Research suggests that cloning may be accompanied by a higher than normal incidence of congenital defects.

Since Dolly was born, other animal clones have been produced and American researchers have cloned the first human embryo – which grew to six cells – with the aim of providing stem cells for therapeutic use. As a result the UK government passed emergency legislation to outlaw human cloning for reproductive purposes.

Clonus
A succession of intermittent muscular relaxations and contractions usually resulting from a sustained stretching stimulus. An example is the clonus stimulated in the calf muscle by maintaining sustained upward pressure on the sole of the foot. The condition is often a sign of disease in the brain or spinal cord.

Clormethiazole
A useful hypnotic, particularly for elderly patients, because of its freedom from hangover effect. It is especially beneficial in the acute withdrawal symptoms of alcoholism and is used to treat STATUS EPILEPTICUS. The drug's sedative effects are an adjunct to regional anaesthesia and may also be of help in ECLAMPSIA. Dependence may occur occasionally and therefore the length of period for which the drug is used should be limited. Side-effects include sneezing, conjunctival irritation and occasional headache.

Clostridium
The genus, or variety, of micro-organisms that produce spores which enable them to survive under adverse conditions. They normally grow in soil, water and decomposing plant and animal matter, where they play an important part in the process of PUTREFACTION. Among the important members of the group, or genus, are *Clostridium welchii*, *Cl. septicum* and *Cl. oedematiens*, the causes of gas gangrene (see GANGRENE); *Cl. tetani*, the cause of TETANUS; and *Cl. botulinum*, the cause of BOTULISM.

Clot
The term applied to any semi-solid mass of blood, lymph or other body fluid. Clotting in the blood is due to the formation of strings of FIBRIN produced by the action of a ferment. Milk clots in a similar manner in the stomach when exposed to the action of the enzyme rennin. Clotting occurs naturally when blood is shed and comes into contact with tissues outside the blood vessels. It occurs also at times in

diseased vessels (THROMBOSIS), producing serious effects upon the tissues supplied or drained by these vessels. Clots sometimes form in the heart when the circulation is failing. (See COAGULATION; EMBOLISM.)

Clotrimazole
A drug of the IMIDAZOLES group used to treat fungal infections of the skin and vagina.

Clotting Time
See COAGULATION.

Clozapine
An antipsychotic drug used to treat schizophrenic patients (see SCHIZOPHRENIA) who have not responded to other treatments or who have suffered serious side-effects from them. Improvement is gradual and it may be several weeks before severe symptoms are relieved. The drug can cause AGRANULOCYTOSIS and so it is given under close hospital supervision.

Clubbing
The term applied to the thickening and broadening of the fingertips – and, less commonly, the tips of the toes – that occurs in certain chronic diseases of the lungs and heart. It is due to interstitial OEDEMA especially at the nail bed, leading to a loss of the acute angle between the nail and the skin of the finger. Clubbing is associated with lung cancer, EMPYEMA, BRONCHIECTASIS and congenital cyanotic heart disease.

Club-Foot
See TALIPES.

Cluster
In statistical terms a group of subjects, closely linked in time and/or place of occurrence. For example, geographical clusters of LEUKAEMIA have been found – that is, an unexpectedly large number of persons with the disease who live in close proximity. Much research goes into trying to discover the cause of clusters but sometimes they appear to have occurred randomly.

Cluster Headaches
A type of MIGRAINE occurring in clusters – that is, a patient may have an attack daily for several days and then none for weeks or months. The pain is on one side of the head, often centred over the eye. The pain is excruciatingly severe and often associated with tearing, nasal discharge and production of thick saliva from the same side of the mouth. It is treated either with

drugs such as SUMATRIPTAN or by breathing 100 per cent oxygen.

CMV
See CYTOMEGALOVIRUS (CMV).

Coagulation
Coagulation of the blood is the process whereby bleeding (or haemorrhage) is normally arrested in the body. Blood starts to clot as soon as the skin (or other tissue) has been cut. Coagulation is part of the process of HAEMOSTASIS which is the arrest of bleeding from an injured or diseased blood vessel. Haemostasis depends on the combined activities of vascular, platelet (see PLATELETS) and PLASMA elements which are offset by processes to restrict the accumulation of platelets and FIBRIN to the damaged area.

The three-stage process of coagulation is complex, involving many different substances. There are two cascading pathways of biochemical reactions for activating coagulation of blood. The extrinsic pathway is the main physiological mechanism, which is triggered when blood vessels are damaged, usually by trauma or surgery. The intrinsic pathway is activated by internal disruption of the wall of a blood vessel. The basic pattern is broadly the same for both and is summarised simply as follows:

prothrombin + calcium + thromboplastin
thrombin + fibrinogen
fibrin

Prothrombin and calcium are normally present in the blood. Thromboplastin is an enzyme which is normally found in the blood platelets and in tissue cells. When bleeding occurs from a blood vessel, there is always some damage to tissue cells and to the blood platelets. As a result of this damage, thromboplastin is released and comes into contact with the prothrombin and calcium in the blood. In the presence of thromboplastin and calcium, prothrombin is converted into thrombin, which in turn interacts with fibrinogen – a protein always present in the blood – to form fibrin. Fibrin consists of needle-shaped crystals which, with the assistance of the blood platelets, form a fine network in which the blood corpuscles become enmeshed. This meshwork, or CLOT as it is known, gradually retracts until it forms a tight mass which, unless the tissue injury is very severe or a major artery has been damaged, prevents any further bleeding. It will thus be seen that clotting, or coagulation, does not occur in the healthy blood vessel because there is no thromboplastin present. There is now evidence suggesting that there is an anti-thrombin substance present in the blood in small amounts, and that this substance antagonises any small amounts of thrombin that may be formed as a result of small amounts of thromboplastin being released.

The clotting or coagulation time is the time taken for blood to clot and can be measured under controlled conditions to ensure that it is normal (3–8 minutes). In certain diseases – HAEMOPHILIA, for example – clotting time is greatly extended and the danger of serious haemorrhage enhanced.

Coagulopathy
Any disorder affecting the coagulability of blood (see COAGULATION). Among acute conditions precipitating the disorder are ABRUPTIO PLACENTA, HAEMOLYSIS following blood transfusions, infection with gram-negative bacteria (see GRAM'S STAIN), HEAT STROKE, SHOCK and snakebite. Chronic disorders linked with coagulopathy are septic ABORTION, TOXAEMIA of pregnancy, certain cancers and LEUKAEMIA.

Coarctation of the Aorta
A narrowing of the AORTA in the vicinity of the insertion of the ductus arteriosus. It is a congenital abnormality but may not be discovered until well into childhood or adolescence. The diagnosis is easily made by discovering a major difference between the blood pressure in the arms and that of the legs. If untreated it leads to hypertension and heart failure, but satisfactory results are now obtained from surgical treatment, preferably in infancy. Paediatricians screen for coarctation by feeling for femoral pulses, which are absent or weak in this condition.

Cobalamins
A group of substances which have an enzyme action (see ENZYME) and are essential for normal growth and nutrition. (See also CYANOCOBALAMIN; HYDROXOCOBALAMIN.)

Cobalt-60
Cobalt-60 is a radioactive isotope of the metallic element cobalt (Co). It is used in the treatment of malignant disease. (See RADIOTHERAPY.)

Cocaine
Coca leaves are obtained from two South American plants, *Erythroxylum coca* and *Erythroxylum truxillense*, and contain an alkaloid, cocaine. Cocaine has marked effects as a stimulant, and, locally applied, as an anaesthetic by paralysing nerves of sensation. The dried leaves have been

used from time immemorial by the South American Indians, who chew them mixed with a little lime. Their effect is to dull the mucous surfaces of mouth and stomach, with which the saliva, produced by chewing them, comes into contact – thus blunting, for long periods, all feeling of hunger. The cocaine, being absorbed, stimulates the central nervous system so that all sense of fatigue and breathlessness vanishes for a time. It was by the use of coca that the Indian post-runners of South America were able to achieve their extraordinary feats of endurance. The continued use of the drug, however, results in emaciation, loss of memory, sleeplessness and general breakdown. DEPENDENCE on cocaine or a derivative, 'crack', is now a serious social problem in many countries.

Uses Before the serious effects that result from its habitual use were realised, the drug was sometimes used by hunters, travellers and others to relieve exhaustion and breathlessness in climbing mountains and to dull hunger. Derivatives of cocaine are used as locally applied analgesics via sprays or injections in dentistry and for procedures in the ear, nose and throat. Because of its serious side-effects and the risk of addiction, cocaine is a strictly controlled Class A drug which can be prescribed only by a medical practitioner with a Home Office licence to do so.

Cocci
Spherical BACTERIA that cause a variety of infections. Staphylococci, streptococci and meningococci (see NEISSERIACEAE) are examples.

Coccydynia
The sensation of severe pain in the COCCYX.

Coccyx
The lower end of the SPINAL COLUMN, resembling a bird's beak and consisting of four fused nodules of bone; these represent vertebrae and correspond to the tail in lower animals. Above the coccyx lies a much larger bone, the SACRUM, and together they form the back wall of the PELVIS, which protects the organs in the lower ABDOMEN.

Cochlea
That part of the inner ear concerned with hearing. (See EAR.)

Cochlear Implants
A cochlear implant is an electronic device, inserted under a general anaesthetic, which stimulates the auditory system, restoring partial hearing in profound sensory deafness. Although there are many types of cochlear implant, they all consist of a microphone, a signal processor, a signal coupler (transmitter and receiver), and an array of electrodes. Most are multi-channel implants. The microphone and signal processor are worn outside the body, like a conventional hearing aid: they receive sound and convert it into an electronic signal which is transmitted through the skin to the receiver. Here the signal is transmitted to the array of electrodes which stimulates the cochlear nerve. Although cochlear implants do not provide normal hearing, most profoundly deaf patients who receive a cochlear implant are able to detect a variety of sounds, including environmental sounds and speech. The duration of hearing-loss and age at implantation are among the many factors which influence the results (see DEAFNESS).

Cochrane Collaboration
A non-profit-making international organisation which systematically finds, appraises and reviews available evidence, mainly from randomised CLINICAL TRIALS, about the consequences of health care. The aim is to help people make well-informed decisions about health care. The main work is done by around 50 review groups, the members of which share an interest in generating reliable, up-to-date evidence on the prevention, treatment and rehabilitation of particular health problems or groups of problems. The UK Cochrane Centre opened in Oxford in 1992 and the International Collaboration launched a year later. Its origins lay in the work of a UK epidemiologist, Dr Archie Cochrane, who in 1979 published a monograph calling for a systematic collection of randomised controlled trials on the effect of health care.

The main output of the Cochrane Collaboration is published electronically as the Cochrane Library, updated quarterly, with free access in many countries. (See CLINICAL TRIALS, EVIDENCE-BASED MEDICINE and Appendix 2.)

Codeine
One of the active principles of OPIUM, codeine is an analgesic (see ANALGESICS) which in the form of codeine phosphate is used to suppress persistent coughs and to relieve pain such as headaches and musculoskeletal discomfort. Side-effects include constipation, nausea and sleepiness. Dependence is rare.

Cod-Liver Oil
Cod-liver oil is derived from the fresh liver of the cod (*Gadus callarius*). It is a rich source of

vitamin D, used in the prevention and treatment of RICKETS, and of vitamin A. Human milk contains more than enough vitamin D for the breast-fed baby, provided the mother has a balanced diet with adequate exposure to sunlight, or is taking vitamin supplements during pregnancy and lactation if considered necessary. All baby foods in the UK contain added vitamins, and therefore supplementation is unnecessary until weaning begins, and the baby starts taking cow's milk, which contains less vitamin D than human milk. (See APPENDIX 5: VITAMINS.)

Coeliac Disease

Around one in 100 people suffers from coeliac disease, a condition in which the small INTESTINE fails to digest and absorb food, but many have no or few symptoms and remain undiagnosed. The intestinal lining is permanently sensitive to the protein gliadin (an insoluble and potentially toxic PEPTIDE protein) which is contained in GLUTEN, a constituent of the germ of wheat, barley and rye. As bread or other grain-based foods are a regular part of most people's diet, the constant presence of gluten in the intestine of sufferers of coeliac disease causes atrophy of the digestive and absorptive cells of the intestine. Children are usually diagnosed when they develop symptoms such as vomiting, diarrhoea, lethargy, ANAEMIA, swollen abdomen and pale, frothy, foul-smelling faeces with failure to thrive. The diagnosis is usually made by a positive blood antibody test such as antiendomysial antibodies. However, because there may be an occasional false positive result, the 'gold standard' is to obtain a biopsy of the JEJUNUM through a tiny metal capsule that can be swallowed, a specimen taken, and the capsule retrieved. Though coeliac disease was long thought to occur in childhood, a second peak of the disorder has recently been identified among people in their 50s.

Not all sufferers from coeliac disease present with gastrointestinal symptoms: doctors, using screening techniques, have increasingly identified large numbers of such people. This is important because researchers have recently discovered that untreated overt and silent coeliac disease increases the risk of sufferers developing osteoporosis (brittle bone disease – see BONE, DISORDERS OF) and cancer. The osteoporosis develops because the bowel fails to absorb the CALCIUM essential for normal bone growth. Because those with coeliac disease lack the enzyme LACTASE, which is essential for digesting milk, they avoid milk – a rich source of calcium.

The key treatment is a strict, lifelong diet free of gluten. As well as returning the bowel lining to normal, this diet results in a return to normal bone density. People with coeliac disease, or parents or guardians of affected children, can obtain help and guidance from the Coeliac Society of the United Kingdom. (See also MALABSORPTION SYNDROME; SPRUE.)

Coelioscopy

A method of viewing the interior of the abdomen in patients in whom a tumour or some other condition requiring operation may be present but cannot with certainty be diagnosed. The examination is carried out by making a minute opening under local anaesthesia, and inserting an ENDOSCOPE – a long flexible instrument bearing an electric lamp and telescopic lenses like that for examining the bladder (CYSTOSCOPE) – into the abdominal cavity. Certain of the abdominal organs can then be directly inspected in turn.

Cognition

The mental processes by which a person acquires knowledge. Among these are reasoning, creative actions and solving problems.

Cognitive Behaviour Therapy

A talking therapy that re-trains the mind to question and banish negative thoughts, change emotional responses and change behaviour. It is based on the theory that some people develop unduly negative and pessimistic thoughts (cognitions) about themselves, their future and the world around them, putting them at risk of depression and other mental-health problems. Put simply, the treatment involves several sessions with a trained therapist who helps to identify the negative patterns of thinking and show that they are not usually realistic.

Research has shown that cognitive therapy is very effective in depression and that it can also help in anxiety, OBSESSIVE COMPULSIVE DISORDER, and EATING DISORDERS such as anorexia and bulimia nervosa. This therapy is also proving useful in helping people cope with HALLUCINATIONS and other symptoms of SCHIZOPHRENIA.

Cohort Study

A systemised follow-up study of people for a specific period of time, or until the occurrence of a defined event such as a particular illness or death. The aim is to follow the disease course and/or the reasons for the participants' deaths. Different cohorts may be compared and conclusions drawn about a particular disease or drug treatment.

Coitus
Coitus is sexual intercourse.

Coitus interruptus (see CONTRACEPTION).

Colchicine
A drug used to treat GOUT in the acute stage. Its use is limited by the development of toxicity at higher doses, but in patients with heart failure it may be preferable to NON-STEROIDAL ANTI-INFLAMMATORY DRUGS (NSAIDS), which tend to cause fluid retention. Colchicine can be given to patients receiving ANTICOAGULANTS. The drug does have side-effects on the gastrointestinal system.

Colchicum
The bulb of *Colchicum autumnale*, or meadow-saffron, has long been used as a remedy for GOUT. How it acts is not quite certain.

Uses Its main use is in gout, for which colchicine, the active principle of colchicum, in doses of 0·5 mg every one or two hours until the pain is relieved, followed by 0·5 mg thrice daily for about a week, is the form generally employed.

Cold, Common
An infection by any one of around 200 viruses, with about half the common-cold infections being caused by RHINOVIRUSES. Certain CORONAVIRUSES, ECHOVIRUSES and COXSACKIE VIRUSES are also culprits. The common cold – traditionally also called a chill – is one of several viral infections that cause respiratory symptoms and systemic illness. Others include PNEUMONIA and GASTROENTERITIS. Colds are commoner in winter, perhaps because people are more likely to be indoors in close contact with others.

Also called acute coryza or upper respiratory infection, the common cold is characterised by inflammation of any or all of the airways – NOSE, sinuses (see SINUS), THROAT, LARYNX, TRACHEA and bronchi (see BRONCHUS). Most common, however, is the 'head cold', which is confined to the nose and throat, with initial symptoms presenting as a sore throat, runny nose and sneezing. The nasal discharge may become thick and yellow – a sign of secondary bacterial infection – while the patient often develops watery eyes, aching muscles, a cough, headache, listlessness and the shivers. PYREXIA (raised temperature) is usual. Colds can also result in a flare-up of pre-existing conditions,

such as asthma, bronchitis or ear infections. Most colds are self-limiting, resolving in a week or ten days, but some patients develop secondary bacterial infections of the sinuses, middle ear (see EAR), trachea, or LUNGS.

Treatment Symptomatic treatment with ANTIPYRETICS and ANALGESICS is usually sufficient; ANTIBIOTICS should not be taken unless there is definite secondary infection or unless the patient has an existing chest condition which could be worsened by a cold. Cold victims should consult a doctor only if symptoms persist or if they have a pre-existing condition, such as asthma which could be exacerbated by a cold.

Most colds result from breathing-in virus-containing droplets that have been coughed or sneezed into the atmosphere, though the virus can also be picked up from hand-to-hand contact or from articles such as hand towels. Prevention is, therefore, difficult, given the high infectivity of the viruses. No scientifically proven, generally applicable preventive measures have yet been devised, but the incidence of the infection falls from about seven to eight years – schoolchildren may catch as many as eight colds annually – to old age, the elderly having few colds. So far, despite much research, no effective vaccines have been produced.

Cold, Injuries from
See CHILBLAIN; FROSTBITE; HYPOTHERMIA.

Cold Sores
See HERPES SIMPLEX.

Cold-Weather Itch
Cold-weather itch is a common form of itchiness that occurs in cold weather. It is characterised by slight dryness of the skin, and is particularly troublesome in the legs of old people. The dryness may be accompanied by some mild inflammation of the skin. Treatment is by the application of emollients such as aqueous cream or zinc ointment.

Colectomy
The operation for removing the COLON.

Cholestyramine
A drug of value in the treatment of the PRURITUS, or itching, which occurs in association with JAUNDICE. It does this by 'binding' the bile salts in the gut and so preventing their being reabsorbed into the bloodstream, where their excess in jaundice is responsible for the itching. It reduces the level of cholesterol and

triglycerides in the blood and thereby, like clofibrate and STATINS, helping to reduce the incidence of coronary artery heart disease. (See HEART, DISEASES OF; HYPERLIPIDAEMIA.)

Colic

This term is generally used for an attack of spasmodic pain in the abdomen.

Simple colic often results from the build-up of indigestible material in the alimentary tract, leading to spasmodic contractions in the muscular lining. Other causes include habitual constipation, with accumulation of faecal material; simple colic also occurs as an accompaniment of neurological disorders. Major risks include sudden obstruction of the bowel from twisting, INTUSSUSCEPTION, or as a result of a tumour or similar condition. (See also INTESTINE, DISEASES OF.)

Lead colic (traditional names include painter's colic, colica pictonum, Devonshire colic, dry belly-ache) is due to the absorption of lead into the system. (See LEAD POISONING.)

Biliary colic and renal colic are the terms applied to that violent pain which is produced, in the one case where a biliary calculus or gall-stone passes down from the gall-bladder into the intestine, and in the other where a renal calculus descends from the kidney along the ureter into the bladder. (See GALL-BLADDER, DISEASES OF and KIDNEYS, DISEASES OF.)

Treatment This consists of means to relieve the spasmodic pain with warmth and analgesics, and removal, where possible, of the underlying cause.

Infantile colic is a common condition in babies under three months, sometimes continuing for a little longer. The babies cry persistently and appear to their parents to have abdominal pain, although this remains unproven. Swaddling and massage can help, as can simply stimulating the child with movement and noise (rocking and singing). Medication is usually unhelpful, although the most severely affected deserve help because of the deleterious effect of infantile colic on family life.

Coliform

Description of a gram-negative bacterium found in the faeces. It covers the bacterial groups *Enterobacter*, *Escherichia*, and *Klebsiella*.

Colistin

A POLYMYXIN antibiotic active against many gram-negative organisms, including *Pseudomonas aeruginosa*. It is not absorbed by mouth and therefore needs to be given by injection to obtain a systemic effect; this is rarely indicated, however, as it has serious adverse effects. Colistin is used by mouth in bowel-sterilisation regimens before surgery in patients. It is given by inhalation of a nebulised solution as an adjunct to some standard antibiotic therapy, and is included in some topical preparations, chiefly for skin, eye and ear infections.

Colitis

Inflammation of the colon, the first part of the large intestine. The subject suffers from diarrhoea, usually passing blood and mucus, abdominal pain or discomfort, and fever. Colitis can be caused by various micro-organisms: for example, CAMPYLOBACTER, CLOSTRIDIUM and SHIGELLA bacteria, viruses or amoeba. Anxiety and antibiotic drugs may also cause colitis, the latter by directly irritating the lining of the gut.

Colitis is classified as an INFLAMMATORY BOWEL DISEASE (IBD) and ULCERATIVE COLITIS is a particularly troublesome form, the cause of which is not known. CROHN'S DISEASE may also cause colitis and is included in the umbrella designation IBD (see also IRRITABLE BOWEL SYNDROME (IBS)).

Collagen

The most abundant protein in the body. It is the major structural component of many parts of the body and occurs in many different forms. Thus it exists as thick fibres in skin and tendons. It is also an important constituent of the heart and blood vessels. With calcium salts it provides the rigid structure of bone. It also occurs as a delicate structure in the cornea of the eye, and in what is known as the basement membrane of many tissues including the glomeruli of the kidneys and the capsule of the lens of the eye. It plays a part in many diseases, hereditary and otherwise. Among the inherited abnormalities of collagen are those responsible for aneurysms of the CIRCLE OF WILLIS and for OSTEOGENESIS IMPERFECTA. On boiling it is converted into gelatin.

Collagen Diseases

A group of diseases affecting CONNECTIVE TISSUE. The term is really outdated since there is no evidence that collagen is primarily involved. Fibrinoid NECROSIS and VASCULITIS are two 'characteristics', and autoimmunity reaction may occur in the connective tissue. The latter affects blood vessels and causes secondary damage in the connective tissue. Such conditions are sometimes described as collagen vascular diseases, examples being RHEUMATOID ARTHRITIS, SYSTEMIC LUPUS ERYTHEMATOSUS (SLE), and SCLERODERMA.

Collapse
See SHOCK.

Collar-Bone
See CLAVICLE.

Colles' Fracture
Colles' fracture is a fracture of the lower end of the radius close to the wrist, caused usually by a fall forwards on the palm of the hand, in which the lower fragment is displaced backwards. (See BONE, DISORDERS OF.)

Collodions
Collodions consist basically of a thick, colourless, syrupy liquid, made by dissolving guncotton (pyroxylin) in a mixture of ether and alcohol or with acetone. When painted on the skin the solvent evaporates, leaving behind a tough protective film that is useful for covering wounds. Flexible collodion – or collodion as it is often known – contains 1·6 per cent of pyroxylin, with colophony, castor oil and alcohol (90 per cent) in solvent ether. It should be kept in a well-sealed container. Being relatively elastic, it does not crack through the movements of the skin.

Colloid
A type of suspension, for instance milk, in which insoluble particles are suspended in a fluid. In medical parlance a colloid preparation is one containing PLASMA proteins and is used to treat patients in SHOCK. The follicles of the thyroid gland also contain a colloid substance.

Coloboma
Coloboma simply means a defect, but its use is usually restricted to congenital defects of the eye. These may involve the lens, the iris, the retina or the eyelid.

Colon
The first part of the large INTESTINE.

Colonic Irrigation
Washing out the large bowel with an ENEMA of water or other medication.

Colonoscope
An ENDOSCOPE for viewing the interior of the COLON. It is made of fibreglass which ensures flexibility, and incorporates a system of lenses for magnification and a lighting system.

Colonoscopy, Virtual
A procedure that links COMPUTED TOMOGRAPHY of the COLON (see also INTESTINE) with techniques that produce three-dimensional views of the mucosa of the large bowel similar to those obtained during traditional colonoscopy. Early experience suggests that the new technique produces better results than barium enemas (see ENEMA) and is almost as effective as conventional colonoscopy. Virtual colonoscopy offers faster results, and image analysis will probably soon be automated. The procedure is easy, non-invasive, safe and complete; once the need for bowel cleansing is eliminated (as seems likely) it will provide a prominent tool in screening for cancer of the colon and RECTUM.

Colostomy
The operation for the establishment of an artificial opening into the COLON. This acts as an artificial ANUS. The operation is carried out when there is an obstruction in the colon or rectum that cannot be overcome, or in cases such as cancer of the rectum in which the rectum and part of the colon have to be removed. A colostomy opening can be trained to function in such a way that the patient can carry on a normal life, eating a more or less normal diet. Anyone desiring help or advice in the practical management of a colostomy should get in touch with the British Colostomy Association. (See also STOMA.)

Colostrum
The first fluid secreted by the mammary glands for two or three days after childbirth. It contains less CASEIN and more albumin (see ALBUMINS) than ordinary milk.

Colour Blindness
See VISION – Defective colour vision.

Colporrhaphy
An operation designed to strengthen the pelvic floor in cases of prolapse of the UTERUS. The surgeon excises redundant tissue from the front vaginal wall (anterior colporrhaphy) or from the rear wall (posterior colporrhaphy), thus narrowing the vagina and tightening the muscles.

Colposcopy
The method of examining the VAGINA and

CERVIX UTERI by means of the binocular instrument known as the colposcope. It is used to screen for cancer of the cervix and in investigation of child sexual abuse.

Coma

A state of profound unconsciousness in which the patient cannot be roused and reflex movements are absent. Signs include long, deep, sighing respirations, a rapid, weak pulse, and low blood pressure. Usually the result of a STROKE, coma may also be due to high fever, DIABETES MELLITUS, glomerulonephritis (see KIDNEYS, DISEASES OF), alcohol, EPILEPSY, cerebral TUMOUR, MENINGITIS, injury to the head, overdose of INSULIN, CARBON MONOXIDE (CO) poisoning, or poisoning from OPIUM and other NARCOTICS. Though usually of relatively short duration (and terminating in death, unless yielding to treatment) it may occasionally last for months or even years. (See UNCONSCIOUSNESS; GLASGOW COMA SCALE.)

Coma Position

See RECOVERY POSITION and APPENDIX 1: BASIC FIRST AID.

Coma Scale

See GLASGOW COMA SCALE.

Comedones

See ACNE.

Commensal

Micro-organisms which live in or on the body (e.g. in the gut or respiratory tract, or on the skin) without doing any harm to the individual.

Comminuted Fracture

See BONE, DISORDERS OF.

Commission for Health Improvement

See HEALTHCARE COMMISSION.

Commissure

Commissure means a joining, and is a term applied to strands of nerve fibres which join one side of the brain to the other; to the band joining one optic nerve to the other; to the junctions of the lips at the corners of the mouth, etc.

Committee on Safety of Medicines (CSM)

An independent advisory committee – launched in 1971 in the United Kingdom – composed of doctors, pharmacists and other specialists. It advises the MEDICINES CONTROL AGENCY in the UK on the safety, efficacy and pharmaceutical quality of MEDICINES for which licences are sought and also reviews reports of ADVERSE REACTIONS TO DRUGS, including spontaneous 'Yellow Card' reports from doctors or pharmacists who suspect that a patient has suffered an adverse reaction from a medicine. Its predecessor, the Committee for Safety of Drugs, was set up in 1963 in response to the THALIDOMIDE disaster.

Common Cold

See COLD, COMMON.

Communicable Disease

This is an infectious or contagious disease which can be passed from one person to another. Direct physical contact, the handling of an infected object, or the transfer by droplets coughed or breathed out are all ways in which micro-organisms can be transmitted. The government produces a list of NOTIFIABLE DISEASES, which includes all the dangerous communicable diseases from anthrax, cholera and diphtheria through meningitis, rabies and smallpox to typhoid fever and whooping-cough (see respective entries). The UK's Public Health (Control of Diseases) Act 1984 and subsequent regulations in 1988 oblige a doctor who suspects that a patient has a notifiable disease to report this to the local consultant in communicable disease. Expert support is provided by the Public Health Laboratory Service via surveillance centres and specialist laboratories.

Communicable Diseases Control

The control of disease caused by infectious agents or their toxic products. Successes in the 19th and 20th centuries in the treatment and control of communicable diseases such as SMALLPOX, CHOLERA, TUBERCULOSIS, gastrointestinal infections, POLIOMYELITIS and SEXUALLY TRANSMITTED DISEASES (STDS) resulted in an erroneous conception that they no longer posed a serious threat to public health, and certainly not in developed countries. As a consequence, the maintenance of effective public health strategies steadily lost out in the competition for resources to the more 'glamorous' developments in medicine, such as improved CANCER treatments, HEART surgery, kidney DIALYSIS and organ TRANSPLANTATION. However, in recent decades the dangers of this approach have become increasingly apparent. Rapidly expanding urban populations, more complex lifestyles, new and resurgent infections (some linked to a spread of antibiotic resistance) such as AIDS/HIV and variant CREUTZFELDT-JAKOB DISEASE (CJD), and the ease with which infection can be spread by the enormous growth of long-distance travel and population migrations are severely straining existing public health measures. The supply of clean water, effective waste- and sewage-disposal measures, the hygienic production and delivery of food and early detection and subsequent prevention of infectious diseases can no longer be taken for granted. Governments will need to strengthen the provision of workable, properly resourced public health facilities, and developing countries will need financial support and expert help from developed nations to achieve this objective. Timely recognition of new and resurgent infectious diseases requires national and international early-warning mechanisms to ensure rapid investigation and implementation of effective control measures. Otherwise, serious breakdowns in public health will occur, and international co-operation is vital to provide and support control measures. (See also COMMUNICABLE DISEASE; NOTIFIABLE DISEASES.)

Community Care

Community care is intended to enable people to lead independent lives at home or in local residential units for as long as they are able to do so. For many years there has been a trend in Britain for care of elderly people and those with mental or physical problems to be shifted from hospitals and into community settings. In 1988 Sir Roy Griffiths's report to the Secretaries of State for Social Services, *Community Care: Agenda for Action*, advised on the best use of public funds to provide effective community care. The White Paper *Caring for People*, published in 1989, outlined the government's ideas for developing these proposals further. The plans were then enshrined in law with the National Health Service and Community Care Act of 1990.

Since April 1993, local social-services departments have been responsible for assessing what help people need from community-care services: these can include home helps, meals on wheels, sheltered housing, etc. Recipients of such services are means-tested and make variable contributions towards the costs. Policies on charging vary from one area to another and there are wide geographical variations in the range of services provided free and the charges levied for others.

People with complex needs may be assigned a case manager to coordinate the care package and ensure that appropriate responses are made to changing circumstances. The success of community care hinges on effective coordin-

ation of the services of an often large number of providers from the health and social-services sectors. Poor communication between sectors and inadequate coordination of services have been among the most common complaints about the community-care reforms.

Health care for people being cared for in the community remains largely free under the NHS arrangements, although there are regular debates about where the boundaries should be drawn between free health services and means-tested social care. A distinction has been made between necessary nursing care (funded by the state) and normal personal care (the responsibility of the patient), but the dividing line often proves hard to define.

As care has shifted increasingly into the community, previous hospital facilities have become redundant. Vast numbers of beds in long-stay geriatric hospitals and in-patient psychiatric wards have been closed. There is now concern that too few beds remain to provide essential emergency and respite services. In some areas, patients fit for discharge are kept in hospital because of delay in setting up community services for the elderly, or because of the inability of the local authority to fund appropriate care in a nursing home or at home with community-care support for other patients; the resulting BED-BLOCKING has an adverse effect on acutely ill patients needing hospital admission.

Community care, if correctly funded and coordinated, is an excellent way of caring for people with long-term needs, but considerable work is still needed in Britain to ensure that all patients have access to high-quality community care when they need it. Problems in providing such are are not confined to the UK.

Community Health Services

Usually managed by NHS trusts, these are a complex variety of services provided to people outside hospital settings. The key parts are the services delivered by district nurses, health visitors and therapists – for example, physiotherapists and speech therapists.

Community Mental Health Teams

Intended as a key part of the NHS's local comprehensive mental health services serving populations of around 50,000, these multidisciplinary, multi-agency teams have been less effective than expected, in part due to varying modes of operation in different districts. Some experts argue that the services they provide – for example, crisis intervention, liaison with primary care services and continuing care for long-term clients – could be delivered more effectively by several specialist teams rather than a single, large generic one comprising psychiatrists, psychologists, community mental health nurses, occupational therapists, support and (sometimes) social workers.

Community Nurses
A term that includes district nurses, health visitors, practice nurses and school nurses. While customarily based in a general practice or a health centre, they are independent health professionals contracted to the NHS (see NURSING).

Community Paediatrician
Formerly entitled consultant paediatrician (community child health), these are specialists dealing with children with chronic problems not involving acute or hospital care. For example, they have a primary role in dealing with disabled children, children with special educational needs and abused children.

Community Physician
A doctor who works in the specialty that encompasses PREVENTIVE MEDICINE, EPIDEMIOLOGY and PUBLIC HEALTH.

Compatibility
The extent to which a person's defence systems will accept invading foreign substances – for example, an injection of a drug, a blood transfusion or an organ transplant. When incompatibility occurs there is usually a rapid antibody attack on the invading antigen with a severe local or system reaction in the individual receiving the antigenic substance. (See IMMUNITY.)

Compensation
In medical parlance, a term applied to the counterbalancing of some defect of structure or function by some other special bodily development. The body possesses a remarkable power of adapting itself even to serious defects, so that disability due to these passes off after a time. The term is most often applied to the ability possessed by the heart to increase in size, and therefore in power, when the need for greater pumping action arises in consequence of a defective valve or some other abnormality in the circulation (see also HEART, DISEASES OF; CIRCULATORY SYSTEM OF THE BLOOD). A heart in this condition is, however, more liable to be prejudicially affected by strains and disease-processes, and the term 'failure of compensation' is applied to the symptoms that result

when this power becomes temporarily insufficient.

Compensation also refers to the financial compensation awarded to an individual who has been injured or made ill as a result of wrongful action or inaction by another individual or organisation. NHS trusts are increasingly being sued for compensation because patients believe that they have had unsatisfactory or damaging treatment. This is costing the NHS over £1 billion a year. (See RISK MANAGEMENT.)

Compensation neurosis Compensation neurosis or 'traumatic' neurosis is a psychological reaction to the prospects of compensation. It is a condition about which specialists disagree. Sufferers complain of a range of symptoms that may be a genuine consequence of their condition or an exaggerated response.

Complement
Complement is a normal constituent of blood serum which plays an important part in the antibody-antigen reaction which is the basis of many immunity processes. (See IMMUNITY.)

Complementary and Alternative Medicine (CAM)
This is the title used for a diverse group of health-related therapies and disciplines which are not considered to be a part of mainstream medical care. Other terms sometimes used to describe them include 'natural medicine', 'non-conventional medicine' and 'holistic medicine'. CAM embraces those therapies which may either be provided alongside conventional medicine (complementary) or which may, in the view of their practitioners, act as a substitute for it. Alternative disciplines purport to provide diagnostic information as well as offering therapy. However, there is a move now to integrate CAM with orthodox medicine and this view is supported by the Foundation for Integrated Medicine in the UK in its report, *A way forward for the next five years? – A discussion paper* (1997).

The University of Exeter Centre for Complementary Health Studies report, published in 2000, estimated that there are probably more than 60,000 practitioners of complementary and alternative medicine in the UK. In addition there are about 9,300 therapist members of organisations representing practitioners who have statutory qualifications, including doctors, nurses (see NURSING), midwives, osteopaths and physiotherapists; chiropractors became fully regulated by statute in

June 2001. There are likely to be many thousands more health staff with an active interest or involvement in the practice of complementary medicine – for example, the 10,000 members of the Royal College of Nursing's Complementary Therapy Forum. It is possible that up to 20,000 statutory health professionals regularly practise some form of complementary medicine including half of all general practices providing access to CAMs – most commonly manipulation therapies. The report from the Centre at Exeter University estimates that up to 5 million patients consulted a practitioner specialising in complementary and alternative medicine in 1999. Surveys of users of complementary and alternative practitioners show a relatively high satisfaction rating and it is likely that many patients will go on to use such therapists over an extended period. The Exeter Centre estimates that, with the increments of the last two years, up to 15–20 million people, possibly 33 per cent of the population of the country, have now sought such treatment.

The 1998 meeting of the British Medical Association (BMA) agreed to 'investigate the scientific basis and efficacy of acupuncture and the quality of training and standards of confidence in its practitioners'. In the resulting report (July 2000) the BMA recommended that guidelines on CAM use for general practitioners, complementary medicine practitioners and patients were urgently needed, and that the Department of Health should select key CAM therapies, including acupuncture, for appraisal by the National Institute for Clinical Medicine (NICE). The BMA also reiterated its earlier recommendation that the main CAM therapies, including acupuncture, should be included in familiarisation courses on CAM provided within medical schools, and that accredited postgraduate education should be provided to inform GPs and other clinicians about the possible benefits of CAM for patients.

Complement System

This is part of the body's defence mechanism that comprises a series of 20 serum peptides (see PEPTIDE). These are sequentially activated to produce three significant effects: firstly, the release of small peptides which provoke inflammation and attract phagocytes (see PHAGOCYTE); secondly, the deposition of a substance (component C3b) on the membranes of invading bacteria or viruses, attracting phagocytes to destroy the microbes; thirdly, the activation of substances that damage cell membranes – called lytic components – which hasten the destruction of 'foreign' cells. (See IMMUNOLOGY.)

Complex

The term applied to a combination of various actions or symptoms. It is particularly applied to a set of symptoms occurring together in mental disease with such regularity as to receive a special name.

Complexion

See   ACNE;   SKIN,   DISEASES   OF; PHOTODERMATOSES.

Compliance

The extent to which a patient follows the advice of a doctor or other health professional, especially in respect of drug or other treatments. This is generally increased if the patient understands both the condition and the basis for the proposed treatment. Assessment of a patient's compliance should be a routine part of treatment review.

Compress

Compress is the name given to a pad of linen or flannel wrung out of water and bound to the body. It is generally wrung out of cold water, and may be covered with a piece of waterproof material. It is used to subdue pain or inflammation. A hot compress is generally called a FOMENTATION.

Compressed Air Illness

Also known as caisson disease, this affects workers operating in compressed-air environments, such as underwater divers and workers in caissons (such as an ammunition wagon, a chest of explosive materials, or a strong case for keeping out the water while the foundations of a bridge are being built; derived from the French *caisse*, meaning case or chest). Its chief symptoms are pains in the joints and limbs (bends); pain in the stomach; headache and dizziness; and paralysis. Sudden death may occur. The condition is caused by the accumulation of bubbles of nitrogen in different parts of the body, usually because of too-rapid decompression when the worker returns to normal atmospheric presure – a change that must be made gradually.

Compression Syndrome

See MUSCLES, DISORDERS OF.

Computed Tomography

Tomography is an X-ray examination technique in which only structures in a particular plane produce clearly focused images. Whole-body computed tomography was introduced in 1977 and has already made a major impact in the investigation and management of medical and surgical disease. The technique is particularly valuable where a mass distorts the contour of an organ (e.g. a pancreatic tumour – see PANCREAS, DISORDERS OF) or where a lesion has a density different from that of surrounding tissue (e.g. a metastasis in the LIVER).

Computed tomography can distinguish soft tissues from cysts or fat, but in general soft-tissue masses have similar appearances, so that distinguishing an inflammatory mass from a malignant process may be impossible. The technique is particularly useful in patients with suspected malignancy; it can also define the extent of the cancer by detecting enlarged lymph nodes, indicating lymphatic spread. The main indications for computed tomography of the body are: mediastinal masses, suspected pulmonary metastases, adrenal disease, pancreatic masses, retroperitoneal lymph nodes, intra-abdominal abscesses, orbital tumours and the staging of cancer as a guide to effective treatment.

Computerised Decision-Support Systems

Also known as 'expert systems', these are computer software systems intended to help doctors make clinical decisions. Primary care medicine is especially noted for its uncertainty by virtue of being most patients' first point of contact with health care, confronting the clinician with many 'undifferentiated' health problems. So far, these systems have not been as effective as expected because of a failure to analyse the needs of primary care. Simple procedures to prompt the delivery of treatment to patients with chronic conditions have improved care quality, but work needs to be done on their cost-effectiveness. The aim of more complex computerised support systems will be to forecast likely future events and the possible effectiveness of proposed interventions, based on available information about the patient and an understanding of the risks and efficacy of interventions by doctors and other experts.

One example, called ISABEL, can be accessed by paediatricians to check on their diagnosis and management of many childhood disorders.

Computerised Tomography

See COMPUTED TOMOGRAPHY.

Conception

Conception signifies the complex set of changes which occur in the OVUM and in the body of the mother at the beginning of pregnancy. The precise moment of conception is that at which the male element, or spermatozoon, and the female element, or ovum, fuse together. Only one-third of these conceptions survive to birth, whilst 15 per cent are cut short by spontaneous abortion or stillbirth. The remainder – over one-half – are lost very early during pregnancy without trace. (See also FETUS.)

Concussion of the Brain

See BRAIN INJURIES.

Conditioned Reflex

The development of a specific response by an individual to a specific stimulus. The best-known conditioned reflex is the one described by Ivan Pavlov, in which dogs that became accustomed to being fed when a bell was sounded salivated on hearing the bell, even if no food was given. The conditioned reflex is an important part of behavioural theory.

Condom

A thin rubber or plastic sheath placed over the erect PENIS before sexual intercourse. It is the most effective type of barrier contraception and is also valuable in preventing the transfer between sexual partners of pathogenic organisms such as gonococci, which cause GONORRHOEA, and human immuno-deficiency virus, which may lead to AIDS (see AIDS/HIV). Sheaths are most effective when properly used and with spermicides.

The female condom might be suitable for contraception when a woman misses a day or two of her contraceptive pill; if there is DYSPAREUNIA; when the perineum needs protection, for example, after childbirth; or in cases of latex allergy to traditional condoms. Used properly with spermicide, it provides an effective barrier both to infections and to spermatozoa. Failure may result if the penis goes alongside the condom, if it gets pushed up into the vagina, or if it falls out. (See CONTRACEPTION.)

Condyle

A rounded prominence at the end of a bone: for example, the prominences at the outer and inner sides of the knee on the thigh-bone (or FEMUR). The projecting part of a condyle is sometimes known as an epicondyle, as in the case of the condyle at the lower end of the HUMERUS where the epicondyles form the prominences on the outer and inner side of the elbow.

Condyloma
A localised, rounded swelling of mucous membrane around the opening of the bowel, and the genital organs, sometimes known as 'genital warts' or 'ano-genital warts'. There are two main forms: condyloma latum, which is syphilitic in origin; and condyloma accuminatum, which often occurs in association with sexually transmitted disease, but is only indirectly due to it, being primarily a virus infection.

Cone
(1) A light-sensitive cell in the retina of the EYE that can also distinguish colours. The other type of light-sensitive cell is called a rod. There are around six million cones in the human retina and these are thought to comprise three types that are sensitive to the three primary colours of red, blue, and green.
(2) A cone biopsy is a surgical technique in which a conical or cylindrical section of the lower part of the neck of the womb is excised.

Confidentiality
The ethical principle that doctors do not reveal information to other people (or to organisations) that their patients have given to them in confidence. Normally the doctor must get permission to release confidential information to an employer (or other authoritative body), insurance company or lawyer. The doctor does have to provide such information if required by a court of law. (See ETHICS.)

Congenital
Congenital deformities, diseases, etc. are those which are either present at birth, or which, being transmitted direct from the parents, show themselves some time after birth.

Congenital Adrenal Hyperplasia
See ADRENOGENITAL SYNDROME and GENETIC DISORDERS.

Congestion
The accumulation of blood or other body fluid in a particular part of the body. The condition may be due to some failure in the circulation, but as a rule is one of the early signs of INFLAMMATION (see also ABSCESS; PNEUMONIA).

Conjoined Twins
Identical twins who are united bodily but are possessed of separate personalities. Their frequency is not known, but it has been estimated that throughout the world, six or more conjoined twins are born every year who are capable of separation. The earliest case on record is that of the 'Biddendon Maids' who were born in England in 1100. The 'Scottish Brothers' lived for 28 years at the court of James III of Scotland. Perhaps the most famous conjoined twins, however, were Chang and Eng, who were born of Chinese parents in Siam in 1811. It was they who were responsible for the introduction of the term, 'Siamese twins', which still remains the popular name for 'conjoined twins'. They were joined together at the lower end of the chest bone, and achieved fame by being shown in Barnum's circus in the United States. They subsequently married English sisters and settled as farmers in North Carolina. They died in 1874.

The earliest attempt at surgical separation is said to have been made by Dr Farius of Basle in 1689. The first successful separation in Great Britain was in 1912: both twins survived the operation and one survived well into adult life. This is said to be the first occasion on which both twins survived the operation. The success of the operation is largely dependent upon the degree of union between the twins. Thus, if this is only skin, subcutaneous tissue and cartilage, the prospects of survival for both twins are good; but if some vital organ such as the liver is shared, the operation is much more hazardous. (See MULTIPLE BIRTHS.)

Conjugate Deviation
The term for describing the persistent and involuntary turning of both eyes in any one direction, and is a sign of a lesion in the brain.

Conjunctiva
See EYE.

Conjunctivitis
See EYE, DISORDERS OF.

Connective Tissue
Sometimes called fibrous tissue, this is one of the most abundant tissues in the body, holding together the body's many different structures. Connective tissue comprises a matrix of substances called mucopolysaccharides in which are embedded various specialist tissues and cells. These include elastic (yellow), collagenous (white) and reticular fibres as well as macrophages (see MACROPHAGE) and MAST CELLS. Assembled in differing proportions, this provides structures with varying functions: bone,

cartilage, tendons, ligaments and fatty and elastic tissues. Collagenous connective tissue binds the muscles together and provides the substance of skin. It is also laid down in wound repair, forming the scar tissue. Contracting with time, connective tissue becomes denser, causing the puckering that is typical in serious wounds or burns. (See ADHESION; SCAR; WOUNDS.)

Connective Tissue Disorders
A group of generalised inflammatory diseases that affect CONNECTIVE TISSUE in almost any system in the body. The term does not include those disorders of genetic origin. RHEUMATIC FEVER and RHEUMATOID ARTHRITIS were traditionally classified in this group, as were those diseases classed under the outdated heading COLLAGEN DISEASES.

Consanguinous
A relationship by blood: siblings are closely consanguinous; cousins, and grandparents and grandchildren, less so. (See INBREEDING.)

Conscientious Objection
See ETHICS.

Consciousness
The state of being aware of physical events or mental concepts. A conscious person is awake and responsive to his or her surroundings. (See also COMA; UNCONSCIOUS; ANAESTHESIA.)

Conservative Treatment
Medical treatment which involves the minimum of active interference by the practitioner. For example, a disc lesion in the back might be treated by bed rest in contrast to surgical intervention to remove the damaged disc.

Consolidation
A term applied to solidification of an organ, especially of a lung. The consolidation may be of a permanent nature due to formation of fibrous tissue, or may be temporary, as in acute pneumonia.

Constipation
A condition in which a person infrequently passes hard FAECES (stools). Patients sometimes complain of straining, a feeling of incomplete evacuation of faeces, and abdominal or perianal discomfort. A healthy individual usually opens his or her bowels once daily but the frequency may vary, perhaps twice daily or once only every two or three days. Constipation is generally defined as fewer than three bowel openings a week. Healthy people may have occasional bouts of constipation, usually reflecting a temporary change in diet or the result of taking drugs – for example, CODEINE – or any serious condition resulting in immobility, especially in elderly people.

Constipation is a chronic condition and must be distinguished from the potentially serious disorder, acute obstruction, which may have several causes (see under INTESTINE, DISEASES OF). There are several possible causes of constipation; those due to gastrointestinal disorders include:

● Dietary: lack of fibre; low fluid consumption.
● Structural: benign strictures (narrowing of gut); carcinoma of the COLON; DIVERTICULAR DISEASE.
● Motility: poor bowel training when young; slow transit due to reduced muscle activity in the colon, occurring usually in women; IRRITABLE BOWEL SYNDROME (IBS); HIRSCHSPRUNG'S DISEASE.
● Defaecation: anorectal disease such as fissures, HAEMORRHOIDS and CROHN'S DISEASE; impaction of faeces.

Non-gastrointestinal disorders causing constipation include:

● Drugs: opiates (preparations of OPIUM), iron supplements, ANTACIDS containing aluminium, ANTICHOLINERGIC drugs.
● Metabolic and endocrine: DIABETES MELLITUS, pregnancy (see PREGNANCY AND LABOUR), hypothyroidism (see under THYROID GLAND, DISEASES OF).
● Neurological: cerebrovascular accidents (STROKE), MULTIPLE SCLEROSIS (MS), PARKINSONISM, lesions in the SPINAL CORD.

Persistent constipation for which there is no obvious cause merits thorough investigation, and people who experience a change in bowel habits – for example, alternating constipation and diarrhoea – should also seek expert advice.

Treatment Most people with constipation will respond to a dietary supplement of fibre, coupled, when appropriate, with an increase in fluid intake. If this fails to work, judicious use of LAXATIVES for, say, a month is justified. Should constipation persist, investigations on the advice of a general practitioner will probably be needed; any further treatment will depend on the outcome of the investigations in which a specialist will usually be involved. Successful treatment of the cause should then return the patient's bowel habits to normal.

Constitution

Constitution, or DIATHESIS, means the general condition of the body, especially with reference to its liability to certain diseases.

Consultant

In Britain's health service a consultant is the senior career post for a fully accredited specialist. He or she normally sees patients referred by general practitioners – hence the historical term 'consultant' – or emergency cases admitted direct to hospital. NHS consultants are also allowed to do a certain amount of private practice if they wish. After qualification and a two-year period of general supervised training, doctors enter onto a specialist training scheme, working in hospitals for 5–8 years before being accredited; many also do research or spend some time working abroad. All must pass difficult higher examinations. In 2004, the number of consultant hospital medical and dental staff in Great Britain was 30,650 (some of these worked part-time, so the whole-time equivalent [w.t.e.] figure was 25,640). The total number of hospital medical and dental staff was 86,996 (w.t.e. 78,462).

Consumption

See TUBERCULOSIS.

Contact a Family

A charity which helps families with disabled children to obtain good-quality information, support and – most of all – contact with other families with children who have the same disorder. This includes children with specific and rare conditions and those with special educational needs. The charity has many local parent groups throughout the UK and publishes a comprehensive directory with brief descriptions of each condition followed by contact addresses, phone numbers and web addresses. It also has a central helpline and a team of parent advisers.

See www.cafamily.org.uk

Contact Lenses

Contact lenses are lenses worn in contact with the EYE, behind the eyelids and in front of the cornea. They may be worn for cosmetic, optical or therapeutic reasons. The commonest reason for wear is cosmetic, many short-sighted people preferring to wear contact lenses instead of glasses. Optical reasons for contact-lens wear include cataract surgery (usually unilateral extraction) and the considerable improvement in overall standard of vision experienced by very short-sighted people when wearing contact lenses instead of glasses. Therapeutic lenses are those used in the treatment of eye disease: 'bandage lenses' are used in certain corneal diseases; contact lenses can be soaked in a particular drug and then put on the eye so that the drug slowly leaks out on to the eye. Contact lenses may be hard, soft or gas permeable. Hard lenses are more optically accurate (because they are rigid), cheaper and more durable than soft. The main advantage of soft lenses is that they are more comfortable to wear. Gas-permeable lenses are so-called because they are more permeable to oxygen than other lenses, thus allowing more oxygen to reach the cornea.

Disposable lenses are soft lenses designed to be thrown away after a short period of continuous use; their popularity rests on the fact that they need not be cleaned. The instructions on use should be followed carefully because the risk of complications, such as corneal infection, are higher than with other types of contact lenses.

Contraindications to the use of contact lenses include a history of ATOPY, 'dry eyes', previous GLAUCOMA surgery and a person's inability to cope with the management of lenses. The best way to determine whether contact lenses are suitable, however, may be to try them out. Good hygiene is essential for wearers so as to minimise the risk of infection, which may lead to a corneal abscess – a serious complication. Corneal abrasions are fairly common and, if a contact-lens wearer develops a red eye, the lens should be removed and the eye tested with fluorescein dye to identify any abrasions. Appropriate treatment should be given and the lens not worn again until the abrasion or infection has cleared up.

Contagion

Contagion means the principle of spread of disease by direct contact with the body of an affected person.

Continued Fevers

Continued fevers-are typhus, typhoid and relapsing fevers, so-called because of their continuing over a more or less definite space of time.

Continuity of Care

A term describing a system of medical care in which individuals requiring advice on their health consult a named primary care physician (GENERAL PRACTITIONER (GP)) or partnership of practitioners. The availability of an individual's medical records, and the doctor's knowledge of his or her medical, family and social history, should facilitate prompt, appropriate decisions about investigations, treatment or referral to specialists. What the doctor(s) know(s) about the patient can, for example, save time, alert hospitals to allergies, avoid the duplication of investigations and provide hospitals with practical domestic information when a patient is ready for discharge. The traditional 24-hours-a-day, 365-days-a-year care by a personal physician is now a rarity: continuity of care has evolved and is now commonly based on a multi-disciplinary health team working from common premises. Changing social structures, population mobility and the complexity and cost of health care have driven this evolution. Some experts have argued that the changes are so great as to make continuity of care an unrealistic concept in the 21st century. Nevertheless, support inside and outside conventional medical practice for HOLISTIC medicine – a related concept for treating the whole person, body and mind – and the fact that many people still appreciate the facility to see their own doctors suggest that continuity of care is still a valid objective of value to the community.

Continuous Autologous Transfusion

See TRANSFUSION.

Continuous Positive Airways Pressure

A method for treating babies who suffer from alveolar collapse in the lung as a result of HYALINE MEMBRANE DISEASE (see also RESPIRATORY DISTRESS SYNDROME).

Contraception

A means of avoiding pregnancy despite sexual activity. There is no ideal contraceptive, and the choice of method depends on balancing considerations of safety, effectiveness and acceptability. The best choice for any couple will depend on their ages and personal circumstances and may well vary with time. Contraceptive techniques can be classified in various ways, but one of the most useful is into 'barrier' and 'non-barrier' methods.

Barrier methods These involve a physical barrier which prevents sperm (see SPERMATOZOON) from reaching the cervix (see CERVIX UTERI). Barrier methods reduce the risk of spreading sexually transmitted diseases, and the

sheath is the best protection against HIV infection (see AIDS/HIV) for sexually active people. The efficiency of barrier methods is improved if they are used in conjunction with a spermicidal foam or jelly, but care is needed to ensure that the preparation chosen does not damage the rubber barrier or cause an allergic reaction in the users.

CONDOM OR SHEATH This is the most commonly used barrier contraceptive. It consists of a rubber sheath which is placed over the erect penis before intromission and removed after ejaculation. The failure rate, if properly used, is about 4 per cent.

DIAPHRAGM OR CAP A rubber dome that is inserted into the vagina before intercourse and fits snugly over the cervix. It should be used with an appropriate spermicide and is removed six hours after intercourse. A woman must be measured to ensure that she is supplied with the correct size of diaphragm, and the fit should be checked annually or after more than about 7 lbs. change in weight. The failure rate, if properly used, is about 2 per cent.

Non-barrier methods These do not provide a physical barrier between sperm and cervix and so do not protect against sexually transmitted diseases, including HIV.

COITUS INTERRUPTUS This involves the man's withdrawing his penis from the vagina before ejaculation. Because some sperm may leak before full ejaculation, the method is not very reliable.

SAFE PERIOD This involves avoiding intercourse around the time when the woman ovulates and is at risk of pregnancy. The safe times can be predicted using temperature charts to identify the rise in temperature before ovulation, or by careful assessment of the quality of the cervical mucus. This method works best if the woman has regular menstrual cycles. If used carefully it can be very effective but requires a highly disciplined couple to succeed. It is approved by the Catholic church.

SPERMICIDAL GELS, CREAMS, PESSARIES, ETC. These are supposed to prevent pregnancy by killing sperm before they reach the cervix, but they are unreliable and should be used only in conjunction with a barrier method.

INTRAUTERINE CONTRACEPTIVE DEVICE (COIL) This is a small metal or plastic shape, placed inside the uterus, which prevents pregnancy by disrupting implantation. Some people regard it as a form of abortion, so it is not acceptable to all religious groups. There is a risk of pelvic infection and eventual infertility in women who have used coils, and in many countries their use has declined substantially. Coils must be inserted by a specially trained health worker, but once in place they permit intercourse at any time with no prior planning. Increased pain and bleeding may be caused during menstruation. If severe, such symptoms may indicate that the coil is incorrectly sited, and that its position should be checked.

HORMONAL METHODS Steroid hormones have dominated contraceptive developments during the past 40 years, with more than 200 million women worldwide taking or having taken 'the pill'. In the past 20 years, new developments have included modifying existing methods and devising more effective ways of delivering the drugs, such as implants and hormone-releasing devices in the uterus. Established hormonal contraception includes the combined oestrogen and progesterone and progesterone-only contraceptive pills, as well as longer-acting depot preparations. They modify the woman's hormonal environment and prevent pregnancy by disrupting various stages of the menstrual cycle, especially ovulation. The combined oestrogen and progesterone pills are very effective and are the most popular form of contraception. Biphasic and triphasic pills contain different quantities of oestrogen and progesterone taken in two or three phases of the menstrual cycle. A wide range of preparations is available and the *British National Formulary* contains details of the commonly used varieties.

The main side-effect is an increased risk of cardiovascular disease. The lowest possible dose of oestrogen should be used, and many preparations are phasic, with the dose of oestrogen varying with the time of the cycle. The progesterone-only, or 'mini', pill does not contain any oestrogen and must be taken at the same time every day. It is not as effective as the combined pill, but failure rates of less than 1-per-100 woman years can be achieved. It has few serious side-effects, but may cause menstrual irregularities. It is suitable for use by mothers who are breast feeding.

Depot preparations include intramuscular injections, subcutaneous implants, and intravaginal rings. They are useful in cases where the woman cannot be relied on to take a pill regularly but needs effective contraception. Their main side-effect is their prolonged action, which means that users cannot suddenly decide that they would like to become pregnant. Skin patches containing a contraceptive that is absorbed through the skin have recently been launched.

HORMONAL CONTRACEPTION FOR MEN There is a growing demand by men worldwide for hormonal contraception. Development of a 'male pill', however, has been slow because of the potentially dangerous side-effects of using high doses of TESTOSTERONE (the male hormone) to suppress spermatogenesis. Progress in research to develop a suitable ANDROGEN-based combination product is promising, including the possibility of long-term STEROID implants.

STERILISATION See also STERILISATION − Reproductive sterilisation. The operation is easier and safer to perform on men than on women. Although sterilisation can sometimes be reversed, this cannot be guaranteed and couples should be counselled in advance that the method is irreversible. There is a small but definite failure rate with sterilisation, and this should also be made clear before the operation is performed.

POSTCOITAL CONTRACEPTION Also known as emergency contraception or the 'morning after pill', postcoital contraception can be effected by two different hormonal methods. Levonorgesterol (a synthetic hormone similar to the natural female sex hormone PROGESTERONE) can be used alone, with one pill being taken within 72 hours of unprotected intercourse, but preferably as soon as possible, and a second one 12 hours after the first. Alternatively, a combined preparation comprising ETHINYLESTRADIOL and levonorgesterol can be taken, also within 72 hours of unprotected intercourse. The single constituent pill has fewer side-effects than the combined version. Neither version should be taken by women with severe liver disease or acute PORPHYRIAS, but the ethinylestradiol/levonorgesterol combination is unsuitable for women with a history of THROMBOSIS.

In the UK the law allows women over the age of 16 to buy the morning-after pill 'over the counter' from a registered pharmacist.

Contracture

The permanent shortening of a muscle or of fibrous tissue. Contraction is the name given to the temporary shortening of a muscle.

Contrast Medium

A material that is used to increase the visibility of the body's tissues and organs during RADIOGRAPHY. A common example is the use of barium which is given by mouth or as an enema to show up the alimentary tract.

Contre-Coup

An injury in which a bone, generally the skull,

is fractured – not at the spot where the violence is applied, but at the exactly opposite point.

Controlled Drugs

In the United Kingdom, controlled drugs are those preparations referred to under the Misuse of Drugs Act 1971. The Act prohibits activities related to the manufacture, supply and possession of these drugs, and they are classified into three groups which determine the penalties for offences involving their misuse. For example, class A includes COCAINE, DIAMORPHINE, MORPHINE, LSD (see LYSERGIC ACID DIETHYL-AMIDE and PETHIDINE HYDROCHLORIDE. Class B includes AMPHETAMINES, BARBITURATES and CODEINE. Class C includes drugs related to amphetamines such as diethylpropion and chlorphentermine, meprobamate and most BENZODIAZEPINES and CANNABIS.

The Misuse of Drugs Regulations 1985 define the classes of person authorised to supply and possess controlled drugs, and lay down the conditions under which these activities may be carried out. In the Regulations, drugs are divided into five schedules specifying the requirements for supply, possession, prescribing and record-keeping. Schedule I contains drugs which are not used as medicines. Schedules II and III contain drugs which are subject to the prescription requirements of the Act (see below). They are distinguished in the *British National Formulary* (BNF) by the symbol CD and they include morphine, diamorphine (heroin), other opioid analgesics, barbiturates, amphetamines, cocaine and diethylpropion. Schedules IV and V contain drugs such as the benzodiazepines which are subject to minimal control. A full list of the drugs in each schedule can be found in the BNF.

Prescriptions for drugs in schedules II and III must be signed and dated by the prescriber, who must give his or her address. The prescription must be in the prescriber's own handwriting and provide the name and address of the patient and the total quantity of the preparation in both words and figures. The pharmacist is not allowed to dispense a controlled drug unless all the information required by law is given on the prescription.

Until 1997 the Misuse of Drugs (Notification and Supply of Addicts) Regulations 1973 governed the notification of addicts. This was required in respect of the following commonly used drugs: cocaine, dextromoramide, diamorphine, dipipanone, hydrocodeine, hydromorphone, levorphanol, methadone, morphine, opium, oxycodone, pethidine, phenazocine and piritranide.

In 1997 the Misuse of Drugs (Supply to Addicts) Regulations 1997 revoked the 1973 requirement for notification. Doctors are now expected to report (on a standard form) cases of drug misuse to their local Drug Misuse Database (DMD). Notification by the doctor should be made when a patient first presents with a drug problem or when he or she visits again after a gap of six months or more. All types of misuse should be reported: this includes opioids, benzodiazepines and central nervous system stimulants. The data in the DMD are anonymised, which means that doctors cannot check on possible multiple prescribing for drug addicts.

The 1997 Regulations restrict the prescribing of diamorphine (heroin), Diconal® (a morphine-based drug) or cocaine to medical practitioners holding a special licence issued by the Home Secretary.

Fuller details about the prescription of controlled drugs are in the *British National Formulary*, updated twice a year, and available on the Internet (see www.bnf.org).

Contusion

See BRUISES.

Convalescence

The condition through which a person passes after having suffered from some acute disease, and before complete health and strength are regained.

Convergence

(1) Inward turning of the eyes to focus on a near point, with the result that a single image is registered by both retinas.
(2) The coming together of various nerve fibres to form a nerve tract that provides a single pathway from different parts of the brain.

Conversion Disorder

A psychological disorder, also called hysterical conversion, in which the affected individual presents with striking neurological symptoms – such as weakness, paralysis, sensory disturbances or memory loss – for which no organic cause can be identified. Up to 4 per cent of patients attending neurological outpatient clinics have been estimated as having conversion disorders. The disorder remains controversial, with theories about its cause unsupported by controlled research results. In clinical practice the physician's experience and intuition are major factors in diagnosis. It has been suggested that the physical symptoms represent guilt about a physical or emotional assault on someone else. Treatment using a COGNITIVE BEHAVIOUR approach may help those with conversion disorders.

Convolutions
See BRAIN.

Convulsions
Rapidly alternating contractions and relaxations of the muscles, causing irregular movements of the limbs or body generally, usually accompanied by unconsciousness.

Causes The most common reason for convulsions is EPILEPSY, and the underlying cause of the latter often remains uncertain. In newborns, convulsions may be due to HYPOXIA following a difficult labour, or to low levels of sugar or calcium in the blood (HYPOGLYCAEMIA; HYPOCALCAEMIA). A sudden rise of body temperature during infective illness may induce convulsions in an infant or young child.

Diseases of the brain, such as meningitis, encephalitis and tumours, or any disturbance of the brain due to bleeding, blockage of a blood vessel, or irritation of the brain by a fracture of the skull, may also be responsible for convulsions (see BRAIN, DISEASES OF).

Asphyxia, for example from choking, may also bring on convulsions.

Treatment Newborns with hypoglycaemia or hypocalcaemia are treated by replacing the missing compound. Infants with febrile convulsions may be sponged with tepid water and fever reduced with paracetamol.

In epilepsy, unless it is particularly severe, the movements seldom need to be restrained. If convulsions persist beyond a few minutes it may be necessary to give BENZODIAZEPINES, either intravenously or rectally. In the UK, paramedics are trained to do this; likewise many parents of epileptic children are capable of administering the necessary treatment. If however this fails to stop the convulsions immediately, hospital admission is needed for further treatment. Once fits are under control, the cause of the convulsions must be sought and the necessary long-term treatment given.

Cooley's Anaemia
See THALASSAEMIA.

Coomb's Test
A sensitive test that detects ANTIBODIES to the body's red cells (see ERYTHROCYTE). There are two methods: one – the direct method – identifies those antibodies that are bound to the cells; the other, indirect, method identifies those circulating unattached in the serum.

Coordination
The governing power exercised by the brain as a whole, or by certain centres in the nervous system, to make various muscles contract in harmony and so produce definite actions (instead of meaningless movements). Coordination is intimately bound up with the complex sense of localisation, which enables a person with their eyes shut to tell, by sensations received from the bones, joints and muscles, the position of the various parts of their body.

The power is impaired in various diseases, such as LOCOMOTOR ATAXIA. It is tested by making the patient shut their eyes, moving their hand in various directions, and then telling them to bring the point of the forefinger steadily to the tip of the nose – or by other simple movements.

Copper
Copper is an essential nutrient for humans, and all tissues in the human body contain traces of it. The total amount in the adult body is 100–150 mg. Many essential enzyme systems are dependent on traces of copper; on the other hand, there is no evidence that dietary deficiency of copper ever occurs in humans. Infants are born with an ample store, and the normal diet for an adult contains around 2 mg of copper a day. It is used in medicine as the two salts, sulphate of copper (blue stone) and nitrate of copper. The former is, in small doses, a powerful astringent, and in larger doses an irritant. Both are caustics when applied externally. Externally, either is used to rub on unhealthy ulcers and growths to stimulate the granulation tissue to more rapid healing.

Coprolalia
An inherited condition, usually beginning in childhood. It presents with motor tics and with irrepressible, explosive, occasionally obscene, verbal ejaculations. (See GILLES DE LA TOURETTE'S SYNDROME.)

Copulation
The act of coitus or sexual intercourse, when the man inserts his erect penis into the woman's vagina and after a succession of thrusting movements ejaculates his semen.

Cordotomy
The surgical operation of cutting the anterolateral tracts of the SPINAL CORD to relieve

otherwise intractable pain. It is also sometimes known as tractotomy.

Cornea

See EYE.

Corneal Graft

Also known as keratoplasty. If the cornea (see EYE) becomes damaged or diseased and vision is impaired, it can be removed and replaced by a corneal graft. The graft is taken from the cornea of a human donor. Some of the indications for corneal grafting include keratoconus (conical-shaped cornea), corneal dystrophies, severe corneal scarring following HERPES SIMPLEX, and alkali burns or other injury. Because the graft is a foreign protein, there is a danger that the recipient's immune system may set up a reaction causing rejection of the graft. Rejection results in OEDEMA of the graft with subsequent poor vision. Once a corneal graft has been taken from a donor, it should be used as quickly as possible. Corneas can be stored for days in tissue-culture medium at low temperature. A small number of grafts are autografts in which a patient's cornea is repositioned.

The Department of Health has drawn up a list of suitable eye-banks to which people can apply to bequeath their eyes, and an official form is now available for the bequest of eyes. (See also DONORS; TRANSPLANTATION.)

Corneal Reflex

Instinctive closing of the eyelids when the surface of the cornea (see EYE) is lightly touched with a fine hair.

Corns and Bunions

A corn is a localised thickening of the cuticle or epidermis (see SKIN) affecting the foot. The thickening is of a conical shape; the point of the cone is directed inwards and is known as the 'eye' of the corn. A general thickening over a wider area is called a callosity. Bunion is a condition found over the joint at the base of the big toe, in which not only is there thickening of the skin, but the head of the metatarsal bone also becomes prominent. Hammer-toe is a condition of the second toe, often caused by short boots, in which the toe becomes bent at its two joints in such a way as to resemble a hammer.

Corns and bunions are caused by badly fitting shoes, hence the importance of children and adults wearing properly fitted footwear. Corns can be pared after softening in warm water, or painted with salicylic acid collodion or other proprietary preparations. Bad corns may need treatment by a chiropodist (see CHIR-OPODY). Bunions may require surgical treatment. Regular foot care is important in patients with DIABETES MELLITUS.

Coronary

A term applied to several structures in the body encircling an organ in the manner of a crown. The coronary arteries are the arteries of supply to the HEART which arise from the aorta, just beyond the aortic valve, and through which the blood is delivered to the muscle of the heart. Disease of the coronary arteries is a very serious condition producing various abnormal forms of heart action and the disorder, ANGINA PECTORIS.

Coronary Angioplasty

A technique of dilating atheromatous obstructions (see ATHEROMA) in CORONARY ARTERIES by inserting a catheter with a balloon on the end into the affected artery (see also CATHETERS). It is passed through the blockage (guided by X-ray FLUOROSCOPY) and inflated. The procedure can be carried out through a percutaneous route.

Coronary Arteries

(See also HEART.) The right coronary artery arises from the right aortic sinus and passes into the right atrio-ventricular groove to supply the right ventricle, part of the intraventricular septum and the inferior part of the left ventricle. The left coronary artery arises from the left sinus and divides into an anterior descending branch which supplies the septum and the anterior and apical parts of the heart, and the circumflex branch which passes into the left atrio-ventricular groove and supplies the lateral posterior surfaces of the heart. Small anastomoses exist between the coronary arteries and they have the potential of enlarging if the blood-flow through a neighbouring coronary artery is compromised. Coronary artery disease is damage to the heart caused by the narrowing or blockage of these arteries. It commonly presents as ANGINA PECTORIS or acute myocardial infarction (see HEART, DISEASES OF).

Coronary Artery Vein Bypass Grafting (CAVBG)

When coronary arteries, narrowed by disease, cannot supply the heart muscle with sufficient blood, the cardiac circulation may be improved by grafting a section of vein from the leg to bypass the obstruction. Around 10,000 people in the United Kingdom have this operation annually and the results are usually good. It is a major procedure that lasts several hours and requires the heart to be stopped temporarily, with blood circulation and oxygenation taken over by a HEART-LUNG MACHINE.

Coronary Care Unit (CCU)

A specialised hospital unit equipped and staffed to provide intensive care (see INTENSIVE THERAPY UNIT (ITU)) for patients who have had severe heart attacks or undergone surgery on the heart.

Coronary Thrombosis

See HEART, DISEASES OF.

Coronaviruses

Coronaviruses – so-called because in electron micrographs the spikes projecting from the virus resemble a crown – are a group of viruses which have been isolated from people with common colds (see COLD, COMMON) and have also been shown to produce common colds under experimental conditions. Their precise significance in the causation of the common cold is still undetermined.

Coroner

An independent legal officer of the Crown who is responsible for deciding whether to hold a POST-MORTEM EXAMINATION and an inquest in cases of sudden or unexpected or unnatural death. He or she presides over an inquest, if held – sometimes with the help of a jury. Coroners are usually lawyers or doctors (some are double-qualified) who have been qualified for at least five years. In Scotland the coroner is known as the procurator fiscal.

Corpulence

See OBESITY.

Cor Pulmonale

Another name for pulmonary heart disease, which is characterised by hypertrophy and failure of the right VENTRICLE of the heart as a result of disease of the LUNGS or disorder of the pulmonary circulation.

Corpuscle

Corpuscle means a small body. (See BLOOD.)

Corpus Luteum

The mass of cells formed in the ruptured Graafian follicle in the ovary (see OVARIES) from which the ovum is discharged about 15 days before the onset of the next menstrual period (see MENSTRUATION). When the ovum escapes, the follicle fills up with blood; this is soon replaced by cells which contain a yellow fatty material. The follicle and its luteal cells constitute the corpus luteum. The corpus luteum begins to disappear after ten days, unless the discharged ovum is fertilised and pregnancy ensues. In pregnancy the corpus luteum persists and grows and secretes the hormone, PROGESTERONE.

Corrigan's Pulse

The name applied to the collapsing pulse found with incompetence of the heart's aortic valve. It is so-called after Sir Dominic John Corrigan (1802–80), the famous Dublin physician, who first described it.

Corrosives

Corrosives are poisonous substances which corrode or eat away the skin or the mucous surfaces of mouth, gullet and stomach with which they come into contact. Examples are strong mineral acids like sulphuric, nitric and hydrochloric acids, caustic alkalis, and some salts like chlorides of mercury and zinc. (See POISONS.)

Corset

A support device worn around the trunk to help in the treatment of backache and spinal injuries or disorders.

Cortex

The tissues that form the outer part of an organ and which are positioned just below the capsule or outer membrane. Examples are the cerebal cortex of the BRAIN and the renal cortex of the KIDNEYS.

Corticosteroids

The generic term for the group of hormones produced by the ADRENAL GLANDS, with a profound effect on mineral and glucose metabolism.

Many modifications have been devised of the basic steroid molecule in an attempt to keep useful therapeutic effects and minimise unwanted side-effects. The main corticosteroid hormones currently available are CORTISONE, HYDROCORTISONE, PREDNISONE, PREDNISOLONE, methyl prednisolone, triamcinolone, dexamethasone, betamethasone, paramethasone and deflazacort.

They are used clinically in three quite distinct circumstances. First they constitute replacement therapy where a patient is unable to produce their own steroids – for example, in adrenocortical insufficiency or hypopituitarism. In this situation the dose is physiological – namely, the equivalent of the normal adrenal output under similar circumstances – and is not

C

associated with any side-effects. Secondly, steroids are used to depress activity of the adrenal cortex in conditions where this is abnormally high or where the adrenal cortex is producing abnormal hormones, as occurs in some hirsute women.

The third application for corticosteroids is in suppressing the manifestations of disease in a wide variety of inflammatory and allergic conditions, and in reducing antibody production in a number of AUTOIMMUNE DISORDERS. The inflammatory reaction is normally part of the body's defence mechanism and is to be encouraged rather than inhibited. However, in the case of those diseases in which the body's reaction is disproportionate to the offending agent, such that it causes unpleasant symptoms or frank illness, the steroid hormones can inhibit this undesirable response. Although the underlying condition is not cured as a result, it may resolve spontaneously. When corticosteroids are used for their anti-inflammatory properties, the dose is pharmacological; that is, higher – often much higher – than the normal physiological requirement. Indeed, the necessary dose may exceed the normal maximum output of the healthy adrenal gland, which is about 250–300 mg cortisol per day. When doses of this order are used there are inevitable risks and side-effects: a drug-induced CUSHING'S SYNDROME will result.

Corticosteroid treatment of short duration, as in angioneurotic OEDEMA of the larynx or other allergic crises, may at the same time be life-saving and without significant risk (see URTICARIA). Prolonged therapy of such connective-tissue disorders, such as POLYARTERITIS NODOSA with its attendant hazards, is generally accepted because there are no other agents of therapeutic value. Similarly the absence of alternative medical treatment for such conditions as autoimmune haemolytic ANAEMIA establishes steroid therapy as the treatment of choice which few would dispute. The use of steroids in such chronic conditions as RHEUMATOID ARTHRITIS, ASTHMA and DERMATITIS needs careful assessment and monitoring.

Although there is a risk of ill-effects, these should be set against the misery and danger of unrelieved chronic asthma or the incapacity, frustration and psychological trauma of rheumatoid arthritis. Patients should carry cards giving details of their dosage and possible complications.

The incidence and severity of side-effects are related to the dose and duration of treatment. Prolonged daily treatment with 15 mg of prednisolone, or more, will cause hypercortisonism; less than 10 mg prednisolone a day may be tolerated by most patients indefinitely. Inhaled steroids rarely produce any ill-effect apart from a propensity to oral thrush (CANDIDA infection) unless given in excessive doses.

General side-effects may include weight gain, fat distribution of the cushingoid type, ACNE and HIRSUTISM, AMENORRHOEA, striae and increased bruising tendency. The more serious complications which can occur during long-term treatment include HYPERTENSION, oedema, DIABETES MELLITUS, psychosis, infection, DYSPEPSIA and peptic ulceration, gastrointestinal haemorrhage, adrenal suppression, osteoporosis (see BONE, DISORDERS OF), myopathy (see MUSCLES, DISORDERS OF), sodium retention and potassium depletion.

Corticotropin
Corticotropin is the *British Pharmacopoeia* name for the adrenocorticotrophic hormone of the PITUITARY GLAND, also known as ACTH. It is so-called because it stimulates the functions of the cortex of the suprarenal glands. This results, among other things, in an increased output of cortisone.

Cortisol
Another name for HYDROCORTISONE.

Cortisone
An early corticosteroid drug (see CORTICOSTEROIDS), now obsolete and replaced by PREDNISOLONE and HYDROCORTISONE.

Corynebacteria
A genus of aerobic and anaerobic gram-positive (see GRAM'S STAIN) bacteria, widely distributed and best known as parasites and pathogens in humans. *C. diphtheria*, a prime example, causes diphtheria.

Coryza
Coryza is the technical name for a 'cold in the head' (see COLD, COMMON).

Costal
Anything pertaining to the ribs.

Costalgia
Pain in the ribs.

Cost of Illness
Traditionally, doctors have been trained to treat a patient on the basis of his or her personal clinical needs. Increasingly, however, the prac-

tice of medicine has been influenced by patients' social circumstances and more recently by community- and government-driven national priorities. One critical aspect of these widening influences has been the cost of medical care which, as medicine becomes more complex, has been rising sharply. Thus health economics has become an integral part of the provision of health care. Cost-of-illness studies now appear commonly in medical publications. Such studies aim to identify and measure all the costs of a particular disease, including, where feasible, the direct, indirect and intangible dimensions. The information obtained is intended to help the development of health policies, nationally and internationally. The application of information from such studies is, however, proving controversial. Firstly, doctors still see their clinical responsibilities to patients as a priority. Secondly, cost-of-care studies are often criticised for excluding broader economic aspects of health care – for example, analyses of the cost-effectiveness of prevention as well as the treatment of illness. This requires assessment of potential and actual outcomes as well as the costs of illnesses. Even so, the increasing complexity of medicine, with its commensurately rising costs affecting both state- and privately funded medical care, makes it inevitable that the cost of maintaining a population's good health will be a growing factor in the provision of health care that seems bound to impinge on how doctors are enabled to treat their individual patients.

Cot Death
See SUDDEN INFANT DEATH SYNDROME (SIDS).

Co-Trimoxazole
This drug – a mixture of trimethoprim and the sulphonamide, sulphamethoxazole – should be used only in the prophylaxis or treatment of pneumocystis PNEUMONIA, and in acute exacerbations of chronic BRONCHITIS, urinary tract infections and otitis media (see EAR, DISEASES OF), where indicated.

Cotton Wool
Cotton wool, or absorbent cotton as it is now technically named by the *British Pharmacopoeia*, is a downy material made from the hairs on cotton plant seeds (*Gossypium herbaceum*). It is used in medicine in wound-dressing packs, skin-cleaning procedures, etc.

Cough
A natural reflex reaction to irritation of the AIR PASSAGES and LUNGS. Air is drawn into the air passages with the GLOTTIS wide open. The inhaled air is blown out against the closed glottis, which, as the pressure builds up, suddenly opens, expelling the air – at an estimated speed of 960 kilometres (600 miles) an hour. This explosive exhalation expels harmful substances from the respiratory tract. Causes of coughing include infection – for example, BRONCHITIS or PNEUMONIA; inflammation of the respiratory tract associated with ASTHMA; and exposure to irritant agents such as chemical fumes or smoke (see also CROUP).

The explosive nature of coughing results in a spray of droplets into the surrounding air and, if these are infective, hastens the spread of colds (see COLD, COMMON) and INFLUENZA. Coughing is, however, a useful reaction, helping the body to rid itself of excess phlegm (mucus) and other irritants. The physical effort of persistent coughing, however, can itself increase irritation of the air passages and cause distress to the patient. Severe and protracted coughing may, rarely, fracture a rib or cause PNEUMOTHORAX. Coughs can be classified as productive – when phlegm is present – and dry, when little or no mucus is produced.

Most coughs are the result of common-cold infections but a persistent cough with yellow or green sputum is indicative of infection, usually bronchitis, and sufferers should seek medical advice as medication and postural drainage (see PHYSIOTHERAPY) may be needed. PLEURISY, pneumonia and lung CANCER are all likely to cause persistent coughing, sometimes associated with chest pain, so it is clearly important for people with a persistent cough, usually accompanied by malaise or PYREXIA, to seek medical advice.

Treatment Treatment of coughs requires treatment of the underlying cause. In the case of colds, symptomatic treatment with simple remedies such as inhalation of steam is usually as effective as any medicines, though ANALGESICS or ANTIPYRETICS may be helpful if pain or a raised temperature are among the symptoms. Many over-the-counter preparations are available and can help people cope with the symptoms. Preparations may contain an analgesic, antipyretic, decongestant or antihistamine in varying combinations. Cough medicines are generally regarded by doctors as ineffective unless used in doses so large they are likely to cause sedation as they act on the part of the brain that controls the cough reflex.

Cough suppressants may contain CODEINE,

DEXTROMETHORPHAN, PHOLCODINE and sedating ANTIHISTAMINE DRUGS. Expectorant preparations usually contain subemetic doses of substances such as ammonium chloride, IPE-CACUANHA, and SQUILL (none of which have proven worth), while demulcent preparations contain soothing, harmless agents such as syrup or glycerol.

A list of systemic cough and decongestant preparations on sale to the public, together with their key ingredients, appears in the *British National Formulary*.

Cough Syncope
Temporary loss of consciousness that may be induced by a severe spasm of coughing. This is the result of the high pressure that may be induced in the chest – over 200 millimetres of mercury – by such a spasm, which prevents the return of blood to the heart. The veins in the neck begin to bulge and the blood pressure falls; this may so reduce the blood flow to the brain that the individual feels giddy and may then lose consciousness. (See FAINTING.)

Council for Healthcare Regulatory Excellence
In 2002 the UK government set up this new statutory council with the aim of improving consistency of action across the eight existing regulatory bodies for professional staff involved in the provision of various aspects of health care. These bodies are: General Medical Council; General Dental Council; General Optical Council; Royal Pharmaceutical Society of Great Britain; General Chiropractic Council; General Osteopathic Council; Health Professions Council; and Nursing and Midwifery Council.

The new Council for Healthcare Regulatory Excellence will help to promote the interests of patients and to improve co-operation between the existing regulatory bodies – providing, in effect, a quality-control mechanism for their activities. The government and relevant professions will nominate individuals for this overarching council. The new council will not have the authority to intervene in the determination by the eight regulatory bodies of individual fitness-to-practise cases unless these concern complaints about maladministration.

Council for Nursing and Midwifery
See APPENDIX 7: STATUTORY ORGANISATIONS.

Counselling
Psychological support and advice provided by a trained therapist or health professional. The aim is to help an individual manage a particular personal or family problem: this may be a diagnosis of cancer, mental and physical trauma following an accident or assault, or a bereavement. Counselling can help people cope with a wide range of demanding circumstances. It is usually done on a one-to-one basis – sometimes in small groups – and needs to be provided with skill and sensitivity or there is a risk of worsening the individual's difficulties. There has been rapid growth in counselling services and it is vital that those providing them have been properly trained.

Cowper's Glands
Also known as the bulbourethral glands, these are a pair of glands whose ducts open into the urethra at the base of the PENIS. They secrete a fluid that is one of the constituents of the SEMEN which carries the spermatozoa and is ejaculated into the VAGINA during coitus (sexual intercourse).

Cowpox
Cowpox is a disease affecting the udders of cows, on which it produces vesicles (see VESICLE; PAPULE). It is communicable to humans, and there has for centuries been a tradition that persons who have caught this disease from cows do not suffer afterwards from SMALLPOX. This formed the basis for Jenner's experiments on VACCINATION.

COX-2 Inhibitors
This stands for cyclo-oxygenase 2 inhibitors – a class of drugs used in treating ARTHRITIS – of which the most well-used is celecoxib. Their main claim is that they are less likely to cause gastrointestinal disturbance than NON-STEROIDAL ANTI-INFLAMMATORY DRUGS (NSAIDS). In 2001, the National Institute for Clinical Excellence (NICE) recommended that they should not be used routinely in rheumatoid arthritis or osteoarthritis but only in patients with a history of peptic ulcer or gastrointestinal bleeding. They should also be considered in persons over the age of 65 taking other drugs which could cause gastrointestinal bleeding, those who are very debilitated, and those who are taking maximum doses of NSAIDs. In 2005, rofecoxib was withdrawn because of concerns about cardiac side-effects.

Coxalgia

Pain in the hip-joint; also referred to as coxodynia.

Coxa Vara

A condition in which the neck of the thigh-bone is bent so that the lower limbs are turned outwards and lameness results.

Coxsackie Viruses

A group of viruses so-called because they were first isolated from two patients with a disease resembling paralytic POLIOMYELITIS, in the village of Coxsackie in New York State. Thirty distinct types have now been identified. They constitute one of the three groups of viruses included in the family of ENTEROVIRUSES, and are divided into two groups: A and B. Despite the large number of types of group A virus (24) in existence, evidence of their role in causing human disease is limited. Some, however, cause aseptic MENINGITIS, non-specicifc upper respiratory infection and MYOCARDITIS, and others cause a condition known as HERPAN-GINA. HAND, FOOT AND MOUTH DISEASE is another disease caused by the A group. All six types of group B virus have been associated with outbreaks of aseptic meningitis, and they are also the cause of BORNHOLM DISEASE. Epidemics of type B$_2$ infections tend to occur in alternate years. (See VIRUS.)

CPR

See CARDIOPULMONARY RESUSCITATION (CPR).

Crab-Louse

Another name for *Pediculus pubis*, a louse that infests the pubic region. (See PEDICULOSIS.)

Cracked-Pot Sound

A peculiar resonance heard sometimes on percussion of the chest over a cavity in the lung, resembling the jarring sound heard on striking a cracked pot or bell. It is also heard on percussion over the skull in patients with diseases of the brain such as haemorrhages and tumours, and in certain cases of fracture of the skull.

Cradle

A cage which is placed over the legs of a patient in bed, in order to take the weight of the bedclothes off the legs.

Cradle Cap

Crusta lactea, or cradle cap as it is technically known, is a form of SEBORRHOEA of the scalp which is not uncommon in nursing infants. It

usually responds to a daily shampoo with cetrimide solution. Warm olive oil gently massaged into the scalp and left overnight, after which the scales can be washed off, also helps with the condition.

Cramp

See MUSCLES, DISORDERS OF.

Cranial Nerves

Cranial nerves are those arising from the BRAIN.

Craniotomy

The removal of part of the SKULL to provide surgical access for an operation on the BRAIN. This may be to obtain a BIOPSY, to remove a tumour or to drain an infection or a blood clot. Following the operation the bone is replaced, along with the membranes, muscle and skin.

Cranium

The part of the skull enclosing the brain as distinguished from the face.

Cream

The oily or fatty part of milk from which butter is prepared. Various medicinal preparations are known also as cream – for example, cold cream, which is a simple ointment containing rosewater, beeswax, borax, and almond oil scented with oil of rose.

Creatine

A nitrogenous substance, methyl-guanidine-acetic acid. The adult human body contains about 120 grams – 98 per cent of which is in the muscles. Much of the creatine in muscles is combined with phosphoric acid as phosphocreatine, which plays an important part in the chemistry of muscular contraction.

Creatine Kinase

An ENZYME which is proving to be of value in the investigation and diagnosis of muscular dystrophy (see MUSCLES, DISORDERS OF – Myopathy), in which it is found in the blood in greatly increased amounts.

Creatinine

Creatinine is the anhydride of CREATINE and is derived from it. It is a metabolic waste product.

Creatinine Clearance

A method of assessing the function of the kidney (see KIDNEYS) by comparing the amount of creatinine – a product of body metabolism which is normally excreted by the kidneys – in the blood with the amount appearing in the urine.

Creeping Eruption

Creeping eruption is a skin condition caused by the invasion of the skin by the larvae of various species of nematode worms. It owes its name to the fact that as the larva moves through and along the skin it leaves behind it a long creeping thin red line. (See STRONGYLOIDIASIS.)

Cremation

See DEAD, DISPOSAL OF THE.

Crenation

Abnormal microscopic appearance of blood cells in which their usually smooth margins appear irregular. It usually occurs after a blood specimen has been stored for a long time, but may occasionally indicate a blood disorder.

Creosote

A clear, yellow liquid, of aromatic smell and burning taste, prepared by distillation from pine-wood or beech-wood. It mixes readily with alcohol, ether, chloroform, glycerin, and oils.

Creosote is a powerful antiseptic and disinfectant; it is also an ingredient of some disinfectant fluids.

Crepitations

Certain sounds which occur along with the breath sounds, as heard by AUSCULTATION, in various diseases of the LUNGS. They are signs of the presence of moist exudations in the lungs or in the bronchial tubes, are classified as fine, medium, and coarse crepitations, and resemble the sound made by bursting bubbles of various sizes.

Crepitus

Crepitus means a grating sound. It is found in cases of fractured bones when the ends rub together; also, in cases of severe chronic arthritis, by the rubbing together of the dried internal surfaces of the joints.

Cresol

An oily liquid obtained from coal tar. It is a powerful antiseptic and disinfectant.

Uses Cresol is used combined with soap to form a clear saponaceous fluid known as lysol, which can be mixed with water in any proportions. For the disinfection of drains it is used at a dilution of one in 20; for heavily infected linen, one in 40; and for floors and walls, one in 100.

Cretinism

An out-of-date name for congenital HYPO-THYROIDISM, a disease caused by defective thyroid function in fetal life or early in infancy.

Creutzfeldt-Jakob Disease (CJD)

A rapidly progressive, fatal, degenerative disease in humans caused by an abnormal PRION protein. There are three aetiological forms of CJD: sporadic, IATROGENIC, and inherited. Sporadic CJD occurs randomly in all countries and has an annual incidence of one per million. Iatrogenic CJD is caused by accidental exposure to human prions through medical and surgical procedures (and cannibalism in the case of the human prion disease known as kuru that occurs in a tribe in New Guinea, where it is called the trembling disease). Inherited or familial CJD accounts for 15 per cent of human prion disease and is caused by a MUTATION in the prion protein gene. In recent years a new variant of CJD has been identified that is caused by BOVINE SPONGIFORM ENCEPHALOPATHY (BSE), called variant CJD. The incubation period for the acquired varieties ranges from four years to 40 years, with an average of 10–15 years. The symptoms of CJD are dementia, seizures, focal signs in the central nervous system, MYO-CLONUS, and visual disturbances.

Abnormal prion proteins accumulate in the brain and the spinal cord, damaging neurones (see NEURON(E)) and producing small cavities. Diagnosis can be made by tonsil (see TONSILS) biopsy, although work is under way to develop a diagnostic blood test. Abnormal prion proteins are unusually resistant to inactivation by chemicals, heat, X-RAYS or ULTRAVIOLET RAYS (UVR). They are resistant to cellular degradation and can convert normal prion proteins into abnormal forms. Human prion diseases, along with scrapie in sheep and BSE in cattle, belong to a group of disorders known as transmissible spongiform encephalopathies. Abnormal prion proteins can transfer from one animal species to another, and variant CJD has occurred as a result of consumption of meat from cattle infected with BSE.

From 1995 to 1999, a scientific study of tonsils and appendixes removed at operation suggested that the prevalence of prion carriage may be as high as 120 per million. It is not known what percentage of these might go on to develop disease.

One precaution is that, since 2003, all surgical instruments used in brain biopsies have had to be quarantined and disposable instruments are now used in tonsillectomy.

Measures have also been introduced to reduce the risk of transmission of CJD from transfusion of blood products.

In the past, CJD has also been acquired from intramuscular injections of human cadaveric pituitary-derived growth hormone and corneal transplantation. The most common form of CJD remains the sporadic variety, although the eventual incidence of variant CJD may not be known for many years.

Crisis

Crisis is a word used with several distinct meanings. (1) The traditional meaning is that of a rapid loss of fever and return to comparative health in certain acute diseases. For example, PNEUMONIA, if allowed to run its natural course, ends by a crisis usually on the eighth day, the temperature falling in 24 hours to normal, the pulse and breathing becoming slow and regular and the patient passing from a partly delirious state into natural sleep. In this sense of the word, the opposite of crisis is lysis: for example, in typhoid fever (see ENTERIC FEVER), where the patient slowly improves during a period of a week or more, without any sudden change. (2) A current use of the word crisis, and still more frequently of critical, is to signify a dangerous state of illness in which it is uncertain whether the sufferer will recover or not.

Crohn's Disease

A chronic inflammatory bowel disease which has a protracted, relapsing and remitting course. An autoimmune condition, it may last for several years. There are many similarities with ULCERATIVE COLITIS; sometimes it can be hard to differentiate between the two conditions. A crucial difference is that ulcerative colitis is confined to the colon (see INTESTINE), whereas Crohn's disease can affect any part of the gastrointestinal tract, including the mouth and anus. The sites most commonly affected in Crohn's disease (in order of frequency) are terminal ILEUM and right side of colon, just the colon, just the ileum and finally the ileum and JEJUNUM. The whole wall of the affected bowel is oedamatous (see OEDEMA) and thickened, with deep ulcers a characteristic feature. Ulcers may even penetrate the bowel wall, with abscesses and fistulas developing. Another unusual feature is the presence in the affected bowel lining of islands of normal tissue.

Crohn's disease is rare in the developing world, but in the western world the incidence is increasing and is now 6–7 per 100,000 population. Around 80,000 people in the UK have the disorder with more than 4,000 new cases occurring annually. Commonly Crohn's disease starts in young adults, but a second incidence surge occurs in people over 70 years of age. Both genetic and environmental factors are implicated in the disease – for example, if one identical twin develops the disease, the second twin stands a high chance of being affected; and 10 per cent of sufferers have a close relative with inflammatory bowel disease. Among environmental factors are low-residue, high-refined-sugar diets, and smoking.

Symptoms and signs of Crohn's disease depend on the site affected but include abdominal pain, diarrhoea (sometimes bloody), ANOREXIA, weight loss, lethargy, malaise, ANAEMIA, and sore tongue and lips. An abdominal mass may be present. Complications can be severe, including life-threatening inflammation of the colon (which may cause TOXAEMIA), perforation of the colon and the development of fistulae between the bowel and other organs in the abdomen or pelvis. If Crohn's disease persists for a decade or more there is an increased risk of the victim developing colon cancer. Extensive investigations are usually necessary to diagnose the disease; these include blood tests, bacteriological studies, ENDOSCOPY and biopsy, and barium X-ray examinations.

Treatment As with ulcerative colitis, treatment is aimed primarily at controlling symptoms. Physicians, surgeons, radiologists and dietitians usually adopt a team approach, while counsellors and patient support groups are valuable adjuncts in a disease that is typically lifelong. Drug treatment is aimed at settling the acute phase and preventing relapses. CORTICOSTEROIDS, given locally to the affected gut or orally, are used initially and the effects must be carefully monitored. If steroids do not work, the immunosuppressant agent AZATHIOPRINE should be considered. Antidiarrhoeal drugs may occasionally be helpful but should not be taken during an acute phase. The anti-inflammatory drug SULFASALAZINE can be beneficial in mild colitis. A new generation of genetically engineered anti-inflammatory drugs is now available, and these selective immunosuppressants may prove of value in the treatment of Crohn's disease.

Diet is important and professional guidance is advisable. Some patients respond to milk- or wheat-free diets, but the best course for most patients is to eat a well-balanced diet, avoiding items that the sufferer knows from experience are poorly tolerated. Of those patients with extensive disease, as many as 80 per cent may require surgery to alleviate symptoms: a section of affected gut may be removed or, as a life-saving measure, a bowel perforation dealt with.

(See APPENDIX 2: ADDRESSES: SOURCES OF INFORMATION, ADVICE, SUPPORT AND SELF-HELP – Colitis; Crohn's disease.)

Crotamiton

A topical cream used to treat pruritus (itch).

Crotch

See PERINEUM.

Croup

Also known as laryngo-tracheo-bronchitis, croup is a household term for a group of diseases characterised by swelling and partial blockage of the entrance to the LARYNX, occurring in children and characterised by crowing inspiration. There are various causes but by far the commonest is acute laryngo-tracheo-bronchitis (see under LARYNX, DISORDERS OF). Croup tends to occur in epidemics, particularly in autumn and early spring, and is almost exclusively viral in origin – commonly due to parainfluenza or other respiratory viruses. It is nearly always mild and sufferers recover spontaneously; however, it can be dangerous, particularly in young children and infants, in whom the relatively small laryngeal airway may easily be blocked, leading to suffocation.

Symptoms Attacks generally come on at night, following a cold caught during the previous couple of days. The breathing is hoarse and croaking (croup), with a barking cough and harsh respiratory noise. The natural tendency for the laryngeal airway to collapse is increased by the child's desperate attempts to overcome the obstruction. Parental anxiety, added to that of the child, only exacerbates the situation. After struggling for up to several hours, the child finally falls asleep. The condition may recur.

Treatment Most children with croup should be looked after at home if the environment is suitable. Severe episodes may require hospital observation, with treatment by oxygen if needed and usually with a single dose of inhaled steroid or oral PREDNISONE. For the very few children whose illness progresses to respiratory obstruction, intubation and ventilation may be needed for a few days. There is little evidence that putting the child in a mist tent or giving antibiotics is of any value. Of greater importance is the reassurance of the child, and careful observation for signs of deterioration, together with the exclusion of other causes such as foreign-body inhalation and bacterial tracheitis.

CRP

Stands for C-Reactive Protein, and refers to a blood measurement which is a marker of inflammation – so offering a clue as to whether infection might be present or, in inflammatory illnesses, being used to track the progress of the condition.

Cruciate Ligaments

Two strong ligaments in the interior of the knee-joint, which cross one another like the limbs of the letter X. They are so attached as to become taut when the lower limb is straightened, and they prevent over-extension or bending forwards at the knee. The cruciate ligaments are sometimes strained or torn as a result of sporting injuries or vehicular accidents; surgery may be needed to repair the damage, but the knee will be permanently weakened.

Crural

Crural means connected with the leg.

Crush Syndrome

A condition in which kidney failure occurs in patients who have been the victims of severe crushing accidents (see also KIDNEYS). The fundamental injury is damage to muscle. The limb swells. The blood volume falls. Blood UREA rises; there is also a rise in the POTASSIUM content of the blood. Urgent treatment in an intensive therapy unit is required and renal dialysis may well be necessary. The patient may survive; or die with renal failure. Post-mortem examination shows degeneration of the tubules of the kidney, and the presence in them of pigment casts.

Crusta Lactea

See CRADLE CAP.

Crutch

(1) An aid to support the weight of the body for a person unable to bear weight on one of his or her legs. Made of wood or metal, usually long enough to reach from the person's armpit to the ground, it has a concave surface that fits under the arm and a cross-bar for the hand. An elbow crutch provides weight-bearing support using the forearm and elbow and is usually recommended when the leg can take some weight.
(2) See PERINEUM.

Crutch Palsy

Crutch palsy is weakness or paralysis of muscles

in the wrist and hand, due to pressure exerted by the CRUTCH head on the nerves that control the affected muscles. It usually occurs because the crutch is too long for the individual, and/or if he or she attempts too much walking. The nerve damage is temporary and symptoms disappear if the crutch is properly used or left aside for a time.

Cryoanalgesia

The induction of analgesia (see ANALGESICS) by the use of cold that is produced by means of a special probe. The use of cold for the relief of pain dates back to the early days of mankind: two millennia ago, Hippocrates was recommending snow and ice packs as a preoperative analgesic. The modern probe allows a precise temperature to be induced in a prescribed area. Among its uses is in the relief of chronic pain which will not respond to any other form of treatment. This applies particularly to chronic facial pain.

Cryoprecipitate

When frozen plasma is allowed to thaw slowly at 4 °C, a proportion of the plasma protein remains undissolved in the cold thawed plasma and stays in this state until the plasma is warmed. It is this cold, insoluble precipitate that is known as cryoprecipitate. It can be recovered quite easily by centrifuging. Its value is that it is a rich source of factor VIII, which is used in the treatment of HAEMOPHILIA.

Cryopreservation

Maintenance at very low temperatures of the viability of tissues or organs that have been excised from the body.

Cryoscopy

The method of finding the concentration of blood, urine, etc., by observing their freezing-point.

Cryosurgery

The use of cold in surgery. Its advantages include little associated pain, little or no bleeding, and excellent healing with little or no scar formation. Hence its relatively wide use in eye surgery, some abdominal surgery, skin cancers and treatment of HAEMORRHOIDS. The coolants used include liquid nitrogen with which temperatures as low as −196 °C can be obtained, carbon dioxide (−78 °C) and nitrous oxide (−88 °C).

Cryotherapy

The treatment of disease by refrigeration. The two main forms in which it is now used are HYPOTHERMIA and refrigeration ANAESTHESIA.

Cryptococcosis

Cryptococcosis is a rare disease due to infection with a yeast known as *Cryptococcus neoformans*. Around 5–10 cases are diagnosed annually in the United Kingdom. It usually involves the lungs in the first instance, but may spread to the MENINGES and other parts of the body, including the skin. As a rule, the disease responds well to treatment with AMPHOTERICIN B, clotrimazole, and flucytosine.

Cryptococcus

A genus of yeasts. *Cryptococcus neoformans* is widespread in nature, and is present in particularly large numbers in the faeces of pigeons. It occasionally infects humans, as a result of the inhalation of dust contaminated by the faeces of pigeons – causing the disease known as CRYPTOCOCCOSIS.

Cryptorchidism

An undescended testis (see TESTICLE). The testes normally descend into the scrotum during the seventh month of gestation; until then, the testis is an abdominal organ. If the testes do not descend before the first year of life, they usually remain undescended until puberty – and even then, descent is not achieved in some instances. Fertility is impaired when one testis is affected and is usually absent in the bilateral cases. The incidence of undescended testis in full-term children at birth is 3·5 per cent, falling to less than 2 per cent at one month and 0·7 per cent at one year. Because of the high risk of infertility, undescended testes should be brought down as early as possible and at the latest by the age of two. Sometimes medical treatment with HUMAN CHORIONIC GONADO-TROPHIN is helpful but frequently surgical interference is necessary. This is the operation of orchidopexy.

CSF

See CEREBROSPINAL FLUID.

CS Gas

A noxious gas used for riot control which causes irritation of the eyes and respiratory tract. Symptoms usually subside within 20 minutes but, if they persist, the victim should be removed to a well-ventilated area, contaminated clothing removed, the affected skin washed with soap and water and the eyes irrigated with water or physiological saline. (CONTACT LENSES should be removed and washed, if hard; discarded, if soft.) If respiratory complications develop, the victim should be admitted to hospital.

CSM
See COMMITTEE ON SAFETY OF MEDICINES (CSM).

CT Scan
See COMPUTED TOMOGRAPHY.

CT Scanner
The machine which combines the use of a computer and X-rays to produce cross-sectional images of the body (see COMPUTED TOMOGRAPHY).

Culdoscopy
Culdoscopy is a method of examining the pelvic organs in women by means of an instrument comparable to a CYSTOSCOPE, inserted into the pelvic cavity through the VAGINA. The instrument used for this purpose is known as a culdoscope.

Curette
A spoon-shaped instrument with a cutting edge, used for scooping out the contents of any body cavity – for example, the uterus – or for removing certain skin lesions, such as verrucae.

Cushing's Syndrome
Described in 1932 by Harvey Cushing, the American neurosurgeon, Cushing's syndrome is due to an excess production of CORTISOL. It can thus result from a tumour of the ADRENAL GLANDS secreting cortisol, or from a PITUITARY GLAND tumour secreting ACTH and stimulating both adrenal cortexes to hypertrophy and secrete excess cortisol. It is sometimes the result of ectopic production of ACTH from non-endocrine tumours in the LUNGS and PANCREAS.

The patient gains weight and the obesity tends to have a characteristic distribution over the face, neck, and shoulder and pelvic girdles. Purple striae develop over the abdomen and there is often increased hairiness or hirsutism. The blood pressure is commonly raised and the bone softens as a result of osteoporosis. The best test to establish the diagnosis is to measure the amount of cortisol in a 24-hourly specimen of urine. Once the diagnosis has been established, it is then necessary to undertake further tests to determine the cause.

Cutaneous
Cutaneous means belonging to the SKIN.

Cuticle
See SKIN.

Cuts
See WOUNDS.

Cyanide Poisoning
Cyanide inhibits cellular RESPIRATION by binding rapidly and reversibly with the ENZYME, cytochrome oxidase. Effects of poisoning are due to tissue HYPOXIA. Cyanide is toxic by inhalation, ingestion and prolonged skin contact, and acts extremely quickly once absorbed. Following inhalation of hydrogen cyanide gas, death can occur within minutes. Ingestion of inorganic cyanide salts may produce symptoms within 10 minutes, again proceeding rapidly to death. On a full stomach, effects may be delayed for an hour or more. Signs of cyanide poisoning are headache, dizziness, vomiting, weakness, ATAXIA, HYPERVENTILATION, DYSPNOEA, HYPOTENSION and collapse. Loss of vision and hearing may occur, then COMA and CONVULSIONS. Other features include cardiac ARRHYTHMIA and PULMONARY OEDEMA. Patients may have a lactic ACIDOSIS. Their arterial oxygen tension is likely to be normal, but their venous oxygen tension high and similar to that of arterial blood.

Treatment Administration of oxygen when available is the most important first-aid management. Rescuers should be trained, must not put themselves at risk, and should use protective clothing and breathing apparatus. In unconscious victims, establish a clear airway and give 100 per cent oxygen. If breathing stops and oxygen is unavailable, initiate expired-air resuscitation. If cyanide salts were ingested, mouth-to-mouth contact must be avoided and a mask with a one-way valve employed instead. Some commercially available first-aid kits contain AMYL NITRATE as an antidote which may be employed if oxygen is unavailable.

Once in hospital, or if a trained physician is on the scene, then antidotes may be administered. There are several different intravenous antidotes that may be used either alone or in combination. In mild to moderate cases, sodium thiosulphate is usually given. In more severe cases either dicobalt edetate or sodium nitrite may be used, followed by sodium thiosulphate. Some of these (e.g. dicobalt edetate) should be given only where diagnosis is certain, otherwise serious adverse reations or toxicity due to the antidotes may occur.

Cyanides

Salts of hydrocyanic or prussic acid. They are highly poisonous, and are also powerful antiseptics. (See CYANIDE POISONING; WOUNDS.)

Cyanocobalamin

The name given by the British Pharmacopoeia Commission to vitamin B$_{12}$, found to be an effective substitute for liver in the treatment of pernicious ANAEMIA. It has now been replaced by HYDROXOCOBALAMIN as the standard treatment for this condition (see also COBALAMINS).

Cyanosis

A condition in which the skin – usually of the face and extremities – takes on a bluish tinge. It accompanies states in which the blood is not properly oxygenated in the lungs, and appears earliest through the nails, on the lips, on the tips of the ears, and over the cheeks. It may be due to blockage of the air passages, or to disease in the lungs, or to a feeble circulation, as in heart disease. (See CHRONIC OBSTRUCTIVE PULMONARY DISEASE (COPD); METHAEMOGLOBINAEMIA.)

Cybernetics

The science of communication and control in the animal and in the machine.

Cyclamates

Artificial sweetening agents which are about 30 times as sweet as cane sugar. After being in use since 1965, they were banned by government decree in 1969 because of adverse reports received from the USA.

Cyclical Oedema

This is a syndrome in women, characterised by irregular intermittent bouts of generalised swelling. Sometimes the fluid retention is more pronounced before the menstrual period (see MENSTRUATION). The eyelids are puffy and the face and fingers feel stiff and bloated. The breasts may feel swollen and the abdomen distended, and ankles may swell. The diurnal weight gain may exceed 4 kg. The underlying disturbance is due to increased loss of fluid from the vascular compartment, probably from leakage of protein from the capillaries increasing the tissue osmotic pressure. Recent evidence suggests that a decrease in the urinary excretion of DOPAMINE may contribute, as this has a natriuretic action (see NATRIURESIS). This may explain why drugs that are dopamine antagonists, such as chlorpromazine, may precipitate or aggravate cyclical oedema. Conversely, bro-mocriptine, a dopamine agonist, may improve the oedema.

Cyclizine Hydrochloride

One of the ANTIHISTAMINE DRUGS which is mainly used for the prevention of sickness, including sea-sickness.

Cyclo-Oxygenase-2 Selective Inhibitors

See COX-2 INHIBITORS.

Cyclophosphamide

A derivative of NITROGEN MUSTARDS used to treat various forms of malignant disease, including HODGKIN'S DISEASE and chronic lymphocytic LEUKAEMIA. (See also ALKYLATING AGENTS; CYTOTOXIC.)

Cycloplegia

Paralysis of the ciliary muscle of the EYE, which results in the loss of the power of ACCOMMODATION in the eye.

Cyclopropane

One of the most potent of the anaesthetics given by inhalation (see ANAESTHESIA). Its advantages are that it acts quickly, causes little irritation to the lungs, and its effects pass off quickly.

Cycloserine

An antibiotic derived from an actinomycete, used to treat certain infections of the genito-urinary tract, and and in combination with other drugs to treat TUBERCULOSIS resistant to first-line drugs.

Cyclothymia

The state characterised by extreme swings of mood from elation to depression, and vice versa. (See also MANIC DEPRESSION; MENTAL ILLNESS.)

Cyclotron

A machine in which positively charged atomic particles are so accelerated that they acquire energies equivalent to those produced by millions of volts. From the medical point of view, its interest is that it is a source of neutrons. (See RADIOTHERAPY.)

Cyesis

Another term for pregnancy (see PREGNANCY AND LABOUR).

Cyproterone Acetate

An antiandrogen. It inhibits the effects of androgens (see ANDROGEN) at receptor level and is therefore useful in the treatment of prostate cancer (see PROSTATE, DISEASES OF), ACNE, HIRSUTISM in women and in the treatment of severe hypersexuality and sexual deviation in men. The drug can have serious side-effects. (See OESTROGENS.)

Cystectomy

The surgical excision of the bladder (see URINARY BLADDER). When this is done – usually to treat cancer of the bladder – an alternative means of collecting urine from the KIDNEYS must be arranged. The URETERS of the kidney can be transplanted into a loop of bowel which is brought to the surface of the abdomen to form a STOMA that exits into an externally worn pouch. The latest surgical technique is to fashion a substitute bladder from a section of intestine and to implant the ureters into it, thus allowing the patient to void urine through the urethra as normal.

Cysteine

An amino acid containing SULPHUR that is an essential constituent of many of the body's enzymes. (See AMINO ACIDS; ENZYME.)

Cystic Duct

The tube that runs from the gall-bladder (see LIVER) and joins up with the hepatic duct (formed from the bile ducts) to form the common BILE DUCT. The BILE produced by the liver cells is drained through this system and enters the small intestine to help in the digestion of food.

Cysticercosis

This disease rarely occurs except in Central Europe, Ethiopia, South Africa, and part of Asia. It results from ova (eggs) being swallowed or regurgitated into the stomach from an adult pork tapeworm in the intestine. In the stomach the larvae escape from the eggs and are absorbed. They are carried in the blood to various parts of the body, most commonly the subcutaneous tissue and skeletal muscle, where they develop and form cysticerci. When superficial, they may be felt under the skin as small pea-like bodies. Although they cause no symptoms here, cysts may also develop in the brain. Five years later the larvae die, and the brain-tissue reaction may result in epileptic fits, obscure neurological disorders, and personality changes. The cysts calcify at this stage, though to a greater degree in the muscles than the brain, allowing them to be seen radiologically. Epilepsy starting in adult life, in anyone who has previously lived in an endemic area, should suggest the possibility of cysticercosis. (See also TAENIASIS.)

Treatment Most important is prevention of the initial tapeworm infection, by ensuring that pork is well cooked before it is eaten. Nurses and others attending to a patient harbouring an adult tapeworm must be careful to avoid ingesting ova from contaminated hands. The tapeworm itself can be destroyed with NICLOSAMIDE. Brain infections are treated with sedatives and anti-convulsants, surgery rarely being necessary. Most patients make a good recovery.

Cystic Fibrosis

This is the most common serious genetic disease in Caucasian children, with an incidence of about one per 2,500 births, and more than 6,000 patients in the UK (30,000 in the USA). It is an autosomal recessive disorder of the mucus-secreting glands of the lungs, the pancreas, the mouth, and the gastrointestinal tract, as well as the sweat glands of the skin. The defective gene is sited on chromosome 7 which encodes for a protein, cystic fibrosis transmembrane conductance regulator (CFTR). Individuals who inherit the gene only on one set of chromosomes can, however, carry the defect into successive generations. Where parents have a child with cystic fibrosis, they have a one-in-four chance of subsequent children having the disease. They should seek GENETIC COUNSELLING.

The disorder is characterised by failure to gain weight in spite of a good appetite, by repeated attacks of bronchitis (with BRONCHIECTASIS developing at a young age), and by the passage of loose, foul-smelling and slimy stools (faeces). AMNIOCENTESIS, which yields amniotic fluid along with cells shed from the fetus's skin, can be used to diagnose cystic fibrosis prenatally. The levels of various enzymes can be measured in the fluid and are abnormal when the fetus is affected by cystic fibrosis. Neonatal screening is possible using a test on blood spots – immunoreactive trypsin (IRT).

In children with symptoms or a positive family history, the disease can be tested for by measuring sweat chloride and sodium. This detects the abnormal amount of salt that is excreted via the sweat glands when cystic fibrosis is present. Confirmation is by genetic testing.

Treatment This consists basically of regular physiotherapy and postural drainage, antibiotics and the taking of pancreatic enzyme tablets and vitamins. Some children need STEROID treatment and all require nutritional support. The earlier treatment is started, the better the results. Whereas two decades ago, only 12 per cent of affected children survived beyond adolescence, today 75 per cent survive into adult life, and an increasing number are surviving into their 40s. Patients with end-stage disease can be treated by heart-lung transplantation (with their own heart going to another recipient). Research is underway on the possible use of GENE THERAPY to control the disorder. Parents of children with cystic fibrosis, seeking help and advice, can obtain this from the Cystic Fibrosis Trust.

Cystitis

Inflammation of the URINARY BLADDER. The presenting symptom is usually dysuria – that is, a feeling of discomfort when urine is passed and frequently a stinging or burning pain in the URETHRA. There is also a feeling of wanting to pass water much more often than usual, even though there is very little urine present when the act is performed. The condition may be associated with a dragging ache in the lower abdomen, and the urine usually looks dark or stronger than normal. It is frequently associated with haematuria, which means blood in the urine and is the result of the inflammation.

Cystitis is a common problem; more than half the women in Britain suffer from it at some time in their lives. The cause of the disease is a bacterial infection of the bladder, the germs having entered the urethra and ascended into the bladder. The most common organism responsible is called *Escherichia coli*. This organism normally lives in the bowel where it causes no harm. It is therefore likely to be present on the skin around the anus so that there is always a potential for infection. The disease is much more common in women because the urethra, vagina and anus are very close together and the urethra is much shorter in the female than it is in the male. It also explains why women commonly suffer cystitis after sexual intercourse and honeymoon cystitis is a very common presentation of bladder inflammation. In most cases the inflammation is more of a nuisance than a danger but the infection can spread up to the kidneys and cause PYELITIS which is a much more serious disorder.

In cases of cystitis the urine should be cultured to grow the responsible organism. The relevant antibiotic can then be prescribed. Fluids should be taken freely not only for an acute attack of cystitis but also to prevent further attacks, because if the urine is dilute the organism is less likely to grow. Bicarbonate of soda is also helpful as this reduces the acidity of the urine and helps to relieve the burning pain, and inhibits the growth of the bacteria. Careful hygiene, in order to keep the PERINEUM clean, is also important. (See URINARY BLADDER, DISEASES OF.)

Cystocoele

A PROLAPSE of the base of the URINARY BLADDER in a woman. The pelvic floor muscles may be weakened after childbirth and, when the woman strains, the front wall of the vagina bulges. Stress incontinence often accompanies a cystocoele and surgical repair is then advisable (see COLPORRHAPHY).

Cystogram

An X-ray picture of the URINARY BLADDER.

Cystometer

An instrument for measuring the pressure in the URINARY BLADDER.

Cystometry

A technique for measuring the pressure in the URINARY BLADDER as part of a URODYNAMIC investigation to assess the functioning of the bladder.

Cystoscope

An instrument for viewing the interior of the URINARY BLADDER. It consists of a narrow tube carrying a small electric lamp at its end; a small mirror set obliquely opposite an opening near the end of the tube; and a telescope which is passed down the tube and by which the reflection of the brightly illuminated bladder wall in the mirror is examined. It is of great value in the diagnosis of conditions like ulcers and small tumours of the bladder.

Fine CATHETERS can be passed along the cystoscope, and by the aid of vision can be inserted into each ureter and pushed up to the kidney, so that the urine from each kidney may be obtained and examined separately in order to diagnose which of these organs is diseased.

Cysts

Hollow tumours (see TUMOUR), containing fluid or soft material. They are almost always simple in nature.

Retention cysts In these, in consequence of

irritation or another cause, some cavity which ought naturally to contain a little fluid becomes distended, or the natural outlet from the cavity becomes blocked. Wens are caused by the blockage of the outlet from sebaceous glands in the skin, so that an accumulation of fatty matter takes place. RANULA is a clear swelling under the tongue, due to a collection of saliva in consequence of an obstruction to a salivary duct. Cysts in the breasts are, in many cases, the result of blockage in milk ducts, due to inflammation; they should be assessed to exclude cancer (see BREASTS, DISEASES OF). Cysts also form in the kidney as a result of obstruction to the free outflow of the urine.

Developmental cysts Of these, the most important are the huge cysts that originate in the OVARIES. The cause is doubtful, but the cyst probably begins at a very early period of life, gradually enlarges, and buds off smaller cysts from its wall. The contents are usually a clear gelatinous fluid. Very often both ovaries are affected, and the cysts may slowly reach a great size – often, however, taking a lifetime to do so.

A similar condition sometimes occurs in the KIDNEYS, and the tumour may have reached a great size in an infant even before birth (congenital cystic kidney).

Dermoid cysts are small cavities, which also originate probably early in life, but do not reach any great size until fairly late in life. They appear about parts of the body where clefts occur in the embryo and close up before birth, such as the corner of the eyes, the side of the neck, and the middle line of the body. They contain hair, fatty matter, fragments of bone, scraps of skin, even numerous teeth.

Hydatid cysts are produced in many organs, particularly in the liver, by a parasite which is the larval stage of a tapeworm found in dogs. They occur in people who keep dogs and allow them to contaminate their food. (See TAENIASIS.)

Cytarabine
An drug used mainly to induce remission of acute myeloblastic LEUKAEMIA. A potent suppressant of myeloblasts, its use requires monitoring by a HAEMATOLOGIST. (See CYTOTOXIC.)

Cyto-
A prefix meaning something connected with a cell or CELLS.

Cytogenetics
The study of the structure and functions of the cells of the body, with particular reference to the CHROMOSOMES.

Cytokines
A family of PROTEIN molecules that carry signals locally between cells. Cytokines are released by cells when activated by antigens (see ANTIGEN), behaving as enhancing mediators for immune response. These proteins include INTERLEUKINS (produced by LEUCOCYTES), lymphokines (produced by lymphocytes – see LYMPHOCYTE), INTERFERON, and tumour necrosis factor, one of whose many functions is killing tumour cells.

Cytology
The study of CELLS.

Cytomegalovirus (CMV)
A commonly occurring virus of the herpes virus group – the name derived from the swollen appearance of infected cells ('cytomegalo' = large cell). The infection is usually asymptomatic (or like mild influenza), but it can cause an illness similar to infectious MONONUCLEOSIS. Most people (80 per cent) will have had CMV infection by the time they are adults, but the virus can remain latent in the body and cause recurrent infections. During an acute infection the virus is excreted in saliva, breast milk and urine as well as from the vagina, and this may continue for years. CMV is transmitted naturally by saliva or during sexual contact, but blood transfusions and organ transplantations are also infection routes. Although CMV rarely causes its host any problems, when it is passed from an infected mother to her fetus *in utero* or to an infant during birth (from vaginal secretions) or via breast milk postnatally, the virus causes a generalised severe infection in the infant. This can involve the central nervous system and liver, causing death of the fetus or neonate. If the infant survives it may be mentally retarded, with motor disabilities, deafness and chronic liver disease. In England and Wales about 400 babies a year are born with CMV-induced disabilities. If an adult is immunodeficient (see IMMUNODEFICIENCY) because of HIV infection/AIDS or as a result of immunosuppressive treatment after an organ transplant, he or she may become seriously ill.

Cytometer
An instrument for counting and measuring CELLS.

Cytoplasm
The PROTOPLASM of the cell body. (See CELLS.)

Cytotoxic

Cytotoxic means destructive to living cells. Cytotoxic drugs possess anti-cancer properties but also have the potential to damage normal tissue. Their use is twofold: to eliminate a cancer and so prolong life; or to alleviate distressing symptoms, especially in patients whose prospects of a cure are poor. In many cases CHEMOTHERAPY with cytotoxic drugs is combined with surgery, RADIOTHERAPY or both. Chemotherapy may be used initially to reduce the size of the primary TUMOUR (a process called neoadjuvant therapy) before using radiotherapy or surgery to eliminate it. Cytotoxic drugs may also be used as adjuvant treatment to prevent or destroy secondary spread of the primary tumour that has either been removed by surgery or treated with radiotherapy. All chemotherapy causes side-effects: the ONCOLOGIST – a specialist in cancer treatment – has to strike a balance between hoped-for benefits and acceptable (for the patient) toxic effects, which include nausea and vomiting, BONE MARROW suppression, ALOPECIA (hair loss) and teratogenic effects (see TERATOGENESIS).

Cytotoxic drugs are used either singly or in combination, when an enhanced response is the aim. Chemotherapy of cancer is a complex process and should be supervised by an oncologist in co-operation with physicians, surgeons, radiotherapists and radiologists as appropriate.

The cytotoxic drugs include:

(1) The alkylating agents which act by damaging DNA, thus interfering with cell reproduction. Cyclophosphamide, ifosfamide, chlorambucil, kelphalan, busulphan, thiotepa and mustine are examples of alkylating agents.

(2) There are a number of cytotoxic antibiotics used in the treatment of cancer – doxorubicin, bleomycin, dactinomycin, mithramycin and amsacrine are examples. They are used primarily in the treatment of acute leukaemia and lymphomas.

(3) Antimetabolites – these drugs combine irreversibly with vital enzyme systems of the cell and hence prevent normal cell division. Methotrexate, cytarabine, fluorouracil, mercaptopurine and azathioprine are examples.

(4) Another group of cytotoxic drugs are the vinca alkaloids such as vincristine, vinblastine and vindesima.

(5) Platinum compounds such as carboplatin, cisplatin and oxaliplatin are effective. All of them are given intravenously, but the latter two tend to have more unpleasant side-effects. Carboplatin and cisplatin are useful in the treatment of solid tumours. Carboplatin, a derivative of cisplatin, is given intravenously in ovarian cancer and in small-cell lung cancer. Better tolerated than cisplatin, the drug causes less nausea and vomiting, nephrotoxicity, neurotoxicity and ototoxicity. Where platinum-containing therapy has failed, intravenous treatment with paclitaxel may be tried. With only a limited success rate, it is relatively toxic and should be carefully supervised; responses, however, are sometimes prolonged.

Also of increasing importance in treating cancer are interferons. These are naturally occurring proteins with complex effects on immunity and cell function. Although toxic, with numerous adverse effects, they have shown some anti-tumour effect against certain lymphomas and solid tumours.

D

D and C
See DILATATION AND CURETTAGE.

Da Costa's Syndrome
See EFFORT SYNDROME.

Dacryocystitis
See EYE, DISORDERS OF.

Dactinomycin
A CYTOTOXIC antibiotic drug principally used for treating cancers such as acute LEUKAEMIA and LYMPHOMA in children. It is given intravenously and treatment normally takes place in hospital. The drug was previously known as actinomycin D. Side-effects are potentially serious.

Dactylitis
Inflammation of a finger or toe.

Danazol
This drug inhibits pituitary gonadotrophin secretion (see PITUITARY GLAND; GONADO-TROPHINS) and is used in the treatment of ENDOMETRIOSIS, MENORRHAGIA and GYNAE-COMASTIA. The dose is usually of the order of 100 mg twice daily and side-effects may include nausea, dizziness, flushing and skeletal muscle pain. It is mildly androgenic (see ANDROGEN).

Dandruff
Also known as scurf. The white scales shed from the scalp, due to increased production of epidermal surface cells. Treatment is regular washing with an antidandruff shampoo. (See also SEBORRHOEA.)

Dangerous Drugs
See CONTROLLED DRUGS.

Dantrolene
A muscle-relaxing drug, indicated for chronic severe spasticity (see SPASTIC) of voluntary muscle such as may occur after a STROKE or in CEREBRAL PALSY and MULTIPLE SCLEROSIS (MS). Unlike most other relaxants, it acts directly on the muscle, thus producing fewer central-nervous-system side-effects. It is contraindicated if liver function is impaired, and is not recommended for children or for acute muscle spasm. It may cause drowsiness, resulting in impaired performance at skilled tasks and driving.

Dapsone
One of the most effective drugs in the treatment of LEPROSY. An antibacterial drug, its use may cause nausea and vomiting; occasionally, it may harm nerves, the liver, and red blood cells. During treatment, blood tests are done to check on liver function and the number of red cells in the blood.

The drug is also used to treat dermatitis herpetiformis, a rare skin disorder.

Dartos
The thin muscle just under the skin of the SCROTUM which enables the scrotum to alter its shape.

Databases
See HEALTH DATABASES.

Data Protection Act 1998
This legislation puts into effect the UK European Directive 95/46/EC on the processing of personal data, whether paper or computer records. The Act is based on eight principles, the first of which stipulates that 'personal data shall be processed fairly and lawfully'. Unfortunately this phrase is open to different interpretations. Clarification is required to determine how the common-law duty of confidentiality affects the health services in the context of using data obtained from patients for research work, especially epidemiological studies (see EPIDEMIOLOGY). Health authorities, trusts and primary care groups in the NHS have appointed 'Caldicott guardians' – named after a review of information that identifies patients. A prime responsibility of the guardians is to agree and review internal protocols for the protection and use of identifiable information obtained from patients. The uncertainties over the interpretation of the legislation require clarification, but some experts have suggested a workable solution: to protect patients' rights, researchers should ensure that data are fully anonymised whenever possible; they should also agree their project design with those responsible for data protection well in advance of its planned starting date. (See ETHICS.)

Date Rape
See DRUG ASSISTED RAPE.

Day Blindness
A condition in which the patient sees better in a

dim light or by night than in daylight. It is only found in conditions in which the light is very glaring, as in the desert and on snow, and is relieved by resting the retina (see EYE) – for example, by wearing coloured glasses for a time.

Daydreams

Daydreams occur when an individual during waking hours imagines enjoyable or exciting events or images. Most people daydream at some stage during their lives, but it tends to occur when someone is stressed or unhappy. Children and teenagers in particular may sometimes daydream a lot. This should not usually worry their parents or teachers unless their work suffers or it affects the individual's personal relationships.

In those circumstances professional advice should be sought from a doctor or counsellor.

Day Surgery

Surgery done in a clinic or a hospital without an overnight stay either before or after the operation. Improvements in surgery – especially the introduction of MINIMALLY INVASIVE SURGERY (MIS) – as well as more effective methods of ANAESTHESIA have simplified many procedures and reduced the physical and mental stress on patients. Patients undergoing day surgery should be accompanied home by a friend or relative. Occasionally a patient may develop complications that require a post-operative stay in hospital.

DDI

Also known as ddI – see DIDANOSINE.

DDT

See DICHLORODIPHENYL TRICHLOROETHANE.

Dead, Disposal of the

Practically, only three methods have been used from the earliest times: burial, embalming and cremation. Burial is perhaps the earliest and most primitive method. It was customary to bury the bodies of the dead in consecrated ground around churches up until the earlier half of the 19th century, when the utterly insanitary state of churchyards led to legislation for their better control. Burials in Britain take place usually upon production of a certificate from a registrar of deaths, to whom notice of the death, accompanied by a medical certificate, must be given without delay by the nearest relatives.

When a death occurs at sea, the captain of the ship has authority to permit burial at sea. If, however, there are any doubts about cause of death, the captain may decide to preserve the body and refer the case to the relevant authorities at the next port of call.

Embalming is still used occasionally. The process consists in removing the internal organs through small openings, and filling the body cavities with various aromatics of antiseptic power – the skin being swathed in bandages or otherwise protected from the action of the air. Bodies are also preserved by injecting the blood vessels with strong antiseptics such as perchloride of mercury.

Cremation or incineration of the body is now the commonest method of disposal of the dead in the UK, where land for burials is increasingly scarce; today it accounts for around 75 per cent of disposals. The process of incineration takes 1–2 hours. Something in the range of 2·3 to 3·2 kg (5–7 lbs) of ash result from the combustion of the body, and there is no admixture with that from the fuel.

Cremation of a body means that it is almost impossible to conduct any meaningful forensic tests should any subsequent doubts be raised about the cause of death. So, before cremation can take place, two doctors have to sign the cremation forms. The first is usually the doctor who was caring for the patient at the time of death – an important exception being cases of sudden death, when the coroner holds an inquest into the cause and authorises the necessary approval for cremation. In 1999, fewer than 3,500 deaths were certified following a post-mortem, out of a total number of deaths in England and Wales of more than 556,000. When the coroner is not involved, the second doctor must have been qualified for five years; he or she must be unconnected with the patient's care and not linked professionally with the first doctor. (For example, if the first doctor is a general practitioner – as in the majority of cases they are – the second doctor should be from another practice.) Before signing the cremation certificate the second doctor must conduct an external examination of the dead person and discuss the circumstances of death with the first doctor.

The two cremation forms are then inspected by crematorium medical referees who must be satisfied that the cause of death has definitely been ascertained. The present death and cremation certification system has been in place in the UK for many years – the legislative framework for cremation was set up in 1902 – and death certification procedures were last reviewed by the government-appointed Brodrick committee in 1971, with no fundamental changes proposed. The case of Harold Shipman, a general practitioner convicted of murdering more than 15 patients, and suspected of murdering many more, has revealed serious weaknesses in the certification system. A comprehensive review of the present procedures was in place at the time of writing (2004).

Dead Fingers
See RAYNAUD'S DISEASE.

Deadly Nightshade
The popular name of *Atropa belladonna*, from which ATROPINE is procured. Its poisonous black berries are sometimes eaten by children.

Dead Space
Gas exchange only occurs in the terminal parts of the pulmonary airways (see LUNGS). That portion of each breath that is taken into the lungs but does not take part in gas exchange is known as dead space. Anatomical dead space describes air in the airways up to the terminal BRONCHIOLES. Physiological dead space also includes gas in alveoli (air sacs) which are unable to take part in gas exchange because of structural abnormalities or disease.

Deafness
Impairment of hearing, which affects about 2 million adults in the UK. In infants, permanent deafness is much less common: about 1–2 per 1,000. It is essential, however, that deafness is picked up early so that appropriate treatment and support can be given to improve hearing and/or ensure that the child can learn to speak.

In most people, deafness is a result of sensorineural hearing impairment, commonly known as nerve deafness. This means that the abnormality is located in the inner ear (the cochlea), in the auditory nerve, or in the brain itself. The prevalence of this type of hearing impairment rises greatly in elderly people, to the extent that more than 50 per cent of the over-70s have a moderate hearing impairment. In most cases no definite cause can be found, but contributory factors include excessive exposure to noise, either at work (e.g. shipyards and steelworks) or at leisure (loud music). Anyone who is exposed to gunfire or explosions is also likely to develop some hearing impairment: service personnel, for example.

Conductive hearing impairment is the other main classification. Here there is an abnormality of the external or middle ear, preventing the normal transmission of sound waves to the inner ear. This is most commonly due to chronic otitis media where there is inflammation of the middle ear, often with a perforation of the ear drum. It is thought that in the majority of cases this is a sequela of childhood middle-ear disease. Many preschool children suffer temporary hearing loss because of otitis media with effusion (glue ear). Wax does not interfere with hearing unless it totally obstructs the ear canal or is impacted against the tympanic membrane. (See also EAR; EAR, DISEASES OF.)

Treatment Conductive hearing impairment can, in many cases, be treated by an operation on the middle ear or by the use of a hearing aid. Sensorineural hearing impairments can be treated only with a hearing aid. In the UK, hearing aids are available free on the NHS. Most NHS hearing aids are ear-level hearing aids – that is, they fit behind the ear with the sound transmitted to the ear via a mould in the external ear. Smaller hearing aids are available which fit within the ear itself, and people can wear such aids in both ears. The use of certain types of hearing aid may be augmented by fittings incorporated into the aid which pick up sound directly from television sets or from telephones, and from wire loop systems in halls, lecture theatres and classrooms. More recently, bone-anchored hearing aids have been developed where the hearing aid is attached directly to the bones of the skull using a titanium screw. This type of hearing aid is particularly useful in children with abnormal or absent ear canals who cannot therefore wear conventional hearing aids. People with hearing impairment should seek audiological or medical advice before purchasing any of the many types of hearing aid available commercially. Those people with a hearing impairment which is so profound ('stone deaf') that they cannot be helped by a hearing aid can sometimes now be fitted with an electrical implant in their inner ear (a cochlear implant).

Congenital hearing loss accounts for a very small proportion of the hearing-impaired population. It is important to detect at an early stage as, if undetected and unaided, it may lead to delayed or absent development of speech. Otitis media with effusion (glue ear) usually resolves spontaneously, although if it persists, surgical intervention has been the traditional treatment involving insertion of a ventilation tube (see GROMMET) into the ear drum, often combined with removal of the adenoids (see NOSE, DISORDERS OF). Recent studies, however, suggest that in many children these operations may provide only transient relief and make no difference to long-term outcome.

Advice and information on deafness and hearing aids may be obtained from the Royal National Institute for Deaf People and other organisations.

Deamination

The process of removal of the amino group, NH_2, from amino acids not required for building up body PROTEIN. This is carried out mainly in the liver by means of an enzyme, deaminase. The fatty acid residue is either burnt up to yield energy, or is converted into glucose.

Death, Causes of

The final cause of death is usually the failure of the vital centres in the brain that control the beating of the heart and the act of breathing. The important practical question, however, is what disease, injury or other agent has led to this failure. Sometimes the cause may be obvious – for example, pneumonia, coronary thrombosis, or brain damage in a road accident. Often, however, the cause can be uncertain, in which case a POST-MORTEM EXAMINATION is necessary.

The two most common causes of death in the UK are diseases of the circulatory system (including strokes and heart disease) and cancer.

Overall annual death rates among women in the UK at the start of the 21st century were 7.98 per 1,000 population, and among men, 5.58 per 1,000. Comparable figures at the start of the 20th century were 16.3 for women and 18.4 for men. The death rates in 1900 among infants up to the age of four were 47.9 per 1,000 females and 57 per 1,000 males. By 2003 these numbers had fallen to 5.0 and 5.8 respectively. All these figures give a crude indication of how the health of Britain's population has improved in the past century.

Death rates and figures on the causes of deaths are essential statistics in the study of EPIDEMIOLOGY which, along with information on the incidence of illnesses and injuries, provides a temporal and geographical map of changing health patterns in communities. Such information is valuable in planning preventive health measures (see PUBLIC HEALTH) and in identifying the natural history of diseases – knowledge that often contributes to the development of preventive measures and treatments for those diseases.

Death, Signs of

There are some minor signs, such as: relaxation of the facial muscles (which produces the staring eye and gaping mouth of the 'Hippocratic countenance'), as well as a loss of the curves of the back, which becomes flat by contact with the bed or table; discoloration of the skin, which takes on a wax-yellow hue and loses its pink transparency at the finger-webs; absence of blistering and redness if the skin is burned (Christison's sign); and failure of a ligature tied round the finger to produce, after its removal, the usual change of a white ring, which, after a few seconds, becomes redder than the surrounding skin in a living person.

The only certain sign of death, however, is that the heart has stopped beating. To ensure that this is permanent, it is necessary to listen over the heart with a stethoscope, or directly with the ear, for at least five minutes. Permanent stoppage of breathing should also be confirmed by observing that a mirror held before the mouth shows no haze, or that a feather placed on the upper lip does not flutter.

In the vast majority of cases there is no difficulty in ensuring that death has occurred. The introduction of organ transplantation, however, and of more effective mechanical means of resuscitation, such as ventilators, whereby an individual's heart can be kept beating almost indefinitely, has raised difficulties in a minority of cases. To solve the problem in these cases the concept of 'brain death' has been introduced. In this context it has to be borne in mind that there is no legal definition of death. Death has traditionally been diagnosed by the irreversible cessation of respiration and heartbeat. In the Code of Practice drawn up in 1983 by a Working Party of the Health Departments of Great Britain and Northern Ireland, however, it is stated that 'death can also be diagnosed by the irreversible cessation of brain-stem function'. This is described as 'brain death'. The brain stem consists of the mid-brain, pons and medulla oblongata which contain the centres controlling the vital processes of the body such as consciousness, breathing and the beating of the heart (see BRAIN). This new concept of death, which has been widely accepted in medical and legal circles throughout the world, means that it is now legitimate to equate brain death with death; that the essential component of brain death is death of the brain stem; and that a dead brain stem can be reliably diagnosed at the bedside. (See GLASGOW COMA SCALE.)

Four points are important in determining the time that has elapsed since death. HYPOSTASIS, or congestion, begins to appear as livid spots on the back, often mistaken for bruises, three hours or more after death. This is due to the blood running into the vessels in the lowest parts. Loss of heat begins at once after death, and the body has become as cold as the surrounding air after 12 hours – although this is delayed by hot weather, death from ASPHYXIA, and some other causes. Rigidity, or rigor mortis, begins in six hours, takes another six to become fully established, remains for 12 hours and passes off during the succeeding 12 hours. It comes on quickly when extreme exertion has been indulged in immediately before death; conversely it is slow in onset and slight in death from wasting diseases, and slight or absent in children. It begins in the small muscles of the eyelid and jaw and then spreads over the body. PUTREFACTION is variable in time of onset, but usually begins in 2–3 days, as a greenish tint over the abdomen.

Death, Sudden

If deaths from accidents are excluded, this term means the unexpected death of an apparently healthy person. CARDIAC ARREST is the most common cause of sudden death. Older people (35 years or above) who suffer cardiac arrest commonly have coronary artery disease (see HEART, DISEASES OF) with restriction or stoppage of blood supply to part of the heart which causes INFARCTION (heart attack). Irregularity of the heartbeat (cardiac ARRHYTHMIA) is another cause. MYOCARDITIS, PNEUMONIA and STROKE can also result in sudden death, as can ASTHMA, anaphylactic shock (see ANAPHYLAXIS), ruptured aortic ANEURYSM and SUICIDE, the incidence of which is rising, especially among young people, and is over 4,000 a year in the UK.

Sudden death sometimes occurs in infants, usually in the first year of life: this is called SUDDEN INFANT DEATH SYNDROME (SIDS) or, colloquially, cot death, the possible causes of which are an ongoing subject for research and debate.

When a person dies unexpectedly the event must be reported to a CORONER, who has the power to decide whether an AUTOPSY is necessary.

Death Certificate

A certificate required by law to be signed by a medical practitioner stating the main and any contributory causes of a person's death.

Death Rate

The death (mortality rate) is the number of deaths per 100,000 – or sometimes 10,000 or 1,000 – of the population per year. In 2001 the population of the UK was 59.8 million, of whom 9 million were over 65 and 4.2 million over 75. Females comprised 30.33 million and males 29.47. In 2003 – the latest year for which figures are available – the death rate was 7.2 per 1,000 population; in 1980 the figure was 11.8. The total mortality comprises individual deaths from different causes: for example, accidents, cancer, coronary artery disease, strokes and suicides. Mortality is often calculated for specific groups in epidemiological (see EPIDEMIOLOGY) studies of particular diseases. Infant mortality measures the deaths of babies born alive who die during the first year of life: infant deaths per 1,000 live births were steady at around 5 from 2003–2005.

Debility

A state of weakness.

Debridement

The surgical removal of foreign material and damaged tissue from a wound.

Decay, Dental

See TEETH, DISORDERS OF – Caries of the teeth.

Decibel

The unit of hearing. One decibel is the least intensity of sound at which a given note can be heard. The usual abbreviation for decibel is dB.

Decidua

The soft coat which lines the interior of the womb during pregnancy and which is cast off at birth.

Decoction

A preparation made by boiling various plants in water and straining the fluid.

Decompensation

A failing condition of the heart in a case of valvular disease (see HEART, DISEASES OF).·

Decongestants

Drugs which relieve nasal congestion and stuffiness. They may be given orally or by nasal spray, and most are SYMPATHOMIMETIC DRUGS which cause vasoconstriction in the nasal mucosa. Too frequent use reduces their effectiveness, and there is a danger of 'rebound' worsening if they are used for more than 10–14 days. A safer option for babies is simple sodium chloride drops. Warm moist air is also a traditional effective decongestant.

Decubitus

Decubitus refers to the positions taken up in

bed by patients suffering from various conditions such as pneumonia, PERITONITIS, or severe exhaustion. Such patients are liable to develop bed sores, or decubitus ulcer (see ULCER).

Decussation
Any point in the nervous system at which nerve fibres cross from one side to the other: for example, the decussation of the pyramidal tracts in the medulla (see BRAIN), where the motor fibres from one side of the brain cross to the other side of the spinal cord.

Deep Vein Thrombosis (DVT)
See THROMBOSIS; VEINS, DISEASES OF.

Defaecation
Opening the bowels. (See CONSTIPATION; DIARRHOEA.)

Defibrillation
If a heart is fibrillating (see VENTRICULAR FIBRILLATION), the application of a large electric shock via paddles applied to the chest wall causes simultaneous electrical depolarisation of all the cardiac cells, and may allow the heart's natural pacemaker to re-establish sinus rhythm. One paddle is placed below the right clavicle and the other over the cardiac apex. Care must be taken that no one is in contact with the patient or the bed when the shock is given, to avoid electrocution.

Defibrillator
Apparatus that delivers a controlled electric shock to restore normal heart rhythm in patients whose hearts have developed VENTRICULAR FIBRILLATION or have stopped beating. The shock is delivered by electrodes placed on the chest wall or directly to the heart after the chest has been surgically opened. Defibrillators are a standard item of equipment for paramedical staff in ambulances, and aeroplanes of some airlines now routinely carry the apparatus. (See also HEART, DISEASES OF.)

Deficiency Disease
Any disease resulting from the absence from the diet of any substance essential to good health: for example, one of the vitamins.

Deformities
Malformations or distortions of part of the body. They may be present at birth, or they may be the result of injuries, or disease, or simply produced by bad posture, like the curved spine occasionally found in children. (See BURNS AND SCALDS; CHEST, DEFORMITIES OF; TALIPES; FLAT-FOOT; JOINTS, DISEASES OF; KNOCK-KNEE; LEPROSY; PALATE, MALFORMATIONS OF; PARALYSIS; RICKETS; SCAR; SKULL; SPINE AND SPINAL CORD, DISEASES AND INJURIES OF.)

Degeneration
A change in structure or in chemical composition of a tissue or organ, by which its vitality is lowered or its function interfered with. Degeneration is of various kinds, the chief being fatty, where cells become invaded by fat globules; calcareous, where calcium is deposited in tissue so that it becomes chalky in consistency; and mucoid, where it becomes semi-liquefied.

Causes of degeneration are, in many cases, very obscure. In some cases heredity plays a part, with particular organs – for example, the kidneys – tending to show fibroid changes in successive generations. Fatty, fibroid, and calcareous degenerations are part of the natural change in old age; defective nutrition may bring them on prematurely, as may excessive and long-continued strain upon an organ like the heart. Various poisons, such as alcohol, play a special part in producing the changes, and so do the poisons produced by various diseases, particularly SYPHILIS and TUBERCULOSIS.

Degenerative Disorders
An umbrella description for a wide variety of conditions in which there is increased deterioration of the structure or function (or both) of the body. Ageing causes a steady degeneration of many tissues and organs – for example, wrinkling of the skin, CATARACT and poor neuromuscular coordination. In degenerative disorders the changes occur earlier in life. The nervous system, muscles, arteries, joints and eyes are all susceptible. Specialised tissues are replaced by CONNECTIVE TISSUE. The commonest example in the nervous system is ALZHEIMER'S DISEASE, which causes dementia; while in HUNTINGTON'S CHOREA, a genetic disorder, dementia is accompanied by incoordination of movements.

Deglutition
Deglutition means the act of swallowing. (See CHOKING.)

Dehiscence
The breaking open of a wound that is partly healed, usually after surgery.

Dehydration
A fall in the water content of the body. Sixty per

cent of a man's body weight is water, and 50 per cent of a woman's; those proportions need to be maintained within quite narrow limits to ensure proper functioning of body tissues. Body fluids contain a variety of mineral salts (see ELECTROLYTES) and these, too, must remain within narrow concentration bands. Dehydration is often accompanied by loss of salt, one of the most important minerals in the body.

The start of 'dehydration' is signalled by a person becoming thirsty. In normal circumstances, the drinking of water will relieve thirst and serious dehydration does not develop. In a temperate climate an adult will lose 1.5 litres or more a day from sweating, urine excretion and loss of fluid through the lungs. In a hot climate the loss is much higher – up to 10 litres if a person is doing hard physical work. Even in a temperate climate, severe dehydration will occur if a person does not drink for two or three days. Large losses of fluid occur with certain illnesses – for example, profuse diarrhoea; POLYURIA in diabetes or kidney failure (see KIDNEYS, DISEASES OF); and serious blood loss from, say, injury or a badly bleeding ULCER in the gastrointestinal tract. Severe thirst, dry lips and tongue, TACHYCARDIA, fast breathing, lightheadedness and confusion are indicative of serious dehydration; the individual can lapse into COMA and eventually die if untreated. Dehydration also results in a reduction in output of urine, which becomes dark and concentrated.

Prevention is important, especially in hot climates, where it is essential to drink water even if one is not thirsty. Replacement of salts is also vital, and a diet containing half a teaspoon of table salt to every litre of water drunk is advisable. If someone, particularly a child, suffers from persistent vomiting and diarrhoea, rehydration therapy is required and a salt-and-glucose rehydration mixture (obtainable from pharmacists) should be taken. For those with severe dehydration, oral fluids will be insufficient and the affected person needs intravenous fluids and, sometimes, admission to hospital, where fluid intake and output can be monitored and rehydration measures safely controlled.

Déjà Vu
A feeling of having already experienced an event which the person is doing or seeing at the moment. French for 'already seen', *déjà vu* is quite common but no satisfactory explanation for the phenomenon has yet been discovered.

Delhi Boil
Delhi boil is a form of chronic body sore occurring in Eastern countries, caused by a protozoan parasite, *Leishmania tropica.* (See LEISHMANIASIS.)

Delinquency
Behaviour by a young person that would be judged a crime if carried out by an adult. Delinquency may also include non-criminal activities – for example, running away from home, missing school lessons, drug or alcohol abuse, and unruly behaviour in public places. Delinquency is now a serious social problem in the UK, especially in deprived areas, and it is increasingly accompanied by alcohol and drug abuse.

Delirium
A condition of altered consciousness in which there is disorientation (as in a confusional state), incoherent talk and restlessness but with hallucination, illusions or delusions also present.

Delirium (confusion) In some old people, acute confusion is a common effect of physical illness. Elderly people are often referred to as being 'confused'; unfortunately this term is often inappropriately applied to a wide range of eccentricities of speech and behaviour as if it were a diagnosis. It can be applied to a patient with the early memory loss of DEMENTIA – forgetful, disorientated and wandering; to the dejected old person with depression, often termed pseudo-dementia; to the patient whose consciousness is clouded in the delirium of acute illness; to the paranoid deluded sufferer of late-onset SCHIZOPHRENIA; or even to the patient presenting with the acute DYSPHASIA and incoherence of a stroke. Drug therapy may be a cause, especially in the elderly.

Delirium tremens is the form of delirium most commonly due to withdrawal from alcohol, if a person is dependent on it (see DEPENDENCE). There is restlessness, fear or even terror accompanied by vivid, usually visual, hallucinations or illusions. The level of consciousness is impaired and the patient may be disorientated as regards time, place and person.

Treatment is, as a rule, the treatment of causes. (See also ALCOHOL.) As the delirium in fevers is due partly to high temperature, this should be lowered by tepid sponging. Careful nursing is one of the keystones of successful treatment, which includes ensuring that ample fluids are taken and nutrition is maintained.

Delivery

The final expulsion of the child in the act of birth. (See PREGNANCY AND LABOUR.)

Delta Waves

Abnormal electrical waves observed in the electroencephalogram (see ELECTROENCEPHALOGRAPHY (EEG)). The frequency of the normal alpha waves is 10 per second; that of the delta waves is 7 or fewer per second. They occur in the region of tumours of the brain, and in the brains of patients with EPILEPSY.

Deltoid

The powerful triangular muscle attached above to the collar-bone and shoulder-blade, and below, by its point, to the humerus, nearly halfway down the outer side of the upper arm. Its action is to raise the arm from the side, and it covers and gives roundness to the shoulder. (See also MUSCLE.)

Delusions

An irrational and usually unshakeable belief (*idée fixe*) peculiar to some individuals. They fail to respond to reasonable argument and the delusion is often paranoid in character with a belief that a person or persons is/are persecuting them. The existence of a delusion, of such a nature as to influence conduct seriously, is one of the most important signs in reaching a decision to arrange for the compulsory admission of the patient to hospital for observation. (See MENTAL ILLNESS.)

Dementia

An acquired and irreversible deterioration in intellectual function. Around 10 per cent of people aged over 65 and 20 per cent of those aged 75 or over are affected to some extent. The disorder is due to progressive brain disease. It appears gradually as a disturbance in problem-solving and agility of thought which may be considered to be due to tiredness, boredom or DEPRESSION. As memory failure develops, the affected person becomes bewildered, anxious and emotional when dealing with new surroundings and complex conversations. In professional skilled workers this is frequently first recognised by family and friends. Catastrophic reactions are usually brief but are commonly associated with an underlying depression which can be mistaken for progressive apathy. The condition progresses relentlessly with loss of recent memory extending to affect distant memory and failure to recognise even friends and family. Physical aggression, unsocial behaviour, deteriorating personal cleanliness and incoherent speech commonly develop. Similar symptoms to those in dementia can occur in curable conditions including depression, INTRACRANIAL tumours, SUBDURAL haematoma, SYPHILIS, vitamin B_1 deficiency (see APPENDIX 5: VITAMINS) and repeated episodes of cerebral ISCHAEMIA. This last may lead to multi-infarct dementia.

Treatment If organic disease is identified, it should, where possible, be treated; otherwise the treatment of dementia is alleviation of its symptoms. The affected person must be kept clean and properly fed. Good nursing care in comfortable surroundings is important and sedation with appropriate drugs may be required. Patients may eventually need institutional care. (See ALZHEIMER'S DISEASE.)

Demography

The study of populations and factors affecting their health.

De Morgan's Spots

De Morgan's spots are a type of small HAEMANGIOMA occuring in the skin of middle-aged people. No more than 3 mm in diameter, they are rarely widespread and are not malignant.

Demyelination

Destruction of the fatty MYELIN sheath around nerve fibres (see NERVE: NEURON(E)) which interferes with the nerve function. It can occur after injury to the nerve, but is particularly associated with MULTIPLE SCLEROSIS (MS).

Dendritic Ulcer

A branching ULCER on the surface of the cornea of the eye, caused by HERPES SIMPLEX infection.

Denervation

Interruption of the nerve supply to an organ or other structure.

Dengue

Also known as dengue fever, breakbone fever, and dandy fever, dengue is endemic and epidemic in tropical and subtropical regions. It is an acute infection caused by a flavivirus (family *togaviridae*) transmitted by mosquitoes – especially *Aedes aegypti*. Incubation period is 5–8 days, and is followed by abrupt onset of symptoms: fever, facial ERYTHEMA with intense itching (which spreads throughout the body), sore throat, running eyes, and painful muscles and joints are common accompaniments. The symptoms subside within a few days and are frequently succeeded by a relapse similar to the first. Further relapses may occur, and joint pains continue for some months. In uncomplicated dengue the mortality rate is virtually zero. Diagnosis is by virus isolation or demonstration of a rising antibody-concentration in the acute phase of infection. There is no specific treatment, but mild analgesics can be used to relieve the pains, and calamine lotion the itching. Prevention can be achieved by reduction of the mosquito-vector population.

Dengue haemorrhagic fever This is a more severe form of the disease which usually occurs in young children; it is largely confined to the indigenous population(s) of south-east Asia. It is accompanied by significant complications and mortality. Immunological status of the host is considered important in pathogenesis.

Dental Emergencies
See TEETH, DISORDERS OF.

Dental Hygienist
A person qualified to carry out the scaling (removal of calculus [deposits]) from the teeth and to advise patients on how to keep their teeth and gums healthy. Hygienists usually work in a qualified dentist's surgery.

Dental Surgeon
A dental surgeon, or dentist, is an individual trained to diagnose and treat disorders of the teeth and gums, as well as to advise on preventive measures to ensure that these areas remain healthy. Dentists qualify after a four-year course at dental school and then register with the GENERAL DENTAL COUNCIL, which is responsible for maintaining educational and professional standards. Around 25,000 dentists practise in the NHS and private sector.

Over the past four decades the financial outlay on NHS dental services has been around 5 per cent of total NHS funding. This contrasts with 10 per cent during the service's early years, when the NHS was coping with decades of 'dental neglect'. The population's dental health has, however, been steadily improving: in 1968 more than one-third of people had no natural teeth; by the late 1990s the proportion had fallen to 13 per cent.

Dentistry is divided into several groupings.

General dental practitioners Concerned with primary dental care, the prevention, diagnosis and treatment of diseases of the gums and teeth – for example, caries (see TEETH, DISORDERS OF). They also deal with difficulties in biting and the effects of trauma, and are aware that oral disorders may reflect disease elsewhere in the body. They will refer to the hospital dental services, patients who require treatment that cannot be satisfactorily carried out in a primary-care setting.

Most routine dental prevention and treatment is carried out in general dental practitioners' surgeries, where the dentists also supervise the work of hygienists and dental auxiliaries. Appliances, such as dentures, crowns, bridges and orthodontic appliances are constructed by dental technicians working in dental laboratories.

There are around 18,800 dentists providing general dental services in the UK. These practitioners are free to accept or reject any potential patient and to practise where they wish. Those dentists treating patients under an NHS contract (a mixture of capitation fees and items of service payments) can also treat patients privately (for an appropriate fee). Some dentists opt for full-time private practice, and their numbers are increasing in the wake of changes in 1990 in the contracts of NHS general dental practitioners.

Community dental practitioner Part of the public-health team and largely concerned with monitoring dental health and treating the young and the handicapped.

In the hospitals and dental schools are those who are involved in only one of the specialities.

Around 2,800 dentists work in NHS hospitals and 1,900 in the NHS's community services. In some parts of the UK, people wanting NHS treatment are having difficulties finding dentists willing to provide such care.

Restorative dentist Concerned with the repair of teeth damaged by trauma and caries, and the replacement of missing teeth.

Orthodontist Correction of jaws and teeth which are misaligned or irregular. This is done with appliances which may be removable or fixed to the teeth which are then moved with springs or elastics.

Oral and maxillo-facial surgeons Perform surgery to the mouth and face. This not only includes removal of buried teeth but also treatment for fractured facial bones, removal of cancers and the repair of missing tissue, and the cosmetic restoration of facial anomalies such as CLEFT PALATE or large or small jaws.

Dentine
See TEETH.

Dentist

See DENTAL SURGEON.

Dentition

See TEETH.

Denture

A plate or frame bearing false teeth. It may be complete (replacing all the teeth in one jaw) or partial.

Deodorants

Substances which remove or lessen objectionable odours. Some, which have a powerful odour, simply cover other smells, but the most effective act by giving off oxygen, so as to convert the objectionable substances into simple and harmless ones.

Varieties Volatile oils of plants, such as eucalyptus and turpentine, chlorine water and chlorinated lime, peroxide of hydrogen and charcoal have been used as deodorants. There are now many commercial products available.

Deoxyribonucleic Acid

See DNA.

Dependence

Physical or psychological reliance on a substance or an individual. A baby is naturally dependent on its parents, but as the child develops, this dependence lessens. Some adults, however, remain partly dependent, making abnormal demands for admiration, love and help from parents, relatives and others.

The dependence that most concerns modern society is one in which individuals become dependent on or addicted to certain substances such as alcohol, drugs, tobacco (nicotine), caffeine and solvents. This is often called substance abuse. Some people become addicted to certain foods or activities: examples of the latter include gambling, computer games and use of the Internet.

The 28th report of the World Health Organisation Expert Committee on Drug Dependence in 1993 defined drug dependence as: 'A cluster of physiological, behavioural and cognitive phenomena of variable intensity, in which the use of a psychoactive drug (or drugs) takes on a high priority. The necessary descriptive characteristics are preoccupation with a desire to obtain and take the drug and persistent drug-seeking behaviour. Psychological dependence occurs when the substance abuser craves the drug's desirable effects. Physical dependence occurs when the user has to continue taking the drug to avoid distressing withdrawal or abstinence symptoms. Thus, determinants and the problematic consequences of drug dependence may be biological, psychological or social and usually interact.'

Different drugs cause different rates of dependence: TOBACCO is the most common substance of addiction; HEROIN and COCAINE cause high rates of addiction; whereas ALCOHOL is much lower, and CANNABIS lower again. Smoking in the western world reached a peak after World War II with almost 80 per cent of the male population smoking. The reports on the link between smoking and cancer in the early 1960s resulted in a decline that has continued so that only around a quarter of the adult populations of the UK and USA smokes. Globally, tobacco consumption continues to grow, particularly in the developing world with multinational tobacco companies marketing their products aggressively.

Accurate figures for illegal drug-taking are hard to obtain, but probably approximately 4 per cent of the population is dependent on alcohol and 2 per cent on other drugs, both legal and illegal, at any one time in western countries.

How does dependence occur? More than 40 distinct theories or models of drug misuse have been put forward. One is that the individual consumes drugs to cope with personal problems or difficulties in relations with others. The other main model emphasises environmental influences such as drug availability, environmental pressures to consume drugs, and sociocultural influences such as peer pressure.

By contrast to these models of why people misuse drugs, models of compulsive drug use – where individuals have a compulsive addiction – have been amenable to testing in the laboratory. Studies at cellular and nerve-receptor levels are attempting to identify mechanisms of tolerance and dependence for several substances. Classical behaviour theory is a key model for understanding drug dependence. This and current laboratory studies are being used to explain the reinforcing nature of dependent substances and are helping to provide an explanatory framework for dependence. Drug consumption is a learned form of behaviour. Numerous investigators have used conditioning theories to study why people misuse drugs. Laboratory studies are now locating the 'reward pathways' in the brain for opiates and stimulants where positive reinforcing mechanisms involve particular sectors of the brain. There is a consensus among experts in addiction that addictive behaviour is amenable to effective treatment, and that the extent to which an addict complies with treatment makes it possible to predict a positive outcome. But there is a long way to go before the mechanisms of drug addiction are properly understood or ways of treating it generally agreed.

Effects of drugs Cannabis, derived from the plant *Cannabis sativa*, is a widely used recreational drug. Its two main forms are marijuana, which comes from the dried leaves, and hashish which comes from the resin. Cannabis may be used in food and drink but is usually smoked in cigarettes to induce relaxation and a feeling of well-being. Heavy use can cause apathy and vagueness and may even cause psychosis. Whether or not cannabis leads people to using harder drugs is arguable, and a national debate is underway on whether its use should be legalised for medicinal use. Cannabis may alleviate the symptoms of some disorders – for example, MULTIPLE SCLEROSIS (MS) – and there are calls to allow the substance to be classified as a prescribable drug.

About one in ten of Britain's teenagers misuses volatile substances such as toluene at some time, but only about one in 40 does so regularly. These substances are given off by certain glues, solvents, varnishes, and liquid fuels, all of which can be bought cheaply in shops, although their sale to children under 16 is illegal. They are often inhaled from plastic bags held over the nose and mouth. Central-nervous-system excitation, with euphoria and disinhibition, is followed by depression and lethargy. Unpleasant effects include facial rash, nausea and vomiting, tremor, dizziness, and clumsiness. Death from COMA and acute cardiac toxicity is a serious risk. Chronic heavy use can cause peripheral neuropathy and irreversible cerebellar damage. (See SOLVENT ABUSE (MISUSE).)

The hallucinogenic or psychedelic drugs include LYSERGIC ACID DIETHYLAMIDE (LSD) or acid, magic mushrooms, ecstasy (MDMA), and phencyclidine (PCP or 'angel' dust, mainly used in the USA). These drugs have no medicinal uses. Taken by mouth, they produce vivid 'trips', with heightened emotions and perceptions and sometimes with hallucinations. They are not physically addictive but can cause nightmarish bad trips during use and flashbacks (vivid reruns of trips) after use, and can probably trigger psychosis and even death, especially if drugs are mixed or taken with alcohol.

Stimulant drugs such as amphetamine and cocaine act like adrenaline and speed up the central nervous system, making the user feel confident, energetic, and powerful for several hours. They can also cause severe insomnia, anxiety, paranoia, psychosis, and even sudden death due to convulsions or tachycardia. Depression may occur on withdrawal of these drugs, and in some users this is sufficiently deterrent to cause psychological dependence. Amphetamine ('speed') is mainly synthesised illegally and may be eaten, sniffed, or injected. Related drugs, such as dexamphetamine sulphate (Dexedrine), are prescribed pills that enter the black market. ECSTASY is another amphetamine derivative that has become a popular recreational drug; it may have fatal allergic effects. Cocaine and related drugs are used in medicine as local anaesthetics. Illegal supplies of cocaine ('snow' or 'ice') and its derivative, 'crack', come mainly from South America, where they are made from the plant *Erythroxylon coca*. Cocaine is usually sniffed ('snorted') or rubbed into the gums; crack is burnt and inhaled.

Opiate drugs are derived from the opium poppy, *Papaver somniferum*. They are described as narcotic because they induce sleep. Their main medical use is as potent oral or injectable analgesics such as MORPHINE, DIAMORPHINE, PETHIDINE HYDROCHLORIDE, and CODEINE. The commonest illegal opiate is heroin, a powdered form of diamorphine that may be smoked, sniffed, or injected to induce euphoria and drowsiness. Regular opiate misuse leads to tolerance (the need to take ever larger doses to achieve the same effect) and marked dependence. A less addictive oral opiate, METHADONE HYDROCHLORIDE, can be prescribed as a substitute that is easier to withdraw.

Some 75,000–150,000 Britons now misuse opiates and other drugs intravenously, and pose a huge public-health problem because injections with shared dirty needles can carry the blood-borne viruses that cause AIDS/HIV and HEPATITIS B. Many clinics now operate schemes to exchange old needles for clean ones, free of charge. Many addicts are often socially disruptive.

For help and advice see APPENDIX 2: ADDRESSES: SOURCES OF INFORMATION, ADVICE, SUPPORT AND SELF-HELP – National Dugs Helpline.

(See ALCOHOL and TOBACCO for detailed entries on those subjects.)

Depigmentation

Also called hypo-pigmentation, this congenital or acquired disorder is one in which the skin loses its pigmentation because of reduced

MELANIN production. It can be classified into three groups: VITILIGO, ALBINISM and post-inflammatory hypopigmentation.

Depilation

The process of destroying hair – substances and processes used for this purpose being known as depilatories. The purpose may be effected in three ways: by removing the hairs at the level of the skin surface; by pulling the hairs out (epilation); and by destroying the roots and so preventing the growth of new hairs.

Shaving is the most effective way of removing superfluous hairs. Rubbing morning and night with a smooth pumice-stone is said to be helpful. Electrolysis and diathermy are also used.

Depression

Depression is a word that is regularly misused. Most people experience days or weeks when they feel low and fed up (feelings that may recur), but generally they get over it without needing to seek medical help. This is not clinical depression, best defined as a collection of psychological symptoms including sadness; unhappy thoughts characterised by worry, poor self-image, self-blame, guilt and low self-confidence; downbeat views on the future; and a feeling of hopelessness. Sufferers may consider suicide, and in severe depression may soon develop HALLUCINATIONS and DELUSIONS.

Doctors make the diagnosis of depression when they believe a patient to be ill with the latter condition, which may affect physical health and in some instances be life-threatening. This form of depression is common, with up to 15 per cent of the population suffering from it at any one time, while about 20 per cent of adults have 'medical' depression at some time during their lives – such that it is one of the most commonly presenting disorders in general practice. Women seem more liable to develop depression than men, with one in six of the former and one in nine of the latter seeking medical help.

Manic depression is a serious form of the disorder that recurs throughout life and is manifested by bouts of abnormal elation – the manic stage. Both the manic and depressive phases are commonly accompanied by psychotic symptoms such as delusions, hallucinations and a loss of sense of reality. This combination is sometimes termed a manic-depressive psychosis or bipolar affective disorder because of the illness's division into two parts. Another psychiatric description is the catch-all term 'affective disorder'.

Symptoms These vary with the illness's severity. Anxiety and variable moods are the main symptoms in mild depression. The sufferer may cry without any reason or be unresponsive to relatives and friends. In its more severe form, depression presents with a loss of appetite, sleeping problems, lack of interest in and enjoyment of social activities, tiredness for no obvious reason, an indifference to sexual activity and a lack of concentration. The individual's physical and mental activities slow down and he or she may contemplate suicide. Symptoms may vary during the 24 hours, being less troublesome during the latter part of the day and worse at night. Some people get depressed during the winter months, probably a consequence of the long hours of darkness: this disorder – SEASONAL AFFECTIVE DISORDER SYNDROME, or SADS – is thought to be more common in populations living in areas with long winters and limited daylight. Untreated, a person with depressive symptoms may steadily worsen, even withdrawing to bed for much of the time, and allowing his or her personal appearance, hygiene and environment to deteriorate. Children and adolescents may also suffer from depression and the disorder is not always recognised.

Causes A real depressive illness rarely has a single obvious cause, although sometimes the death of a close relative, loss of employment or a broken personal relationship may trigger a bout. Depression probably has a genetic background; for instance, manic depression seems to run in some families. Viral infections sometimes cause depression, and hormonal disorders – for example, HYPOTHYROIDISM or postnatal hormonal disturbances (postnatal depression) – will cause it. Difficult family or social relations can contribute to the development of the disorder. Depression is believed to occur because of chemical changes in the transmission of signals in the nervous system, with a reduction in the neurochemicals that facilitate the passage of messages throughout the system.

Treatment This depends on the type and severity of the depression. These are three main forms.

PSYCHOTHERAPY either on a one-to-one basis or as part of a group: this is valuable for those whose depression is the result of lifestyle or personality problems. Various types of psychotherapy are available.

DRUG TREATMENT is the most common method and is particularly helpful for those with physical symptoms. ANTIDEPRESSANT DRUGS are divided into three main groups: TRICYCLIC ANTIDEPRESSANT DRUGS (amitriptyline, imipramine and dothiepin are examples); MONOAMINE OXIDASE INHIBITORS (MAOIS) (phenelzine, isocarboxazid and tranylcypromine are examples); and SELECTIVE SEROTONIN REUPTAKE INHIBITORS (SSRIS) (fluoxetine – well known as Prozac®, fluvoxamine and paroxetine are examples). For manic depression, lithium carbonate is the main preventive drug and it is also used for persistent depression that fails to respond to other treatments. Long-term lithium treatment reduces the likelihood of relapse in about 80 per cent of manic depressives, but the margin between control and toxic side-effects is narrow, so the drug must be carefully supervised. Indeed, all drug treatment for depression needs regular monitoring as the substances have powerful chemical properties with consequential side-effects in some people. Furthermore, the nature of the illness means that some sufferers forget or do not want to take the medication.

ELECTROCONVULSIVE THERAPY (ECT) If drug treatments fail, severely depressed patients may be considered for ECT. This treatment has been used for many years but is now only rarely recommended. Given under general anaesthetic, in appropriate circumstances, ECT is safe and effective and may even be life-saving, though temporary impairment of memory may occur. Because the treatment was often misused in the past, it still carries a reputation that worries patients and relatives; hence careful assessment and counselling are essential before use is recommended.

Some patients with depression – particularly those with manic depression or who are a danger to themselves or to the public, or who are suicidal – may need admission to hospital, or in severe cases to a secure unit, in order to initiate treatment. But as far as possible patients are treated in the community (see MENTAL ILLNESS).

Depressor

(1) A muscle that lowers or flattens a part of the body.

(2) The name given to a nerve by whose stimulation motion, secretion, or some other function is restrained or prevented: for example, the depressor nerve of the heart slows the beating of this organ.

Deprivation Score

A measure of an individual's or group's lack of normal social amenities such as proper housing, diet and warmth. It was devised in the 1980s to help assess the medical services needed by a socially deprived population.

Dermabrasion

Dermabrasion, or 'skin planing', is a method of removing the superficial layers of the skin, useful in the treatment of tattoos and acne scars.

Dermatitis

Synonymous with eczema in all respects. Although the lay term 'eczema' usually refers to atopic (see ATOPY) or endogenous eczema, there are many other causes. Susceptibility to dermatitis is genetically determined in some cases; in others, environmental irritants and allergens are implicated. Symptoms typically include itching, dryness or cracking and, occasionally, soreness of the skin. Physical signs include redness (erythema), scaling, and vesiculation (tiny blisters just beneath the surface of the skin). (See also SKIN, DISEASES OF.)

Dermatofibroma

Also known as histiocytoma. A firm, painless nodule in the skin, typically on a leg, due to excessive formation of COLLAGEN. A common disorder, it is often a slow response to an insect bite and persists indefinitely.

Dermatoglyphics

Dermatoglyphics is the study of the patterns made by the ridges and crevices of the hands and the soles of the feet.

Dermatologist

A medically qualified specialist who diagnoses and treats disorders of the skin (see SKIN, DISEASES OF).

Dermatology

In essence, this is the study of the skin. As well as being an organ in its own right, the skin is a stage on which other organs as well as the emotions most visibly play out their roles. Changes in its blood vessels – and hence blood flow through the skin – may indicate a major immunological response to a range of potential factors (see SKIN, DISEASES OF).

Dermatome

(1) Embryological tissue which has developed from the somites to become the dermis and subcutaneous tissue. The cutaneous area that is derived from each dermatome is supplied by a single dorsal spinal nerve root.

(2) A surgical instrument for removing very thin slices of skin for grafting.

Dermatomyositis

A rare disease, possibly caused by an auto-immune reaction, in which muscle inflammation and weakness is associated with a characteristic heliotrope ERYTHEMA of the face and backs of the hands. In adults it may be associated with underlying malignancy. Tissue changes are similar to those in POLYMYOSITIS.

Dermatophytes

Fungi which can infect skin, hair and nails. About 30 species in three genera are PATHO-GENIC to humans (see RINGWORM).

Dermographism

Dermographism, or factitious URTICARIA, refers to transient ERYTHEMA and wealing caused by trauma to the skin.

Dermoid Cyst

See CYSTS.

Desensitisation

In psychiatry, a method for treating phobias used in BEHAVIOUR THERAPY. The affected individual is slowly acclimatised to the cause of his or her fear. (See also ALLERGY.)

Desferrioxamine

An agent which binds to heavy metals, used in the treatment of iron poisoning and THALASSAEMIA.

Designer Drugs

A group of chemical substances produced illegally whose properties and effects are similar to those of drugs of abuse. They may be derived from narcotic ANALGESICS, AMPHET-AMINES or HALLUCINOGENS. Ecstasy is a widely used designer drug and has caused deaths among teenagers. Designer drugs are potentially dangerous, especially if taken with alcohol.

Desquamation

The scaling-off of the superficial layer of the epidermis (see SKIN).

Detached Retina

Separation of the retina from the choroid in the EYE. It may be due to trauma or be secondary to tumour or inflammation of the choroid, and causes blindness in the affected part of the retina. It can be treated surgically using PHOTOCOAGULATION.

Detergents

Substances which clean the skin surface. This means that, strictly speaking, any soap, or soap-like substance used in washing, is a detergent. At the present day, however, the term is largely used for the synthetic detergents which are now used on such a large scale. These are prepared by the cracking and oxidation of high-petroleum waxes with sulphuric acid. The commoner ones in commercial preparations are aryl alkyl sulphate or sulphonate and secondary alkyl sulphate.

In view of their widespread use, such detergents appear to cause relatively little trouble with the skin, but more trouble has been reported with the so-called 'biological' detergents – named because they contain an ENZYME which destroys protein. As a result they are claimed to remove proteins (stains such as blood, chocolate, milk or gravy) which are relatively difficult for ordinary detergents to remove. Unfortunately these 'biological' detergents may cause dermatitis. In addition, they have been reported to cause asthma in those using them, and even more so in workers manufacturing them.

Detoxication

Also called detoxification, this is a process whereby toxic agents are removed from the body and toxic effects neutralised. (See POISONS and TOXINS.)

Deviance

Variation from normal. Often used to describe unusual sexual behaviour.

Dexamethasone

A CORTICOSTEROIDS derivative. As an anti-inflammatory agent it is approximately 30 times as effective as cortisone and eight times as effective as prednisolone. On the other hand, it has practically none of the salt-retaining properties of cortisone.

Dexamphetamine

A drug that stimulates the central nervous system. It can be used to treat NARCOLEPSY and hyperactive children but should not be used to combat obesity or treat depression. It is also a drug of abuse.

Dextran

The name given to a group of polysaccharides first discovered in sugar-beet preparations which had become infected with certain bacteria. A homogenous preparation of dextran, with a consistent molecular weight and free from PROTEIN, is in appropriate clinical circumstances used as a substitute for plasma for TRANSFUSION purposes. Dextran is often used as an immediate transfusion measure to treat severe bleeding or certain types of shock until properly cross-matched blood is available. A blood sample for cross-matching must be taken before intravenous dextran is given.

Dextrocardia

A condition in which a person's heart is situated on the right of the chest in a mirror image of its usual position. This may be associated with similar inversion of the abdominal organs – *situs inversus*.

Dextromethophan

An over-the-counter drug used to relieve dry, irritating, persistent coughs, this opioid acts as a cough suppressant. It is available either alone or in combination with other drugs in linctus, lozenges and syrups prepared to provide symptomatic relief for coughs and colds.

Dextrose

Another name for purified grape sugar or glucose. A common constituent of intravenous fluids.

Dia-

Dia- is a prefix meaning through or thoroughly.

Diabetes Insipidus

Diabetes insipidus is a relatively rare condition and must be differentiated from DIABETES MELLITUS which is an entirely different disease.

It is characterised by excessive thirst and the passing of large volumes of urine which have a low specific gravity and contain no abnormal constituents. It is either due to a lack of the antidiuretic hormone normally produced by the HYPOTHALAMUS and stored in the posterior PITUITARY GLAND, or to a defect in the renal tubules which prevents them from responding to the antidiuretic hormone VASOPRESSIN. When the disorder is due to vasopressin insufficiency, a primary or secondary tumour in the area of the pituitary stalk is responsible for one-third of cases. In another one-third of cases there is no apparent cause, and such IDIO-PATHIC cases are sometimes familial. A further one-third of cases result from a variety of lesions including trauma, basal MENINGITIS and granulomatous lesions in the pituitary-stalk area. When the renal tubules fail to respond to vasopressin this is usually because of a genetic defect transmitted as a sex-linked recessive characteristic, and the disease is called nephrogenic dia-

betes insipidus. Metabolic abnormalities such as HYPERCALCAEMIA and potassium depletion render the renal tubule less sensitive to vasopressin, and certain drugs such as lithium and tetracycline may have a similar effect.

If the disease is due to a deficiency of vasopressin, treatment should be with the analogue of vasopressin called desmopressin which is more potent than the natural hormone and has less pressor activity. It also has the advantage in that it is absorbed from the nasal mucosa and so does not need to be injected.

Nephrogenic diabetes insipidus cannot be treated with desmopressin. The urine volume can, however, usually be reduced by half by a thiazide diuretic (see THIAZIDES).

Diabetes Mellitus

Diabetes mellitus is a condition characterised by a raised concentration of glucose in the blood due to a deficiency in the production and/or action of INSULIN, a pancreatic hormone made in special cells called the islet cells of Langerhans.

Insulin-dependent and non-insulin-dependent diabetes have a varied pathological pattern and are caused by the interaction of several genetic and environmental factors.

Insulin-dependent diabetes mellitus (IDDM) (juvenile-onset diabetes, type 1 diabetes) describes subjects with a severe deficiency or absence of insulin production. Insulin therapy is essential to prevent KETOSIS – a disturbance of the body's acid/base balance and an accumulation of ketones in the tissues. The onset is most commonly during childhood, but can occur at any age. Symptoms are acute and weight loss is common.

Non-insulin-dependent diabetes mellitus (NIDDM) (maturity-onset diabetes, type 2 diabetes) may be further sub-divided into obese and non-obese groups. This type usually occurs after the age of 40 years with an insidious onset. Subjects are often overweight and weight loss is uncommon. Ketosis rarely develops. Insulin production is reduced but not absent.

A new hormone has been identified linking obesity to type 2 diabetes. Called resistin – because of its resistance to insulin – it was first found in mice but has since been identified in humans. Researchers in the United States believe that the hormone may, in part, explain how obesity predisposes people to diabetes. Their hypothesis is that a protein in the body's fat cells triggers insulin resistance around the body. Other research suggests that type 2 diabetes may now be occurring in obese children; this could indicate that children should be eating a more-balanced diet and taking more exercise.

Diabetes associated with other conditions (*a*) Due to pancreatic disease – for example, chronic pancreatitis (see PANCREAS, DISORDERS OF); (*b*) secondary to drugs – for example, GLUCOCORTICOIDS (see PANCREAS, DISORDERS OF); (*c*) excess hormone production – for example, growth hormone (ACROMEGALY); (*d*) insulin receptor abnormalities; (*e*) genetic syndromes (see GENETIC DISORDERS).

Gestational diabetes Diabetes occurring in pregnancy and resolving afterwards.

Aetiology Insulin-dependent diabetes occurs as a result of autoimmune destruction of beta cells within the PANCREAS. Genetic influences are important and individuals with certain HLA tissue types (HLA DR3 and HLA DR4) are more at risk; however, the risks associated with the HLA genes are small. If one parent has IDDM, the risk of a child developing IDDM by the age of 25 years is 1·5–2·5 per cent, and the risk of a sibling of an IDDM subject developing diabetes is about 3 per cent.

Non-insulin-dependent diabetes has no HLA association, but the genetic influences are much stronger. The risks of developing diabetes vary with different races. Obesity, decreased exercise and ageing increase the risks of disease development. The risk of a sibling of a NIDDM subject developing NIDDM up to the age of 80 years is 30–40 per cent.

Diet Many NIDDM diabetics may be treated with diet alone. For those subjects who are overweight, weight loss is important, although often unsuccessful. A diet high in complex carbohydrate, high in fibre, low in fat and aiming towards ideal body weight is prescribed. Subjects taking insulin need to eat at regular intervals in relation to their insulin regime and missing meals may result in hypoglycaemia, a lowering of the amount of glucose in the blood, which if untreated can be fatal (see below).

Oral hypoglycaemics are used in the treatment of non-insulin-dependent diabetes in addition to diet, when diet alone fails to control blood-sugar levels. (*a*) SULPHONYLUREAS act mainly by increasing the production of insulin; (*b*) BIGUANIDES, of which only metformin is available, may be used alone or in addition to sulphonylureas. Metformin's main actions are to lower the production of glucose by the liver and improve its uptake in the peripheral tissues.

Complications The risks of complications increase with duration of disease.

Diabetic hypoglycaemia occurs when amounts of glucose in the blood become low. This may occur in subjects taking sulphonylureas or insulin. Symptoms usually develop when the glucose concentration falls below 2·5 mmol/l. They may, however, occur at higher concentrations in subjects with persistent hyperglycaemia – an excess of glucose – and at lower levels in subjects with persistent hypoglycaemia. Symptoms include confusion, hunger and sweating, with coma developing if blood-sugar concentrations remain low. Refined sugar followed by complex carbohydrate will return the glucose concentration to normal. If the subject is unable to swallow, glucagon may be given intramuscularly or glucose intravenously, followed by oral carbohydrate, once the subject is able to swallow.

Although it has been shown that careful control of the patient's metabolism prevents late complications in the small blood vessels, the risk of hypoglycaemia is increased and patients need to be well motivated to keep to their dietary and treatment regime. This regime is also very expensive. All risk factors for the patient's cardiovascular system – not simply controlling hyperglycaemia – may need to be reduced if late complications to the cardiovascular system are to be avoided.

Diabetes is one of the world's most serious health problems. Recent projections suggest that the disorder will affect nearly 240 million individuals worldwide by 2010 – double its prevalence in 1994. The incidence of insulin-dependent diabetes is rising in young children; they will be liable to develop late complications.

Although there are complications associated with diabetes, many subjects live normal lives and survive to an old age. People with diabetes or their relatives can obtain advice from Diabetes UK (www.diabetes.org.uk).

Increased risks are present of (*a*) heart disease, (*b*) peripheral vascular disease, and (*c*) cerebrovascular disease.

Diabetic eye disease (*a*) retinopathy, (*b*) cataract. Regular examination of the fundus enables any abnormalities developing to be detected and treatment given when appropriate to preserve eyesight.

Nephropathy Subjects with diabetes may develop kidney damage which can result in renal failure.

Neuropathy (*a*) Symmetrical sensory polyneuropathy; damage to the sensory nerves that commonly presents with tingling, numbness of pain in the feet or hands. (*b*) Asymmetrical motor diabetic neuropathy, presenting as progressive weakness and wasting of the proximal muscles of legs. (*c*) Mononeuropathy; individual motor or sensory nerves may be affected. (*d*) Autonomic neuropathy, which affects the autonomic nervous system, has many presentations including IMPOTENCE, diarrhoea or constipation and postural HYPOTENSION.

Skin lesions There are several skin disorders associated with diabetes, including: (*a*) necrobiosis lipoidica diabeticorum, characterised by one or more yellow atrophic lesions on the legs; (*b*) ulcers, which most commonly occur on the feet due to peripheral vascular disease, neuropathy and infection. Foot care is very important.

Diabetic ketoacidosis occurs when there is insufficient insulin present to prevent KETONE production. This may occur before the diagnosis of IDDM or when insufficient insulin is being given. The presence of large amounts of ketones in the urine indicates excess ketone production and treatment should be sought immediately. Coma and death may result if the condition is left untreated.

Symptoms Thirst, POLYURIA, GLYCOSURIA, weight loss despite eating, and recurrent infections (e.g. BALANITIS and infections of the VULVA) are the main symptoms.

However, subjects with non-insulin-dependent diabetes may have the disease for several years without symptoms, and diagnosis is often made incidentally or when presenting with a complication of the disease.

Treatment of diabetes aims to prevent symptoms, restore carbohydrate metabolism to as near normal as possible, and to minimise complications. Concentration of glucose, fructosamine and glycated haemoglobin in the blood are used to give an indication of blood-glucose control.

Insulin-dependent diabetes requires insulin for treatment. Non-insulin-dependent diabetes may be treated with diet, oral HYPOGLYCAEMIC AGENTS or insulin.

Insulin All insulin is injected – mainly by syringe but sometimes by insulin pump – because it is inactivated by gastrointestinal enzymes. There are three main types of insulin preparation: (*a*) short action (approximately six hours), with rapid onset; (*b*) intermediate action (approximately 12 hours); (*c*) long action, with slow onset and lasting for up to 36 hours. Human, porcine and bovine preparations are available. Much of the insulin now used is prepared by genetic engineering techniques from micro-organisms. There are many regimens of insulin treatment involving different combinations of insulin; regimens vary depending on the requirements of the patients, most of whom administer the insulin themselves. Carbohydrate intake, energy expenditure and the presence of infection are important determinants of insulin requirements on a day-to-day basis.

A new treatment for diabetes, pioneered in Canada and entering its preliminary clinical trials in the UK, is the transplantation of islet cells of Langerhans from a healthy person into a patient with the disorder. If the transplantation is successful, the transplanted cells start producing insulin, thus reducing or eliminating the requirement for regular insulin injections. If successful the trials would be a significant advance in the treatment of diabetes.

Scientists in Israel have developed a drug, Dia Pep 277, which stops the body's immune system from destroying pancratic β cells as happens in insulin-dependent diabetes. The drug, given by injection, offers the possibility of preventing type 1 diabetes in healthy people at genetic risk of developing the disorder, and of checking its progression in affected individuals whose β cells are already perishing. Trials of the drug are in progress.

Diagnosis

The skill of distinguishing one disease from another; it is essential to scientific and successful treatment. The name is also given to the opinion arrived at as to the nature of a disease. It is in diagnosis more than in treatment that the highest medical skill is required, and, for a diagnosis, the past and hereditary history of a case, the symptoms complained of, and the signs of disease found upon examination are all weighed. Many methods of laboratory examination are also used at the present day in aiding diagnosis. Computers are also being used to help clinical and laboratory diagnostic procedures.

Dialysis

A procedure used to filter off waste products from the blood and remove surplus fluid from the body in someone who has kidney failure (see KIDNEYS, DISEASES OF). The scientific process involves separating crystalloid and COLLOID substances from a solution by interposing a semi-permeable membrane between the solution and pure water. The crystalloid substances pass through the membrane into the water until a state of equilibrium, so far as the crystalloid substances are concerned, is established between the two sides of the membrane. The colloid substances do not pass through the membrane.

Dialysis is available as either haemodialysis or peritoneal dialysis.

Haemodialysis Blood is removed from the circulation either through an artificial arterio-venous fistula (junction) or a temporary or permanent internal catheter in the jugular vein (see CATHETERS). It then passes through an artificial kidney ('dialyser') to remove toxins (e.g. potassium and urea) by diffusion and excess salt and water by ultrafiltration from the blood into dialysis fluid prepared in a 'proportionator' (often referred to as a 'kidney machine'). Dialysers vary in design and performance but all work on the principle of a semi-permeable membrane separating blood from dialysis fluid. Haemodialysis is undertaken two to three times a week for 4–6 hours a session.

Peritoneal dialysis uses the peritoneal lining (see PERITONEUM) as a semi-permeable membrane. Approximately 2 litres of sterile fluid is run into the peritoneum through the permanent indwelling catheter; the fluid is left for 3–4 hours; and the cycle is repeated 3–4 times per day. Most patients undertake continuous ambulatory peritoneal dialysis (CAPD), although a few use a machine overnight (continuous cycling peritoneal dialysis, CCPD) which allows greater clearance of toxins.

Disadvantages of haemodialysis include cardiovascular instability, HYPERTENSION, bone disease, ANAEMIA and development of periarticular AMYLOIDOSIS. Disadvantages of peritoneal dialysis include peritonitis, poor drainage of fluid, and gradual loss of overall efficiency as endogenous renal function declines. Haemodialysis is usually done in outpatient dialysis clinics by skilled nurses, but some patients can carry out the procedure at home. Both haemodialysis and peritoneal dialysis carry a relatively high morbidity and the ideal treatment for patients with end-stage renal failure is successful renal TRANSPLANTATION.

Diamorphine

Diamorphine is another name for HEROIN.

Diaphoresis

Another name for sweating (see PERSPIRATION).

Diaphragm

The diaphragm is the thin, dome-shaped muscular partition which separates the cavity of the abdomen from that of the chest. It is of great importance in respiration, playing the chief part in filling the lungs. During deep respiration its movements are responsible for 60 per cent of the total amount of air breathed, and in the horizontal posture, or in sleep, an even greater percentage.

The description 'diaphragm' is also used for the hemispherical rubber ('dutch') cap used in conjunction with a chemical spermicide as a contraceptive. It fits over the neck of the uterus (cervix) inside the vagina. (See CONTRACEPTION.)

Diaphysectomy

The operation whereby a part of the shaft of a long bone (e.g. humerus, femur) is excised.

Diaphysis

The shaft of a long bone.

Diarrhoea

Diarrhoea or looseness of the bowels is increased frequency, fluidity or volume of bowel movements compared to usual. Most people have occasional attacks of acute diarrhoea, usually caused by contaminated food or water or excessive alcohol consumption. Such attacks normally clear up within a day or two, whether or not they are treated. Chronic diarrhoea, on the other hand, may be the result of a serious intestinal disorder or of more general disease.

The commonest cause of acute diarrhoea is food poisoning, the organisms involved usually being STAPHYLOCOCCUS, CLOSTRIDIUM bacteria, salmonella, *E. coli* O157 (see ESCHERICHIA), CAMPYLOBACTER, cryptosporidium, and Norwalk virus. A person may also acquire infective diarrhoea as a result of droplet infections from adenoviruses or echoviruses. Interference with the bacterial flora of the intestine may cause acute diarrhoea: this often happens to someone who travels to another country and acquires unfamiliar intestinal bacteria. Other infections include bacillary dysentery, typhoid fever and paratyphoid fevers (see ENTERIC FEVER). Drug toxicity, food allergy, food intolerance and anxiety may also cause acute diarrhoea, and habitual constipation may result in attacks of diarrhoea.

Treatment of diarrhoea in adults depends on the cause. The water and salts (see ELECTRO-LYTES) lost during a severe attack must be replaced to prevent dehydration. Ready-prepared mixtures of salts can be bought from a pharmacist. Antidiarrhoeal drugs such as codeine phosphate or loperamide should be used in infectious diarrhoea only if the symptoms are disabling. Antibacterial drugs may be used under medical direction. Persistent diarrhoea – longer than a week – or blood-stained diarrhoea must be investigated under medical supervision.

Diarrhoea in infants can be such a serious condition that it requires separate consideration. One of its features is that it is usually accompanied by vomiting; the result can be rapid dehydration as infants have relatively high fluid requirements. Mostly it is causd by acute gastroenteritis caused by various viruses, most commonly ROTAVIRUSES, but also by many bacteria. In the developed world most children recover rapidly, but diarrhoea is the single greatest cause of infant mortality worldwide. The younger the infant, the higher the mortality rate.

Diarrhoea is much more rare in breast-fed babies, and when it does occur it is usually less severe. The environment of the infant is also important: the condition is highly infectious and, if a case occurs in a maternity home or a children's hospital, it tends to spread quickly. This is why doctors prefer to treat such children at home but if hospital admission is essential, isolation and infection-control procedures are necessary.

Treatment An infant with diarrhoea should not be fed milk (unless breast-fed, when this should continue) but should be given an electrolyte mixture, available from pharmacists or on prescription, to replace lost water and salts. If the diarrhoea improves within 24 hours, milk can gradually be reintroduced. If diarrhoea continues beyond 36–48 hours, a doctor should be consulted. Any signs of dehydration require urgent medical attention; such signs include drowsiness, lack of response, loose skin, persistent crying, glazed eyes and a dry mouth and tongue.

Diastase

A mixture of enzymes obtained from malt. These enzymes have the property of converting starch into sugar. Diastase is used in the preparation of predigested starchy foods, and in the treatment of DYSPEPSIA, particularly that due to inability to digest starch adequately. It is also used for the conversion of starch to fermentable sugars in the brewing and fermentation industries.

Diastasis

A term applied to separation of the end of a growing bone from the shaft. The condition resembles a fracture, but is more serious because of the damage done to the growing cartilage through which the separation takes place, so that the future growth of the bone is considerably diminished.

Diastole

The relaxation of a hollow organ. The term is applied in particular to the HEART, to indicate the resting period between the beats (systole), while blood is flowing into the organ.

Diastolic Pressure

The pressure exerted by the blood against the arterial wall during DIASTOLE. This is the lowest blood pressure in the cardiac cycle. A normal reading of diastolic pressure in a healthy adult at rest is 70 mm Hg. (See HEART.)

Diathermy

A process by which electric currents can be passed into the deeper parts of the body so as to produce internal warmth and relieve pain; or, by using powerful currents, to destroy tumours and diseased parts bloodlessly. The form of electricity used consists of high-frequency oscillations, the frequency of oscillation ranging from 10 million to 25,000 million oscillations per second. The current passes between two electrodes placed on the skin.

The so-called ultra-short-wave diathermy (or short-wave diathermy, as it is usually referred to) has replaced the original long-wave diathermy, as it is produced consistently at a stable wave-length (11 metres) and is easier to apply. In recent years microwave diathermy has been developed, which has a still higher oscillating current (25,000 million cycles per second, compared with 500 million for short-wave diathermy).

When the current passes, a distinct sensation of increasing warmth is experienced and the temperature of the body gradually rises; the heart's action becomes quicker; there is sweating with increased excretion of waste products. The general blood pressure is also distinctly lowered. The method is used in painful rheumatic conditions, both of muscles and joints.

By concentrating the current in a small electrode, the heating effects immediately below this are very much increased. The diathermy knife utilises this technique to coagulate bleeding vessels and cauterise abnormal tissue during surgery.

Diathesis

An archaic term meaning constitutional or inherited state giving an individual a predisposition towards a disease, a group of diseases or a structural or metabolic abnormality. An example is HAEMOPHILIA, a bleeding disorder.

Diazepam

See TRANQUILLISERS; BENZODIAZEPINES.

Dicephalus

The term applied to symmetrical CONJOINED TWINS with two separate heads.

Dichlorodiphenyl Trichloroethane

DDT is the generally used abbreviation for the compound which has been given the official name of dicophane. It was first synthesised in 1874, but it was not until 1940 that, as a result of research work in Switzerland, its remarkable toxic action on insects was discovered. This work was taken up and rapidly expanded in Great Britain and the USA, and one of its first practical applications was in controlling the spread of TYPHUS FEVER. This disease is transmitted by the louse, one of the insects for which DDT is most toxic. Its toxic action against the mosquito has also been amply proved, and it thus rapidly became one of the most effective measures in controlling MALARIA. DDT is toxic to a large range of insects in addition to the louse and the mosquito; these include houseflies, bed-bugs, clothes-moths, fleas, cockroaches, and ants. It is also active against many agricultural and horticultural pests, including weevils, flour beetles, pine sawfly, and most varieties of scale insect.

DDT has thus had a wide use in medicine, public health, veterinary medicine, horticulture, and agriculture. Unfortunately, the indiscriminate use of DDT is potentially hazardous, and its use is now restricted or banned in several countries, including the United Kingdom.

The danger of DDT is that it enters the bio-logical food chain with the result that animals at the end of the food chain such as birds or predators may build up lethal concentrations of the substance in their tissues.

In any case, an increasing number of species of insects were becoming resistant to DDT. Fortunately, newer insecticides have been introduced which are toxic to DDT-resistant insects, but there are doubts whether this supply of new insecticides can be maintained as insects develop resistance to them.

Dicrotism

A condition in which the PULSE occurs as a beat each time the heart contracts. A dicrotic wave is naturally present in a tracing of any pulse as recorded by an instrument for the purpose, but in health it is imperceptible to the finger. In fevers, a dicrotic pulse is a serious sign in which the heart continues to beat violently while the small blood vessels have lost their tone.

Didanosine

Didanosine (ddI, DDI) is a nucleoside reverse transcriptase inhibitor used to treat progressive or advanced HIV infection (see AIDS/HIV). Preferably it should be given in combination with other antiretroviral drugs. This drug has a range of potentially serious side-effects such as pancreatitis (see PANCREAS, DISEASES OF), peripheral NEUROPATHY, DIABETES MELLITUS and liver failure. Its use requires monitoring and patients taking it should receive counselling.

Dieldrin

An effective insecticide toxic to a wide range of insects. It attacks the insects' nervous system and is more toxic to humans than DDT (see DICHLORODIPHENYL TRICHLOROETHANE), so must therefore be handled with care. Its use in the UK is restricted.

Diencephalon

Part of the forebrain (see BRAIN).

Dienoestrol

A synthetic oestrogen closely related to STILBOESTROL. It is not as potent as stilboestrol, but is less toxic and is used as a cream to treat vaginal dryness.

Diet

The mixture of food and drink consumed by an individual. Variations in morbidity and mortality between population groups are believed to be due, in part, to differences in diet. A balanced diet was traditionally viewed as one which provided at least the minimum requirement of energy, protein, vitamins and minerals needed by the body. However, since nutritional deficiencies are no longer a major problem in developed countries, it seems more appropriate to consider a 'healthy' diet as being one which provides all essential nutrients in sufficient quantities to prevent deficiencies but which also avoids health problems associated with nutrient excesses.

Major diet-related health problems in prosperous communities tend to be the result of dietary excesses, whereas in underdeveloped, poor communities, problems associated with dietary deficiencies predominate. Excessive intakes of dietary energy, saturated fats, sugar, salt and alcohol, together with an inadequate intake of dietary fibre, have been linked to the high prevalence of OBESITY, cardiovascular disease, dental caries, HYPERTENSION, gall-stones (see GALL-BLADDER, DISEASES OF), non-insulin-dependent DIABETES MELLITUS and certain cancers (e.g. of the breast, endometrium, intestine and stomach) seen in developed nations. Health-promotion strategies in these countries generally advocate a reduction in the intake of fat, particularly saturated fat, and salt, the avoidance of excessive intakes of alcohol and simple sugars, an increased consumption of starch and fibre and the avoidance of obesity by taking appropriate physical exercise. A maximum level of dietary cholesterol is sometimes specified.

Undernutrition, including protein-energy malnutrition and specific vitamin and mineral deficiencies, is an important cause of poor health in underdeveloped countries. Priorities here centre on ensuring that the diet provides enough nutrients to maintain health.

In healthy people, dietary requirements depend on age, sex and level of physical activity. Pregnancy and lactation further alter requirements. The presence of infections, fever, burns, fractures and surgery all increase dietary energy and protein requirements and can precipitate undernutrition in previously well-nourished people.

In addition to disease prevention, diet has a role in the treatment of certain clinical disorders, for example, obesity, diabetes mellitus, HYPERLIPIDAEMIA, inborn errors of metabolism, food intolerances and hepatic and renal diseases. Therapeutic diets increase or restrict the amount and/or change the type of fat, carbohydrate, protein, fibre, vitamins, minerals and/or water in the diet according to clinical indications. Additionally, the consistency of the food eaten may need to be

altered. A commercially available or 'homemade' liquid diet can be used to provide all or some of a patient's nutritional needs if necessary. Although the enteral (by mouth) route is the preferred route for feeding and can be used for most patients, parenteral or intravenous feeding is occasionally required in a minority of patients whose gastrointestinal tract is unavailable or unreliable over a period of time.

A wide variety of weight-reducing diets are well publicised. People should adopt them with caution and, if in doubt, seek expert advice.

Dietetics

Dietitians apply dietetics, the science of nutrition, to the feeding of groups and individuals in health and disease. Their training requires a degree course in the nutritional and biological sciences. The role of the dietitian can be divided as follows.

Preventive By liaising with health education departments, schools and various groups in the community. They plan and provide nutrition education programmes including in-service training and the production of educational material in nutrition. They are encouraged to plan and participate in food surveys and research projects which involve the assessment of nutritional status.

Therapeutic Their role is to advise patients who require specific dietary therapy as all or part of their treatment. They teach patients in hospitals to manage their own dietary treatment, and ensure a supportive follow-up so that patients and their families can be seen to be coping with the diet. Therapeutic dietitians further advise catering departments on the adaptation of menus for individual diets and on the nutritional value of the food supplied to patients and staff. They advise social-services departments so that meals-on-wheels provision has adequate nutritional value.

Industry The advice of dietitians is sought by industry in the production of product information literature, data sheets and professional leaflets for manufacturers of ordinary foods and specialist dietetic food. They give advice to the manufacturers on nutritional and dietetic requirements of their products.

Diethylcarbamazine Citrate

A FILARICIDE derived from PIPERAZINE used to

treat FILARIASIS – a group of diseases caused by parasitic worms called nematode filariae.

Dietitian

See DIETETICS.

Differential Diagnosis

A list of the possible diagnoses that might explain a patient's symptoms and signs, and from which the correct DIAGNOSIS will be extracted after further investigations.

Differentiation

The gradual diversification of the STEM CELLS of the early EMBRYO into the specialised cells, tissues and organs that go to make up the fully developed organism.

Digestion

The three processes by which the body incorporates food are digestion, ABSORPTION, and ASSIMILATION. In digestion, food is softened and converted into a form soluble in the watery fluids of the body; or, in the case of fat, into minute globules. The substances formed are then absorbed from the bowels and carried throughout the body by the blood. In assimilation, these substances, deposited from the blood, are used by the various tissues for their growth and repair.

Digoxin

One of a number of drugs known as CARDIAC GLYCOSIDES. They increase the contractility of heart muscle, depress the conducting tissue while increasing myocardial excitability, and increase activity of the VAGUS nerve. Digoxin is usually given orally for the treatment of atrial FIBRILLATION and heart failure. The adverse effects of overdosage (which occur more commonly in people with HYPOKALAEMIA, the elderly, and those with renal failure – see KIDNEYS, DISEASES OF) are vomiting, DYSRHYTHMIA, muscle weakness, and visual disturbances. The ELECTROCARDIOGRAM (ECG) has a characteristic appearance.

Dihydrocodeine

An analgesic drug with similar efficacy to CODEINE.

Dilatation and Curettage

Commonly referred to as D and C, a gynaecological operation to scrape away the lining of the UTERUS (ENDOMETRIUM). The procedure may be used to diagnose and treat heavy bleeding from the womb (ENDOMETRIOSIS) as well as other uterine disorders. It can be used to terminate a pregnancy or to clean out the uterus after a partial miscarriage. D and C is increasingly being replaced with a LASER technique using a hysteroscope – a type of ENDOSCOPE.

Dilator

(1) A muscle which has the action of increasing the diameter of an organ or vessel.
(2) A drug which usually acts by relaxing smooth muscle to increase the diameter of blood vessels, the bronchial tree, or other organs.
(3) An instrument used to increase the diameter of an orifice or organ, either to treat a stricture or to allow surgical access.

Diltiazem

One of the CALCIUM-CHANNEL BLOCKERS, effective in most types of ANGINA; however, it should not be given to patients with heart failure. A longer-acting version of the drug can be used in HYPERTENSION.

Diluents

Diluents are watery fluids of a non-irritating nature, which are given to increase the amount of perspiration or of urine, and carry solids with them from the system. Examples are water, milk, barley-water, and solutions of alkaline salts.

Dimenhydrinate

Dimenhydrinate, or dramamine, is an antihistamine drug, obtainable without prescription, to prevent and treat travel sickness.

Dimercaprol

Also called British Anti-Lewisite (BAL), this is a chelating agent used in the treatment of metal poisoning (e.g. arsenic, lead, mercury). It has a high incidence of side-effects and is now only rarely used as it has been superseded by less toxic chelating agents.

Dioctyl Sodium Sulphosuccinate

See DOCUSATE SODIUM.

Diodone

A complex, radio-opaque, organic, iodine-containing preparation, used for contrast radiography of parts of the body – in particular, the urinary tract (see PYELOGRAPHY).

Dioptre

A term used in the measurement of the refractive or focusing power of lenses; one dioptre is the power of a lens with a focal distance of one metre and is the unit of refractive power. As a stronger lens has a greater refractive power, this means that the focal distance will be shorter. The strength in dioptres therefore is the reciprocal of the focal length expressed in metres.

Diphenhydramine

A widely used antihistamine (see ANTI-HISTAMINE DRUGS) with sedative effects.

Diphenoxylate

Also known as cophentrope or Lomotil®. When mixed with ATROPINE sulphate, it is used as tretament for adult patients with DIAR-RHOEA, particularly if chronic. It has no anti-bacterial properties but is sometimes used to treat traveller's diarrhoea.

Diphtheria

Diphtheria is an acute infectious disease of the respiratory tract. Rarely seen in the UK since the introduction of inoculation in 1940, it is still an important cause of disease in many parts of the world. The infection is caused by the *Corynebacterium diphtheriae* and is spread by water droplets. It usually presents with a sore throat, and there is a slightly raised membrane on the tonsils surrounded by an inflammatory zone. There may be some swelling of the neck and lymph nodes, though the patient's temperature is seldom much raised. Occasionally the disease occurs in the eye or genital tract, or it may complicate lesions of the skin. More serious consequences follow the absorption of TOXINS which damage the heart muscle and the nervous system.

Treatment Provided that the patient is not allergic to horse serum, an injection of the antitoxin is given immediately. A one-week course of penicillin is started (or erythromycin if the patient is allergic to penicillin). Diphtheria may cause temporary muscle weakness or paralysis, which should resolve without special treatment; if the respiratory muscles are involved, however, artificial respiration may be necessary.

All infants should be immunised against diphtheria; for details see table under IMMUNISATION.

Diplegia

Extensive PARALYSIS on both sides of the body but affecting the legs more than the arms.

Diplo-

A prefix meaning twofold.

Diplococcus

A group of spherical bacterial organisms which usually occur in pairs: for example, pneumo-cocci. (See BACTERIA.)

Diploë

The layer of spongy bone which intervenes between the compact outer and inner tables of the skull.

Diploid

An adjective describing cells, nuclei or organisms in which every chromosome – apart from the Y sex one – is represented twice.

Diplopia

Double vision. It is due to some irregularity in action of the muscles which move the eyeballs, in consequence of which the eyes are placed so that rays of light from one object do not fall upon corresponding parts of the two retinae, and two images are produced. It is a symptom of several nervous diseases, and often a temporary attack follows an injury to the eye, intoxication, or some febrile disease like DIPHTHERIA.

Diprosopus

The term applied to a FETUS which has two faces instead of one.

Dipsomania

A morbid and insatiable craving for ALCOHOL.

Dipygus

A FETUS with a double PELVIS.

Disability

An observable mental or physical loss or impairment which is measurable and which may be permanent or temporary. If the disability is serious enough to affect a person's normal function adversely, it is described as a handicap.

Disabled Persons

Disabled persons in the United Kingdom have a range of services and financial support available to help them to lead as normal and active a life as possible. Officially, the disabled include those with significant impairment of any kind, including impairment of sight and hearing, learning difficulties, and chronic illness as well as disablement due to accidents and the like.

Social services are provided by local-authority social-services departments. They include: practical help in the home (usually through home helps or aids to daily living); assistance in taking advantage of available educational facilities; help with adaptations to the disabled person's house; provision of meals ('Meals on Wheels' or luncheon centres); and help in obtaining a telephone. Many of these facilities will involve the disabled person in some expense, but full details can be obtained from the local social-services department which will, if necessary, send a social worker to discuss the matter in the disabled person's home. Owing to lack of funds and staff, many local-authority social-services departments are unable to provide the full range of services.

Aids to daily living There is now a wide range of aids for the disabled. Full details and addresses of local offices can be obtained from: Disabled Living Foundation and British Red Cross.

Aids to mobility and transport Some car manufacturers make specially equipped or adapted cars, and some have official systems for discounts. Details can be obtained from local dealers. Help can also be obtained from Motability, which provides advice.

Disarticulation
The amputation of a bone by cutting through the joint of which the bone forms a part.

Disc
An anatomical term describing a rounded flattened structure. Examples are the cartilagenous disc positioned between two vertebrae (see SPINAL COLUMN) and the optic disc (see EYE).

Discharge
Abnormal emission or emissions from any part of the body. It usually applies to purulent material – for example, the septic material which comes away from an infected ear, or nose – but can be the result of excess secretions from the mucous linings of the vagina or rectum.

Discission
The term applied to an operation for destroying a structure by tearing it without removal: for example, the operation of needling the lens of the eye for cataract (see EYE, DISORDERS OF).

Discoid Lupus Erythematosus (DLE)
See under LUPUS.

Disease
Any abnormality of bodily structure or func-

tion, other than those arising directly from physical injury.

Disinfectants
Substances that destroy micro-organisms, thus preventing them from causing infections. The name is usually applied to powerful chemicals that are also capable of destroying tissue and so are used only to sterilise inanimate surfaces. ANTISEPTICS are used to cleanse living tissues.

Disinfection
Processes by which vegetative organisms, excluding spores, are killed in order to prevent the items disinfected from passing on infection. Equipment, bedlinen and hard surfaces may all be disinfected – the method chosen will depend on the material and size of the object. One of the most important procedures in preventing the spread of infection is the careful washing of hands before handling equipment and between treating different patients. STERILISATION is different from disinfection in that the methods used kill all living organisms and spores.

Methods of disinfection (1) Skin, wounds, etc. – chlorhexidine (with detergent or spirit); iodine (with detergent or spirit); cetrimide; ethyl alcohol; all must stay in contact with the skin for long enough for bacteria to be killed. (2) Hard surfaces (floors, walls, etc.) – hypochlorites (i.e. bleaches) with or without detergent; cetrimide; iodine-containing solutions; ethyl alcohol. (3) Equipment – wet or dry heat (e.g. boiling for more than 5 minutes); submersion in liquid disinfectants for the appropriate time (e.g. glutaraldehyde 2·5 per cent), chlorhexidine in spirit 70 per cent, formaldehyde (irritant), chlorhexidine (0·1 per cent aqueous), hypochlorites.

Disinfestation
The destruction of insect pests, especially lice, whether on the person or in dwelling-places.

Dislocations
Injuries to joints of such a nature that the ends of the opposed bones are forced more or less out of connection with one another. Besides displacement of the bones, there is bruising of the tissues around them, and tearing of the ligaments which bind the bones together.

Dislocations, like fractures (see BONE, DISORDERS OF), are divided into simple and compound, the bone in the latter case being forced through the skin. This seldom occurs, since the round head of the bone has not the same power to wound as the sharp end of a broken bone. Dislocations are also divided according to whether they are (1) congenital, i.e. present at birth in consequence of some malformation, or (2) acquired at a later period in consequence of injury, the great majority falling into the latter class. The reduction of a dislocated joint is a skilled procedure and should be done by an appropriately trained professional.

Disodium Cromoglycate

A drug used in the prophylactic (preventive) treatment of allergic disorders (see ALLERGY), particularly ASTHMA, conjunctivitis (see EYE, DISORDERS OF), nasal allergies, and food allergies – especially in children. Although inappropriate for the treatment of acute attacks of asthma, regular inhalations of the drug can reduce its incidence, and allow the dose of BRONCHODILATORS and oral CORTICO-STEROIDS to be cut.

Disopyramide

One of the ANTIARRHYTHMIC DRUGS given by intravenous injection after myocardial infarction to restore supraventricular and ventricular arrhythmias to normal, particularly when patients have not responded to lidocaine (lignocaine). It can impair the contractility of heart muscle and it does have an antimuscarinic effect (see ANTIMUSCARINE); consequently its administration has to be undertaken with care, especially in patients with GLAUCOMA or enlargement.

Disorientation

Orientation in a clinical sense includes a person's awareness of time and place in relation to him- or herself and others, the recognition of personal friends and familiar places, and the ability to remember at least some past experience and to register new data. It is therefore dependent on the ability to recall all learned memories and make effective use of memory. Disorientation can be the presenting feature of both DELIRIUM (confusion) and DEMENTIA; delirium is reversible, developing dramatically and accompanied by evidence of systemic disease, while dementia is a gradually evolving, irreversible condition.

Displacement

A term used in psychological medicine to describe the mental process of attaching to one object, painful emotions associated with another object.

Dyspraxia

See APRAXIA.

Dissection

(1) The cutting of tissue to separate the structural components for identification or removal during an operation or the study of anatomy. (2) Dissection of an artery involves tearing of the inner part of the wall, allowing blood to track through the media occluding the origins of smaller arteries and often leading to vessel rupture (see also ARTERIES).

Disseminated

Spread of disease from its original site throughout an organ or the body. Often used to describe the spread of CANCER.

Disseminated Sclerosis

See MULTIPLE SCLEROSIS (MS).

Dissociation

A psychiatric term describing the process whereby an individual separates his or her ideas and thoughts from consciousness, thus allowing them to function independently. The result may be that the individual holds contrary views on the same subject.

Dissociative Disorder

A collection of psychological disorders in which a particular mental function becomes cut off from a person's mind. Hysterical AMNESIA is one example, when the person forgets his or her personal history but can still absorb and talk about new events. Other examples are FUGUE, depersonalisation (detachment from self and environment), and MULTIPLE PERSONALITY DISORDER.

Distal

An adjective applied to a body part that is further away from another part, with reference, for example, to the trunk.

Distichiasis

Distichiasis is the term applied to the condition in which there are two complete rows of eyelashes in one eyelid (or in both).

Distoma

Distoma is a general term including various forms of trematodes, or fluke-worms, parasitic in the intestine, lung and other organs.

Disulfiram

Disulfiram is used as an adjunct in the treatment of alcoholism. It is relatively non-toxic by itself, but when taken in conjunction with alcohol it produces most unpleasant effects: for example, flushing of the face, palpitations, a sense of oppression and distress, and ultimately sickness and vomiting. The rationale of treatment therefore is to give the alcoholic subject a course of disulfiram and then demonstrate, by letting him or her take some alcoholic liquor, how unpleasant are the effects. If the patient is co-operative, the treatment may be effective, but there is some risk so it must be given under skilled medical supervision.

Disuse Atrophy
The wasting of muscles after prolonged immobility. This can be seen after lengthy immobilisation in a plaster cast, and is particularly severe following paralysis of a limb through nerve injury. (See ATROPHY.)

Dithranol
A drug used to treat PSORIASIS. It is usually very effective, being applied normally for short contact periods of up to 1 hour. Dithranol can cause severe skin irritation so must be used with care and at appropriate concentrations. Hands should be thoroughly washed after use.

Diuresis
An increase in the production of urine. This may result from increased fluid intake, decreased levels of antidiuretic hormone, renal disease, or the use of drugs (see DIURETICS).

Diuretics
Substances which increase urine and solute production by the KIDNEYS. They are used in the treatment of heart failure, HYPERTENSION, and sometimes for ASCITES secondary to liver failure. They may work by extra-renal or renal mechanisms.

The potential side-effects of diuretics are HYPOKALAEMIA, DEHYDRATION, and GOUT (in susceptible individuals).

Extra-renal mechanisms (*a*) Inhibiting release of antidiuretic hormone (e.g. water, alcohol); (*b*) increased renal blood flow (e.g. dopamine in renal doses).

Renal mechanisms (*a*) Osmotic diuretics act by 'holding' water in the renal tubules and preventing its reabsorption (e.g. mannitol); (*b*) loop diuretics prevent sodium, and therefore water, reabsorption (e.g. FRUSEMIDE); (*c*) drugs acting on the cortical segment of the Loop of Henle prevent sodium reabsorption, but are 'weaker' than loop diuretics (e.g. THIAZIDES);

(*d*) drugs acting on the distal tubule prevent sodium reabsorption by retaining potassium (e.g. spironalactone).

Diverticular Disease
The presence of numerous diverticula (sacs or pouches) in the lining of the COLON accompanied by spasmodic lower abdominal pain and erratic bowel movements. The sacs may become inflamed causing pain (see DIVERTICULITIS).

Diverticulitis
Inflammation of diverticula (see DIVERTICULUM) in the large intestine. It is characterised by pain in the left lower side of the abdomen, which has been aptly described as 'left-sided appendicitis' as it resembles the pain of appendicitis but occurs in the opposite side of the abdomen. The onset is often sudden, with fever and constipation. It may, or may not, be preceded by DIVERTICULOSIS. Treatment consists of rest, no solid food but ample fluid, and the administration of tetracycline. Complications are unusual but include ABSCESS formation, perforation of the colon, and severe bleeding.

Diverticulosis
The presence of diverticula (see DIVERTICULUM) or sacs in the large intestine. Such diverticula are not uncommon over the age of 40, increasing with age until over the age of 70 they may be present in one-third to one-half of the population. They mostly occur in the lower part of the COLON, and are predominantly due to muscular hyperactivity of the bowel forcing the lining of the bowel through weak points in the bowel wall, just as the inner tube of a pneumatic tyre bulges through a defective tyre. There is increasing evidence that the low-residue diet of western civilisation is a contributory cause. The condition may or may not produce symptoms. If it does, these consist of disturbance of the normal bowel function and pain in the left side in the lower abdomen. If diverticulosis is causing symptoms, treatment consists of a high-residue diet (see CONSTIPATION) and an AGAR or METHYLCELLULOSE preparation.

Diverticulum
A pouch or pocket leading off a main cavity or tube. The term is especially applied to protrusions from the intestine, which may be present either at the time of birth as a developmental peculiarity, or which develop in numbers upon the large intestine during the course of life.

Dizygotic Twins
Two people born at the same time to the same parents after fertilisation of two separate

oöcytes (see OÖCYTE). They may be of different sexes and are no more likely to resemble each other than any other sibling pairs.

Dizziness

This means different things to different people, so it is important to establish what the individual means by dizziness. It may encompass a feeling of disequilibrium; it may be lightheadedness, faintness, a sensation of swimming or floating, an inbalance or unsteadiness, or episodes of mental confusion. It may be true VERTIGO, which is an hallucination of movement. These symptoms may be due to diseases of the ear, eye, central nervous system, cardiovascular system, or endocrine system, or they may be a manifestation of psychiatric disease. Dizziness is a common symptom in the elderly and by the age of 80, two-thirds of women and one-third of men have suffered from the condition.

DLE

See LUPUS – Discoid lupus erythematosus (DLE).

DMSA

See LEAD POISONING – Treatment.

DNA

DNA is the abbreviation for deoxyribonucleic acid, one of the two types of NUCLEIC ACID that occur in nature. It is the fundamental genetic material of all CELLS, and is present in the nucleus of the cell where it forms part of the CHROMOSOMES and acts as the carrier of genetic information. The molecule is very large, with a molecular weight of several millions, and consists of two single chains of nucleotides (see NUCLEIC ACID) which are twisted round each other to form a double helix (or spiral). The genetic information carried by DNA is encoded along one of these strands. A gene, which represents the genetic information needed to form protein, is a stretch of DNA containing, on average, around 1,000 nucleotides paired in these two strands (see GENES).

To allow it to fulfil its vitally important function as the carrier of genetic information in living cells, DNA has the following properties. It is stable, so that successive generations of species maintain their individual characteristics, but not so stable that evolutionary changes cannot take place. It must be able to store a vast amount of information: for example, an animal cell contains genetic information for the synthesis of over a million proteins. It must be duplicated exactly before each cell division to ensure that both daughter cells contain an accurate copy of the genetic information of the parent cells (see GENETIC CODE).

DNR

An acronym for 'do not resuscitate' – advice sometimes written on a patient's hospital notes to indicate that if he or she suffers, say, a life-threatening complication (such as a CARDIAC ARREST) to an existing serious illness, the patient should not be given emergency life-saving treatment. The use of DNR is an emotive and controversial issue, even if the patient (or the relatives), when a serious illness such as spreading cancer is concerned, may have indicated a wish not to be resuscitated in the event of organ failures. (See ETHICS.)

Dobutamine

A cardiac stimulant drug of the inotropic sympathomimetic group (see SYMPATHOMIMETIC DRUGS), dobutamine acts on sympathetic receptors in cardiac muscle, increasing the contractility and hence improving the cardiac output but with little effect on the cardiac rate. It is particularly useful in cardiogenic shock. It must be given by intravenous infusion. (See also HEART.)

Docetaxel

A member of the group of antitumour drugs known as TAXANES, docetaxel is used to treat advanced or metastatic cancer arising in the breast (see BREASTS, DISEASES OF). It is also used to treat non-small cancer of the LUNGS. The NATIONAL INSTITUTE FOR CLINICAL EXCELLENCE (NICE) has recommended that both docetaxel and PACLITAXEL should be available for the treatment of advanced breast cancer where initial anticancer CHEMOTHERAPY (including one of the ANTHRACYCLINES) has failed or is inappropriate.

Doctor

The academic title granted to someone who has a university degree higher than a master's degree. Some UK universities grant a medical doctorate (MD) for a research thesis of approved standard. In Britain, 'doctor' is also the title given to a qualified medical practitioner registered by the General Medical Council, usually after he or she has obtained a bachelor's degree or a diploma in medicine and surgery. In the UK a doctor has to spend a year of supervised practice in a recognised hospital post before he or she is registered as fully qualified, but specialists have to obtain further training and higher qualifications before they can be accredited and therefore practise as specialists in the NHS. General practitioners must complete a three-year vocational training course before practising as an independent GP. In Britain, surgical specialists are customarily addressed as 'Mr'. Other countries have different regulations.

Docusate Sodium
A faecal-softening agent used to treat constipation in old people. It can be given orally or as a rectal suppository.

Dog Bites
See BITES AND STINGS; RABIES.

Dolichocephalic
Dolichocephalic means long-headed, and is a term applied to skulls the breadth of which is less than four-fifths of the length.

Dominant Gene
See GENETIC DISORDERS.

Donepezil
A drug used for the symptomatic treatment of mild to moderate DEMENTIA only in ALZHEIMER'S DISEASE. Around four in ten patients may benefit by a reduction in the rate of cognitive and non-cognitive deterioration.

Donor Insemination
Use of the SEMEN of an anonymous donor to produce fertilisation in cases of INFERTILITY where the male partner has OLIGOSPERMIA or IMPOTENCE. The donor is chosen for ethnic and physiognomic similarity to the male partner and is screened for transmissible diseases (e.g. HIV, syphilis, hepatitis, gonorrhoea, and genetic disorders). Insemination is performed at the time of ovulation by introducing the semen into the upper vagina. Semen may be fresh or have been stored frozen in liquid nitrogen. (See ARTIFICIAL INSEMINATION.)

Donors
People who donate parts of their bodies for use in other people. Many organs and tissues can be donated – most commonly blood, but skin, corneas, kidneys, livers and hearts can all be used. Combined heart and lung transplants are being increasingly used for patients with severe lung diseases, and, if the recipients have a condition such as CYSTIC FIBROSIS in which the heart is normal, it is sometimes possible for them to receive a heart and lungs from one donor and to donate their own heart to someone else. Recent work has explored the possibility of using pancreatic transplants. Apart from blood, it is unusual for tissue to be taken from living donors. Skin, small pieces of liver, and a kidney can, in theory, be obtained from living donors, but the ETHICS of this are hotly debated and the situations under which it may be done are tightly controlled. Because transplanted organs are seen by the receiving body as 'foreign bodies', careful matching before transplantation is necessary to avoid rejection, and immunosuppressive drugs may be required for some time after the operation to prevent this from occurring.

There are strict regulations about how death should be diagnosed before organs can be removed for transplantation, and potential donors must satisfy the BRAIN-STEM DEATH criteria, performed twice by two doctors who are independent of the transplant team. There is a great shortage of suitable organs for donation – partly because they must be in excellent condition if the operation is to be a success. Some medical conditions or modes of death make people unsuitable as organ donors; this makes it all the more important that people should be encouraged to donate their organs. People who wish to do so can carry a special card indicating their willingness to become donors in the event of their death. These cards can be obtained from various sources, including hospitals, GPs' surgeries and many public buildings such as libraries. In the UK, informed positive approval from the patient, or relatives, is required.

Information about becoming a blood donor can be obtained by telephoning 0845–7 711 711. Those who wish to bequeath their bodies for dissection purposes should get in touch with HM Inspector of Anatomy. Other would-be organ donors may contact the British Organ Donor Society.

Dopa
A precursor of DOPAMINE and NORADRENALINE. Levodopa is a drug used in the treatment of PARKINSONISM. It can cross the blood–brain barrier and increase the concentration of dopamine in the basal ganglia. It also inhibits prolactin secretion and may be used to treat GALACTORRHEA.

Dopamine
Dopamine is one of the CATECHOLAMINES and a precursor of NORADRENALINE. Its highest concentration is in that portion of the brain known as the basal nuclei (see BRAIN) where its function is to convey inhibitory influences to the extrapyramidal system. There is good evidence that dopamine deficiency is one of the causative factors in PARKINSONISM.

Dopamine is given by intravenous infusion

as treatment for cardiogenic shock in cardiac infarction or cardiac surgery.

Dorsal Root Ganglia

These are swellings on the dorsal roots of spinal nerves just proximal to the union of the dorsal and ventral nerve roots. They are situated in the inter-vertebral foramina and contain the cell bodies of sensory neurones. (See SPINAL COLUMN; SPINAL CORD.)

Dorsum

(Adjective: dorsal.) The back or posterior part of an organ or structure. The dorsum of the hand is the opposite surface to the palm.

Dorzolamide

A carbonic anhydrase-inhibitor drug restricted to use in patients with raised intraocular pressure in ocular hypertension or open-angle GLAUCOMA. It can be used alone or as an adjunct to a topical beta blocker (see BETA-ADRENOCEPTOR-BLOCKING DRUGS).

Dosage

Many factors influence the activity with which drugs operate. Among the factors which affect the necessary quantity are age, weight, sex, idiosyncrasy, genetic disorders, habitual use, disease, fasting, combination with other drugs, the form in which the drug is given, and the route by which it is given.

Normally, a young child requires a smaller dose than an adult. There are, however, other factors than age to be taken into consideration. Thus, children are more susceptible than adults to some drugs such as MORPHINE, whilst they are less sensitive to others such as ATROPINE. The only correct way to calculate a child's dose is by reference to texts supplying a recommended dose in milligrams per kilogram. However, many reference texts simply quote doses for certain age-ranges.

Old people, too, often show an increased susceptibility to drugs. This is probably due to a variety of factors, such as decreased weight; diminished activity of the tissues and therefore diminished rate at which a drug is utilised; and diminished activity of the KIDNEYS resulting in decreased rate of excretion of the drug.

Weight and sex have both to be taken into consideration. Women require slightly smaller doses than men, probably because they tend to be lighter in weight. The effect of weight on dosage is partly dependent on the fact that much of the extra weight of a heavy individual is made up of fatty tissue which is not as active

as other tissues of the body. In practice, the question of weight seldom makes much difference unless the individual is grossly over- or underweight.

Idiosyncrasy occasionally causes drugs administered in the ordinary dose to produce unexpected effects. Thus, some people are but little affected by some drugs, whilst in others, certain drugs – for example, psychoactive preparations such as sedatives – produce excessive symptoms in normal or even small doses. In some cases this may be due to hypersensitivity, or an allergic reaction, to the drug, which is a possibility that must always be borne in mind (e.g. with PENICILLIN). An individual who is known to be allergic to a certain medication is strongly advised to carry a card to this effect, and always to inform medical and dental practitioners and/or a pharmacist before accepting a new prescription or buying an over-the-counter preparation.

Habitual use of a drug is perhaps the influence that causes the greatest increase in the dose necessary to produce the requisite effect. The classical example of this is with OPIUM and its derivatives.

Disease may modify the dose of medicines. This can occur in several ways. Thus, in serious illnesses the patient may be more susceptible to drugs, such as narcotics, that depress tissue activity, and therefore smaller doses must be given. Again, absorption of the drug from the gut may be slowed up by disease of the gut, or its effect may be enhanced if there is disease of the kidneys, interfering with the excretion of the drug.

Fasting aids the rapidity of absorption of drugs, and also makes the body more susceptible to their action. Partly for this reason, as well as to avoid irritation of the stomach, it is usual to prescribe drugs to be taken after meals, and diluted with water.

Combination of drugs is to be avoided if possible as it is often difficult to assess what their combined effect may be. In some cases they may have a mutually antagonistic effect, which means that the patient will not obtain full benefit. Sometimes a combination may have a deleterious effect.

Form, route and frequency of administration Drugs are now produced in many forms, though tablets are the most common and, usually, convenient. In Britain, medicines are given by mouth whenever possible, unless there is some degree of urgency, or because the drug is either destroyed in, or is not absorbed from, the gut. In these circumstances, it is given intravenously, intra-muscularly or subcutaneously. In some cases, as in cases of ASTHMA or BRONCHITIS, the drug may be given in the form of an inhalant (see INHALANTS), in order to get the maximum concentration at the point where it is wanted: that is, in the lungs. If a local effect is wanted, as in cases of diseases of the skin, the drug is applied topically to the skin. In some countries there is a tendency to give medicines in the form of a suppository which is inserted in the rectum.

Recent years have seen developments whereby the assimilation of drugs into the body can be more carefully controlled. These include, for example, what are known as transdermals, in which drugs are built into a plaster that is stuck on the skin, and the drug is then absorbed into the body at a controlled rate. This method is now being used for the administration of GLYCERYL TRINITRATE in the treatment of ANGINA PECTORIS, and of hyoscine hydrobromide in the treatment of MOTION (TRAVEL) SICKNESS. Another is a new class of implantable devices. These are tiny polymers infused with a drug and implanted just under the skin by injection. They can be tailored so as to deliver drugs at virtually any rate – from minutes to years. A modification of these polymers now being investigated is the incorporation of magnetic particles which allow an extra burst of the incorporated drug to be released in response to an oscillating magnetic field which is induced by a magnetic 'watch' worn by the patient. In this way the patient can switch on an extra dose of drug when this is needed: insulin, for instance, in the case of diabetics. In yet another new development, a core of drug is enclosed in a semi-permeable membrane and is released in the stomach at a given rate. (See also LIPOSOMES.)

Dothiepin

A drug used in the treatment of depression, particularly when the patient needs sedation. (See ANTIDEPRESSANT DRUGS.)

Double Blind Trial

A scientific study in which different patients receive a different drug, the same drug at a different dose, or a placebo – with neither the investigators assessing the outcome nor the subjects being treated knowing which of these the latter are receiving. The aim is to remove any hint of bias due to the investigators' or patients' preferences or preconceptions. The results are analysed after all the data have been collected and the code has been broken. Trials should have a separate supervising committee, the members of which know the code but do not take part in the study. Their job is to check the results at intervals so they can stop the trial if one arm of treatment is clearly better than another. Otherwise, it would be unethical to continue. (See INTERVENTION STUDY.)

Double Vision

See SQUINT.

Douche

An application to the body of a jet of fluid via a pipe or tube. It may be used to clean any part of the body but is used most commonly with reference to the vagina (although used as a method of contraception it is ineffective).

Down's (Down) Syndrome

A genetic disorder in which the affected person usually carries an extra chromosome – 47 instead of the usual 46. The extra chromosome occurs in the no. 21 group, hence the disorder is described as trisomy 21. The condition was named after Dr J L H Down, the London doctor who first described it in 1866. The incidence is around one in 600 births. The disorder is characterised by a particular physical appearance and learning difficulties, with the affected individuals having an INTELLIGENCE QUOTIENT (IQ) ranging from 30 to 80 (normal is 100). Most people with the syndrome have eyes that slope up at the outer corners with skin folds that cover the inner ones. The face and features are smaller than normal, while the tongue is larger; the back of the head is flattened and the hands are usually short and broad. The facial features led to the syndrome being described as 'mongolism', a term that is no longer used.

Children with Down's syndrome are usually friendly and fit in well with the family. Despite their learning disabilities, some learn to read and, if they have appropriate educational and environmental stimulation, can make the most of their abilities.

A heart defect is present in around 25 per cent of the children at birth, and deafness and acute LEUKAEMIA occur more frequently than in unaffected youngsters. Those with the syndrome are particularly prone to developing ear infections. ATHEROSCLEROSIS often develops early in adults and ALZHEIMER'S DISEASE tends to occur as early as 40 years of age. A friendly home environment helps them to enjoy life, but a few individuals with the syndrome may eventually require institutional care. Improved social and medical care means that many now live until their 60s.

Routine screening tests early in pregnancy, starting with blood analysis but going on if necessary to AMNIOCENTESIS and chorionic villus sampling (see PRENATAL SCREENING OR DIAGNOSIS), can identify fetuses likely to develop the disorder. If a sample of fetal cells confirms the chromosome defect (triple marker test – see PREGNANCY AND LABOUR), the parents may consider termination of the pregnancy. In the UK, screening is normally offered to women over 35 because of their increased risk. When younger parents have a child with Down's syndrome, the chances of a subsequent child with the disorder are relatively high as it is probable that both parents carry a chromosome abnormality insufficient to cause ill-health until combined. So they may wish to discuss with their medical advisers the question of further pregnancies.

Parents who have a child with Down's syndrome will understandably feel a combination of strong emotions, including anger and guilt, and constructive counselling can be valuable. Among societies offering advice and support is the Down's Syndrome Association.

Doxorubicin

A successful and widely used antitumour drug. It is used in the treatment of acute LEUKAEMIA, LYMPHOMA, and various forms of sarcoma and CANCER, including cancer of the bladder. (See CYTOTOXIC.)

Doxycycline

A wide-spectrum, long-acting antibiotic which is active against a range of micro-organisms, including the causative organisms of scrub typhus (see under TYPHUS FEVER), TRACHOMA, PSITTACOSIS, LYME DISEASE and some influenzas.

DPT Vaccine

Often called the TRIPLE VACCINE, the injections produce immunity against DIPHTHERIA, whooping cough (PERTUSSIS) and TETANUS. The vaccine is given as a course of three injections to infants around the ages of two, three and four months, together with haemophilus influenza B and meningococcal C vaccine as well as oral polio vaccine. A booster injection is given at school entry (see schedule in IMMUNISATION).

Dracontiasis

Dracontiasis, or dracunculiasis, is a nematode infection caused by *Dracunculus medinensis*

(guinea-worm). The major clinical problem is secondary infection of the worm track, causing CELLULITIS, SYNOVITIS, epididymo-ORCHITIS, periarticular FIBROSIS, and ARTHRITIS; TETANUS is a potentially lethal complication. CHEMO-THERAPY is unsatisfactory and the time-honoured method of extracting the female adult by winding it around a matchstick remains in use. Surgical treatment may be necessary. Ultimate prevention consists of removing *Cyclops* spp. from drinking water.

Dracunculiasis

See DRACONTIASIS.

Dramamine

See DIMENHYDRINATE.

Draught

A draught is a small mixture intended to be taken at one dose. It consists generally of two or four tablespoonfuls of fluid.

Dreams

See SLEEP.

Drepanocytosis

Another term for sickle-cell anaemia (see ANAEMIA), which is characterised by the presence in the blood of red blood corpuscles that are sickle-like in shape. The anaemia is a severe one and afflicts black people and to a lesser extent people of Mediterranean background.

Dressings

See WOUNDS.

Drop Attack

A brief episode affecting the nervous system that causes the person to fall suddenly. There is no loss of consciousness. The loss of tone in the muscles, responsible for the fall, may persist for several hours; in such cases moving the patient or applying pressure to the soles of the feet may restore muscle tone. In most cases, however, recovery is immediate. The cause is probably a temporary interference with the blood supply to the brain. In others there may be some disturbance of the vestibular apparatus which controls the balance of the body. (See EAR, DISEASES OF; TRANSIENT ISCHAEMIC ATTACKS OR EPISODES (TIA, TIE).)

Drop Foot

This is the inability to dorsiflex the foot at the ankle. The foot hangs down and has to be swung clear of the ground while walking. It is commonly caused by damage to the lateral popliteal nerve or the peroneal muscles.

Drop Wrist
This is the inability to extend the hand at the wrist. It is usually due to damage to the radial nerve which supplies the extensor muscles.

Drowning
See APPENDIX 1: BASIC FIRST AID.

Drug Absorption
Drugs are usually administered distant to their site of action in the body; they must then pass across cell membranes to reach their site of action. For example, drugs given by mouth must pass across the gut membrane to enter the bloodstream and then pass through the endothelium of vessel walls to reach the site of action in the tissues. This process is called absorption and may depend on lipid diffusion, aqueous diffusion, active transport, or pinocytosis – a process in which a cell takes in small droplets of fluid by cytoplasmic engulfment.

Drug Addiction
See DEPENDENCE.

Drug Assisted Rape
Also known as 'date rape', this is an unwelcome phenomenon in which an intending rapist undermines a potential victim's resistance by giving her a hypnotic drug such as benzodiazepine. The *British National Formulary* warns that flunitrazepam (Rohypnol®) tablets may be particularly subject to abuse – perhaps given to the unsuspecting victim in an alcoholic drink so the sedative effect is greatly enhanced.

Drug Binding
The process of attachment of a drug to a receptor or plasma protein, fat, mucopolysaccharide or other tissue component. This process may be reversible or irreversible.

Drug Clearance
The volume of blood from which a drug is completely removed in one minute is known as clearance. Renal clearance of a drug is the amount of blood completely cleared of the drug by the kidney in one minute.

Drug Interactions
Many patients are on several prescribed drugs, and numerous medicines are available over the counter, so the potential for drug interaction is large. A drug may interact with another by inhibiting its action, potentiating its action, or by simple summation of effects.

The interaction may take place:

(1) Prior to absorption or administration – for example, antacids bind tetracycline in the gut and prevent absorption.

(2) By interfering with protein binding – one drug may displace another from binding sites on plasma proteins. The action of the displaced drug will be increased because more drug is now available; for example, anticoagulants are displaced by analgesics.

(3) During metabolism or excretion of the drug – some drugs increase or decrease the activity of liver enzymes which metabolise drugs, thus affecting their rate of destruction; for example, barbiturates, nicotine, and alcohol all activate hepatic enzymes. Altering the pH of urine will affect the excretion of drugs via the kidney.

(4) At the drug receptor – one drug may displace another at the receptor, affecting its efficacy or duration of action.

Drug Metabolism
A process by which the body destroys and excretes drugs, so limiting their duration of action. Phase 1 metabolism consists of transformation by oxidation, reduction, or hydrolysis. In phase 2 this transformed product is conjugated (joined up) with another molecule to produce a water-soluble product which is easier to excrete.

Drugs
These are natural products or synthetic chemicals that can alter the way in which the body works, or be used to prevent or treat disease. One or more drugs, combined with stabilisers, colourings, and other ingredients, make(s) up a medicine for practical use in treating patients. (See DEPENDENCE; MEDICINES.) In Britain, the supply of drugs is controlled by the Medicines Act. Some drugs are available only on prescription; some both on prescription and over the counter; and some are not available on NHS prescription. When enquiring about drugs that a patient is taking, it is essential to ask about all items bought over the counter and any herbal or traditional remedies that might be used, as these can interact with other prescribed drugs (see DRUG INTERACTIONS) or affect the patient's presenting complaints. Each drug has a single generic name, but many will also have several proprietary (brand) names. It is often much cheaper to prescribe the generic form of a drug, and many doctors do so. Many hospitals and general practices in the United Kingdom now

provide a list of suggested drugs for doctors to prescribe. If a doctor wishes to use a drug not on the list, he or she must give a valid reason.

Prescriptions for drugs should be printed or written clearly in ink and signed and dated by the prescriber (computer-generated facsimile signatures do not meet legal requirements). They should include the patient's name, address and age (obligatory for children under 12), the name of the drug to be supplied, the dose and dose frequency, and the total quantity to be supplied. Any special instructions (e.g. 'after food') should be stated. There are special regulations about the prescription of drugs controlled under the Misuse of Drugs Regulations 1985 (see CONTROLLED DRUGS). A pharmacist can advise about which drugs are available without prescription, and is able to recommend treatment for many minor complaints. Information about exemption from prescription charges in the NHS can be obtained from health visitors, general practitioners, or social security offices.

Drugs in Pregnancy

Unnecessary drugs during pregnancy should be avoided because of the adverse effect of some drugs on the fetus which have no harmful effect on the mother. Drugs may pass through the PLACENTA and damage the fetus because their pharmacological effects are enhanced as the enzyme systems responsible for their degradation are undeveloped in the fetus. Thus, if the drug can pass through the placenta, the pharmacological effect on the fetus may be great whilst that on the mother is minimal. WARFARIN may thus induce fetal and placental haemorrhage and the administration of THIAZIDES may produce THROMBOCYTOPENIA in the newborn. Many progestogens have androgenic side-effects and their administration to a mother for the purpose of preventing recurrent abortion may produce VIRILISATION of the female fetus. Tetracycline administered during the last trimester commonly stains the deciduous teeth of the child yellow.

The other dangers of administering drugs in pregnancy are the teratogenic effects (see TERATOGENESIS). It is understandable that a drug may interfere with a mechanism essential for growth and result in arrested or distorted development of the fetus and yet cause no disturbance in the adult, in whom these differentiation and organisation processes have ceased to be relevant. Thus the effect of a drug upon a fetus may differ qualitatively as well as quantitatively from its effect on the mother. The susceptibility of the embryo will depend on the stage of development it has reached when the drug is given. The stage of early differentiation – that is, from the beginning of the third week to the end of the tenth week of pregnancy – is the time of greatest susceptibility. After this time the risk of congenital malformation from drug treatment is less, although the death of the fetus can occur at any time.

Drunkenness
See ALCOHOL; DEPENDENCE.

Duchenne Muscular Dystrophy
An X-linked recessive disorder (that is, the abnormal gene is carried on the X chromosome). This means that the disease occurs almost exclusively in males, as its presence in a female is counteracted by the normal gene likely to be in her other X chromosome. The disorder is characterised by progressive muscular weakness and wasting. It is the most common form of muscular dystrophy, ocurring in 30 per 100,000 live male births, often – but not always – in families with other members having the disorder.

The disease usually appears within the first three years of life, beginning in the pelvic girdle and lower limbs and later spreading to the shoulder girdle. The calf muscles become bulky (pseudohypertrophy). The weakness gives rise to a characteristic waddling gait and, when rising from the supine position, the child rolls on to his face and then uses his arms to push himself up. Death usually occurs by the middle of the second decade from respiratory infections. Prenatal screening of female carriers using gene probes is increasingly available. (See DYSTROPHY; MUSCLES, DISORDERS OF – Myopathy.)

Duct
The name applied to a passage leading from a gland into some hollow organ, or on to the surface of the body, by which the secretion of the gland is discharged: for example, the pancreatic duct and the bile duct opening into the duodenum, and the sweat ducts opening on the skin surface.

Ductless Gland
Any one of certain glands in the body the secretion of which goes directly into the bloodstream and so is carried to different parts of the body. These glands – the pituitary, thyroid, parathyroid, adrenal and reproductive – are also known as the ENDOCRINE GLANDS. Some glands may be both duct glands and ductless glands. For example, the PANCREAS manu-

factures a digestive juice which passes by a duct into the small intestine. It also manufactures, by means of special cells, a substance called INSULIN which passes straight into the blood.

Ductus Arteriosus

The blood vessel in the fetus through which blood passes from the pulmonary artery to the aorta, thereby bypassing the lungs, which do not function during intra-uterine life. (See CIRCULATORY SYSTEM OF THE BLOOD.) The ductus normally ceases to function soon after birth and within a few weeks is converted into a fibrous cord. Occasionally this obliteration does not occur: a condition known as patent ductus arteriosus. This is one of the more common congenital defects of the heart, and one which responds particularly well to surgical treatment. Closure of the duct can also be achieved in some cases by the administration of indomethacin. (See HEART, DISEASES OF.)

Ductus Deferens

Ductus deferens, or VAS DEFERENS, is the tube which carries spermatozoa from the epididymis to the seminal vesicles. (See TESTICLE.)

Dumbness

See SPEECH DISORDERS.

Dumping Syndrome

A sensation of weakness and sweating after a meal in patients who have undergone GASTRECTOMY. Rapid emptying of the stomach and the drawing of fluid from the blood into the intestine has been blamed, but the exact cause is unclear.

Duodenal Ileus

Dilatation of the DUODENUM due to its chronic obstruction, caused by an abnormal position of arteries in the region of the duodenum pressing on it.

Duodenal Ulcer

This disorder is related to gastric ulcer (see STOMACH, DISEASES OF), both being a form of chronic peptic ulcer. Although becoming less frequent in western communities, peptic ulcers still affect around 10 per cent of the UK population at some time. Duodenal ulcers are 10–15 times more common than gastric ulcers, and occur in people aged from 20 years onwards. The male to female ratio for duodenal ulcer varies between 4:1 and 2:1 in different communities. Social class and blood groups are also influential, with duodenal ulcer being more common among the upper social classes, and those of blood group O.

Causes It is likely that there is some abrasion, or break, in the lining membrane (or mucosa) of the stomach and/or duodenum, and that it is gradually eroded and deepened by the acidic gastric juice. The bacterium helicobacter pylori is present in the antrum of the stomach of people with peptic ulcers; 15 per cent of people infected with the bacterium develop an ulcer, and the ulcers heal if *H. pylori* is eradicated. Thus, this organism has an important role in creating ulcers. Mental stress may possibly be a provocative factor. Smoking seems to accentuate, if not cause, duodenal ulcer, and the drinking of alcohol is probably harmful. The apparent association with a given blood group, and the fact that relatives of a patient with a peptic ulcer are unduly likely to develop such an ulcer, suggest that there is some constitutional factor.

Symptoms and signs Peptic ulcers may present in different ways, but chronic, episodic pain lasting several months or years is most common. Occasionally, however, there may be an acute episode of bleeding or perforation, or obstruction of the gastric outlet, with little previous history. Most commonly there is pain of varying intensity in the middle or upper right part of the abdomen. It tends to occur 2–3 hours after a meal, most commonly at night, and is relieved by some food such as a glass of milk; untreated it may last up to an hour. Vomiting is unusual, but there is often tenderness and stiffness ('guarding') of the abdominal muscles. Confirmation of the diagnosis is made by radiological examination ('barium meal'), the ulcer appearing as a niche on the film, or by looking at the ulcer directly with an endoscope (see FIBREOPTIC ENDOSCOPY). Chief complications are perforation of the ulcer, leading to the vomiting of blood, or HAEMATEMESIS; or less severe bleeding from the ulcer, the blood passing down the gut, resulting in dark, tarry stools (see MELAENA).

Treatment of a perforation involves initial management of any complications, such as shock, haemorrhage, perforation, or gastric outlet obstruction, usually involving surgery and blood replacement. Medical treatment of a chronic ulcer should include regular meals, and the avoidance of fatty foods, strong tea or coffee and alcohol. Patients should also stop smoking and try to reduce the stress in their lives. ANTACIDS may provide symptomatic relief. However, the mainstay of treatment involves four- to six-week courses with drugs such as CIMETIDINE and RANITIDINE. These are H2 RECEPTOR ANTAGONISTS which heal peptic ulcers by reducing gastric-acid output. Of those relapsing after stopping this treatment, 60–95 per cent have infection with *H. pylori*. A combination of BISMUTH chelate, amoxycillin (see PENICILLIN; ANTIBIOTICS) and METRONIDAZOLE – 'triple regime' – should eliminate the infection: most physicians advise the triple regime as first-choice treatment because it is more likely to eradicate *Helicobacter* and this, in turn, enhances healing of the ulcer or prevents recurrence. Surgery may be necessary if medical measures fail, but its use is much rarer than before effective medical treatments were developed.

Duodenum
The first part of the INTESTINE immediately beyond the stomach, so-named because its length is about 12 fingerbreadths.

Dupuytren's Contracture
A condition of unknown aetiology in which there is progressive thickening and contracture of the FASCIA in the palm of the hand with adherence of the overlying skin. A clawing deformity of the fingers, particularly the little and ring fingers, develops. It is associated with liver disease, diabetes, epilepsy, and gout. Treatment is surgical to excise the affected fascia. Recurrence is not uncommon.

Dura Mater
The outermost and strongest of the three membranes or meninges which envelop the brain and spinal cord. In it run vessels which nourish the inner surface of the skull. (See BRAIN.)

DVT
See DEEP VEIN THROMBOSIS (DVT).

Dwarfism
Dwarfism, or short stature, refers to underdevelopment of the body. The condition, which has various causes, is not common. All children who by the age of five years are at least what is technically known as 'three standard deviations below the mean' – well below average size for children of that age – should be referred for specialist advice. Among the causes are:
- **genetic**: familial; abnormalities of chromosomes, for example, TURNER'S SYNDROME; abnormal skeletal development; and failure of primary growth.

- **intrauterine growth retardation**: maternal disorders; placental abnormalities; multiple fetuses.
- **constitutional delay in normal growth**.
- **systemic conditions**: nutritional deficiencies; gastrointestinal absorption disorders; certain chronic diseases; psychosocial deprivation; endocrine malfunctions, including HYPOTHYROIDISM, CUSHING'S SYNDROME, RICKETS, dysfunction of the PITUITARY GLAND which produces growth hormone, the endocrine growth controller.

Treatment of short stature is, where possible, to remedy the cause: for example, children with hypothyroidism can be given THYROXINE. Children who are not growing properly should be referred for expert advice to determine the diagnosis and obtain appropriate curative or supportive treatments.

Dynamometer
An elliptical ring of steel to which is attached a dial and moving index. It is used to test the strength of the muscles of the forearm, being squeezed in the hand, and registering the pressure in pounds or kilograms.

Dys-
A prefix meaning difficult or painful.

Dysarthria
A general term applied when weakness or incoordination of the speech musculature prevents clear pronunciation of words. The individual's speech may sound as if it is slurred or weak. It may be due to damage affecting the centres in the brain which control movements of the speech muscles, or damage to the muscles themselves.

Examples of dysarthria may be found in strokes, CEREBRAL PALSY and the latter stages of PARKINSONISM, MULTIPLE SCLEROSIS (MS) and MOTOR NEURONE DISEASE (MND). Whatever the cause, a speech therapist can assess the extent of the dysarthria and suggest exercises or an alternative means of communication.

Dyscalculia
A condition commonly seen when the brain's PARIETAL LOBE is diseased or injured, in which an individual finds it hard to carry out simple mathematical calculations.

Dyschezia
Constipation due to retention of FAECES in the rectum. This retention is the outcome of irregular habits, which damp down the normal reflex causing defaecation.

Dysdiadochokinesia

Loss of the ability to perform rapid alternate movements, such as winding up a watch. It is a sign of a lesion in the cerebellum. (See BRAIN.)

Dysentery

A clinical state arising from invasive colo-rectal disease; it is accompanied by abdominal colic, diarrhoea, and passage of blood/mucus in the stool. Although the two major forms are caused by *Shigella* spp. (bacillary dysentery) and *Entamoeba histolytica* (amoebic dysentery), other organisms including entero-haemorrhagic *Escherichia coli* (serotypes 0157:H7 and 026:H11) and *Campylobacter* spp. are also relevant. Other causes of dysentery include *Balantidium coli* and that caused by schistosomiasis (bilharzia) – *Schistosoma mansoni* and *S. japonicum* infection.

Shigellosis This form is usually caused by *Shigella dysenteriae*-1 (Shiga's bacillus), *Shigella flexneri*, *Shigella boydii*, and *Shigella sonnei*; the latter is the most benign and occurs in temperate climates also. It is transmitted by food and water contamination, by direct contact, and by flies; the organisms thrive in the presence of overcrowding and insanitary conditions. The incubation is between one and seven days, and the severity of the illness depends on the strain responsible. Duration of illness varies from a few days to two weeks and can be particularly severe in young, old, and malnourished individuals. Complications include perforation and haemorrhage from the colo-rectum, the haemolytic uraemic syndrome (which includes renal failure), and REITER'S SYNDROME. Diagnosis is dependent on demonstration of *Shigella* in (a) faecal sample(s) – before or usually after culture.

If dehydration is present, this should be treated accordingly, usually with an oral rehydration technique. *Shigella* is eradicated by antibiotics such as trimethoprim-sulphamethoxazole, trimethoprim, ampicillin, and amoxycillin. Recently, a widespread resistance to many antibiotics has developed, especially in Asia and southern America, where the agent of choice is now a quinolone compound, for example, ciprofloxacin; nalidixic acid is also effective. Prevention depends on improved hygiene and sanitation, careful protection of food from flies, fly destruction, and garbage disposal. A *Shigella* carrier must not be allowed to handle food.

Entamoeba histolytica infection Most cases occur in the tropics and subtropics. Dysentery may be accompanied by weight loss, anaemia, and occasionally DYSPNOEA. *E. histolytica* contaminates food (e.g. uncooked vegetables) or drinking water. After ingestion of the cyst-stage, and following the action of digestive enzymes, the motile trophozoite emerges in the colon causing local invasive disease (amoebic colitis). On entering the portal system, these organisms may gain access to the liver, causing invasive hepatic disease (amoebic liver 'abscess'). Other sites of 'abscess' formation include the lungs (usually right) and brain. In the colo-rectum an amoeboma may be difficult to differentiate from a carcinoma. Clinical symptoms usually occur within a week, but can be delayed for months, or even years; onset may be acute – as for *Shigella* spp. infection. Perforation, colo-rectal haemorrhage, and appendicitis are unusual complications. Diagnosis is by demonstration of *E. histolytica* trophozoites in a fresh faecal sample; other amoebae affecting humans do not invade tissues. Research techniques can be used to differentiate between pathogenic (*E. dysenteriae*) and non-pathogenic strains (*E. dispar*). Alternatively, several serological tests are of value in diagnosis, but only in the presence of invasive disease.

Treatment consists of one of the 5-nitroimidazole compounds – metronidazole, tinidazole, and ornidazole; alcohol avoidance is important during their administration. A five- to ten-day course should be followed by diloxanide furoate for ten days. Other compounds – emetine, chloroquine, iodoquinol, and paromomycin – are now rarely used. Invasive disease involving the liver or other organ(s) usually responds favourably to a similar regimen; aspiration of a liver 'abscess' is now rarely indicated, as controlled trials have indicated a similar resolution rate whether this technique is used or not, provided a 5-nitroimidazole compound is administered.

Dysidrosis

Disturbance of sweat secretion.

Dyskinesia

Abnormal movements of the muscles resulting from disorder of the brain. Movements are uncoordinated and involuntary and occur in facial as well as limb muscles. They include athetosis (writhing movements), CHOREA (jerking movements predominate), choreoathetosis (a combined type), myoclonus (spasms), tics and tremors.

Dyslexia

Dyslexia is difficulty in reading or learning to

read. It is always accompanied by difficulty in writing, and particularly by difficulties in spelling. Reading difficulties might be due to various factors – for example, a general learning problem, bad teaching or understimulation, or a perceptive problem such as poor eyesight. Specific dyslexia ('word blindness'), however, affects 4–8 per cent of otherwise normal children to some extent. It is three times more common in boys than in girls, and there is often a family history. The condition is sometimes missed and, when a child has difficulty with reading, dyslexia should be considered as a possible cause.

Support and advice may be obtained from the British Dyslexia Association.

Dysmenorrhoea
Painful MENSTRUATION.

Dyspareunia
Dyspareunia means painful or difficult COITUS. In women the cause may be physical – for example, due to local inflammation or infection in the vagina – or psychological; say, a fear of intercourse. In men the cause is usually physical, such as prostatitis (see PROSTATE, DISEASES OF) or a tight foreskin (see PREPUCE).

Dyspepsia
This is another name for indigestion. It describes a sensation of pain or discomfort in the upper abdomen or lower chest following eating. There may be additional symptoms of heartburn, flatulence, or nausea. There are many causes of dyspepsia including oesophagitis (see OESOPHAGUS, DISEASES OF), PEPTIC ULCER, gallstones (see under GALL-BLADDER, DISEASES OF), HIATUS HERNIA, malignancy of the stomach or oesophagus, and hepatic or pancreatic disease. Occasionally it may be psychological in origin. Treatment depends on the underlying cause but, if there is no specific pathology, avoidance of precipitating foods may be helpful. ANT-ACIDS may relieve discomfort and pain if taken when symptoms occur or are expected.

Dysphagia
Difficulty in swallowing. This may be caused by narrowing of the oesophagus because of physical disease such as cancer or injury. Disturbance to the nervous control of the swallowing mechanism – for example, in STROKE or MOTOR NEURONE DISEASE (MND) – can also cause dysphagia.

Dysphasia
Dysphasia is the term used to describe the difficulties in understanding language and in self-expression, most frequently after STROKE or other brain damage. When there is a total loss in the ability to communicate through speech or writing, it is known as global aphasia. Many more individuals have a partial understanding of what is said to them; they are also able to put their own thoughts into words to some extent. The general term for this less severe condition is dysphasia. Individuals vary widely, but in general there are two main types of dysphasia. Some people may have a good understanding of spoken language but have difficulty in self-expression; this is called expressive or motor dysphasia. Others may have a very poor ability to understand speech, but will have a considerable spoken output consisting of jargon words; this is known as receptive or sensory dysphasia. Similar difficulties may occur with reading, and this is called DYSLEXIA (a term more commonly encountered in the different context of children's reading disability). Adults who have suffered a stroke or another form of brain damage may also have difficulty in writing, or dysgraphia. The speech therapist can assess the finer diagnostic pointsand help them adjust to the effects of the stroke on communication. (See SPEECH THERAPY.)

Dysphasia may come on suddenly and last only for a few hours or days, being due to a temporary block in the circulation of blood to the brain. The effects may be permanent, but although the individual may have difficulty in understanding language and expressing themselves, they will be quite aware of their surroundings and may be very frustrated by their inability to communicate with others.

Further information may be obtained from Speakability.

Dysphonia
Abnormal vocal sounds when speaking. It is caused by injury or disease of the LARYNX or of the nerves suplying the laryngeal muscles.

Dysplasia
Abnormal development of cells, tissues or structures in the body.

Dyspnoea
Difficulty in breathing (see BREATHLESSNESS; ORTHOPNOEA).

Dyspraxia
See APRAXIA.

Dysrhythmia

Disturbance in the rhythmical contractions of the heart. It is also called ARRHYTHMIA.

Dystocia

Slow or painful birth of a child. This may occur because the baby is large and/or the mother's pelvis is small or wrongly shaped for the baby to pass through easily. Abnormal presentation of the baby is another cause (see PREGNANCY AND LABOUR; BREECH PRESENTATION).

Dystonia

Dystonia refers to a type of involuntary movement characterised by a sustained muscle contraction, frequently causing twisting and repetitive movements or abnormal postures, and caused by inappropriate instructions from the brain. It is sometimes called torsion spasm, and may be synonymous with ATHETOSIS when the extremities are involved. Often the condition is of unknown cause (idiopathic), but an inherited predisposition is increasingly recognised among some cases. Others may be associated with known pathology of the brain such as CEREBRAL PALSY or WILSON'S DISEASE.

The presentation of dystonia may be focal (usually in adults) causing blepharospasm (forceful eye closure), oromandibular dystonia (spasms of the tongue and jaw), cranial dystonia/Meige syndrome/Brueghel's syndrome (eyes and jaw both involved), spastic or spasmodic dysphonia/laryngeal dystonia (strained or whispering speech), spasmodic dysphagia (difficulty swallowing), spasmodic torti/latero/ante/retrocollis (rotation, sideways, forward or backward tilting of the neck), dystonic writer's cramp or axial dystonia (spasms deviating the torso). Foot dystonia occurs almost exclusively in children and adolescents. In adults, the condition usually remains focal or involves at most an adjacent body part. In children, it may spread to become generalised. The condition has always been considered rare, but commonly is either not diagnosed or mistakenly thought to be of psychological origin. It may, in fact, be half as common as MULTIPLE SCLEROSIS (MS). Similar features can occur in some subjects treated with major tranquillising drugs, in whom a predisposition to develop dystonia may be present.

One rare form, called dopa-responsive dystonia, can be largely abolished by treatment with LEVODOPA. Particularly in paediatric practice this drug will often be tried on a child with dystonia.

Dystrophia Myotonica

A type of muscular dystrophy (see MUSCLES, DISORDERS OF) in which the affected person has weakness and wasting of the muscles, particularly those in the face and neck. Other effects are CATARACT, ptosis (see EYE, DISORDERS OF), baldness and malfunctioning of the endocrine system (see ENDOCRINE GLANDS). Both sexes may be affected by this inherited disorder.

Dystrophy

Dystrophy means defective or faulty nutrition, and is a term applied to a group of developmental changes occurring in the muscles, independently of the nervous system (see MUSCLES, DISORDERS OF). The best-known form is progressive muscular dystrophy, a group of hereditary disorders characterised by symmetrical wasting and weakness, with no sensory loss. There are three types: Duchenne (usually occurring in boys within the first three years of life); limb girdle (occurring in either sex in the second or third decade); and facio-scapulo-humeral (either sex, any age). The three types have different prognoses, but may lead to severe disability and premature death, often from respiratory failure. The third type progresses very slowly, however, and is compatible with a long life.

Diagnosis may be confirmed by ELECTRO-MYOGRAPHY (EMG) or muscle biopsy. Although genetic research is pointing to possible treatment or prevention, at present no effective treatment is known, and deterioration may occur with excessive confinement to bed. Physio-therapeutic and orthopaedic measures may be necessary to counteract deformities and contractures, and may help in coping with some disabilities.

Dysuria

Difficulty or pain in urination. The condition is commonly associated with frequency and urgency of MICTURITION if caused by infection of the bladder (CYSTITIS) or urethra (see URETHRA, DISEASES OF). A burning feeling is common and relief is achieved by treating the underlying cause. Drinking large amounts of water may help to alleviate symptoms. If these persist, medical advice should be sought.

Ear

The ear is concerned with two functions. The more evident is that of the sense of hearing; the other is the sense of equilibration and of motion. The organ is divided into three parts: (1) the external ear, consisting of the auricle on the surface of the head, and the tube which leads inwards to the drum; (2) the middle ear, separated from the former by the tympanic membrane or drum, and from the internal ear by two other membranes, but communicating with the throat by the Eustachian tube; and (3) the internal ear, comprising the complicated labyrinth from which runs the vestibulocochlear nerve into the brain.

External ear The auricle or pinna consists of a framework of elastic cartilage covered by skin, the lobule at the lower end being a small mass of fat. From the bottom of the concha the external auditory (or acoustic) meatus runs inwards for 25 mm (1 inch), to end blindly at the drum. The outer half of the passage is surrounded by cartilage, lined by skin, on which are placed fine hairs pointing outwards, and glands secreting a small amount of wax. In the inner half, the skin is smooth and lies directly upon the temporal bone, in the substance of which the whole hearing apparatus is enclosed.

Middle ear The tympanic membrane, forming the drum, is stretched completely across the end of the passage. It is about 8 mm (one-third of an inch) across, very thin, and white or pale pink in colour, so that it is partly transparent and some of the contents of the middle ear shine through it. The cavity of the middle ear is about 8 mm (one-third of an inch) wide and 4 mm (one-sixth of an inch) in depth from the tympanic membrane to the inner wall of bone. Its important contents are three small bones – the malleus (hammer), incus (anvil) and stapes (stirrup) – collectively known as the auditory ossicles, with two minute muscles which regulate their movements, and the chorda tympani nerve which runs across the cavity. These three bones form a chain across the middle ear, connecting the drum with the internal ear. Their function is to convert the air-waves, which strike upon the drum, into mechanical movements which can affect the fluid in the inner ear.

The middle ear has two connections which are of great importance as regards disease (see EAR, DISEASES OF). In front, it communicates by a passage 37 mm (1.5 inches) long – the Eustachian (or auditory) tube – with the upper part of the throat, behind the nose; behind and above, it opens into a cavity known as the mastoid antrum. The Eustachian tube admits air from the throat, and so keeps the pressure on both sides of the drum fairly equal.

Internal ear This consists of a complex system of hollows in the substance of the temporal bone enclosing a membranous duplicate. Between the membrane and the bone is a fluid known as perilymph, while the membrane is distended by another collection of fluid known as endolymph. This membranous labyrinth, as it is called, consists of two parts. The hinder part, comprising a sac (the utricle) and three short semicircular canals opening at each end into it, is the part concerned with the balancing sense; the forward part consists of another small bag (the saccule), and of a still more important part, the cochlear duct, and is the part concerned with hearing. In the cochlear duct is placed the spiral organ of Corti, on which sound-waves are finally received and by which the sounds are communicated to the cochlear nerve, a branch of the vestibulocochlear nerve, which ends in filaments to this organ of Corti. The essential parts in the organ of Corti are a double row of rods and several rows of cells furnished with fine hairs of varying length which respond to differing sound frequencies.

The act of hearing When sound-waves in the air reach the ear, the drum is alternately pressed in and pulled out, in consequence of which a to-and-fro movement is communicated to the chain of ossicles. The foot of the stapes communicates these movements to the perilymph. Finally these motions reach the delicate filaments placed in the organ of Corti, and so affect the auditory nerve, which conveys impressions to the centre in the brain.

Ear, Diseases of

Diseases may affect the EAR alone or as part of a more generalised condition. The disease may affect the outer, middle or inner ear or a combination of these.

Examination of the ear includes inspection of the external ear. An auriscope is used to

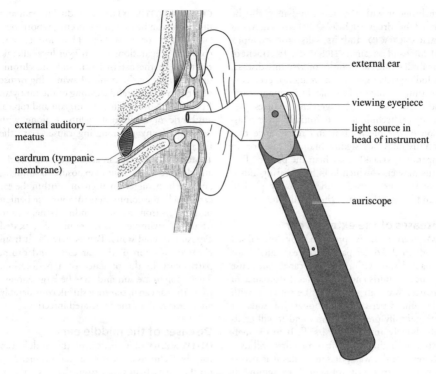

external ear

viewing eyepiece

light source in
head of instrument

external auditory
meatus

eardrum (tympanic
membrane)

auriscope

Auriscope positioned in external auditory meatus of left ear for viewing ear drum.

examine the external ear canal and the ear drum. If a more detailed inspection is required, a microscope may be used to improve illumination and magnification.

Tuning-fork or Rinne tests are performed to identify the presence of DEAFNESS. The examiner tests whether the vibrating fork is audible at the meatus, and then the foot of the fork is placed on the mastoid bone of the ear to discover at which of the two sites the patient can hear the vibrations for the longest time. This can help to differentiate between conductive and nerve deafness.

Hearing tests are carried out to determine the level of hearing. An audiometer is used to deliver a series of short tones of varying frequency to the ear, either through a pair of headphones or via a sound transducer applied directly to the skull. The intensity of the sound is gradually reduced until it is no longer heard and this represents the threshold of hearing, at that frequency, through air and bone respectively. It may be necessary to play a masking noise into the opposite ear to prevent that ear from hearing the tones, enabling each ear to be tested independently.

General symptoms The following are some of the chief symptoms of ear disease:

DEAFNESS (see DEAFNESS).

EARACHE is most commonly due to acute inflammation of the middle ear. Perceived pain in this region may be referred from other areas, such as the earache commonly experienced after tonsillectomy (removal of the TONSILS) or that caused by carious teeth (see TEETH, DISORDERS OF). The treatment will depend on the underlying cause.

TINNITUS or ringing in the ear often accompanies deafness, but is sometimes the only symptom of ear disease. Even normal people sometimes experience tinnitus, particularly if put in soundproofed surroundings. It may be described as hissing, buzzing, the sound of the sea, or of bells. The intensity of the tinnitus usually fluctuates, sometimes disappearing altogether. It may occur in almost any form of ear disease, but is particularly troublesome in nerve deafness due to ageing and in noise-induced deafness.

The symptom seems to originate in the brain's subcortical regions, high in the central nervous system. It may be a symptom of general diseases such as ANAEMIA, high blood pressure and arterial disease, in which cases it is often synchronous with the pulse, and may also be caused by drugs such as QUININE, salicylates (SALICYLIC ACID and its salts, for example, ASPIRIN) and certain ANTIBIOTICS. Treatment of any underlying ear disorder or systemic disease, including DEPRESSION, may reduce or even cure the tinnitus, but unfortunately in many cases the noises persist. Management involves psychological techniques and initially an explanation of the mechanism and reassurance that tinnitus does not signify brain disease, or an impending STROKE, may help the person. Tinnitus maskers – which look like hearing aids – have long been used with a suitably pitched sound helping to 'mask' the condition.

Diseases of the external ear

WAX (cerumen) is produced by specialised glands in the outer part of the ear canal only. Impacted wax within the ear canal can cause deafness, tinnitus and sometimes disturbance of balance. Wax can sometimes be softened with olive oil, 5-per-cent bicarbonate of soda or commercially prepared drops, and it will gradually liquefy and 'remove itself'. If this is ineffective, syringing by a doctor or nurse will usually remove the wax but sometimes it is necessary for a specialist (otologist) to remove it manually with instruments. Syringing should not be done if perforation of the tympanic membrane (eardrum) is suspected.

FOREIGN BODIES such as peas, beads or buttons may be found in the external ear canal, especially in children who have usually introduced them themselves. Live insects may also be trapped in the external canal causing intense irritation and noise, and in such cases spirit drops are first instilled into the ear to kill the insect. Except in foreign bodies of vegetable origin, where swelling and pain may occur, syringing may be used to remove some foreign bodies, but often removal by a specialist using suitable instrumentation and an operating microscope is required. In children, a general anaesthetic may be needed.

ACUTE OTITIS EXTERNA may be a diffuse inflammation or a boil (furuncle) occurring in the outer ear canal. The pinna is usually tender on movement (unlike acute otitis media – see below) and a discharge may be present. Initially treatment should be local, using magnesium sulphate paste or glycerine and 10-per-cent ichthaminol. Topical antibiotic drops can be used and sometimes antibiotics by mouth are necessary, especially if infection is acute. Clotrimazole drops are a useful antifungal treatment. Analgesics and locally applied warmth should relieve the pain.

CHRONIC OTITIS EXTERNA producing pain and discharge, can be caused by eczema, seborrhoeic DERMATITIS or PSORIASIS. Hair lotions and cosmetic preparations may trigger local allergic reactions in the external ear, and the chronic disorder may be the result of swimming or use of dirty towels. Careful cleaning of the ear by an ENT (Ear, Nose & Throat) surgeon and topical antibiotic or antifungal agents – along with removal of any precipitating cause – are the usual treatments.

TUMOURS of the ear can arise in the skin of the auricle, often as a result of exposure to sunlight, and can be benign or malignant. Within the ear canal itself, the commonest tumours are benign outgrowths from the surrounding bone, said to occur in swimmers as a result of repeated exposure to cold water. Polyps may result from chronic infection of the ear canal and drum, particularly in the presence of a perforation. These polyps are soft and may be large enough to fill the ear canal, but may shrink considerably after treatment of the associated infection.

Diseases of the middle ear

OTITIS MEDIA or infection of the middle ear, usually occurs as a result of infection spreading up the Eustachian tubes from the nose, throat or sinuses. It may follow a cold, tonsillitis or sinusitis, and may also be caused by swimming and diving where water and infected secretions are forced up the Eustachian tube into the middle ear. Primarily it is a disease of children, with as many as 1.5 million cases occurring in Britain every year. Pain may be intense and throbbing or sharp in character. The condition is accompanied by deafness, fever and often TINNITUS.

In infants, crying may be the only sign that something is wrong – though this is usually accompanied by some localising manifestation such as rubbing or pulling at the ear. Examination of the ear usually reveals redness, and sometimes bulging, of the ear drum. In the early stages there is no discharge, but in the later stages there may be a discharge from perforation of the ear drum as a result of the pressure created in the middle ear by the accumulated pus. This is usually accompanied by an immediate reduction in pain.

Treatment consists of the immediate administration of an antibiotic, usually one of the penicillins (e.g. amoxicillin). In the majority of cases no further treatment is required, but if this does not quickly bring relief then it may be necessary to perform a myringotomy, or incision of the ear drum, to drain pus from the middle ear. When otitis media is treated immediately with sufficient dosage of the appropriate antibiotic, the chances of any permanent damage to the ear or to hearing are reduced to a negligible degree, as is the risk of any complications such as mastoiditis (discussed later in this section).

CHRONIC OTITIS MEDIA WITH EFFUSION or glue ear, is the most common inflammatory condition of the middle ear in children, to the extent that one in four children in the UK entering school has had an episode of 'glue ear'. It is characterised by a persistent sticky fluid in the middle ear (hence the name); this causes a conductive-type deafness. It may be associated with enlarged adenoids (see NOSE, DISORDERS OF) which impair the function of the Eustachian tube. If the hearing impairment is persistent and causes problems, drainage of the fluid, along with antibiotic treatment, may be needed – possibly in conjunction with removal of the adenoids. The insertion of grommets (ventilation tubes) was for a time standard treatment, but while hearing is often restored, there may be no long-term gain and even a risk of damage to the tympanic membrane, so the operation is less popular than it was a decade or so ago.

MASTOIDITIS is a serious complication of inflammation of the middle ear, the incidence of which has been dramatically reduced by the introduction of antibiotics. Inflammation in this cavity usually arises by direct spread of acute or chronic inflammation from the middle ear. The signs of this condition include swelling and tenderness of the skin behind the ear, redness and swelling inside the ear, pain in the side of the head, high fever, and a discharge from the ear. The management of this condition in the first instance is with antibiotics, usually given intravenously; however, if the condition fails to improve, surgical treatment is necessary. This involves draining any pus from the middle ear and mastoid, and removing diseased lining and bone from the mastoid.

Diseases of the inner ear

MENIÈRE'S DISEASE is a common idiopathic disorder of ENDOLYMPH control in the semicircular canals (see EAR), characterised by the triad of episodic VERTIGO with deafness and tinnitus. The cause is unknown and usually one ear only is affected at first, but eventually the opposite ear is affected in approximately 50 per cent of cases. The onset of dizziness is often sudden and lasts for up to 24 hours. The hearing loss is temporary in the early stages, but with each attack there may be a progressive nerve deafness. Nausea and vomiting often occur. Treatment during the attacks includes rest and drugs to control sickness. Vasodilator drugs such as betahistine hydrochloride may be helpful. Surgical treatment is sometimes required if crippling attacks of dizziness persist despite these measures.

OTOSCLEROSIS A disorder of the middle ear that results in progressive deafness. Often running in families, otosclerosis affects about one person in 200; it customarily occurs early in adult life. An overgrowth of bone fixes the stapes (the innermost bone of the middle ear) and stops sound vibrations from being transmitted to the inner ear. The result is conductive deafness. The disorder usually affects both ears. Those affected tend to talk quietly and deafness increases over a 10–15 year period. Tinnitus often occurs, and occasionally vertigo.

Abnormal hearing tests point to the diagnosis; the deafness may be partially overcome with a hearing aid but surgery is eventually needed. This involves replacing the stapes bone with a synthetic substitute (stapedectomy). (See also OTIC BAROTRAUMA.)

Eating Disorders

The term 'eating disorders' covers OBESITY, feeding problems in childhood, anorexia nervosa, and bulimia nervosa. The latter two are described here.

Anorexia nervosa Often called the slimmer's disease, this is a syndrome characterised by the loss of at least a quarter of a person's normal body weight; by fear of normal weight; and, in women, by AMENORRHOEA. An individual's body image may be distorted so that the sufferer cannot judge real weight and wants to diet even when already very thin.

Anorexia nervosa usually begins in adolescence, affecting about 1–2 per cent of teenagers and college students at any time. It is 20 times more common among women than men. Up to 10 per cent of sufferers' sisters also have the syndrome. Anorexia may be linked with episodes of bulimia (see below).

The symptoms result from secretive self-starvation, usually with excessive exercise, self-induced vomiting, and misuse of laxatives. An anorexic (or anorectic) person may wear layers of baggy clothes to keep warm and to hide the figure. Starvation can cause serious problems such as ANAEMIA, low blood pressure, slow heart rate, swollen ankles, and osteoporosis. Sudden death from heart ARRHYTHMIA may occur, particularly if the sufferer misuses DIURETICS to lose weight and also depletes the body's level of potassium.

E

There is probably no single cause of anorexia nervosa. Social pressure to be thin seems to be an important factor and has increased over the past 20–30 years, along with the incidence of the syndrome. Psychological theories include fear of adulthood and fear of losing parents' attention.

Treatment should start with the general practitioner who should first rule out other illnesses causing similar signs and symptoms. These include DEPRESSION and disorders of the bowel, PITUITARY GLAND, THYROID GLAND, and OVARIES.

If the diagnosis is clearly anorexia nervosa, the general practitioner may refer the sufferer to a psychiatrist or psychologist. Moderately ill sufferers can be treated by COGNITIVE BEHAVIOUR THERAPY. A simple form of this is to agree targets for daily calorie intake and for acceptable body weight. The sufferer and the therapist (the general practitioner or a member of the psychiatric team) then monitor progress towards both targets by keeping a diary of food intake and measuring weight regularly. Counselling or more intensely personal PSYCHOTHERAPY may help too. Severe life-threatening complications will need urgent medical treatment in hospital, including rehydration and feeding using a nasogastric tube or an intravenous drip.

About half of anorectic sufferers recover fully within four years, a quarter improve, and a quarter remain severely underweight with (in the case of women) menstrual abnormalities. Recovery after ten years is rare and about 3 per cent die within that period, half of them by suicide.

Bulimia nervosa is a syndrome characterised by binge eating, self-induced vomiting and laxative misuse, and fear of fatness. There is some overlap between anorexia nervosa and bulimia but, unlike the former, bulimia may start at any age from adolescence to 40 and is probably more directly linked with ordinary dieting. Bulimic sufferers say that, although they feel depressed and guilty after binges, the 'buzz' and relief after vomiting and purging are addictive. They often respond well to cognitive behaviour therapy.

Bulimia nervosa does not necessarily cause weight loss because the binges – for example of a loaf of bread, a packet of cereal, and several cans of cold baked beans at one sitting – are cancelled out by purging, by self-induced vomiting and by brief episodes of starvation. The full syndrome has been found in about 1 per cent of women but mild forms may be much more common. In one survey of female college students, 13 per cent admitted to having had bulimic symptoms.

Bulimia nervosa rarely leads to serious physical illness or death. However, repeated vomiting can cause oesophageal burns, salivary gland infections, small tears in the stomach, and occasionally dehydration and chemical imbalances in the blood. Inducing vomiting using fingers may produce two tell-tale signs – bite marks on the knuckles and rotten, pitted teeth.

Those suffering from this condition may obtain advice from the Eating Disorders Association.

Ebola Virus Disease

Ebola virus disease is another name for VIRAL HAEMORRHAGIC FEVER. The ebola virus is one of the most virulent micro-organisms known. Like the marburg virus (see MARBURG DISEASE), it belongs to the filovirus group which originates in Africa. Increased population mobility and wars have meant that the infection occasionally occurs elsewhere, with air travellers developing symptoms on returning home.

Treatment As the disease can be neither prevented nor cured, treatment is supportive, with strict anti-infection procedures essential as human-to-human transmission can occur via skin and mucous-membrane contacts. Incubation period is 5–10 days. Fever with MYALGIA and headache occur initially, often accompanied by abdominal and chest symptoms. Haemorrhagic symptoms soon develop and the victim either starts to improve in the second week or develops multi-organ failure and lapses into a coma. Mortality ranges from 25 to 90 per cent.

Eburnation

Eburnation is a process of hardening and polishing which takes place at the ends of bones, giving them an ivory-like appearance. It is caused by the wearing away, in consequence of OSTEOARTHRITIS, of the smooth plates of cartilage which in health cover the ends of the bones.

Ecchymosis

The development of a discoloured skin patch resulting from escape of blood into the tissues just under the skin, often from bruising.

ECG

See ELECTROCARDIOGRAM (ECG).

Echinococcus

The immature form of a small tapeworm, *Taenia echinococcus*, found in dogs, wolves and jackals and from which human beings become infected, so that they harbour the immature parasite in the form known as hydatid cyst. (See TAENIASIS.)

Echocardiography

The use of ultrasonics (see ULTRASOUND) for the purpose of examining the HEART. By thus recording the echo (hence the name) from the heart of ultrasound waves, it is possible to study, for example, the movements of the heart valves as well as the state of the interior of the heart. Safe, reliable and painless, the procedure cuts the need for the physically interventionist procedure of CARDIAC CATHETERISATION.

Echolalia

Echolalia is the meaningless repetition, by a person suffering from mental deterioration, of words and phrases addressed to him/her.

Echoviruses

Echoviruses, of which there are more than 30 known types, occur in all parts of the world. Their full name is Enteric Cytopathogenic Human Orphan (ECHO – hence the acronym). They are more common in children than in adults, and have been responsible for outbreaks of MENINGITIS, common-cold-like illnesses, gastrointestinal infections, and infections of the respiratory tract. They are particularly dangerous when they infect premature infants, and there have been several outbreaks of such infection in neonatal units, in which premature infants and other seriously ill small babies are nursed. The virus is introduced to such units by mothers, staff and visitors who are unaware that they are carriers of the virus.

Eclampsia

A rare disorder in which convulsions occur during late pregnancy (see also PREGNANCY AND LABOUR – Increased blood pressure). This condition occurs in around 50 out of every 100,000 pregnant women, especially in the later months and at the time of delivery, but in a few cases only after delivery has taken place. The cause is not known, although cerebral OEDEMA is thought to occur. In practically all cases the KIDNEYS are profoundly affected. Effective antenatal care should identify most women at risk of developing eclampsia.

Symptoms Warning symptoms include dizziness, headache, oedema, vomiting, and the secretion of albumin (protein) in the urine. These are normally accompanied by a rise in blood pressure, which can be severe. Pre-eclamptic symptoms may be present for some days or weeks before the seizure takes place, and, if a woman is found to have these during antenatal care, preventive measures must be taken. Untreated, CONVULSIONS and unconsciousness are very likely, with serious migraine-like frontal headache and epigastric pain the symptoms.

Treatment Prevention of eclampsia by dealing with pre-eclamptic symptoms is the best management, but even this may not prevent convulsions. Hospital treatment is essential if eclampsia develops, preferably in a specialist unit. The treatment of the seizures is that generally applicable to convulsions of any kind, with appropriate sedatives given such as intravenous DIAZEPAM. HYDRALLAZINE intravenously should also be administered to reduce the blood pressure. Magnesium sulphate given intramuscularly sometimes helps to control the fits. The baby's condition should be monitored throughout.

Urgent delivery of the baby, if necessary by CAESAREAN SECTION, is the most effective 'treatment' for a mother with acute eclampsia. (See PREGNANCY AND LABOUR.)

Women who have suffered from eclampsia are liable to suffer a recurrence in a further preganancy. Careful monitoring is required. There is a self-help organisation, Action on Pre-eclampsia (APEC), to advise on the condition.

Ecstasy

Ecstasy refers to a morbid mental condition, associated with an extreme sense of well-being, with a feeling of rapture, and temporary loss of self-control. It often presents as a form of religious obsession, with a feeling of direct communication with God, saintly voices and images being perceived. In milder cases the patient may preach as though with a divine mission to help others. Ecstasy may occur in happiness PSYCHOSIS, SCHIZOPHRENIA, certain forms of EPILEPSY, and abnormal personalities.

The term is also a street drug name for an amphetamine derivative, 3, 4-methylenedioxymethamphetamine or MDMA, increasingly used as a 'recreational' drug. It is classified as a class A drug under the Misuse of Drugs Act 1971. MDMA is structurally similar to endogenous CATECHOLAMINES and produces central and peripheral sympathetic stimulation of alpha and beta ADRENERGIC RECEPTORS. It is taken into nerve terminals by the serotonin transporter and causes release of the NEURO-TRANSMITTER substances serotonin and dopamine. Following this, SEROTONIN depletion is prolonged. As serotonin plays a major part in mood control, this leads to the characteristic 'midweek depression' experienced by MDMA users.

Several fatalities in young people have been attributed to adverse reactions resulting from MDMA use/abuse and possibly accompanying alcohol consumption. The principal effects are increase in pulse, blood pressure, temperature and respiratory rate. Additional complications such as cardiac ARRHYTHMIA, heatstroke-type syndrome, HYPONATRAEMIA and brain haemorrhage may occur. There is also concern over possible effects on the mental concentration and memory of those using ecstasy.

Management of patients who get to hospital is largely symptomatic and supportive but may include gastric decontamination, and use of DIAZEPAM as the first line of treatment as it reduces central stimulation which may also reduce TACHYCARDIA, HYPERTENSION and PYREXIA.

ECT

See ELECTROCONVULSIVE THERAPY (ECT).

Ectasia

A term that means widening, usually referring to a disorder of a duct bearing secretions from a gland or organ (e.g. mammary duct ectasia).

Ecthyma

In debilitated or immunodepressed subjects, staphylococcal IMPETIGO or folliculitis (inflammation of hair follicles [see SKIN]) may become ulcerated. This is called ecthyma and is seen in vagrants, drug addicts, and individuals with AIDS/HIV or uncontrolled DIABETES MELLITUS.

Ecto-

Ecto- is a prefix meaning on the outside.

Ectoderm

The outer of the three germ layers of the EMBRYO during its early development. The ectoderm develops into the nervous systems, organs of sensation, teeth and lining of mouth, and the SKIN and its associated structures such as hair and nails.

Ectopic

Ectopic means out of the usual place. For example, the congenital displacement of the heart outside the thoracic cavity is said to be ectopic. An 'ectopic gestation' means a pregnancy outside of the womb (see ECTOPIC PREGNANCY).

Ectopic Beat

A heart muscle contraction that is outside the normal sequence of the cardiac cycle (see HEART). The impulse is generated outside the usual focus of the SINOATRIAL NODE. Also known as extrasystoles, ectopic beats are called ventricular if they arise from a focus in the ventricles and supraventricular if they arise in the atria. They may cause no symptoms and the affected subject may be unaware of them. The beat may, however, be the result of heart disease or may be caused by NICOTINE or CAFFEINE. If persistent, the individual may suffer from irregular rhythm or ventricular fibrillation and need treatment with anti-arrhythmic drugs.

Ectopic Pregnancy

An ectopic pregnancy most commonly develops in one of the FALLOPIAN TUBES. Occasionally it may occur in one of the OVARIES, and rarely in the uterine cervix or the abdominal cavity. Around one in 200 pregnant women have an ectopic gestation. As pregnancy proceeds, surrounding tissues may be damaged and, if serious bleeding happens, the woman may present as an 'abdominal emergency'. A life-threatening condition, this needs urgent surgery. Most women recover satisfactorily and can have further pregnancies despite the removal of one Fallopian tube as a result of the ectopic gestation. Death is unusual. This disorder of pregnancy may occur because infection or a previous abdominal injury or operation may have damaged the normal descent of an ovum from the ovary to the womb. The first symptoms usually appear during the first two months of pregnancy, perhaps before the woman realises she is pregnant. Severe lower abdominal pain and vaginal bleeding are common presenting symptoms. Ultrasound can be used to diagnose the condition and laparoscopy can be used to remove the products of conception. (See PREGNANCY AND LABOUR.)

Ectromelia

Ectromelia means the absence of a limb or limbs, from congenital causes.

Ectropion

See EYE, DISORDERS OF.

Eczema
See DERMATITIS.

Edentulous
Lacking teeth: this may be because teeth have not developed or because they have been removed or fallen out.

EDTA
Ethylenediamine tetra-acetic acid is used to treat poisoning with metals such as lead and strontium. One of the CHELATING AGENTS, EDTA is used in the form of sodium or calcium salts. The stable chelate compounds resulting from the treatment are excreted in the urine.

EEG
See ELECTROENCEPHALOGRAPHY (EEG).

Efavirenz
A drug known as a non-nucleoside reverse transcriptase inhibitor, used in the treatment of HIV infection in combination with other antiretroviral drugs (see VIRUSES; AIDS/HIV). It should not be used in patients with severe kidney impairment or liver damage. Pregnant women and older people should not take efavirenz. The drug has a wide range of side-effects.

Efferent
The term applied to vessels which convey away blood or a secretion from a body part, or to nerves which carry nerve impulses outwards from the nerve-centres. (Opposite: AFFERENT.)

Effort Syndrome
Also known as Da Costa's syndrome, this is a condition in which symptoms occur, such as palpitations and shortness of breath, which are attributed by the patient to disorder of the heart. There is no evidence, however, of heart disease, and psychological factors are thought to be of importance. (See PSYCHOSOMATIC DISEASES.)

Effusion
The passage of fluid through the walls of a blood vessel into a tissue or body cavity. It commonly occurs as a result of inflammation or damage to the blood vessel. A pleural effusion may occur in heart failure (as a result of increased blood pressure in the veins forcing out fluid) or as a result of inflammation in the lung tissue (PNEUMONIA). Effusions may also develop in damaged joints.

Egg
See OVUM.

Ego
A psychoanalytical term to describe that part of the mind which develops as a result of the individual's interactions with the outside world. Freud (see FREUDIAN THEORY) describes the Ego as reconciling the demands of the Id (a person's unconscious, instinctive mind), the Superego (moral conscience) and the reality of the outside world.

Eisenmenger Syndrome
A condition in which the subject suffers from a defect in one of the dividing walls (septum) of the HEART and this is accompanied by PULMONARY HYPERTENSION. The defect allows blood low in oxygen to flow from the right to the left side of the heart and be pumped into the aorta, which normally carries oxygenated blood to the body. The patient has a dusky blue appearance, becomes breathless and has a severely restricted exercise tolerance. There is an increase in red blood cells as the body attempts to compensate for the lowered oxygen delivery. The condition may be avoided by early surgical repair of the septal defect, but once it is evident, surgery may not be possible.

Ejaculation
The expulsion of SEMEN from the PENIS during ORGASM. The stimulation of sexual intercourse (coitus) or masturbation produces a spinal reflex action that causes ejaculation. As well as containing spermatozoa (male germ cells), the semen comprises several constituents arising from COWPER'S GLANDS, the PROSTATE GLAND, the testicles and seminal vesicles (see TESTICLES) and these are discharged in sequence. (See also PREMATURE EJACULATION.)

Elastic Tissue
CONNECTIVE TISSUE which contains a profusion of yellow elastic fibres. Long, slender and branching, these fibres (made up of elastin, an albumin-like PROTEIN) ensure that the elastic tissue is flexible and stretchable. The dermis layer of the skin, arterial walls and the alveolar walls in the LUNGS all contain elastic tissue.

Electrical Injuries
These are usually caused by the passage through the body of an electric current of high voltage owing to accidental contact with a live wire or to a discharge of lightning. The general effects produced are included under the term electric

shock, but vary greatly in degree. The local effects include spasmodic contraction of muscles, fracture of bones, and in severe cases more or less widespread destruction of tissues which may amount simply to burns of the skin or may include necrosis of masses of muscle and internal organs. Fright due to the unexpectedness of the shock, and pain due to the sudden cramp of muscles, are the most common symptoms and in most cases pass off within a few minutes. In more severe cases – especially when the person has remained in contact with a live wire for some time, or has been unable to let go of the electrical contact owing to spasmodic contraction of the muscles – the effects are more pronounced and may include concussion or compression of the brain (see BRAIN, DISEASES OF). In still more severe cases, death may ensue either from paralysis of the respiration or stoppage of the heart's action. If prompt measures are taken for treatment, the victim can often be resuscitated.

In Britain there are an average of 110 deaths a year from electrocution, half of these occurring in the home.

Treatment No electrical apparatus or switch should be touched by anyone who is in metallic contact with the ground, such as through a metal pipe, especially, for example, from a bath. The first action is to break the current. This can sometimes be done by turning off a switch. If the victim is grasping or in contact with a live wire, the contact may be severed with safety only by someone wearing rubber gloves or rubber boots; but as these are not likely to be immediately available, the rescuer's hands may be protected by a thick wrapping of dry cloth, or the live wire may be hooked or pushed out of the way with a long wooden stick such as a broom-handle. If the injured person is unconscious, and especially if breathing has stopped, artificial respiration should be applied as described in APPENDIX 1: BASIC FIRST AID – Electrocution. When the patient begins to breathe again, he or she must be treated for shock and professional help obtained urgently.

Electrocardiogram (ECG)

A record of the variations in electric potential which occur in the HEART as it contracts and relaxes. Any muscle in use produces an electric current, but when an individual is at rest, the main muscular current in the body is that produced by the heart. This can be recorded by connecting the outside of the body by electrodes with an instrument known as an electro-

cardiograph. The patient is connected to the electrocardiograph by leads from either the arms and legs or different points on the chest. The normal electrocardiogram of each heartbeat shows one wave corresponding to the activity of the atria and four waves corresponding to the phases of each ventricular beat. Various readily recognisable changes are seen in cases in which the heart is acting in an abnormal manner, or in which one or other side of the heart is enlarged. This record therefore forms a useful aid in many cases of heart disease (see HEART, DISEASES OF). The main applications of the electrocardiogram are in the diagnosis of myocardial infarction and of cardiac ARRHYTHMIA.

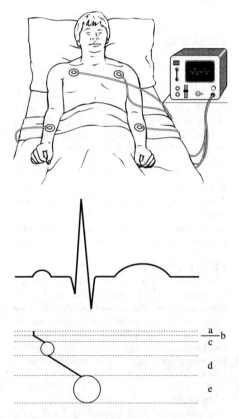

(a) origin of the sinus impulse
(b) conduction through the sino-atrial junction
(c) atrial activation
(d) conduction through the atrioventricular junction
(e) spread of activation within the ventricles

Tracing of normal electrical impulse that initiates heartbeat (after *The Cardiac Arrhythmias Pocket Book*, Boehrringer, Ingelheim).

Electrocardiography

A method of recording the electrical activity of the heart muscles. Electrodes from a recording machine (electrocardiograph) are placed on the skin of the chest wall, arms and legs. The record of the electrical changes is called an ECG (electrocardiogram). The number of electrodes used depends on the complexity of the heart disorder being monitored. The procedure can be done in hospital, doctors' surgeries and the patient's home, and should not cause any discomfort.

In certain circumstances – for example, where a person has had bouts of chest pain – an exercise ECG may be performed under medical supervision. The patient walks on a treadmill while the ECG is recorded continuously.

Electrocautery

The use of an electrically heated needle or loop to destroy diseased or unwanted tissue. Benign growths, warts and polyps can be removed with this technique.

Electrocoagulation

A method of sealing blood vessels using heat generated by high-frequency electric current through fine needles or a surgical knife. The procedure is used during surgery to close newly cut vessels. It can also be used to stop nosebleeds and to stop vascular deformities such as naevi (see NAEVUS).

Electrocochleography

Electrocochleography is a method of recording the activity of the cochlea, the part of the inner ear concerned with hearing. (See EAR.)

Electroconvulsive Therapy (ECT)

A controversial but sometimes rapidly effective treatment for cases of severe DEPRESSION, particularly where psychotic features are present (see PSYCHOSIS), or in high-risk patients such as suicidal or post-partum patients. ECT is only indicated after antidepressants have been tried and shown to be ineffective; the full procedure of treatment should be explained to the patient, whose consent must be obtained.

Before treatment, the patient will have been fasted for at least eight hours. After checking for any potential drug ALLERGY or interactions, the patient is given a general anaesthetic and muscle relaxants. Depending on the side of the patient's dominance, either unilateral (on the side of the non-dominant hemisphere of the BRAIN) or bilateral (if dominance is uncertain, e.g. in left-handed people) positioning of elec-

trodes is used. Unilateral ECT has the advantage of being associated with less anterograde AMNESIA. When the current passes, the muscles will contract for approximately 10 seconds, with further tonic spasms lasting up to a minute. The patient should then be put in the COMA or recovery position and observed until fully conscious. Up to 12 treatments may be given over a month, improvement usually showing after the third session. Widely used at one time, the treatment is now given only rarely. It can be extremely frightening for patients and relatives and is not recommended for children.

Electroencephalography (EEG)

In the BRAIN there is a regular, rhythmical change of electric potential, due to the rhythmic discharge of energy by nerve cells. These changes can be recorded graphically and the 'brain waves' examined – a procedure introduced to medicine in the 1920s. These records – electroencephalograms – are useful in DIAGNOSIS: for example, the abnormal electroencephalogram occurring in EPILEPSY is characteristic of this disease. The normal waves, known as alpha waves, occur with a frequency of 10 per second. Abnormal waves, with a frequency of 7 or fewer per second, are known as delta waves and occur in the region of cerebral tumours and in the brains of epileptics. An electroencephalogram can assess whether an individual is awake, alert or asleep. It may also be used during surgery to monitor the depth of unconsciousness in anaesthetised patients.

Electrolysis

The use of short-wave electric currents to destroy the roots of hairs (see SKIN) and so remove unwanted hair from the skin surface. If used by a trained operator, the procedure is safe, but care must be taken in the vicinity of the eyes and, as electrolysis of hair on the legs is such a lengthy process, it is best avoided there.

Electrolytes

Substances, for example, potassium chloride, whose molecules split into their constituent electrically charged particles, known as ions, when dissolved in fluid. In medicine the term is customarily used to describe the ion itself. The description 'serum electrolyte concentration' means the amounts of separate ions – for example, sodium and chloride in the case of salt – present in the serum of the circulating blood. Various diseases alter the amounts of electrolytes in the blood, either because more than normal are lost through vomiting or diarrhoea, or because electrolytes may be retained as the kidney fails to excrete them properly. Measurements of electrolytes are valuable clues to the type of disease, and provide a means of monitoring a course of treatment. Electrolyte imbalances can be corrected by administering appropriate substances orally or intravenously, or by DIALYSIS. (See APPENDIX 6: MEASUREMENTS IN MEDICINE.)

Electromyography (EMG)

The recording of electrical activity in a muscle using electrodes placed in the fibres. The procedure is used to diagnose muscle and nerve disorders and to assess recovery in certain types of paralysis.

Electron

One of the negatively charged subatomic particles distributed around a positive nucleus (positron) to form an atom. (See RADIOTHERAPY.)

Electronic Monitoring Devices

Electronically driven equipment that will constantly monitor the physiological status of patients and the effects of medical intervention on that status. Such devices should relieve hospital staff of time-consuming 'human monitoring' procedures and in some instances will enable patients to carry monitoring devices during their daily living activities. An example would be the regular assessment of blood-sugar concentration in subjects with DIABETES MELLITUS or the routine checking on the blood or tissue concentrations of administered drugs.

Electron Microscope

See MICROSCOPE.

Electro-Oculography

A method of recording movements of the eyes, which is of value in assessing the function of the retina (see EYE.)

Electrophoresis

The migration of charged particles between electrodes. A simple method of electrophoresis, known as paper electrophoresis, has been introduced to analyse PROTEIN in body fluids. This method consists in applying the protein-containing solution as a spot or a streak to a strip of filter paper which has been soaked in buffer solution and across the ends of which a potential difference is then applied for some hours. Comparison is made between filter strips of normal fluids and that of the patient under investigation. Identification and quantification

of proteins in the blood are possible using this method.

Electroretinogram

An electroretinogram is the record of an electrical response of visual receptors in the retina (see EYE), which can be measured with corneal electrodes.

Elephantiasis

Chronically oedematous (see OEDEMA) and thickened tissue, especially involving the lower extremities and genitalia, which arises from repeated attacks of inflammation of the skin and subcutaneous tissue, with concurrent obstruction of lymphatic vessels. In a tropical country, the usual cause is lymphatic FILARIASIS.

Filarial elephantiasis *Wuchereria bancrofti* and *Brugia malayi* are conveyed to humans by a mosquito bite. Resultant lymphatic obstruction gives rise to enlargement and disfiguration, with thickening of the skin (resembling that of an elephant) in one or both lower limbs and occasionally genitalia (involving particularly the SCROTUM). By the time the condition is recognised, lymphatic damage is irreversible. However, if evidence of continuing activity exists, a course of diethylcarbamazine should be administered (see FILARIASIS). Relief can be obtained by using elastic bandaging, massage, rest, and elevation of the affected limb. Surgery is sometimes indicated. For prevention, destruction of mosquitoes is important.

ELISA

See ENZYME-LINKED IMMUNOSORBENT ASSAY (ELISA).

Elixir

A liquid preparation of a potent or nauseous drug made pleasant to the taste by the addition of aromatic substances and sugar.

Emaciation

Pronounced wasting; a common symptom of many diseases, particularly those which are associated with a prolonged or repeated rise of temperature, such as TUBERCULOSIS. It is also associated with diseases of the alimentary system in which digestion is inefficient, or in which the food is not fully absorbed: for example, in long-standing diarrhoea, whatever its cause. It is also a marked feature of severe malnutrition and malignant disease.

Embalming

See DEAD, DISPOSAL OF THE.

Embolectomy

Surgical removal of a clot or EMBOLUS to clear an obstruction in an artery (see ARTERIES, DISEASES OF). The obstruction may be cleared by inserting a balloon (Fogarty) catheter (see CATHETERS) into the blood vessel or by surgical incision through the arterial wall. Embolectomy may be a life-saving operation when a patient has a PULMONARY EMBOLISM.

Embolism

The plugging of a small blood vessel by an EMBOLUS which has been carried through the larger vessels by the bloodstream. It is due usually to fragments of a clot which has formed in some vessel, or to small portions carried off from the edge of a heart-valve when this organ is diseased. However, the plug may also be a small mass of bacteria, or a fragment of a tumour, or even a mass of air bubbles sucked into the veins during operations on the neck. The result is usually more or less destruction of the organ or part of an organ supplied by the obstructed vessel. This is particularly the case in the BRAIN, where softening of the brain, with APHASIA or a STROKE, may be the result. If the plug is a fragment of malignant tumour, a new growth develops at the spot; if it is a mass of bacteria, an ABSCESS forms there. Air-embolism occasionally causes sudden death in the case of wounds in the neck, the air bubbles completely stopping the flow of blood. Fat-embolism is a condition which has been known to cause death – masses of fat, in consequence of such an injury as a fractured bone, finding their way into the circulation and stopping the blood in its passage through the lungs. (See also PULMONARY EMBOLISM.)

Embolus

Substances – for example, air, AMNIOTIC FLUID, blood clot, fat or foreign body – that are carried by the blood from a vessel (or vessels) in one part of the body to another part where the matter lodges in a blood vessel causing a blockage (see EMBOLISM).

Embrocations

Embrocations are mixtures, usually of an oily nature, intended for external application in cases of rheumatism, sprains, and other painful conditions. Their action is due mainly to the massage employed in rubbing in the embrocations, in part to the counter-irritant action of the drugs which they contain. (See LINIMENTS.)

Embryo

The FETUS in the womb prior to the end of the second month.

Embryology

The study of the growth and development of an EMBRYO and subsequently the FETUS from the fertilisation of the OVUM by the SPERMATOZOON through the gestational period until birth. Embryology is valuable in the understanding of adult anatomy, how the body works and the occurrence of CONGENITAL deformities.

Embryo Research

When a woman is treated for infertility it is necessary to nurture human embryos for a few days (until the first cell divisions of the fertilised egg have occurred) in a specialised laboratory. More eggs are fertilised than are usually needed because not all fertilisations are successful. Surplus embryos may be frozen for use in later attempts to implant an embryo in the womb. Research has been done on very early embryos but the practice is controversial and some countries have either forbidden it or imposed tight restrictions. In the UK such research is controlled by the government Human Fertilisation & Embryology Authority (see ASSISTED CONCEPTION).

Embryo Transfer

Embryo transfer is the process whereby the initial stages of procreation are produced outside the human body and completed in the uterus or womb. The procedure is also known as 'embryo transplantation' and 'in vitro fertilisation' (IVF). It consists of extracting an ovum (or egg) from the prospective mother's body and placing this in a dish where it is mixed with the male partner's SEMEN and special nutrient fluids. After the ovum is fertilised by the sperm it is transferred to another dish containing a special nutrient solution. Here it is left for several days while the normal early stages of development (see FETUS) take place. The early EMBRYO, as it has then become, is then implanted in the mother's uterus, where it 'takes root' and develops as a normal fetus.

The first 'test-tube baby' – to use the popular, and widely used, term for such a child – was born by CAESAREAN SECTION in England on 25 July 1978. Many other children conceived in this manner have since been born, and, though only 10 per cent of women conceive at the first attempt, the overall success rate is improving. Embryo transplantation and research are controversial procedures and in many countries, including the UK, are controlled by legislation. Embryo transfer and research using embryos are regulated by the Human Fertilisation & Embryology Authority (see ASSISTED CONCEPTION; APPENDIX 7: STATUTORY ORGANISATIONS).

Emergency

A condition that needs urgent medical care. Examples include life-threatening injuries involving blood loss or damage to major organs, cardiac arrest or sudden loss of consciousness from, say, a blow or an epileptic fit. Emergency is a term also applied to any resuscitative procedure that must be undertaken immediately – for instance, cardiopulmonary resuscitation (see APPENDIX 1: BASIC FIRST AID – Cardiac/respiratory arrest) or TRACHEOSTOMY. Patients with an emergency condition may initially be treated on the spot by suitably qualified paramedical staff before being transported by road or air ambulance to a hospital Accident and Emergency department, also known as an A&E or Casualty department. These departments are staffed by doctors and nurses experienced in dealing with emergencies; their first job when an emergency arrives is to conduct a TRIAGE assessment to decide the seriousness of the emergency and what priority the patient should be given in the context of other patients needing emergency care.

As their title shows, A&E departments (and the 999 and 112 telephone lines) are for patients who are genuine emergencies: namely, critical or life-threatening circumstances such as:
- unconsciousness.
- serious loss of blood.
- suspected broken bones.
- deep wound(s) such as a knife wound.
- suspected heart attack.
- difficulty in breathing.
- suspected injury to brain, chest or abdominal organs.
- fits.

To help people decide which medical service is most appropriate for them (or someone they are caring for or helping), the following questions should be answered:
- Could the symptoms be treated with an over-the-counter (OTC) medicine? If so, visit a pharmacist.
- Does the situation seem urgent? If so, call NHS Direct or the GP for telephone advice, and a surgery appointment may be the best action.
- Is the injured or ill person an obvious emergency (see above)? If so, go to the local A&E department or call 999 for an ambu-

lance, and be ready to give the name of the person involved, a brief description of the emergency and the place where it has occurred.

Emesis

Emesis means VOMITING.

Emetics

An emetic is a substance which induces VOMITING (emesis). Emetics were previously used for gut decontamination in the treatment of poisoning but are now considered obsolete. This is because the efficacy of emesis as a means of gut decontamination is unproved; there is a delay between administration and actual emesis, during which time continued absorption of the poison may occur; and some emetics have effects other than vomiting which may mask the clinical features of the ingested poison. The most commonly used emetic was syrup of ipecacuanha (ipecac). Salt (sodium chloride) water emetics were also used but there are many cases of fatal HYPERNATRAEMIA resulting from such use and salt water emetics should never be given. The most common method of gut decontamination currently used is the administration of activated CHARCOAL.

Emetine

The active principles of IPECACUANHA.

EMG

See ELECTROMYOGRAPHY (EMG).

Emission

A discharge. The term is commonly used to describe the orgasmic flow of SEMEN from the erect PENIS that occurs during sleep. Described as a nocturnal emission or, colloquially, as a 'wet dream', it is a common event in late PUBERTY.

EMLA

This is a proprietary brand of topical cream (the abbreviation stands for Eutectic Mixture of Local Anaesthetics). EMLA has revolutionised the care of children in hospital in the last decade by allowing blood-taking, lumbar puncture and other invasive procedures to be conducted relatively painlessly. It is applied to the skin and covered. After one hour the skin is anaesthetised.

Emmetropia

The normal condition of the EYE as regards refraction of light rays. When the muscles in the eyeball are completely relaxed, the focusing power is accurately adjusted for parallel rays, so that vision is perfect for distant objects.

Emollients

Emollients are substances which have a softening and soothing effect upon the skin. They include dusting powders such as French chalk, oils such as olive oil and almond oil, and fats such as the various pharmacopoeial preparations of paraffin, suet, and lard. Glycerin is also an excellent emollient.

Uses They are used in various inflammatory conditions such as eczema (see DERMATITIS), when the skin becomes hard, cracked, and painful. They may be used in the form of a dusting powder, an oil or an ointment.

Emotion

Mental arousal that the individual may find enjoyable or unpleasant. The three components are subjective, physiological and behavioural. The instinctive fear and flee response in animals comprises physiological reaction – raised heart rate, pallor and sweating – to an unpleasant event or stimulus. The loving relationship between mother and child is another well-recognised emotional event. If this emotional bond is absent or inadequate, the child may suffer emotional deprivation, which can be the trigger for behavioural problems ranging from attention-craving to aggression. Emotional problems are common in human society, covering a wide spectrum of psychological disturbances. Upbringing, relationships or psychiatric illnesses such as anxiety and DEPRESSION may all contribute to the development of emotional problems (see MENTAL ILLNESS).

Empathy

The facility to understand and be sympathetic to the feelings and thoughts of another individual. Empathy in the therapist is an essential component of successful psychotherapy and is a valuable characteristic in anyone who is a member of a caring profession.

Emphysema

The presence of air in the body's tissues. Divided into two types, surgical and pulmonary emphysema, the former occurs when air escapes from leaks in the LUNGS and OESOPHAGUS – perhaps as the result of injury or infection – and collects in the tissues of the chest and neck. Air occasionally escapes into other tissues as a result of surgery or injury, and bacterial infection can also produce gas in soft tissues (see gas gangrene under GANGRENE). Air or gas gives the affected

tissue an unmistakable crackling feel when touched. X-rays of an affected area will usually show the presence of air. Such air is generally absorbed by the body when the leak has been sealed.

The second type of emphysema affects the lung tissue and is called pulmonary emphysema. It is now grouped with other lung disorders such as chronic BRONCHITIS and some types of ASTHMA under the umbrella heading CHRONIC OBSTRUCTIVE PULMONARY DISEASE (COPD). See under this entry for further information.

Empirical

Method of treatment founded simply on experience rather than on scientific evidence from, for example, clinical trials. Because a given remedy has been successful in the treatment of a certain group of symptoms, it is assumed, by those who uphold this principle, that it will be successful in the treatment of other cases presenting similar groups of symptoms, without any inquiry as to the cause of the symptoms or reason underlying the action of the remedy. It is the contrary of 'rational' or 'scientific' treatment. Sometimes empirical treatment is a reasonable course of action where there is no known proven effective treatment for a condition.

Empyema

An accumulation of PUS within a cavity, the term being generally reserved for collections of pus within one of the pleural cavities (see LUNGS). Since the advent of antibiotics, the condition is relatively uncommon in developed countries. The condition is virtually an ABSCESS, and therefore gives rise to the general symptoms accompanying that condition. However, on account of the thick, unyielding wall of the chest, it is unlikely to burst through the surface, and therefore it is of particular importance that the condition should be recognised early and treated adequately.

The condition most commonly follows an attack of PNEUMONIA; it may also occur in the advanced stage of pulmonary TUBERCULOSIS. Empyema also occurs at times through infection from some more serious disease in neighbouring organs, such as cancer of the GULLET, or follows upon wounds penetrating the chest wall.

Treatment may be by surgery or by drainage through a tube inserted into the pleural cavity, combined with instillation of agents which break down the secretions.

Emulsions

Emulsions are oil-in-water or water-in-oil dispersions. Therapeutic emulsions (creams) require an added stabilising substance.

Enamel

See TEETH.

Encephalin

A naturally occurring brain PEPTIDE, the effects of which resemble those of MORPHINE or other opiates (see ENDORPHINS; ENKEPHALINS).

Encephalitis

Encephalitis means inflammation or infection of the brain, usually caused by a virus; it may also be the result of bacterial infection. It occurs throughout the world and affects all racial groups and ages. Rarely it occurs as a complication of common viral disease such as measles, mumps, glandular fever, or chickenpox. It may occur with no evidence of infection elsewhere, such as in HERPES SIMPLEX encephalitis, the most common form seen in Europe and America. RABIES is another form of viral encephalitis, and the HIV virus which causes AIDS invades the brain to cause another form of encephalitis (see AIDS/HIV). In some countries – North and South America, Japan and east Asia and Russia – there may be epidemics spread by the bite of mosquitoes or ticks.

The clinical features begin with influenza-like symptoms – aches, temperature and wretchedness; then the patient develops a headache with drowsiness, confusion and neck stiffness. Severely ill patients develop changes in behaviour, abnormalities of speech, and deterioration, sometimes with epileptic seizures. Some develop paralysis and memory loss. CT (see COMPUTED TOMOGRAPHY) and MRI brain scans show brain swelling, and damage to the temporal lobes if the herpes virus is involved. ELECTROENCEPHALOGRAPHY (EEG), which records the brainwaves, is abnormal. Diagnosis is possible by an examination of the blood or other body fluids for antibody reaction to the virus, and modern laboratory techniques are very specific.

In general, drugs are not effective against viruses – antibiotics are of no use. Herpes encephalitis does respond to treatment with the antiviral agent, aciclovir. Treatment is supportive: patients should be given painkillers, and fluid replacement drugs to reduce brain swelling and counter epilepsy if it occurs. Fortunately, most sufferers from encephalitis make a complete recovery, but some are left severely disabled with physical defects, personality and memory

disturbance, and epileptic fits. Rabies is always fatal and the changes found in patients with AIDS are almost always progressive. Except in very specific circumstances, it is not possible to be immunised against encephalitis.

Encephalitis lethargica is one, now rare, variety that reached epidemic levels after World War I. It was characterised by drowsiness and headache leading on to COMA. The disease occasionally occurs as a complication after mumps and sometimes affected individuals subsequently develop postencephalitic PARKINSONISM.

Encephaloid

A form of cancer which, to the naked eye, resembles the tissue of the brain.

Encephalomyelitis

Inflammation of the substance of both brain and spinal cord.

Encephalopathy

The term covering certain conditions in which there are signs of cerebral irritation without any localised lesion to account for them. Examples are HYPERTENSIVE ENCEPHALOPATHY, SPONGIFORM ENCEPHALOPATHY, WERNICKE'S ENCEPHALOPATHY and lead encephalopathy. In the first, which occurs in the later stages of chronic glomerulonephritis (see KIDNEYS, DISEASES OF), or URAEMIA, the headache, convulsions and delirium which constitute the main symptoms are supposed to be due to a deficient blood supply to the brain.

Enchondroma

A TUMOUR formed of cartilage.

Encysted

Enclosed within a bladder-like wall. The term is applied to parasites, collections of pus, etc., which are shut off from surrounding tissues by a membrane or by adhesions.

Endarterectomy

Surgical reopening of an artery obstructed by ATHEROMA. If a blood clot is present, the reboring process is called thromboendarterectomy. Restored patency allows arterial blood supply to restart. The carotid arteries and arteries to the legs are those most commonly operated on.

Endarteritis

Inflammation of the inner coat of an artery. (See ARTERIES, DISEASES OF.)

Endemic

A term applied to diseases which exist in particular localities or among certain races. Some diseases, which are at times EPIDEMIC over wide districts, have a restricted area where they are always endemic, and from which they spread. For example, both CHOLERA and PLAGUE are endemic in certain parts of Asia.

Endo-

Prefix meaning situated inside.

Endocarditis

Inflammation of the lining, valves and muscle of the HEART. The main causes are bacterial and virus infections and rheumatic fever, and the condition occurs most often in patients whose ENDOCARDIUM is already damaged by congenital deformities or whose immune system has been suppressed by drugs. Infection may be introduced into the bloodstream during dental treatment or surgical procedures, especially on the heart or on the gastrointestinal system. The condition is potentially very serious and treatment is with large doses of antibiotic drugs. (See HEART, DISEASES OF.)

Endocardium

A thin membrane consisting of flat endothelial cells; it lines the four chambers of the HEART and is continuous with the lining of arteries and veins. The endocardium has a smooth surface which helps the blood to flow easily. The valves at the openings of the heart's chambers are made from folded-up membranes. Inflammation of the endocardium is called ENDOCARDITIS.

Endocrine Glands

Organs whose function it is to secrete into the blood or lymph, substances known as HORMONES. These play an important part in general changes to or the activities of other organs at a distance. Various diseases arise as the result of defects or excess in the internal secretions of the different glands. The chief endocrine glands are:

Adrenal glands These two glands, also known as suprarenal glands, lie immediately above the kidneys. The central or medullary portion of the glands forms the secretions known as ADRENALINE (or epinephrine) and NORADRENALINE. Adrenaline acts upon structures innervated by sympathetic nerves. Briefly, the blood vessels of the skin and of the abdominal viscera (except the intestines) are constricted, and at the same time the arteries of the muscles and the coronary arteries are dilated; systolic blood pressure rises; blood sugar increases; the metabolic rate rises; muscle fatigue is diminished. The superficial or cortical part of the glands produces steroid-based substances such as aldosterone, cortisone, hydrocortisone, and deoxycortone acetate, for the maintenance of life. It is the absence of these substances, due to atrophy or destruction of the suprarenal cortex, that is responsible for the condition known as ADDISON'S DISEASE. (See CORTICOSTEROIDS.)

Ovaries and testicles The ovary (see OVARIES) secretes at least two hormones – known, respectively, as oestradiol (follicular hormone) and progesterone (corpus luteum hormone). Oestradiol develops (under the stimulus of the anterior pituitary lobe – see PITUITARY GLAND below, and under separate entry) each time an ovum in the ovary becomes mature, and causes extensive proliferation of the ENDOMETRIUM lining the UTERUS, a stage ending with shedding of the ovum about 14 days before the onset of MENSTRUATION. The corpus luteum, which then forms, secretes both progesterone and oestradiol. Progesterone brings about great activity of the glands in the endometrium. The uterus is now ready to receive the ovum if it is fertilised. If fertilisation does not occur, the corpus luteum degenerates, the hormones cease acting, and menstruation takes place.

The hormone secreted by the testicles (see TESTICLE) is known as TESTOSTERONE. It is responsible for the growth of the male secondary sex characteristics.

Pancreas This gland is situated in the upper part of the abdomen and, in addition to digestive enzymes, it produces INSULIN within specialised cells (islets of Langerhans). This controls carbohydrate metabolism; faulty or absent insulin production causes DIABETES MELLITUS.

Parathyroid glands These are four minute glands lying at the side of, or behind, the thyroid (see below). They have a certain effect in controlling the absorption of calcium salts by the bones and other tissues. When their secretion is defective, TETANY occurs.

Pituitary gland This gland is attached to the base of the brain and rests in a hollow on the base of the skull. It is the most important of all endocrine glands and consists of two embryologically and functionally distinct lobes.

The function of the anterior lobe depends on the secretion by the HYPOTHALAMUS of certain 'neuro-hormones' which control the secretion of the pituitary trophic hormones. The hypothalamic centres involved in the control of specific pituitary hormones appear to be anatomically separate. Through the pituitary trophic hormones the activity of the thyroid, adrenal cortex and the sex glands is controlled. The anterior pituitary and the target glands are linked through a feedback control cycle. The liberation of trophic hormones is inhibited by a rising concentration of the circulating hormone of the target gland, and stimulated by a fall in its concentration. Six trophic (polypeptide) hormones are formed by the anterior pituitary. Growth hormone (GH) and prolactin are simple proteins formed in the acidophil cells. Follicle-stimulating hormone (FSH), luteinising hormone (LH) and thyroid-stimulating hormone (TSH) are glycoproteins formed in the basophil cells. Adrenocorticotrophic hormone (ACTH), although a polypeptide, is derived from basophil cells.

The posterior pituitary lobe, or neurohypophysis, is closely connected with the hypothalamus by the hypothalamic-hypophyseal tracts. It is concerned with the production or storage of OXYTOCIN and vasopressin (the antidiuretic hormone).

PITUITARY HORMONES Growth hormone, gonadotrophic hormone, adrenocorticotrophic hormone and thyrotrophic hormones can be assayed in blood or urine by radio-immunoassay techniques. Growth hormone extracted from human pituitary glands obtained at autopsy was available for clinical use until 1985, when it was withdrawn as it is believed to carry the virus responsible for CREUTZFELDT-JAKOB DISEASE (COD). However, growth hormone produced by DNA recombinant techniques is now available as somatropin. Synthetic growth hormone is used to treat deficiency of the natural hormone in children and adults, TURNER'S SYNDROME and chronic renal insufficiency in children.

Human pituitary gonadotrophins are readily obtained from post-menopausal urine. Commercial extracts from this source are available and are effective for treatment of infertility due to gonadotrophin insufficiency.

The adrenocorticotrophic hormone is extracted from animal pituitary glands and has been available therapeutically for many years. It is used as a test of adrenal function, and, under certain circumstances, in conditions for which corticosteroid therapy is indicated (see CORTI-

COSTEROIDS). The pharmacologically active polypeptide of ACTH has been synthesised and is called tetracosactrin. Thyrotrophic hormone is also available but it has no therapeutic application.

HYPOTHALAMIC RELEASING HORMONES which affect the release of each of the six anterior pituitary hormones have been identified. Their blood levels are only one-thousandth of those of the pituitary trophic hormones. The release of thyrotrophin, adrenocorticotrophin, growth hormone, follicle-stimulating hormone and luteinising hormone is stimulated, while release of prolactin is inhibited. The structure of the releasing hormones for TSH, FSH-LH, GH and, most recently, ACTH is known and they have all been synthesised. Thyrotrophin-releasing hormone (TRH) is used as a diagnostic test of thyroid function but it has no therapeutic application. FSH-LH-releasing hormone provides a useful diagnostic test of gonadotrophin reserve in patients with pituitary disease, and is now used in the treatment of infertility and AMENORRHOEA in patients with functional hypothalamic disturbance. As this is the most common variety of secondary amenorrhoea, the potential use is great. Most cases of congenital deficiency of GH, FSH, LH and ACTH are due to defects in the hypothalamic production of releasing hormone and are not a primary pituitary defect, so that the therapeutic implication of this synthesised group of releasing hormones is considerable.

GALACTORRHOEA is frequently due to a microadenoma (see ADENOMA) of the pituitary. DOPAMINE is the prolactin-release inhibiting hormone. Its duration of action is short so its therapeutic value is limited. However, BROMOCRIPTINE is a dopamine agonist with a more prolonged action and is effective treatment for galactorrhoea.

Thyroid gland The functions of the thyroid gland are controlled by the pituitary gland (see above) and the hypothalamus, situated in the brain. The thyroid, situated in the front of the neck below the LARYNX, helps to regulate the body's METABOLISM. It comprises two lobes each side of the TRACHEA joined by an isthmus. Two types of secretory cells in the gland – follicular cells (the majority) and parafollicular cells – secrete, respectively, the iodine-containing hormones THYROXINE (T_4) and TRI-IODOTHYRONINE (T_3), and the hormone CALCITONIN. T_3 and T_4 help control metabolism and calcitonin, in conjunction with parathyroid hormone (see above), regulates the body's calcium balance. Deficiencies in thyroid function produce HYPOTHYROIDISM and, in children, retarded development. Excess thyroid activity causes thyrotoxicosis. (See THYROID GLAND, DISEASES OF.)

Endocrinology
The study of the endocrine system, the substances (hormones) it secretes and its disorders (see ENDOCRINE GLANDS.)

Endoderm
The inner layer of the three germ layers of the EMBRYO during its early development. The endoderm develops into the lining of the gastrointestinal tract and associated glands (LIVER; gall-bladder – see LIVER; PANCREAS), the lining of the bronchi and alveoli of the LUNGS and much of the URINARY TRACT.

Endogenous
Coming from within the body. Endogenous depression, for instance, occurs as a result of causes inside a person.

Endolymph
The fluid that fills the membranous labyrinth of the inner ear (see EAR).

Endometriosis
The condition in which the endometrium (the cells lining the interior of the UTERUS) is found in other parts of the body. The most common site of such misplaced endometrium is the muscle of the uterus. The next most common site is the ovary (see OVARIES), followed by the PERITONEUM lining the PELVIS, but it also occurs anywhere in the bowel. The cause is not known. Endometriosis never occurs before puberty and seldom after the menopause. The main symptoms it produces are MENOR-RHAGIA, DYSPAREUNIA, painful MENSTRUATION and pelvic pain. Treatment is usually by removal of the affected area, but in some cases satisfactory results are obtained from the administration of a PROGESTOGEN such as NORETHISTERONE, norethynodrel and DANAZOL.

Endometritis
Inflammation of the mucous membrane lining the womb. (See UTERUS, DISEASES OF.)

Endometrium
The mucous membrane which lines the interior of the UTERUS.

End Organ
A structure at the end of a peripheral nerve that acts as receptor for a sensation. For example, the olfactory nerves have end organs that identify smells.

Endorphins
Peptides (see PEPTIDE) produced in the brain which have a pain-relieving action; hence their alternative name of opiate peptides. Their name is derived from endogenous MORPHINE. They have been defined as endogenous opiates or any naturally occurring substances in the brain with pharmacological actions resembling opiate alkaloids such as morphine. There is some evidence that the pain-relieving action of ACU-PUNCTURE may be due to the release of these opiate peptides. It has also been suggested that they may have an antipsychotic action and therefore be of value in the treatment of major psychotic illnesses such as SCHIZOPHRENIA.

Endoscope
A tube-shaped instrument inserted into a cavity in the body to investigate and treat disorders. It is flexible and equipped with lenses and a light source. Examples of endoscopes are the CYSTO-SCOPE for use in the bladder, the GASTROSCOPE for examining the stomach and the ARTHRO-SCOPE for looking into joints (see also FIBREOP-TIC ENDOSCOPY).

Endoscopic Retrograde Cholangiopancreatography (ERCP)
This is a procedure in which a catheter (see CATHETERS) is passed via an ENDOSCOPE into the AMPULLA OF VATER of the common BILE DUCT. The duct is then injected with a radio-opaque material to show up the ducts radio-logically. The technique is used to diagnose pancreatic disease as well as obstructive jaundice.

Endoscopy
Examination of a body cavity – for example, PLEURAL CAVITY, GASTROINTESTINAL TRACT, BILE DUCT and URINARY BLADDER – using an ENDOSCOPE in order to diagnose or treat a disorder in the cavity. The development of endoscopy has reduced the need for major surgery, as many diagnostic procedures can be performed with an endoscope (as can MINIMALLY INVASIVE SURGERY (MIS)). The development of fibre optics (the transmission of light along bundles of glass or plastic fibres) has greatly advanced the practice of endoscopy and hospitals now routinely run endoscopy clinics on

E

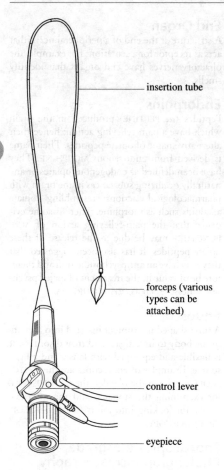

insertion tube

forceps (various types can be attached)

control lever

eyepiece

an out-patient basis, often without the necessity for a general anaesthetic.

Endothelium

The membrane lining various vessels and cavities of the body, such as the pleura (lining the lung), the pericardium (lining the heart), the peritoneum (lining the abdomen and abdominal organs), the lymphatic vessels, blood vessels, and joints. It consists of a fibrous layer covered with thin flat cells, which render the surface perfectly smooth and secrete the fluid for its lubrication.

Endotoxin

A poison produced by certain gram-negative bacteria that is released after the microorganisms die. Endotoxins can cause fever and shock, the latter by rendering the walls of blood vessels permeable so that fluid leaks into the tissues, with a consequent sharp fall in blood pressure. (See EXOTOXIN.)

Endotracheal Intubation

Insertion of a rubber or plastic tube through the nose or mouth into the TRACHEA. The tube often has a cuff at its lower end which, when inflated, provides an airtight seal. This allows an anaesthetist to supply oxygen or anaesthetic gases to the lungs with the knowledge of exactly how much the patient is receiving. Endotracheal intubation is necessary to undertake artificial ventilation of a patient (see ANAESTHESIA).

Enema

Introduction of fluid into the RECTUM via the

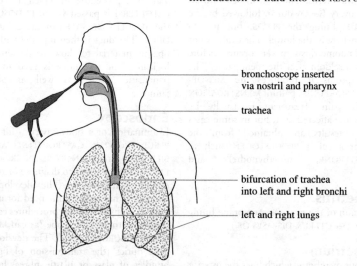

bronchoscope inserted via nostril and pharynx

trachea

bifurcation of trachea into left and right bronchi

left and right lungs

A fibreoptic bronchoscope used to examine the larger bronchial tubes of the lungs to determine, for example, whether a tumour is present.

E

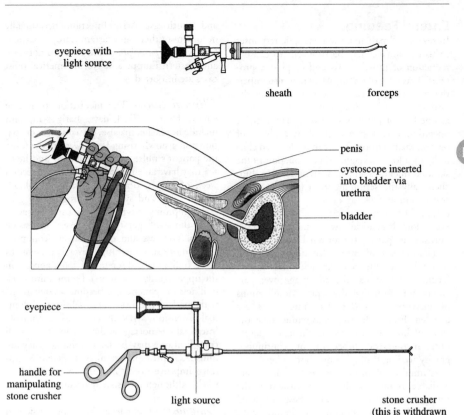

eyepiece with light source

sheath

forceps

penis

cystoscope inserted into bladder via urethra

bladder

eyepiece

handle for manipulating stone crusher

light source

stone crusher (this is withdrawn to enable operator to view pelvis)

Percutaneous nephroscope used for examining the interior of the kidney. It is passed into the pelvis of the kidney through a track from the surface of the skin. (The track is made with a needle and guide wire.) Instruments can be passed through the nephroscope under direct vision to remove calculi.

ANUS. Enemas may be given to clear the intestine of faeces prior to intestinal surgery or to relieve severe constipation. They may also be used to give barium for diagnostic X-rays as well as drugs such as CORTICOSTEROIDS, used to treat ULCERATIVE COLITIS. The patient is placed on his or her side with a support under the hips. A catheter (see CATHETERS) with a lubricated end is inserted into the rectum and warmed enema fluid gently injected. Disposable enemas and miniature enemas, which can be self-administered, are widely used; they contain preprepared solution.

Enflurane
A volatile inhalational anaesthetic similar to HALOTHANE but less potent and less likely to have toxic effects on the LIVER.

Engagement
The event during pregnancy when the present-ing part of the baby, usually the head, moves down into the mother's pelvis. (See PREGNANCY AND LABOUR.)

Enkephalins
Peptides (see PEPTIDE) that have a pain-killing effect similar to that of ENDORPHINS. Produced by certain nerve endings and in the brain, enkephalins (also spelt encephalins) are also believed to act as a sedative and mood-changer.

Enophthalmos
Abnormal retraction of the eye into its socket: for example, when the sympathetic nerve in the neck is paralysed.

Entamoeba
See AMOEBA.

ENT Disorders
See OTORHINOLARYNGOLOGY.

Enteral Feeding

In severely ill patients, the metabolic responses to tissue damage may be sufficient to cause a reduction of muscle mass and of plasma proteins. This state of CATABOLISM may also impair the immune response to infection and delay the healing of wounds. It is probable that as many as one-half of patients who have had a major operation a week previously show evidence of protein malnutrition. This can be detected clinically by a loss of weight and a reduction in the skinfold thickness and arm circumference. Biochemically the serum-albumin (see ALBUMINS) concentration falls, as does the LYMPHOCYTE count. The protein reserves of the body fall even more dramatically when there are SEPSIS, burns, acute pancreatitis or renal failure.

The purpose of enteral feeding is to give a liquid, low-residue food through a naso-gastric feeding tube. It has the advantage over parenteral nutrition that the septic complications of insertion of CATHETERS into veins are avoided. Enteral feeding may either take the form of intermittent feeding through a large-bore naso-gastric tube, or of continuous gravity-feeding through a fine-bore tube.

A number of proprietary enteral foods are available. Some contain whole protein as the nitrogen source; others – and these are called elemental diets – contain free amino acids. DIARRHOEA is the most common problem with enteral feeding and it tends to occur when enteral feeding is introduced too rapidly or with too strong a preparation.

Enteralgia

Another name for COLIC.

Enteric-Coated

A description of tablets covered in material that allows them to pass through the stomach and enter the intestine unaltered. Drugs coated in this way are those whose action is reduced or stopped by acid in the stomach.

Enteric Fever

Enteric fever is caused by bacterial infection with either *Salmonella typhi* or *Salmonella paratyphi* A, B or C. These infections are called typhoid fever, or paratyphoid fever respectively. Transmission usually occurs by ingestion of water or food that has been contaminated with human faeces – for example, by drinking water contaminated with sewage, or eating foods prepared by a cook infected with or carrying the organisms. Enteric fever is ENDEMIC in many areas of the world, including Africa, Central and South America, the Indian subcontinent and south-east Asia. Infection occasionally occurs in southern and eastern Europe, particularly with *S. paratyphi* B. However, in northern and western Europe and North America, most cases are imported.

Clinical course The incubation period of enteric fever is 7–21 days. Early symptoms include headache, malaise, dry cough, constipation and a slowly rising fever. Despite the fever, the patient's pulse rate is often slow and he or she may have an enlarged SPLEEN. In the second week of illness, organisms invade the bloodstream again and symptoms progress. In general, symptoms of typhoid fever are more severe than those of paratyphoid fever: increasing mental slowness and confusion are common, and a more sustained high fever is present. In some individuals, discrete red spots appear on the upper trunk (rose spots). By the third week of illness the patient may become severely toxic, with marked confusion and delirium, abdominal distension, MYOCARDITIS, and occasionally intestinal haemorrage and/or perforation. Such complications may be fatal, although they are unusual if prompt treatment is given. Symptoms improve slowly into the fourth and fifth weeks, although relapse may occur.

Diagnosis Enteric fever should be considered in any traveller or resident in an ENDEMIC area presenting with a febrile illness. The most common differential diagnosis is MALARIA. Diagnosis is usually made by isolation of the organism from cultures of blood in the first two weeks of illness. Later the organisms are found in the stools and urine. Serological tests for ANTIBODIES against *Salmonella typhi* antigens (see ANTIGEN) (the Widal test) are less useful due to cross-reactions with antigens on other bacteria, and difficulties with interpretation in individuals immunised with typhoid vaccines.

Treatment Where facilities are available, hospital admission is required. Antibiotic therapy with chloramphenicol or amoxycillin is effective. However, the potential toxicity of the former and the widespread resistance that has developed to both these antibiotics has led to the use of QUINOLONES such as CIPROFLOXACIN as the initial therapy for enteric fever in the UK and in areas where resistant organisms are common. A few individuals become chronic carriers of the organisms after they have recovered from the symptoms. These people are a potential source of spread to others and should be excluded from occupations that involve handling food or drinking-water.

Prolonged courses of antibiotic therapy may be required to eradicate carriage.

Prevention Worldwide, the most important preventive measure is improvement of sanitation and maintenance of clean water supplies. Vaccination is available for travellers to endemic areas.

Enteritis

Enteritis means inflammation of the intestines. (See DIARRHOEA; INTESTINE, DISEASES OF.)

Enterobiasis

Infection with *Enterobius vermicularis*, the threadworm (or pinworm as it is known in the USA). It is the most common of all the intestinal parasites in Britain, and the least harmful. The male is about 6 mm (¼ inch) in length and the female about 12 mm (½ inch) in length. Each resembles a little piece of thread. These worms live in considerable numbers in the lower bowel, affecting children particularly. They usually cause no symptoms but can result in great irritation round the anus or within the female genitalia, especially at night when the female worm emerges from the anus to lay its eggs and then die. The most effective form of treatment is either viprynium embonate or piperazine citrate, which needs to be taken by the whole family. Bedclothes must then be laundered.

Enterocele

A HERNIA of the bowel.

Enterogastrone

A hormone derived from the mucosal lining of the small intestine which inhibits the movements and secretion of the stomach.

Enterokinase

The ENZYME secreted in the DUODENUM and jejunum (see INTESTINE) which converts the enzyme, trypsinogen, secreted by the PANCREAS, into TRYPSIN. (See also DIGESTION.)

Enteroptosis

A condition in which, owing to a lax condition of the mesenteries (see MESENTERY) and ligaments which support the intestines, the latter descend into the lower part of the abdominal cavity.

Enterostomy

An operation by which an artificial opening is formed into the intestine and joined to another part of the intestine or brought to the exterior via the abdominal wall.

Enterotoxin

A type of toxin (see TOXINS) that causes inflammation of the intestinal lining and results in vomiting and diarrhoea (see FOOD POISONING).

Enteroviruses

A family of VIRUSES which include the POLIO-MYELITIS, COXSACKIE and ECHO (see ECHOVIRUSES) groups of viruses. Their importance lies in their tendency to invade the central nervous system. They receive their name from the fact that their mode of entry into the body is through the gut.

Entonox

A proprietary analgesic drug taken by inhalation and comprising half nitrous oxide and half oxygen. It is valuable in providing relief to casualties who are in pain, as it provides analgesia without making them unconscious. Entonox is also used in obstetric practice to ease the pains of childbirth.

Entropion

See EYE, DISORDERS OF.

Enuresis

Bed-wetting, or the involuntary passage of urine at night. It can occur at all ages but is a particular problem with children and the elderly. In general, paediatricians prefer not to treat enuresis much before the age of six, as it may be a normal phenomenon and usually stops as the child grows older. However, when the condition persists, the child (and parents) need advice. Treatment is by positive reinforcement of bladder control, alarm systems such as the 'pad and bell', or ocasionally by drugs such as Desmopressin, which reduces night-time urinary output. Some children have an 'irritable bladder' and can be helped by drugs which relieve this. Enuresis is often a result of psychological disturbance, particularly where family relationships are disrupted. In this circumstance medication is unlikely to be effective.

Constipation is a common cause of urinary incontinence – and hence bed-wetting – in the elderly and should be treated. Enuresis in the elderly may also be due to organic disease or to mental deterioration and confusion. Appropriate investigation, treatment and nursing should be arranged. (See NOCTURNAL ENURESIS.)

Advice is available from the Enuresis Resource and Information Centre (ERIC) whose weekday helpline is 0117 960 3060. Also www.eric.org.uk

Environmental Health Officer

A local-authority health official specially qualified in aspects of environmental health such as clean air, food hygiene, housing, pollution, sanitation and water supplies. He or she is responsible for running the authority's environmental health department and, when epidemiological advice is needed, the relevant public-health physician acts in a consultative capacity (see EPIDEMIOLOGY; PUBLIC HEALTH).

Environmental Medicine

The study of the consequences for people's health of the natural environment. This includes the effects of climate, geography, sunlight and natural vegetation.

Environment and Health

Environment and Health concerns those aspects of human health, including quality of life, that are determined by physical, biological, social and psychosocial factors in the environment. The promotion of good health requires not only public policies which support health, but also the creation of supportive environments in which living and working conditions are safe, stimulating and enjoyable.

Health has driven much of environmental policy since the work of Edwin Chadwick in the early 1840s. The first British public-health act was introduced in 1848 to improve housing and sanitation with subsequent provision of purified water, clean milk, food hygiene regulations, vaccinations and antibiotics. In the 21st century there are now many additional environmental factors that must be monitored, researched and controlled if risks to human health are to be well managed and the impact on human morbidity and mortality reduced.

Environmental impacts on health include:
- noise
- air pollution
- water pollution
- dust
- odours
- contaminated ground
- loss of amenities
- vermin
- vibration
- animal diseases

Environmental risk factors Many of the major determinants of health, disease and death are environmental risk factors. Some are natural hazards; others are generated by human activities. They may be directly harmful, as in the examples of exposure to toxic chemicals at work, pesticides, or air pollution from road transport, or to radon gas penetrating domestic properties. Environmental factors may also alter people's susceptibility to disease: for example, the availability of sufficient food. In addition, they may operate by making unhealthy choices more likely, such as the availability and affordability of junk foods, alcohol, illegal drugs or tobacco.

Populations at risk Children are among the populations most sensitive to environmental health hazards. Their routine exposure to toxic chemicals in homes and communities can put their health at risk. Central to the ability to protect communities and families is the right of people to know about toxic substances. For many, the only source of environmental information is media reporting, which often leaves the public confused and frustrated. To benefit from public access to information, increasingly via the Internet, people need basic environmental and health information, resources for interpreting, understanding and evaluating health risks, and familiarity with strategies for prevention or reduction of risk.

Risk assessment Environmental health experts rely on the principles of environmental toxicology and risk assessment to evaluate the environment and the potential effects on individual and community health. Key actions include:
- identifying sources and routes of environmental exposure and recommending methods of reducing environmental health risks, such as exposure to heavy metals, solvents, pesticides, dioxins, etc.
- assessing the risks of exposure-related health hazards.
- alerting health professionals, the public, and the media to the levels of risk for particular potential hazards and the reasons for interventions.
- ensuring that doctors and scientists explain the results of environmental monitoring studies – for example, the results of water fluoridation in the UK to improve dental health.

National policies In the United Kingdom in 1996, an important step in linking environment and health was taken by a government-initiated joint consultation by the Departments of Health and Environment about adding 'environment' as a key area within the *Health of*

the Nation strategy. The first UK Minister of State for Public Health was appointed in 1997 with responsibilities for health promotion and public-health issues, both generally and within the NHS. These responsibilities include the implementation of the *Health of the Nation* strategy and its successor, *Our Healthy Nation*. The aim is to raise the priority given to human health throughout government departments, and to make health and environmental impact assessment a routine part of the making, implementing and assessing the impact of policies.

Global environmental risks The scope of many environmental threats to human health are international and cannot be regulated effectively on a local, regional or even national basis. One example is the Chernobyl nuclear reactor accident, which led to a major release of radiation, the effects of which were felt in many countries. Some international action has already been taken to tackle global environmental problems, but governments should routinely measure the overall impacts of development on people and their environments and link with industry to reduce damage to the environment. For instance, the effects of global warming and pollution on health should be assessed within an ecological framework if communities are to respond effectively to potential new global threats to the environment.

Enzyme

A protein that acts as a catalyst for the body's metabolic processes. The body contains thousands of enzymes, with each cell producing several varieties. The first enzyme was obtained in a reasonably pure state in 1926. Since then, several hundred enzymes have been obtained in pure crystalline form. They are present in the digestive fluids and in many of the tissues, and are capable of producing in small amounts the transformation on a large scale of various compounds. Examples of enzymes are found in the PTYALIN of saliva and DIASTASE of pancreatic juice which split up starch into sugar; the PEPSIN of the gastric juice and the trypsin of pancreatic juice which break proteins into simpler molecules and eventually into the constituent amino acids; and the thrombin of the blood which causes coagulation.

The diagnosis of certain disorders can be helped by measuring the concentrations of various enzymes in the blood. After a heart attack (myocardial infarction – see HEART, DISEASES OF), raised levels of heart enzymes occur as a result of damage to the cells of the heart muscle. Some inherited diseases such as GALACTOSAEMIA and PHENYLKETONURIA are the result of deficiencies of certain enzymes.

Enzymes can be a useful part of treatment for some disorders. STREPTOKINASE, for example, is used to treat THROMBOSIS; wound-dressings containing papain from the pawpaw fruit – this contains protein-digesting enzymes – assist in the healing process; and pancreatic enzymes can be of value to patients with malabsorption caused by disorders of the PANCREAS.

Enzyme-Linked Immunosorbent Assay (ELISA)

This is a sensitive method for measuring the quantity of a substance. An antibody to the substance is prepared along with an ENZYME which binds to the antibody and which can be accurately measured using colour changes that occur as a result of the chemical reaction.

Eosinophil

Any cell in the body with granules in its substance that stain easily with the dye, eosin. Granulocytes which form about 2 per cent of the white cells of the blood are eosinophils.

Eosinophilia

Eosinophilia means an abnormal increase in the number of eosinophils (see EOSINOPHIL) in the blood. It occurs in Hodgkin's disease (see LYMPHOMA), in ASTHMA and hay fever, in some skin diseases, and in parasitic infestation.

Ephedrine

An alkaloid (see ALKALOIDS) derived from a species of *Ephedra* or prepared synthetically. A BRONCHODILATOR, it was once widely used to treat asthma, but has now been superseded by the much safer (and more effective) selective beta-2-adrenoceptor stimulants (see ADRENERGIC RECEPTORS). Ephedrine is a constituent of several decongestant cold and cough remedies available to the general public.

Ephelides

The technical term for FRECKLES.

Ephelis

See EPHELIDES.

Epi-

A prefix meaning situated on or outside of.

Epicanthic Fold

A vertical skinfold that runs from the upper eyelid to the side of the nose. These folds are normal in oriental races but uncommon in others, although babies may have a temporary fold that disappears. Folds are present in people with DOWN'S (DOWN) SYNDROME.

Epicondyle

The protuberance above a CONDYLE at the end of a bone with an articulating joint – for example, at the bottom of the humerus, the bone of the upper arm.

Epidemic

Epidemic is a term applied to a disease which affects a large number of people in a particular locality at one time. The term is, in a sense, opposed to ENDEMIC, which means a disease always found in the locality in question. A disease may, however, be endemic as a rule – for example, MALARIA in swampy districts – and may become at times epidemic, when an unusually large number of people are affected. The rapid expansion of air travel has extended the scope for the spread of epidemic and endemic disease.

An epidemic disease is usually infectious from person to person, but not necessarily so since many persons in a locality may simply be exposed to the same cause at one time; for example, outbreaks of lead-poisoning are epidemic in this sense.

The conditions which govern the outbreak of epidemics are poorly understood, but include infected food supplies, such as drinking water contaminated by waste from people with CHOLERA or typhoid fever (see ENTERIC FEVER); milk infected with TUBERCLE bacillus; or 'fast food' products contaminated with salmonella. The migrations of certain animals, such as rats, are in some cases responsible for the spread of PLAGUE, from which these animals die in great numbers. Certain epidemics occur at certain seasons: for example, whooping-cough occurs in spring, whereas measles produces two epidemics – as a rule, one in winter and one in March. Influenza, the common cold, and other infections of the upper respiratory tract, such as sore throat, occur predominantly in the winter.

There is another variation, both as regards the number of persons affected and the number who die in successive epidemics: the severity of successive epidemics rises and falls over periods of five or ten years.

Epidemiology

The study of disease as it affects groups of people. Originating in the study of epidemics of diseases like CHOLERA, PLAGUE and SMALLPOX, epidemiology is an important discipline which contributes to the control not only of infectious diseases but also of conditions such as heart disease and cancer. Their distributions in populations can provide important pointers to possible causes. The relation between the environment and disease is an essential part of epidemiology. (See ENVIRONMENT AND HEALTH; PUBLIC HEALTH.)

Epidermis

The outer layer of the SKIN, which forms the protective covering of the body.

Epidermophyton

A fungus infection of the skin causing RINGWORM or tinea.

Epididymis

An oblong body attached to the upper part of each TESTICLE, composed of convoluted vessels and ducts, that connects the VASA EFFERENTIA to the VAS DEFERENS. Sperm cells produced in the testis pass along the epididymis, maturing as they go, to be stored in the seminal vesicles until EJACULATION occurs. The epididymis may be damaged by trauma or infection resulting sometimes in sterility. Cysts may also occur.

Epidural Anaesthesia

See ANAESTHESIA.

Epigastrium

The region lying in the middle of the ABDOMEN over the stomach.

Epigenetics

The science of how the activity of DNA (deoxyribonucleic acid, which is the fundamental genetic material of cells) can be altered semipermanently by chemical processes rather than by natural MUTATION. Genes contain instructions for making proteins. The natural process of implementing these instructions – gene expression – can be altered by chemical groups attaching themselves to the chemical bases that make up a strand of DNA. This, in turn, affects the generation of proteins from the genes so tagged. Some chemical groups can even stop a gene from being expressed. Recently, research in Australia showed that such a chemically induced alteration could be inherited, at least in mice. This points to the possibility that inherited epigenetic characteristics could cause 'inherited diseases' in the same way that natural genetic mutations do. These developments suggest that epigenetics will be an important part of genetic studies and research. Not all geneticists, however, believe that this developing aspect of genetics is so important and this debate will continue.

Epiglottis

A leaf-like piece of elastic CARTILAGE covered with mucous membrane, which stands upright between the back of the tongue and the glottis, or entrance to the LARYNX. In the act of swallowing, it prevents fluids and solids from passing off the back of the tongue into the larynx.

Epiglottitis

Acute epiglottitis is a septicaemic illness which includes an acute inflammatory OEDEMA of the EPIGLOTTIS, due to *Haemophilus influenzae*. It progresses very rapidly and a child can be dangerously ill or even die within hours of onset. Once recognised, however, it is easily and successfully treated by immediate transfer to hospital for emergency intubation and ventilation and use of antibiotics and steroids. Fortunately it is now very rare as a result of the introduction of haemophilus vaccine into the primary vaccination course of infants. (See LARYNGO-TRACHEO-BRONCHITIS.)

Epignathus

Maldevelopment of the FETUS in which the deformed remains of one twin are united to the upper jaw of the other.

Epilation

Removal of hair by the roots. (See DEPILATION.)

Epilepsy

(See also FIT; SEIZURE.) Epilepsy is the name given to any condition in which a person suffers repeated fits or seizures. It is present in one in 200 (0·5 per cent) of the population and up to 5 per cent of all children will have had a fit by the age of 12, although most of these are harmless accompaniments of an acute feverish illness.

It is a recurrent and paroxysmal disorder starting suddenly and ceasing spontaneously due to occasional sudden excessive rapid and local discharge of the nerve cells in the grey matter (cortex) of the BRAIN. Epilepsy always arises in this way from the brain, but its origin is often of microscopic size. It is diagnosed by the clinical symptoms based on the observations of witnesses. Its cause can sometimes be established by laboratory tests, and brain scanning. Fits can be the first sign of a tumour, or follow a stroke, brain injury or infection, but in the large majority no underlying cause is found – so-called idiopathic epilepsy.

A single epileptic fit is not epilepsy. Of those people who have a single seizure, a significant minority (20 per cent) have no further attacks.

Major (generalised) seizures have a sudden, often unprovoked onset; the patient emits a cry, then falls to the ground, rigid, blue, and then twitching or jerking both sides of the body: the tonic-clonic convulsion. Drowsiness and confusion may last for some hours after recovering consciousness. Some experience a momentary warning (AURA): a smell, or sensation in the head or abdomen, vision, or *déjà vu*.

Partial seizures: focal motor (Jacksonian) begin with twitching of the angle of the mouth, the thumb, or the big toe. If the seizure discharge then spreads, the twitching or jerking spreads gradually through the limbs. Consciousness is preserved unless the seizure spreads to produce a secondary generalised fit. In some attacks the eyes and head may turn, the arm may rise, and the body may turn, while some patients feel tingling in the limbs.

Complex partial seizures (temporal lobe epilepsy) The patient usually appears blank, vacant and may be unable to talk, or may mumble or chatter – though later they often have no memory of this period. They may be able to carry out complex tasks, taking off gloves or clothes, and may smack their lips or rub repeatedly on one limb (automatisms). A sense of strangeness supervenes: unreality, or a feeling of having experienced it all before (*déja vu*). There may be a sense of panic. Strange unpleasant smells and tastes are olfactory and gustatory hallucinations. The visual hallucinations evoke complex scenes. An initial rising sense of warmth or discomfort in the stomach, or 'speeding-up' of thoughts are common psychomotor symptoms. All these strange symptoms are brief, disappearing within a few seconds or up to 3–4 minutes.

Minor seizures (petit mal) Attacks start in childhood. They last a few seconds. The child ceases what he or she is doing, stares, looks a little pale, and may flutter the eyelids. The head may drop forwards. Attacks are commonly provoked by overbreathing. The child and parents may be unaware of the attacks – 'just daydreaming'. Major fits develop in one-third of subjects. By contrast with other types of epilepsy, the ELECTROENCEPHALOGRAM (EEG) is diagnostic.

Precautions Children with epilepsy should take normal school exercises and games, and can swim under supervision. Adults must avoid working at heights, with exposed dangerous machinery, and driving vehicles on public roads. Current legislation allows driving after two years of complete freedom from attacks during waking hours; those who for more than three years have had a history of attacks only while asleep may also drive.

Treatment identifies, and avoids where possible, any factors (such as shortage of sleep or excessive fluids) which aggravate or trigger attacks. If fits are very infrequent, treatment may not be recommended. However, frequent fits may be embarassing, may cause injury or may cause long-term brain damage so treatment is advisable. Anti-epileptic drugs are usually necessary for several years under medical supervision. Carbamazepine and sodium valproate are the most frequently prescribed. The dose is governed by the degree of control of fits and sometimes drug levels can be monitored by blood tests to check on dosage. Strict adherence to the drug schedule gives a reasonable chance of total suppression of fits, especially in younger patients whose fits have started recently. The table summarises anticonvulsant drugs in use. Interactions can occur between anti-epileptics and, if drug treatment is changed, the patient needs careful monitoring. In particular, abrupt withdrawal of a drug should be avoided as this may precipitate severe rebound seizures.

	Indications
First-choice drugs:	
Ethosuximide	PM, JME
Phenobarbitone	M, P
Phenytoin	M, P, CP
Carbamazepine	M, P, CP
Valproate	M, PM, JME
Second-line drugs:	
Primidone	M, P, CP
Clobazam	M, CP
Vigabatrin	M, P, CP
Lamotrigine	M, P, CP
Gabapentin	M, P, CP
Topirimate	P

M = major generalised tonic-clonic; P = partial or focal; CP = complex partial (temporal lobe); PM = petit mal; JME = juvenile myoclonic epilepsy.

Anticonvulsant drugs

As all anticonvulsant drugs have an effect on the brain, it is not surprising that there may be side-effects, especially inolving alertness or behaviour. In each case careful assessment is necessary for doctor and patient to agree on the best compromise between stopping fits and avoiding ill-effects of medication.

Patients who have an epileptic seizure should not be restrained or have a gag or anything else placed in their mouths; nor should they be moved unless in danger of further injury. Any tight clothing around the neck should be loosened and, when the seizure has passed, the person should be placed in the recovery position to facilitate a return to consciousness (see APPENDIX 1: BASIC FIRST AID).

Patients with epilepsy and their relatives can obtain further advice and information from the British Epilepsy Association or Epilepsy Action Scotland.

Epiloia
See TUBEROUS SCLEROSIS.

Epiphora
Inadequate drainage of tears in the eyes with the result that they 'overflow' down the cheeks. The condition is caused by an abnormality of the tear ducts which drain away the normal secretions that keep the eyeball moist (see EYE).

Epiphysis
See BONE – Growth of bones.

Epiphysitis
Inflammation of an epiphysis (see BONE – Growth of bones).

Epirubicin
A cytotoxic anthracycline antibiotic drug used in the treatment of solid tumours, acute LEUKAEMIA and LYMPHOMA. It is related structurally to DOXORUBICIN and is given intravenously, and by instillation into the URINARY BLADDER to treat bladder cancer under specialist supervision.

Episclera
The most superficial layer of the sclera of the EYE. It sometimes becomes inflamed (episcleritis) but the condition usually clears without treatment.

Episiotomy
A cut made in the PERINEUM to enlarge the vaginal opening and facilitate childbirth during a difficult birth when the baby's head (or in a breech delivery, the buttocks) is making slow progress down the birth canal, or when forceps have to be applied. (See PREGNANCY AND LABOUR.)

Epispadias
An inherited abnormality of the PENIS in which the opening of the URETHRA is on the upper

surface instead of at the end of the organ. Surgical correction carried out in infancy has a high success rate.

Epistasis
(1) Stopping a flow or discharge of, for example, blood from a wound. (2) In genetics the term describes a type of gene action (see GENES) where a gene is able to block the action of another one.

Epistaxis
Bleeding from the nose. (See HAEMORRHAGE.)

Epithelioma
Epithelioma is a tumour of malignant nature arising in the EPITHELIUM covering the surface of the body. (See CANCER.)

Epithelium
Epithelium is the cellular layer which forms the epidermis on the skin, covers the inner surface of the bowels, and forms the lining of ducts and hollow organs, like the bladder. It consists of one or more layers of cells which adhere to one another, and is one of the simplest tissues of the body. It is of several forms: for example, the epidermis is formed of scaly epithelium, the cells being in several layers and more or less flattened. (See SKIN.) The bowels are lined by a single layer of columnar epithelium, the cells being long and narrow in shape. The air passages are lined by ciliated epithelium: that is to say, each cell is provided with flagellae (lashes) which drive the fluid upon the surface of the passages gradually upwards.

Epizoötic
Any disease in animals which diffuses itself widely. The term corresponds to the word EPIDEMIC as applied to human beings. In plague, for example, an epizoötic in rats usually precedes the epidemic in human beings.

Eponym
A species, structure or disorder named after a particular individual, customarily the one who first described or discovered it. The use of eponyms has been widespread in medicine, but more descriptive – and so more practical – terms are replacing them.

Epsom Salts
The popular name for magnesium sulphate, which was used as a saline purgative.

Epstein Barr Virus
The virus that causes glandular fever or infectious MONONUCLEOSIS. It is similar to the viruses that cause herpes and is associated with BURKITT'S LYMPHOMA. It has been suggested as precipitating some attacks of MYALGIC ENCEPHALOMYELITIS (ME), also known as CHRONIC FATIGUE SYNDROME (CFS).

Eptifibitide
An antiplatelet drug, best given under the supervision of a specialist. It inhibits the aggregation of PLATELETS in the blood that occurs in THROMBUS formation, and is used with HEPARIN and ASPIRIN to prevent early myocardial infarction (heart attack – see HEART, DISEASES OF) in patients with unstable ANGINA PECTORIS.

Epulis
Epulis is a term applied to any tumour connected with the jaws. (See MOUTH, DISEASES OF.)

Equine Oestrogens
See OESTROGENS.

Erb's Paralysis
Erb's paralysis is a form of paralysis of the arm due to stretching or tearing of the fibres of the brachial nerve plexus. Such damage to the brachial plexus may occur during birth, especially when the baby is unusually large, and it is found that the arm lies by the side of the body with elbow extended, forearm pronated, and the fingers flexed. The infant is unable to raise the arm.

ERCP
See ENDOSCOPIC RETROGRADE CHOLANGIO-PANCREATOGRAPHY (ERCP).

Erection
The rigid state of the PENIS when it responds to sexual stimulus. An erection is necessary for effective penetration of the VAGINA. As a result of sexual arousal, the three cylinders of erectile tissue in the penis become engorged with blood, lengthening, raising and hardening the penis. Muscles surrounding the blood vessels contract and retain the blood in the penis. Erections also occur during sleep and in young boys. Inability to have or maintain an erection is one cause of IMPOTENCE (see also SILDENAFIL CITRATE).

Erg-
A prefix indicating activity or work.

Ergocalciferol
A combination of CALCIFEROL and vitamin D_2 (see APPENDIX 5: VITAMINS) given to prevent or

cure RICKETS, a deficiency disorder caused by the lack of calcium and vitamin D in the diet.

Ergometrine

An active constituent of ergot, it has a powerful action in controlling the excessive bleeding from the UTERUS which may occur after childbirth. The official *British Pharmacopoeia* preparation is ergometrine maleate.

Ergonomics

A broad science involving the application of psychological and physiological principles to the study of human beings in relation to their work and working surroundings. It includes the design of buildings, machinery, vehicles, and anything else with which people have contact in the course of their work.

Ergosterol

A sterol found in yeasts and fungi and in plant and animal fat. Under the action of sunlight or ultraviolet rays it produces vitamin D_2. The substance produced in this way is known as calciferol, and is used for the prevention and cure of RICKETS and OSTEOMALACIA. A similar change in the ergosterol of the skin is produced when the body is freely exposed to sunlight. Calciferol is probably not so active as, and differs chemically from, the vitamin D occurring in fish-liver oils. (See APPENDIX 5: VITAMINS.)

Ergot Poisoning

Ergot poisoning, or ergotism, occasionally results from eating bread made from rye infected with the fungus, *Claviceps purpurea*. Several terrible epidemics (St Anthony's Fire), characterised by intense pain and hallucinations, occurred in France and Germany during the Middle Ages (see ERYSIPELAS). Its symptoms are the occurrence of spasmodic muscular contractions, and the gradual production of gangrene in parts like the fingers, toes and tips of the ears because of constriction of blood vessels and therefore the blood supply.

Ergotamine

One of the alkaloids in ergot. In the form of ergotamine tartrate it is usually given orally to treat MIGRAINE, but treatment carries a risk and should be medically supervised.

Ergotism

See ERGOT POISONING.

Erogenous

A term to describe those parts of the body – for example, the mouth, breasts and genitals – which, when stimulated, result in the individual's sexual arousal.

Erosion

Erosion means a process of gradual wearing down of structures in the body. The term is applied to the effect of tumours, when they cause destruction of tissue in their neighbourhood without actually growing into the latter: for example, an ANEURYSM may erode bones in its neighbourhood. The term is also applied to minute ulcers – for example, erosions of the stomach, caused by extreme acidity of the gastric juice.

Dental erosion is the loss of tooth substance due to a cause other than decay or trauma. This is usually as a result of the presence of acid; for example, frequent vomiting or the excessive intake of citrus fruits. The teeth appear very smooth and later develop saucer-shaped depressions.

Eroticism

The emotional nature and characteristics of sexual arousal. This may occur as a result of visual, auditory or physical stimuli and also as a result of sexually oriented memories or imaginings.

Eructation

Eructation, or belching, is the sudden escape of gas or of portions of half-digested food from the stomach up into the mouth.

Eruption

Eruption, or rash, means an outbreak, in a scattered form, upon the surface of the skin. The skin is usually raised and red, or it may be covered with scales, or crusts, or vesicles containing fluid. Eruptions differ in appearance: for example, the eruption of MEASLES is always distinguishable from that of CHICKENPOX. But the same disease may also produce different eruptions in different people; or in the same person in different states of health; or even on different parts of the body at one time.

Eruptions may be acute or chronic. Most of the acute eruptions belong to the exanthemata (see EXANTHEM): that is, they are bright in colour and burst out suddenly like a flower. These are the eruptions of SCARLET FEVER, measles, German measles (see RUBELLA), SMALLPOX and chickenpox. In general, the severity of these diseases can be measured by the amount of eruption. Some eruptions are very transitory, like nettle-rash, appearing and vanishing again in the course of a few hours. (See also SKIN, DIS-EASES OF.)

Erysipelas
A streptococcal infection (see STREPTOCOCCUS) of the skin characterised by an acute onset with fever, malaise and a striking, usually unilateral, rash (see ERUPTION) almost always on a lower leg or the face. Shivering, local pain and tenderness are associated with a sharply defined, spreading, bright red swollen zone of skin inflammation. On the leg, blistering and PURPURA may follow. The bacteria enter the skin through a fissure in a toe cleft (often associated with tinea pedis [RINGWORM]) or via a crack in the skin behind an ear or in a nostril.

Treatment PENICILLIN in full dosage should be given orally for ten days. In those allergic to penicillin, ERYTHROMYCIN can be substituted. Recurrent attacks are common and may cause progressive lymphatic damage leading to chronic OEDEMA. Such recurrences can be prevented by long-term prophylactic oral penicillin.

Erythema
Redness of the skin due to dilatation of dermal blood vessels. It may be transient or chronic, localised or widespread, and it can be blanched by pressure. Erythema may be caused by excessive exposure to heat or ultraviolet light, or by inflammation of the skin due to infection, DERMATITIS, and various allergic reactions – for example, to drugs. It may be emotional (e.g. as in flushing), mediated by the autonomic nervous system.

Erythema ab igne is a fixed redness of the skin caused by chronic exposure to heat from a domestic fire or radiator.

Erythema pernio (See CHILBLAIN.) Redness induced by spasm of the skin arterioles due to cold. It affects the hands, feet or calves in winter. The red swollen areas are cooler than normal.

Erythema nodosum A singular pattern of red, tender nodules occurring on the shins, often lasting several weeks. It may be caused by a streptococcal throat infection, primary tuberculosis, SARCOIDOSIS, or may be drug-induced.

Erythema multiforme is an acute allergic eruption of the extremities characterised by circular areas of erythema, purpura and blistering, which resolve over two or three weeks, caused by infections or drugs. In severe forms the mucous membranes of the eyes, mouth and genitalia may be involved.

Erythema infectiosum is an acute contagious disease of children caused by a parvovirus (see PARVOVIRUSES). In young children a bright erythema of the face gives a 'slapped cheek' appearance.

Erythrasma
A superficial mild infection of the skin caused by CORYNEBACTERIA. It produces pink or slightly brown flaky areas of skin usually on the upper inner thighs or axillae. Toe clefts may be affected with thickened, white, macerated skin. The affected areas fluoresce coral pink under ultraviolet light. CLOTRIMAZOLE or KETOCONAZOLE cream clears the rash rapidly. Very extensive erythrasma responds to oral ERYTHROMYCIN given for seven days.

Erythroblastosis Fetalis
See HAEMOLYTIC DISEASE OF THE NEWBORN.

Erythroblasts
A series of nucleated cells in the bone marrow that go through various stages of development until they form ERYTHROCYTES. They may appear in the blood in certain diseases.

Erythrocytes
The biconcave red blood cells that carry oxygen from the lungs to the tissues, and return carbon dioxide (see also RESPIRATION). They have an excess of membrane, some of which may be lost in various disorders, as a result of which they become progressively more spherical and rigid. Erythrocytes, which have no nuclei, are formed during ERYTHROPOEISIS from ERYTHROBLASTS in the BONE MARROW, and each mm^3 of blood contains 5 million of them. They are by far the largest constituent among the blood cells and they contain large amounts of the oxygen-carrier HAEMOGLOBIN. They have a life of about 120 days after which they are absorbed by macrophages (see MACROPHAGE), the blood's scavenging cells. Most components of the erythrocytes, including the red pigment haemoglobin, are re-used, though some of the pigment is broken down to the waste product BILIRUBIN.

Erythrocyte Sedimentation Rate
See ESR.

Erythroderma
A rare inflammation of the skin which causes universal itching. The skin is red, thickened

and scaly. It is also called generalised exfoliative dermatitis (see SKIN, DISEASES OF). It may complicate chronic eczema (see DERMATITIS) or PSORIASIS, particularly in men, in the second half of life. It may also result from HYPERSENSITIVITY to a drug, such as gold injections used in RHEUMATOID ARTHRITIS. Rarely, it may be a manifestation of T-cell LYMPHOMA.

Universal inflammation of the skin may cause heart failure, particularly in elderly people with pre-existing heart disease. It may lead to HYPOTHERMIA due to excessive heat loss from the skin and protein deficiency caused by the shedding of large quantities of skin scales containing keratin. Rarely, these complications can be fatal.

Treatment depends on the cause, but in eczematous erythroderma, oral CORTICO-STEROIDS (PREDNISOLONE) in full dosage may be needed.

Erythromelalgia
A condition in which the fingers or toes, or even larger portions of the limbs, become purple and bloated in appearance, and very painful. In people suffering from the condition – which is not a common one – the attacks come and go, being worse in summer (unlike chilblains), and worse on exertion or when the affected parts are warmed or allowed to hang down. The condition may appear without apparent cause, but is often associated with vascular diseases, such as HYPERTENSION and POLYCYTHAEMIA VERA. It also occurs in association with certain diseases of the central nervous system, and in cases of metallic poisoning (e.g. arsenic, mercury and thallium). Treatment is unsatisfactory but aspirin provides sympomatic relief.

Erythromycin
One of the MACROLIDES, it has an antibacterial spectrum similar, but not identical, to that of penicillin. The drug is a valuable alternative for patients who are allergic to penicillin. Erythromycin is used for respiratory infections, including spread within a family of WHOOPING-COUGH, and also CHLAMYDIA, LEGIONNAIRE'S DISEASE, SYPHILIS and enteritis caused by CAMPYLOBACTER. It is also used with neomycin when preparing for bowel surgery. Though often active against penicillin-resistant staphylococci, these bacteria are now sometimes resistant to erythromycin. The drug may be given orally, intravenously or topically (for acne).

Erythropoeisis
The process by which ERYTHROCYTES or red blood cells are produced. The initiating cell is the haemopoietic stem cell from which an identifiable proerythroblast develops. This goes through several stages as a normoblast before losing its nucleus to become an erythrocyte. This process takes place in the blood-forming bone-marrow tissue.

Erythropoietin
The protein, produced mainly in the kidney, that is the major stimulus for the production of ERYTHROCYTES, or red blood corpuscles. It is used when treating ANAEMIA dure to end-stage kidney failure and in premature newborns with anaemia. (See also BLOOD.)

Eschar
Hard adherent crust caused by tissue killed by heat, chemicals or disease.

Escherichia
The generic name for the group of gram-negative, usually motile, rod-shaped BACTERIA that can ferment CARBOHYDRATE. They occur naturally in the intestines of humans and some animals. *E. coli*, which ferments lactose, is not normally harmful but some varieties, particularly *E. coli* O157, cause gastrointestinal infections which may be severe in old people. *E. coli* is also used in laboratory experiments for genetic and bacteriological research.

Eserine
Another name for PHYSOSTIGMINE.

Esmarch's Bandage
A rubber bandage which is applied to a limb before surgery from below upwards, in order to drive blood from the limb. The bandage is removed after an inflated pneumatic TOURNIQUET has been placed round the limb; the operation can then proceed.

ESP
See EXTRASENSORY PERCEPTION (ESP).

ESR
The ESR or erythrocyte sedimentation rate is a test that measures the rate at which red blood cells settle out of suspension in blood PLASMA. In certain diseases, such as infection and malignancy, the amount of proteins in the plasma increases; the result is that red cells settle out more quickly and this test is used to show whether inflammation is present and, to some extent, its severity.

Essential Amino Acids
See INDISPENSABLE AMINO ACIDS.

Essential (Benign) Hypertension
See HYPERTENSION.

Essential Fatty Acids
Three acids – arachidonic, linolenic and tinoleic – which are essential for life, but which the body cannot produce. They are found in natural vegetable and fish oils and their functions are varied. EFAs have a vital function in fat metabolism and transfer and they are also precursors of PROSTAGLANDINS.

Ester
An organic compound formed from an alcohol and an acid by the removal of water.

Ethacrynic Acid
A potent diuretic, with a rapid onset, and a short duration (4–6 hours), of action. (See THIAZIDES; DIURETICS.)

Ethambutol
Ethambutol is a synthetic drug, often included in the treatment regimen of TUBERCULOSIS when the infection is thought to be resistant to other drugs. The main side-effects are visual disturbances, chiefly loss of acuity and colour blindness. Such toxic effects are more common when excessive dosages are used, or the patient has some renal impairment, in which case the drug should be avoided – as it should be in young children.

Ethanol
Ethanol is another name for ethyl alcohol. (See ALCOHOL.)

Ether
A colourless, volatile, highly inflammable liquid, formed by the action of sulphuric acid on alcohol. Ether boils below body temperature and therefore rapidly evaporates when sprayed over the skin. Dissolving many substances such as fats, oils and resins better than alcohol or water, it is used in the preparation of many drugs. Formerly used as an anaesthetic, it has been replaced by safer and more efficient drugs.

Etherified Starch
Along with DEXTRAN and GELATIN, this is a substance with a large molecular structure used to treat shocked patients with burns (see BURNS AND SCALDS) or SEPTICAEMIA in order to expand and maintain their blood volume. Like other plasma substitutes, this form of starch can be used as an emergency, short-term treatment for severe bleeding until blood for transfusion is available. Plasma substitutes must be used with caution in patients who have heart disease or impairment of their kidney function. Patients should be monitored for hypersensitivity reactions and for changes in their BLOOD PRESSURE (see SHOCK).

Ethics
Within most cultures, care of the sick is seen as entailing special duties, codified as a set of moral standards governing professional practice. Although these duties have been stated and interpreted in differing ways, a common factor is the awareness of an imbalance of power between doctor and patient and an acknowledgement of the vulnerability of the sick person. A function of medical ethics is to counteract this inevitable power imbalance by encouraging doctors to act in the best interests of their patients, refrain from taking advantage of those in their care, and use their skills in a manner which preserves the honour of their profession. It has always been accepted, however, that doctors cannot use their knowledge indiscriminately to fulfil patients' wishes. The deliberate ending of life, for example, even at a patient's request, has usually been seen as alien to the shared values inherent in medical ethics. It is, however, symptomatic of changing concepts of ethics and of the growing power of patient choice that legal challenges have been mounted in several countries to the prohibition of EUTHANASIA. Thus ethics can be seen as regulating individual doctor-patient relationships, integrating doctors within a moral community of their professional peers and reflecting societal demands for change.

Medical ethics are embedded in cultural values which evolve. Acceptance of abortion within well-defined legal parameters in some jurisdictions is an example of how society influences the way in which perceptions about ethical obligations change. Because they are often linked to the moral views predominating in society, medical ethics cannot be seen as embodying uniform standards independent of cultural context. Some countries which permit capital punishment or female genital mutilation (FGM – see CIRCUMCISION), for example, expect doctors to carry out such procedures. Some doctors would argue that their ethical obligation to minimise pain and suffering obliges them to comply, whereas others would deem their ethical obligations to be the complete opposite. The medical community attempts to address such variations by establishing globally applicable ethical principles through debate within bodies such as the World Medical Association (WMA) or World Psychiatric Association (WPA). Norm-setting bodies increasingly reflect accepted concepts of human rights and patient rights within professional ethical codes.

Practical changes within society may affect the perceived balance of power within the doctor-patient relationship, and therefore have an impact on ethics. In developed societies, for example, patients are increasingly well informed about treatment options: media such as the Internet provide them with access to specialised knowledge. Social measures such as a well-established complaints system, procedures for legal redress, and guarantees of rights such as those set out in the NHS's *Patient's Charter* appear to reduce the perceived imbalance in the relationship. Law as well as ethics emphasises the importance of informed patient consent and the often legally binding nature of informed patient refusal of treatment. Ethics reflect the changing relationship by emphasising skills such as effective communication and generation of mutual trust within a doctor-patient partnership.

A widely known modern code is the WMA's *International Code of Medical Ethics* which seeks to provide a modern restatement of the Hippocratic principles.

Traditionally, ethical codes have sought to establish absolutist positions. The WMA code, for example, imposes an apparently absolute duty of confidentiality which extends beyond the patient's death. Increasingly, however, ethics are perceived as a tool for making morally appropriate decisions in a sphere where there is rarely one 'right' answer. Many factors – such as current emphasis on autonomy and the individual values of patients; awareness of social and cultural diversity; and the phenomenal advance of new technology which has blurred some moral distinctions about what constitutes a 'person' – have contributed to the perception that ethical dilemmas have to be resolved on a case-by-case basis.

An approach adopted by American ethicists has been moral analysis of cases using four fundamental principles: autonomy, beneficence, non-maleficence and justice. The 'four principles' provide a useful framework within which ethical dilemmas can be teased out, but they are criticised for their apparent simplicity in the face of complex problems and for the fact that the moral imperatives implicit in each principle often conflict with some or all of the other three. As with any other approach to problem-solving, the 'four principles' require interpretation. Enduring ethical precepts such as the obligation to benefit patients and avoid harm (beneficence and non-maleficence) may be differently interpreted in cases where prolongation of life is contrary to a patient's wishes or where sentience has been irrevocably lost. In such cases, treatment may be seen as constituting a 'harm' rather than a 'benefit'.

The importance accorded to ethics in daily practice has undergone considerable development in the latter half of the 20th century. From being seen mainly as a set of values passed on from experienced practitioners to their students at the bedside, medical ethics have increasingly become the domain of lawyers, academic philosophers and professional ethicists, although the role of experienced practitioners is still considered central. In the UK, law and medical ethics increasingly interact. Judges resolve cases on the basis of established medical ethical guidance, and new ethical guidance draws in turn on common-law judgements in individual cases. The rapid increase in specialised journals, conferences and postgraduate courses focused on ethics is testimony to the ever-increasing emphasis accorded to this area of study. Multidisciplinary practice has stimulated the growth of the new discipline of 'health-care ethics' which seeks to provide uniformity across long-established professional boundaries. The trend is to set common standards for a range of health professionals and others who may have a duty of care, such as hospital chaplains and ancillary workers. Since a primary function of ethics is to find reasonable answers in situations where different interests or priorities conflict, managers and health-care purchasers are increasingly seen as potential partners in the effort to establish a common approach. Widely accepted ethical values are increasingly applied to the previously unacknowledged dilemmas of rationing scarce resources.

In modern debate about ethics, two important trends can be identified. As a result of the increasingly high profile accorded to applied ethics, there is a trend for professions not previously subject to widely agreed standards of behaviour to adopt codes of ethical practice. Business ethics or the ethics of management are comparatively new. At the same time, there is some debate about whether professionals, such as doctors, traditionally subject to special ethical duties, should be seen as simply doing a job for payment like any other worker. As some doctors perceive their power and prestige eroded by health-care managers deciding on how and when to ration care and pressure for patients to exercise autonomy about treatment decisions, it is sometimes argued that realistic limits must be set on medical obligations. A logical implication of patient choice and rejection of medical paternalism would appear to be a concomitant reduction in the freedom of doctors to carry out their own ethical obligations. The concept of conscientious objection, incorporated to some extent in law (e.g. in relation to abortion) ensures that doctors are not obliged to act contrary to their own personal or professional values.

Ethics Committees

(In the USA, Institutional Review Boards.) Various types of ethics committee operate in the UK, fulfilling four main functions: the monitoring of research; debate of difficult patient cases; establishing norms of practice; and publishing ethical guidance.

The most common – Local Research Ethics Committees (LRECs) – have provided a monitoring system of research on humans since the late 1960s. Established by NHS health authorities, LRECs were primarily perceived as exercising authority over research carried out on NHS patients or on NHS premises or using NHS records. Their power and significance, however, developed considerably in the 1980s and 90s when national and international guidance made approval by an 'appropriately constituted' ethics committee obligatory for any research project involving humans or human tissue. The work of LRECs is supplemented by so-called 'independent' ethics committees usually set up by pharmaceutical companies, and since 1997 by multicentre research ethics committees (MRECs). An MREC is responsible for considering all health-related research which will be conducted within five or more locations. LRECs have become indispensable to the conduct of research, and are doubtless partly responsible for the lack of demand in the UK for legislation governing research. A plethora of guidelines is available, and LRECs which fail to comply with recognised standards could incur legal liability. They are increasingly governed by international standards of practice. In 1997, guidelines produced by the International Committee on Harmonisation of Good Clinical Practice (ICH-GCP) were introduced into the UK. These provide a unified standard for research conducted in the European Union, Japan and United States to ensure the mutual acceptance of clinical data by the regulatory authorities in these countries.

Other categories of ethics committee include Ethics Advisory Committees, which debate difficult patient cases. Most are attached to specialised health facilities such as fertility clinics or children's care facilities. The 1990s have seen a greatly increased interest in professional ethics and the establishment of many new ethics committees, including some like that of the National Council for Hospice and Specialist Palliative Care Services which cross professional boundaries. Guidance on professional and ethical standards is produced by these new bodies and by the well-established ethics committees of regulatory or representative bodies, such as the medical and nursing Royal Colleges, the General Medical Council, United Kingdom Central Council for Nursing, Midwifery and Health Visiting, British Medical Association (see APPENDIX 8: PROFESSIONAL ORGANISATIONS) and bodies representing paramedics and professions supplementary to medicine. Their guidance ranges from general codes of practice to detailed analysis of single topics such as EUTHANASIA or surrogacy.

LRECs are now supervised by a central body – COREC (www.corec.gov.org.uk).

Ethinylestradiol

A highly active oestrogen – about 20 times more active than STILBOESTROL; it is active when given by mouth. (See OESTROGENS.)

Ethmoid

A bone in the base of the SKULL which separates the cavity of the nose from the membranes of the brain. It is a spongy bone with numerous cavities or sinuses.

Suppuration in the ethmoidal sinuses is sometimes responsible for inflammation in neighbouring parts such as the eye.

Ethosuximide

A drug used in the treatment of the form of EPILEPSY known as petit mal.

Ethyl Chloride

A flammable, colourless liquid that is extremely volatile, and rapidly produces freezing of a surface when sprayed upon it. Now occasionally used to deaden pain for small and short operations, ethyl chloride was once used as an inhalant general anaesthetic for brief operations, and to induce ANAESTHESIA in patients in whom the anaesthesia is subsequently to be maintained by some other anaesthetic such as nitrous oxide or ether.

Ethylene

A colourless, flammable gas occasionally used as an inhalant anaesthetic.

Ethyloestrenol
See ANABOLIC STEROIDS.

Etidronate
Also known as disodium etidronate, this is one of a group of substances called biphosphates used mainly to treat PAGET'S DISEASE OF BONE. The drug is given orally and, when combined with calcium carbonate (Didrone®), it is used to treat osteoporosis (see under BONE, DISORDERS OF) and to prevent bone loss in postmenopausal women, especially if hormone replacement therapy (HRT – see under MENOPAUSE) is not appropriate.

Etiology
Etiology, or AETIOLOGY, means the group of conditions which form the cause of any disease.

Etomidate
An intravenous agent for inducing general ANAESTHESIA prior to surgery or other procedures that require patients to be unconscious. When the drug is injected intravenously, pain sometimes occurs, but this can be minimised by premedication with an opioid analgesic (see ANALGESICS).

Eu-
A prefix meaning satisfactory or beneficial.

Eucalyptus
Eucalyptus (*Eucalyptus globulus*) is a tree, originally a native of Australia and now grown all over the world. Its important constituent, oil of eucalyptus, is an oil of pleasant smell and spicy taste, which is obtained by distillation from the leaves of the tree. The oil may be used as a disinfectant and deodorant.

Eugenics
The study and cultivation of conditions that may improve the human race, in particular the detection and elimination of genetic disease.

Eukaryote
A cell that has a NUCLEUS bounded by a membrane and with chromosomes containing DNA, RNA and proteins. The cell divides by MITOSIS and also contains MITOCHONDRIA. Animals, plants and cellular organisms made up of this type of cell are included in the biological superkingdom of Eukaryote.

Eunuch
A man whose testes (see TESTICLE) have been removed or seriously damaged so that he is unable to produce male hormones and thus is sterile. A male castrated before puberty will have a feminine appearance and underdeveloped secondary sexual characteristics. The term was historically used to describe boys, castrated to make them suitable for working in harems, or boy singers, castrated to retain their higher-register voices (castrati singers).

Euphoria
A feeling of well-being. This may occur normally; for instance, when someone has passed an examination. In some neurological or psychiatric conditions, however, patients may have an exaggerated and quite unjustified feeling of euphoria. This is then a symptom of the underlying condition. Euphoria may also be drug-induced – by drugs of addiction or by therapeutic drugs such as CORTICOSTEROIDS.

Euphoriants
Drugs which induce a state of EUPHORIA or well-being.

Eustachian Tubes
The passages, one on each side, leading from the throat to the middle ear. Each is about 38 mm (1½ inches) long and is large at either end, though at its narrowest part it only admits a fine probe. The tubes open widely in the act of swallowing or yawning. The opening into the throat is situated just behind the lower part of the nose, so that a catheter can be passed through the corresponding nostril into the tube for inflation of the middle ear. (See also EAR; NOSE.)

Euthanasia
Literally meaning the procuring of an easy and painless death, euthanasia (or 'mercy killing') has come to be understood as a deliberate act or omission whose primary intention is to end another person's life. The qualifiers 'voluntary', 'involuntary' and 'non-voluntary' are used to indicate the degree of patient involvement in the decision. Much debate has centred on whether individuals should be entitled to manage their own death or appoint others to do so for them (voluntary euthanasia). UK public-opinion surveys appear to indicate substantial support for such a proposal but this partly reflects the way in which the issue is broached. Predictably, if the choice is portrayed as one between euthanasia and an inevitably drawn-out, painful or distressing death, many agree that competent, terminally ill patients who ask for euthanasia should be helped to die. Difficult issues arise, however, when attempts are made to set limits and safeguards. This has generally been seen as a major stumbling block to any

proposal to change the law prohibiting euthanasia in the UK. Such pragmatic rather than ethical or legal arguments were a key feature of the conclusions of the House of Lords Select Committee on Medical Ethics in 1994. There has also been much debate about whether euthanasia should attract a lesser penalty than other forms of murder which carry a mandatory life sentence. Nevertheless, in the UK, killing a person intentionally is still classified as murder, even if that person consents to the killing.

Most of the detailed information available about the practice of euthanasia comes from the Netherlands, where court rulings in the 1970s and 1980s began to permit voluntary euthanasia under certain circumstances (although both euthanasia and assisted suicide remain technically illegal). The difficulty of maintaining limits was highlighted in 1994–5 when it became clear that a small percentage of Dutch patients undergoing euthanasia had previously expressed an interest but not specifically requested it (involuntary euthanasia) or had no known desire for it and may have been opposed to it (non-voluntary euthanasia). The relevance of terminal illness and physical suffering was tested in Holland in 1994 when a patient received euthanasia who was not physically ill and subject to mental rather than physical suffering. Nevertheless, Dutch doctors risk prosecution if they fail to follow rules of careful conduct when carrying out euthanasia or assisted suicide. (See also ETHICS; SUICIDE.)

Euthyroid

The descriptive term for a person with a normally functioning THYROID GLAND, or someone who has had successful treatment for an underactive (hypothyroid) or overactive (hyperthyroid) gland.

Evacuant

Evacuant is a name for a purgative medicine (see LAXATIVES).

Evacuator

A device for extracting fluid from a cavity. In its basic form it comprises a hollow flexible bulb attached (using a valve system) to a tube inserted into the cavity. Another valve leads to the discharge tube. One use of an evacuator is to empty the urinary bladder of extraneous material during surgery for removal of CALCULI or for PROSTATECTOMY.

Evaluation

See PUBLIC HEALTH.

Evidence

See EVIDENCE-BASED MEDICINE.

Evidence-Based Medicine

The process of systematically identifying, appraising and using the best available research findings, integrated with clinical expertise, as the basis for clinical decisions about individual patients. The aim is to encourage clinicians, health-service managers and consumers of health care to make decisions, taking account of the best available evidence, on the likely consequences of alternative decisions and actions. Evidence-based medicine has been developing internationally for the past 25 years, but since around 1990 its development has accelerated. The International COCHRANE COLLABORATION finds and reviews relevant research. Several other centres have been set up to look at the clinical application of research results, including the Centre for Evidence-Based Medicine in Oxford.

Evisceration

Extrusion of the abdominal VISCERA or internal organs, usually as the result of serious injury. (Usually described as disembowelment when deliberately carried out by one person on another.) In surgery the term refers to partremoval of the viscera, and in OPHTHALMOLOGY it is an operation to remove the contents of the eyeball (see also EYE).

Evolution

An uninterrupted process of change from one condition, form or state to another. In biological evolution, all varieties of living things are seen as having developed by inheritable, incremental changes from unicellular structures to complex organisms such as humankind. Although the likelihood of some form of evolution had been postulated by scientists in the late 18th and early 19th centuries, the prime contribution to the development of biological evolutionary doctrine came from the British scientist, Charles Darwin, who argued in his book *The Origin of Species by Means of Natural Selection* (1859) that natural selection resulted in the survival of the fittest organisms. The precise biological mechanism of evolution was not unravelled until the 20th century, with the discovery of CHROMOSOMES and GENES and the development of the science of genetics. Charles Darwin's theory was based on his studies of the varied and unique animal life in the Galapagos Islands in the 19th century. He believed that the diversity of life on the planet could be ascribed to the combined effects of random variation in living things, inherited by succeeding generations.

Ewing's Sarcoma

An uncommon but very malignant cancer of the bone in children and young adults, the condition was first identified as being different from OSTEOSARCOMA by Dr J Ewing in 1921. It usually occurs in the limbs or pelvis and soon spreads to other parts of the body. Treatment is by RADIOTHERAPY and CYTOTOXIC drugs. Since the use of the latter, the number of patients who survive for five years or more has much improved.

Ex- (Exo-)

Prefix meaning outer or outside.

Exanthem

Rash caused by a systemic infection. Several childhood infections – for example, MEASLES and RUBELLA – have characteristic exanthemata.

Exchange Transfusion

A method of treating newborn infants with HAEMOLYTIC DISEASE. Blood is taken out of the baby through the umbilical vein and is replaced with the same quantity of blood from a donor that is compatible with the mother's blood. The procedure is repeated several times to get rid of damaged cells while maintaining the infant's blood volume and keeping its red cell count constant. (See also TRANSFUSION.)

Excimer Laser

A type of laser that is used to remove thin sheets of tissue from the surface of the cornea (see EYE), thus changing the curvature of the eye's corneal surface. The procedure is used to excise diseased tissue or to correct myopia (see REFRACTION), when it is known as photorefractive keratectomy or lasik.

Excipient

An inert substance added to a prescription in order to make the remedy as prescribed more suitable in bulk, consistence, or form for administration.

Excision

A term applied to the removal of any structure from the body, when such removal necessitates a certain amount of separation from surrounding parts: for example, the excision of a tumour, of a gland or of a joint. When an opening is simply made into the body, the term incision is used; when a limb, or part of one, is removed, the term AMPUTATION is employed.

Excitation

When used in neurophysiology, the term means the triggering of a conducted electrical impulse in the membrane of a muscle cell or the nerve fibre controlling it.

Excitement

See DELIRIUM; ECSTASY; HYSTERIA; MENTAL ILLNESS.

Excoriation

Excoriation means the destruction of small pieces of the surface of skin or mucous membrane.

Excreta

Waste material, especially FAECES.

Excretion

The process by which the residue of undigested food in the gastrointestinal tract (faeces) and the waste products of the body's metabolism – mainly as urine via the kidneys, but also as sweat from the skin, and water and carbon dioxide from the lungs – are eliminated.

Exercise

An activity requiring physical exertion. Everyone should take regular exercise: this keeps muscles in tone, maintains the CARDIO-VASCULAR SYSTEM in good shape, helps to keep weight at an optimum level and promotes relaxation and sleep. When an individual is at rest, the heart's output is 5 litres of blood per minute. When running at 12 km (7½ miles) per hour, this rises to around 25 litres, obliging the heart and lungs to operate more efficiently and speeding up the metabolism of food to provide the necessary energy. Lack of exercise by children may lead to faulty posture and flabby muscles; in adults it results in an increase in weight and poorly functioning respiratory and cardiovascular system, with an increased chance of heart disease later in life. Adolescents and adults, participating regularly in sporting activities, should train regularly, preferably under expert supervision, to ensure that they do not place potentially damaging demands on their cardiovascular, respiratory and musculoskeletal systems. Those wanting to participate in demanding sports would be wise to have a medical examination before embarking on training programmes (see SPORTS MEDICINE).

Exfoliation

The separation, in layers, of pieces of dead bone or skin.

Exhalation
Also called expiration, this is the act of breathing air from the lungs out through the bronchi, trachea, mouth and nose. (See also RESPIRATION.)

Exhibitionism
Public flaunting of a person's characteristics. Also a term describing the public exposure of genitals to another person, regarded as a form of sexual deviation, colloquially called 'flashing'.

Exocrine Gland
A gland that secretes its products through a duct to the surface of the body or of an organ. The sweat glands in the skin and the salivary glands in the mouth are examples. The secretion is set off by a hormone (see HORMONES) or a NEUROTRANSMITTER.

Exogenous
Arising outside the body. For example, exogenous DEPRESSION is an illness caused by an outside factor such as the death of a close relative; an exogenous illness may occur because of something eaten in the diet.

Exomphalos
The term applied to a congenital HERNIA formed by the projection of abdominal organs through the UMBILICUS.

Exophthalmometer
Also known as a proptometer. An instrument used to measure the extent of protrusion of the eyeball – a development that occurs in certain disorders such as GOITRE, TUMOUR, OEDEMA, injuries, orbital inflammation or cavernous venous thrombosis (a blood clot in the cavernous sinus in the base of the skull behind each eye). (See EXOPHTHALMOS.)

Exophthalmos
Exophthalmos, or PROPTOSIS, refers to forward displacement of the eyeball and must be distinguished from retraction of the eyelids, which causes an illusion of exophthalmos. Lid retraction usually results from activation of the autonomic nervous sytem. Exophthalmos is a more serious disorder caused by inflammatory and infiltrative changes in the retro-orbital tissues and is essentially a feature of Graves' disease, though it has been described in chronic thyroiditis (see THYROID GLAND, DISEASES OF). Exophthalmos commonly starts shortly after the development of thyrotoxicosis but may occur months or even years after hyperthyroidism has been successfully treated. The degree of exophthalmos is not correlated with the severity of hyperthyroidism even when their onset is simultaneous. Some of the worst examples of endocrine exophthalmos occur in the euthyroid state and may appear in patients who have never had thyrotoxicosis; this disorder is named ophthalmic Graves' disease. The exophthalmos of Graves' disease is due to autoimmunity (see IMMUNITY). Antibodies to surface antigens on the eye muscles are produced and this causes an inflammatory reaction in the muscle and retro-orbital tissues.

Exophthalmos may also occur as a result of OEDEMA, injury, cavernous venous THROMBOSIS or a tumour at the back of the eye, pushing the eyeball forwards. In this situation it is always unilateral.

Exopththalmic Goitre
Sometimes called Graves' disease, this is a disorder in which there is overactivity of the thyroid gland, protrusion of the eyes, and other symptoms. (See HYPERTHYROIDISM.)

Exostosis
An outgrowth from a bone: it may be due to chronic inflammation, constant pressure or tension on the bone, or tumour-formation. (See BONE, DISORDERS OF.)

Exotoxin
A powerful poison produced by a bacterial cell and secreted into its surrounding environment. Exotoxins are often damaging to only few tissues and they are usually inactivated by chemicals, heat and light. Bacteria causing BOTULISM, DIPHTHERIA and TETANUS all produce exotoxins. (See ENDOTOXIN.)

Expectant
A form of treatment in which the cure of the patient is left mainly to nature, while the physician simply watches for any unsatisfactory developments or symptoms, and relieves them if they occur.

Expectorants
Drugs which are claimed to help the removal of secretions from the AIR PASSAGES – although there is no convincing evidence that they do this. A simple expectorant may, however, be a useful placebo. Most preparations are available without a doctor's prescription and pharmacists will advise on which might be helpful for particular patients with dry or congestive coughs.

Expectoration
Expectoration means either material brought

up from the chest by the AIR PASSAGES, or the act by which it is brought up.

Expiration
(1) Breathing out air from the lungs.
(2) The act of dying.

Exploration
A surgical operation to investigate the cause of a patient's illness.

Exposure
(1) A term used in BEHAVIOUR THERAPY to describe a method of treating fears and phobias (see PHOBIA). The subject is confronted by the circumstances that he or she fears, either gradually or suddenly, with the aim of defusing the fear or phobia.
(2) The term is also a colloquialism for public exposure by a man of his genitals to achieve sexual gratification.

Exsanguinate
The removal of blood from the body. This may occur as the result of a serious accident in which the victim bleeds extensively. Rarely, it may happen that bleeding becomes uncontrollable during an operation.

Extension
Extension is the process of straightening or stretching a limb. When used in the natural sense, it involves the contraction of the muscles opposing those used in FLEXION. In cases of fractured limbs (see BONE, DISORDERS OF – Bone fractures), extension is employed during the application of splints, in order to reduce the displacement caused by the fracture, and prevent movement of the broken ends of bone. It is effected by gently and steadily pulling upon the part of the limb beyond the fracture. Extension of a more permanent type is used in the after-treatment of some fractures, as well as in diseases of the spine, by placing the patient upon an inclined bed and affixing weights to his or her lower limbs, or to his or her head by means of adhesive plaster or of straps.

Exteriorisation
In surgery, the procedure to transfer an organ from its normal place in the body to the skin surface. It may be temporary or permanent. A common example is when the intestine is brought to the abdominal surface as a COLOSTOMY: this may be permanent because of serious disease in the lower part of the COLON, or temporary to allow a disorder in the colon to be treated.

Extinction
(1) In behavioural psychology, the lessening of a conditioned reflex that occurs when it is not regularly reinforced. An example is in the treatment of unsatisfactory behaviour such as violence, when by preventing the individual from enjoying the rewards of violent acts – namely, the attention he or she attracts – the conditioned reflex that is part of the cycle of violence is reduced in strength.
(2) Elimination of life or of a biological species.

Extirpation
The total removal of a growth, organ or tissue by surgery.

Extra-
Extra- is the Latin prefix meaning outside of, or in addition – such as extracapsular, meaning outside the capsule of a joint, and extrasystole, meaning an additional contraction of the heart.

Extracellular
An adjective that describes an object or event outside a cell. An example is extracellular fluid, the medium surrounding a cell.

Extracts
Extracts are preparations, usually of a semi-solid consistency, containing the active parts of various plants extracted in one of several ways. In the case of some extracts, the juice of the fresh plant is simply pressed out and purified; in the case of others the active principles are dissolved out in water, which is then to a great extent driven off by evaporation. Other extracts are similarly made by the help of alcohol, and in some cases ether is the solvent.

Extradural
Outside the DURA MATER, the outermost of the three membranes that cover the BRAIN and SPINAL CORD. The extradural or epidural space is the space between the vertebral canal and the dura mater of the spinal cord. (See ANAESTHESIA – Local anaesthetics: epidural.)

Extrapyramidal System
This is a complex part of the nervous system, extending from the cortex to the medulla in the BRAIN, from which emerge descending spinal pathways which influence voluntary motor activity throughout the body. Although the normal functions of the system are poorly understood, there are characteristic signs of an extrapyramidal LESION. These include disturbance of voluntary movements, notably slowness and 'poverty' of movement; disturbance of

muscular tone, which may be increased or decreased; and involuntary movements, such as a tremor, irregular jerking movements, or slow writhing movements.

Diseases There are several diseases that result from lesions to the extrapyramidal system, of which the most common is PARKINSONISM. Others include WILSON'S DISEASE, KERN-ICTERUS, CHOREA and ATHETOSIS.

Extrasensory Perception (ESP)

An alleged way of perceiving current events (clairvoyance), future events (precognition) or the thoughts of other people (telepathy). ESP has never been scientifically proven and does not involve the use of any known senses.

Extrasystole

Extrasystole is a term applied to premature contraction of one or more of the chambers of the heart. A beat of the heart occurs sooner than it should do in the ordinary rhythm and is followed by a longer rest than usual before the next beat. In an extrasystole, the stimulus to contraction arises in a part of the heart other than the usual. Extrasystoles often give rise to an unpleasant sensation as of the heart stumbling over a beat, but their occurrence is not usually serious.

Extrauterine Pregnancy

See ECTOPIC PREGNANCY.

Extravasation

An escape of fluid from the vessels or passages which ought to contain it. Extravasation of blood due to tearing of vessel walls is found in STROKE, and in the commoner condition known as a bruise. Extravasation of urine takes place when the bladder or the URETHRA is ruptured by a blow on the abdomen or on the crutch (PERINEUM), or torn in a fracture of the pelvis. Intravenous infusions frequently extravasate.

Extrinsic

(1) Originating outside the body.
(2) An extrinsic muscle is one whose origin is some way from the part of the body it acts upon – for example, the muscles controlling the movement of the eyeball which are attached to the bony orbit in which the eye sits.

Extrovert

A person who is outgoing, enjoys mixing with others and looks for fresh activities to take part in. Tends to act emotionally rather than intellectually.

Exudation

The process in which some of the constituents of the blood pass slowly through the walls of the small vessels in the course of inflammation, and also means the accumulation resulting from this process. For example, in PLEURISY the solid, rough material deposited on the surface of the lung is an exudation.

Eye

The eye is the sensory organ of sight. It is an elaborate photoreceptor detecting information, in the form of light, from the environment and transmitting this information by a series of electrochemical changes to the BRAIN. The visual cortex is the part of the brain that processes this information (i.e. the visual cortex is what 'sees' the environment). There are two eyes, each a roughly spherical hollow organ held within a bony cavity (the orbit). Each orbit is situated on the front of the skull, one on each side of the nose. The eye consists of an outer wall of three main layers and a central cavity divided into three.

The outer coat consists of the sclera and the cornea; their junction is called the limbus.
SCLERA This is white, opaque, and constitutes the posterior five-sixths of the outer coat. It is made of dense fibrous tissue. The sclera is visible anteriorly, between the eyelids, as the 'white of the eye'. Posteriorly and anteriorly it is covered by Tenons capsule, which in turn is covered by transparent conjunctiva. There is a hole in the sclera through which nerve fibres from the retina leave the eye in the optic nerve. Other smaller nerve fibres and blood vessels also pass through the sclera at different points.
CORNEA This constitutes the transparent, colourless anterior one-sixth of the eye. It is transparent in order to allow light into the eye and is more steeply curved than the sclera. Viewed from in front, the cornea is roughly circular. Most of the focusing power of the eye is provided by the cornea (the lens acts as the 'fine adjustment'). It has an outer epithelium, a central stroma and an inner endothelium. The cornea is supplied with very fine nerve fibres which make it exquisitely sensitive to pain. The central cornea has no blood supply – it relies mainly on aqueous humour for nutrition. Blood vessels and large nerve fibres in the cornea would prevent light from entering the eye.
LIMBUS is the junction between cornea and sclera. It contains the trabecular meshwork, a

sieve-like structure through which aqueous humour leaves the eye.

The middle coat (uveal tract) consists of the choroid, ciliary body and iris.

CHOROID A highly vascular sheet of tissue lining the posterior two-thirds of the sclera. The network of vessels provides the blood supply for the outer half of the retina. The blood supply of the choroid is derived from numerous ciliary vessels which pierce the sclera in front and behind.

CILIARY BODY A ring of tissue extending 6 mm back from the anterior limitation of the sclera. The various muscles of the ciliary body by their contractions and relaxations are responsible for changing the shape of the lens during ACCOMMODATION. The ciliary body is lined by cells that secrete aqueous humour. Posteriorly, the ciliary body is continuous with the choroid; anteriorly it is continuous with the iris.

IRIS A flattened muscular diaphragm that is attached at its periphery to the ciliary body, and has a round central opening – the pupil. By contraction and relaxation of the muscles of the iris, the pupil can be dilated or constricted (dilated in the dark or when aroused; constricted in bright light and for close work). The iris forms a partial division between the anterior chamber and the posterior chamber of the eye. It lies in front of the lens and forms the back wall of the anterior chamber. The iris is visible from in front, through the transparent cornea, as the 'coloured part of the eye'. The amount and distribution of iris pigment determine the colour of the iris. The pupil is merely a hole in the centre of the iris and appears black.

The inner layer The retina is a multilayered tissue (ten layers in all) which extends from the edges of the optic nerve to line the inner surface of the choroid up to the junction of ciliary body and choroid. Here the true retina ends at the ora serrata. The retina contains light-sensitive cells of two types: (i) cones – cells that operate at high and medium levels of illumination; they subserve fine discrimination of vision and colour vision; (ii) rods – cells that function best at low light intensity and subserve black-and-white vision.

The retina contains about 6 million cones and about 100 million rods. Information from them is conveyed by the nerve fibres which are in the inner part of the retina, and leave the eye in the optic nerve. There are no photoreceptors at the optic disc (the point where the optic nerve leaves the eye) and therefore there is no light perception from this small area. The optic disc thus produces a physiological blind spot in the visual field.

The retina can be subdivided into several areas:

PERIPHERAL RETINA contains mainly rods and a few scattered cones. Visual acuity from this area is fairly coarse.

MACULA LUTEA So-called because histologically it looks like a yellow spot. It occupies an area 4·5 mm in diameter lateral to the optic disc. This area of specialised retina can produce a high level of visual acuity. Cones are abundant here but there are few rods.

FOVEA CENTRALIS A small central depression at the centre of the macula. Here the cones are tightly packed; rods are absent. It is responsible for the highest levels of visual acuity.

The chambers of the eye There are three: the anterior and posterior chambers, and the vitreous cavity.

ANTERIOR CHAMBER Limited in front by the inner surface of the cornea, behind by the iris and pupil. It contains a transparent clear watery fluid, the aqueous humour. This is constantly being produced by cells of the ciliary body and constantly drained away through the trabecular meshwork. The trabecular meshwork lies in the angle between the iris and inner surface of the cornea.

POSTERIOR CHAMBER A narrow space between the iris and pupil in front and the lens behind. It too contains aqueous humour in transit from the ciliary epithelium to the anterior chamber, via the pupil.

VITREOUS CAVITY The largest cavity of the eye. In front it is bounded by the lens and behind by the retina. It contains vitreous humour.

Lens Transparent, elastic and biconvex in cross-section, it lies behind the iris and in front of the vitreous cavity. Viewed from the front it is roughly circular and about 10 mm in diameter. The diameter and thickness of the lens vary with its accommodative state. The lens consists of:

CAPSULE A thin transparent membrane surrounding the cortex and nucleus.

CORTEX This comprises newly made lens fibres that are relatively soft. It separates the capsule on the outside from the nucleus at the centre of the lens.

NUCLEUS The dense central area of old lens fibres that have become compacted by new lens fibres laid down over them.

ZONULE Numerous radially arranged fibres attached between the ciliary body and the lens around its circumference. Tension in these zonular fibres can be adjusted by the muscles of the ciliary body, thus changing the shape of the lens and altering its power of accommodation.

VITREOUS HUMOUR A transparent jelly-like structure made up of a network of collagen fibres suspended in a viscid fluid. Its shape conforms to that of the vitreous cavity within which it is contained: that is, it is spherical except for a shallow concave depression on its anterior surface. The lens lies in this depression.

Eyelids

These are multilayered curtains of tissue whose functions include spreading of the tear film over the front of the eye to prevent desiccation; protection from injury or external irritation; and to some extent the control of light entering the eye. Each eye has an upper and lower lid which form an elliptical opening (the palpebral fissure) when the eyes are open. The lids meet at the medial canthus and lateral canthus respectively. The inner medial canthus is fixed; the lateral canthus more mobile. An epicanthus is a fold of skin which covers the medial canthus in oriental races.

Each lid consists of several layers. From front to back they are: very thin skin; a sheet of muscle (orbicularis oculi, whose fibres are concentric around the palpebral fissure and which produce closure of the eyelids); the orbital septum (modified near the lid margin to form the tarsal plates); and finally, lining the back surface of the lid, the conjunctiva (known here as tarsal conjunctiva). At the free margin of each lid are the eyelashes, the openings of tear glands which lie within the lid, and the lacrimal punctum. Toward the medial edge of each lid is an elevation known as the papilla: the lacrimal punctum opens into this papilla. The punctum forms the open end of the cannaliculus, part of the tear-drainage mechanism.

Orbit

The bony cavity within which the eye is held. The orbits lie one on either side of the nose, on the front of the skull. They afford considerable protection for the eye. Each is roughly pyramidal in shape, with the apex pointing backwards and the base forming the open anterior part of the orbit. The bone of the anterior orbital margin is thickened to protect the eye from injury. There are various openings into the posterior part of the orbit – namely the optic canal, which allows the optic nerve to leave the orbit en route for the brain, and the superior orbital and inferior orbital fissures, which allow passage of nerves and blood vessels to and from the orbit. The most important structures holding the eye within the orbit are the extra-ocular muscles, a suspensory ligament

of connective tissue that forms a hammock on which the eye rests and which is slung between the medial and lateral walls of the orbit. Finally, the orbital septum, a sheet of connective tissue extending from the anterior margin of the orbit into the lids, helps keep the eye in place. A pad of fat fills in the orbit behind the eye and acts as a cushion for the eye.

Conjunctiva

A transparent mucous membrane that extends from the limbus over the anterior sclera or 'white of the eye'. This is the bulbar conjunctiva. The conjunctiva does not cover the cornea. Conjunctiva passes from the eye on to the inner surface of the eyelid at the fornices and is continuous with the tarsal conjunctiva. The semilunar fold is the vertical crescent of conjunctiva at the medial aspect of the palpebral fissure. The caruncle is a piece of modified skin just within the inner canthus.

Eye muscles

The extra-ocular muscles. There are six in all, the four rectus muscles (superior, inferior, medial and lateral rectus muscles) and two oblique muscles (superior and inferior oblique muscles). The muscles are attached at various points between the bony orbit and the eyeball. By their combined action they move the eye in horizontal and vertical gaze. They also produce torsional movement of the eye (i.e. clockwise or anticlockwise movements when viewed from the front).

Lacrimal apparatus

There are two components: a tear-production system, namely the lacrimal gland and accessory lacrimal glands; and a drainage system.

Tears keep the front of the eye moist; they also contain nutrients and various components to protect the eye from infection. Crying results from excess tear production. The drainage system cannot cope with the excess and therefore tears overflow on to the face. Newborn babies do not produce tears for the first three months of life.

LACRIMAL GLAND Located below a small depression in the bony roof of the orbit. Numerous tear ducts open from it into predominantly the upper lid. Accessory lacrimal glands are found in the conjunctiva and within the eyelids: the former open directly on to the surface of the conjunctiva; the latter on to the eyelid margin.

LACRIMAL DRAINAGE SYSTEM This consists of:

PUNCTUM An elevated opening toward the medial aspect of each lid. Each punctum opens into a canaliculus.

CANALICULUS A fine tube-like structure running within the lid, parallel to the lid margin. The canaliculi from upper and lower lid join to form a common canaliculus which opens into the lacrimal sac.

LACRIMAL SAC A small sac on the side of the nose which opens into the nasolacrimal duct. During blinking, the sac sucks tears into itself from the canaliculus. Tears then drain by gravity down the nasolacrimal duct.

NASOLACRIMAL DUCT A tubular structure which runs down through the wall of the nose and opens into the nasal cavity.

Visual pathway

Light stimulates the rods and cones of the retina. Electrochemical messages are then passed to nerve fibres in the retina and then via the optic nerve to the optic chiasm. Here information from the temporal (outer) half of each retina continues to the same side of the brain. Information from the nasal (inner) half of each retina crosses to the other side within the optic chiasm. The rearranged nerve fibres then pass through the optic tract to the lateral geniculate body, then the optic radiation to reach the visual cortex in the occipital lobe of the brain.

Eyeball

See EYE.

Eye, Disorders of

Arcus senilis The white ring or crescent which tends to form at the edge of the cornea with age. It is uncommon in the young, when it may be associated with high levels of blood lipids (see LIPID).

Astigmatism (See ASTIGMATISM.)

Blepharitis A chronic inflammation of the lid margins. SEBORRHOEA and staphylococcal infection are likely contributors. The eyes are typically intermittently red, sore and gritty over months or years. Treatment is difficult and may fail. Measures to reduce debris on the lid margins, intermittent courses of topical antibiotics, steroids or systemic antibiotics may help the sufferer.

Blepharospasm Involuntary closure of the eye. This may accompany irritation but may also occur without an apparent cause. It may be severe enough to interfere with vision. Treatment involves removing the source of irritation, if present. Severe and persistent cases may respond to injection of *Botulinum* toxin into the orbicularis muscle.

Cataract A term used to describe any opacity in the lens of the eye, from the smallest spot to total opaqueness. The prevalence of cataracts is age-related: 65 per cent of individuals in their sixth decade have some degree of lens opacity, while all those over 80 are affected. Cataracts are the most important cause of blindness worldwide. Symptoms will depend on whether one or both eyes are affected, as well as the position and density of the cataract(s). If only one eye is developing a cataract, it may be some time before the person notices it, though reading may be affected. Some people with cataracts become shortsighted, which in older people may paradoxically 'improve' their ability to read. Bright light may worsen vision in those with cataracts.

The extent of visual impairment depends on the nature of the cataracts, and the first symptoms noticed by patients include difficulty in recognising faces and in reading, while problems watching television or driving, especially at night, are pointers to the condition. Cataracts are common but are not the only cause of deteriorating vision. Patients with cataracts should be able to point to the position of a light and their pupillary reactions should be normal. If a bright light is shone on the eye, the lens may appear brown or, in advanced cataracts, white (see diagram).

While increasing age is the commonest cause of cataract in the UK, patients with DIABETES MELLITUS, UVEITIS and a history of injury to the eye can also develop the disorder. Prolonged STEROID treatment can result in cataracts. Children may develop cataracts, and in them the condition is much more serious as vision may be irreversibly impaired because development of the brain's ability to interpret visual signals is hindered. This may happen even if the cataracts are removed, so early referral for treatment is essential. One of the physical signs which doctors look for when they suspect cataract in adults as well as in children is the 'red reflex'. This is observable when an ophthalmoscopic examination of the eye is made (see OPHTHALMOSCOPE). Identification of this red reflex (a reflection of light from the red surface of the retina –see EYE) is a key diagnostic sign in children, especially young ones.

There is no effective medical treatment for established cataracts. Surgery is necessary and the decision when to operate depends mainly on how the cataract(s) affect(s) the patient's vision. Nowadays, surgery can be done at any time with limited risk. Most patients with a vision of 6/18 – 6/10 is the minimum standard for driving – or worse in both eyes should

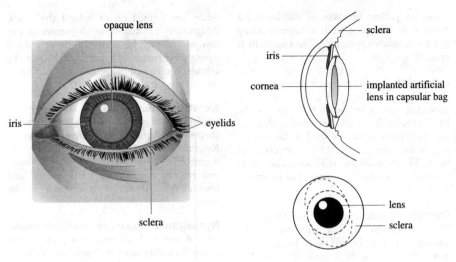

Cataract: the opaque lens of any eye with cataract (left) is replaced with an implanted artificial lens (right).

benefit from surgery, though elderly people may tolerate visual acuity of 6/18 or worse, so surgery must be tailored to the individual's needs. Younger people with a cataract will have more demanding visual requirements and so may opt for an 'earlier' operation. Most cataract surgery in Britain is now done under local anaesthetic and uses the 'phaco-emulsification' method. A small hole is made in the anterior capsule of the lens after which the hard lens nucleus is liquified ultrasonically. A replacement lens is inserted into the empty lens bag (see diagram). Patients usually return to their normal activities within a few days of the operation. A recent development under test in the USA for children requiring cataract operations is an intra-ocular flexible implant whose magnifying power can be altered as a child develops, thus precluding the need for a series of corrective operations as happens now.

Chalazion A firm lump in the eyelid relating to a blocked meibomian gland, felt deep within the lid. Treatment is not always necessary; a proportion spontaneously resolve. There can be associated infection when the lid becomes red and painful requiring antibiotic treatment. If troublesome, the chalazion can be incised under local anaesthetic.

Conjunctivitis Inflammation of the conjunctiva (see EYE) which may affect one or both eyes. Typically the eye is red, itchy, sticky and gritty but is not usually painful. Redness is not always present. Conjunctivitis can occasionally be painful, particularly if there is an associated

keratitis (see below) – for example, adenovirus infection, herpetic infection.

The cause can be infective (bacteria, viruses or CHLAMYDIA), chemical (e.g. acids, alkalis) or allergic (e.g. in hay fever). Conjunctivitis may also be caused by contact lenses, and preservatives or even the drugs in eye drops may cause conjunctival inflammation. Conjunctivitis may addtionally occur in association with other illnesses – for example, upper-respiratory-tract infection, Stevens-Johnson syndrome (see ERYTHEMA – erythema multiforme) or REITER'S SYNDROME. The treatment depends on the cause. In many patients acute conjunctivitis is self-limiting.

Dacryocystitis Inflammation of the lacrimal sac. This may present acutely as a red, painful swelling between the nose and the lower lid. An abscess may form which points through the skin and which may need to be drained by incision. Systemic antibiotics may be necessary. Chronic dacryocystitis may occur with recurrent discharge from the openings of the tear ducts and recurrent swelling of the lacrimal sac. Obstruction of the tear duct is accompanied by watering of the eye. If the symptoms are troublesome, the patient's tear passageways need to be surgically reconstructed.

Ectropion The lid margin is everted – usually the lower lid. Ectropion is most commonly associated with ageing, when the tissues of the lid become lax. It can also be caused by shortening of the skin of the lids such as happens with scarring or mechanical factors – for example,

E

a tumour pulling the skin of the lower lid downwards. Ectropion tends to cause watering and an unsightly appearance. The treatment is surgical.

Entropion The lid margin is inverted – usually the lower lid. Entropion is most commonly associated with ageing, when the tissues of the lid become lax. It can also be caused by shortening of the inner surfaces of the lids due to scarring – for example, TRACHOMA or chemical burns. The inwardly directed lashes cause irritation and can abrade the cornea. The treatment is surgical.

Episcleritis Inflammation of the EPISCLERA. There is usually no apparent cause. The inflammation may be diffuse or localised and may affect one or both eyes. It sometimes recurs. The affected area is usually red and moderately painful. Episcleritis is generally not thought to be as painful as scleritis and does not lead to the same complications. Treatment is generally directed at improving the patient's symptoms. The inflammation may respond to NON-STEROIDAL ANTI-INFLAMMATORY DRUGS (NSAIDS) or topical CORTICOSTEROIDS.

Errors of refraction (Ametropia.) These will occur when the focusing power of the lens and cornea does not match the length of the eye, so that rays of light parallel to the visual axis are not focused at the fovea centralis (see EYE). There are three types of refractive error:
HYPERMETROPIA or long-sightedness. The refractive power of the eye is too weak, or the eye is too short so that rays of light are brought to a focus at a point behind the retina. Long-sighted people can see well in the distance but generally require glasses with convex lenses for reading. Uncorrected long sight can lead to headaches and intermittent blurring of vision following prolonged close work (i.e. eye strain). As a result of ageing, the eye becomes gradually long-sighted, resulting in many people needing reading glasses in later life: this normal process is known as presbyopia. A particular form of long-sightedness occurs after cataract extraction (see above).
MYOPIA (Short sight or near sight.) Rays of light are brought to a focus in front of the retina because the refractive power of the eye is too great or the eye is too short. Short-sighted people can see close to but need spectacles with concave lenses in order to see in the distance.
ASTIGMATISM The refractive power of the eye is not the same in each meridian. Some rays of light may be focused in front of the retina while others are focused on or behind the retina. Astigmatism can accompany hypermetropia or myopia. It may be corrected by cylindrical lenses: these consist of a slice from the side of a cylinder (i.e. curved in one meridian and flat in the meridian at right-angles to it).

Keratitis Inflammation of the cornea in response to a variety of insults – viral, bacterial, chemical, radiation, or mechanical trauma. Keratitis may be superficial or involve the deeper layers, the latter being generally more serious. The eye is usually red, painful and photophobic. Treatment is directed at the cause.

Nystagmus Involuntary rhythmic oscillation of one or both eyes. There are several causes including nervous disorders, vestibular disorders, eye disorders and certain drugs including alcohol.

Ophthalmia Inflammation of the eye, especially the conjunctiva (see conjunctivitis, above). Ophthalmia neonatorum is a type of conjunctivitis that occurs in newborn babies. They catch the disease when passing through an infected birth canal during their mother's labour (see PREGNANCY AND LABOUR). CHLAMYDIA and GONORRHOEA are the two most common infections. Treatment is effective with antibiotics: untreated, the infection may cause permanent eye damage.

Pinguecula A benign degenerative change in the connective tissue at the nasal or temporal limbus (see EYE). This is visible as a small, flattened, yellow-white lump adjacent to the cornea.

Pterygium Overgrowth of the conjunctival tissues at the limbus on to the cornea (see EYE). This usually occurs on the nasal side and is associated with exposure to sunlight. The pterygium is surgically removed for cosmetic reasons or if it is thought to be advancing towards the visual axis.

Ptosis Drooping of the upper lid. May occur because of a defect in the muscles which raise the lid (levator complex), sometimes the result of ageing or trauma. Other causes include HORNER'S SYNDROME, third cranial nerve PALSY, MYASTHENIA GRAVIS, and DYSTROPHIA MYOTONICA. The cause needs to be determined and treated if possible. The treatment for a severely drooping lid is surgical, but other measures can be used to prop up the lid with varying success.

Retina, disorders of The retina can be damaged by disease that affects the retina alone, or by diseases affecting the whole body.

Retinopathy is a term used to denote an abnormality of the retina without specifying a cause. Some retinal disorders are discussed below.

DIABETIC RETINOPATHY Retinal disease occurring in patients with DIABETES MELLITUS. It is the commonest cause of blind registration in Great Britain of people between the ages of 20 and 65. Diabetic retinopathy can be divided into several types. The two main causes of blindness are those that follow: first, development of new blood vessels from the retina, with resultant complications and, second, those following 'water logging' (oedema) of the macula. Treatment is by maintaining rigid control of blood-sugar levels combined with laser treatment for certain forms of the disease – in particular to get rid of new blood vessels.

HYPERTENSIVE RETINOPATHY Retinal disease secondary to the development of high blood pressure. Treatment involves control of the blood pressure (see HYPERTENSION).

SICKLE CELL RETINOPATHY People with sickle cell disease (see under ANAEYIA) can develop a number of retinal problems including new blood vessels from the retina.

RETINOPATHY OF PREMATURITY (ROP) Previously called retrolental fibroplasia (RLF), this is a disorder affecting low-birth-weight premature babies exposed to oxygen. Essentially, new blood vessels develop which cause extensive traction on the retina with resultant retinal detachment and poor vision.

RETINAL ARTERY OCCLUSION; RETINAL VEIN OCCLUSION These result in damage to those areas of retina supplied by the affected blood vessel: the blood vessels become blocked. If the peripheral retina is damaged the patient may be completely symptom-free, although areas of blindness may be detected on examination of field of vision. If the macula is involved, visual loss may be sudden, profound and permanent. There is no effective treatment once visual loss has occurred.

SENILE MACULAR DEGENERATION ('Senile' indicates age of onset and has no bearing on mental state.) This is the leading cause of blindness in the elderly in the western world. The average age of onset is 65 years. Patients initially notice a disturbance of their vision which gradually progresses over months or years. They lose the ability to recognise fine detail; for example, they cannot read fine print, sew, or recognise people's faces. They always retain the ability to recognise large objects such as doors and chairs, and are therefore able to get around and about reasonably well. There is no effective treatment in the majority of cases.

RETINITIS PIGMENTOSA A group of rare, inherited diseases characterised by the development of night blindness and tunnel vision. Symptoms start in childhood and are progressive. Many patients retain good visual acuity, although their peripheral vision is limited. One of the characteristic findings on examination is collections of pigment in the retina which have a characteristic shape and are therefore known as 'bone spicules'. There is no effective treatment.

RETINAL DETACHMENT usually occurs due to the development of a hole in the retina. Holes can occur as a result of degeneration of the retina, traction on the retina by the vitreous, or injury. Fluid from the vitreous passes through the hole causing a split within the retina; the inner part of the retina becomes detached from the outer part, the latter remaining in contact with the choroid. Detached retina loses its ability to detect light, with consequent impairment of vision. Retinal detachments are more common in the short-sighted, in the elderly or following cataract extraction. Symptoms include spots before the eyes (floaters), flashing lights and a shadow over the eye with progressive loss of vision. Treatment by laser is very effective if caught early, at the stage when a hole has developed in the retina but before the retina has become detached. The edges of the hole can be 'spot welded' to the underlying choroid. Once a detachment has occurred, laser therapy cannot be used; the retina has to be repositioned. This is usually done by indenting the wall of the eye from the outside to meet the retina, then making the retina stick to the wall of the eye by inducing inflammation in the wall (by freezing it). The outcome of surgery depends largely on the extent of the detachment and its duration. Complicated forms of detachment can occur due to diabetic eye disease, injury or tumour. Each requires a specialised form of treatment.

Scleritis Inflammation of the sclera (see EYE). This can be localised or diffuse, can affect the anterior or the posterior sclera, and can affect one or both eyes. The affected eye is usually red and painful. Scleritis can lead to thinning and even perforation of the sclera, sometimes with little sign of inflammation. Posterior scleritis in particular may cause impaired vision and require emergency treatment. There is often no apparent cause, but there are some associated conditions – for example, RHEUMATOID ARTHRITIS, GOUT, and an autoimmune disease affecting the nasal passages and lungs called Wegener's granulomatosis. Treatment depends on severity but may involve NON-STEROIDAL ANTI-INFLAMMATORY DRUGS (NSAIDS), topical CORTICOSTEROIDS or systemic immunosuppressive drugs.

Stye Infection of a lash follicle. This presents as a painful small red lump at the lid margin. It often resolves spontaneously but may require antibiotic treatment if it persists or recurs.

Sub-conjunctival haemorrhage Haemorrhage between the conjunctiva and the underlying episclera. It is painless. There is usually no apparent cause and it resolves spontaneously.

Trichiasis Inward misdirection of the lashes. Trichiasis occurs due to inflammation of or trauma to the lid margin. Treatment involves removal of the patient's lashes. Regrowth may be prevented by electrolysis, by CRYOTHERAPY to the lid margin, or by surgery.

For the subject of artificial eyes, see under PROSTHESIS; also GLAUCOMA, SQUINT and UVEITIS.

Eye Drops

Eye drops and ointment are used extensively in the treatment of eye disease. They should be used as instructed by the prescribing physician. Most can be used for one month after the bottle has been opened but should then be discarded and a repeat prescription obtained if necessary. Any eye drops or ointment can have side-effects, and any difficulty with them should be referred to the prescribing physician.

Eye Injuries

Victims of eye injuries are advised to seek prompt medical advice if the injury is at all serious or does not resolve with simple first-aid measures – for example, by washing out a foreign body using an eye bath.

Blunt injuries These may cause haemorrhage inside the eye, cataract, retinal detachment or even rupture of the eye (see also EYE, DISORDERS OF). Injuries from large blunt objects – for example, a squash ball – may also cause a 'blow-out fracture' of the orbital floor resulting in double vision. Surgical treatment may be required depending on the patient's specific problems.

Chemical burns Most chemical splashes cause conjunctivitis and superficial keratitis in the victim (see EYE, DISORDERS OF); both conditions are self-limiting. Alkalis are, however, more likely to penetrate deeper into the eye and cause permanent damage, particularly to the cornea. Prompt irrigation is important. Further treatment may involve testing the pH of the tears, topical antibiotics and CORTICOSTEROIDS, and vitamin C (drops or tablets – see APPENDIX 5: VITAMINS), depending on the nature of the injury.

Corneal abrasion Loss of corneal epithelium (outermost layer). Almost any sort of injury to the eye may cause this. The affected eye is usually very painful. In the absence of other problems, the epithelium heals rapidly: small defects may close within 24 hours. Treatment conventionally consists of antibiotic ointment and sometimes a pad over the injured eye.

Foreign bodies Most foreign bodies which hit the eye are small and are found in the conjunctival sac or on the cornea; most are superficial and can be easily removed. A few foreign bodies penetrate deeper and may cause infection, cataract, retinal detachment or haemorrhage within the eye. The foreign body is usually removed and the damage repaired; nevertheless the victim's sight may have been permanently damaged. Particularly dangerous activities include hammering or chiselling on metal or stone; people carrying out these activities (and others, such as hedge-cutting and grass-strimming) should wear protective goggles.

Fabricated and Induced Illness
See MUNCHAUSEN'S SYNDROME.

Face Lift
An operation to reduce wrinkles and lift 'loose' skin on the face of mature persons with the aim of making them look younger. It can be performed under local anaesthetic as an outpatient or with general anaesthesia as an inpatient. The operation is regarded as cosmetic and is usually done in the private health-care sector in the UK.

Facial Nerve
The seventh cranial nerve (arising from the BRAIN), supplying the muscles of expression in the face, being purely a motor nerve. It enters the face immediately below the ear after splitting up into several branches. (See BELL'S PALSY.)

Facies
Facies is a term applied to the expression or appearance of the face.

Factitious Urticaria
See DERMOGRAPHISM.

Factor VIII
A coagulative blood protein that is a constituent of the COAGULATION cascade – an essential component in the clotting of blood. Those people with the inherited disorder, HAEMO-PHILIA, have abnormally low amounts of factor VIII and so bleed more when cut. They are treated with a concentrated version to reduce the tendency to bleed.

Faeces
Faeces, or stools, consist of the remainder of the food after it has passed through the alimentary canal and been subjected to the action of the digestive juices, and after the nutritious parts have been absorbed by the intestinal mucous membrane. The stools also contain various other matters, such as pigment derived from BILE, and large quantities of bacteria which are the main component of human stools. The stools are passed once daily by most people, but infants have several evacuations of the bowels in 24 hours and some adults may defaecate only two or three times weekly. Sudden changes in bowel habit, persistent diarrhoea or a change from the normal dark brown (caused by the bile pigment, stercobilin) to very pale or very dark stools are reasons for seeking medical advice. Blood in the stools may be due to HAEMOR-RHOIDS or something more serious, and anyone with such symptoms should see a doctor.

Incontinence of the bowels, or inability to retain the stools, is found in certain diseases in which the sphincter muscles – those muscles that naturally keep the bowel closed – relax. It is also a symptom of disease in, or injury to, the SPINAL CORD.

Pain on defaecation is a characteristic symptom of a FISSURE at the ANUS or of inflamed haemorrhoids, and is usually sharp. Pain of a duller character associated with the movements of the bowels may be caused by inflammation in the other pelvic organs.

CONSTIPATION and DIARRHOEA are considered under separate headings.

Fainting
Fainting, or SYNCOPE, is a temporary loss of consciousness caused by inadequate supply of blood to the brain. It may be preceded by nausea, sweating, loss of vision, and ringing in the ears (see TINNITUS). It is most often caused by pooling of blood in the extremities, which reduces venous return (see CIRCULATORY SYSTEM OF THE BLOOD) and thus cardiac output: this may be due to hot weather or prolonged standing. Occasionally, fainting on standing occurs in people with low blood pressure (see HYPOTENSION), autonomic neuropathy (in which normal vasomotor reflexes are absent), or those taking antihypertensive drugs. A prolonged rise in intrathoracic pressure caused by coughing, MICTURITION, or VALSALVA'S MANOEUVRE also impedes venous return and may cause fainting. HYPOVOLAEMIA produced by bleeding, prolonged diarrhoea, or vomiting may also cause fainting, and the condition can be produced by severe pain or emotional upset. Cardiac causes, such as severe stenotic valve disease or rhythm disturbances (particularly complete heart block or very rapid tachycardias), may result in fainting (see HEART, DISEASES OF). Treatment must be directed towards the underlying cause, but immediate first aid consists of laying the patient down and elevating the legs.

Faith Healing
The facility, claimed by some people, to cure disease by a healing force present in their

make-up. The healer 'transmits' the force by direct contact with the person seeking treatment. Strong religious beliefs are usually the characteristics of the healer and his or her subject. The force is inexplicable to science but some medically qualified doctors have been convinced of its beneficial effect in certain individuals.

Fallen Arches
Weakness in the muscles that support the bony arches of the foot. The result is flat feet, a condition that can adversely affect a person's ability to walk and run normally.

Falling Sickness
An old name for EPILEPSY.

Fallopian Tubes
Tubes, one on each side, lying in the pelvic area of the abdomen, which are attached at one end to the UTERUS, and have the other unattached but lying close to the ovary (see OVARIES). Each is 10–12.5 cm (4–5 inches) long, large at the end next to the ovary, but communicating with the womb by an opening which admits only a bristle. These tubes conduct the ova (see OVUM) from the ovaries to the interior of the womb. Blockage of the Fallopian tubes by a chronic inflammatory process resulting from infection is a not uncommon cause of infertility in women. (See ECTOPIC PREGNANCY; REPRODUCTIVE SYSTEM.)

Fallot's Tetralogy
See TETRALOGY OF FALLOT.

False-Memory Syndrome
See REPRESSED MEMORY THERAPY.

Familial
A description of a disorder, illness or characteristic that runs in families.

Famotidine
One of the H2 RECEPTOR ANTAGONISTS used to heal gastric ulcers (see STOMACH, DISEASES OF) and DUODENAL ULCER. The drug works by blocking H_2 receptors and so cutting the output of gastric acid. It is taken orally; side-effects may include dizziness, changed bowel habit, fatigue, rashes, confusion, reversible liver damage and headache.

Fansidar
A combination of PYRIMETHAMINE and sulfadoxine used in conjunction with other antimalarial drugs to treat *falciparum* malaria (see MALARIA).

Farmer's Lung
A form of external allergic ALVEOLITIS caused by the inhalation of dust from mouldy hay or straw.

Fascia
Sheets or bands of fibrous tissue which enclose the body tissues beneath the skin and connect the muscles.

Fasciitis
Inflammation of FASCIA. The most common site is the sole of the foot, where it is known as plantar fasciitis. It is characterised by gnawing pain. There is no specific treatment, but the condition usually clears up spontaneously – though over a considerable time.

Fascioliasis
Disease caused by the liver fluke, *Fasciola hepatica*. This is found in sheep, cattle and other herbivorous animals, in which it is the cause of the condition known as liver rot. It measures about 35×13 mm, and is transmitted to humans from the infected animals by snails. In Britain it is the most common disease found in animal slaughterhouses. The danger to humans is in eating vegetables – particularly wild watercress – that have been infected by snails; there have been several outbreaks of fascioliasis in Britain due to eating contaminated wild watercress, and much larger outbreaks from the same cause have been reported in France. The disease is characterised by fever, dyspepsia (indigestion), heavy sweating, loss of appetite, abdominal pain, URTICARIA, and a troublesome cough. In the more serious cases there may be severe damage to the LIVER, with or without JAUNDICE. The diagnosis is clinched by the finding of the eggs of the fluke in the stools. The two drugs used in treatment are bithionol and chloroquine. Even though many cases are quite mild and recover spontaneously, prevention is particularly important. This consists primarily of never eating wild watercress, as this is the main cause of infestation. Lettuces have also been found to be infested.

Fasciotomy
An operation to relieve pressure on muscles caused by tight surrounding FASCIA or fibrous CONNECTIVE TISSUE. The fascia is slit with an incision.

Fasting
Fasting is the abstention from, or deprivation of, food and drink. It may result from a genuine desire to lose weight – in an attempt to improve

one's health and/or appearance – or from a MENTAL ILLNESS such as DEPRESSION, or from one of the EATING DISORDERS. Certain religious customs and practices may demand periods of fasting. Forced fasting, often extended, has been used for many years as an effective means of torture.

Without food and drink the body rapidly becomes thinner and lighter as it draws upon its stored energy reserves, initially mainly fat. Body temperature gradually falls, and muscle is progressively broken down as the body struggles to maintain its vital functions. Dehydration, leading to cardiovascular collapse, inevitably follows unless a basic amount of water is taken – particularly if the body's fluid output is high, such as may occur with excessive sweating.

After prolonged fasting the return to food should be gradual, with careful monitoring of blood-pressure levels and concentrations of serum ELECTROLYTES. Feeding should consist mainly of liquids and light foods at first, with no heavy meals being taken for several days.

Fat

A food that has more energy-producing power, weight for weight, than any other. Animal fat is a mixture in varying proportions of stearic, palmitic, and oleic acids combined with glycerin. Butter contains about 80 per cent of fat; ordinary cream, 20 per cent; and rich cream 40 per cent – whilst olive oil is practically a pure form of fat. When taken to a large extent in the diet, fat requires to be combined with a certain proportion of either CARBOHYDRATE or PROTEIN in order that it may be completely consumed, otherwise harmful products, known as ketones, may form in the blood. Each gram of fat has an energy-producing equivalent of 9·3 Calories (see CALORIE).

Fats are divided into saturated fats – that is, animal fats and dairy produce; and unsaturated fats, which include vegetable oils from soya bean, maize and sunflower, and marine oils from fish (e.g. cod-liver oil). (See also ADIPOSE TISSUE; LIPID; OBESITY.)

Body fat Most of the body's fat is stored in ADIPOSE TISSUE which is mainly sited beneath the skin and around various internal organs. Some, however, is stored in liver, muscle and other cellular structures such as bone marrow (see BONE). Various methods can be used to estimate the body's fat content but all are indirect and not very accurate, depending as they do on hard-to-measure differences in composition between fat and lean tissues. The average body fat of healthy young men and women is below 20 per cent and 25 per cent respectively of their body weight. In economically developed countries, middle-aged men and women usually undergo a steady increase in body fat. This is probably not a feature of ageing, however, since in developing nations, which have different diets and greater levels of physical activity, increased age does not bring with it an increase in body fat. One widely used means to estimate whether a person has excess fat is to measure his or her skinfold thickness on the arms and torso. The distribution of fat can be a pointer to certain disorders: those adults, for example, who deposit their fat abdominally rather than on their hips – an android rather than a gynaecoid distribution – are particularly susceptible to disease of the CARDIOVASCULAR SYSTEM and to DIABETES MELLITUS.

Adipose tissue comprises fat deposited as a result of eating more food than is metabolised by exercise and the body's basic energy needs. Surplus fat can in some circumstances be a useful energy store. For example, hibernating animals 'burn off' the fat stored during the summer months and are much leaner when they wake up in the spring. Excessive quantities of adipose tissue result in OBESITY, an increasingly serious problem among all age groups, including children, in countries with developed economies.

Fatigue

Tiredness: a physiological state in which muscles become fatigued by the LACTIC ACID accumulating in them as the result of their activity. For the removal of lactic acid in the recovery phase of muscular contraction, oxygen is needed. If the supply of oxygen is not plentiful enough, or cannot keep pace with the work the muscle is doing, then lactic acid accumulates and fatigue results. There is also a nervous element in muscular fatigue: it is diminished by stimulation of the sympathetic nervous system. (See also MUSCLE.)

Chronic fatigue is a symptom of some illnesses such as ANAEMIA, CHRONIC FATIGUE SYNDROME (CFS), HYPOTHYROIDISM, MONONUCLEOSIS, MOTOR NEURONE DISEASE (MND), MYASTHENIA GRAVIS, MYALGIC ENCEPHALOMYELITIS (ME) and others. Some drugs may also produce a feeling of fatigue.

Fat Necrosis

In injury to, or inflammation of, the PANCREAS, the fat-splitting enzyme in it may escape into the abdominal cavity, causing death of fat-containing cells.

Fatty Degeneration

As a result of ANAEMIA, interference with blood or nerve supply, or because of the action of various poisons, body cells may undergo abnormal changes accompanied by the appearance in their substance of fat droplets.

Fauces

The somewhat narrowed opening between the mouth and throat. It is bounded above by the soft palate, below by the tongue, and on either side by the tonsil. In front of, and behind, the tonsil are two ridges of mucous membrane, the anterior and posterior pillars of the fauces.

Favism

A type of haemolytic ANAEMIA, attacks of which occur within an hour or two of eating broad beans (*Vicia fava*). It is a hereditary disease due to lack of an essential ENZYME called glucose-6-phosphate dehydrogenase, which is necessary for the continued integrity of the red cell. This defect is inherited as a sex-linked dominant trait, and the red cells of patients with this abnormality have a normal life-span until challenged by certain drugs or fava beans when the older cells are rapidly destroyed, resulting in haemolytic anaemia. Fourteen per cent of African-Americans are affected and 60 per cent of Yemenite Jews in Israel. The perpetuation of the gene is due to the greater resistance against MALARIA that it carries. Severe and even fatal HAEMOLYSIS has followed the administration of the antimalarial compounds pamaquine and primaquine in sensitive individuals. These red cells are sensitive not only to fava beans and primaquine but also to sulphonamides, acetanilide, phenacetin, para-aminosalicyclic acid, nitrofurantoin, probenecid and vitamin K analogues.

Favus

Another name for honeycomb ringworm. (See RINGWORM.)

Fear

An emotional condition provoked by danger and usually characterised by unpleasant subjective feelings accompanied by physiological and behavioural changes. The heart rate increases, sweating occurs and the blood pressure rises. Sometimes fear of certain events or places may develop into a phobia: for example, agoraphobia, a fear of open spaces.

Febrile

Having a FEVER. Describes a patient whose body temperature is greater than normal (36.9–37.8 °C).

Febrile Convulsion

Convulsion occurring in a child aged six months to six years with a high temperature in which the limbs twitch; he or she may lose consciousness. The condition is common, with one child in 20 suffering from it. It is a result of immature homeostatic control (see HOMEO-STASIS) and is not usually serious, occurring generally during an infection such as measles or tonsillitis. The brain and nervous system are normal in most cases. Treatment is tepid sponging and attention to the underlying cause, with the child placed in the recovery position. It is important to rule out more serious illness, such as MENINGITIS, if the child seems particularly ill.

Feedback Mechanism

Many glands which produce HORMONES are influenced by other hormones, particularly those secreted by the HYPOTHALAMUS (a controlling centre in the brain) and the PITUITARY GLAND. If the amount of hormone produced by a gland rises, negative feedback mechanisms operate by instructing the pituitary gland, via the hypothalamus, to produce less of the stimulating hormones. This cuts activity in the target gland. Should the amount of hormone produced fall, the feedback mechanism weakens with the result that the output of stimulating hormones increases.

Female Genital Mutilation (FGM)

See CIRCUMCISION.

Feminisation

The development of a feminine appearance in a man, often the result of an imbalance in the sex hormones. Castration, especially before puberty, causes feminisation, as may the use of hormones to treat an enlarged PROSTATE GLAND.

Femoral

Adjective relating to the FEMUR or the region of the thigh. For example, the femoral nerve, artery, vein and canal.

Femur

The thigh bone, which is the longest and strongest bone in the body. As the upper end is set at an angle of about 120 degrees to the rest of the bone, and since the weight of the body is entirely borne by the two femora, fracture of one of these bones close to its upper end is a common accident in old people, whose bones are often weakened by osteoporosis (see under BONE, DISORDERS OF). The femur fits, at its upper end, into the acetabulum of the pelvis, forming the hip-joint, and, at its lower end, meets the tibia and patella in the knee-joint.

Fenestration

A largely obsolete surgical operation to form a new opening in the bony LABYRINTH of the inner ear in the treatment of deafness caused by otosclerosis (see under EAR, DISEASES OF). Nowadays the disorder is usually surgically treated by STAPEDECTOMY.

Fertilisation

The process by which male and female gametes (spermatozoa and oöcytes respectively) fuse to form a zygote which develops, by a complex process of cell division and differentiation, into a new individual of the species. In humans, fertilisation occurs in the FALLOPIAN TUBES. Sperm deposited in the upper vagina traverse the cervix and uterus to enter the Fallopian tube. Many sperm attempt to penetrate the zona pellucida surrounding the oöcyte, but only one is able to penetrate the oöcyte proper and this prevents any other sperm from entering. Once the sperm has entered the oöcyte, the two nuclei fuse before the zygote begins to divide.

Fertility Rate

The number of live births that occur in a year for every 1,000 women of childbearing age (this is usually taken as 15–44 years of age). The fertility rate in the UK (all ages) was 54.9 in 2002 (*UK Health Statistics*, 2001 edition, The Stationery Office).

Fester

A popular, not a medical, term used to mean any collection or formation of pus. It is applied to both abscesses and ulcers. (See ABSCESS; ULCER; WHITLOW.)

Festination

The involuntary quickening of gait seen in some nervous diseases, especially in PARKINSONISM.

Fetal Alcohol Syndrome

A disorder of newborn infants that is caused by the toxic effects on the growing FETUS of excessive amounts of alcohol taken by the mother. Low birth-weight and retarded growth are the main consequences, but affected babies may have hand and facial deformities and are sometimes mentally retarded.

Fetal Blood Sampling

A procedure performed during a mother's labour in which a blood sample is taken from a vein in the scalp of the FETUS. This enables tests to be performed that indicate whether the fetus is, for example, suffering from a shortage of oxygen (HYPOXIA). If so, the obstetrician will usually accelerate the baby's birth.

Fetal Transplant

A procedure in which cells – for example, from the pancreas – are taken from an aborted FETUS and then transplanted into the malfunctioning organ (pancreas) of an individual with a disorder of that organ (in this case, diabetes). The cells from the fetus are intended to take over the function of the host's diseased or damaged cells. Fetal brain cells have also been transplanted into brains of people suffering from PARKINSONISM. These treatments are at an experimental stage.

Fetishism

This is a form of sexual deviation in which the person becomes sexually stimulated by parts of the body, such as the feet, which are not usually regarded as erotogenic. Some people are sexually aroused by items of clothing or shoes.

Fetoscopy

Inspection of a FETUS by passing a fibreoptic instrument called a fetoscope through the abdominal wall of a pregnant woman into her UTERUS. The procedure is usually conducted in the 18th to 20th week of pregnancy to assess the fetus for abnormalities and to take blood samples to preclude diseases such as HAEMOPHILIA, DUCHENNE MUSCULAR DYSTROPHY and sickle-cell ANAEMIA. The procedure should be used only if there is a serious possibility of abnormality, the presence of which will usually have been indicated by other screening tests such as ULTRASOUND and tests of blood obtained by (intrauterine) cordocentesis (withdrawal of blood by syringe inserted into the umbilical cord).

Fetus

The name given to the unborn child after the eighth week of development. Humans, like all animals, begin as a single cell, the OVUM, in the ovary (see OVARIES). After FERTILISATION with a SPERMATOZOON, the ovum becomes embedded in the mucous membrane of the UTERUS, its covering being known as the decidua. Increase in size is rapid, and development of complexity is still more marked. The original cell divides repeatedly to form new cells, and these become arranged in three layers known as the ectoderm, mesoderm and endoderm. The first produces the skin, brain and spinal cord, and the nerves; the second the bones, muscles, blood vessels and connective tissues; while the third develops into the lining of the digestive system and the various glands attached to it.

The embryo develops upon one side of the ovum, its first appearance consisting of a groove, the edges of which grow up and join to form a tube, which in turn develops into the brain and spinal cord. At the same time, a part of the ovum beneath this is becoming pinched off to form the body, and within this the endoderm forms a second tube, which in time is changed in shape and lengthened to form the digestive canal. From the gut there grows out very early a process called the allantois, which attaches itself to the wall of the uterus, developing into the PLACENTA (afterbirth), a structure well supplied with blood vessels which draws nourishment from the mother's circulation via the wall of the womb.

The remainder of the ovum – which within two weeks of conception has increased to about 2 mm (1/12 inch) in size – splits into an outer and inner shell, from the outer of which are developed two covering membranes, the chorion and amnion; while the inner constitutes the yolk sac, attached by a pedicle to the developing gut of the embryo. From two weeks after conception onwards, the various organs and limbs appear and grow. The human embryo at this stage is almost indistinguishable in appearance from the embryo of other animals. After around the middle of the second month, it begins to show a distinctly human form and then is called the fetus. The property of 'life' is present from the very beginning, although the movements of the fetus are not usually felt by the mother until the fifth month.

During the first few days after conception the eye begins to be formed, beginning as a cup-shaped outgrowth from the mid-brain, its lens being formed as a thickening in the skin. It is very soon followed by the beginnings of the nose and ear, both of which arise as pits on the surface, which increase in complexity and are joined by nerves that grow outward from the brain. These three organs of sense have practically their final appearance as early as the beginning of the second month.

The body closes in from behind forwards,

the sides growing forwards from the spinal region. In the neck, the growth takes the form of five arches, similar to those which bear gills in fishes. From the first of these the lower jaw is formed; from the second the hyoid bone, all the arches uniting, and the gaps between them closing up by the end of the second month. At this time the head and neck have assumed quite a human appearance.

The digestive canal begins as a simple tube running from end to end of the embryo, but it grows in length and becomes twisted in various directions to form the stomach and bowels. The lungs and the liver arise from this tube as two little buds, which quickly increase in size and complexity. The kidneys also appear very early, but go through several changes before their final form is reached.

The genital organs appear late. The swellings, which form the ovary in the female and the testicle (or testis) in the male, are produced in the region of the loins, and gradually descend to their final positions. The external genitals are similar in the two sexes till the end of the third month, and the sex is not clearly distinguishable till late in the fourth month.

The blood vessels appear in the ovum even before the embryo. The heart, originally double, forms as a dilatation upon the arteries which later produce the aorta. These two hearts later fuse into one.

The limbs appear at about the end of the third week, as buds which increase quickly in length and split at their ends into five parts, for fingers or toes. The bones at first are formed of cartilage, in which true bone begins to appear during the third month. The average period of human gestation is 266 days – or 280 days from the first day of the last menstrual period. The average birth weight of an infant born of a healthy mother (in the UK) is 3,200 g (see table).

The following table gives the average size and weight of the fetus at different periods:

Age	Length	Weight
4 weeks	5 mm	1·3 grams
3 months	8 to 9 cm	30 to 60 grams
5 months	15 to 25 cm	170 to 340 grams
7 months	32 to 35 cm	1,360 to 1,820 grams
Birth	45 to 60 cm	3,200 grams

(See also PREGNANCY AND LABOUR.)

Fever

Fever, or PYREXIA, is the abnormal rise in body TEMPERATURE that frequently accompanies disease in general.

Causes The cause of fever is the release of fever-producing proteins (pyrogens) by phago-cytic cells called monocytes and macrophages, in response to a variety of infectious, immuno-logical and neoplastic stimuli. The lymphocytes (see LYMPHOCYTE) play a part in fever produc-tion because they recognise the antigen and release substances called lymphokines which promote the production of endogenous pyro-gen. The pyrogen then acts on the thermo-regulatory centre in the HYPOTHALAMUS and this results in an increase in heat generation and a reduction in heat loss, resulting in a rise in body temperature.

The average temperature of the body in health ranges from 36·9 to 37·5 °C (98·4 to 99·5 °F). It is liable to slight variations from such causes as the ingestion of food, the amount of exercise, the menstrual cycle, and the temperature of the surrounding atmosphere. There are, moreover, certain appreciable daily variations, the lowest temperature being between the hours of 01.00 and 07.00 hours, and the highest between 16.00 and 21.00 hours, with trifling fluctuations during these periods.

The development and maintenance of heat within the body depends upon the metabolic oxidation consequent on the changes continu-ally taking place in the processes of nutrition. In health, this constant tissue disintegration is exactly counterbalanced by the consumption of food, whilst the uniform normal temperature is maintained by the adjustment of the heat developed, and of the processes of exhalation and cooling which take place, especially from the lungs and skin. During a fever this balance breaks down, the tissue waste being greatly in excess of the food supply. The body wastes rap-idly, the loss to the system being chiefly in the form of nitrogen compounds (e.g. urea). In the early stage of fever a patient excretes about three times the amount of urea that he or she would excrete on the same diet when in health.

Fever is measured by how high the tempera-ture rises above normal. At 41.1 °C (106 °F) the patient is in a dangerous state of hyperpy-rexia (abnormally high temperature). If this persists for very long, the patient usually dies.

The body's temperature will also rise if exposed for too long to a high ambient tem-perature. (See HEAT STROKE.)

Symptoms The onset of a fever is usually marked by a RIGOR, or shivering. The skin feels hot and dry, and the raised temperature will often be found to show daily variations – namely, an evening rise and a morning fall.

There is a relative increase in the pulse and breathing rates. The tongue is dry and furred; the thirst is intense, while the appetite is gone; the urine is scanty, of high specific gravity and containing a large quantity of solid matter, particularly urea. The patient will have a head-ache and sometimes nausea, and children may develop convulsions (see FEBRILE CONVULSION).

The fever falls by the occurrence of a CRISIS – that is, a sudden termination of the symptoms – or by a more gradual subsidence of the temperature, technically termed a lysis. If death ensues, this is due to failure of the vital centres in the brain or of the heart, as a result of either the infection or hyperpyrexia.

Treatment Fever is a symptom, and the cor-rect treatment is therefore that of the under-lying condition. Occasionally, however, it is also necessary to reduce the temperature by more direct methods: physical cooling by, for example, tepid sponging, and the use of anti-pyretic drugs such as aspirin or paracetamol.

Fibre, Dietary
See ROUGHAGE.

Fibreoptic Endoscopy
A visualising technique enabling the operator to examine the internal organs with the minimum of disturbance or damage to the tissues. The procedure has transformed the management of, for example, gastrointestinal disease. In chest disease, fibreoptic bronchoscopy has now replaced the rigid wide-bore metal tube which was previously used for examination of the tracheo-bronchial tree.

The principle of fibreoptics in medicine is that a light from a cold light source passes down a bundle of quartz fibres in the endoscope to illuminate the lumen of the gastrointestinal tract or the bronchi. The reflected light is returned to the observer's eye via the image bundle which may contain up to 20,000 fibres. The tip of the instrument can be angulated in both directions, and fingertip controls are pro-vided for suction, air insufflation and for water injection to clear the lens or the mucosa. The oesophagus, stomach and duodenum can be visualised; furthermore, visualisation of the pancreatic duct and direct endoscopic cannula-tion is now possible, as is visualisation of the bile duct. Fibreoptic colonoscopy can visualise the entire length of the colon and it is now possible to biopsy polyps or suspected carcin-omas and to perform polypectomy.

The flexible smaller fibreoptic bronchoscope

has many advantages over the rigid tube, extending the range of view to all segmental bronchi and enabling biopsy of pulmonary parenchyma. Biopsy forceps can be directed well beyond the tip of the bronchoscope itself, and the more flexible fibreoptic instrument causes less discomfort to the patient.

Fibreoptic laparoscopy is a valuable technique that allows the direct vizualisation of the abdominal contents: for example, the female pelvic organs, in order to detect the presence of suspected lesions (and, in certain cases, effect their subsequent removal); check on the development and position of the fetus; and test the patency of the Fallopian tubes.

(See also ENDOSCOPE; BRONCHOSCOPE; LARYNGOSCOPE; LAPAROSCOPE; COLONOSCOPE.)

Fibrillation

A term applied to rapid contraction or TREMOR of muscles, and especially to a form of abnormal action of the heart muscle in which individual bundles of fibres take up independent action. It is believed to be due to a state of excessive excitability in the muscle associated with the stretching which occurs in dilatation of the heart. The main causes are ATHEROSCLEROSIS, chronic rheumatic heart disease and hypertensive heart disease (see HEART, DISEASES OF). Fibrillation is distinguished as atrial or ventricular, depending on whether the muscle of the atria or of the ventricles is affected. In atrial fibrillation, the heartbeats and the pulse become extremely irregular, both as regards time and force; when the atrium is fibrillating there is no significant contraction of the atrial muscle but the cardiac output is maintained by ventricular contraction. In ventricular fibrillation there is no significant contractile force, so that there is no cardiac output. The commonest cause is myocardial infarction. Administration of DIGOXIN, timolol or verapamil may restore normal rhythm, and in some patients, CARDIOVERSION – a controlled direct-current electric shock given via a modified defibrillator placed on the chest wall – is effective.

Fibrin

A substance formed in the BLOOD as it clots: indeed, its formation causes clotting. The substance is produced in threads; after the threads have formed a close meshwork through the blood, they contract, and produce a dense, felted mass. The substance is formed not only from shed blood but also from LYMPH which exudes from the lymph vessels. Thus fibrin is found in all inflammatory conditions within

serous cavities like the PLEURA, PERITONEUM, and PERICARDIUM, and forms a thick coat upon the surface of the inflamed membranes. It is also found in inflamed joints, and in the lung as a result of pneumonia. (See COAGULATION.)

Fibrinogen

The soluble protein in the blood which is the precursor of FIBRIN, the substance in blood clot.

Fibrinolysis

The way in which blood clots are removed from the circulation. The insoluble protein FIBRIN is broken down by the enzyme plasmin (see PLASMINOGEN) which is activated at the same time as the COAGULATION process of blood. There is normally a balance between coagulation and fibrinolysis; an abnormal increase in the latter causes excessive bleeding.

Fibrinolytic Drugs

A group of drugs, also known as thrombolytics, with the ability to break down the protein FIBRIN, the prime constituent of blood clots (see THROMBUS; THROMBOSIS). They are used to disperse blood clots that have formed in the vessels of the circulatory system. The group includes STREPTOKINASE, alteplase and reteplase. The drugs work by activating PLASMINOGEN to form PLASMIN which degrades fibrin and breaks up the blood clot (see COAGULATION).

Fibroadenoma

A benign tumour of glandular EPITHELIUM containing fibrous elements. The commonest benign tumour is of the breast, often occurring in young women.

Fibroblasts

Cells distributed widely throughout CONNECTIVE TISSUE that produce the precursor substances of COLLAGEN, elastic fibres and reticular fibres.

Fibrocystic Disease of the Pancreas

See CYSTIC FIBROSIS.

Fibroid

Fibroid, or fibromyoma, is the commonest form of tumour of the uterus (see UTERUS, DISEASES OF), and one of the most common tumours of the human body. It is composed of a mixture of muscular and fibrous tissue. The tumour may be small or as large as a grapefruit. Fibroids may cause pain and heavy menstrual bleeding and usually occur in women over 30 years of age. In some women the fibroid may be small enough to remove surgically but, if it is large, a HYSTERECTOMY is often necessary. Small, symptomless fibroids are no danger and can be left untreated.

Fibroma
A benign tumour comprising mainly CONNECTIVE TISSUE – the substance that surrounds body structures, binding them together. Examples are neurofibroma, affecting connective tissue around nerves, and ovarian fibroma which develops around the follicles from which eggs (ova) develop in the OVARIES. Unless the fibroma is causing symptoms (as a result of pressure on surrounding tissues) it does not require treatment. If symptoms occur, the tumour is removed surgically.

Fibromyalgia Syndrome
Symptoms These vary, with pain and fatigue generally prominent, sometimes causing considerable disability. Patients can usually dress and wash independently but cannot cope with a job or household activities. Pain is mainly axial, but may affect any region. ANALGESICS, NON-STEROIDAL ANTI-INFLAMMATORY DRUGS (NSAIDS) and local physical treatments are generally ineffective.

Patients often have a poor sleep pattern, waking exhausted. Unexplained headache, urinary frequency and abdominal symptoms are common, but no cause has been found. Patients generally score highly on measures of anxiety and DEPRESSION. Fibromyalgia is not an ideal description; idiopathic diffuse-pain syndrome and non-restorative sleep disorder are increasingly preferred terms.

Clinical findings are generally unremarkable; most important is the presence of multiple hyperalgesic tender sites (e.g. low cervical spine, low lumbar spine, suboccipital muscle, mid upper trapezius, tennis-elbow sites, upper outer quadrants of buttocks, medial fat pad of knees). In fibromyalgia, hyperalgesia (excessive discomfort) is widespread and symmetrical, but absent at sites normally non-tender. Claims by patients to be tender all over are more likely to be due to fabrication or psychiatric disturbance. OSTEOARTHRITIS and periarticular syndrome are much more common and should be excluded, together with other conditions, such as hypothyroidism (see THYROID GLAND, DISEASES OF), SYSTEMIC LUPUS ERYTHEMATOSUS (SLE) and inflammatory myopathy (see MUSCLES, DISORDERS OF), which may present with similar symptoms.

Cause There is no investigational evidence of inflammatory, metabolic or structural abnormality, and the problem seems functional rather than pathological. SEROTONIN deficiency has a significant role in fibromyalgia syndrome.

Management Controlled trials have confirmed the usefulness of low-dose AMITRIPTYLINE or DOTHIEPIN together with a graded exercise programme to increase aerobic fitness. How this works is still unclear; its efficacy may be due to its normalising effects on the sleep centre or 'pain gating' (reduction of pain sensation) at the spinal-cord level. Prognosis is often poor. Nevertheless, suitable advice and training can help most patients to learn to cope better with their condition and avoid unnecessary investigations and drug treatments.

Fibrosarcoma
A cancer of the CONNECTIVE TISSUE arising in the fibroblasts, stem cells that produce connective tissue cells. The tumours can develop in bone or in soft tissue and occur most commonly in the limbs. Treatment is by surgery or RADIOTHERAPY.

Fibrosing Alveolitis
See ALVEOLITIS.

Fibrosis
The formation of fibrous or scar tissue, which is usually due to infection, injury or surgical operation.

Fibrositis
Pain, muscular stiffness and inflammation affecting the soft tissues of the arm, legs and trunk. The cause is unknown but may include immunological factors, muscular strain and psychological stress. Treatment is usually palliative.

Fibrous Dysplasia
A rare disease in which areas of bone are replaced by fibrous tissue (see CONNECTIVE TISSUE). This renders the bone fragile and liable to fracture. It may involve only one bone – usually the thigh bone or FEMUR – or several bones. This latter form of the disease may be accompanied by pigmentation of the skin and the early onset of PUBERTY.

Fibrous Tissue
See CONNECTIVE TISSUE.

Fibula
The slender outer bone of the leg. The head of

this bone articualtes with the TIBIA just below the knee, and at the ANKLE it articulates with the TALUS bone.

Filariasis

The term used to describe several clinical entities caused by one or other of the nematode filariae; these include *Wuchereria bancrofti/Brugia malayi, Onchocerca volvulus, Loa loa, Dracunculus medinensis* (DRACONTIASIS or guineaworm disease), *Mansonella perstans*, etc. These organisms have widely differing geographical distributions. Whereas lymphatic filariasis is present throughout much of the tropics and subtropics, ONCHOCERCIASIS (river-blindness) is largely confined to west and central Africa and southern America. Loaiasis is an infection of west and central Africa, and dracontiasis involves west and central Africa and western India only.

Clinically, the lymphatic filariases characteristically cause ELEPHANTIASIS (lymphoedema); onchocerciasis gives rise to ophthalmic complications (river-blindness), rashes and subcutaneous nodules; loaiasis causes subcutaneous 'Calabar swellings' and subconjunctival involvement; and dracontiasis predisposes to secondary bacterial infections (usually involving the lower limbs). Diagnosis is by finding the relevant filarial nematode, either in blood (day and night films should be examined), or in one or other of the body fluids. An EOSINOPHILIA is often present in peripheral blood. Serological diagnosis is also of value. In onchocerciasis, skin-snips and the Mazotti reaction are valuable adjuncts to diagnosis.

The mainstay of chemotherapy consists of diethylcarbamazine (aimed predominantly at the larval stage of the parasite). However, ivermectin (not available in the UK) is effective in onchocerciasis, and metronidazole or one of the benzimidazole compounds have limited value in dracontiasis. Suramin has been used to kill adult filarial worms. Prevention consists of eradication of the relevant insect vector.

Filaricide

A generic term for drugs used to treat filarial infections (see FILARIASIS).

Filling

The insertion, in denistry, of a specially prepared material into a cavity drilled into a tooth, usually for the treatment of dental caries (see TEETH, DISORDERS OF).

Finasteride

Finasteride is a drug which inhibits the ENZYME that metabolises TESTOSTERONE into the more potent ANDROGEN, dihydrotestosterone. This action results in a reduction of prostate tissue. The drug is used to treat an enlarged PROSTATE GLAND, thus improving urinary flow. Its side-effects include reduced LIBIDO, and IMPOTENCE. Finasteride offers an alternative to PROSTATECTOMY for some men but a significant minority do not improve. Women of childbearing age should not handle broken or crushed tablets.

Fingerprint

The unique pattern of fine ridges in the outer horny layer of the skin at the front of the tip of each finger and thumb. The ridges are of three types: loops (70 per cent), whorls (25 per cent) and arches (5 per cent). Fingerprint patterns are used as a routine forensic test by police forces to identify individuals. Some patterns can indicate that the subject has an inherited disorder.

First Aid

Emergency procedures to help an ill or injured person before he or she receives expert medical attention or is admitted to hospital. Courses of instruction in first aid comprise 6–12 sessions, each of about 2 hours' duration. Syllabuses of instruction are published by various organisations, the principal ones being the British Red Cross, the St John Ambulance Association, and the St Andrew's Ambulance Association. (See APPENDIX 1: BASIC FIRST AID; APPENDIX 2: ADDRESSES: SOURCES OF INFORMATION, ADVICE, SUPPORT AND SELF-HELP.)

Fissure

A term applied both to clefts of normal anatomical structure and also to small narrow ulcers occurring in skin and mucous membrane. The latter type of fissure occurs especially at the corners of the mouth and at the anus. (See LIPS; RECTUM, DISEASES OF.)

Fistula

An unnatural, narrow channel leading from some natural cavity – such as the duct of a gland, or the interior of the bowels – to the surface. Alternatively a fistula may be a communication between two such cavities where none should exist – as, for example, a direct communication between the bladder and bowel.

Cause Fistulas may be congenital or develop as a result of injury or infection. A SALIVARY fistula may develop between the salivary gland

and the outside of the cheek because of a blockage in the duct from the gland to the mouth. A urinary fistula may be one consequence of a fracture of the PELVIS which has damaged the URETHRA. Fistulas of the anus are one of the most common forms, usually the result of infection and ABSCESS formation.

Treatment As a rule, a fistula is extremely difficult to close, especially after it has persisted for some time. The treatment consists in an operation to restore the natural channel, be it salivary duct, or urethra, or bowel. This is effected by appropriate means in each locality, and when it is attained the fistula heals quickly under simple dressings.

Fit
A popular name for a sudden convulsive SEIZURE, although the term is also extended to include sudden seizures of every sort. During the occurrence of a fit of any sort, the chief object should be to prevent the patient from doing any harm to him or herself as a result of the convulsive movements. The person should therefore be laid flat, and the head supported on a pillow or other soft material. (See CONVULSIONS; ECLAMPSIA; EPILEPSY; FAINTING; HYSTERIA; STROKE; URAEMIA; APPENDIX 1: BASIC FIRST AID.)

Fitness
An ability to perform daily activities without becoming overtired. Fitness is dependent on strength, flexibility and endurance, and the level of an individual's fitness will often depend on their type of employment and the extent to which they indulge in physical exercise, whether training in the local health club or at home or regularly participating in sports. Regular fitness improves one's health and well-being. Fitness exercises should be matched to a person's age and abilities and there is a health danger if someone regularly exercises beyond their capabilities.

5-Hydroxytryptamine
See SEROTONIN.

Flaccid
Relaxed or lacking in stiffness. Used to describe muscles that are not contracting (or following DENERVATION), and organs – for example, the penis – that are lying loose, empty, or with wrinkles. (Opposite: firm or erect.)

Flap
A section of tissue (usually skin) separated from underlying structures but still attached at its distal end by a PEDICLE through which it receives its blood supply. The free end may then be sutured into a new position to cover a defect caused by trauma or excision of diseased tissue. A free flap involves detachment of a section of tissue, often including bone and muscle, to a distant site where the artery and vein supplying it are anastomosed to adjacent vessels and the tissue is sutured into place. (See RECONSTRUCTIVE (PLASTIC) SURGERY.)

Flat-Foot
Flat-foot, or pes planus, is a deformity of the foot in which its arch sinks down so that the inner edge of the foot comes to rest upon the ground.

Causes The disorder may develop in infancy or occur in adult life, usually resulting from a combination of obesity and/or an occupation involving long periods of standing.

Symptoms Often none, but there may be pain along the instep and beneath the outer ankle. The foot is stiff and broad, walking is tiresome, and the toes turn far out.

Treatment A change of occupation may be necessary, to one which allows sitting. In early cases the leg muscles may be strengthened by tiptoe exercises performed for ten minutes night and morning. A pad to support the arch may have to be worn inside the shoe. Rarely, children may require surgery.

Flatulence
A collection of gas in the stomach or bowels. In the former case the gas is expelled from time to time in noisy eructations (see ERUCTATION) by the mouth; in the latter it may produce rumblings in the bowels, or be expelled from the ANUS.

Causes When gas is found in large amount in the bowels, its production is usually due to fermentation set up by bacteria.

Treatment Flatulence in the stomach is treated by relieving the DYSPEPSIA which causes it. It may also be relieved, or eased, by the administration of CARMINATIVES. Flatulence may be aggravated by anxiety. If the flatulence is due to, or aggravated by, the habit of swallowing air, the patient must try and break the habit. To reduce intestinal flatulence, a sufferer may require a change of diet to easily digestible foods.

Flatus

Gas from the intestines (see INTESTINE) that is passed out via the ANUS and formed in the large intestine as a result of bacteria breaking down carbohydrate and amino acids in digested food.

Flavine

See ANTISEPTICS.

Flexible Training

A term applied to the system of postgraduate medical training that allows young doctors to integrate their domestic commitments with the training requirements necessary to become a fully qualified specialist, usually by working part-time.

Flexion

The bending of a joint in the SAGITTAL plane. Usually an anterior movement, it is occasionally posterior, as in the case of the knee-joint. Lateral flexion refers to the bending of the spine in the coronal plane – that is, from side to side.

Flexor

A MUSCLE that causes bending of a limb or other body part.

Flexure

A bend in an organ or body part. The term is used, for example, to describe the skin on the inner aspect of the elbow or knee, as in the 'hepatic flexure' of the COLON.

Floaters

Particles that appear to be floating in a person's field of vision. They move quickly as the eye moves, but when the eye is still they seem to drift. Vision is not usually affected. Most floaters are shadows on the retina from minute particles in the vitreous humour (see EYE) which lies in the main part of the eyeball behind the lens. As a person ages, the jelly-like vitreous humour usually shrinks a little and becomes detached from the retina; this produces floaters which vanish over time. If a person notices a sudden cloud of floaters, sometimes accompanied by flashes of light, it is likely that a tear in or detachment of the retina has occurred. This requires prompt medical attention (see EYE, DISORDERS OF – Retinal detachment).

Flooding

A popular name for an excessive blood-stained discharge from the womb (UTERUS). (See MEN-STRUATION; MENORRHAGIA.) In the majority of cases, flooding is the sign of a miscarriage (see ABORTION).

Flucloxacillin

A PENICILLINASE-resistant PENICILLIN used to treat penicillin-resistant staphylococci infection (see also STAPHYLOCOCCUS; ANTIBIOTICS).

Fluconazole

An oral triazole antifungal drug used to treat local and systemic infections.

Fluctuation

A sign obtained from collections of fluid by laying the fingers of one hand upon one side of the swelling, and, with those of the other, tapping or pressing suddenly on a distant point of the swelling. The 'thrill' communicated from one hand to the other through the fluid is one of the most important signs of the presence of an ABSCESS, or of effusion of fluid into joints or into the peritoneal cavity (see PERITONEUM).

Flucytosine

A synthetic drug used as an intravenous adjunct to amphotericin to treat severe systemic fungal infections such as candidiasis (see CANDIDA) and cryptococcosis.

Fluid Balance

The appropriate balance of fluid input and output (along with dissolved salts essential for life) over 24 hours. During this period, about 2,500 millilitres (ml) of fluid should be taken in by a 70-kg man and the same amount excreted; of this, 1,500 ml will be drunk, 800 ml will be in the food eaten, and 200 ml produced by food metabolism. Excreted water is made up of 1,500 ml of urine, 800 ml insensible loss and 200 ml in the faeces. A 70-kg man's total body fluid is 42 litres – 60 per cent of body weight. Intracellular fluid comprises 28 litres, extracellular, 14 litres and blood, 5 litres. Water is controlled mainly by the sodium concentration in the body fluids via the release of antidiuretic hormone (ADH – see VASOPRESSIN) from the posterior part of the PITUITARY GLAND. In seriously ill people, close monitoring of fluid intake and output, along with measurements of PLASMA sodium and calcium concentrations, is an essential factor in treatment.

Flukes

Flukes are a variety of parasitic worms. (See FASCIOLIASIS.)

Flunitrazepam

A drug with the trade name Rohypnol®, fluni-trazepam is one of the BENZODIAZEPINES with a prolonged action prescribed as a hypnotic (see HYPNOTICS). The *British National Formulary* warns that the drug may be particularly subject to abuse (see DRUG-ASSISTED RAPE).

Fluocinolone

Fluocinolone is one of the CORTICOSTEROIDS and is applied to the skin as a cream, lotion or ointment. It is more potent than hydro-cortisone. It must not be given by mouth.

Fluorescein

A dye which has the special property of absorb-ing blue-light energy and emitting this energy as green light. This property is made use of in examining the cornea for scratches or ulcera-tion; it is also used to detect abnormally perme-able (or leaking) blood vessels in the retina and iris – especially in diabetic retinopathy and dis-eases of the macula (see EYE; EYE, DISORDERS OF).

Fluoridation

See FLUORINE.

Fluorine

One of the halogen series of elements. In the form of fluoride it is one of the constituents of bone and teeth. Supplementing the daily intake of fluorine diminishes the incidence of dental caries (see TEETH, DISORDERS OF). In America and in Britain, evidence indicates that people who, throughout their lives, have drunk water with a natural fluorine content of 1 part per million have less dental caries than those whose drinking water is fluorine-free. All the available evidence indicates that this is the most satisfactory way of giving fluorine, and that if the concentration of fluorine in drink-ing water does not exceed 1 part per million, there are no toxic effects. Several water com-panies in the UK have added fluoride to the public water supply, but opponents of this pol-icy, who claim that fluoride has serious side-effects, have prevented fluoridation being introduced nationwide.

Fluoroscope

An apparatus for rendering X-rays visible after they have passed through the body, by project-ing them on a screen of calcium tungstate. The technique is known as fluoroscopy. It provides a method of being able to watch, for instance, the beating of the heart, or the movements of the intestine after the administration of a barium meal. (See also X-RAYS.)

Fluorouracil

An drug of the antimetabolite group – a group that disrupts normal cell division. Fluorouracil is used intravenously to treat recurrent and inoperable carcinoma of the colon and rectum, as well as secondaries from cancer of the breast. It can be used topically for some malignant and premalignant skin lesions. (See CYTOTOXIC.)

Fluoxetine

Better known by its trade name Prozac®, this drug – one of the SELECTIVE SEROTONIN-REUPTAKE INHIBITORS (SSRIS) – has been widely used, especially in North America, for the treatment of depression and anxiety (see MEN-TAL ILLNESS). Though causing fewer side-effects than TRICYCLIC ANTIDEPRESSANT DRUGS (the first such drugs widely used), SSRI drugs should be prescribed with care and should not be stopped abruptly. Unlike benzodiazepine tranquillisers such as Valium®, fluoxetine is not addictive, but there have been rare reports of it allegedly provoking people to acts of violence. The drug acts by modifying the activities of neurotransmitters, notably DOPAMINE and SEROTONIN in the brain, thus prolonging the effects of these chemical messengers.

Flupenthixol

A tranquilliser used in the treatment of schizo-phrenia (see MENTAL ILLNESS).

Fluphenazine

One of the phenothiazine derivatives, of value as an antipsychotic drug. (See also NEUROLEPTICS.)

Flurazepam

See BENZODIAZEPINES.

Flutamide

An antiandrogen (see ANDROGEN) drug used in the treatment of cancer of the PROSTATE GLAND, sometimes in conjunction with GONADORELIN.

Fluticasone

An aerosol corticosteroid drug used in the prevention and treatment of attacks of ASTHMA. Inhaled corticosteroids have few or no systemic side-effects unless given in excessive dosage.

Flutter

The term applied to a form of abnormal cardiac rhythm, in which the atria contract at a rate of 200–400 beats a minute, and the ventricles more slowly. The abnormal rhythm is the result of a diseased heart. (See HEART, DISEASES OF; FIBRILLATION.)

Fluvastatin

One of the STATINS group of drugs used to reduce the levels of LDL-CHOLESTEROL in the blood and thus help to prevent coronary heart disease, which is more prevalent in people with raised blood cholesterol levels (see HEART, DISEASES OF).

Foetus

See FETUS.

Folic Acid

One of the constituents of the vitamin B complex, folic acid derives its name from the fact that it is found in many green leaves, including spinach and grass. It has also been obtained from liver, kidney and yeasts. It has proved to be of value in the treatment of macrocytic anaemias (see ANAEMIA), particularly those associated with SPRUE and nutritional deficiencies.

In order to prevent NEURAL TUBE defects and cleft lip or palate (see CLEFT PALATE), all women planning to become pregnant should be advised to have a diet rich in folic acid in the months before conception until 13 weeks' gestation, or to take folic acid tablets.

Recent research has suggested that adequate levels of folic acid can prevent the build-up of homocysteine, a compound in the blood closely associated with heart attacks and strokes. It has been suggested that the official recommendation of 200 micrograms a day in the diet should be doubled. (See APPENDIX 5: VITAMINS.)

Folium

(Plural: folia.) Latin term for leaf: for example, digitalis folium is digitalis leaf.

Follicle

Follicle is the term applied to a very small sac or gland: for example, small collections of adenoid tissue in the throat, and the small digestive glands on the mucous membrane of the intestine.

Follicle-Stimulating Hormone

A hormone produced by the anterior PITUITARY GLAND which stimulates the formation of follicles in the ovary each menstrual cycle (see OVARIES; MENSTRUATION) and of spermatocytes in the testis (see TESTICLE). It is under hypothalamic control (see HYPOTHALAMUS) and in the female there is feedback inhibition by oestrogens from the developing follicle.

Follicular Hormone

See OESTRADIOL.

Fomentation

(See also POULTICES.) Any warm application to the surface of the body in the form of a cloth. Usually, the fomentation cloth is heated by being wrung out of hot water.

Fomites

A traditional term used to include all articles which have been brought into sufficiently close contact with a person sick of some infectious disease to retain the infective material and spread the disease. For example, clothes, bedding, carpets, toys and books may all be fomites until they are disinfected.

Fontanelle

Areas on the head on which bone has not yet formed. The chief of these is the anterior fontanelle, situated on the top of the head between the frontal and two parietal bones. In shape it is four-sided, about 25 mm (1 inch) square at the time of birth, gradually diminishing until it is completely covered by bone, which should happen by the age of 18 months. The pulsations of the brain can be readily felt through it. Delay in its closure is particularly found in cases of RICKETS, as well as in other states of defective development. The fontanelle bulges in raised intracranial pressure from HYDROCEPHALUS and MENINGITIS, and depressed in DEHYDRATION.

Food

Mixture of substances containing CARBOHYDRATE, FAT, PROTEIN, VITAMINS, TRACE ELEMENTS and water consumed by animals, including humans, to provide the necessary nutrients to maintain the body's METABOLISM.

Food Intolerance

This is divided into food aversion, where a person simply avoids a food they dislike; food intolerance, where taking the food causes symptoms; and food allergy, where the symptoms are due to an immunological reaction. Some cases of food intolerance are due to idiosyncrasy – that is, a genetic defect in the patient, such as alactasia, where the intestine lacks the enzyme that digests milk sugar, with the result that individuals so affected develop diarrhoea when they drink milk. Intolerance to specific foods, as distinct from allergy, is probably quite common and may be an important factor in the aetiology of the IRRITABLE BOWEL SYNDROME (IBS).

For the diagnosis of true food allergy, it is

necessary to demonstrate that there is a reproducible intolerance to a specific food; also, that there is evidence of an abnormal immunological reaction to it. Occasionally the allergic response may not be to the food itself but to food contaminants such as penicillin, or to food additives such as tartrazine. There may also be reactions to foods which have pharmacological effects, such as caffeine in strong coffee or histamine in fermented cheese, or such reactions may be due to the irritant effect on the intestinal mucosa (especially if it is already diseased) by, say, highly spiced curries.

Testing blood and skin for food allergy is beloved of some alternative practitioners but, in practice, the results of tests do not necessarily agree with what happens when the food is taken. Therefore, a careful history is as useful as any test in making a diagnosis.

Food Poisoning

This illness is characterised by vomiting, diarrhoea and abdominal pain, and results from eating food contaminated with metallic or chemical poisons, certain micro-organisms or microbial products. Alternatively, the foods – such as undercooked red kidney beans or fish of the scombroid family (mackerel and tuna) – may contain natural posions. Food poisoning caused by chemical or metallic substances usually occurs rapidly, within minutes or a few hours of eating. Among micro-organisms, bacteria are the leading cause of food poisoning, particularly *Staphylococcus aureus, Clostridium perfringens* (formerly *Cl. welchii*), *Salmonella spp., Campylobacter jejuni,* and *Escherichia coli* O157.

Staphylococcal food poisoning occurs after food such as meat products, cold meats, milk, custard and egg products becomes contaminated before or after cooking, usually through incorrect handling by humans who carry *S. aureus*. The bacteria produce an ENTEROTOXIN which causes the symptoms of food poisoning 1–8 hours after ingestion. The toxin can withstand heat; thus, subsequent cooking of contaminated food will not prevent illness.

Heat-resistant strains of *Cl. perfringens* cause food poisoning associated with meat dishes, soups or gravy when dishes cooked in bulk are left unrefrigerated for long periods before consumption. The bacteria are anaerobes (see ANAEROBE) and form spores; the anaerobic conditions in these cooked foods allow the germinated spores to multiply rapidly during cooling, resulting in heavy contamination. Once ingested the bacteria produce enterotoxin in the intestine, causing symptoms within 8–24 hours.

Many different types of Salmonella (about 2,000) cause food poisoning or ENTERITIS, from eight hours to three days after ingestion of food in which they have multiplied. *S. brendeny, S. enteritidis, S. heidelberg, S. newport* and *S. thompson* are among those commonly causing enteritis. Salmonella infections are common in domesticated animals such as cows, pigs and poultry whose meat and milk may be infected, although the animals may show no symptoms. Duck eggs may harbour Salmonella (usually *S. typhimurium*), arising from surface contamination with the bird's faeces, and foods containing uncooked or lightly cooked hen's eggs, such as mayonnaise, have been associated with enteritis. The incidence of human *S. enteritidis* infection has been increasing, by more than 15-fold in England and Wales annually, from around 1,100 a year in the early 1980s to more than 32,000 at the end of the 1990s, but has since fallen to about 10,000. A serious source of infection seems to be poultry meat and hen's eggs.

Although Salmonella are mostly killed by heating at 60 °C for 15 minutes, contaminated food requires considerably longer cooking and, if frozen, must be completely thawed beforehand, to allow even cooking at a sufficient temperature.

Enteritis caused by *Campylobacter jejuni* is usually self-limiting, lasting 1–3 days. Since reporting of the disease began in 1977, in England and Wales its incidence has increased from around 1,400 cases initially to nearly 13,000 in 1982 and to over 42,000 in 2004. Outbreaks have been associated with unpasteurised milk: the main source seems to be infected poultry.

ESCHERICHIA COLI O157 was first identified as a cause of food poisoning in the early 1980s, but its incidence has increased sharply since, with more than 1,000 cases annually in the United Kingdom in the late 1990s. The illness can be severe, with bloody diarrhoea and life-threatening renal complications. The reservoir for this pathogen is thought to be cattle, and transmission results from consumption of raw or undercooked meat products and raw dairy products. Cross-infection of cooked meat by raw meat is a common cause of outbreaks of *Escherichia coli* O157 food poisoning. Water and other foods can be contaminated by manure from cattle, and person-to-person spread can occur, especially in children.

Food poisoning associated with fried or boiled rice is caused by *Bacillus cereus,* whose heat-resistant spores survive cooking. An enterotoxin is responsible for the symptoms, which occur 2–8 hours after ingestion and resolve after 8–24 hours.

Viruses are emerging as an increasing cause of some outbreaks of food poisoning from shellfish (cockles, mussels and oysters).

The incidence of food poisoning in the UK rose from under 60,000 cases in 1991 to nearly 79,000 in 2004. Public health measures to control this rise include agricultural aspects of food production, implementing standards of hygiene in abattoirs, and regulating the environment and process of industrial food production, handling, transportation and storage.

Food Standards Agency

An independent agency recently set up by the UK government. The aim is for the agency to protect consumers' interests in every aspect of food safety and nutrition. The agency advises ministers and the food industry, conducts research and surveillance, and monitors enforcement of food safety and hygiene laws.

Foramen

The Latin term for a hole. It is especially applied to natural openings in bones, such as the foramen magnum, the large opening in the base of the skull through which the brain and spinal cord are continuous.

Forced Diuresis

A means of encouraging EXCRETION via the KIDNEYS of a compound by altering the pH and increasing the volume of the urine. Forced diuresis is occasionally used after drug overdoses, but is potentially dangerous and so only suitable where proper intensive monitoring of the patient is possible. Excretion of acid compounds, such as salicylates, can be encouraged by raising the pH of the urine to 7·5–8·5 by the administration of an alkali such as bicarbonate (forced alkali diuresis) and that of bases, such as AMPHETAMINES, by lowering the pH of the urine to 5·5–6·5 by giving an acid such as ammonium chloride (forced acid diuresis).

Forced Feeding

See ENTERAL FEEDING.

Forceps

Surgical instruments with a pincer-like action which are used, for example, during operations, for grasping tissues and other materials. There are many different designs for different uses.

Obstetric forceps are designed to fit around the infant's head and allow traction to be applied to aid its delivery or to protect the soft skull of a very premature baby. (See PREGNANCY AND LABOUR.)

Forensic Medicine

That branch of medicine concerned with matters of law and the solving of crimes, for example, by determining the cause of a death in suspicious circumstances or identifying a criminal by examining tissue found at the scene of a crime. The use of DNA identification to establish who was present at the 'scene of the crime' is now a widely used procedure in forensic medicine.

Foreskin

See PREPUCE.

Formaldehyde

The *British Pharmacopoeia* preparation, formaldehyde solution, contains 34–38 per cent formaldehyde in water. It is a powerful antiseptic, and also has the power to harden the tissues. The vapour is very irritating to the eyes and nose.

Uses For disinfection it is largely used in the form of a spray; it can also be vaporised by heat. One of its advantages is that it does not damage metals or fabrics. In 3 per cent solution in water it is used for the treatment of warts on the palms of the hands and the soles of the feet.

Formestane

One of the steroidal AROMATASE INHIBITORS recently introduced for the treatment of patients with advanced postmenopausal breast cancer. It is better tolerated than non-steroidal aromatase inhibitors and acts by blocking the conversion of androgens (see ANDROGEN) to OESTROGEN in peripheral tissue.

Formulary

A list of formulae used as drugs and other medical preparations. The *British National Formulary* is an authoritative six-monthly publication containing information and advice on medicines and drugs. Published jointly by the British Medical Association and the Royal Pharmaceutical Society of Great Britain, with input from the Department of Health, it is distributed to all NHS doctors by the government. In 2005 a *BNF* for children was published and many hospitals and general practices produce formularies for use by doctors working in those facilities.

Fossa

A term applied to various depressions or holes, both on the surface of the body and in internal parts, such as the iliac fossa in each lower corner of the abdomen, and the fossae within the skull which lodge the different parts of the brain.

Fovea

A small depression. In the EYE this is an area near the fundus which contains predominantly cones and is the area with greatest visual acuity (see also VISION).

Fractures

See BONE, DISORDERS OF – Bone fractures.

Fraenum

See FRENUM.

Framycetin

A broad-spectrum antibiotic derived from *Streptomyces decaris*. It is active against a wide range of organisms, and is used in drops to treat infections of the eyes and ears.

Freckles

Also known as ephelides, these are small, brown, flat spots on the skin. They occur mostly in blonde or red-haired subjects in exposed areas, and darken on exposure to the sun. Melanocytes (see MELANOCYTE) are not increased in the basal layer of the EPIDERMIS.

Free Association

A psychoanalytic technique in which the therapist encourages the patient to follow up a specific line of thought and ideas as they enter his or her consciousness.

Freeze Drying

A technique for fixating specimens of tissue, involving a minimum of chemical and physical alteration. The histological specimen is immersed in a chemical, isopentane, which has been cooled in liquid air to a temperature just below 200 °C. This preserves the tissue instantly without large ice crystals forming – these would result in structural damage. The specimen is then dehydrated in a vacuum for three days, after which it can be examined using a MICROSCOPE.

Fremitus

Tremors or vibrations in an area of the body, detected by palpating (feeling) with the fingers or the hand or by auscultation (listening). The procedure is most commonly used when examining the chest and assessing what happens when the patient breathes, coughs or speaks. This helps the doctor to diagnose whether disorders such as fluid in the pleural cavity or solidification of a section of the lung have occurred.

Friction fremitus is a grating feeling communicated to the hand by the movements of lungs or heart when the membrane covering them is roughened, as in PLEURISY or PERICARDITIS. Vocal fremitus means the sensation felt by the hand when a person speaks; it is increased when the lung is more solid than usual. The 'thrills' felt over a heart affected by valvular disease are also varieties of fremitus.

Frenum

Also known as the fraenum or frenulum, this comprises the folds of mucous membrane that anchor the bottom of the tongue to the floor of the mouth.

Frequency

(1) The number of regular recurrences of an event during a given period of time. Examples in medicine are the heartbeat, and sound vibrations in the EAR or vocal cords.

(2) The word is also used to describe frequent passage of urine, a symptom that is usually caused by disorders in the urinary tract – for example, an infection; or any systemic disease which increases the daily output of urine – for example, DIABETES MELLITUS and DIABETES INSIPIDUS or disorders of the kidney.

Freudian Theory

A theory that emotional and allied diseases are due to a psychic injury or trauma, generally of a sexual nature, which did not produce an adequate reaction when it was received and therefore remains as a subconscious or 'affect' memory to trouble the patient's mind. As an extension of this theory, Freudian treatment consists of encouraging the patient to tell everything that happens to be associated with trains of thought which lead up to this memory, thus securing a 'purging' of the mind from the original 'affect memory' which is the cause of the symptoms. This form of treatment is also called psychocatharsis or abreaction.

The general term, psychoanalysis, is applied, in the first place, to the method of helping the patient to recover buried memories by free association of thoughts. In the second place, the term is applied to the body of psychological knowledge and theory accumulated and devised by Sigmund Freud (1856–1939) and his followers. The term 'psychoanalyst' has traditionally been applied to those who have undergone

Freudian training, but Freud's ideas are being increasingly questioned by some modern psychiatrists.

Friction

The name given either to the FREMITUS felt, or to the grating noise heard, when two rough surfaces of the body move over one another. It is characteristically obtained over the chest in cases of dry PLEURISY.

Friedreich's Ataxia

A hereditary disease resembling LOCOMOTOR ATAXIA, and due to degenerative changes in nerve tracts and nerve cells of the spinal cord and the brain. It occurs usually in children, or at any rate before the 20th year of life, and affects often several brothers and sisters. Its chief symptoms are unsteadiness of gait, with loss of the knee jerks, followed later by difficulties of speech, tremors of the hands, head and eyes, deformity of the feet, and curvature of the spine. There is often associated heart disease. The sufferer gets gradually worse, but may live, with increasing disability, for 20–30 years.

Frigidity

A term used to describe a lack of interest in sexual intercourse (COITUS) or the inability to achieve intercourse or ORGASM. Though applicable to both sexes, frigidity is usually applied to women with these sexual problems.

Fringe Medicine

See COMPLEMENTARY AND ALTERNATIVE MEDICINE (CAM).

Fröhlich's Syndrome

A condition in children characterised by obesity, physical sluggishness, and retarded sexual development. It is the result of disturbed PITUITARY GLAND function.

Frontal

Describing the anterior part of a body or organ.

Frontal Bone

The bone which forms the forehead and protects the frontal lobes of the brain. Before birth, the frontal bone consists of two halves, and this division may persist throughout life – a deep groove remaining down the centre of the forehead. Above each eye is a heavy ridge in the bone, most marked in men; behind this, in the substance of the bone, is a cavity on each side (the frontal sinus) which communicates with the nose. CATARRH in these cavities produces the frontal headache characteristic of a 'cold in

the head', and sometimes infection develops known as SINUSITIS (see NOSE, DISORDERS OF).

Frontal Lobe

The anterior part of the cerebral hemisphere as far back as the central sulcus. It contains the motor cortex and the parts of the brain concerned with personality, behaviour and learning. (See BRAIN.)

Frontal Sinus

One of the airspaces that form the paranasal sinuses (see SINUS) within some of the frontal bones of the skull. These sinuses are lined with mucous membrane and open into the nasal cavity.

Frostbite

This results from the action of extreme cold (below 0 °C) on the skin. VASOCONSTRICTION results in a reduced blood – and hence, oxygen – supply, leading to NECROSIS of the skin and, in severe cases, of the underlying tissues. Chiefly affecting exposed parts of the body, such as the face and the limbs, frostbite occurs especially in people exercising at high altitudes, or in those at risk of peripheral vascular disease, such as diabetics (see DIABETES MELLITUS), who should take particular care of their fingers and toes when in cold environments.

In mild cases – the condition sometimes known as frostnip – the skin on exposed parts of the body, such as the cheeks or nose, becomes white and numb with a sudden and complete cessation of cold and discomfort. In more severe cases, blisters develop on the frozen part, and the skin then gradually hardens and turns black until the frozen part, such as a finger, is covered with a black shell of dead tissue. Swelling of the underlying tissue occurs and this is accompanied by throbbing and aching. If, as is often the case, only the skin and the tissues immediately under it are frozen, then in a matter of months the dead tissue peels off. In the most severe cases of all, muscles, bone and tendon are also frozen, and the affected part becomes cold, swollen, mottled and blue or grey. There may be no blistering in these severe cases. At first there is no pain, but in time shooting and throbbing pains usually develop.

Prevention This consists of wearing the right clothing and never venturing on even quite short expeditions in cold weather, particularly on mountains, without taking expert advice as to what should be worn.

Treatment Frostnip is the only form of frostbite that should be treated on the spot. As it usually occurs on exposed parts, such as the face, each member of the party should be on the lookout for it in another. The moment that whitening of the skin is seen, the individual should seek shelter and warm the affected part by covering it with his or her warm hand or a glove until the normal colour and consistency of the affected part are restored. In more severe cases, treatment should only be given in hospital or in a well-equipped camp. In essence this consists of warming the affected part, preferably in warm water, against a warm part of the body or warm air. Rewarming should be done for spells of 20 minutes at a time. The affected part should never be placed near an open fire. Generalised warming of the whole body may also be necessary, using hot drinks, and putting the victim in a sleeping bag.

Frozen Shoulder

A painful condition of the shoulder accompanied by stiffness and considerable limitation of movement. The usual age-incidence is between 50 and 70. The cause is inflammation and contracture of the ligaments and muscles of the shoulder joint, probably due to overuse. Treatment is physiotherapy and local steroid infections. There is practically always complete recovery, even though this may take 12–18 months.

Fructose

Fructose is another name for laevulose, or fruit sugar, which is found along with glucose in most sweet fruits. It is sweeter than sucrose (cane or beet sugar) and this has led to its use as a sweetener.

Frusemide

A potent loop diuretic with a rapid onset (30 minutes), and short duration, of action. (See THIAZIDES, DIURETICS.)

Fugue

The term literally means flight, and it is used to describe the mental condition in which an individual is suddenly seized with a subconscious motivation to flee from some intolerable reality of everyday existence: this usually involves some agonising interpersonal relationship. As a rule, fugue lasts for a matter of hours or days, but may go on for weeks or even months. During the fugue the individual seldom behaves in a particularly odd manner – though he or she may be considered somewhat eccentric. When it is over there is no remembrance of events during the fugue.

Three types of fugue have been identified: (*a*) acute anxiety; (*b*) a manifestation of DEPRESSION; (*c*) a manifestation of organic mental state such as occurs after an epileptic seizure (see EPILEPSY).

Fumigation

A means of DISINFECTION by the vapour of powerful antiseptics.

Functional Diseases

See PSYCHOSOMATIC DISEASES.

Fundus

(1) The base of an organ, or that part remote from its opening.

(2) Point on the retina opposite the pupil through which nerve fibres and blood vessels traverse the retina (see EYE).

Fungal and Yeast Infections

These infections, also called mycoses (see MYCOSIS), are common and particularly affect the skin or mucosal membranes in, for example, the mouth, anus or vagina. Fungi consist of threadlike hyphae which form tangled masses or mycelia – common mould. In what is called dermatophyte (multicellular fungi) fungal infection of the hair, nails and SKIN, these hyphae invade the KERATIN. This is usually described as 'RINGWORM', although no worm is present and the infection does not necessarily occur in rings. PITYRIASIS versicolor and candidosis (monoliasis – see CANDIDA), called thrush when it occurs in the vulva, vagina and mouth, are caused by unicellular fungi which reproduce by budding and are called yeasts. Other fungi, such as ACTINOMYCOSIS, may cause deep systemic infection but this is uncommon, occurring mainly in patients with immunosuppressive disorders or those receiving prolonged treatment with ANTIBIOTICS.

Diagnosis and treatment Any person with isolated, itching, dry and scaling lesions of the skin with no obvious cause – for example, no history of eczema (see DERMATITIS) – should be suspected of having a fungal infection. Such lesions are usually asymmetrical. Skin scrapings or nail clippings should be sent for laboratory analysis. If the lesions have been treated with topical steroids they may appear untypical. Ultraviolet light filtered through glass (Wood's light) will show up microsporum infections, which produce a green-blue fluorescence.

Fungal infections used to be treated quite effectively with benzoic-acid compound ointment; it has now been superseded by new IMI-

DAZOLES preparations, such as CLOTRIMAZOLE, MICONAZOLE and terbinafine creams. The POLYENES, NYSTATIN and AMPHOTERICIN B, are effective against yeast infections. If the skin is macerated it can be treated with magenta (Castellani's) paint or dusting powder to dry it out.

Refractory fungal infection can be treated systematically provided that the diagnosis of the infection has been confirmed. Terbinafine, imidazoles and GRISEOFULVIN can all be taken by mouth and are effective for yeast infections. (Griseofulvin should not be taken in pregnancy or by people with liver failure or porphyria.) (See also FUNGUS; MICROBIOLOGY.)

Fungus

A simple plant that is parasitic on other plants and animals. Included in this group are mildews, moulds, mushrooms, toadstools and yeasts. Unlike other plants, they do not contain the green pigment chlorophyll. Most of the world's 100,000 different species of fungus are harmless or even beneficial to humans. Yeasts are used in the preparation of food and drinks, and antibiotics are obtained from some fungi. A few, however, can cause fatal disease and illness in humans (see FUNGUS POISONING).

Fungus Poisoning

Around 2,000 mushrooms (toadstools) grow in England, of which 200 are edible and a dozen are classified as poisonous. Not all the poisonous ones are dangerous. It is obviously better to prevent mushroom poisoning by ensuring correct identification of those that are edible; books and charts are available. If in doubt, do not eat a fungus.

Severe poisoning from ingestion of fungi is very rare, since relatively few species are highly toxic and most species do not contain toxic compounds. The most toxic species are those containing amatoxins such as death cap (*Amanita phalloides*); this species alone is responsible for about 90 per cent of all mushroom-related deaths. There is a latent period of six hours or more between ingestion and the onset of clinical effects with these more toxic species. The small intestine, LIVER and KIDNEYS may be damaged – therefore, any patient with gastro-intestinal effects thought to be due to ingestion of a mushroom should be referred immediately to hospital where GASTRIC LAVAGE and treatment with activated charcoal can be carried out, along with parenteral fluids and haemodialysis if the victim is severely ill. In most cases where effects occur, these are early-onset gastrointestinal effects due to ingestion of mushrooms containing gastrointestinal irritants.

Muscarine is the poisonous constituent of some species. Within two hours of ingestion, the victim starts salivating and sweating, has visual disturbances, vomiting, stomach cramps, diarrhoea, vertigo, confusion, hallucinations and coma, the severity of symptoms depending on the amount eaten and type of mushroom. Most people recover in 24 hours, with treatment.

'Magic' mushrooms are a variety that contains psilocybin, a hallucinogenic substance. Children who take such mushrooms may develop a high fever and need medical care. In adults the symptoms usually disappear within six hours.

Treatment If possible, early gastric lavage should be carried out in all cases of suspected poisoning. Identification of the mushroom species is a valuable guide to treatment. For muscarine poisoning, ATROPINE is a specific antidote. As stated above, hospital referral is advisable for people who have ingested poisonous fungi.

Funiculitis

Inflammation of the SPERMATIC CORD, usually arising in men with epididymitis (inflammation of the EPIDIDYMIS in the TESTICLE). The condition can be painful. ANTIBIOTICS and ANALGESICS are effective treatment.

Funnel Chest

See CHEST DEFORMITIES.

Funnybone

Colloquial name for the small area at the back of the elbow where the ULNAR NERVE goes over a prominence at the lower end of the HUMERUS bone. If the nerve is hit, acute pain results, accompanied by tingling in the forearm and hand.

Furuncle

Another term for a boil.

Fusidic Acid

A valuable antistaphylococcal antibiotic used both orally and topically. It is particularly useful in osteomyelitis (see BONE, DISORDERS OF).

Fusobacterium

A species of gram-negative, rod-shaped BACTERIA. It occurs among the normal flora of the human mouth, COLON and reproductive tract. Occasionally, fusobacterium is isolated from abscesses occurring in the lungs, abdomen and pelvis. One variety occurs in patients with VINCENT'S ANGINA (trench mouth).

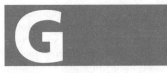

GABA

GABA, or gamma aminobutyric acid, is an amino acid (see AMINO ACIDS) that occurs in the central nervous system, mainly in the brain tissue. It is a chemical substance that transmits inhibitory impulses from nerve endings across synapses to other nerves or tissues.

Gag

A device that, when placed between a person's teeth, keeps the mouth open.

Gag Reflex

Assessment of victims of major trauma must include maintenance of their airways and breathing. Any false teeth, vomitus and foreign bodies should be removed, and the response to digital stimulation of the posterior pharyngeal wall – the 'gag reflex' – assessed. Even with a normal gag reflex, the airway may be seriously threatened if vomiting occurs. During the initial stages of resuscitation, careful and constant supervision of the airway is essential, with a high-volume sucker immediately available. If the gag reflex is absent or impaired, an endotracheal tube should be inserted (see ENDOTRACHEAL INTUBATION).

Gait

The way in which an individual walks. Gait may be affected by inherited disorders; by illness – especially neurological disorders; by injury; or by drug and alcohol abuse. Children, as a rule, begin to walk between the ages of 12 and 18 months, having learned to stand before the end of the first year. If a normal-sized child shows no ability to make movements by this time, the possibility of mental retardation must be borne in mind, and if the power of walking is not gained by the time the child is a year and a half old, RICKETS, CEREBRAL PALSY, or a malformation of the hip-joint must be excluded.

In hemiplegia, or PARALYSIS down one side of the body following a STROKE, the person drags the paralysed leg.

Steppage gait occurs in certain cases of alcoholic NEURITIS, tertiary SYPHILIS (tabes) and other conditions where the muscles that raise the foot are weak so that the toes droop. The person bends the knee and lifts the foot high, so that the toes may clear obstacles on the ground. (See DROP-FOOT.)

In LOCOMOTOR ATAXIA or tabes dorsalis, the sensations derived from the lower limbs are blunted, and consequently the movements of the legs are uncertain and the heels planted upon the ground with unnecessary force. When the person tries to turn or stands with the eyes shut, he or she may fall over. When they walk, they feel for the ground with a stick or keep their eyes constantly fixed upon it.

In spastic paralysis the limbs are moved with jerks. The foot first of all clings to the ground and then leaves it with a spasmodic movement, being raised much higher than is necessary.

In PARKINSONISM the movements are tremulous, and as the person takes very short steps, he or she has the peculiarity of appearing constantly to fall forwards, or to be chasing themselves.

In CHOREA the walk is bizarre and jerky, the affected child often seeming to leave one leg a step behind, and then, with a screwing movement on the other heel, go on again.

Psychologically based idiosyncrasies of gait are usually of a striking nature, quite different from those occuring in any neurological conditions. They tend to draw attention to the patient, and are worse when he or she is observed.

Galactocele

A cyst-like swelling in the breast which forms as a result of obstruction in the milk-duct draining the swollen area.

Galactorrhoea

This term may refer to unusually copious secretion of milk from the mammary glands when a mother is feeding her baby. It is also used to describe secretion of milk after the mother has stopped breast feeding.

Galactosaemia

A very rare, recessively inherited disease, with an incidence of around one in 75,000 births. Its importance lies in the disastrous consequences of it being overlooked, and results from the deficiency of an ENZYME essential for the metabolism of GALACTOSE. Normal at birth, affected infants soon develop jaundice, vomiting, diarrhoea, and fail to thrive on starting milk feeds. If the disorder remains unrecognised, liver disease, cataracts (see EYE, DISORDERS OF) and mental retardation result. Treatment consists of a lactose-free diet, and special lactose-free milks are now available.

Galactose

A constituent of lactose, galactose is a simple

sugar that is changed in the liver to glucose. A rare genetic metabolic disease, GALACTOSAE-MIA, results in infants being unable to achieve this conversion because the enzyme necessary for the reaction is absent.

Gall
Another name for BILE.

Gall-Bladder
See LIVER.

Gall-Bladder, Diseases of
The gall-bladder rests on the underside of the LIVER and joins the common hepatic duct via the cystic duct to form the common BILE DUCT. The gall-bladder acts as a reservoir and concentrator of BILE, alterations in the composition of which may result in the formation of gall-stones, the most common disease of the gall-bladder.

Gall-stones affect 22 per cent of women and 11 per cent of men. The incidence increases with age, but only about 30 per cent of those with gall-stones undergo treatment as the majority of cases are asymptomatic. There are three types of stone: cholesterol, pigment and mixed, depending upon their composition; stones are usually mixed and may contain calcium deposits. The cause of most cases is not clear but sometimes gall-stones will form around a 'foreign body' within the bile ducts or gall-bladder, such as suture material.
BILIARY COLIC Muscle fibres in the biliary system contract around a stone in the cystic duct or common bile duct in an attempt to expel it. This causes pain in the right upper quarter of the abdomen, with nausea and occasionally vomiting.
JAUNDICE Gall-stones small enough to enter the common bile duct may block the flow of bile and cause jaundice.
ACUTE CHOLECYSTITIS Blockage of the cystic duct may lead to this. The gall-bladder wall becomes inflamed, resulting in pain in the right upper quarter of the abdomen, fever, and an increase in the white-blood-cell count. There is characteristically tenderness over the tip of the right ninth rib on deep inhalation (Murphy's sign). Infection of the gall-bladder may accompany the acute inflammation and occasionally an EMPYEMA of the gall-bladder may result.
CHRONIC CHOLECYSTITIS A more insidious form of gall-bladder inflammation, producing non-specific symptoms of abdominal pain, nausea and flatulence which may be worse after a fatty meal.

Diagnosis Stones are usually diagnosed on the basis of the patient's reported symptoms, although asymptomatic gall-stones are often an incidental finding when investigating another complaint. Confirmatory investigations include abdominal RADIOGRAPHY – although many gall-stones are not calcified and thus do not show up on these images; ULTRASOUND scanning; oral CHOLECYSTOGRAPHY – which entails a patient's swallowing a substance opaque to X-rays which is concentrated in the gall-bladder; and endoscopic retrograde cholangiopancreatography (ERCP) – a technique in which an ENDOSCOPE is passed into the duodenum and a contrast medium injected into the biliary duct.

Treatment Biliary colic is treated with bed rest and injection of morphine-like analgesics. Once the pain has subsided, the patient may then be referred for further treatment as outlined below. Acute cholecystitis is treated by surgical removal of the gall-bladder. There are two techniques available for this procedure: firstly, conventional cholecystectomy, in which the abdomen is opened and the gall-bladder cut out; and, secondly, laparoscopic cholecystectomy, in which fibreoptic instruments called endoscopes (see FIBREOPTIC ENDOSCOPY) are introduced into the abdominal cavity via several small incisions (see MINIMALLY INVASIVE SURGERY (MIS)). Laparoscopic surgery has the advantage of reducing the patient's recovery time. Gall-stones may be removed during ERCP; they can sometimes be dissolved using ultrasound waves (lithotripsy) or tablet therapy (dissolution chemotherapy). Pigment stones, calcified stones or stones larger than 15 mm in diameter are not suitable for this treatment, which is also less likely to succeed in the overweight patient. Drug treatment is prolonged but stones can disappear completely after two years. Stones may re-form on stopping therapy. The drugs used are derivatives of bile salts, particularly chenodeoxycholic acid; side-effects include diarrhoea and liver damage.

Other disorders of the gall-bladder
These are rare.
POLYPS may form and, if symptomatic, should be removed. Malignant change is rare.
CARCINOMA of the gall-bladder is a disease of the elderly and is almost exclusively associated with gall-stones. By the time such a cancer has produced symptoms, the prognosis is bleak: 80 per cent of these patients die within one year of diagnosis. If the tumour is discovered early, 60 per cent of patients will survive five years.

Gall-Stones
See under GALL-BLADDER, DISEASES OF.

Gamete
A sexual or germ cell: for example, an OVUM or SPERMATOZOON.

Gamete Intrafallopian Transfer (GIFT)
See ASSISTED CONCEPTION.

Gamgee Tissue
A surgical dressing composed of a thick layer of cotton-wool between two layers of absorbent gauze, introduced by the Birmingham surgeon, Sampson Gamgee (1828–1886). Gamgee tissue has been a registered trademark since 1911.

Gamma Aminobutyric Acid
See GABA.

Gamma Benzene Hexachloride
A drug that is used in the treatment of PEDICULOSIS and SCABIES.

Gamma-Globulin
Gamma-globulin describes a group of proteins present in the blood PLASMA. They are characterised by their rate of movement in an electrical field, and can be separated by the process of ELECTROPHORESIS. Most gamma-globulins are IMMUNOGLOBULINS. Gamma-globulin injection provides passive or active immunity against HEPATITIS A. (See also GLOBULIN; IMMUNITY; IMMUNOLOGY.)

Gamma Rays
Short-wavelength penetrating electromagnetic rays produced by some radioactive compounds. More powerful than X-rays, they are used in certain RADIOTHERAPY treatments and to sterilise some materials.

Gammexane
The proprietary name for a synthetic insecticide which is a formulation of benzene hexachloride. It is active against a large range of insects and pests, including mosquitoes, fleas, lice, cockroaches, house-flies, clothes moths, bed-bugs, ants, and grain pests.

Ganciclovir
A drug used in the treatment of life- or sight-threatening infection with CYTOMEGALOVIRUS (CMV) in patients whose immune systems (see IMMUNITY) are compromised. Administered by intravenous transfusion, the drug is toxic and should be prescribed only when the potential benefits outweigh the risks. It is also used for the prevention of cytomegalovirus infection in patients who have had a liver transplant.

Ganglion
This term is used in two senses. In anatomy, it means an aggregation of nerve cells found in the course of certain nerves. In surgery, it means an enlargement of the sheath of a tendon, containing fluid. The latter occurs particularly in connection with the tendons in front of, and behind, the wrist.

Causes The cause of these dilatations on the tendon-sheaths is either some irregular growth of the SYNOVIAL MEMBRANE which lines them and secretes the fluid that lubricates their movements, or the forcing-out of a small pouch of this membrane through the sheath in consequence of a strain. In either case a bag-like swelling forms, whose connection with the synovial sheath becomes cut off, so that synovial fluid collects in it and distends it more and more.

Symptoms A soft, elastic, movable swelling forms, most often on the back of the wrist. It is usually small and gives no problems. Sometimes weakness and discomfort may develop. A ganglion which forms in connection with the flexor tendons in front of the wrist sometimes attains a large size, and extends down to form another swelling in the palm of the hand.

Treatment Sudden pressure with the thumbs may often burst a ganglion and disperse its contents beneath the skin. If this fails, surgical excision is necessary but, as the ganglion may disappear spontaneously, there should be no rush to remove it unless it is causing inconvenience or pain.

Gangrene
The death and decay of body tissues caused by a deficiency or cessation of the blood supply. There are two types: dry and moist. The former is a process of mummification, with the blood supply of the affected area of tissue stopping and the tissue withering up. Moist gangrene is characterised by putrefactive tissue decay caused by bacterial infection. The dead part, when formed of soft tissues, is called a slough and, when part of a bone, is called a sequestrum.

Causes These include injury – especially that sustained in war – disease, FROSTBITE, severe burns, ATHEROMA in large blood vessels, and diseases such as DIABETES MELLITUS and RAYNAUD'S DISEASE. Gas gangrene is a form that occurs when injuries are infected with soil contaminated with gas-producing bacilli such as *Clostridium welchii*, which are found in well-cultivated ground.

Treatment Dry gangrene must be kept dry, and AMPUTATION of the dead tissue performed when a clear demarcation line with healthy tissue has formed. Wet gangrene requires urgent surgery and prompt use of appropriate antibiotics.

Gargles
Gargling is a process by which various substances in solution are brought into contact with the throat without being swallowed. The watery solutions used for the purpose are called gargles. Gargles are used in the symptomatic treatment of infections of the throat: for example, 'sore throat', pharyngitis and tonsillitis.

Gargoylism
Also known as Hurler's syndrome, gargoylism is a rare condition due to lack of a specific ENZYME. It is a progressive disorder usually leading to death before the age of 10 years. The affected child is usually normal during the first few months of life; mental and physical deterioration then set in. The characteristic features include coarse facial features (hence the name of the condition), retarded growth, chest deformity, stiff joints, clouding of the cornea (see EYE), enlargement of the liver and spleen, deafness, and heart murmurs, with mental deterioration. It occurs in about one in 100,000 births.

Gas
See ANAESTHESIA; CARBON MONOXIDE (CO); NITROUS OXIDE GAS.

Gas Gangrene
See GANGRENE.

Gastrectomy
A major operation to remove the whole or part of the STOMACH. Total gastrectomy is a rare operation, usually performed when a person has cancer of the stomach; the OESPHAGUS is then connected to the DUODENUM. Sometimes cancer of the stomach can be treated by doing a partial gastrectomy: the use of partial gastrectomy to treat PEPTIC ULCER used to be common before the advent of effective drug therapy.

The operation is sometimes still done if the patient has failed to respond to dietary treatment and treatment with H_2-blocking drugs (see CIMETIDINE; RANITIDINE) along with antibiotics to combat *Helicobacter pylori*, an important contributary factor to ulcer development. Partial gastrectomy is usually accompanied by VAGOTOMY, which involves cutting the VAGUS nerve controlling acid secretion in the stomach. Among the side-effects of gastrectomy are fullness and discomfort after meals; formation of ulcers at the new junction between the stomach and duodenum which may lead to GASTRITIS and oesophagitis (see OESOPHAGUS, DISEASES OF); dumping syndrome (nausea, sweating and dizziness because the food leaves the stomach too quickly after eating); vomiting and diarrhoea. The side-effects usually subside but may need dietary and drug treatment.

Gastric
Relating to or affecting the STOMACH: for example, gastric ulcer.

Gastric Lavage
A method of gastric decontamination used in the treatment of poisoning. It is not used routinely. Lavage involves the passage of a lubricated tube via the mouth and OESOPHAGUS into the stomach. Patients are positioned on their side with the head lower than the feet. A small quantity of fluid (300 ml) is passed into the stomach and the contents then drained out (by gravity) by lowering the end of the tube. This is repeated until the solution is clear of particulate matter. The procedure should be done only by an experienced health professional.

Gastric Ulcer
See STOMACH, DISEASES OF.

Gastrin
A hormone produced by the MUCOUS MEMBRANE in the pyloric part of the STOMACH. The arrival of food stimulates production of the hormone which in turn stimulates the production of gastric juice.

Gastritis
Inflammation of the STOMACH lining. This may take an acute form when excess alcohol or other irritating substances have been taken, resulting in vomiting. Chronic gastritis may be the result of regular smoking and chronic alcoholism, or the condition may be caused by the back flow of BILE from the DUODENUM. The common cause, however, is chronic infection

with HELICOBACTER PYLORI. Symptoms are vague but victims are likely to develop gastric ulcers or sometimes cancer. Atrophic gastritis, when the mucosal lining of the stomach withers away, may follow chronic gastritis but sometimes occurs as an autoimmune disorder.

Gastrocnemius
The large double muscle which forms the chief bulk of the calf, and ends below in the tendo calcaneus.

Gastroduodenostomy
A surgical operation to join the DUODENUM to a hole made in the STOMACH wall to circumvent an obstruction in the gut – for example, PYLORIC STENOSIS – or to improve the passage of food from the stomach into the duodenum.

Gastroenteritis
Inflammation of the STOMACH and intestines (see INTESTINE), usually resulting from an acute bacterial or viral infection. The main symptoms are diarrhoea and vomiting, often accompanied by fever and – especially in infants – DEHYDRATION. Although generally a mild disease in western countries, it is the number-one killer of infants in the developing world, with more than 1·5 million children dying annually from the disease in India – a situation exacerbated by early weaning and malnutrition. Complications may include CONVULSIONS, kidney failure, and, in severe cases, brain damage.

Treatment This involves the urgent correction of dehydration, using intravenous saline and dextrose feeds initially, with continuing replacement as required. Antibiotics are not indicated unless systemic spread of bacterial infection is likely. (See also FOOD POISONING.)

Gastroenterostomy
An operation performed usually in order to relieve some obstruction to the outlet from the STOMACH. One opening is made in the lower part of the stomach; another in a neighbouring loop of the small intestine. The two are then stitched together.

Gastrointestinal Tract
The passage along which the food passes, in which it is digested (see DIGESTION), and from which it is absorbed by lymphatics and blood vessels into the circulation. The tract consists of the mouth, pharynx or throat, oesophagus or gullet, stomach, small intestine, and large intestine, in this order. For details, see articles under

these headings. The total length in humans is about 9 metres.

Gastro-Oesophageal Reflux
A disorder in which the contents of the STOMACH back up into the OESOPHAGUS because the usual neuromuscular mechanisms for preventing this are intermittently or permanently failing to work properly. If persistent, the failure may cause oesophagitis (see OESOPHAGUS, DISEASES OF). If a person develops HEARTBURN, regurgitation, discomfort and oesophagitis, the condition is called gastro-oesophageal reflux disease (GORD) and sometimes symptoms are so serious as to warrant surgery. Gastro-oesophageal reflux is sometimes associated with HIATUS HERNIA.

Gastro-oesophageal disease should be diagnosed in those patients who are at risk of physical complications from the reflux. Diagnosis is usually based on the symptoms present or by monitoring the production of acid using a pH probe inserted into the oesophagus through the mouth, since lesions are not usually visible on ENDOSCOPY. Severe heartburn, caused by the lining of the oesophagus being damaged by acid and PEPSIN from the stomach, is commonly confused with DYSPEPSIA. Treatment should start with graded doses of one of the PROTON PUMP INHIBITORS; if this is not effective after several months, surgery to remedy the reflux may be required, but the effects are not easily predictable.

Gastroscope
An endoscopic instrument (see ENDOSCOPE) for viewing the interior of the STOMACH. Introduced into the stomach via the mouth and OESOPHAGUS, the long flexible instrument (also called an oesophagogastroduodenoscope) transmits an image through a fibreoptic bundle or by a small video camera. The operator can see and photograph all areas of the stomach and also take biopsy specimens when required. (See also FIBREOPTIC ENDOSCOPY.)

Gastrostomy
An operation on the STOMACH by which, when the gullet is blocked by a tumour or other cause, an opening is made from the front of the abdomen into the stomach, so that fluid food can be passed into the organ.

Gaucher's Disease
A disease characterised by abnormal storage of LIPID, particularly in the SPLEEN, central nervous system, BONE MARROW, and LIVER. This results in enlargement of the spleen and the

liver – particularly of the former – and ANAEMIA. It runs a chronic course. Diagnosis is usually by skin fibroblast glucocerebrosidase assay. Death often results from PNEUMONIA or bleeding. Infantile Gaucher's often presents with marked neurological signs of rigid neck DYSPHAGIA, CATATONIA, hyper-reflexia and low IQ. The disease can now be treated with enzyme replacement using alglucerase. The annual cost per patient is substantial – several thousand pounds.

Gel

The term applied to a COLLOID substance which is firm in consistency although it contains much water: for example, ordinary GELATIN.

Gelatin

This is derived from COLLAGEN, the chief constituent of CONNECTIVE TISSUE. It is a colourless, transparent substance which dissolves in boiling water, and on cooling sets.into a jelly. Such a jelly is a pleasant addition to the invalid diet, especially when suitably flavoured, but it is of relatively little nutritive value as not more than one ounce can be taken in the day (i.e. the amount required to make one pint of jelly). Although it is a protein, it is lacking in several of the vital amino acids. The ordinary household 'stock' made from boiling bones contains gelatin. Mixed with about two and a half times its weight of glycerin, gelatin forms a soft substance used as the basis for many pastilles and suppositories. Partially degraded gelatin is sometimes given as a PLASMA-substitute transfusion for short-term emergency treatment for patients in SHOCK as a result of a.severe blood or fluid loss from burns or SEPTICAEMIA.

Gemeprost

One of the PROSTAGLANDINS administered vaginally as pessaries for the medical induction of late therapeutic ABORTION. Gemeprost also softens the cervix before surgical abortion, being particularly useful for women in their first pregnancy. Prostaglandins induce contractions of the UTERUS while keeping blood loss to a minimum.

Gender Identity Disorders

Gender identity is the inner sense of masculinity or femininity, and gender role is an individual's public expression of being male, female, or a 'mix' (androgynous). Most people have no difficulty because their gender identity and role are congruous. A person with a gender identity disorder, however, has a conflict between anatomical sex and gender identity.

Gender is determined by a combination of genetic and environmental factors, in which the influence of family upbringing is an important factor. When physical sexual characteristics are ambiguous, the child's gender identity can usually be established if the child is reared as being clearly male or female. Should, however, the child be confused about its sexual identity, the uncertainty may continue into adult life. Transsexuals generally experience conflicts of identity in childhood, and such problems usually occur by the age of two years. In this type of identity disorder, which occurs in one in 30,000 male births and one in 100,000 female births, the person believes that he or she is the victim of a biological accident, trapped in a body different from what is felt to be his or her true sex.

Treatment is difficult: psychotherapy and hormone treatment may help, but some affected individuals want surgery to change their body's sexual organs to match their innately felt sexual gender. The decision to seek a physical sex change raises major social problems for individuals, and ethical problems for their doctors. Surgery, which is not always successful in the long term, requires careful assessment, discussion and planning. It is important to preclude mental illness; results in homosexual men who have undergone surgery are not usually satisfactory. Advice and information may be obtained from Gender Identity Consultancy Services.

General Dental Council

A statutory body set up by the *Dentists Act* which maintains a register of dentists (see DENTAL SURGEON), promotes high standards of dental education, and oversees the professional conduct of dentists. Membership comprises elected and appointed dentists and appointed lay members. Like other councils responsible for registering health professionals, the General Dental Council now comes under the umbrella of the new Council for Regulatory Excellence, a statutory body. (See APPENDIX 7: STATUTORY ORGANISATIONS.)

General Dental Services

See DENTAL SURGEON.

General Medical Council (GMC)

A statutory body of elected and appointed medical practitioners and appointed lay members with the responsibility of protecting patients and guiding doctors in their professional practice. Set up by parliament in 1858 – at the request of the medical profession, which was concerned by the large numbers of untrained people practising as doctors – the GMC is responsible for setting educational and professional standards; maintaining a register of qualified practitioners; and disciplining doctors who fail to maintain appropriate professional standards, cautioning them or temporarily or permanently removing them from the Medical Register if they are judged unfit to practise.

The Council is funded by doctors' annual fees and is responsible to the Privy Council. Substantial reforms of the GMC's structure and functions have been and are still being undertaken to ensure that it operates effectively in today's rapidly evolving medical and social environment. In particular, the Council has strengthened its supervisory and disciplinary functions, and among many changes has proposed the regular revalidation of doctors' professional abilities on a periodic basis. The Medical Register, maintained by the GMC, is intended to enable the public to identify whom it is safe to approach to obtain medical services. Entry on the Register shows that the doctor holds a recognised primary medical qualification and is committed to upholding the profession's values. Under revalidation requirements being finalised, in addition to holding an initial qualification, doctors wishing to stay on the Register will have to show their continuing fitness to practise according to the professional attributes laid down by the GMC.

Once revalidation is fully established, there will be four categories of doctor:

● Those on the Register who successfully show their fitness to practise on a regular basis.
● Those whose registration is limited, suspended or removed as a result of the Council's disciplinary procedures.
● Those who do not wish to stay on the Register or retain any links with the GMC.
● Those, placed on a supplementary list, who do not wish to stay on the main Register but who want to retain a formal link with the medical profession through the Council. Such doctors will not be able to practise or prescribe.

General Optical Council

The statutory body that regulates the professions of ophthalmic OPTICIAN (optometrist) and dispensing optician. It promotes high standards of education and professional conduct and was set up by the Opticians Act 1958.

General Paralysis of the Insane

An outdated term for the tertiary stage of SYPHILIS.

General Practitioner (GP)

A general practitioner ('family doctor'; 'family practitioner') is a doctor working in primary care, acting as the first port of professional contact for most patients in the NHS. There are approximately 35,000 GPs in the UK and their services are accessed by registering with a GP practice – usually called a surgery or health centre. Patients should be able to see a GP within 48 hours, and practices have systems to try to ensure that urgent problems are dealt with immediately. GPs generally have few diagnostic or treatment facilities themselves, but can use local hospital diagnostic services (X-rays, blood analysis, etc.) and can refer or admit their patients to hospital, where they come under the supervision of a CONSULTANT. GPs can prescribe nearly all available medicines directly to their patients, so that they treat 90 per cent of illnesses without involving specialist or hospital services.

Most GPs work in groups of self-employed individuals, who contract their services to the local Primary Care Trust (PCT) – see below. Those in full partnership are called principals, but an increasing number now work as non-principals – that is, they are employees rather than partners in a practice. Alternatively, they might be salaried employees of a PCT. The average number of patients looked after by a full-time GP is 1,800 and the average duration of consultation about 10 minutes. GPs need to be able to deal with all common medical conditions and be able to recognise conditions that require specialist help, especially those requiring urgent action.

Until the new General Medical Services Contract was introduced in 2004, GPs had to take individual responsibility for providing 'all necessary medical services' at all times to their patient list. Now, practices rather than individuals share this responsibility. Moreover, the contract now applies only to the hours between 8.00 a.m. and 6.30 p.m., Mondays to Fridays; out-of-hours primary care has become the responsibility of PCTs. GPs still have an obligation to visit patients at home on weekdays in case of medical need, but home-visiting as a proportion of GP work has declined steadily since the NHS began. By contrast, the amount of time spent attending to preventive care and organisational issues has steadily increased. The 2004 contract for the first time introduced payment for specific indicators of good clinical care in a limited range of conditions.

A telephone advice service, NHS Direct, was launched in 2000 to give an opportunity for patients to 'consult' a trained nurse who guides the caller on whether the symptoms indicate that self-care, a visit to a GP or a hospital Accident & Emergency department, or an ambulance callout is required. The aim of this service is to give the patient prompt advice and to reduce misuse of the skills of GPs, ambulance staff and hospital facilities.

Training of GPs Training for NHS general practice after qualification and registration as a doctor requires a minimum of two years' post-registration work in hospital jobs covering a variety of areas, including PAEDIATRICS, OBSTETRICS, care of the elderly and PSYCHIATRY. This is followed by a year or more working as a 'registrar' in general practice. This final year exposes registrars to life as a GP, where they start to look after their own patients, while still closely supervised by a GP who has him- or herself been trained in educational techniques. Successful completion of 'summative assessment' – regular assessments during training – qualifies registrars to become GPs in their own right, and many newly qualified GPs also sit the membership exam set by the Royal College of General Practitioners (see APPENDIX 8: PROFESSIONAL ORGANISATIONS).

A growing number of GP practices offer educational attachments to medical students. These attachments provide experience of the range of medical and social problems commonly found in the community, while also offering them allocated time to learn clinical skills away from the more specialist environment of the hospital.

In addition to teaching commitments, many GPs are also choosing to spend one or two sessions away from their practices each week, doing other kinds of work. Most will work in, for example, at least one of the following: a hospital specialist clinic; a hospice; occupational medicine (see under OCCUPATIONAL HEALTH, MEDICINE AND DISEASES); family-planning clinics; the police or prison services. Some also become involved in medical administration, representative medicopolitics or journalism. To help them keep up to date with advances and changes in medicine, GPs are required to produce personal-development plans that outline any educational activities they have completed or intend to pursue during the forthcoming year.

NHS GPs are allowed to see private patients, though this activity is not widespread (see PRIVATE HEALTH CARE).

Primary Care Trusts (PCTs) Groups of GPs (whether working alone, or in partnership with others) are now obliged by the NHS to link communally with a number of other GPs in the locality, to form Primary Care Trusts (PCTs). Most have a membership of about 30 GPs, working within a defined geographical area, in addition to the community nurses and practice counsellors working in the same area; links are also made to local council social services so that health and social needs are addressed together. Some PCTs also run ambulance services.

One of the roles of PCTs is to develop primary-care services that are appropriate to the needs of the local population, while also occupying a powerful position to influence the scope and quality of secondary-care services. They are also designed to ensure equity of resources between different GP surgeries, so that all patients living in the locality have access to a high quality and uniform standard of service.

One way in which this is beginning to happen is through the introduction of more overt CLINICAL GOVERNANCE. PCTs devise and help their member practices to conduct CLINICAL AUDIT programmes and also encourage them to participate in prescribing incentive schemes. In return, practices receive payment for this work, and the funds are used to improve the services they offer their patients.

Generic Drug

A medicinal drug that is sold under its official (generic) name instead of its proprietary (patented brand) name. NHS doctors are advised to prescribe generic drugs where possible as this enables any suitable drug to be dispensed, saving delay to the patient and sometimes expense to the NHS. (See APPROVED NAMES FOR MEDICINES.)

Genes

Humans possess around 30,000 genes which are the biological units of heredity. They are arranged along the length of the 23 pairs of CHROMOSOMES and, like the chromosomes, therefore come in pairs (see GENETIC CODE). Human beings have 46 chromosomes, comprising two sex chromosomes and 44 autosomes, but there is also a mitochondrial chromosome outside the cell nucleus (see CELLS) which is inherited from the mother.

Half of a person's genes come from the father and half from the mother, and this mix determines the offspring's characteristics. (A quarter of a person's genes come from each of the four grandparents.) Genes fulfil their functions by controlling the manufacture of particular proteins in the body. The power that genes have to influence the body's characteristics varies: broadly, some are dominant (more powerful); others are recessive (less powerful) whose functions are overridden by the former. Genes are also liable to change or mutate, giving the potential for the characteristics of individuals or their offspring to be altered. (See GENETIC CODE; GENETIC DISORDERS; GENE THERAPY; HUMAN GENOME.)

Gene Testing
See GENETIC SCREENING.

Gene Therapy
Gene therapy is the transfer of normal GENES into a patient to combat the effects of abnormal genes which are causing disease(s). The GENETIC ENGINEERING technique used is SOMATIC cell gene therapy in which the healthy gene is put into somatic cells that produce other cells – for example, stem cells that develop into BONE MARROW. Descendants of these altered cells will be normal and, when sufficient numbers have developed, the patient's genetic disorder should be remedied. The abnormal gene, however, will still be present in the treated individual's germ cells (eggs or sperm) so he or she can still pass the inherited defect on to succeeding generations.

Gene therapy is currently used to treat disorders caused by a fault in a single recessive gene, when the defect can remedied by introducing a normal ALLELE. Treating disorders caused by dominant genes is more complicated. CYSTIC FIBROSIS is an example of a disease caused by a recessive gene, and clinical trials are taking place on the effectiveness of using LIPOSOMES to introduce the normal gene into the lungs of someone with the disorder. Trials are also underway to test the effectiveness of introducing tumour-suppressing genes into cancer cells to check their spread.

Gene therapy was first used in 1990 to treat an American patient. Eleven European medical research councils (including the UK's) recommended in 1988 that gene therapy should be restricted to correcting disease or defects, and that it should be limited to somatic cells. Interventions in germ-line cells (the sperm and egg) to effect changes that would be inherited, though technically feasible, is not allowed (see CLONING; HUMAN GENOME).

Genetic Code
The message set out sequentially along the human CHROMOSOMES. The human gene map is being constructed through the work of the international, collaborative HUMAN GENOME project; so far, only part of the code has been translated and this is the part that occurs in the GENES. Genes are responsible for the PROTEIN synthesis of the cell (see CELLS): they instruct the cell how to make a particular polypeptide chain for a particular protein.

Genes carry, in coded form, the detailed specifications for the thousands of kinds of protein molecules required by the cell for its existence, for its enzymes, for its repair work and for its reproduction. These proteins are synthesised from the 20 natural AMINO ACIDS, which are uniform throughout nature and which exist in the cell cytoplasm as part of the metabolic pool. The protein molecule consists of amino acids joined end to end to form long polypeptide chains. An average chain contains 100–300 amino acids. The sequence of bases in the nucleic acid chain of the gene corresponds in some fundamental way to the sequence of amino acids in the protein molecule, and hence it determines the structure of the particular protein. This is the genetic code. Deoxyribonucleic acid (see DNA) is the bearer of this genetic information.

DNA has a long backbone made up of repeating groups of phosphate and sugar deoxyribose. To this backbone, four bases are attached as side groups at regular intervals. These four bases are the four letters used to spell out the genetic message: they are adenine, thymine, guanine and cystosine. The molecule of the DNA is made up of two chains coiled round a common axis to form what is called a double helix. The two chains are held together by hydrogen bonds between pairs of bases. Since adenine only pairs with thymine, and guanine only with cystosine, the sequences of bases in one chain fixes the sequence in the other. Several hundred bases would be contained in the length of DNA of a typical gene. If the message of the DNA-based sequences is a continuous succession of thymine, the RIBOSOME will link together a series of the amino acid, phenylalanine. If the base sequence is a succession of cytosine, the ribosome will link up a series of prolines. Thus, each amino acid has its own particular code of bases. In fact, each amino acid is coded by a word consisting of three adjacent bases. In addition to carrying genetic information, DNA is able to synthesise or replicate itself and so pass its information on to daughter cells.

All DNA is part of the chromosome and so remains confined to the nucleus of the cell (except in the mitochondrial DNA). Proteins are synthesised by the ribosomes which are in the cytoplasm. DNA achieves control over pro-

G

tein production in the cytoplasm by directing the synthesis of ribonucleic acid (see RNA). Most of the DNA in a cell is inactive, otherwise the cell would synthesise simultaneously every protein that the individual was capable of forming. When part of the DNA structure becomes 'active', it acts as a template for the ribonucleic acid, which itself acts as a template for protein synthesis when it becomes attached to the ribosome.

Ribonucleic acid exists in three forms. First 'messenger RNA' carries the necessary 'message' for the synthesis of a specific protein, from the nucleus to the ribosome. Second, 'transfer RNA' collects the individual amino acids which exist in the cytoplasm as part of the metabolic pool and carries them to the ribosome. Third, there is RNA in the ribosome itself. RNA has a similar structure to DNA but the sugar is ribose instead of deoxyribose and uracil replaces the base thymine. Before the ribosome can produce the proteins, the amino acids must be lined up in the correct order on the messenger RNA template. This alignment is carried out by transfer RNA, of which there is a specific form for each individual amino acid. Transfer RNA can not only recognise its specific amino acid, but also identify the position it is required to occupy on the messenger RNA template. This is because each transfer RNA has its own sequence of bases and recognises its site on the messenger RNA by pairing bases with it. The ribosome then travels along the chain of messenger RNA and links the amino acids, which have thus been arranged in the requisite order, by peptide bonds and protein is released.

Proteins are important for two main reasons. First, all the enzymes of living cells are made of protein. One gene is responsible for one enzyme. Genes thus control all the biochemical processes of the body and are responsible for the inborn difference between human beings. Second, proteins also fulfil a structural role in the cell, so that genes controlling the synthesis of structural proteins are responsible for morphological differences between human beings.

Genetic Counselling

The procedure whereby advice is given about the risks of a genetic disorder and the various options that are open to the individual at risk. This may often involve establishing the diagnosis in the family, as this would be a prerequisite before giving any detailed advice. Risks can be calculated from simple Mendelian inheritance (see MENDELISM) in many genetic disorders. However, in many disorders with a genetic element, such as cleft lip or palate (see CLEFT PALATE), the risk of recurrence is obtained from population studies. Risks include not only the likelihood of having a child who is congenitally affected by a disorder, but also, for adults, that of being vulnerable to an adult-onset disease.

The options for individuals would include taking no action; modifying their behaviour; or taking some form of direct action. For those at risk of having an affected child, where prenatal diagnosis is available, this would involve either carrying on with reproduction regardless of risk; deciding not to have children; or deciding to go ahead to have children but opting for prenatal diagnosis. For an adult-onset disorder such as a predisposition to ovarian cancer, an individual may choose to take no action; to take preventive measures such as use of the oral contraceptive pill; to have screening of the ovaries with measures such as ultrasound; or to take direct action such as removing the ovaries to prevent ovarian cancer from occurring.

There are now regional genetics centres throughout the United Kingdom, and patients can be referred through their family doctor or specialists.

Genetic Disorders

These are caused when there are mutations or other abnormalities which disrupt the code of a gene or set of GENES. These are divided into autosomal (one of the 44 CHROMOSOMES which are not sex-linked), dominant, autosomal recessive, sex-linked and polygenic disorders.

Dominant genes A dominant characteristic is an effect which is produced whenever a gene or gene defect is present. If a disease is due to a dominant gene, those affected are heterozygous – that is, they only carry a fault in the gene on one of the pair of chromosomes concerned. Affected people married to normal individuals transmit the gene directly to one-half of the children, although this is a random event just like tossing a coin. HUNTINGTON'S CHOREA is due to the inheritance of a dominant gene, as is neurofibromatosis (see VON RECKLINGHAUSEN'S DISEASE) and familial adenomatous POLYPOSIS of the COLON. ACHONDROPLASIA is an example of a disorder in which there is a high frequency of a new dominant mutation, for the majority of affected people have normal parents and siblings. However, the chances of the children of a parent with the condition being affected are one in two, as with any other dominant characteristic. Other diseases inherited as dominant characteristics include spherocytosis, haemorrhagic telangiectasia and adult polycystic kidney disease.

Recessive genes If a disease is due to a recessive gene, those affected must have the faulty gene on both copies of the chromosome pair (i.e. be homozygous). The possession of a single recessive gene does not result in overt disease, and the bearer usually carries this potentially unfavourable gene without knowing it. If that person marries another carrier of the same recessive gene, there is a one-in-four chance that their children will receive the gene in a double dose, and so have the disease. If an individual sufferer from a recessive disease marries an apparently normal person who is a heterozygous carrier of the same gene, one-half of the children will be affected and the other half will be carriers of the disease. The commonest of such recessive conditions in Britain is CYSTIC FIBROSIS, which affects about one child in 2,000. Approximately 5 per cent of the population carry a faulty copy of the gene. Most of the inborn errors of metabolism, such as PHENYLKETONURIA, GALACTOSAEMIA and congenital adrenal hyperplasia (see ADRENOGENITAL SYNDROME), are due to recessive genes.

There are characteristics which may be incompletely recessive – that is, neither completely dominant nor completely recessive – and the heterozygotus person, who bears the gene in a single dose, may have a slight defect whilst the homozygotus, with a double dose of the gene, has a severe illness. The sickle-cell trait is a result of the sickle-cell gene in single dose, and sickle-cell ANAEMIA is the consequence of a double dose.

Sex-linked genes If a condition is sex-linked, affected males are homozygous for the mutated gene as they carry it on their single X chromosome. The X chromosome carries many genes, while the Y chromosome bears few genes, if any, other than those determining masculinity. The genes on the X chromosome of the male are thus not matched by corresponding genes on the Y chromosome, so that there is no chance of the Y chromosome neutralising any recessive trait on the X chromosome. A recessive gene can therefore produce disease, since it will not be suppressed by the normal gene of the homologous chromosome. The same recessive gene on the X chromosome of the female will be suppressed by the normal gene on the other X chromosome. Such sex-linked conditions include HAEMOPHILIA, CHRISTMAS DISEASE, DUCHENNE MUSCULAR DYSTROPHY (see also MUSCLES, DISORDERS OF – Myopathy) and nephrogenic DIABETES INSIPIDUS.

If the mother of an affected child has another male relative affected, she is a heterozygote carrier; half her sons will have the disease and half her daughters will be carriers. The sister of a haemophiliac thus has a 50 per cent chance of being a carrier. An affected male cannot transmit the gene to his son because the X chromosome of the son must come from the mother; all his daughters, however, will be carriers as the X chromosome for the father must be transmitted to all his daughters. Hence sex-linked recessive characteristics cannot be passed from father to son. Sporadic cases may be the result of a new mutation, in which case the mother is not the carrier and is not likely to have further affected children. It is probable that one-third of haemophiliacs arise as a result of fresh mutations, and these patients will be the first in the families to be affected. Sometimes the carrier of a sex-linked recessive gene can be identified. The sex-linked variety of retinitis pigmentosa (see EYE, DISORDERS OF) can often be detected by ophthalmoscopic examination.

A few rare disorders are due to dominant genes carried on the X chromosome. An example of such a condition is familial hypophosphataemia with vitamin-D-resistant RICKETS.

Polygenic inheritance In many inherited conditions, the disease is due to the combined action of several genes; the genetic element is then called multi-factorial or polygenic. In this situation there would be an increased incidence of the disease in the families concerned, but it will not follow the Mendelian (see MENDELISM; GENETIC CODE) ratio. The greater the number of independent genes involved in determining a certain disease, the more complicated will be the pattern of inheritance. Furthermore, many inherited disorders are the result of a combination of genetic and environmental influences. DIABETES MELLITUS is the most familiar of such multi-factorial inheritance. The predisposition to develop diabetes is an inherited characteristic, although the gene is not always able to express itself: this is called incomplete penetrance. Whether or not the individual with a genetic predisposition towards the disease actually develops diabetes will also depend on environmental factors. Diabetes is more common in the relatives of diabetic patients, and even more so amongst identical twins. Non-genetic factors which are important in precipitating overt disease are obesity, excessive intake of carbohydrate foods, and pregnancy.

SCHIZOPHRENIA is another example of the combined effects of genetic and environmental influences in precipitating disease. The risk of schizophrenia in a child, one of whose parents has the disease, is one in ten, but this figure is modified by the early environment of the child.

Genetic Engineering

Genetic engineering, or recombinant DNA technology, has only developed in the past decade or so; it is the process of changing the genetic material of a cell (see CELLS). GENES from one cell – for example, a human cell – can be inserted into another cell, usually a bacterium, and made to function. It is now possible to insert the gene responsible for the production of human INSULIN, human GROWTH HORMONE and INTERFERON from a human cell into a bacterium. Segments of DNA for insertion can be prepared by breaking long chains into smaller pieces by the use of restriction enzymes. The segments are then inserted into the affecting organism by using PLASMIDS and bacteriophages (see BACTERIOPHAGE). Plasmids are small packets of DNA that are found within bacteria and can be passed from one bacterium to another.

Already genetic engineering is contributing to easing the problems of diagnosis. DNA analysis and production of MONOCLONAL ANTIBODIES are other applications of genetic engineering. Genetic engineering has significantly contributed to horticulture and agriculture with certain characteristics of one organism or variant of a species being transfected (a method of gene transfer) into another. This has given rise to higher-yield crops and to alteration in colouring and size in produce. Genetic engineering is also contributing to our knowledge of how human genes function, as these can be transfected into mice and other animals which can then act as models for genetic therapy. Studying the effects of inherited mutations derived from human DNA in these animal models is thus a very important and much faster way of learning about human disease.

Genetic engineering is a scientific procedure that could have profound implications for the human race. Manipulating heredity would be an unwelcome activity under the control of maverick scientists, politicians or others in positions of power.

Genetic Fingerprinting

This technique shows the relationships between individuals: for example, it can be used to prove maternity or paternity of a child. The procedure is also used in FORENSIC MEDICINE whereby any tissue left behind by a criminal at the scene of a crime can be compared genetically with the tissue of a suspect. DNA, the genetic material in living cells, can be extracted from blood, semen and other body tissues. The technique, pioneered in Britain in 1984, is now widely used.

Genetics

The science which deals with the origin of the characteristics of an individual or the study of HEREDITY.

Genetic Screening

A screening procedure that tests whether a person has a genetic make-up that is linked with a particular disease. If so, the person may either develop the disease or pass it on to his or her offspring. When an individual has been found to carry a genetically linked disease, he or she should receive genetic counselling from an expert in inherited diseases.

Genetic screening is proving to be a controversial subject. Arguments are developing over whether the results of such screenings should be made available to employers and insurance companies – a move that could have adverse consequences for some individuals with potentially harmful genetic make-ups. (See GENES; GENETIC DISORDERS.)

Genital Herpes

See HERPES GENITALIS.

Genitalia

The external organs of reproduction. The term is usually applied to the external parts of the reproductive system: the VULVA in females and PENIS and SCROTUM in males. Rarely the sex of an individual may not be apparent from the genitalia. Genitals develop from a common embryonic structure, and disturbances in the hormone controls of the developing genitalia may produce an individual whose external genitalia are ambiguous. The condition is known as intersex. The individual may be HERMAPHRODITE or PSEUDOHERMAPHRODITE.

Genito-Urinary Medicine

The branch of medicine that deals with the effects of SEXUALLY TRANSMITTED DISEASES (STDS) on the URINARY TRACT, REPRODUCTIVE SYSTEM and other systems in the body. The specialty overlaps with GYNAECOLOGY (women's urinary and reproductive systems) and UROLOGY (men's urinary and reproductive system).

Genito-Urinary Tract

This consists of the KIDNEYS, ureters (see URETER), URINARY BLADDER and URETHRA – and, in the male, also the genital organs.

Genome

A complete set of CHROMOSOMES derived from one parent, or the total gene complement of a set of chromosomes. An international study is well underway to produce a complete map of the HUMAN GENOME.

Genotype

All of an individual's genetic information that is encoded in his or her CHROMOSOMES. It also means the genetic information carried by a pair of alleles which controls a particular characteristic. (See GENES.)

Gentamicin

An antibiotic derived from a species of micro-organisms, *Micromonospora purpurea*. Its main value is that it is active against certain micro-organisms such as *Pseudomonas pyocyanea*, *E. coli* and *Aerobacter aerogenes* which are not affected by other antibiotics, as well as staphylococci which have become resistant to PENICILLIN.

Gentian Violet

A dye belonging to the rosaniline group. It is a useful superficial antiseptic for use on unbroken skin.

Genu Valgum

The medical term for knock-knee – a deformity of the lower limbs in such a direction that when the limbs are straightened, the legs diverge from one another. As a result, in walking, the knees knock against each other. The amount of knock-knee is measured by the distance between the medial malleoli of the ankles, with the inner surfaces of the knee touching and the knee-caps facing forwards. The condition is so common in children between the ages of 2–6 years that it may almost be regarded as a normal phase in childhood. When marked, or persisting into later childhood, it can be corrected by surgery (osteotomy).

Genu Varum

Genu varum is the medical term for BOW LEG.

Geriatrics

Now increasingly termed 'medicine of the elderly', this is a branch of medicine that deals with disorders and diseases associated with old age, and particularly their social consequences (see also AGEING).

German Measles

See RUBELLA.

Germ Cell

Those embryonic cells with the potential to develop into ova (see OVUM) or spermatozoa (see SPERMATOZOON).

Germ Layer

Any one of the three discrete varieties of body tissue that develop in the early stages of growth of the EMBRYO. Development of the layers can be followed throughout the embryo's stages of growth and specialisation into the body's full range of tissues and organs (see ECTODERM; ENDODERM; MESODERM).

Germs

See MICROBIOLOGY.

Gerontology

The study of alterations in the body and mind that occur as a person ages, and the problems that result (see AGEING).

Gestaltism

A school of psychology based on the concept that an individual's sense of wholeness is more valuable than a piecemeal approach to perception and behaviour. Founded in Germany early in the 20th century, the school's practitioners regarded the whole as more than a sum of its parts. Aimed at resolving personal problems, the therapy increased subjects' self-awareness of all aspects of themselves in their environment.

Gestation

Gestation is another name for pregnancy (see PREGNANCY AND LABOUR).

GFR

See GLOMERULAR FILTRATION RATE (GFR).

Giardiasis

A condition caused by a parasitic organism known as *Giardia lamblia*, which is found in the duodenum (see INTESTINE) and the upper part of the small intestine. This organism is usually harmless, but is sometimes responsible for causing diarrhoea. The illness develops one or two weeks after exposure to infection, and usually starts as an explosive diarrhoea, with the passage of pale fatty stools, abdominal pain and nausea. It responds well to METRONIDAZOLE or MEPACRINE.

Giddiness
See VERTIGO.

GIFT
See ASSISTED CONCEPTION.

Gigantism
Excessive growth (mainly in height) caused by overproduction, during childhood or adolescence, of GROWTH HORMONE by a tumour of the PITUITARY GLAND. Untreated, the affected individual may die in early adulthood. Sometimes the tumour appears after the individual has stopped growing and the result then is ACROMEGALY rather than gigantism.

Gilles De La Tourette's Syndrome
Also known as Tourette's syndrome, this is a hereditary condition of severe and multiple tics (see TIC) of motor or vocal origin. It usually starts in childhood and becomes chronic (with remissions). With a prevalance of one in 2,000, a dominant gene (see GENES) with variable expression may be responsible. The disorder is associated with explosive vocal tics and grunts, occasionally obscene (see COPROLALIA). The patient may also involuntarily repeat the words or imitate the actions of others (see PALILALIA). HALOPERIDOL, pimozide (an oral antipsychotic drug similar to CHLORPROMAZINE hydrochloride) and clonidine are among drugs that may help to control this distressing, but fortunately rare, disorder.

Gingivitis
Inflammation of the gums (see TEETH, DISORDERS OF).

Gland
A collection of CELLS or an ORGAN with a specialised ability to make and secrete chemical substances such as enzymes and hormones essential for the normal functioning of the body. Glands are classified into two groups: ENDOCRINE and EXOCRINE. The former secrete their products, hormones, straight into the bloodstream; the latter's secretions are discharged through ducts. (These functional differences are the reason why glands have been defined as ductless and ducted.) Examples of endocrine glands are the adrenals, PITUITARY GLAND and THYROID GLAND. Exocrine glands include SEBACEOUS GLANDS (in the skin) and the SALIVARY GLANDS in the mouth whose enzymes start the digestion of food. The BREASTS or mammary glands are exocrine glands that secrete milk. Though strictly speaking not a gland, LYMPH nodes (part of the lymphatic system) are sometimes called that. While they do not produce secretions, lymph glands do release white blood cells, an essential part of the body's defence system.

Glandular Fever
See MONONUCLEOSIS.

Glans
The term applied to the ends of the PENIS and the CLITORIS. In the penis the glans is the distal, helmet-shaped part that is formed by the bulbous corpus spongiosum (erectile tissue). In an uncircumcised man the glans is covered by the foreskin or PREPUCE when the penis is flaccid.

Glasgow Coma Scale
A method developed by two doctors in Glasgow that is used to assess the depth of COMA or unconsciousness suffered by an individual. The scale is split into three groups – eye opening, motor response, and verbal response – with the level of activity within each group given a score. A person's total score is the sum of the numbers scored in each group, and this provides a reasonably objective assessment of the patient's coma state – particularly useful when monitoring people who have suffered a head injury. (See also PERSISTENT VEGETATIVE STATE (PVS).)

Glaucoma
A group of disorders of the eye characterised by the intraocular pressure being so high as to damage the nerve fibres in the retina and the optic nerve (see EYE) as it leaves the eye en route to the brain. The affected person suffers limitation of the field of vision and on examination the optic disc can be seen to be cupped. The clinical signs depend on the rate and extent of rise in pressure.

Individuals most at risk have a family history of GLAUCOMA (especially among siblings), are myopic (short-sighted), or have diabetic or thyroid eye disease. People with a strong family history of the disease should have regular eye checks, including tonometry, from the age of 35 years.

Glaucoma is usually classified as being either open-angle glaucoma or narrow-angle glaucoma.

Open-angle glaucoma is a chronic, slowly progressive, usually bilateral disorder. It occurs in one in 200 of people over 40 and accounts for 20 per cent of those registered blind in Great Britain. Symptoms are virtually non-existent until well into the disease, when the patient may experience visual problems. It is not painful. The characteristic findings are that the intraocular pressure is raised (normal pressure is up to 21 mm Hg) causing cupping of the optic disc and a glaucomatous visual-field loss. The angle between the iris and the cornea remains open. Treatment is aimed at decreasing the intraocular pressure initially by drops, tablets and intravenous drug administration. Surgery may be required later. A trabeculectomy is an operation to create a channel through which fluid can drain from the eye in a controlled fashion in order to bring the pressure down.

Narrow-angle glaucoma affects one in 1,000 people over 40 years of age and is more common in women. Symptoms may start with coloured haloes around street lights at night. These may then be followed by rapid onset of severe pain in and around the eye accompanied by a rapid fall in vision. One eye is usually affected first; this alerts the surgeon so that action can be taken to prevent a similar attack in the other eye. Treatment must be started as an emergency with a topical beta blocker (see BETA-ADRENOCEPTOR-BLOCKING DRUGS) in eye drops with other drugs such as ADRENALINE or pilocarpine added as necessary. Dorzolamide, a topical anhydrase inhibitor, can also be used. ACETAZOLAMIDE, also an anhydrase inhibitor, can be given by mouth. In an emergency before surgery, MANNITOL can be given through an intravenous infusion; this is followed by surgery to prevent recurrence. Acute narrow-angle glaucoma occurs because the peripheral iris is pushed against the back of the cornea. This closes off the angle between iris and cornea through which aqueous humour drains out of the eye. Since the aqueous humour cannot drain away, it builds up inside the eye causing a rapid increase in pressure.

Various types of LASER treatment – trabeculoplasty ('burning' the trabecular network); iridotomy (cutting holes to relieve pressure); and ciliary-body ablation by 'burning' – are sometimes used in preference to surgery.

Gleet
Gleet means a chronic form of GONORRHOEA.

Glenoid
The term applied to the shallow socket on the shoulder-blade into which the HUMERUS fits, forming the shoulder-joint.

Glia
Also called neuroglia, this is the specialised connective tissue of the CENTRAL NERVOUS SYSTEM. Providing support and nutrition to neurones (see NEURON(E)), glia comprises various cells including oligodendrocytes, astrocytes and ependymal cells. There are around ten times as many glial cells as neurons and they form about 40 per cent of the total volume of the brain and spinal cord, playing an essential role in the neurochemical transmission function of neurons (see BRAIN).

Glibenclamide
A drug which stimulates the beta cells of the PANCREAS to liberate INSULIN, and is used to treat some patients with DIABETES MELLITUS. (See also SULPHONYLUREAS.)

Gliclazide
See SULPHONYLUREAS.

Gliobastoma
A type of brain tumour arising from tissue. It grows rapidly, destroying brain cells and causing a progressive loss of brain function. The patient suffers from headache as a result of raised cranial pressure, eventually vomiting regularly and becoming increasingly drowsy. The prognosis is poor and palliative treatment is required as surgical removal, radiotherapy and chemotherapy are not effective.

Glioma
A tumour in the brain or spinal cord, composed of neuroglia, which is the special connective tissue that supports the nerve cells and nerve fibres (see GLIA). Low-grade malignant gliomas cause symptoms by putting pressure on surrounding tissues and organs. Highly malignant gliomas are usually invasive. Gliomas, like other space-occupying tumours in the brain, may present with headaches, seizures, neurological symptoms or symptoms of mental disturbance. Treatment may include surgery, radiotherapy and chemotherapy and should be done in a specialist neurological centre. Gliomas tend to spread within the brain and can be difficult to remove surgically.

Glipizide
See SULPHONYLUREAS.

Gliquidone
See SULPHONYLUREAS.

Globin
A protein which, when it combines with haem, forms HAEMOGLOBIN – the molecule found in the red blood cell that carries oxygen and carbon dioxide.

Globulin

A class of proteins which are insoluble in water and alcohol and soluble in weak salt solution. (See also GAMMA-GLOBULIN.)

Globus

A term applied generally to any structures of ball shape, but especially to the sensation of a ball in the throat causing choking, which forms a common symptom of acute anxiety (globus hystericus).

Glomerular Filtration Rate (GFR)

Each of the two KIDNEYS filters a large volume of blood – 25 per cent of cardiac output, or around 1,300 ml – through its two million glomeruli (see GLOMERULUS) every minute. The glomeruli filter out cell, protein, and fat-free fluid which, after reabsorption of certain chemicals, is excreted as urine. The rate of this ultra-filtration process, which in health is remarkably constant, is called the glomerular filtration rate (GFR). Each day nearly 180 litres of water plus some small molecular-weight constituents of blood are filtrated. The GFR is thus an indicator of kidney function. The most widely used measurement is CREATININE clearance and this is assessed by measuring the amount of creatinine in a 24-hour sample of urine and the amount of creatinine in the plasma; a formula is applied that gives the GFR.

Glomerulitis

See KIDNEYS, DISEASES OF.

Glomerulonephritis

See KIDNEYS, DISEASES OF.

Glomerulus

A small knot of blood vessels about the size of a grain of sand, of which around 1,000,000 are found in each of the two KIDNEYS, and from which the excretion of fluid out of the blood into the tubules of the kidney takes place.

Glossitis

Inflammation of the tongue. Causes include ANAEMIA, CANDIDA infection and dietary (particularly vitamin) deficiencies. The condition may also occur as a result of friction of the tongue against the sharp edge of a tooth.

Glossopharyngeal

The glossopharyngeal nerve is the ninth cranial nerve, which in the main is a SENSORY nerve, being the nerve of taste in the posterior third of the tongue and the nerve of general sensation for the whole upper part of the throat and

middle ear. It also supplies the PAROTID GLAND and one of the muscles on the side of the throat.

Glottis

The narrow opening at the upper end of the LARYNX. The glottis is made up of the true vocal cords. (See AIR PASSAGES; CHOKING.)

Glucagon

A hormone secreted by the alpha cells of the islets of Langerhans in the PANCREAS, which increases the amount of glucose in the blood. This it does by promoting the breakdown of liver GLYCOGEN (glycogenolysis). It is secreted in response to a lowered blood sugar and is used therapeutically to treat HYPOGLYCAEMIA.

Glucocorticoids

One of the two main groups of CORTICO-STEROIDS. CORTISOL, CORTISONE and corticosterone are part of this group and are essential for the body to utilise CARBOHYDRATE, FAT and PROTEIN – in particular, when the body is reacting to stress. Glucocorticoids occur naturally but can be synthesised, and they have strong anti-inflammatory properties, being used to treat conditions in which inflammation is a part.

Gluconeogenesis

The formation of sugar from amino acids in the LIVER.

Glucose

Glucose, also known as dextrose or grape sugar, is the form of sugar found in honey and in grapes and some other fruits. It is also the form of sugar circulating in the bloodstream, and the form into which all sugars and starches are converted in the small INTESTINE before being absorbed. Glucose is a yellowish-white crystalline substance soluble in water and having the property of turning a ray of polarised light to the right. It is often given to patients orally or, sometimes, intravenously as an easily assimilated form of CARBOHYDRATE. It has the further practical advantage in this context of not being nearly as sweet-tasting as cane sugar and therefore relatively large amounts can be consumed without sickening the patient.

Glucose-6-Phosphate Dehydrogenase

An ENZYME that performs an essential function in the metabolism of CARBOHYDRATE. A deficiency in this enzyme – acronym G6PD – results in the breakdown of ERYTHROCYTES

(HAEMOLYSIS), usually in the presence of oxidants (see OXIDANT) such as infections or drugs. The deficiency disorder is a hereditary condition in which the enzyme is absent. The condition, characterised by pallor, rigors and pain in the loin, is divided into African, European (including FAVISM) and Oriental types. Sufferers should avoid substances that trigger haemolysis. Acute episodes are best treated symptomatically.

Glucose-Tolerance Test
A way of assessing the body's efficiency at metabolising GLUCOSE. The test is used in the diagnosis of DIABETES MELLITUS. The patient is starved for up to 16 hours, after which he or she is fed glucose by mouth. The concentrations of glucose in the blood and urine are then measured at half-hour intervals over a period of two hours.

Glucoside
A GLYCOSIDE formed from GLUCOSE.

Glue Ear
Another name for secretory otitis media (see EAR, DISEASES OF).

Glue Sniffing
See SOLVENT ABUSE.

Glutamate
An amino acid (see AMINO ACIDS) which, along with aspartate, is a major excitatory chemical neurotransmitter – method of communication between neurones (see NEURON(E)) – in the central nervous system. The two amino acids are found in the cortex and cerebellum of the BRAIN and in the SPINAL CORD.

Glutaminase
An ENZYME occurring in the KIDNEYS which catalyses the breakdown of glutamine (see AMINO ACIDS) to ammonia – a phase in the production of the metabolic waste product, UREA.

Gluteal
The region of the buttock and the structures situated in it, such as the gluteal muscles (see GLUTEUS), arteries, and nerves.

Gluten
The constituent of wheat-flour which forms an adhesive substance on addition of water, and allows the 'raising' of bread. It can be separated from the starch of flour, and being of a protein nature is used to make bread for those diabetics who are debarred from starchy and sugary foods.

It is also responsible for certain forms of what is now known as the MALABSORPTION SYNDROME. In patients with this condition, an essential part of treatment is a gluten-free diet. (See also COELIAC DISEASE.)

Gluteus
Three gluteal muscles form each buttock. The gluteus maximus is the large, powerful muscle that gives the buttocks their rounded shape. The remaining two muscles are the gluteus medius and gluteus minimus; together the three muscles are responsible for moving the thigh.

Glycerin
Glycerin, or glycerol, is an alcohol, $C_3H_8O_3$, which occurs naturally in combination with organic acids in the form of fats or triglycerides. It is a clear, colourless, thick liquid of sweet taste. It dissolves many substances, and absorbs water effectively.

Uses Glycerin has many and varied uses. Numerous substances, such as carbolic acid, tannic acid, alum, borax, boric acid and starch, are dissolved in it for application to the body. It is frequently applied along with other remedies to inflamed areas for its action in extracting fluid and thus diminishing inflammation.

Glycerol
Another name for GLYCERIN.

Glyceryl Trinitrate
Also known as trinitrin and nitroglycerin, this is a drug used in the treatment of ANGINA PECTORIS and left ventricular failure of the heart. It is normally given as a sublingual tablet or spray, though percutaneous preparations may be useful in the prophylaxis of angina – particularly for patients who suffer attacks at rest, and especially at night. Sublingually it provides rapid symptomatic relief of angina, but is only effective for 20–30 minutes. It is a potent vasodilator, and this may lead to unwanted side-effects such as flushing, headache, and postural HYPOTENSION. Its antispasmodic effects are also valuable in the treatment of ASTHMA, biliary and renal colic, and certain cases of VOMITING. (See also COLIC.)

Glyco-
A prefix meaning of the nature of, or containing, sugar.

Glycogen

Glycogen, or animal starch, is a CARBO-HYDRATE substance found specially in the liver, as well as in other tissues. It is the form in which carbohydrates taken in the food are stored in the liver and muscles before they are converted into GLUCOSE as the needs of the body require.

Glycoproteins

Compounds comprising a PROTEIN and a CARBOHYDRATE, such as mucins, mucoid and amyloid.

Glycoside

A compound of a sugar and a non-sugar unit. Glycosides are widespread throughout nature and include many important drugs such as DIGOXIN.

Glycosylated Haemoglobin (HbA1c)

This forms a small proportion of the total HAEMOGLOBIN in the blood. It differs from the major component, HbA, in that it has a glucose group attached. The rate of synthesis of HbA1c is a function of the blood-glucose concentration, and since it accumulates throughout the life span of the red blood cell – normally 120 days – the concentration of HbA1c is related to the mean blood-glucose concentration over the past 3–4 months. It is thus a useful indicator of medium-term diabetic control (see DIABETES MELLITUS) – a good target range would be a concentration of 5–8 per cent. When interpreting the HbA1c level, however, it is important to remember that wide fluctuations in blood-glucose concentration, together with ANAEMIA or a reduced ERYTHROCYTES life span, may give misleading results.

Glycosuria

The presence of sugar in the urine. By far the most common cause of glycosuria is DIABETES MELLITUS, but it may also occur as a result of a lowered renal threshold for sugar when it is called renal glycosuria, and is not indicative of disease. Measurements of the amounts of sugar in the urine is a standard method used by patients (and health professionals) to assess the stability of treatment for diabetes mellitus, indicating whether adjustment is required in the hypoglycaemic (sugar-lowering) agents they are taking.

Goblet Cell

A columnar secretory cell occurring in the EPI-THELIUM of the respiratory and intestinal tracts. The cells produce the main constituents of MUCUS.

Goitre

Goitre is a term applied to a swelling in the front of the neck caused by an enlargement of the THYROID GLAND. The thyroid lies between the skin and the front of the windpipe and in health is not large enough to be seen. The four main varieties of goitre are the simple goitre, the nodular, the lymphadenoid goitre and the toxic goitre. (See THYROID GLAND, DISEASES OF.)

Gold Salts

These are used in the treatment of RHEUMA-TOID ARTHRITIS. Gold may be administered in various forms – for example, sodium aurothiomalate. It is injected in very small doses intramuscularly and produces a reaction in the affected tissues which leads to their scarring and healing. Auranofin is a gold preparation that can be given orally; if no response has been achieved within six months the drug should be stopped. It is less effective than gold given by intramuscular injection. If gold is administered in too large quantities, skin eruptions, albuminuria (see PROTEINURIA), metallic taste in the mouth, JAUNDICE, and feverishness may be produced, so that it is necessary to prolong a course of this remedy over many months in minute doses. Routine blood and urine tests are also necessary in order to detect any adverse or toxic effect at an early stage.

Golfer's Elbow

A term applied to a condition comparable to tennis elbow. It is not uncommon in the left elbow of right-handed golfers who catch the head of their club in the ground when making a duff shot.

Gonad

A gland which produces a gamete – that is, an ovary (see OVARIES) or a testis (see TESTICLE).

Gonadorelin

A hormone that stimulates the PITUITARY GLAND to secrete three hormones: gonadotrophic, luteinising and follicle-stimulating. Gonadorelin can be made artificially and given by intravenous injection. It is used to stimulate the OVARIES when treating infertile women, and to investigate suspected disease of the HYPO-THALAMUS. Analogues of the hormone (buserelin and goserelin) are chemically similar and can be used to suppress release of gonadorelin, so cutting the production of pituitary hormones. The two analogues are given to treat

ENDOMETRIOSIS, breast cancer (see BREASTS, DISEASES OF) and prostate cancer (see PROSTATE GLAND, DISEASES OF).

Gonadotrophins

Gonadotrophins, or gonadotrophic hormones, are hormones that control the activity of the gonads (i.e. the testes and ovaries). In the male they stimulate the secretion of TESTOSTERONE and the production of spermatozoa (see SPERMATOZOON); in the female they stimulate the production of ova (see OVUM) and the secretion of OESTROGENS and PROGESTERONE. There are two gonadotrophins produced by the PITUITARY GLAND. CHORIONIC GONADOTROPHIC HORMONE is produced in the PLACENTA and excreted in the urine.

Gonococci

A bacterium of the species responsible for the sexually transmitted disease GONORRHOEA.

Gonorrhoea

Gonorrhoea is an inflammatory disease caused by *Neisseria gonococcus*, affecting especially the mucous membrane of the URETHRA in the male and that of the VAGINA in the female, but spreading also to other parts. It is the most common of the SEXUALLY TRANSMITTED DISEASES (STDS). According to the WHO, 200 million new cases are notified annually in the world. In the UK the incidence has been declining since 1991; in 1999 the rate per million of population was 385 for males (599.4 in 1991) and 171.3 for females (216.5 in 1991).

Causes The disease is directly contagious from another person already suffering from it – usually by sexual intercourse, but occasionally conveyed by the discharge on sponges, towels or clothing as well as by actual contact. The gonococcus is found in the discharge expressed from the urethra, which may be spread as a film on a glass slide, suitably stained, and examined under the microscope; or a culture from the discharge may be made on certain bacteriological media and films from this, similarly examined under the microscope. Since discharges resembling that of gonorrhoea accompany other forms of inflammation, the identification of the organism is of great importance. A gram-stained smear of urethral discharge enables rapid identification of the gonococcus in around 90 per cent of men.

Symptoms These differ considerably, according to whether the disease is in an acute or a chronic stage.

MEN After an incubation period of 2–10 days, irritation in the urethra, scalding pain on passing water, and a viscid yellowish-white discharge appear; the glands in the groin often enlarge and may suppurate. The urine when passed is hazy and is often found to contain yellowish threads of pus visible to the eye. After some weeks, if the condition has become chronic, the discharge is clear and viscid, there may be irritation in passing urine, and various forms of inflammation in neighbouring organs may appear – the TESTICLE, PROSTATE GLAND and URINARY BLADDER becoming affected. At a still later stage the inflammation of the urethra is apt to lead to gradual formation of fibrous tissue around this channel. This contracts and produces narrowing, so that urination becomes difficult or may be stopped for a time altogether (the condition known as stricture). Inflammation of some of the joints is a common complication in the early stage – the knee, ankle, wrist, and elbow being the joints most frequently affected – and this form of 'rheumatism' is very intractable and liable to lead to permanent stiffness. The fibrous tissues elsewhere may also develop inflammatory changes, causing pain in the back, foot, etc. In occasional cases, during the acute stage, SEPTICAEMIA may develop, with inflammation of the heart-valves (ENDOCARDITIS) and abscesses in various parts of the body. The infective matter occasionally is inoculated accidentally into the eye, producing a very severe form of conjunctivitis: in the newly born child this is known as ophthalmia neonatorum and, although now rare in the UK. has in the past been a major cause of blindness (see EYE, DISORDERS OF).

WOMEN The course and complications of the disease are somewhat different in women. It begins with a yellow vaginal discharge, pain on urination, and very often inflammation or abscess of the Bartholin's glands, situated close to the vulva or opening of the vagina. The chief seriousness, however, of the disease is due to the spread of inflammation to neighbouring organs, the UTERUS, FALLOPIAN TUBES, and OVARIES, causing permanent destructive changes in these, and leading occasionally to PERITONITIS through the Fallopian tube with a fatal result. Many cases of prolonged ill-health and sterility or recurring miscarriages are due to these changes.

Treatment The chances of cure are better the earlier treatment is instituted. PENICILLIN is the antibiotic of choice but unfortunately the gonococcus is liable to become resistant to this. In patients who are infected with penicillin-resistant organisms, one of the other antibiotics (e.g. cefotaxime, ciprofloxacin or spectinomycin) is used. In all cases it is essential that bacteriological investigation should be carried out at weekly intervals for three or four weeks, to make sure that the patient is cured. Patients attending with gonorrhoea are asked if they will agree to tests for other sexually transmitted infections, such as HIV (see AIDS/HIV) and for assistance in contact tracing.

Good Medical Practice
Guidelines for doctors on the provision of good medical care laid down by the GENERAL MEDICAL COUNCIL (GMC).

Gout
A term used to describe several disorders associated with a raised concentration of URIC ACID in the blood, of which various forms of inflammatory disease and kidney disease are the most important. The condition has an overall prevalence in the UK of around 0·6 per cent.

Causes The cardinal feature of gout is the presence of an excessive amount of uric acid in PLASMA and various body tissues, and its deposition in the joints in the form of sodium monourate. The cause of this excess is not known, but there is an hereditary element and there is a family history of the disease in 50–80 per cent of cases. Inadequate exercise, habitual over-indulgence in animal food and rich dishes, and excess of alcohol have been indicated as precipitating factors, but the disease can occur in vegetarians and teetotallers.

Gout is infrequent before the age of 40, but it may occasionally affect very young people in whom there is a strong family history. About 95 per cent of patients are males. In women it most often appears during the menopause.

Symptoms An attack of gout may appear without warning, or there may be premonitory symptoms. The affected joint is swollen and the symptoms come and go, usually being worse at night. Tophi (see TOPHUS) may develop around an affected joint. Urinary CALCULI (urate-based) often occur in patients with gout.

Treatment and prevention NON-STEROIDAL ANTI-INFLAMMATORY DRUGS (NSAIDS) such as NAPROXEN should be started as soon as possible for an acute attack. After the attack subsides, a lower dose should be continued for at least a week. Salicylates (such as aspirin) and diuretics should be avoided.

In patients prone to recurrent or particularly severe attacks, long-term prophylaxis with ALLOPURINOL is indicated, especially when associated with kidney disease. This drug, which has few side-effects, lowers the serum urate concentration by preventing the formation of uric acid. A sensible weight-reducing diet is usually helpful.

GP
See GENERAL PRACTITIONER (GP).

Graft
The term applied to a piece of tissue removed from one person or animal and implanted in another, or the same, individual in order to remedy some defect. Skin grafts are commonly used, and artificial skin for grafting has recently been developed. Bone grafts are also used to replace bone which has been lost by disease: for example, a portion of rib is sometimes removed in order to furnish support for a spine weakened by disease, after removal of the damaged bone. Also, the bone of young animals is used to afford additional growth and strength to a limb-bone which it has been necessary to remove in part on account of disease or injury. Research is also underway on artifical bone. Vein grafts are used to replace stretches of arteries which have become blocked, particularly in the heart and lower limbs. The veins most commonly used for this purpose are the saphenous veins of the individual in question, provided they are healthy. An alternative is specially treated umbilical vein. (See SKIN-GRAFTING.)

When a replacement organ, such as kidney, heart or liver, is 'grafted' into someone's body, it called a 'transplant' (see TRANSPLANTATION).

Graft Versus Host Disease (GVHD)
A condition that is a common complication of BONE MARROW transplant (see TRANSPLANTATION). It results from certain LYMPHOCYTES in the transplanted marrow attacking the transplant recipient's tissues, which they identify as 'foreign'. GVHD may appear soon after a transplant or develop several months later. The condition, which is fatal in about a third of victims, may be prevented by immunosuppressant drugs such as ciclosporin.

Gram
The unit of weight in the metric system, equal to a little over 15·4 grains. For the purposes of weighing food, 30 grams are usually taken as being approximately equal to an

ounce. (See APPENDIX 6: MEASUREMENTS IN MEDICINE.)

Gram-Positive/Negative

See GRAM'S STAIN.

Gram's Stain

Bacteria can be stained with an iodine-based chemical dye called Gram's stain (after the scientist who discovered the technique). Different bacteria react differently to exposure to the stain. Broadly, the bacterial specimens are stained first with gentian violet, then with Gram's stain, and finally counterstained with a red dye after a decolorising process. Bacteria that retain the gentian stain are called gram-positive; those that lose it but absorb the red stain are called gram-negative. Some species of staphylococcus, streptococcus and clostridium are gram-positive, whereas salmonella and *Vibrio cholerae* are gram-negative.

Grand Mal

An out-of-date and now colloquial name for a tonic-clonic seizure (in contrast to petit mal) – see EPILEPSY.

Granisetron

One of several serotonin antagonists used to treat nausea and vomiting induced by CYTOTOXIC chemotherapy.

Granulations

Small masses of formative cells containing loops of newly formed blood vessels which spring up over any raw surface, as the first step in the process of healing of wounds. (See ULCER; WOUNDS.)

Granulocytes

A variety of white blood cells, also called polymorphonuclear LEUCOCYTES, which, when stained with Romanowsky stains containing thiazine dyes and eosin, are found to contain granules in their cytoplasm. The colour of the granules enables the cells to be further classified as basophils, eosinophils, and neutrophils. Neutrophils isolate and destroy invading bacteria – pus comprises mostly neutrophils. Eosinophils are also involved in the body's allergic response to foreign proteins, and basophils are involved in inflammatory and allergic reactions.

Granuloma

A non-malignant or new growth made up of granulation tissue. This is caused by various forms of chronic inflammation, such as SYPHILIS and TUBERCULOSIS.

Gravel

The name applied to any sediment which precipitates in the urine, but particularly to small crystal masses of uric acid. It produces DYSURIA and other urinary symptoms. (See URINARY BLADDER, DISEASES OF; GOUT; URINE.)

Graves' Disease

See THYROID GLAND, DISEASES OF.

Gravid

Pregnant (see PREGNANCY AND LABOUR).

Greenstick Fracture

An incomplete fracture, in which the bone is not completely broken across. It occurs in the long bones of children and is usually due to indirect force. (See BONE, DISORDERS OF – Bone fractures.)

Grey Matter

Those parts of the BRAIN and SPINAL CORD that comprise mainly the interconnected and tightly packed nuclei of neurons (nerve cells). The tissue is darker than that of the white matter, which is made of axons from the nerve cells. In the brain, grey matter is mainly found in the outer layers of the cerebrum, which is the zone responsible for advanced mental functions. The inner core of the spinal cord is made up of grey matter.

Griseofulvin

An antibiotic obtained from *Penicillium griseofulvum Diercke*, used to treat various forms of RINGWORM.

Groin

The region which includes the upper part of the front of the thigh and lower part of the abdomen. A deep groove runs obliquely across it, which corresponds to the inguinal ligament, and divides the thigh from the abdomen. The principal diseased conditions in this region are enlarged glands (see GLAND), and HERNIA.

Grommet

A small bobbin-shaped tube used to keep open the incision made in the ear drum in the treatment of secretory otitis media. It acts as a ventilation tube by allowing the Eustachian tube to recover its normal function. The operation is now less commonly performed than 20 years ago. (See EAR, DISEASES OF; EUSTACHIAN TUBES.)

Group Therapy

Psychotherapy in which at least two, but more commonly up to ten, patients, as well as the therapist, take part. The therapist encourages the patients to analyse their own and the others' emotional and psychological difficulties. Group therapy is also used to help patients sharing the same condition – for instance, alcoholism or compulsive gambling. They discuss their problems for perhaps an hour twice a week and explore ways of resolving them.

Growing Pains

Ill-defined discomfort and pains that occur in the limbs of some children. They occur mainly at night between the ages of 6–12 years. The cause is unknown, but the condition is not significant and does not require treatment once other more important conditions have been ruled out.

Growth

A popular term applied to any new formation in any part of the body. (See CANCER; CYSTS; GANGLION; TUMOUR.) For growth of children, see WEIGHT AND HEIGHT.

Growth Hormone

A product of the anterior part of the PITUITARY GLAND that promotes normal growth and development in the body by changing the chemical activity in the cells. The hormone activates protein production in the muscle cells as well as the release of energy from the metabolism of fats. Its release is controlled by the contrasting actions of growth-hormone releasing factor and somatostatin. If the body produces too much growth hormone before puberty GIGANTISM results; in adulthood the result is ACROMEGALY. Lack of growth hormone in children retards growth.

For many years growth hormone was extracted from human corpses and very rarely this caused CREUTZFELDT-JAKOB DISEASE (CJD) in the recipients. The hormone is now genetically engineered, so safe.

Guillain-Barré Syndrome

A disease of the peripheral nerves causing weakness and numbness in the limbs. It customarily occurs up to three weeks after an infection – for example, CAMPYLOBACTER infection of the gastrointestinal tract provoking an allergic response in the nerves. It may begin with weakness of the legs and gradually spread up the body. In the worst cases the patient may become totally paralysed and require to be arti-ficially ventilated. Despite this, recovery is the rule.

Guinea-Worm

See DRACONTIASIS.

Gulf War Syndrome

A collection of varying symptoms, such as persistent tiredness, headaches, muscle pain and poor concentration, reported by members of the Coalition Armed Forces who served in the 1991 Gulf War. Whilst there is strong evidence for a health effect related to service, there is no evidence of a particular set of signs and symptoms (the definition of a 'syndrome') unique to those who served in the Gulf War. Symptoms have been blamed on multiple possible hazards, such as exposure to depleted uranium munitions, smoke from oil-well fires and use of pesticides. However, the only clearly demonstrated association is with the particular pattern of vaccinations used to protect against biological weapons. Many conflicts in the past have generated their own 'syndromes', given names such as effort syndrome and shell-shock, suggesting a link to the psychological stress of being in the midst of warfare.

Gullet

Gullet, or OESOPHAGUS, is the tube down which food passes from the throat to the stomach.

Gum

(*a*) The soft tissue surrounding the TEETH. Also called the gingiva, this tissue protects underlying structures and helps to keep the teeth tightly in the jawbones. Inflammation of the gum is called gingivitis and may be due to dental PLAQUE or to systemic disorders such as LEUKAEMIA and SCURVY.

(*b*) A complex viscid substance which exudes from the stems and branches of various trees, and consists principally of arabin or bassorin. The two best-known gums are gum acacia and gum tragacanth. Gum-resins such as asafoetida, galbanum and myrrh also contain resin.

Gumboil

A painful condition of inflammation, ending sometimes as an ABSCESS, situated in the gum about the root of a carious tooth (see TEETH, DISORDERS OF – Caries of the teeth).

Gumma

A hard swelling, or GRANULOMA, characteristic of tertiary SYPHILIS. It normally develops in the skin or subcutaneous tissue, mucous membranes or submucosa, and the long bones. Although often painless, it may produce marked symptoms by interfering with the brain or other internal organs in which it may be located. Treatment with penicillin (or tetracycline if the patient is allergic) usually ensures a rapid disappearance of the gumma.

Gums, Diseases of
See MOUTH, DISEASES OF; TEETH, DISEASES OF.

GVHD
See GRAFT VERSUS HOST DISEASE (GVHD).

Gynaecology
The branch of medicine dealing with the female pelvic and urogenital organs, in both the normal and diseased states. It encompasses aspects of CONTRACEPTION, ABORTION, and *in vitro* fertilisation or IVF (see under ASSISTED CONCEPTION). Covering the full age range, it is closely related to OBSTETRICS, while involving aspects of both surgery and psychiatry.

Gynaecomastia
An abnormal increase in size of the male breast.

Gypsum
Plaster of Paris used to stabilise and externally splint fractured bones. It is applied wet and moulded to the appropriate shape to immobilise the broken bone (see BONE, DISORDERS OF – Bone fractures.)

Gyrus
Gyrus is the term applied to a convolution of the BRAIN.

H2 Receptor Antagonists

These are drugs that block the action of HISTAMINE at the H_2 receptor (which mediates the gastric and some of the cardiovascular effects of histamine). By reducing the production of acid by the stomach, these drugs – chiefly cimetidine, ranitidine, famotidine and nizatidine – are valuable in the treatment of peptic ulcers (healing when used in high dose; preventing relapse when used as maintenance therapy in reduced dose), reflux oesophagitis (see OESOPHAGUS, DISEASES OF), and the ZOLLINGER-ELLISON SYNDROME. These drugs are now being supplanted by PROTON-PUMP INHIBITORS and HELICOBACTER PYLORI eradication therapy. (See also DUODENAL ULCER.)

Habit

A behavioural response or practice that is established by the individual frequently repeating the same act. The process is called habituation, and the more a person is exposed to a particular stimulus, the less is he or she aroused by it. People may also become habituated to certain drugs, requiring more and more of a substance to produce the same effect – a process known as TOLERANCE.

Habituation

See HABIT.

Haem

An iron-containing porphyrin (see PORPHYRINS) compound that combines with the protein GLOBULIN to make HAEMOGLOBIN, a constituent of erythrocytes (red blood cells).

Haemangioma

These can be acquired or congenital. The acquired type presents as a red PAPULE which bleeds easily; treatment is normally by cautery. A 'strawberry NAEVUS' is a 'capillary-cavernous' haemangioma appearing at or soon after birth, which may grow to a large size. Treatment is not usually required, as most of them fade – although this may take a few years. Where a haemangioma is disfiguring or interfering with vision or breathing, treatment is necessary: this may be by laser, by using CORTICOSTEROIDS or INTERFERON treatment, or by surgery.

Haemarthrosis

Haemarthrosis is the process of bleeding into, or the presence of blood in, a joint. It may occur as a result of major trauma (for example, fracture of the patella may lead to bleeding into the knee-joint), or, more commonly, following minor trauma. It may even occur spontaneously, in cases of HAEMOPHILIA or other disorders of blood clotting. If repeated several times, haemarthrosis may lead to FIBROSIS of the joint-lining and inflammation of the cartilage, causing marked stiffness and deformity.

Haematemesis

Haematemesis means the vomiting of blood. Blood brought up from the stomach is generally dark in colour and may have been so far digested as to form small brown granules resembling coffee grounds. Vomiting of blood is one of the main symptoms of PEPTIC ULCER, but it may occur in GASTRITIS, from VARICOCOELES in the OESOPHAGUS, or, rarely, in cancer of the stomach. Gastritis caused by an irritant poison, sustained intake of ALCOHOL, or the regular use of certain drugs such as ASPIRIN and NON-STEROIDAL ANTI-INFLAMMATORY DRUGS (NSAIDS) may cause bleeding. Blood may also originate from the nose and throat, be swallowed and then vomited. Persistent haematemesis or a sudden severe bleed is a potentially serious medical emergency and the patient should be referred urgently to hospital (see HAEMORRHAGE).

Haematinic

A drug that raises the quantity of HAEMOGLOBIN in the blood. Ferrous sulphate is a common example of iron-containing compounds given to anaemic (see ANAEMIA) patients whose condition is due to iron deficiency. Traditionally, haematinics have been used to prevent anaemia in pregnant women, but nowadays a maternal diet containing iron-rich foods and regular antenatal checks of haemoglobin concentrations in the blood should make the routine use of haematinics unnecessary.

Haematocoele

A cavity containing blood. Generally as the result of an injury which ruptures blood vessels, blood is effused into one of the natural cavities of the body, or among loose cellular tissue, producing a haematocoele.

Haematocolpos

The condition in which menstrual blood cannot drain from the VAGINA because of an imperforate HYMEN.

Haematocrit

Also known as packed cell volume, this is an expression of the fraction of blood volume occupied by the ERYTHROCYTES. It is determined by centrifuging a sample of blood in a capillary tube and measuring the height of the resulting packed cells as a percentage of the total sample height.

Normal values:
males 42–53 per cent or 0.42–0.53 mL/dL
females 32–48 per cent or 0.36–0.48 mL/dL

Haematogenous

An adjective applied to a biological process which produces blood, or to an agent produced in or coming from blood. For example, a haematogenous infection is one resulting from contact with blood that contains a virus or bacterium responsible for the infection.

Haematologist

A doctor or scientist who specialises in the study and treatment of blood and blood disorders.

Haematology

The study of diseases of the blood.

Haematoma

Haematoma means a collection of blood forming a definite swelling. It is found often upon the head of newborn children after a protracted and difficult labour (cephalhaematoma). It may occur as the result of any injury or operation.

Haematuria

Blood in the URINE. The blood may come from any part of the urinary tract. When the blood comes from the kidney or upper part of the urinary tract, it is usually mixed throughout the urine, giving the latter a brownish or smoky tinge. This condition is usually the result of glomerulonephritis, or it may be present in persons suffering from high blood pressure or PYELITIS. Blood may also appear in the urine when a stone or gravel is present in the pelvis of the kidney setting up irritation, especially after exercise. The blood may also originate from a bladder that is inflamed or infected or which contains benign growths (papilloma) or malignant growths. Inflammation or injury to the URETHRA can also cause haematuria. Someone with haematuria should seek medical advice. (See also KIDNEYS, DISEASES OF.)

Haemic Murmur

Unusual sounds heard over the heart and large blood vessels in severe cases of ANAEMIA. They disappear as the condition improves.

Haemochromatosis

A disease in which cirrhosis of the liver (see LIVER, DISEASES OF), enlargement of the SPLEEN, pigmentation of the skin, and DIABETES MELLITUS are associated with the abnormal and excessive deposit in the organs of the body of the iron-containing pigment, haemosiderin. It is caused by an increase in the amount of iron absorbed from the gastrointestinal tract.

Haemodialysis

A method of removing waste products or poisons from the circulating blood using the principle of DIALYSIS. The procedure is used on patients with malfunctioning or nonfunctioning KIDNEYS. It is done using an artificial kidney or dialyser which restores blood to its normal state. The process has to be repeated, sometimes for many months, until a donor kidney is available for transplantation to replace the patient's failing one.

Haemofiltration

A technique similar to HAEMODIALYSIS. Blood is dialysed using ultrafiltration through a membrane permeable to water and small molecules (molecular weight <12,000). Physiological saline solution is simultaneously reinfused.

Haemoglobin

The colouring compound which produces the red colour of blood. Haemoglobin is a chromoprotein, made up of a protein called globin and the iron-containing pigment, haemin. When separated from the red blood corpuscles – each of which contains about 600 million haemoglobin molecules – it is crystalline in form.

Haemoglobin exists in two forms: simple haemoglobin, found in venous blood; and oxyhaemoglobin, which is a loose compound with oxygen, found in arterial blood after the blood has come into contact with the air in the lungs. This oxyhaemoglobin is again broken down as the blood passes through the tissues, which take up the oxygen for their own use. This is the main function of haemoglobin: to act as a carrier of oxygen from the lungs to all the tissues of the body. When the haemoglobin leaves the lungs, it is 97 per cent saturated with oxygen; when it comes back to the lungs in the venous blood, it is 70 per cent saturated. The oxygen content of 100 millilitres of blood leaving the lungs is 19·5 millilitres, and that of venous blood returning to the lungs, 14·5 millilitres. Thus, each 100 millilitres of blood delivers 5 millilitres of oxygen to the tissues of the body. Human male blood contains 13–18 grams of haemoglobin per 100 millilitres; in women, there are 12–16 grams per 100 millilitres. A man weighing 70 kilograms (154 pounds) has around 770 grams of haemoglobin circulating in his red blood corpuscles.

Haemoglobinopathies

Abnormal HAEMOGLOBIN formation occurs in the haemoglobinopathies, which are hereditary haemolytic anaemias, genetically determined and related to race. The haemoglobin may be abnormal because: (1) there is a defect in the synthesis of normal adult haemoglobin as in THALASSAEMIA, when there may be an absence of one or both of the polypeptide chains characteristic of normal adult haemoglobin; or (2) there is an abnormal form of haemoglobin such as haemoglobin S which results in sickle-cell disease (see ANAEMIA). This abnormality may involve as little as one amino acid of the 300 in the haemoglobin molecule. In sickle-cell haemoglobin, one single amino-acid molecule – that of glutamic acid – is replaced by another – that of valine; this results in such a deficient end product that the ensuing disease is frequently severe.

Haemoglobinuria

The presence of blood pigment in the URINE caused by the destruction of blood corpuscles in the blood vessels or in the urinary passages. It turns urine a dark red or brown colour. In some people this condition, known as intermittent haemoglobinuria, occurs from time to time, especially on exposure to cold. It is also produced by various poisonous substances taken in the food. It occurs in malarious districts in the form of one of the most fatal forms of MALARIA: BLACKWATER FEVER. (See also MARCH HAEMOGLOBINURIA.)

Haemolysis

The destruction of red blood corpuscles by the action of poisonous substances, usually of a protein nature, circulating in the blood, or by certain chemicals. It occurs, for example, gradually in some forms of ANAEMIA and rapidly in poisoning by snake venom.

Haemolytic Disease of the Newborn

A potentially serious disease of the newborn, characterised by haemolytic ANAEMIA (excessive destruction of red blood cells) and JAUNDICE. If severe, it may be obvious before birth because the baby becomes very oedematous (see OEDEMA) and develops heart failure – so-called hydrops fetalis. It may first present on the first day of life as jaundice and anaemia. The disease

is due to blood-group incompatibility between the mother and baby, the commoneset being rhesus incompatibility (see BLOOD GROUPS). In this condition a rhesus-negative mother has been previously sensitised to produce rhesus antibodies, either by the delivery of a rhesus-positive baby, a miscarriage or a mismatched blood transfusion. These antibodies cross over into the fetal circulation and attack red blood cells which cause HAEMOLYSIS.

Treatment In severely affected fetuses, a fetal blood transfusion may be required and/or the baby may be delivered early for further treatment. Mild cases may need observation only, or the reduction of jaundice by phototherapy alone (treatment with light, involving the use of sunlight, non-visible ULTRAVIOLET light, visible blue light, or LASER).

Whatever the case, the infant's serum BILIRUBIN – the bilirubin present in the blood – and its HAEMOGLOBIN concentration are plotted regularly so that treatment can be given before levels likely to cause brain damage occur. Safe bilirubin concentrations depend on the maturity and age of the baby, so reference charts are used.

High bilirubin concentrations may be treated with phototherapy; extra fluid is given to prevent dehydration and to improve bilirubin excretion by shortening the gut transit time. Severe jaundice and anaemia may require exchange TRANSFUSION by removing the baby's blood (usually 10 millilitres at a time) and replacing it with rhesus-negative fresh bank blood. Haemolytic disease of the newborn secondary to rhesus incompatibility has become less common since the introduction of anti-D (Rho) immunoglobulin. This antibody should be given to all rhesus-negative women at any risk of a fetomaternal transfusion, to prevent them from mounting an antibody response. Anti-D is given routinely to rhesus-negative mothers after the birth of a rhesus-positive baby, but doctors should also give it after threatened abortions, antepartum haemorrhages, miscarriages, and terminations of pregnancy.

Occasionally haemolytic disease is caused by ABO incompatibility or that of rarer blood groups.

Haemolytic Uraemic Syndrome

A disease of children resulting in acute RENAL failure. A febrile illness of the gastrointestinal or respiratory tracts is followed by intravascular COAGULATION of blood which results in HAEMOLYSIS, ANAEMIA, THROMBOCYTOPAENIA and renal failure (resulting from fibrin deposition in renal arterioles and glomerular capillaries).

The death rate is 2–10 per cent and the majority of patients survive without renal failure. The longer the period of OLIGURIA, the greater the risk of chronic renal failure.

Treatment is supportive, with replacement of blood and clotting factors, control of HYPERTENSION, and careful observation of fluid balance.

Haemopericardium
The presence of blood in the PERICARDIUM, the membranous sac which surrounds the heart. The condition may result from a myocardial infarction (see HEART, DISEASES OF), leaking ANEURYSM, injury, or tumour. Because the pericardial blood compresses the heart, the latter's pumping action is impeded, reducing the blood pressure and causing cardiac failure. Urgent surgical drainage of the blood may be required.

Haemophilia
An inherited disorder of blood COAGULATION which results in prolonged bleeding even after minor injury. There is a deficiency of factor VIII, an essential clotting factor in the coagulation cascade – the complex series of biochemical events that leads from injury of the wall of a blood vessel to the formation of a blood clot that checks bleeding. Haemophilia is a sex-linked recessive disorder (though a small number of cases arise by spontaneous mutation), so that, if females carry the disease, one-half of their sons will be affected and one-half of their daughters will be carriers. The sons of haemophiliacs are unaffected but one-half of their daughters will be carriers.

Haemophilia affects approximately 1:4,000 of the UK population but only 1:20,000 is severely affected. Severity of the disease depends upon the percentage, compared with normal, of factor VIII activity present. Less than 1 per cent and there will be spontaneous bleeding into joints and muscles; 1–5 per cent and there will be occasional spontaneous bleeding and severe bleeding after minor injury; 5–25 per cent and there will only be severe bleeding after major injury. Before treatment was available, severe haemophiliacs suffered from acute pain and deformity from bleeds into joints and muscles. Bleeding also occurred into the gut, kidneys and brain, and few survived past adolescence.

Freeze-dried factor VIII may be kept in domestic refrigerators. Haemophiliacs can use it to abort minor bleeds by reconstituting it and injecting it intravenously. More major bleeding or preparation for surgery involves raising factor VIII levels to 30–100 per cent by giving cryoprecipitate.

With treatment, most haemophiliacs lead normal lives, although obviously dangerous or contact sports should be avoided. Before donors of blood were screened for HEPATITIS B and C or for HIV infection (see AIDS/HIV), some individuals with haemophilia receiving factor VIII were unwittingly infected with those diseases. Today's screening procedures make such infections very unlikely.

There is a National Haemophilia Register and each registered sufferer carries a card with details about his or her condition. Information may also be obtained from NHS haemophilia centres and the Haemophilia Society.

Haemophilus
Gram-negative (see GRAM'S STAIN), rod-like, aerobic, non-sporing and non-motile parasitic bacteria. Mostly found in the respiratory tract, they may be part of the normal flora, but may also be responsible for several diseases. The main pathogenic species of haemophilus is *H. influenzae*, which may cause severe exacerbations of chronic BRONCHITIS, as well as MENINGITIS, EPIGLOTTITIS, SINUSITIS, and otitis media (see EAR, DISEASES OF). Other species may cause conjunctivitis (see EYE, DISORDERS OF) or CHANCROID. Haemophilus species are sensitive to a wide range of antibiotics, though generally resistant to penicillin. Infants are routinely immunised with Haemophilus B vaccine to prevent meningitis, septicaemia and epiglottitis – all potentially fatal disesases.

Haemopoietic Stem Cell
This is the basic cell from which all types of blood cells originate. Its appearance is believed to be similar to that of a LYMPHOCYTE.

Haemopoiesis
The formation of blood cells and PLATELETS – a continuous process throughout life. As ageing cells are removed from the circulation, new ones, generated in the BONE MARROW, replace them.

Haemoptysis
The coughing-up of blood from the lungs. The blood is usually bright red and frothy, thus distinguishing it from blood brought up from the stomach. It is a potentially serious sign of lung disease, although in elderly people haemoptysis may be due to a varicose condition of the small veins in the throat. In young people this condition is often due to bleeding from the nose, in which, owing to the position of the head, the

blood happens to run backwards instead of forwards through the nostrils. (See also HAEMORRHAGE; TUBERCULOSIS.)

Haemorrhage

The escape of blood from any of the blood vessels, normally in response to some trauma, or as a result of a clotting disorder such as HAEMOPHILIA. The bleeding may be external – for example, following a skin laceration; or it may be internal – for example, haematemesis (bleeding into the stomach), haemoptysis (bleeding from the lungs), or haematuria (bleeding from the kidneys or urinary tract). For more information about these conditions, see separate entries.

Bleeding into or around the brain is a major concern following serious head injuries, or in newborn infants following a difficult labour. Haemorrhage is classified as arterial – the most serious type, in which the blood is bright red and appears in spurts (in severe cases the patient may bleed to death within a few minutes); venous – less serious (unless from torn varicose veins) and easily checked, in which the blood is dark and wells up gradually into the wound; and capillary, in which the blood slowly oozes out of the surface of the wound and soon stops spontaneously. Haemorrhage is also classified as primary, reactionary, and secondary (see WOUNDS). Severe haemorrhage causes SHOCK and ANAEMIA, and blood TRANSFUSION is often required.

When a small artery is cut across, the bleeding stops in consequence of changes in the wall of the artery on the one hand, and in the constitution of the blood on the other. Every artery is surrounded by a fibrous sheath, and when cut, the vessel retracts some little distance within this sheath and a blood clot forms, blocking the open end (see COAGULATION). When a major blood vessel is torn, such spontaneous closure may be impossible and surgery is required to stop the bleeding.

Three main principles are applicable in the control of a severe external haemorrhage: (*a*) direct pressure on the bleeding point or points; (*b*) elevation of the wounded part; (*c*) pressure on the main artery of supply to the part.

Control of internal haemorrhage is more difficult than that of external bleeding. First-aid measures should be taken while professional help is sought. The patient should be laid down with legs raised, and he or she should be reassured and kept warm. The mouth may be kept moist but no fluids should be given. (See APPENDIX 1: BASIC FIRST AID.)

Haemorrhoids

Haemorrhoids, or piles, are varicose (swollen) veins in the lining of the ANUS. They are very common, affecting nearly half of the UK population at some time in their lives, with men having them more often and for a longer time.

Varieties Haemorrhoids are classified into first-, second- and third-degree, depending on how far they prolapse through the anal canal. First-degree ones do not protrude; second-degree piles protrude during defaecation; third-degree ones are trapped outside the anal margin, although they can be pushed back. Most haemorrhoids can be described as internal, since they are covered with glandular mucosa, but some large, long-term ones develop a covering of skin. Piles are usually found at the three, seven and eleven o'clock sites when viewed with the patient on his or her back.

Causes The veins in the anus tend to become distended because they have no valves; because they form the lowest part of the PORTAL SYSTEM and are apt to become overfilled when there is the least interference with the circulation through the portal vein; and partly because the muscular arrangements for keeping the rectum closed interfere with the circulation through the haemorrhoidal veins. An absence of fibre from western diets is probably the most important cause. The result is that people often strain to defaecate hard stools, thus raising intra-abdominal pressure which slows the rate of venous return and engorges the network of veins in the anal mucosa. Pregnancy is an important contributory factor in women developing haemorrhoids. In some people, haemorrhoids are a symptom of disease higher up in the portal system, causing interference with the circulation. They are common in heart disease, liver complaints such as cirrhosis or congestion, and any disease affecting the bowels.

Symptoms Piles cause itching, pain and often bleeding, which may occur whenever the patient defaecates or only sometimes. The piles may prolapse permanently or intermittently. The patient may complain of aching discomfort which, with the pain, may be worsened.

Treatment Prevention is important; a high-fibre diet will help in this, and is also necessary after piles have developed. Patients should not spend a long time straining on the lavatory. Itching can be lessened if the PERINEUM is properly washed, dried and powdered. Prolapsed piles can be replaced with the finger. Local anaesthetic and steroid ointments can help to relieve symptoms when they are relatively mild, but do not remedy the underlying disorder. If conservative measures fail, then surgery may be required. Piles may be injected, stretched or excised according to the patient's particular circumstances.

Where haemorrhoids are secondary to another disorder, such as cancer of the rectum or colon, the underlying condition must be treated – hence the importance of medical advice if piles persist.

Haemosiderosis
An increase in the amount of iron stored in the body. Rarely, it may be due to ingestion of too much iron, but a more likely cause is repeated blood transfusions. The extra iron may affect the function of the heart and liver.

Haemostasis
The process by which bleeding stops. It involves constriction of blood vessels, the formation of a platelet plug, and blood clotting. The term is also used for surgical interventions to stop bleeding – for example, the use of diathermy. (See COAGULATION; HAEMORRHAGE.)

Haemostatics
A group of drugs used to treat bleeding disorders such as HAEMOPHILIA. Factor VIII is one of the clotting factors available for treatment: preparations of it are injected after abnormal bleeding or before surgery. Vitamin K preparations are another haemostatic group used to treat an overdose of ANTICOAGULANTS.

Haemostatic preparations of gelatine and cellulose are used to stem bleeding from the skin and gums, or as a result of tooth extractions.

Haemothorax
An effusion of blood into the PLEURAL CAVITY.

Hair, Removal of
See DEPILATION.

Hair
See SKIN; WHITE HAIR.

Half Life
The time taken for the PLASMA concentration of an administered drug to decline by half as a result of redistribution, METABOLISM and EXCRETION.

Halfway House
A residential home for mentally ill individuals where they can live under supervision after discharge from hospital. They may be fit to work but cannot manage an independent life.

Halibut-Liver Oil
The oil expressed from fresh, or suitably preserved, halibut liver. It is a particularly rich source of vitamin A (30,000 international units per gram), and also contains vitamin D (2,300–2,500 units per gram). It is available in capsules as a means of providing the two vitamins. (See APPENDIX 5: VITAMINS.)

Halitosis
Bad breath. This may be a sign of illness – for example, lung disease or SINUSITIS; and a person with DIABETES MELLITUS may have breath tainted with acetone if his or her sugar metabolism is poorly controlled. Usually, however, halitosis is caused by smoking, drinking alcohol, eating certain foods (garlic or onions), or inadequate oral and dental hygiene.

Hallucinations
False perceptions arising without an adequate external stimulus, as opposed to illusions, which are misinterpretations of stimuli arising from an external object. Hallucinations come from 'within', although the affected individual may see them as coming from 'without'. Nevertheless, they may occur at the same time as real perceptions, and may affect any sense (vision, hearing, smell, taste, touch, etc.).

Causes They may be the result of intense emotion or suggestion, sensory deprivation (for example, overwork or lack of sleep), disorders of sense organs, or disorders of the central nervous system. Although hallucinations may occur in perfectly sane people, they are more commonly an indication of a MENTAL ILLNESS. They may be deliberately induced by the use of HALLUCINOGENS.

Hallucinogens
Compounds characterised by their ability to produce distortions of perception, emotional changes, depersonalisation, and a variety of effects on memory and learned behaviour. They include CANNABIS, LYSERGIC ACID DIETHYLAMIDE (LSD) and MESCALINE. (See also DEPENDENCE.)

Hallux
The anatomical name of the great toe.

Hallux Rigidus
Stiffness of the joint between the great toe and the foot, which induces pain on walking. It is usually due to a crush injury or stubbing of the toe. Such stubbing is liable to occur in adolescents with a congenitally long toe. If trouble-

some, the condition is treated by an operation to create a false joint.

Hallux Valgus

Outward displacement of the great toe – always associated with a bunion (see CORNS AND BUN-IONS). It is due to the pressure of footwear on an unduly broad foot. In adolescents, this broad foot is inherited; in adults it is due to splaying of the foot as a result of loss of muscle tone. The bunion is produced by pressure of the footwear on the protruding base of the toe. In mild cases the wearing of comfortable shoes may be all that is needed. In more severe cases the bunion may need to be removed, while in the most severe the operation of ARTHROPLASTY may be needed.

Halo

A coloured circle seen around a bright light in some eye conditions. When accompanied by headache, it is especially likely to be caused by GLAUCOMA.

Haloperidol

One of the butyrophenone group of drugs used to treat patients with psychoses (see PSYCHOSIS). Its action is similar to that of the PHENOTHI-AZINES. It is also used in depot form, being administered by deep intramuscular injection for maintenance control of SCHIZOPHRENIA and other psychoses. The drug may help to control tics and intractable hiccups.

Halothane

A volatile liquid anaesthetic, used for many years as a potent inhalant anaesthetic. It provides smooth induction of ANAESTHESIA and is non-irritant and pleasant to inhale. A few patients have an idiosyncracy to halothane, putting them at risk if it is used frequently, so a careful history is essential before it is administered to a patient (see HALOTHANE HEPATITIS).

Halothane Hepatitis

A very rare form of HEPATITIS following exposure to HALOTHANE during anaesthesia (1:35,000 halothane anaesthetics). Jaundice develops three to four days after exposure and will occasionally develop into a fatal massive hepatic necrosis. It is of unknown aetiology but probably has an immunological basis. It is more common following multiple exposures in a short time (less than 28 days), and in obesity, middle age and females. It is rare in children.

Hamartoma

These are benign tumours, usually in the lung, containing normal components of pulmonary tissue such as smooth muscle and connective tissue.

Hamate

One of the carpal bones of the HAND that articulate between the METATARSAL BONES and the RADIUS and ulnar bones of the forearm.

Hammer-Toe

The deformity in which there is permanent flexion, or bending, of the middle joint of the toe. The condition may affect all the toes, as in CLAW-FOOT; more commonly it affects one toe, usually the second. It is due to a relatively long toe and the pressure on it of the footwear. A painful bunion usually develops on it (see CORNS AND BUNIONS). In mild cases, relief is obtained by protecting the toe with adhesive pads. If this does not suffice then an operation is necessary.

Hamstrings

The name given to the tendons at the back of the knee – two on the inner side and one on the outer side – which bend this joint. They are attached to the tibia below. Strains, or 'pulls', and tears of the hamstring are common in people taking part in strenuous sports such as athletics, football, rugby and tennis (see SPORTS MEDICINE).

Hand

In structure, the hand has a bony basis of eight small carpal bones in the wrist, five metacarpal bones in the fleshy part of the hand, and three phalanges in each finger – two only in the thumb. From the muscles of the forearm, 12 strong tendons run in front of the wrist. Of these, nine go to the fingers and thumb and are bound down by a strong band, the flexor retinaculum, in front of the wrist. They are enclosed in a complicated synovial sheath, and pass through the palm and down the fingers. Behind the wrist, 12 tendons likewise cross from forearm to hand.

Forming the ball of the thumb and that of the little finger, and filling up the gaps between the metacarpal bones, are other muscles, which act to separate and bring together the fingers, and to bend them at their first joints (knuckles).

Hand, Foot and Mouth Disease

A contagious disease due to infection with coxsackie A16 virus (see COXSACKIE VIRUSES). Most common in children, the incubation period is 3–5 days. It is characterised by an eruption of blisters on the palms and the feet (often the toes), and in the mouth. The disease

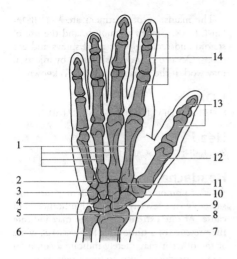

1 metatarsal bones of the finger
2 hamate (c)
3 pisiform (c)
4 triquetrum (c)
5 lunate (c)
6 ulna
7 radius
8 capitate (c)
9 scaphoid (c)
10 trapezium (c)
11 trapezoid (c)
12 metatarsal bone of the thumb
13 phalanges of the thumb
14 phalanges of the index finger

The bones of the right hand and wrist (anterior view). Bones marked '(c)' form the carpal group of bones.

has no connection with foot and mouth disease in cattle, deer, pigs and sheep.

Handicap
The inability to carry out a social, occupational or other activity that could normally be done by a person without such a handicap. The handicap may be partial or complete, physical or mental, and may result from disease, injury or inherited disorder. The extent of the handicap is measured against the normal function of those in a peer group. The impairment may be functionally rather than physically based, in which case the affected person may not always be aware of it until revealed by a clinical examination. Considerable government and voluntary community efforts have been made to lessen the day-to-day difficulties of living faced by disabled people. Increasingly, public buildings, houses and vehicles are being modified to ensure that these are user-friendly to such individuals. The health and social-work professions also contribute to reducing the impact of handicaps on the affected individuals.

Hanging
Hanging is a form of death due to suspension of the body from the neck – either suddenly, as in judicial hanging (although not in the United Kingdom, as the death penalty is not used in the UK justice system), so as to damage the spinal column and cord, or in such a way as to constrict the AIR PASSAGES and the blood vessels to the brain. Death is, in any case, speedy, resulting in 2–3 minutes if not instantaneously. Apart from judicial hanging, and in the absence of any signs of a struggle, hanging is usually due to SUICIDE. The resuscitation of people found hanging is similar to that for drowning. (See APPENDIX 1: BASIC FIRST AID – Cardiac/respiratory arrest.)

Hang-Nail
A splitting of the skin (cuticle) at the side of a fingernail. In manual workers it is usually caused by trauma, but ISCHAEMIA of the fingers (see also RAYNAUD'S DISEASE) may predispose to the condition. Secondary infection and inflammation may make hang-nail a very tender condition; treatment consists of reducing trauma, and the use of EMOLLIENTS and ANTIBIOTICS if necessary.

Hansen's Disease
See LEPROSY.

Hantavirus
A group of viruses that infect mice, rats and voles and can also infect humans who come into contact with the excreta or secretions of these animals. Widely distributed in Asia, the USA and Europe, in Britain hantavirus usually affects rural and sewage workers, as well as people engaged in watersports. Many victims have a mild feverish illness; severe cases are characterised by headache, high temperature, nausea, vomiting and even shock, accompanied by skin PETECHIAE. The kidneys and sometimes the lungs are affected, and in severely affected patients mortality is high.

Haploid
An adjective describing organisms, cells or nuclei that have a single set of unpaired CHROMOSOMES. Human beings have haploid gametes (see GAMETE) following MEIOSIS.

Hapten
See ANTIGEN.

Hard Water

The term applied to water that contains a large amount of calcium and magnesium salts (lime salts). These form an insoluble curd with soap and thus interfere with the use of the water for washing. Hard water is especially found in districts where the soil is chalky. Temporary hardness, which is due mainly to the presence of bicarbonates of lime, can be remedied by boiling, when the lime is precipitated as carbonate of lime. Permanent hardness is not remedied by boiling, and is due to the presence of a large amount of sulphate of lime. It may be removed by the addition of sodium carbonate (washing soda) or by the Permutit process which involves the use of various combinations of silicate of alumina and soda. In the past, hard water was often blamed for many ills – without any convincing evidence. Epidemiologists suggest that drinking soft water may lead to a greater risk of heart disease.

Hare-Lip

See PALATE, MALFORMATIONS OF.

Hartmann's Solution

A solution commonly used as a means of fluid replacement in dehydrated patients (see also DEHYDRATION). Each litre contains 3·1 grams of sodium lactate, 6 grams of sodium chloride, 0·4 grams of potassium chloride, and 0·7 grams of calcium chloride.

Hashimoto's Disease

A condition in which the whole of the THYROID GLAND is diffusely enlarged and firm. It is one of the diseases produced by AUTOIMMUNITY. The enlargement is due to diffuse infiltration of lymphocytes and increase of fibrous tissue. This form of GOITRE appears in middle-aged women, does not give rise to symptoms of thyrotoxicosis (see THYROID GLAND, DISEASES OF – Thyrotoxicosis), and tends to produce myxoedema (see THYROID GLAND, DISEASES OF – Hypothyroidism).

Haversian Canals

The fine canals in BONE which carry the blood vessels, lymphatics and nerves necessary for the maintenance and repair of bone.

Hay Fever

Also known as allergic rhinitis, this is caused by an ALLERGY to the pollen of grasses, trees and other plants. Contact with the particular pollen to which the sufferer is allergic causes HISTAMINE release, resulting in a blocked, runny nose and itchy, watering eyes. It affects approximately 3 million people each year in the UK.

The mainstays of treatment are ANTIHISTAMINE DRUGS, taken by mouth, and the use of steroid and cromoglycate nasal sprays and eye drops. Occasionally desensitisation by injection may work if the particular allergen is known.

HDA

See HEALTH DEVELOPMENT AGENCY (HDA).

Head

See BRAIN; FACE; SCALP; SKULL.

Headache

A very common condition which may vary considerably in severity, type, significance and cause. At one extreme, headache may indicate the presence of a tumour or MENINGITIS, while at the other it may merely indicate a common cold or tiredness. Even so, persistent or recurrent headaches should always be taken seriously. Although the brain itself is insensitive to pain, the surrounding membranes – meninges – are very sensitive, and changes in intracranial arteries, or spasm of the neck or scalp muscles, which may occur for various reasons, may cause considerable pain. In most cases a clinical diagnosis should be possible; further investigations should only be necessary following head injury, if headaches recur, or if neurological signs such as drowsiness, vomiting, confusion, seizures or focal signs develop.

Stress and anxiety are probably the most common causes of headache and, where possible, the reasons – overwork, family problems, unemployment, financial difficulties, etc. – should be tackled. An unpleasant environment such as traffic pollution or badly ventilated or overcrowded working conditions may provoke headaches in some people, as may excessive smoking or caffeine intake. MIGRAINE is a characteristic and often disabling type of headache; high blood pressure may cause the condition (see HYPERTENSION); and, occasionally, refractive errors of the eyes (see EYE, DISORDERS OF) are associated with headaches. SINUS infections are often characterised by frontal headaches. Rheumatism in the muscles of the neck and scalp produce headaches; fever is commonly accompanied by a headache; and sunstroke and HEAT STROKE customarily result in headaches. Finally, diseases in the brain such as meningitis, tumours and HAEMORRHAGE may first manifest themselves as persistent or recurrent headaches.

Treatment Obtaining a reliable diagnosis – with the help of further investigations, including CT (see COMPUTED TOMOGRAPHY) or MRI scanning when indicated – should always be the initial aim; treatment in most cases should then be aimed at the underlying condition. Particular concerns include headache that worsens at night or in the early morning; ever-increasing headaches; those associated with abnormal neurological signs on examination; or those associated with fits (see FIT).

Whether the cause is physical or stress-induced, used sensibly and for a limited period a low dose of aspirin or paracetamol may be helpful. In many cases of stress-induced headache, however, the most effective treatment is relaxation. There are many specific treatments for migraine and hypertension. Sinusitis is treated with antibiotics and sometimes by surgery.

Head Injury

Any injury to the head, whether associated with a skull fracture (see BONE, DISORDERS OF – Bone fractures) or not. Patients with head injuries should be assessed for signs of neurological damage, which may not develop at once. Patients who after a head injury are or have been UNCONSCIOUS or who are drowsy, vomiting, confused or have any focal neurological signs – for example, blurred vision or a motor or sensory malfunction – should be seen by a doctor. Particular care should be taken with individuals who have consumed alcohol and sustained a head injury in a fight, fall or vehicle accident. Symptoms indicative of a severe head injury may be attributed (wrongly) to the effects of alcohol, and crucial time thus lost in treating the injury.

In hospital the possible need for urgent action is monitored by use of the GLASGOW COMA SCALE.

People suffering the results of such injuries and their relatives can obtain help and advice from Headway – the brain injury association.

Heaf Test

A skin test to find out if a person is immune to TUBERCULOSIS. TUBERCULIN (a preparation derived from the TUBERCLE bacillus) is injected via punctures in the skin of the forearm, using a spring-loaded gunlike instrument with six very short needles set in circular form. A positive test is indicated by a red raised reaction of the skin: this means that the subject is immune. If the result is negative, the subject can be given BCG VACCINE.

Healing

See WOUNDS.

Health

The state of health implies much more than freedom from disease, and good health may be defined as the attainment and maintenance of the highest state of mental and bodily vigour of which any given individual is capable. Environment, including living and working conditions, plays an important part in determining a person's health. The UK government is now placing much greater emphasis on health promotion and the prevention of disease, and has published national targets for reducing the incidence of some major diseases. The 1978 World Health Organisation statement declares that primary care should 'be made universally accessible to individuals and families in the community, by means acceptable to them, through their full participation, and at the cost that the community and country can afford to maintain in the spirit of self-reliance . . . [and] addresses the main health problems in the community, providing promotive, preventative, curative and rehabilitative services accordingly'. Factors affecting access to health include finance, ideology, and education. (See ENVIRONMENT AND HEALTH; PUBLIC HEALTH.)

Health and Safety Executive (HSE)

The statutory body in Britain responsible for the health and safety of workers. The address of the HSE can be found in APPENDIX 7: STATUTORY ORGANISATIONS.

Health-Care Priorities

As the needs and demands of patients, and the costs of health care of populations, have risen sharply in recent years, governments and health-care providers – whether tax-funded, insurance-based, employer-provided or a mix of these – have had increasingly to face the dilemma of what services a country or a community can afford to provide. As a result, various techniques for deciding priorities of care and treatment are evolving. In the United Kingdom, priorities were for many years based on the decisions of individual clinicians who had wide freedom to prescribe the most appropriate care. Increasingly, this clinical freedom is being circumscribed by managerial, community and political decisions driven in part by the availability of resources and by what people want. Rationing services, however, is not popular and as yet no broadly agreed consensus has emerged, either in western Europe or in North America, as to how priorities can be decided that have broad community support and which can be afforded. (See CLINICAL GOVERNANCE; EVIDENCE-BASED MEDICINE.)

Health Centre

An imprecise term that may refer to a group of doctors and supporting staff operating from one building owned or leased by the doctors, or to a building owned or leased by a health authority that contains staff or services from one or more sections of the National Health Service.

Health Databases

The centralised collection and storage of information about the health of individuals. Recent advances in GENETICS have raised concerns about the potential for abuse of all health databases, whether maintained for scientific research – which has long used them – or for government or community health planning, or by groups of professionals (or individuals) to help in the treatment of patients. The public is concerned about whether their rights to privacy and confidentiality are threatened by databases and whether information about them could be disclosed and misused.

Health Development Agency (HDA)

Appointed by the UK government to help improve the NHS in England (Scotland, Wales and Northern Ireland have similar bodies), HDA replaced the long-established Health Education Authority in April 2000. The agency supports government priorities to improve public health and to tackle health inequalities. Among its key functions are:

● Maintaining an up-to-date evidence base of 'what works' in public health and health improvements.
● Providing useful information to health practitioners.
● Commissioning research to remedy the gaps in the evidence base for medical practice.
● Improving health promotion and advising on the standards for (and implementation of) public-health activities.

(See APPENDIX 7: STATUTORY ORGANISATIONS.)

Health Education

The process of educating the public to adopt a healthy lifestyle and abandon dangerous or unhealthy behaviour. With the rising cost of health care and the increasing amount of illness and injury resulting from preventable causes, health professionals, governments and the World Health Organisation are strongly supporting more and better health education for everyone from schoolchildren to the elderly. Information on all aspects of health education in the United Kingdom can be obtained from the HEALTH DEVELOPMENT AGENCY (HDA) (see also APPENDIX 7: STATUTORY ORGANISATIONS).

Health Impact Assessment

This is a structured, multi-disciplinary process for assessing and improving the health consequences of projects and policies in the non-health sector. It combines a range of qualitative and quantitative evidence in preparing conclusions. Applications of the assessments include appraisal of national policies, local urban planning, and the progress of transport, water and agricultural projects.

Health Promotion

A surveillance plan based on a community, and aimed at maintaining an optimum state of health and quality of life for those who make up the community – both as individuals and as a group. Programmes would include immunisation targets, health education and screening tests, as well as environmental procedures such as monitoring atmosphere, improving housing, water and food supplies, and encouraging safe and healthy working practices. (See ENVIRONMENT AND HEALTH; PUBLIC HEALTH.)

Health Service Commissioner

An official, responsible to the United Kingdom's parliament, appointed to protect the interests of National Health Service patients in matters concerning the administration of the health service and the delivery of health care (excluding clinical judgements). Known colloquially as the health ombudsman, the Commissioner presents regular reports on the complaints dealt with.

Health-Service Management

The administrative machinery for planning, delivering and monitoring health care provided by health professionals and their supporting staff. This may range from running a small primary-care centre to organising a large hospital or being responsible for meeting the health needs of a region or a nation. Whether the overall structure for proving care is state-funded, insurance-based, private-practice or a mixture of these, health-service management is essential in an era of rapidly evolving and expensive scientific medicine. Health-service managers are administrators with special training and skills in managing health care; sometimes they are doctors, nurses or other health professionals, but many have been trained in management in commercial, civil service or industrial environments.

Health Visitors

Health visitors are community nurses with a special training who form an important part of the primary health-care team. Working in close conjunction with general practitioners, they are primarily responsible for illness prevention and health screening and education of children and elderly people in the community.

Healthcare Commission (Commission for Health Improvement)

Launched in 1999 in England and Wales as CHI, this is an inspectorate charged with protecting patients from 'unacceptable failings in the National Health Service'. A statutory body under the 1999 Health Act, it evaluates and refines local systems designed to safeguard standards of clinical quality. Working separately from the NHS and the health departments, it offers an independent safeguard that provides systems to monitor and improve clinical quality in primary care, community services and hospitals. As of 2004 it became responsible for dealing with patients' complaints if they could not be settled by the trust concerned. The board members include health professionals, academics and eight lay members. Scotland has set up a similar statutory body. (See APPENDIX 7: STATUTORY ORGANISATIONS.)

Hearing

See DEAFNESS; EAR.

Hearing Aids

Nearly two-thirds of people aged over 70 have some degree of hearing impairment (see DEAFNESS). Hearing aids are no substitute for definitive treatment of the underlying cause of poor hearing, so examination by an ear, nose and throat surgeon and an audiologist is sensible before a hearing aid is issued (and is essential before one can be given through the NHS). The choice of aid depends on the age, manipulative skills, and degree of hearing impairment of the patient and the underlying cause of the deafness. The choice of hearing aid for a deaf child is particularly important, as impaired hearing can hinder speech development.

Electronic aids consist, essentially, of a microphone, an amplifier, and an earphone. In postural aids the microphone and amplifier are contained in a small box worn behind the ear or attached to spectacles. The earphone is on a specially moulded earpiece. Some patients find it difficult to manipulate the controls of an aid worn behind the ear, and they may be better off with a device worn on the body. Some hearing aids are worn entirely within the ear and are very discreet. They are particularly useful for people who have to wear protective headgear such as helmets.

The most sophisticated aids sit entirely within the ear canal so are virtually invisible. They may be tuned so that only the frequencies the wearer cannot hear are amplified.

Many have a volume control and a special setting for use with telephone and in rooms fitted with an inductive coupler that screens out background noise.

In making a choice therefore from the large range of effective hearing aids now available, the expert advice of an ear specialist must be obtained. The RNID (Royal National Institute for Deaf People) provides a list of clinics where such a specialist can be consulted. It also gives reliable advice concerning the purchase and use of hearing aids – a worthwhile function, as some aids are very expensive.

Heart

A hollow muscular pump with four cavities, each provided at its outlet with a valve, whose function is to maintain the circulation of the blood. The two upper cavities are known as atria; the two lower ones as ventricles. The term auricle is applied to the ear-shaped tip of the atrium on each side.

Shape and size In adults the heart is about the size and shape of a clenched fist. One end of the heart is pointed (apex); the other is broad (base) and is deeply cleft at the division between the two atria. One groove running down the front and up the back shows the division between the two ventricles; a circular, deeper groove marks off the atria above from the ventricles below. The capacity of each cavity is somewhere between 90 and 180 millilitres.

Structure The heart lies within a strong fibrous bag, known as the pericardium. Since the inner surface of this bag and the outer surface of the heart are both covered with a smooth, glistening membrane faced with flat cells and lubricated by a little serous fluid (around 20 ml), the movements of the heart are accomplished almost without friction. The main thickness of the heart wall consists of bundles of muscle fibres, some of which run in circles right around the heart, and others in loops, first round one cavity, then round the corresponding cavity of the other side. Within all the cavities is a smooth lining membrane, continuous with that lining the vessels which open into the heart. The investing smooth membrane is known as epicardium; the muscular substance as myocardium; and the smooth lining membrane as endocardium.

Important nerves regulate the heart's action, especially via the vagus nerve and with the sympathetic system (see NERVOUS SYSTEM). In the near part of the atria lies a collection of nerve cells and connecting fibres, known as the sinuatrial node or pacemaker, which forms the starting-point for the impulses that initiate the beats of the heart. In the groove between the ventricles and the atria lies another collection of similar nerve tissue, known as the atrioventricular node. Running down from there into the septum between the two ventricles is a band of special muscle fibres, known as the atrioventricular bundle, or the bundle of His. This splits up into a right and a left branch for the two ventricles, and the fibres of these distribute themselves throughout the muscular wall of the ventricles and control their contraction.

Openings There is no direct communication between the cavities on the right side and those on the left; but the right atrium opens into the right ventricle by a large circular opening, and similarly the left atrium into the left ventricle. Into the right atrium open two large veins, the superior and inferior venae cavae, with some smaller veins from the wall of the heart itself, and into the left atrium open two pulmonary veins from each lung. One opening leads out of each ventricle – to the aorta in the case of the left ventricle, to the pulmonary artery from the right.

Before birth, the FETUS's heart has an opening (foramen ovale) from the right into the left atrium through which the blood passes; but when the child first draws air into his or her lungs this opening closes and is represented in the adult only by a depression (fossa ovalis).

Valves The heart contains four valves. The mitral valve consists of two triangular cusps; the tricuspid valve of three smaller cusps. The aortic and pulmonary valves each consist of three semilunar-shaped segments. Two valves are placed at the openings leading from atrium into ventricle, the tricuspid valve on the right side, the mitral valve on the left, so as completely to prevent blood from running back into the atrium when the ventricle contracts. Two more, the pulmonary valve and the aortic valve, are at the entrance to these arteries, and prevent regurgitation into the ventricles of blood which has been driven from them into the arteries. The noises made by these valves in closing constitute the greater part of what are known as the heart sounds, and can be heard by anyone who applies his or her ear to the front of a person's chest. Murmurs heard accompanying these sounds indicate defects in the valves, and may be a sign of heart disease (although many murmurs, especially in children, are 'innocent').

Action At each heartbeat the two atria contract and expel their contents into the ventricles, which at the same time they stimulate to contract together, so that the blood is driven into the arteries, to be returned again to the atria after having completed a circuit in about 15 seconds through the body or lungs as the case may be. The heart beats from 60 to 90 times a minute, the rate in any given healthy person being about four times that of the respirations. The heart is to some extent regulated by a nerve centre in the MEDULLA, closely connected with those centres which govern the lungs and stomach, and nerve fibres pass to it in the vagus nerve. The heart rate and force can be diminished by some of these fibres, by others increased, according to the needs of the various organs of the body. If this nerve centre is injured or poisoned – for example, by lack of oxygen – the heart stops beating in human beings; although in some of the lower animals (e.g. frogs, fishes and reptiles) the heart may under favourable conditions go on beating for hours even after its entire removal from the body.

Heart, Artificial

A mechanical device in the chest that enhances or takes over the pumping action of the HEART, thus maintaining the necessary level of circulation of blood through the lungs and other body structures. An artificial heart was first used in humans in 1985 and the three types in use are: an intra-aortic balloon pump, driven by compressed air, which inflates a balloon in the AORTA with every heartbeat, increasing the volume of circulating blood; an electrical device that assists the left VENTRICLE by pumping blood into the abdominal aorta; and a mechanical artificial heart that replaces a diseased heart that has been removed. As yet there is no artificial heart suitable for long-term use. Existing devices are intended to tide over a patient who is extremely ill until a live heart can be transplanted from a donor. The results from artificial hearts have been disappointing because of complications and also because the patients have usually been already dangerously ill.

Heart, Diseases of

Heart disease can affect any of the structures of the HEART and may affect more than one at a time. Heart attack is an imprecise term and may refer to ANGINA PECTORIS (a symptom of pain originating in the heart) or to coronary artery thrombosis, also called myocardial infarction.

Arrhythmias An abnormal rate or rhythm of the heartbeat. The reason is a disturbance in the electrical impulses within the heart. Sometimes a person may have an occasional irregular heartbeat: this is called an ECTOPIC beat (or an extrasystole) and does not necessarily mean that an abnormality exists. There are two main types of arrhythmia: bradycardias, where the rate is slow – fewer than 60 beats a minute and sometimes so slow and unpredictable (heartblock) as to cause blackouts or heart failure; and tachycardia, where the rate is fast – more than 100 beats a minute. A common cause of arrhythmia is coronary artery disease, when vessels carrying blood to the heart are narrowed by fatty deposits (ATHEROMA), thus reducing the blood supply and damaging the heart tissue. This condition often causes myocardial infarction after which arrhythmias are quite common and may need correcting by DEFIBRILLATION (application of a·short electric shock to the heart). Some tachycardias result from a defect in the electrical conduction system of the heart that is commonly congenital. Various drugs can be used to treat arrhythmias (see ANTIARRHYTHMIC DRUGS). If attacks constantly recur, the arrhythmia may be corrected by electrical removal of dead or diseased tissue that is the cause of the disorder. Heartblock is most effectively treated with an artificial CARDIAC PACE-MAKER, a battery-activated control unit implanted in the chest.

Cardiomyopathy Any disease of the heart muscle that results in weakening of its contractions. The consequence is a fall in the efficiency of the circulation of blood through the lungs and remainder of the body structures. The myopathy may be due to infection, disordered metabolism, nutritional excess or deficiency, toxic agents, autoimmune processes, degeneration, or inheritance. Often, however, the cause is not identified. Cardiomyopathies are less common than other types of heart diseases, and the incidence of different types of myopathy (see below) is not known because patients or doctors are sometimes unaware of the presence of the condition.

The three recognised groups of cardiomyopathies are hypertrophic, dilated and restrictive.

● Hypertrophic myopathy, a familial condition, is characterised by great enlargement of the muscle of the heart ventricles. This reduces the muscle's efficiency, the ventricles fail to relax properly and do not fill sufficiently during DIASTOLE.

● In the dilated type of cardiomyopathy, both ventricles overdilate, impairing the efficiency of contraction and causing congestion of the lungs.

● In the restrictive variety, proper filling of the ventricles does not occur because the muscle walls are less elastic than normal. The result is raised pressure in the two atria (upper cavities) of the heart: these dilate and develop FIBRILLATION. Diagnosis can be difficult and treatment is symptomatic, with a poor prognosis. In suitable patients, heart TRANSPLAN-TATION may be considered.

Disorders of the heart muscle may also be caused by poisoning – for example, heavy consumption of alcohol. Symptoms include tiredness, palpitations (quicker and sometimes irregular heartbeat), chest pain, difficulty in breathing, and swelling of the legs and hands due to accumulation of fluid (OEDEMA). The heart is enlarged (as shown on chest X-ray) and ECHOCARDIOGRAPHY shows thickening of the heart muscle. A BIOPSY of heart muscle will show abnormalities in the cells of the heart muscle.

Where the cause of cardiomyopathy is unknown, as is the case with most patients, treatment is symptomatic using DIURETICS to control heart failure and drugs such as DIGOXIN to return the heart rhythm to normal. Patients should stop drinking alcohol. If, as often happens, the patient's condition slowly deteriorates, heart transplantation should be considered.

Congenital heart disease accounts for 1–2 per cent of all cases of organic heart disease. It may be genetically determined and so inherited; present at birth for no obvious reason; or, in rare cases, related to RUBELLA in the mother. The most common forms are holes in the heart (atrial septal defect, ventricular septal defect – see SEPTAL DEFECT), a patent DUCTUS ARTERIOSUS, and COARCTATION OF THE AORTA. Many complex forms also exist and can be diagnosed in the womb by fetal echocardiography which can lead to elective termination of pregnancy. Surgery to correct many of these abnormalities is feasible, even for the most severe abnormalities, but may only be palliative giving rise to major difficulties of management as the children become older. Heart transplantation is now increasingly employed for the uncorrectable lesions.

Coronary artery disease Also known as ischaemic heart disease, this is a common cause of symptoms and death in the adult population. It may present for the first time as sudden death, but more usually causes ANGINA PEC-TORIS, myocardial infarction (heart attack) or heart failure. It can also lead to a disturbance of heart rhythm. Factors associated with an increased risk of developing coronary artery disease include diabetes, cigarette smoking, high blood pressure, obesity, and a raised concentration of cholesterol in the blood. Older males are most affected.

Coronary thrombosis or acute myocardial infarction is the acute, dramatic manifestation of coronary-artery ischaemic heart disease – one of the major killing diseases of western civilisation. In 1999, ischaemic heart disease was responsible for about 115,000 deaths in England and Wales, compared with 153,000 deaths in 1988. In 1999 more than 55,600 people died of coronary thrombosis. The underlying cause is disease of the coronary arteries which carry the blood supply to the heart muscle (or myocardium). This results in narrowing of the arteries until finally they are unable to transport sufficient blood for the myocardium to function efficiently. One of three things may happen. If the narrowing of the coronary arteries occurs gradually, then the individual concerned will develop either angina pectoris or signs of a failing heart: irregular rhythm, breathlessness, CYANOSIS and oedema.

If the narrowing occurs suddenly or leads to complete blockage (occlusion) of a major branch of one of the coronary arteries, then the victim collapses with acute pain and distress. This is the condition commonly referred to as a coronary thrombosis because it is usually due to the affected artery suddenly becoming completely blocked by THROMBOSIS. More correctly, it should be described as coronary occlusion, because the final occluding factor need not necessarily be thrombosis.

Causes The precise cause is not known, but a wide range of factors play a part in inducing coronary artery disease. Heredity is an important factor. The condition is more common in men than in women; it is also more common in those in sedentary occupations than in those who lead a more physically active life, and more likely to occur in those with high blood pressure than in those with normal blood pressure (see HYPERTENSION). Obesity is a contributory factor. The disease is more common among smokers than non-smokers; it is also often

associated with a high level of CHOLESTEROL in the blood, which in turn has been linked with an excessive consumption of animal, as opposed to vegetable, fats. In this connection the important factors seem to be the saturated fatty acids (low-density and very low-density lipo-proteins [LDLs and VLDLs] – see CHOLES-TEROL) of animal fats which would appear to be more likely to lead to a high level of cholesterol in the blood than the unsaturated fatty acids of vegetable fats. As more research on the subject is carried out, the arguments continue about the relative influence of the different factors. (For advice on prevention of the disease, see APPENDIX 2: ADDRESSES: SOURCES OF INFORMATION, ADVICE, SUPPORT AND SELF-HELP.)

Symptoms The presenting symptom is the sudden onset, often at rest, of acute, agonising pain in the front of the chest. This rapidly radiates all over the front of the chest and often down over the abdomen. The pain is frequently accompanied by nausea and vomiting, so that suspicion may be aroused of some acute abdominal condition such as biliary colic (see GALL-BLADDER, DISEASES OF) or a perforated PEPTIC ULCER. The victim soon goes into SHOCK, with a pale, cold, sweating skin, rapid pulse and difficulty in breathing. There is usually some rise in temperature.

Treatment is immediate relief of the pain by injections of diamorphine. Thrombolytic drugs should be given as soon as possible ('rapid door to needle time') and ARRHYTHMIA corrected. OXYGEN is essential and oral ASPIRIN is valuable. Treatment within the first hour makes a great difference to recovery. Subsequent treatment includes the continued administration of drugs to relieve the pain; the administration of ANTIARRHYTHMIC DRUGS that may be necessary to deal with the heart failure that commonly develops, and the irregular action of the heart that quite often develops; and the continued administration of oxygen. Patients are usually admitted to coronary care units, where they receive constant supervision. Such units maintain an emergency, skilled, round-the-clock staff of doctors and nurses, as well as all the necessary resuscitation facilities that may be required.

The outcome varies considerably. The first (golden) hour is when the patient is at greatest risk of death: if he or she is treated, then there is a 50 per cent reduction in mortality compared with waiting until hospital admission. As each day passes the prognosis improves with a first coronary thrombosis, provided that the patient does not have a high blood pressure and is not overweight. Following recovery, there should be a gradual return to work, care being taken to avoid any increase in weight, unnecessary stress and strain, and to observe moderation in all things. Smoking must stop. In uncomplicated cases patients get up and about as soon as possible, most being in hospital for a week to ten days and back at work in three months or sooner.

Valvular heart disease primarily affects the mitral and aortic valves which can become narrowed (stenosis) or leaking (incompetence). Pulmonary valve problems are usually congenital (stenosis) and the tricuspid valve is sometimes involved when rheumatic heart disease primarily affects the mitral or aortic valves. RHEUMATIC FEVER, usually in childhood, remains a common cause of chronic valvular heart disease causing stenosis, incompetence or both of the aortic and mitral valves, but each valve has other separate causes for malfunction.

Aortic valve disease is more common with increasing age. When the valve is narrowed, the heart hypertrophies and may later fail. Symptoms of angina or breathlessness are common and dizziness or blackouts (syncope) also occur. Replacing the valve is a very effective treatment, even with advancing age. Aortic stenosis may be caused by degeneration (senile calcific), by the inheritance of two valvular leaflets instead of the usual three (bicuspid valve), or by rheumatic fever. Aortic incompetence again leads to hypertrophy, but dilatation is more common as blood leaks back into the ventricle. Breathlessness is the more common complaint. The causes are the same as stenosis but also include inflammatory conditions such as SYPHILIS or ANKYLOSING SPONDYLITIS and other disorders of connective tissue. The valve may also leak if the aorta dilates, stretching the valve ring as with HYPERTENSION, aortic ANEURYSM and MARFAN'S SYNDROME – an inherited disorder of connective tissue that causes heart defects. Infection (endocarditis) can worsen acutely or chronically destroy the valve and sometimes lead to abnormal outgrowths on the valve (vegetations) which may break free and cause devastating damage such as a stroke or blocked circulation to the bowel or leg.

Mitral valve disease leading to stenosis is rheumatic in origin. Mitral incompetence may be rheumatic but in the absence of stenosis can be due to ISCHAEMIA, INFARCTION, inflamma-

tion, infection and a congenital weakness (prolapse). The valve may also leak if stretched by a dilating ventricle (functional incompetence). Infection (endocarditis) may affect the valve in a similar way to aortic disease. Mitral symptoms are predominantly breathlessness which may lead to wheezing or waking at night breathless and needing to sit up or stand for relief. They are made worse when the heart rhythm changes (atrial fibrillation) which is frequent as the disease becomes more severe. This leads to a loss of efficiency of up to 25 per cent and a predisposition to clot formation as blood stagnates rather than leaves the heart efficiently. Mitral incompetence may remain mild and be of no trouble for many years, but infection must be guarded against (endocarditis prophylaxis).

Endocarditis is an infection of the heart which may acutely destroy a valve or may lead to chronic destruction. Bacteria settle usually on a mild lesion. Antibiotics taken at vulnerable times can prevent this (antibiotic prophylaxis) – for example, before tooth extraction. If established, lengthy intravenous antibiotic therapy is needed and surgery is often necessary. The mortality is 30 per cent but may be higher if the infection settles on a replaced valve (prosthetic endocarditis). Complications include heart failure, shock, embolisation (generation of small clots in the blood), and cerebral (mental) confusion.

PERICARDITIS is an inflammation of the sac covering the outside of the heart. The sac becomes roughened and pain occurs as the heart and sac rub together. This is heard by stethoscope as a scratching noise (pericardial rub). Fever is often present and a virus the main cause. It may also occur with rheumatic fever, kidney failure, TUBERCULOSIS or from an adjacent lung problem such as PNEUMONIA or cancer. The inflammation may cause fluid to accumulate between the sac and the heart (effusion) which may compress the heart causing a fall in blood pressure, a weak pulse and circulatory failure (tamponade). This can be relieved by aspirating the fluid. The treatment is then directed at the underlying cause.

Heart-Lung Machine

A device that temporarily takes over the function of the heart and lungs. It is used in certain operations in the chest, giving the surgeon more time for operations such as open-heart surgery, heart transplants and heart-lung transplants. The machine also ensures an operating area largely free of blood, which helps the surgeon to work more quickly. A pump replaces the heart and an oxygenator replaces the lungs. When connected up, the machine in effect bypasses normal cardiopulmonary activity. It also contains a heat exchanger to warm or cool the patient's blood according to the requirements of the operation. The patient is given an anticoagulant (HEPARIN) to counteract clotting which may occur when blood cells get damaged during the machine's use. Patients are on the machine for a few hours only, because blood supply to vital organs begins to be reduced.

Heart-Lung Transplant

An operation in which a patient's diseased lungs and heart are removed and replaced with donor organs from someone who has been certified as 'brain dead' (see BRAIN-STEM DEATH). As well as the technical difficulties of such an operation, rejection by the recipient's tissues of donated heart and lungs has proved hard to overcome. Since the early 1990s, however, immunosuppressant drug therapy (see CICLOSPORIN; TRANSPLANTATION) has facilitated the regular use of this type of surgery. Even so, patients receiving transplanted hearts and lungs face substantial risks such as lung infection and airway obstruction as well as the long-term problems of transplant rejection.

Heart Surgery

Open-heart surgery permits the treatment of many previously inoperable conditions that were potentially fatal, or which made the patient chronically disabled. CORONARY ARTERY VEIN BYPASS GRAFTING (CAVBG), used to remedy obstruction of the arteries supplying the heart muscle, was first carried out in the mid-1960s and is now widely practised. Constricted heart valves today are routinely dilated by techniques of MINIMALLY INVASIVE SURGERY (MIS), such as ANGIOPLASTY and laser treatment, and faulty valves can be replaced with mechanical alternatives (see VALVULOPLASTY).

Heart transplant Replacement of a person's unhealthy heart with a normal heart from a healthy donor. The donor's heart needs to be removed immediately after death and kept chilled in saline before rapid transport to the recipient. Heart transplants are technically demanding operations used to treat patients with progressive untreatable heart disease but whose other body systems are in good shape. They usually have advanced coronary artery disease and damaged heart muscle (CARDIO-MYOPATHY). Apart from the technical difficulties of the operation, preventing rejection of the transplanted heart by the recipient's immune

system requires complex drug treatment. But once the patient has passed the immediate postoperative phase, the chances of five-year survival is as high as 80 per cent in some cardiac centres. A key difficulty in doing heart transplants is a serious shortage of donor organs.

Heartburn

A burning sensation experienced in the region of the heart and up the back to the throat. It is caused by an excessive acidity of the gastric juice – often aggravated by dietary indiscretions – and is relieved temporarily by taking alkaline substances, such as 1·2 grams of bicarbonate of soda, or commercial preparations such as aluminium-containing antacid tablets (e.g. Aluminium Hydroxide Tablets) or prescribed drugs such as lansoprazole. The frequency of heartburn attacks can be lessened by eating a sensible diet, avoiding fatty or indigestible foods and restricting alcohol consumption.

Persistent heartburn may be a sign of more serious oesophageal disease and medical advice should be sought.

Heat Cramps

Painful cramps in the muscles occurring in workers, such as stokers, who labour in hot conditions. The cramps are the result of loss of salt in the sweat, and can be cured by giving the sufferer salty water to drink. (See also HEAT STROKE.)

Heat Spots

A vague term applied to small inflamed and congested areas which appear especially upon the skin of the face, neck and chest or other parts of the body in warm weather.

Heat Stroke

A condition resulting from environmental temperatures which are too high for compensation by the body's thermo-regulatory mechanism(s). It is characterised by hyperpyrexia, nausea, headache, thirst, confusion, and dry skin. If untreated, COMA and death ensue. The occurrence of heat stroke is sporadic: whereas a single individual may be affected (occasionally with fatal consequences), his or her colleagues may remain unaffected. Predisposing factors include unsatisfactory living or working conditions, inadequate acclimatisation to tropical conditions, unsuitable clothing, underlying poor health, and possibly dietetic or alcoholic indiscretions. The condition can be a major problem during pilgrimages – for example, the Muslim Hadj. Four clinical syndromes are recognised:

Heat collapse is characterised by fatigue, giddiness, and temporary loss of consciousness. It is accompanied by HYPOTENSION and BRADYCARDIA; there may also be vomiting and muscular cramps. Urinary volume is diminished. Recovery is usual.

Heat exhaustion is characterised by increasing weakness, dizziness and insomnia. In the majority of sufferers, sweating is defective; there are few, if any, signs of dehydration. Pulse rate is normal, and urinary output good. Body temperature is usually 37·8–38·3 °C.

Heat cramps (usually in the legs, arms or back, and occasionally involving the abdominal muscles) are associated with hard physical work at a high temperature. Sweating, pallor, headache, giddiness and intense anxiety are present. Body temperature is only mildly raised.

Heat hyperpyrexia is heralded by energy loss and irritability; this is followed by mental confusion and diminution of sweating. The individual rapidly becomes restless, then comatose; body temperature rises to 41–42 °C or even higher. The condition is fatal unless expertly treated as a matter of urgency.

Treatment With the first two syndromes, the affected individual must be removed immediately to a cool place, and isotonic saline administered – intravenously in a severe case. The fourth syndrome is a medical emergency. The patient should be placed in the shade, stripped, and drenched with water; fanning should be instigated. He or she should be wrapped in a sheet soaked in cool water and fanning continued. When rectal temperature has fallen to 39 °C, the patient is wrapped in a dry blanket. Immediately after consciousness returns, normal saline should be given orally; this usually provokes sweating. The risk of circulatory collapse exists. Convalescence may be protracted and the patient should be repatriated to a cool climate. Prophylactically, personnel intended for work in a tropical climate must be very carefully selected. Adequate acclimatisation is also essential; severe physical exertion must be avoided for several weeks, and light clothes should be worn. The diet should be light but nourishing, and fluid intake adequate. Those performing hard physical work at a very high ambient temperature should receive sodium chloride supplements. Attention to ventilation and air-conditioning is essential; fans are also of value.

Hebephrenia
A form of SCHIZOPHRENIA that comes on in youth and is marked by depression and gradual failure of mental faculties with egotistic and self-centred delusions.

Heberden's Nodes
Small hard knobs which appear at the sides of the last phalanges of the fingers in people who have OSTEOARTHRITIS.

Heel
The heel is the hind part of the foot, formed by the CALCANEUS and the especially thick skin covering it. It is not subject to many diseases. Severe pain in the heel is sometimes a sign of gout or rheumatism.

Height
See WEIGHT AND HEIGHT.

Helicobacter Pylori
A bacterium which colonises the stomach. While it may cause no disease, it has a tendency to produce inflammation – gastritis. This may progress in some people to peptic ulceration (see PEPTIC ULCER), and even to gastric cancer. The bacterium can be identified on blood testing or, more accurately, by obtaining a biopsy of the stomach wall by ENDOSCOPY. It can be eradicated by treatment with PROTON-PUMP INHIBITORS and antibiotics.

Heliotherapy
Sunbathing; the exposure of the body to sunlight to promote healing.

Helium
This is the lightest gas known, with the exception of hydrogen. This property renders it of value in ANAESTHESIA, as its addition to the anaesthetic means that it can be inhaled with less effort by the patient. Thus it can be used in the presence of any obstruction to the entry of air to the lungs.

HELLP Syndrome
A type of severe PRE-ECLAMPSIA (a disorder affecting some pregnant women) that affects various systems in the body. HAEMOLYSIS, raised concentration of the enzymes in the LIVER, and a low blood platelet count are among the characteristics (and explain the name HELLP); patients are acutely ill and immediate termination of pregnancy is necessary. (See also PREGNANCY AND LABOUR.)

Helminths

Another name for parasitic worms such as FLUKES, tapeworms (see TAENIASIS) and nematodes (see ASCARIASIS).

Hemianaesthesia

Loss of the sense of touch down one side of the body.

Hemianopia

A term meaning loss of half the usual area of vision. The affected person may see everything clearly to the left or to the right, the field of vision stopping abruptly at the middle line; they may see things only when straight ahead of them; or, thirdly, they may see objects far out on both sides, although there is a wide area straight in front for which they are quite blind. The position of the blind area is important in localising the position in the brain of the disease responsible for the condition.

Hemiatrophy

Atrophy of one side of the body, or of part of the body on one side: for example, facial hemiatrophy, in which one-half of the face is smaller than the other, either in the course of development or as a result of some nervous disorder.

Hemiballismus

Involuntary movements similar to choreiform (see CHOREA) movements, but of much greater amplitude and force. The violent, throwing movements of the limbs are usually unilateral, and tend to occur acutely as a result of vascular damage to the mid-brain.

Hemicolectomy

An operation to remove the right or left half of the COLON, usually with end-to-end ANASTO-MOSIS of the remaining portion of the intestine. This is often used for the treatment of malignant or inflammatory diseases of the colon.

Hemicrania

A headache limited to one side of the head. (See also MIGRAINE.)

Hemimelia

This consists of defects in the distal part of the extremities: for example, the absence of a forearm or hand. Hemimelia is a congenital defect; large numbers of cases resulted from the administration of THALIDOMIDE during pregnancy (see also PHOCOMELIA; TERATOGENESIS).

Hemiparesis

Paralysis affecting the muscles of one side of the body. This most commonly follows a STROKE and occurs when parts of the brain serving motor function on the opposite side of the body are damaged.

Hemiplegia

PARALYSIS that is limited to one side of the body.

Hemp

See CANNABIS.

Henle, Loop of

That part of the nephron (see KIDNEYS) between the proximal and distal convoluted tubules. It extends into the renal medulla as a hairpin-shaped loop. The ascending link of the loop actively transports sodium from the lumen of the tube to the interstitium, and this, combined with the 'counter-current' flow of fluid through the two limbs of the loop, plays a part in concentrating the urine.

Henoch-Schönlein Purpura

This is an inflammatory condition of the small blood vessels, the cause of which is not known but may be an allergic response to food or drugs. Most common among young children, the inflammation causes blood to leak into joints, kidneys, intestine and skin. The child presents with a purpuric rash and stomach pains which may come and go for weeks. Paracetamol alone is often sufficient to alleviate the condition, but severely ill patients may need corticosteroid drugs. All sufferers need follow-up for 12 months to ensure that they have not developed kidney disease.

Heparin

Heparin is one of the naturally produced ANTI-COAGULANTS with a rapid effect, which is thought to act by neutralising thrombin (see COAGULATION). Inactive when taken orally, it is normally given intravenously – it may be given for a few days, combined with an oral anticoagulant such as warfarin, to initiate anticoagulation. Low-dose heparin may be given by subcutaneous injection for longer periods, for the prophylaxis of DEEP VEIN THROMBOSIS (DVT) or PULMONARY EMBOLISM in 'high-risk' patients, such as those with obesity or a history of thrombosis, or post-operatively. If haemorrhage occurs, withdrawal of heparin is usually sufficient, but protamine sulphate is a rapidly active and specific antidote. Prolonged treatment with heparin may cause osteoporosis (see under BONE, DISORDERS OF).

Hepatectomy

The operation for removal of the LIVER, or part of it.

Hepatic Encephalopathy

A neuropsychiatric syndrome caused by disease of the LIVER, and occurring most often in patients with CIRRHOSIS – see also LIVER, DISEASES OF; it also occurs in acute form in acute failure of liver function. The disorder is believed to be the result of biochemical disturbance of brain function, because the condition is reversible and pathological changes in brain tissue are rarely found. The patient's intellect, personality, emotions and consciousness are altered but neurological signs may or may not be identified. Apathy, confusion, drowsiness, sometimes CONVULSIONS, speech disturbance and eventually COMA mark the progress of the condition. The principles of treatment are to remove the precipitating causes. These include: URAEMIA; sedative, antidepressant and hypnotic drugs; gastrointestinal bleeding; too much protein in the diet; infection; and trauma (including surgical operations).

Hepatitis

Inflammation of the LIVER which damages liver cells and may ultimately kill them. Acute injury of the liver is usually followed by complete recovery, but prolonged inflammation after injury may result in FIBROSIS and CIRRHOSIS. Excluding trauma, hepatitis has several causes:

● Viral infections by any of hepatitis A, B, C, D, or E viruses and also CYTOMEGALOVIRUS (CMV), EPSTEIN BARR VIRUS, and HERPES SIMPLEX.
● Autoimmune disorders such as autoimmune chronic hepatitis, toxins, alcohol and certain drugs – ISONIAZID, RIFAMPICIN, HALOTHANE and CHLORPROMAZINE.
● WILSON'S DISEASE.

Acute viral hepatitis causes damage throughout the liver and in severe infections may destroy whole lobules (see below).

Chronic hepatitis is typified by an invasion of the portal tract by white blood cells (mild hepatitis). If these mononuclear inflammatory cells invade the body (parenchyma) of the liver tissue, fibrosis and then chronic disease or cirrhosis can develop. Cirrhosis may develop at any age and commonly results in prolonged ill health. It is an important cause of premature death, with excessive alcohol consumption commonly the triggering factor. Sometimes, cirrhosis may be asymptomatic, but common symptoms are weakness, tiredness, poor appetite, weight loss, nausea, vomiting, abdominal discomfort and production of abnormal amounts of wind. Initially, the liver may enlarge, but later it becomes hard and shrunken, though rarely causing pain. Skin pigmentation may occur along with jaundice, the result of failure to excrete the liver product BILIRUBIN. Routine liver-function tests on blood are used to help diagnose the disease and to monitor its progress. Spider telangiectasia (caused by damage to blood vessels – see TELANGIECTASIS) usually develop, and these are a significant pointer to liver disease. ENDOCRINE changes occur, especially in men, who lose their typical hair distribution and suffer from atrophy of their testicles. Bruising and nosebleeds occur increasingly as the cirrhosis worsens, and portal hypertension (high pressure of venous blood circulation through the liver) develops due to abnormal vascular resistance. ASCITES and HEPATIC ENCEPHALOPATHY are indications of advanced cirrhosis.

Treatment of cirrhosis is to tackle the underlying cause, to maintain the patient's nutrition (advising him or her to avoid alcohol), and to treat any complications. The disorder can also be treated by liver transplantation; indeed, 75 per cent of liver transplants are done for cirrhosis. The overall prognosis of cirrhosis, however, is not good, especially as many patients attend for medical care late in the course of the disease. Overall, only 25 per cent of patients live for five years after diagnosis, though patients who have a liver transplant and survive for a year (80 per cent do) have a good prognosis.

Autoimmune hepatitis is a type that most commonly occurs in women between 20 and 40 years of age. The cause is unknown and it has been suggested that the disease has several immunological subtypes. Symptoms are similar to other viral hepatitis infections, with painful joints and AMENORRHOEA as additional symptoms. Jaundice and signs of chronic liver disease usually occur. Treatment with CORTICOSTEROIDS is life-saving in autoimmune hepatitis, and maintenance treatment may be needed for two years or more. Remissions and exacerbations are typical, and most patients eventually develop cirrhosis, with 50 per cent of victims dying of liver failure if not treated. This figure falls to 10 per cent in treated patients.

Viral hepatitis The five hepatic viruses (A to E) all cause acute primary liver disease, though each belongs to a separate group of viruses.
● Hepatitis A virus (HAV) is an ENTEROVIRUS

which is very infectious, spreading by faecal contamination from patients suffering from (or incubating) the infection; victims excrete viruses into the faeces for around five weeks during incubation and development of the disease. Overcrowding and poor sanitation help to spread hepatitis A, which fortunately usually causes only mild disease.

- Hepatitis B (HBV) is caused by a hepadna virus, and humans are the only reservoir of infection, with blood the main agent for transferring it. Transfusions of infected blood or blood products, and injections using contaminated needles (common among habitual drug abusers), are common modes of transfer. Tattooing and ACUPUNCTURE may spread hepatitis B unless high standards of sterilisation are maintained. Sexual intercourse, particularly between male homosexuals, is a significant infection route.
- Hepatitis C (HCV) is a flavivirus whose source of infection is usually via blood contacts. Effective screening of blood donors and heat treatment of blood factors should prevent the spread of this infection, which becomes chronic in about 75 per cent of those infected, lasting for life. Although most carriers do not suffer an acute illness, they must practise life-long preventive measures.
- Hepatitis D (HDV) cannot survive independently, needing HBV to replicate, so its sources and methods of spread are similar to the B virus. HDV can infect people at the same time as HBV, but it is capable of superinfecting those who are already chronic carriers of the B virus. Acute and chronic infection of HDV can occur, depending on individual circumstances, and parenteral drug abuse spreads the infection. The disease occurs worldwide, being endemic in Africa, South America and the Mediterranean littoral.
- Hepatitis E virus (HEV) is excreted in the stools, spreading via the faeco-oral route. It causes large epidemics of water-borne hepatitis and flourishes wherever there is poor sanitation. It resembles acute HAV infection and the patient usually recovers. HEV does not cause chronic infection.

The clinical characteristics of the five hepatic viruses are broadly similar. The initial symptoms last for up to two weeks (comprising temperature, headache and malaise), and JAUNDICE then develops, with anorexia, nausea, vomiting and diarrhoea common manifestations. Upper abdominal pain and a tender enlarged liver margin, accompanied by enlarged cervical lymph glands, are usual.

As well as blood tests to assess liver function, there are specific virological tests to identify the five infective agents, and these are important contributions to diagnosis. However, there is no specific treatment of any of these infections. The more seriously ill patients may require hospital care, mainly to enable doctors to spot at an early stage those developing acute liver failure. If vomiting is a problem, intravenous fluid and glucose can be given. Therapeutic drugs – especially sedatives and hypnotics – should be avoided, and alcohol must not be taken during the acute phase. Interferon is the only licensed drug for the treatment of chronic hepatitis B, but this is used with care.

Otherwise-fit patients under 40 with acute viral hepatitis have a mortality rate of around 0.5 per cent; for those over 60, this figure is around 3 per cent. Up to 95 per cent of adults with acute HBV infection recover fully but the rest may develop life-long chronic hepatitis, particularly those who are immunodeficient (see IMMUNODEFICIENCY).

Infection is best prevented by good living conditions. HVA and HVB can be prevented by active immunisation with vaccines. There is no vaccine available for viruses C, D and E, although HDV is effectively prevented by immunisation against HBV. At-risk groups who should be vaccinated against HBV include:

- Parenteral drug abusers.
- Close contacts of infected individuals such as regular sexual partners and infants of infected mothers.
- Men who have sex with men.
- Patients undergoing regular haemodialysis.
- Selected health professionals, including laboratory staff dealing with blood samples and products.

Hepatocyte

The main cell type present in the LIVER. A large cell, it has several important metabolic functions: these include synthesis and storage of biochemical products; detoxification of poisons and unwanted substances; and the manufacture of BILE, the liver secretion that passes through the bile ducts to the small intestine and helps in the digestion of fat.

Hepatolenticular Degeneration

See WILSON'S DISEASE.

Hepatoma

A primary malignant tumour of LIVER cells. It has marked geographical variation, being most common in parts of Africa and the Far East. It is more common in men and with those who have pre-existing CIRRHOSIS.

Hepatomegaly

Enlargement of the LIVER. This may be caused by congestion (e.g. in heart failure), infection (e.g. HEPATITIS), malignancy, inflammation, or early CIRRHOSIS.

Hepolenticular Degeneration

See WILSON'S DISEASE.

Herbal Medicine

The use of herbs as medicines is probably as old as mankind; every culture has its own traditions. Herbalism was formally established in England by an Act of Parliament during Henry VIII's reign. Different parts of a variety of plants are used to treat symptoms and to restore functions.

Heredity

The principle on which various peculiarities of bodily form or structure, or of physical or mental activity, are transmitted from parents to offspring. (See also GENES.)

Hermaphrodite

An individual in whom both ovarian (see OVARIES) and testicular (see TESTICLE) tissue is present. Hermaphrodites may have a testis on one side and an ovary on the other; or an ovotestis on one side and an ovary or testis on the other; or there may be an ovotestis on both sides. Both gonads are usually intra-abdominal. The true hermaphrodite usually has a UTERUS and at least one Fallopian tube (see FALLOPIAN TUBES) on the side of the ovary, and on the side of the testis there is usually a VAS DEFERENS. Most true hermaphrodites are raised as males, but external virilisation is not usually complete. Even when significant phallic development is present, HYPOSPADIAS and CRYPTORCHIDISM are common. At puberty, GYNAECOMASTIA develops and MENSTRUATION is common, as ovarian function is usually more nearly normal than testicular function. The condition is rare. A more common condition is pseudohermaphroditism: these are individuals who possess the gonads of only one sex but whose external genitalia may be ambiguous. The cause is a hormonal imbalance and can usually be corrected by hormone treatment.

Hernia

The protrusion of an organ, or part of an organ, through the wall of the cavity that normally contains it. The most common types of hernia involve the organs of the abdomen which can herniate externally through the abdominal wall, or internally usually through a defect in the diaphragm. External hernias appear as a swelling, covered with skin, which bulges out on coughing or straining but which can normally be made to disappear with gentle pressure.

Types Inguinal hernia appears in the groin; less common is femoral hernia, which appears just below the groin. Incisional hernia may occur through a defect in any abdominal surgical scar, a paraumbilical hernia arising just to the side of the umbilicus and an epigastric hernia in the mid line above the umbilicus. In children, herniation may occur through the umbilicus itself, which is a natural weak spot. The commonest internal hernia is a hiatus hernia, when part of the stomach slips upwards into the chest through the DIAPHRAGM (see diagram).

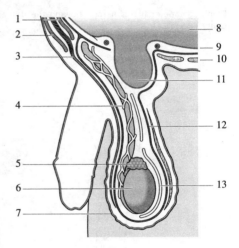

1 transverse abdominis muscle
2 external oblique muscle
3 internal oblique muscle
4 spermatic cord
5 epidydimis
6 testis
7 scrotum
8 abdominal contents
9 abdominal peritoneum
10 rectus femoris
11 abdominal peritoneum
    intruding to form hernial sac
12 internal spermatic fascia
13 tunica vaginalis

Anatomy of indirect inguinal hernia: area 11 is where the displaced loop of intestine intrudes into scrotum.

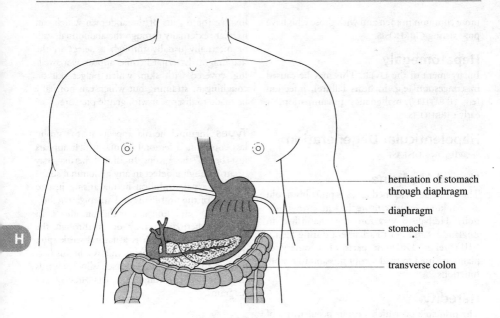

Diaphragmatic or hiatus hernia showing the stomach pushing through the diaphragm into the chest cavity.

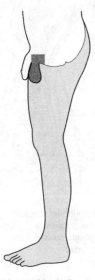

Site of inguinal hernia (shaded).

Causes Hernias may be due to a defect present at birth (congenital), or may develop later in life (acquired). Acquired hernias arise due to the development of a defect or injury of the abdominal wall or due to increased pressure within the abdominal cavity, which forces the organ through a potential weakness. Such causes include chronic coughing or excessive straining due to constipation.

Complications Small hernias may cause no problems at all. However, some may be large and cumbersome, or may give rise to a dragging sensation or even pain.

Although most reduce spontaneously under the effects of gravity or gentle pressure, any organs that may have been displaced inside some hernias may become stuck, when they are said to be irreducible. If the contents become so trapped that their blood supply is cut off, then strangulation occurs. This is a surgical emergency because the strangulated organs will soon die or rupture. When strangulation – usually of a loop of intestine – does occur, the hernia becomes irreducible, red, and very painful. If the hernia contains bowel, then the bowel may also become obstructed.

Treatment Conservative treatment with a compression belt, or truss, is now used only for those unfit for surgery or while awaiting surgery. Surgical repair can be at an open operation or by laparoscope, and consists of returning the herniated organs to their proper place and then repairing the defect through which the hernia occurred. This may be done safely under local or general anaesthetic, often as a day-case procedure, and most operative repairs result in a permanent cure.

Hernioplasty
A surgical technique for repair of a HERNIA.

The abnormal opening is sewn up or the weakness strengthened with sutures or the insertion of a polypropylene mesh.

Herniorraphy

Surgical repair of a HERNIA. This may be done as an open operation or as MINIMALLY INVASIVE SURGERY (MIS) using a LAPAROSCOPE.

Herniotomy

The surgical removal of the sac of connective tissue surrounding a HERNIA. In children or healthy young adults with an inguinal hernia, a herniotomy is usually sufficient to cure the condition.

Heroin

Also known as diacetyl morphine or diamorphine, this Class A controlled drug is an opiate – a group which includes morphine, codeine, pethidine and methadone. It is a powerful analgesic and cough suppressant, but its capacity to produce euphoria rapidly induces DEPENDENCE. Popular with addicts, its mostly pleasant effects soon produce TOLERANCE; the need to inject the drug, with associated risks of HIV infection, has affected its use by addicts. Withdrawal symptoms include restlessness, insomnia, muscle cramps, vomiting and diarrhoea; signs include dilated pupils, raised pulse rate, and disturbed temperature control. Although rarely life-threatening, the effects of withdrawal may cause great distress, and for this reason methadone, which has a slower and less severe withdrawal syndrome, is commonly used when weaning addicts off heroin. Legally still available to doctors in the UK, heroin is normally only used in patients with severe pain, or to comfort the dying.

Herpangina

Herpangina is a short febrile illness in which minute vesicles or punched-out ulcers develop in the posterior parts of the mouth. It is due to infection with the group A COXSACKIE VIRUSES.

Herpes Genitalis

An infection of the genitals (see GENITALIA) of either sex, caused by HERPES SIMPLEX virus type 2. It is mostly acquired as a result of sexual activity; some cases are caused by simplex type 1. After initial infection the virus lies latent in the dorsal nerve root ganglion (of the spinal cord) which enervates the affected area of the skin. Latent virus is never cured and reactivation results in either a recurrence of symptoms or in asymptomatic shedding of the virus which then infects a sexual partner. Around 30,000 cases of genital herpes are reported annually from clinics dealing with SEXUALLY TRANSMITTED DISEASES (STDS) in England, but there are also many unrecognised (by either patient or doctor) infections. Patients may have a history of painful attacks of ulceration of the genitals for many years before seeking medical advice. All patients with a first episode of the infection should be given oral antiviral treatment, and those who suffer more than six attacks a year should be considered for suppressive antiviral treatment. ACICLOVIR, valaciclovir and famciclovir are all effective antiviral drugs. If a woman in the final three months of her pregnancy contracts herpes genitalis, this can have serious consequences for the baby as he or she will be at risk of herpes encephalitis after delivery.

Herpes Simplex

An acute infectious disease, characterised by the development of groups of superficial vesicles, or blebs, in the skin and mucous membrane. It is due to either simplex type 1 or 2 virus, and infection can occur at any time from birth onwards; however the usual time for primary infection with type 1 is between the second and 15th year. Once an individual is infected, the virus persists in the body for the rest of their life. It is one of the causes of scrum-pox. Type 2 causes HERPES GENITALIS.

Symptoms Symptoms vary with the age of infection. In young infants, herpes simplex may cause a generalised infection which is sometimes fatal. In young children the infection is usually in the mouth, and this may be associated with enlargement of the glands in the neck, general irritability and fever. The condition usually settles in 7–10 days. In adults the vesicles may occur anywhere in the skin or mucous membranes: the more common sites are the lips, mouth and face, where they are known as cold sores. The vesicles may also appear on the genitalia (herpes genitalis) or in the conjunctiva or cornea of the EYE, and the brain may be infected, causing ENCEPHALITIS or MENINGITIS. The first sign is the appearance of small painful swellings; these quickly develop into vesicles which contain clear fluid and are surrounded by a reddened area of skin. Some people are particularly liable to recurrent attacks, and these often tend to be associated with some debilitating condition or infection, such as pneumonia.

Except in the case of herpes of the cornea, the eruption clears completely unless it becomes contaminated with some other organism. In the case of the cornea, there may be residual scarring, which may impair vision.

Treatment Aciclovir is effective both topically as cream or eye drops or orally. In severe systemic infections it can be given intravenously.

Herpes Viruses

One member of a group of viruses containing DNA which cause latent infections in animals and humans. Viruses from this group cause HERPES SIMPLEX, HERPES ZOSTER (shingles) and CHICKENPOX, and include CYTOMEGALOVIRUS (CCMV) and EPSTEIN-BARR VIRUS.

Herpes Zoster

Herpes zoster, or shingles, is a skin eruption of acute nature, closely related to CHICKENPOX and consisting in the appearance of small yellow vesicles, which spread over an area, dry up, and heal by scabbing. It receives its name from the Greek word for a 'circingle' or girdle, because it spreads in a zone-like manner along the intercostal nerves around half the chest. Herpes of the face also occurs, particularly on the brow and around the eye.

Causes Shingles is due to the same virus that causes chickenpox. This invades the ganglia of the nerves, particularly the spinal nerves of the chest and the fifth cranial nerve which supplies the face. Despite being due to the same virus as chickenpox, it is rare for herpes zoster to occur as a result of contact with a case of chickenpox. On the other hand, it is not unusual for a patient with herpes zoster to infect a child with chickenpox. It is a disease of adults rather than children, and the older the person, the more likely he or she is to develop the disease. Thus in adults under 50, the incidence is around 2·5 per 1,000 people a year; between 50 and 60 it is around 5 per 1,000; whilst in octogenarians it is 10 per 1,000. Occasionally it may be associated with some serious underlying disease such as LEUKAEMIA, LYMPHADENOMA, or multiple myeloma (see MYELOMATOSIS).

Symptoms The first symptoms are much like those of any feverish attack. The person feels unwell for some days, has a slight rise of temperature, and feels vague pain in the side or in various other parts. Often the area of skin to be affected feels hypersensitive (hyperaesthesia) as though something were rubbing on it. The pain finally settles at a point in the side, and, two or three days after the first symptoms, the rash appears. Minute yellow blebs – or vesicles, as they are known – are seen on the skin of the back, of the side, or of the front of the chest, or simultaneously on all three, the points corresponding to the space between one pair of ribs right around. These blebs increase in number for some days, and spread until there is often a complete half-girdle around one side of the chest. The pain in this stage is severe, but it appears to vary a good deal with age, being slight in children and very severe in old people, in whom indeed herpes sometimes forms a serious illness. After one or two weeks, most of the vesicles have dried up and formed scabs. The pain may not pass off when the eruption disappears, but may remain for weeks or even months – a condition known as post-herpetic NEURALGIA. Old people are prone to develop this condition.

Treatment ACICLOVIR or famciclovir can be given orally, and are effective if started in large doses early in the attack. Later, topical antibiotics may be required. Analgesics may be necessary if neuralgia is severe.

Hertz

The SI (International System of Units) unit of frequency. It indicates the number of cycles per second (c/s). The abbreviation for hertz is Hz.

Heterograft

A transplant from one animal to another of a different species. It is also known as a xenograft.

Heterosexual

Sexual attraction to individuals of the opposite sex. (See also HOMOSEXUALITY.)

Heterozygous

An individual having dissimilar members of the pair of genes coding for a given characteristic (see GENES).

Hexachlorophene

A widely used antiseptic (see ANTISEPTICS) which is active against a range of micro-organisms, including gram-positive and gram-negative organisms (see GRAM'S STAIN), *Shigella dysenteriae*, and *Salmonella typhi*. One of its advantages is that it retains its activity in the presence of soap, and is therefore often used in soaps and creams in a concentration of 1–2 per cent. It must be used with caution in babies as it can be absorbed through the skin and prove harmful. Hexachlorophene must not be used on burned or excoriated skin.

Hexamine

A substance which, when excreted by the kidneys, releases formaldehyde which has an antiseptic action. It is given to patients with recurrent CYSTITIS. It acts only in urine with an acid reaction, and, if the urine is alkaline, ascorbic acid may acidify it. Hexamine is used prophylactically and for long-term treatment of recurrent urinary-tract infections.

Hg

The chemical symbol for mercury. BLOOD PRESSURE was traditionally measured in millimetres (mm) of mercury using a SPHYGMOMANOMETER consisting of an inflatable cuff (usually wrapped round the upper arm) connected by a rubber tube to a column of mercury calibrated in mm of mercury.

Hiatus Hernia

A displacement of a portion of the stomach through the opening in the diaphragm through which the oesophagus passes from the chest to the abdominal cavity (see HERNIA).

Hiccup

An involuntary spasmodic contraction of the DIAPHRAGM which produces an indrawing of breath during which there is a sudden closure of the vocal cords. This results in the well-known sound and sensation. It is usually of benign cause (e.g. indigestion) but may be a symptom of medullary brain damage, URAEMIA, typhoid fever (see ENTERIC FEVER) or ENCEPHALITIS lethargica. There are many folk remedies for hiccups, but most cases subside spontaneously. Prolonged hiccups due to disease may respond to treatment with CHLORPROMAZINE or HALOPERIDOL.

High Dependency Unit

A hospital unit equipped and staffed to nurse patients who require a high level of technically supported care. Patients are usually moved to such units when they have made satisfactory progress in an INTENSIVE THERAPY UNIT (ITU) and do not require the one-to-one nursing necessary in ITUs. Patients who have undergone major surgery are often transferred from the recovery ward to a high dependency unit until they are well enough to be cared for in a standard ward.

Hilum

A term applied to the depression on organs such as the lung, kidney, and spleen, at which the vessels and nerves enter it and around which the lymphatic glands cluster. The hilum of the lung is also known as its root.

Hindbrain

That part of the BRAIN comprising the cerebellum, pons and medulla oblongata.

Hip

That part of the body on each side of the pelvis where it articulates with the head of the femur (thigh bone).

Hip-Joint

The joint formed by the head of the thigh bone and the deep, cup-shaped hollow on the side of the pelvis which receives it (acetabulum). The joint is of the ball-and-socket variety, is dislocated only by very great violence, and is correspondingly difficult to reduce to its natural state after dislocation. It is enclosed by a capsule of fibrous tissue, strengthened by several bands, of which the principal is the ilio-femoral or Y-shaped ligament placed in front of the joint. A round ligament also unites the head of the thigh bone to the margin of the acetabulum.

For hip-joint disease, see under JOINTS, DISEASES OF.

Hippocrates

A famous Greek physician who lived from c.460 to 377 BC and who taught students at the medical school in Cos. Often called the 'father of medicine', he is renowned for drawing up the HIPPOCRATIC OATH, some of which may have been derived from the ancient oath of the Aesclepiads. Apart from his oath, Hippocrates has about 60 other medical works attributed to him, forming a corpus which was collected around 250 BC in the famous library of Alexandria in Egypt. Hippocratic medicine appealed 'to reason rather than to rules or to supernatural forces' is how the late Roy Porter, the English social historian, summed up its ethos in his medical history, *The Greatest Benefit to Mankind* (Harper Collins, 1997). Porter also commended Hippocrates as being patient-centred rather than disease-orientated in his practice of medicine.

Hippocratic Oath

An oath once (but no longer) taken by doctors on qualification, setting out the moral precepts of their profession and binding them to a code of behaviour and practice aimed at protecting the interests of their patients. The oath is named after HIPPOCRATES (460–377 BC), the Greek 'father of medicine'. Almost half of British medical students and 98 per cent of American ones make a ceremonial commitment to assume the responsibilities and obligations of the medical profession, but not by reciting this oath.

Hippus

Hippus is a tremor of the iris which produces alternating contraction and dilatation of the pupil (see EYE).

Hirschsprung's Disease

Hirschsprung's disease, or MEGACOLON, is a rare congenital disorder characterised by great hypertrophy and dilatation of the colon (see INTESTINE). The RECTUM and lower colon have failed to develop a normal nerve network, thus disturbing normal contraction and expansion of these structures. Treatment is surgical removal of the affected sections, with the remaining colon being joined to the anus.

Hirsutism

The growth of hair of the male type and distribution in women. It is due either to the excess production of androgens (see ANDROGEN), or to undue sensitivity of the hair follicle to normal female levels of circulating androgens. The latter is called idiopathic hirsutism, because the cause is unknown. The increased production of androgens in the female may come from the ovary (see OVARIES) and be due to POLYCYSTIC OVARY SYNDROME or an ovarian tumour, or the excess androgen may come from the adrenal cortex (see ADRENAL GLANDS) and be the result of congenital adrenal HYPERPLASIA, an adrenal tumour or CUSHING'S SYNDROME. However, there is a wide range of normality in the distribution of female body hair. It varies with different racial groups: the Mediterranean races have more body hair than Nordic women, and the Chinese and Japanese have little body hair. It is not abnormal for many women, especially those with dark hair, to have hair apparent on the upper lip, and a few coarse hairs on the chin and around the nipples are not uncommon. Extension of the pubic hair towards the umbilicus is also frequently found. Dark hair is much more apparent than fair hair, and this is why bleaching is of considerable benefit in the management of hirsutism.

The treatment of hirsutism is that of the primary cause. Idiopathic hirsutism must be managed by simple measures such as bleaching the hair and the use of depilatory waxes and creams. Coarse facial hairs can be removed by electrolysis, although this is time-consuming. Shaving is often the most effective remedy and neither increases the rate of hair growth nor causes the hairs to become coarser.

Histamine

An amine (see AMINES) derived from HISTIDINE. It is widely distributed in the tissues of plants and animals, including humans. It is a powerful stimulant of gastric juice, a constrictor of smooth muscle including that of the bronchi, and a dilator of arterioles and capillaries. It is this last action which is responsible for the eruption of URTICARIA.

Histidine

An amino acid from which HISTAMINE is derived.

Histiocytoma

See DERMATOFIBROMA.

Histology

The study of the minute structure of the tissues using special staining processes which are combined with electron and light microscopy. The specialty is staffed by medically qualified pathologists (histologists) and scientifically qualified technicians.

Histoplasmosis

A disease due to a yeast-like fungus known as *Histoplasma capsulatum*. Most cases have been reported from the USA. In infants it is characterised by fever, ANAEMIA, enlargement of the liver and spleen, and involvement of the lungs and gastrointestinal tract. In older children it may resemble pulmonary tuberculosis, whilst in adults it may be confined to involvement of the skin.

HIV

Human immunodeficiency virus: the virus that is responsible for AIDS (see AIDS/HIV). It is one of the family of human T-cell lymphocytotrophic viruses, others of which may cause lymphomas (see LYMPHOMA) in humans.

Hives

A popular term applied to eruptions of URTICARIA.

HLA System

The major histocompatibility complex, or human leucocyte antigen (HLA) region, consists of genetically determined antigens, situated on chromosome 6. Found in most tissues, though to a differing extent, the four gene loci are known as A, B, C, D, while the individual alleles at each locus are numbered 1, 2, 3, etc. The number of possible combinations is thus enormous, and the chance of two unrelated people being identical for HLA is very low.

HLA incompatibility causes the immune response, or rejection reaction, that occurs with unmatched tissue grafts. Strong associations between HLA and susceptibility to certain diseases – notably the AUTOIMMUNE DISORDERS such as rheumatoid arthritis, insulin-dependent diabetes, and thyrotoxicosis – have been described. Certain HLA antigens occur together more frequently than would be expected by chance (linkage disequilibrium), and may have a protective effect, conferring resistance to a disease. (See IMMUNITY.)

Hodgkin's Disease
See LYMPHOMA.

Holistic
A term used for a method of medical care in which patients are treated as a whole, and which takes into account their physical and mental state as well as social background rather than just treating the disease alone.

Homatropine
Homatropine is an alkaloid derived from ATROPINE, which is used to produce dilatation of the pupil (see EYE) and to paralyse ACCOMMODATION temporarily for the purpose of examining the interior of the eye. It is used in 1 per cent solution, and its effects last a few hours.

Homeopathy
A system of medicine founded by Hahnemann at the end of the 18th century. It is based upon the theory that diseases are curable by those drugs which produce effects on the body similar to symptoms caused by the disease (similia similibus curantur). In administering drugs, the theory is also held that their effect is increased by giving them in minute doses obtained by substantially diluting them.

Homeostasis
The normal physiological process which ensures that the body's internal systems, such as its metabolism, blood pressure and body temperature, maintain an equilibrium whatever the conditions of the outside environment. For example, the body temperature remains at around 37 °C (98.4 °F) in a cold or a hot climate.

Homocysteine
An intermediate product in the body's synthesis of the amino acid CYSTEINE.

Homocystinuria
Homocystinuria is a congenital disease due to the inability of the affected individual to metabolise, or to utilise properly, one of the essential AMINO ACIDS known as methionine. The main features of the condition are abnormality of the lens of the EYE, learning disability, and a tendency to thromboses (blood clots).

Homograft
A piece of tissue or an organ, such as a kidney, transplanted from one animal to another of the same species: for example, from person to person. It is also known as an allograft.

Homosexuality
Sexual activity with a member of the same sex. There has been considerable debate among psychiatrists as to whether homosexuality should be regarded as a normal sexual variant or as a psycho-pathological development or deviation. Although homosexuality is found in virtually every society and culture, there is no society in which it is the predominant or preferred mode of sexual activity. Various attempts have been made to link homosexuality to hormonal factors, particularly lowered TESTOSTERONE levels, or to find a genetic explanation, but there is no evidence for either. Psychoanalytic theories link homosexuality to early child-rearing influences, in particular the close-binding and intimate mother.

The number of homosexual men and women in the UK is unknown. Re-analysis of the Kinsey report suggests that only 3 per cent of adult men have exclusively homosexual leanings and a further 3 per cent have extensive homosexual and heterosexual experience. Homosexuality among women (lesbianism) seems to be less common. Some homosexual men have high rates of sexual activity and multiple partners and, as with heterosexual men and women, this increases the risk of acquiring sexually transmitted diseases, unless appropriate precautionary measures are taken – for example, the use of condoms for penetrative sex, whether vaginal or anal. It was in homosexual males that the virus responsible for AIDS (see AIDS/HIV) was first identified, but the infection now occurs in both sexes.

Homozygous
An individual having identical members of the pair of genes coding for a given characteristic (see GENES).

Hookworm
See ANCYLOSTOMIASIS.

Hormone Replacement Therapy (HRT)
See under MENOPAUSE.

Hormones
These are 'chemical messengers' that are dispersed by the blood and act on target organs to produce effects distant from their point of release. The main organs involved in hormone production are the PITUITARY GLAND, PANCREAS, ovary (see OVARIES), testis (see TESTICLE), THYROID GLAND, and ADRENAL GLANDS. The release of many hormones is, ultimately, under the control of the central nervous system via a series of inhibiting and releasing factors from the HYPOTHALAMUS. Hormones are involved in maintaining homeostasis: for example, insulin regulates the concentration of glucose in the blood. They also participate in growth and maturation: for example, growth hormone promotes growth and helps to regulate fat, carbohydrate, and protein metabolism; and the sex hormones promote sexual maturation and reproduction. (See also ENDOCRINE GLANDS.)

Horner's Syndrome
This is the description given to a combination of changes resulting from paralysis of the sympathetic nerve in the neck. They are: a small pupil; a drooping upper lid; and an apparently (though not actually) sunken eye.

Horseshoe Kidney
See KIDNEYS, DISEASES OF.

Hospice
A hospital that cares only for the terminally ill and dying. The emphasis is on providing quality of life, and special care is taken in providing pain relief by whichever methods are deemed best suited to the person's needs. Hospice care in the United Kingdom has been greatly developed, in particular with the leadership of Dr (Dame) Cicely Saunders. Many hospices are funded by charitable funds and their activities supported by voluntary workers.

Hospital
An institution providing treatment for sick and injured persons. This may be done on an inpatient or outpatient basis. A hospital provides investigative and therapeutic services which are not available on a domiciliary basis.

Hospitals are broadly divided into general hospitals (available in each district in the United Kingdom) and hospitals specialising in particular ailments (e.g. ophthalmology; ear,

nose and throat; neurology, etc.). In addition there are teaching hospitals which have the dual function of patient care and the education of medical staff. (See NATIONAL HEALTH SERVICE (NHS).)

In the UK all patients are entitled to hospital care provided by their NHS trust when referred by their GENERAL PRACTITIONER (GP) or admitted via the Accident & Emergency department. (In exceptional cases, patients with severe mental illness can be compulsorily admitted by the authorities.) Admission will depend on clinical priority, as demand commonly exceeds supply of beds in some localities. Private hospital care is available under the care of a consultant of choice, provided that the patient is covered by appropriate private medical insurance or can pay direct the substantial hospital and medical fees.

The future development of hospital medicine is controversial, but the long-term future may well see many fewer, much better equipped, highly specialised hospitals for patients requiring high-technology-based treatments. These might be backed up with a range of smaller general (or halfway) hospitals caring for patients with less demanding clinical needs who nevertheless require some bed-based care. Many more patients requiring routine specialist treatment will be treated as day patients than is the case now, and there will (or should) be much greater emphasis (with appropriate resources) on PREVENTIVE MEDICINE.

Britain is experimenting with a prototype 'virtual hospital'. The project will target hospital patients who need to remain under the care of specialists but whose condition can be managed at home. Suitable NHS patients will be provided with monitoring equipment that enables them, for example, to read their own blood pressure, lung and heart functions, with the results transferred electronically to the office of relevant specialists who will prescribe and monitor treatment.

Hospital-Acquired Infection
An infection acquired by a patient while in hospital. Because of the high level of antibiotic use in hospitals, some bacteria become resistant – for example, METHICILLIN-RESISTANT STAPHYLOCOCCUS AUREUS (MRSA). This makes hospital-acquired infections potentially dangerous and sometimes life-threatening, and is one of the developments that is prompting calls for greater care in the prescribing of antibiotics as well as higher standards of cleanliness.

Hospital Chaplaincy

A service provided by a religious denomination, primarily aimed at meeting the spiritual and religious needs of patients in hospitals. In the UK, NHS hospital trusts employ both full-time and part-time chaplains, usually representing the mainline Christian churches (Anglican, Free and Roman Catholic). Their duties vary but always at the least involve meeting the specifically religious needs of patients as well as of relatives and staff who may ask for help. Public services in chapels, the bedside administration of the Word and Sacraments, and prayers and radio services are among chaplains' duties. When requested by patients, chaplains also liaise with representatives of other world faiths.

Chaplains have a broad responsibility for the spiritual health care of all in hospital. They share this with other staff members, particularly the nursing staff, for whom the chaplains can be a resource. Chaplains also train and use volunteers from local churches to help with ward visiting and other chaplaincy duties. Much of the time spent with patients takes the form of a listening ministry, helping patients to find their own answers to what is happening to them in hospital and in life generally. Spiritual health can be seen as a quest for the right relationships in four areas – with other people; with oneself; with the world around; and with 'Life' itself. The religious person subsumes all that in his/her relationship to God.

The link between spiritual disease and physical ill-health is well established; the chaplain therefore helps a hospital to provide a HOLISTIC approach to health care. Chaplains also give time to the care of staff who face increasing levels of stress at work, making use of support groups, counselling, meditation, etc. Chaplains support patients' relatives facing a crisis, for example, by being with them over the period of a death, and by providing regular bereavement services for those who have lost babies. Some chaplains have a particular expertise in ETHICS and are members of the various hospital ethics committees. A chaplain may have a 'non-management' view of the health of the hospital itself, which can be of use to hospital management. (See also SPIRITUAL PAIN.)

Host

An organism on which a parasite lives.

Hour-Glass Stomach

The term given to the X-ray appearance of a stomach which is constricted in its middle part due either to spasm of the stomach muscle or to contraction of scar tissue from a gastric ulcer.

Housemaid's Knee

An inflammation of the bursa in front of the knee-cap, often mistaken for some disease in the joint itself (see BURSITIS).

HRT

Hormone Replacement Therapy – see under MENOPAUSE.

HSE

See HEALTH AND SAFETY EXECUTIVE (HSE).

Human Chorionic Gonadotrophin

A glycoprotein hormone secreted by the PLACENTA in early pregnancy, and stimulating the CORPUS LUTEUM within the ovary (see OVARIES) to secrete OESTROGENS, PROGESTERONE, and relaxin. The hormone is essential for the maintenance of pregnancy up to about 6–8 weeks of gestation. A RADIOIMMUNOASSAY can be used to detect its presence, and pregnancy can be diagnosed as early as six days after conception by testing for it in the urine. Some tumours also secrete human chorionic gonadotrophin, particularly HYDATIDIFORM MOLE, which produces large amounts.

Human Fertilisation & Embryology Act 1990

See ASSISTED CONCEPTION.

Human Fertilisation & Embryology Authority (HFEA)

See ASSISTED CONCEPTION.

Human Genome

In simple terms, this is the genetic recipe for making a human being. GENOME is a combination of the words gene and chromosome, and a genome is defined as all the genetic material – known as deoxyribonucleic acid, or DNA – in a cell. Most genes encode sequences of AMINO ACIDS, the constituents of proteins, thus initiating and controlling the replication of an organism. The identification and characterisation of the human genetic puzzle have been a key bioscience research target. The Human Genome Project was launched in 1990 (and completed in 2003) to produce a full sequence of the three million base pairs that make up the human genome.

Carried out as two separate exercises – one by a privately funded American team; another by an international joint venture between tax-funded American laboratories, a charitably funded British one and several other smaller research teams from around the world – the first results were announced on 26 June 2000. In February 2001 the privately funded American group, known as Celera Genomics, announced that it had identified 26,558 genes. At the same time the Human Genome Project consortium reported that it had identified 31,000. Allowing for margins of error, this gives a figure much lower than the 100,000 or more human genes previously forecast by scientists. Interestingly, genes were found to make up only 3 per cent of the human genome. The remaining 97 per cent of the genome comprises non-coding DNA which, though not involved in producing the protein-initiating genetic activity, does have significant roles in the structure, function and evolution of the genome.

One surprise from the Project so far is that the genetic differences between humans and other species seem much smaller than previously expected. For example, the Celera team found that people have only 300 genes that mice do not have; yet, the common ancestor of mice and men probably lived 100 million years or more in the past. Mice and humans, however, have around twice as many genes as the humble fruit fly.

Cells die out when they become redundant during embryonic development: genes also die out during evolution, according to evidence from the Genome Project – a finding that supports the constant evolutionary changes apparent in living things; the Darwinian concept of survival of the fittest.

Apart from expanding our scientific knowledge, the new information – and promise of much more as the Genome Project continues – should enhance and expand the use of genetic engineering in the prevention and cure of disease. Studies are in progress on the gene for a receptor protein in the brain which will shed light on how the important neurotransmitter SEROTONIN in the brain works, and this, for example, should help the development of better drugs for the treatment of DEPRESSION. Another gene has been found that is relevant to the development of ASTHMA and yet another that is involved in the production of amyloid, a complex protein which is deposited in excessive amounts in both DOWN'S (DOWN) SYNDROME and ALZHEIMER'S DISEASE.

Human Immunodeficiency Virus
See AIDS/HIV.

Human Leucocyte Antigen (HLA)
See HLA SYSTEM.

Human Organs Transplants Act
UK legislation that lays down the framework and rules governing organ transplantation. The UK Transplant Support Service Authority (UKTSSA), a special health authority set up in 1991, is responsible for administering the NHS Organ Donor Registry and the Act (see APPENDIX 7: STATUTORY ORGANISATIONS).

Humerus
The bone of the upper arm. It has a rounded head, which helps to form the shoulder-joint, and at its lower end presents a wide pulley-like surface for union with the radius and ulna. Its epicondyles form the prominences at the sides of the elbow.

Humidification
The air we breathe must be moist for the efficient working of the lungs (see RESPIRATION). Humidification, or moistening of the air, is achieved largely by the NOSE, which acts as an air-conditioner, warming, moistening and filtering the 10,000 litres of air which we inhale daily – in the process of which, incidentally, it produces around 1·5 litres of secretion daily.

Humidity is expressed as relative humidity (RH). This is the amount of moisture in the air expressed as a percentage of the maximum possible at that temperature. If the temperature of a room is raised without increasing the moisture content, the RH falls. The average outdoor RH in Britain is around 70–80 per cent; with central heating it may drop to 25 per cent or lower. This is why humidification, as it is known, of the air is essential in buildings heated by modern heating systems. The aim should be to keep the RH at around 30–50 per cent. In houses this may be achieved quite satisfactorily by having a jug or basin of water in the room, or some receptacle that can be attached to the heater. In offices, some more elaborate form of humidifier is necessary. Those suffering from chronic BRONCHITIS are particularly susceptible to dry air, as are those individuals with disorders of the EYE because the secretions that bathe the eyes and keep them moist are unnaturally dried out. (See also VENTILATION.)

Humidifier Fever
A form of ALVEOLITIS caused by contamination of the water used to humidify, or moisten, the air in air-conditioning plants. The breathing of the contaminated air results in infection of the lung, which is characterised by fever, cough, shortness of breath and malaise – worse on Monday and tending to improve during the

course of the week. (See also LEGIONNAIRE'S DISEASE.)

Humour

An archaic term once used for a theory regarding the causation of disease as due to an improper mixture in the body of blood, bile, phlegm and black bile. The term remains in describing some body fluids, such as the aqueous and vitreous humours of the EYE.

Hunger

A craving for food or other substance necessary to bodily activity. Hunger for food is supposed to be directly produced by strong contractions of the stomach which occur when it is empty, or nearly so. (See also THIRST.)

Air hunger is an instinctive craving for oxygen resulting in breathlessness, either when a person ascends to great heights where the pressure of air is low, or in some diseases such as pneumonia and DIABETES MELLITUS which affect the body's METABOLISM and therefore its need for oxygen – an essential constituent in this process.

Huntington's Chorea

A hereditary disease characterised by involuntary movements and DEMENTIA. Each child of a parent with the disease has a 50:50 chance of developing it. Onset is most common between the ages of 35 and 45, but 10 per cent of cases occur under the age of 20. Some patients show more severe mental disturbance; others more severe disturbances of movement; but in all it pursues an inexorable downward course over a period of 10–20 years to a terminal state of physical and mental helplessness. It is estimated that there are around 6,000 cases in Britain. The defective gene (located on chromosome no. 4) has now been identified and GENETIC SCREENING is possible for those at risk. People with Huntington's chorea and their relatives can obtain help and guidance from Huntington's Disease Association.

Hurler's Syndrome

See GARGOYLISM.

Hutchinson's Teeth

The term applied to the narrowed and notched permanent incisor teeth which occur in congenital SYPHILIS. They are so-named after Sir Jonathan Hutchinson (1828–1913), the London physician who first described them.

Hyaline

Tissue material that has a glass-like appearance when stained and viewed under the microscope. It occurs in a variety of tissues and diseases, particularly ACUTE RESPIRATORY DISTRESS SYNDROME (ARDS), hyaline degeneration of arterioles, and alcoholic liver disease.

Hyaline Membrane Disease

A form of ACUTE RESPIRATORY DISTRESS SYNDROME (ARDS) found in premature infants and some of those born by CAESAREAN SECTION, characterised by the onset of difficulty in breathing a few hours after birth. Most require extra oxygen and many need mechanical ventilation for a few days or even weeks. Recovery is the rule, although the most severely affected may die or suffer damage from oxygen lack. In this condition the ALVEOLITIS and the finer BRONCHIOLES of the lungs are lined with a dense membrane. The cause of the condition is a deficiency of SURFACTANT in the lung passages which adversely affects gas exchanges in the alveoli.

Treatment includes the full gamut of neonatal intensive care, as well as specific therapy with PULMONARY SURFACTANT.

Hyaluronidase

Hyaluronidase is an ENZYME which hydrolyses hyaluronic acid. The latter is a gel-like substance which is widely distributed throughout the body and which helps to bind together the tissue cells and also acts as a lubricant in joints. By virtue of its action in hydrolysing hyaluronic acid, hyaluronidase is now used in subcutaneous injections of fluid as it facilitates the spread of the injected fluid and therefore its absorption.

Hydatid

A cyst produced by the growth of immature forms of a tapeworm. (See TAENIASIS.)

Hydatidiform Mole

A rare complication of pregnancy, in which there is tremendous proliferation of the epithelium of the chorion (the outer of the two fetal membranes). It seldom occurs during a first pregnancy. Treatment consists of immediate evacuation of the womb.

Hydradenitis Suppurativa

A chronic inflammatory disease of the apocrine sweat glands (see PERSPIRATION). It is more common in women – in whom it usually occurs in the armpit – than in men, in whom it is most common in the perineum of the drivers of lorries and taxis. It occurs in the form of painful, tender lumps underneath the skin, which burst often in a week or so. Treatment consists of removal by operation.

Hydrallazine

A vasodilator hypotensive drug, useful as an adjunct to other treatment for HYPERTENSION.

Hydramnios

A condition characterised by excess of fluid in the amniotic cavity (see AMNION).

Hydrocarbamide

A drug used to treat chronic myeloid leukaemia (see MYELOID; LEUKAEMIA).

Hydrocephalus

An abnormal accumulation of CEREBROSPINAL FLUID, or CSF, within the skull, as a result of one or more of three main causes: (i) excessive CSF production; (ii) defective CSF absorption; (iii) blockage of the circulation of CSF. Such disturbances in the circulation of the fluid may be due to congenital reasons (most commonly associated with SPINA BIFIDA), to MENINGITIS, or to a tumour.

Symptoms In children, the chief symptoms observed are the gradual increase in size of the upper part of the head, out of all proportion to the face or the rest of the body. The head is globular, with a wide anterior FONTANELLE and separation of the bones at the sutures. The veins in the scalp are prominent, and there is a 'crackpot' note on percussion. The normal infant's head should not grow more than 2·5 cm (1 inch) in each of the first two months of life, and much more slowly subsequently; growth beyond this rate should arouse suspicions of hydrocephalus, so medical professionals caring for infants use centile charts for this purpose.

The cerebral ventricles are widely distended, and the convolutions of the brain flattened, while occasionally the fluid escapes into the cavity of the cranium, which it fills, pressing down the brain to the base of the skull. As a consequence of such changes, the functions of the brain are interfered with, and in general the mental condition of the patient is impaired. Untreated, the child is dull and listless, irritable and sometimes suffers from severe mental subnormality. The special senses become affected as the disease advances, especially vision, and sight is often lost, as is also hearing. Towards the end, paralysis is apt to occur.

Treatment Numerous ingenious operations have been devised for the treatment of hydro-cephalus. The most satisfactory of these utilise unidirectional valves and shunts (tubes), whereby the cerebrospinal fluid is bypassed from the brain into the right atrium of the heart or the peritoneal cavity. The shunt may have to be left in position indefinitely.

Hydrochloric Acid

A colourless, pungent, fuming liquid. Secreted by the parietal cells in the lining of the stomach, it aids in the digestion of the food.

Hydrochlorothiazide

See THIAZIDES.

Hydrocoele

A collection of fluid connected with the testis (see TESTICLE) or spermatic cord. When there is no obvious cause, it is classified as primary: such hydrocoeles are usually large and tense, and are commonly found in middle-aged and younger men, presenting as a large, painless scrotal swelling. Congenital hydrocoeles may occur in infants, when they are often associated with a hernial sac (see HERNIA). Hydrocoele of the cord is rare. Secondary hydrocoele is generally smaller and lax; it is usually secondary to a tumour or inflammation of the underlying testis or epididymis.

Treatment Congenital hydrocoeles usually disappear spontaneously and may be safely watched; surgery is only indicated when there is a hernia, or if the condition persists after the first year. Hydrocoeles in adults should be tapped and the testis palpated to exclude primary lesions. Primary hydrocoeles may be managed by intermittent tapping, or, preferably, by surgical removal. Secondary hydrocoeles require treatment of the underlying condition.

Hydrocortisone

Hydrocortisone has the chemical formula, 17-hydroxycorticosterone. It is closely allied to CORTISONE both in its structure (cortisone is an oxidation product of hydrocortisone) and in its action. Available in tablet, topical or injection form, hydrocortisone is used in adrenocortical insufficiency, for the suppression of local and systemic inflammatory and allergic disorders, and in the treatment of shock. Its mineralo-corticoid effects – control of salt and water balance – mean that the drug should not be used long term except as replacement therapy in the treatment of ADDISON'S DISEASE or following adrenalectomy when hydrocortisone should be given with the mineral corticoid fludrocortisone (see ADRENAL GLANDS; CORTICOSTEROIDS).

Hydrogen Peroxide

A thick colourless liquid with the formula H_2O_2 (water is H_2O, possessing only one oxygen atom in its molecule). Available in solution with water and as a cream, it is readily reduced to water – giving up oxygen in the process, which causes the characteristic frothing seen when used. H_2O_2 has antiseptic and deodorising properties; thus it is used as a mouthwash, to clean wounds and ulcers, and occasionally to disinfect body cavities at operation. It is also a bleach.

Hydromorphone Hydrochloride

A recently introduced opioid analgesic drug used to relieve severe pain in cancer. A controlled drug, it is taken in capsule form or the powder may be sprinkled over soft food.

Hydronephrosis

See KIDNEYS, DISEASES OF.

Hydrophobia

Another name for RABIES.

Hydrops Fetalis

See HAEMOLYTIC DISEASE OF THE NEWBORN.

Hydrotherapy

Treatment using water in the form of baths, douches, etc.

Hydrothorax

A collection of fluid in the pleural cavities of the lungs.

Hydroxocobalamin

Hydroxocobalamin, or vitamin B_{12}, has now replaced CYANOCOBALAMIN in the treatment of pernicious ANAEMIA. It has the practical advantage that fewer injections are required than in the case of cyanocobalamin. Like cyanocobalamin, it belongs to the group of substances known as cobalamins which have an ENZYME action in practically every metabolic system in the body and are essential for normal growth and nutrition. (See APPENDIX 5: VITAMINS.)

Hygiene

The science of health and the study of ways of its preservation, particularly by widespread education and promotion of cleanliness. Especially valuable in developing countries, where it plays a vital role in helping to limit the spread of infectious diseases.

Hymen

The thin membranous fold partially closing the lower end of the virginal VAGINA. If the opening is small, the hymen will tear at the time of first intercourse, usually with a little bleeding.

Hyoid

A U-shaped bone at the root of the tongue. The hyoid can be felt from the front of the neck, lying about 2·5 cm above the prominence of the thyroid cartilage.

Hyoscine

Also called scopalamine, this is an alkaloid (see ALKALOIDS) obtained from the plant henbane (hyoscyamus). It is an ANTICHOLINERGIC drug sometimes used as a premedicant in patients undergoing ANAESTHESIA for its sedative and antiemetic effects and for its ability to reduce saliva production. It may cause confusion in the elderly.

Hyper-

Prefix denoting abnormally increased or excessive.

Hyperactivity

A pattern of behaviour, usually in children, characterised by inability to concentrate, accompanied by overactivity. (See also ATTENTION DEFICIT DISORDER (HYPERACTIVITY SYNDROME).)

Hyperacusis

Hyperacusis means an abnormally acute sense of hearing.

Hyperaemia

Congestion or presence of an excessive amount of blood in a body part.

Hyperaesthesia

Oversensitivity of a part of the body – as found, for example, in certain neurological diseases such as HERPES ZOSTER or shingles. (See also TOUCH.)

Hyperalgesia

Excessive sensitivity to PAIN; see also TOUCH.

Hyperbaric

A pressure that is greater than that of the standard atmosphere at sea level (1,013 millibars). Hyperbaric oxygenation is a procedure in which the patient is exposed to high-pressure oxygen. The technique is used for the treatment of people suffering from CARBON MONOXIDE (CO) poisoning, compressed-air illness, gas GANGRENE and serious breathing disorders. Occasionally it is used for patients undergoing cardiac surgery.

Hypercalcaemia

A state in which the PLASMA calcium concentration is significantly raised. The most important causes are HYPERPARATHYROIDISM, malignant bone disease and other (non-metastatic) cancers, and chronic renal failure. Less common causes include SARCOIDOSIS, MYELOMATOSIS, vitamin D overdosage (see APPENDIX 5: VITAMINS), hyperthyroidism (see THYROID GLAND, DISEASES OF), and immobilisation.

Signs and symptoms A general malaise and depression are common, with generalised muscular weakness, anorexia and vomiting. Disturbed renal function causes increased urine output and thirst, with calcium deposits eventually leading to renal stones. Primary bone disease may cause pain and weakness, with an increased incidence of fractures, and there may be gritty deposits of calcium in the eyes. Severe hypercalcaemia produces ANURIA, with confusion and COMA leading to death.

Treatment The patient should be rehydrated and a diuretic (see DIURETICS) given. Attention should then be focused on the underlying cause – usually a parathyroid adenoma or bone tumour – and surgical removal should produce complete clinical cure, provided that advanced renal disease is not already present.

Hypercalciuria

An abnormally large amount of calcium in the urine. It is the most common single cause of stones in the KIDNEYS in Britain. (See HYPERCALCAEMIA.)

Hypercapnia

An abnormal increase in the amount of carbon dioxide in the blood or in the lungs (see BLOOD GASES). It may be caused by a reduced respiratory rate or effort, diseases of the chest wall and lung (affecting breathing), and cyanotic heart disease.

Hyperchlorhydria

Excessive production of hydrochloric acid in the stomach. It is a characteristic finding in certain forms of DYSPEPSIA, particularly that associated with a duodenal ulcer, and causes HEARTBURN and WATERBRASH. (See also DUODENAL ULCER; STOMACH, DISEASES OF.)

Hypercholesterolaemia
See CHOLESTEROL; HYPERLIPIDAEMIA.

Hyperemesis Gravidarum

A rare condition (less than 0·2 per cent) of pregnancy, in which there is severe vomiting. If untreated it can result in severe dehydration, ketoacidosis (an excess of KETONE acids) and liver damage. More common in multiple pregnancy, it may recur in subsequent pregnancies.

Hyperglycaemia

An excess of sugar in the blood that may occur in various diseases, typically in DIABETES MELLITUS. The normal blood glucose level in the fasting state is between 3.5 and 5.5 mmol/l blood (see APPENDIX 6: MEASUREMENTS IN MEDICINE); four or five times that amount is found in diabetes, owing to insufficient insulin in the blood, possibly accompanied by an excessive carbohydrate intake. Untreated, it may lead to diabetic coma.

Hyperidrosis
Excessive sweating (see PERSPIRATION).

Hyperkalaemia

A concentration of POTASSIUM in the PLASMA that is above the normal range. It is often caused by renal failure or by excessive intake of potassium – perhaps in a drug – and may cause cardiac dysrhythmia (abnormal rhythm of the heart).

Hyperkeratosis

Thickening of the horny (outer) layer of skin, affecting the palms of the hands and soles of the feet. The disorder may be inherited.

Hyperkinetic Syndrome
See HYPERACTIVITY.

Hyperlipidaemia

An excess of fat in the blood, characterising a group of metabolic disorders. The two most important fats circulating in the blood are CHOLESTEROL and TRIGLYCERIDE. Raised blood levels of cholesterol predispose to ATHEROMA and coronary artery disease (see HEART, DISEASES OF); raised triglycerides predispose to pancreatitis (see PANCREAS, DISORDERS OF). Six types of hyperlipidaemia have been identified, and diagnosis of the different types depends upon blood tests to discover lipid levels. Some of the hyperlipidaemias are familial, and some are secondary to other diseases such as hypothyroidism (see THYROID GLAND, DISEASES OF), DIABETES MELLITUS, nephrotic syndrome and alcoholism.

Treatment There is evidence that therapy which lowers the lipid concentration reduces the progression of premature atheroma, particularly in those who suffer from the familial disorder. Treatment should include appropriate diets, usually food that is low in cholesterol and saturated fats. There are a number of drugs available for lowering the lipid content of the plasma, but these should be reserved for patients in whom severe hyperlipidaemia is inadequately controlled by weight reduction. Anion-exchange resins – clofibrate, bezafibrate and gemfibrozil, for example – and statins such as atorvastatin and simvastatin, as well as nicotinic acid, all lower plasma cholesterol and plasma triglyceride concentration through their effect on reducing the hepatic production of lipoproteins. Cholestyramine and colestipol, both of which are anion-exchange resins, bind bile salts in the gut and so decrease the absorption of the cholesterol that these bile salts contain – hence lowering plasma cholesterol concentrations. Probucol lowers plasma cholesterol concentrations by increasing the metabolism of low-density lipoproteins.

The statins (atorvastatin, cerivastatin, fluvastatin, pravastatin and simvastatin) inhibit an enzyme involved in synthesising cholesterol, especially in the liver. They are more effective than anion-exchange resins in lowering LDL (low-density lipoprotein) cholesterol – a form of low-density cholesterol carried in the bloodstream, high levels of which are believed to be the main cause of atheroma. Statins are, however, less effective than the clofibrate group in reducing triglycerides and raising HDL (high-density lipoprotein) cholesterol (high-density cholesterol).

Hypermetropia

Hypermetropia, or hyperopia, is a term applied to long-sightedness, in which the eye is too flat from front to back and rays of light are brought to a focus behind the retina. (See EYE; VISION.)

Hypernatraemia

A SERUM sodium concentration that is above normal. The condition is usually caused by dehydration (either from inadequate intake or excessive loss of water); occasionally it may be caused by excessive sodium intake, and rarely by a raised level of ALDOSTERONE hormone.

Hypernephroma

Now named renal cell carcinoma, this is a malignant tumour resembling the tissue of the suprarenal gland and occurring in the KIDNEYS. Fever, loin pain, HAEMATURIA and swelling are among the presenting symptoms, but the tumour may be symptomless for many years. Surgical removal is the initial treatment; hypernephromas are fairly insensitive to CYTOTOXIC drugs and RADIOTHERAPY – although hormone treatment may help – and are prone to spread via the bloodstream, for example, to the lungs.

Hyperparathyroidism

Increased activity of the PARATHYROID gland. Parathyroid hormone increases SERUM calcium. Hyperparathyroidism may be primary (due to an ADENOMA or HYPERPLASIA of the gland), secondary (in response to HYPOCALCAEMIA) or tertiary (when secondary hyperparathyroidism causes the development of an autonomous adenoma).

Hyperpituitarism

Overactivity of the anterior lobe of the PITUITARY GLAND, causing ACROMEGALY (GIGANTISM).

Hyperplasia

Hyperplasia means an abnormal increase in the number of cells in a tissue.

Hyperprolactinaemia

Overproduction of the hormone PROLACTIN, usually as a result of a tumour of the PITUITARY GLAND (prolactinoma).

Hyperpyrexia

High FEVER. (See also TEMPERATURE.)

Hypersensitivity

An abnormal immunological reaction produced by some people when re-exposed to antigens that are innocuous to normal individuals. An antigen or allergen is a protein that stimulates an allergic response. This may mean that the next time the person is exposed to that antigen, there may be a dramatic health- or life-threatening reaction, such as ANAPHYLAXIS. (See also ALLERGY; IMMUNITY.)

Hypertension

Means high BLOOD PRESSURE (raised pressure of the circulating blood), but since there is a wide range of 'normal' blood pressure in the population, a precise level of pressure above which an individual is deemed hypertensive is arbitrary. (A healthy young adult would be expected to have a systolic pressure of around 120 mm Hg and a diastolic of 80 mm Hg, recorded as 120/80.) Hypertension is not a disease as such but a quantitative deviation from the norm. A person with a pressure higher than the average for his or her age group is usually symptomless – although sometimes such people may develop headaches. The identification of people with hypertension is important because it is a signal that they will be more likely to have a STROKE or myocardial infarct (coronary thrombosis or heart attack) than someone whose pressure is in the 'normal' range. Preventive steps can then be taken to lessen the likelihood of their developing these potentially life-threatening conditions.

Blood pressure is measured using two values. The systolic pressure – the greater of the two – represents the pressure when blood is pumped from the left VENTRICLE of the heart into the AORTA. The diastolic pressure is the measurement when both ventricles relax between beats. The pressures are measured in millimetres (mm) of mercury (Hg). Despite the grey area between normal and raised blood pressure, the World Health Organisation (WHO) has defined hypertension as a blood pressure consistently greater than 160 mm Hg (systolic) and 95 mm Hg (diastolic). Young children have readings well below these, but blood pressure rises with age and a healthy person may well live symptom free with a systolic pressure above the WHO figure. A useful working definition of hypertension is the figure at which the benefits of treating the condition outweigh the risks and costs of the treatment.

Between 10 and 20 per cent of the adult population in the UK has hypertension, with more men than women affected. Incidence is highest in the middle-aged and elderly. Because most people with hypertension are symptomless, the condition is often first identified during a routine medical examination, otherwise a diagnosis is usually made when complications occur. Many people's blood pressure rises when they are anxious or after exercise, so if someone's pressure is above normal at the first testing, it should be taken again after, say, 10 minutes' rest, by which time the reading should have settled to the person's regular level. BP measurements should then be taken on two subsequent occasions. If the pressure is still high, the cause needs to be determined: this is done using a combination of personal and family histories (hypertension can run in families), a physical examination and investigations, including an ECG and blood tests for renal disease.

Over 90 per cent of hypertensive people have no immediately identifiable cause for their condition. They are described as having essential hypertension. In those patients with an identifiable cause, the hypertension is described as secondary. Among the causes of secondary hypertension are:

- Lifestyle factors such as smoking, alcohol, stress, excessive dietary salt and obesity.
- Diseases of the KIDNEYS.
- Pregnancy (ECLAMPSIA).
- Various ENDOCRINE disorders – for example, PHAEOCHROMOCYTOMA, CUSHING'S DISEASE, ACROMEGALY, thyrotoxicosis (see under THYROID GLAND, DISEASES OF).
- COARCTATION OF THE AORTA.
- Drugs – for example, oestrogen-containing oral contraceptives (see under CONTRACEPTION), ANABOLIC STEROIDS, CORTICOSTEROIDS, NON-STEROIDAL ANTI-INFLAMMATORY DRUGS (NSAIDS).

Treatment People with severe hypertension may need prompt admission to hospital for urgent investigation and treatment. Those with a mild to moderate rise in blood pressure for which no cause is identifiable should be advised to change their lifestyle: smokers should stop the habit, and those with high alcohol consumption should greatly reduce or stop their drinking. Obese people should reduce their food consumption, especially of animal fats, and take more exercise. Everyone with hypertension should follow a low-salt diet and take regular exercise. Patients should also be taught how to relax, which helps to reduce blood pressure and, if they have a stressful life, working patterns should be modified if possible. If these lifestyle changes do not reduce a person's blood pressure sufficiently, drugs to achieve this will be needed. A wide range of anti-hypertensive drugs are available on prescription.

A first-line treatment is one of the THIAZIDES, effective at a low dosage and especially useful in the elderly. Beta blockers (see BETA-ADRENOCEPTOR-BLOCKING DRUGS), such as oxprenolol, acebutol or atenolol, are also first-line treatments. ACE inhibitors (see ANGIOTENSIN-CONVERTING ENZYME (ACE) INHIBITORS) and CALCIUM-CHANNEL BLOCKERS can be used if the first-line choices are not effective. The drug treatment of hypertension is complex, and sometimes various drugs or combinations of drugs have to be tried to find what regimen is effective and suits the patient. Mild to moderate hypertension can usually be treated in general practice, but patients who do not respond or have complications will normally require specialist advice. Patients on anti-hypertensive treatments require regular monitoring, and, as treatment may be necessary for several years, particular attention should be paid to identifying side-effects. Nevertheless, effective treatment of hypertension does enable affected individuals to live longer and more comfortable lives than would otherwise be the case. Older people with moderately raised blood pressure are often able to live with the condition, and treatment with anti-hypertensive drugs may produce symptoms of HYPOTENSION.

In summary, hypertension is a complex disorder, with different patients responding differently to treatment. So the condition sometimes requires careful assessment before the most effective therapy for a particular individual is identified, and continued monitoring of patients with the disorder is advisable.

Complications Untreated hypertension may eventually result in serious complications. People with high blood pressure have blood vessels with thickened, less flexible walls, a narrowed LUMEN and convoluted shape. Sometimes arteries become rigid. ANEURYSM may develop and widespread ATHEROMA (fat deposits) is apparent in the arterial linings. Such changes adversely affect the blood supply to body tissues and organs and so damage their functioning. Patients suffer STROKE (haemorrhage from or thrombosis in the arteries of the BRAIN) and heart attacks (coronary thrombosis – see HEART, DISEASES OF). Those with hypertension may suffer damage to the retina of the EYE and to the OPTIC DISC. Indeed, the diagnosis of hypertension is sometimes made during a routine eye test, when the doctor or optician notices changes in the retinal arteries or optic disc. Kidney function is often affected, with patients excreting protein and excessive salt in their urine. Occasionally someone with persistent hypertension may suffer an acceleration of damage to the blood vessels – a condition described as 'malignant' hypertension, and one requiring urgent hospital treatment.

Hypertension is a potentially dangerous disease because it develops into a cycle of self-perpetuating damage. Faulty blood vessels lead to high blood pressure which in turn aggravates the damage in the vessels and thus in the tissues and organs they supply with blood; this further raises the affected individual's blood pressure and the pathological cycle continues.

Hypertensive Encephalopathy
A complication of severe HYPERTENSION, this serious but uncommon condition is characterised by neurological symptoms which include transient verbal and visual disturbances, PARAESTHESIA, disorientation, fits and sometimes loss of consciousness. It also affects the eyes,

causing PAPILLOEDEMA. Haemorrhages may occur in the brain, usually in the area of the BASAL GANGLIA. Neurological symptoms can usually be treated effectively by controlling the patient's hypertension.

Hyperthermia
Hyperthermia means abnormally high body temperature. A rapid rise of temperature to dangerous levels – called malignant hyperthermia – may be precipitated by general ANAESTHESIA but the condition is rare (1:50,000 operations) and is usually inherited. The anaesthetic is stopped and icepacks are used to cool the patient. Pure oxygen and intravenous sodium choride are also administered.

It is also the name given to the treatment of disease by the artificial production of FEVER. This can be achieved by various methods, such as radiation heat cabinets boosted with radio frequency (RF); immersion in a hot wax bath; heated suits or blankets; techniques using electromagnetic waves (e.g. RF, MICROWAVES); and ULTRASOUND of appropriate frequencies. Hyperthermia is sometimes of help as an adjunct to surgery, CHEMOTHERAPY, or RADIOTHERAPY in the treatment of cancer.

Hyperthyroidism
Excessive activity of the thyroid gland. (See THYROID GLAND, DISEASES OF.)

Hypertonic
(1) Referring to one solution which has a greater osmotic pressure (see OSMOSIS) than another. Physiologically it is used to describe solutions which have a greater osmotic pressure than body fluids.
(2) Muscles with abnormally increased tone (e.g. following a STROKE).

Hypertrophy
The increase in size which takes place in an organ as the result of an increased amount of work demanded of it by the bodily economy. For example, when valvular disease of the heart is present, compensation occurs by an increase in thickness of the heart muscle, and the organ, by beating more powerfully, is able to overtake the strain thrown upon it. Similarly, if one kidney is removed, the other hypertrophies or grows larger to take over the double workload.

Hyperventilation
An abnormally rapid resting respiratory rate (see RESPIRATION). If voluntarily induced, it causes lightheadedness and then unconsciousness by lowering the blood tension of carbon dioxide.

Hyperventilation is a manifestation of chest and heart diseases which raise carbon dioxide tension or cause HYPOXIA (e.g. severe CHRONIC OBSTRUCTIVE PULMONARY DISEASE (COPD) or PULMONARY OEDEMA). Mechanically ventilated patients may be hyperventilated to lower carbon dioxide tension in order to reduce INTRACRANIAL PRESSURE. (See also HYPOCAPNIA.)

Hypervolaemia

An increase in the volume of circulating blood above the normal range.

Hypnotics

These are drugs that induce SLEEP. Before a hypnotic is prescribed, it is vital to establish – and, where possible, treat – the cause of the insomnia (see under SLEEP, DISORDERS OF). Hypnotics are most often needed to help an acutely distressed patient (for example, following bereavement), or in cases of jet lag, or in shift workers.

If required in states of chronic distress, whether induced by disease or environment, it is especially important to limit the drugs to a short time to prevent undue reliance on them, and to prevent the use of hypnotics and sedatives from becoming a means of avoiding the patient's real problem. In many cases, such as chronic depression, overwork, and alcohol abuse, hypnotics are quite inappropriate; some form of counselling and relaxation therapy is preferable.

Hypnotics should always be chosen and prescribed with care, bearing in mind the patient's full circumstances. They are generally best avoided in the elderly (confusion is a common problem), and in children – apart from special cases. Barbiturates should not now be used as they tend to be addictive. The most commonly used hypnotics are the BENZODIAZEPINES such as nitrazepam and temazepam; chloral derivatives, while safer for the few children who merit them, are generally second choice and should be used in the lowest possible dose for the minimum period.

Side-effects include daytime drowsiness – which may interfere with driving and other skilled tasks – and insomnia following withdrawal, especially after prolonged use, is a hazard. Occasionally benzodiazepines will trigger hostility and aggression. Zolpidem and zopiclone are two drugs similar to the benzodiazepines, indicated for short-term treatment of insomnia in the elderly. Adverse effects include confusion, incoordination and unsteadiness, and falls have been reported.

FLUNITRAZEPAM is a tranquilliser/hypnotic that has been misused as a recreational drug.

Hypnotism

The process of producing a state of mind known as hypnosis. Although recognised for hundreds of years, the precise nature of this process is still poorly understood. One modern writer has defined hypnosis as 'a temporary condition of altered attention, the most striking feature of which is greatly increased suggestibility'. There is no evidence, as has been claimed, that women can be more easily hypnotised than men; in fact, children and young adults are the more easily hypnotised, with middle-aged people being more resistant.

Hypnosis is induced by various methods, but the basis of all is some rhythmic stimulus accompanied by the repetition of carefully worded suggestions. The most commonly used method is to ask the patient to fix his or her eye on a given spot, or light, and then to keep on repeating, in a quiet and soothing voice, that the patient's eyes will gradually become tired and that he or she will want to close them.

There are various levels of hypnosis, usually classified as light, medium, and deep, and it has been estimated that 10 per cent of people cannot be hypnotised; 35 per cent can be taken into light hypnosis; 35 per cent into medium hypnosis; and 20 per cent into deep hypnosis.

Hypnosis can be used as a treatment for some psychiatric patients and in some people with psychosomatic conditions in which emotional or psychological disturbances precipitate physical disorders such as skin lesions or headaches. Hypnosis may help to relieve pain in childbirth; asthma may also respond to it. Some people may find hypnosis to be of help in overcoming addictions to smoking, alcohol or gambling. The process has associated risks, and its use in treatment should be by doctors trained in the technique.

Hypo-

A prefix meaning below, under, or less than normal: for example, hypotension (low blood pressure) and hypodermic (under the skin).

Hypocalcaemia

A SERUM concentration of calcium below the normal range (between 2.33 and 3.05 mmol of calcium per 100 ml of serum). This may cause TETANY, acutely; chronically it may give rise to RICKETS, OSTEOMALACIA or osteoporosis (see BONE, DISORDERS OF). It may be caused by hypoparathyroidism (see THYROID GLAND, DISEASES OF), vitamin D deficiency (see APPENDIX

5: VITAMINS), malabsorption, renal failure or acute pancreatitis (see PANCREAS, DISORDERS OF).

Hypocapnia

A blood tension of carbon dioxide below normal. It is produced by HYPERVENTILATION which may be voluntary, mechanical (if the patient is on a ventilator) or in response to a physiological insult such as metabolic acidosis or brain injury.

Hypochlorhydria

An insufficient secretion of HYDROCHLORIC ACID from the digestive cells of the stomach lining.

Hypochondriasis

Obsession with the body's functions and a DELUSION of ill health, often severe, such that patients may believe they have a brain tumour or incurable insanity. Furthermore, patients may believe that they have infected others, or that their children have inherited the condition. It is a characteristic feature of DEPRESSION, but may also occur in SCHIZOPHRENIA, when the delusions may be secondary to bodily HALLUCINATIONS, and a sense of subjective change. Chronic hypochondriasis may be the result of an abnormal personality development: for example, the insecure, bodily-conscious person. Delusional preoccupations with the body – usually the face – may occur, such that the patient is convinced that his or her face is twisted, or disfigured with acne.

Treatment Hypochondriacal patients may also develop physical illness, and any new symptoms must always be carefully evaluated. In most patients the condition is secondary, and treatment should be directed to the underlying depression or schizophrenia. In the rare cases of primary hypochondriasis, supportive measures are the mainstay of treatment.

Hypodermic

A term pertaining to the region immediately under the skin. Thus, a hypodermic injection means an injection given underneath the skin. A hypodermic syringe is a small syringe which, fitted with a fine needle, is used to give such injections.

Hypogammaglobulinaemia

A lower-than-normal amount of the protein GAMMA-GLOBULIN in the blood. The origin may be genetic – several types are inherited – or an acquired defect (for instance, some lymphomas cause the condition). Gamma-globulin largely comprises antibodies (IMMUNO-GLOBULINS) so deficiency of the protein reduces an individual's natural resistance to infection (see IMMUNOLOGY).

Hypogastric

A term means pertaining to the lower middle part of the abdomen, just above the pubis.

Hypoglossal Nerve

The 12th cranial nerve, which supplies the muscles of the tongue, together with some others lying near it. This nerve is responsible for movements required for swallowing and talking. (See also NERVOUS SYSTEM.)

Hypoglycaemia

A deficiency of glucose in the blood – the normal range being 3·5–7·5 mmol/l (see DIABETES MELLITUS). It most commonly occurs in diabetic patients – for example, after an excessive dose of INSULIN and heavy exercise, particularly with inadequate or delayed meals. It may also occur in non-diabetic people, however: for example, in very cold situations or after periods of starvation. Hypoglycaemia is normally indicated by characteristic warning signs and symptoms, particularly if the blood glucose concentration is falling rapidly. These include anxiety, tremor, sweating, breathlessness, raised pulse rate, blurred vision and reduced concentration, leading – in severe cases – to unconsciousness. Symptoms may be relieved by taking some sugar, some sweet biscuits or a sweetened drink. In emergencies, such as when the patient is comatose (see COMA), an intramuscular injection of GLUCAGON or intravenous glucose should be given. Early treatment is vital, since prolonged hypoglycaemia, by starving the brain cells of glucose, may lead to irreversible brain damage.

Hypoglycaemic Agents

These oral agents reduce the excessive amounts of GLUCOSE in the blood (HYPERGLYCAEMIA) in people with type 2 (INSULIN-resistant) diabetes (see DIABETES MELLITUS). Although the various drugs act differently, most depend on a supply of endogenous (secreted by the PANCREAS) insulin. Thus they are of no value in treating patients with type 1 diabetes (insulin-dependent diabetes mellitus (IDDM), in which the pancreas produces little or no insulin and the patient's condition is stabilised using insulin injections). The traditional oral hypoglycaemic drugs have been the sulphonylureas and biguanides; new agents are now available – for example, thiazolidine-diones (insulin-enhancing agents) and alpha-glucosidase inhibitors, which delay the digestion of CARBOHYDRATE and the absorption of glucose. Hypoglycaemic agents should not be prescribed until diabetic patients have been shown not to respond adequately to at least three months' restriction of energy and carbohydrate intake.

Sulphonylureas The main group of hypoglycaemic agents, these act on the beta cells to stimulate insulin release; consequently they are effective only when there is some residual pancreatic beta-cell activity (see INSULIN). They also act on peripheral tissues to increase sensitivity, although this is less important. All sulphonylureas may lead to HYPOGLYCAEMIA four hours or more after food, but this is relatively uncommon, and usually an indication of overdose.

There are several different sulphonylureas; apart from some differences in their duration or action (and hence in their suitability for individual patients) there is little difference in their effectiveness. Only chlorpropamide has appreciably more side-effects – mainly because of its prolonged duration of action and consequent risk of hypoglycaemia. There is also the common and unpleasant chlorpropamide/alcohol-flush phenomenon when the patient takes alcohol. Selection of an individual sulphonylurea depends on the patient's age and renal function, and often just on personal preference. Elderly patients are particularly prone to the risks of hypoglycaemia when long-acting drugs are used. In these patients chlorpropamide, and preferably glibenclamide, should be avoided and replaced by others such as gliclazide or tolbutamide.

These drugs may cause weight gain and are indicated only if poor control persists despite adequate attempts at dieting. They should not be used during breast feeding, and caution is necessary in the elderly and in those with renal or hepatic insufficiency. They should also be avoided in porphyria (see PORPHYRIAS). During surgery and intercurrent illness (such as myocardial infarction, COMA, infection and trauma), insulin therapy should be temporarily substituted. Insulin is generally used during pregnancy and should be used in the presence of ketoacidosis.

Side-effects Chiefly gastrointestinal disturbances and headache; these are generally mild and infrequent. After drinking alcohol, chlorpropamide may cause facial flushing. It also may enhance the action of antidiuretic hormone (see VASOPRESSIN), very rarely causing HYPONATRAEMIA.

Sensitivity reactions are very rare, usually occurring in the first six to eight weeks of therapy. They include transient rashes which rarely progress to erythema multiforme (see under ERYTHEMA) and exfoliate DERMATITIS, fever and jaundice; chlorpropamide may also occasionally result in photosensitivity. Rare blood disorders include THROMBOCYTOPENIA, AGRANULOCYTOSIS and aplastic ANAEMIA.

Biguanides Metformin, the only available member of this group, acts by reducing GLUCONEOGENESIS and by increasing peripheral utilisation of glucose. It can act only if there is some residual insulin activity, hence it is only of value in the treatment of non-insulin dependent (type 2) diabetics. It may be used alone or with a sulphonylurea, and is indicated when strict dieting and sulphonylurea treatment have failed to control the diabetes. It is particularly valuable in overweight patients, in whom it may be used first. Metformin has several advantages: hypoglycaemia is not usually a problem; weight gain is uncommon; and plasma insulin levels are lowered. Gastrointestinal side-effects are initially common and persistent in some patients, especially when high doses are being taken. Lactic acidosis is a rarely seen hazard occurring in patients with renal impairment, in whom metformin should not be used.

Other antidiabetics Acarbose is an inhibitor of intestinal alpha glucosidases (enzymes that process GLUCOSIDES), delaying the digestion of starch and sucrose, and hence the increase in blood glucose concentrations after a meal containing carbohydrate. It has been introduced for the treatment of type 2 patients inadequately controlled by diet or diet with oral hypoglycaemics.

Guar gum, if taken in adequate doses, acts by delaying carbohydrate absorption, and therefore reducing the postprandial blood glucose levels. It is also used to relieve symptoms of the DUMPING SYNDROME.

Hypoglycaemic Coma

Hypoglycaemia or low blood sugar occurs when a patient with DIABETES MELLITUS suffers an imbalance between carbohydrate/glucose intake and INSULIN dosage. If there is more insulin than is needed to help metabolise the available carbohydrate, it causes a range of symptoms such as sweating, trembling, pounding heartbeat, anxiety, hunger, nausea, tiredness and headache. If the situation is not quickly remedied by taking oral sugar – or, if severe, giving glucose by injection – the patient may become confused, drowsy and uncoordinated, finally lapsing into a COMA. Hypoglycaemia is infrequent in people whose diabetes is controlled with diet and oral HYPOGLYCAEMIC AGENTS.

Treatment of acute hypoglycaemia depends upon the severity of the condition. Oral carbohydrate, such as a sugary drink or chocolate, may be effective if the patient is conscious enough to swallow; if not, glucose or GLUCAGON by injection will be required. Comatose patients who recover after an injection should then be given oral carbohydrates. An occasional but dangerous complication of coma is cerebral oedema (see BRAIN, DISEASES OF – Cerebral oedema), and this should be considered if coma persists. Emergency treatment in hospital is then needed. When the patient has recovered, management of his or her diabetes should be assessed in order to prevent further hypoglycaemic attacks.

Hypogonadism

A condition characterised by underactivity of the testes (see TESTICLE) or OVARIES – the gonads. The condition may be caused by a genetically based disorder resulting in an abnormally functioning gonad (primary hypogonadism) or by a malfunctioning PITUITARY GLAND that fails to produce an adequate amount of gonadotrophin hormone (see GONADOTROPHINS) – secondary hypogonadism. Those affected may fail to develop adequately the secondary characteristics of their sex: males will have delayed puberty, erectile impotence and infertility and also develop GYNAECOMASTIA; females also have delayed puberty, infertility, and sometimes HIRSUTISM.

Hypokalaemia

An abnormally low concentration of potassium in the blood.

Hypomania

Hypomania is a modest manifestation of mania (see under MENTAL ILLNESS). The individual is elated to an extent that he or she may make unwise decisions, and social behaviour may become animated and uninhibited. To the casual observer individuals may, however, seem normal. Treatment is advisable to prevent them from harming their own or their family's interests. Treatment is as for mania.

Hyponatraemia

A SERUM concentration of sodium below the normal range. It may be produced by dilution of blood (giving large volumes of salt-poor solu-

tions intravenously), excessive water retention (inappropriate secretion of antidiuretic hormone), excessive sodium loss, and, rarely, by inadequate salt intake.

Hypoparathyroidism

Underactivity of the parathyroid glands (see under ENDOCRINE GLANDS). Thus there is a lack of parathyroid hormone resulting in HYPOCALCAEMIA. It may be caused by inadvertent removal of the glands when the thyroid gland is surgically removed, or by failure of the glands because of autoimmune disease.

Hypophysectomy

Surgical excision of the PITUITARY GLAND. This can be done by opening the skull, by inserting very low-temperature needles (CRYOSURGERY) into the gland, or by inserting needles of radioactive YTTRIUM-90.

Hypophysis

Another name for the PITUITARY GLAND.

Hypopiesis

The condition, or state, characterised by HYPOTENSION, or abnormally low blood pressure.

Hypopituitarism

Underactivity of the PITUITARY GLAND. It can cause dwarfism, delayed puberty, impotence, infertility, AMENORRHOEA, hypothyroidism (see THYROID GLAND, DISEASES OF), and hypoadrenalism. Causes include tumours, irradiation of the gland, SARCOIDOSIS, and necrosis associated with post-partum haemorrhage (Sheehan's syndrome).

Hypoplasia

Excessive smallness of an organ or part, arising from imperfect development.

Hypoproteinaemia

A fall in the amount of PROTEIN in the blood. This may be caused by malnutrition, loss of protein from kidney disorders, or faulty production of protein which occurs in some liver disorders. Hypoproteinaemia causes OEDEMA because fluid accumulates in the tissues as a consequence of the metabolic abnormalities. Patients' resistance to infections is also impaired.

Hypoprothrombinaemia

A deficiency of PROTHROMBIN (clotting factor) in the blood. As a result the affected individual tends to bleed more easily. The defect may be inherited or be the consequence of liver disease or a deficiency in vitamin K.

H

Anticoagulant therapy will also cause a fall in prothrombin levels.

Hypospadias

A developmental abnormality in the male, in which the URETHRA opens on the undersurface of the penis or in the PERINEUM. The condition is treatable with surgery, but several operations over a period of years may be required to ensure normal urinary and sexual functions.

Hypostasis

The term applied to the condition in which blood accumulates in a dependent part of the body as a result of poor circulation. Congestion of the base of the lungs in old people from this cause, and infection, is called hypostatic PNEUMONIA.

Hypotension

Low blood pressure (see HYPERTENSION for raised blood pressure). Some healthy individuals with a normal cardiovascular system have a permanently low arterial blood pressure for their age. What blood-pressure reading constitutes hypotension is arguable, but a healthy young person with figures below 100 mm Hg systolic and 65 mm Hg diastolic could be described as hypotensive. For a healthy 60 year old, comparative figures might be 120/80. The most common type of hypotension is called postural, with symptoms occurring when a person suddenly stands up, particularly after a period of rest or a hot bath. It results from the muscular tone of blood vessels becoming relaxed and being unable to respond quickly enough to the changing posture, the consequence being a temporary shortage of arterial blood to the brain and organs in the chest. Symptoms of dizziness, occasionally fainting, and nausea occur. Older people are especially vulnerable and may fall as a result of the sudden hypotension. Some drugs – anti-hypertensives and antidepressant ones – cause hypotension. People with DIABETES MELLITUS occasionally develop hypotension because of nerve damage that affects the reflex impulses controlling blood pressure. Any severe injury or burn that results in serious loss of blood or body fluid will cause hypotension and SHOCK. Myocardial infarction (see HEART, DISEASES OF) or failure of the ADRENAL GLANDS can cause hypotension and shock. A severe emotional event that causes shock may also result in hypotension and fainting.

Hypotension in healthy people does not require treatment, although affected individuals should be advised not to stand up suddenly or get out of a bath quickly. Someone who faints as a result of a hypotensive incident should be laid down for a few minutes to allow the circulation to return to normal. Hypotension resulting from burns, blood loss, heart attack or adrenal failure (shock) requires medical attention for the causative condition.

Hypothalamus

That part of the fore-brain situated beneath and linked with the THALAMUS on each side and forming the floor of the third ventricle (see BRAIN). Also linked to the PITUITARY GLAND beneath it, the hypothalamus contains collections of nerve cells believed to form the controlling centres of (1) the sympathetic and (2) the parasympathetic nervous systems (see under NERVOUS SYSTEM). The hypothalamus is the nervous centre for primitive physical and emotional behaviour. It contains nerve centres for the regulation of certain vital processes: the metabolism of fat, carbohydrate and water; sleep; body temperature and sexual functions.

Hypothermia

A core body temperature of less than 35 °C. As the temperature of the body falls, there is increasing dysfunction of all the organs, particularly the central nervous and cardiovascular systems. The patient becomes listless and confused, with onset of unconsciousness between 33–28 °C. Cardiac output at first rises with shivering but then falls progressively, as do the oxygen requirements of the tissues. Below 17–26 °C, cardiac output is insufficient even to supply this reduced demand for oxygen by the tissues. The heart is susceptible to spontaneous ventricular FIBRILLATION below 28 °C. Metabolism is disturbed and the concentration of blood GLUCOSE and POTASSIUM rises as the temperature falls. Cooling of the kidneys produces a DIURESIS and further fluid loss from the circulation to the tissues causes HYPOVOLAEMIA.

Severe hypothermia is sometimes complicated by gastric erosions and haemorrhage, as well as pancreatitis (see PANCREAS, DISORDERS OF). Infants and the elderly are less efficient at regulating temperature and conserving heat than other age groups, and are therefore more at risk from accidental hypothermia during cold weather if their accommodation is not warm enough. Approximately half a million elderly people are at risk in Britain each winter from hypothermia. The other major cause of accidental hypothermia is near-drowning in icy water. Deliberate hypothermia is sometimes used to reduce metabolic rate so that prolonged periods of cardiac arrest may occur without tissue HYPOXIA developing. This technique is used for some cardiac and neurosurgical operations and is produced by immersion of the anaesthetised patient in iced water or by cooling an extracorporeal circulation.

Treatment of hypothermia is by warming the patient and treating any complications that arise. Passive warming is usual, with conservation of the patient's own body heat with insulating blankets. If the core temperature is below 28 °C, then active rewarming should be instituted by means of warm peritoneal, gastric or bladder lavage or using an extracorporeal circulation. Care must be taken in moving hypothermic patients, as a sudden rush of cold peripheral blood to the heart can precipitate ventricular fibrillation. Prevention of hypothermia in the elderly is important. Special attention must be paid to diet, heating the home and adequate clothing in several layers to limit heat loss.

Hypothyroidism
Underactivity of the thyroid gland (see THYROID GLAND, DISEASES OF).

Hypotonic
(1) Referring to a solution which has a lower osmotic pressure (see OSMOSIS) than another. Physiologically it describes a solution with a lower osmotic pressure than body fluids.
(2) Muscles with abnormally reduced tone.

Hypoventilation
Shallow and/or slow breathing, often caused by the effects of injury or drugs on the respiratory centre. It causes HYPERCAPNIA and HYPOXIA.

Hypovolaemia
A reduced circulating blood volume. Acutely, it is caused by unreplaced losses from bleeding, sweating, diarrhoea, vomiting or diuresis. Chronically it may be caused by inadequate fluid intake.

Hypoxaemia
A fall in the concentration of OXYGEN in the arterial blood. Symptoms are those of CYANOSIS and, if severe, the affected individual will show signs of respiratory failure.

Hypoxia
A shortage of OXYGEN in the body tissues. It may be caused by low inspired concentration of oxygen, an abnormal breathing pattern, lung disease or heart disease. If severe and prolonged

it will cause organ damage and death, as cellular function is dependent on oxygen. (See also HYPOXAEMIA.)

Hysterectomy
Surgical removal of the UTERUS. Hystero-oophorectomy is the term applied to removal of the uterus and OVARIES. (See also UTERUS, DISEASES OF.)

Hysteria
An out-of-date description for a symptom (or symptoms) with no obvious organic cause, which is an unconscious reaction and from which the person may benefit. It is now recognised as a dissociative disorder: such disorders – AMNESIA, FUGUE, multiple personality states and trancelike conditions – are powerful defence mechanisms against severe stress when a patient is unable to cope with a particular problem or problems. Symptoms can also mimic physical conditions: for example, apparent paralysis or inability to speak (mutism). Mass hysteria is a phenomenon characterised by extreme suggestibility in a group of often emotionally charged people.

The name originates from the ancient idea that hysteria – a Greek-based word for 'UTERUS' – was in some way associated with the womb. Hence the old-fashioned association of hysteria with women, and with supposed sexual disturbances. Doctors should make sure there is not a physical disease present to explain the symptoms before diagnosing a dissociative disorder. Most subside spontaneously, but if not, the individual needs psychiatric advice. Treatment is difficult. Reasons for stress should be explored and, if possible, resolved. Hypnosis (see HYPNOTISM) to help the person to relive stressful episodes – known as ABREACTION – may be of value.

Hysteroscopy
Hysteroscopy is the direct visualisation of the interior of the UTERUS using FIBREOPTIC ENDOSCOPY. The technique, which allows minor surgical procedures to be carried out at the same time, has transformed the management of uterine disorders.

Hysterotomy
An operation in which the UTERUS is opened to remove a FETUS before 28 weeks' gestation. After 28 weeks it would be called a CAESAREAN SECTION. It is now seldom used as a means of abortion.

Iatric
Anything pertaining to a physician (see also DOCTOR).

Iatrogenic Disease
Disease induced by a physician: most commonly a drug-induced disease.

IBD
See INFLAMMATORY BOWEL DISEASE (IBD).

IBS
See IRRITABLE BOWEL SYNDROME (IBS).

Ibuprofen
One of the NON-STEROIDAL ANTI-INFLAMMATORY DRUGS (NSAIDS) with analgesic properties, Ibuprofen is used to treat rheumatoid arthritis and other forms of rheumatism as well as headaches and muscular pains. It can cause gastric irritation and bleeding in susceptible individuals if used regularly.

ICD
See INTERNATIONAL CLASSIFICATION OF DISEASE (ICD).

Ichthammol
Ichthammol is ammonium ichthosulphonate – an almost black, thick liquid of fishy smell, prepared from a bituminous shale. It is used in chronic eczema (see DERMATITIS).

Ichthyosis
A disorder in which the skin is permanently dry and scaly. It is usually genetically determined and several different forms are recognised:

Ichthyosis vulgaris Common and inherited as a dominant trait. Beginning in early childhood, it is often associated with atopic eczema (see DERMATITIS). The limb flexures and face are spared.

X-linked ichthyosis is much less common, more severe and appears earlier than ichthyosis vulgaris. The fish-like scales are larger and darker and do not spare the flexures and face.

Ichthyosiform erythroderma Of two types and very rare: in the recessive form, the

appearance at birth is of the so-called 'collodion baby'; in the dominant form the baby is born with universally red, moist and eroded skin with an unpleasant smell. Gradually, over several months, thick scales replace the ERYTHEMA.

Treatment Minor forms are helped by constant use of EMOLLIENTS and moisturising applications. Cream containing UREA can be valuable. The rare erythrodermic patterns in the neonate require skilled intensive care as thermoregulation is disturbed and massive fluid loss occurs through the skin. Later in childhood, oral RETINOIDS are useful.

Icterus
Icterus is another name for JAUNDICE.

Ictus
Ictus is another term for a STROKE.

Identical Twins
See MULTIPLE BIRTHS.

Idiopathic
Idiopathic is a term applied to diseases to indicate that their cause is unknown.

Idiopathic Facial Nerve Palsy
See BELL'S PALSY.

Idiopathic Thrombocytopenic Purpura (ITP)
Sometimes described as thrombocytopenia, this is an autoimmune disorder in which blood PLATELETS are destroyed. This disturbs the blood's coagulative properties (see COAGULATION) and spontaneous bleeding (PURPURA) occurs into the skin. The disease may be acute in children but most recover without treatment. Adults may develop a more serious, chronic variety which requires treatment with CORTICOSTEROIDS and sometimes SPLENECTOMY. Should the disease persist despite these treatments, intravenous immunoglobulin or immunosuppressive drugs (see IMMUNOSUPPRESSION) are worth trying. Should the bleeding be or become life-threatening, concentrates of platelets should be administered.

Idiosyncrasy
A generally unexpected, so unpredictable, abnormal reaction to a drug caused by a constitutional defect in the patient. In some cases the underlying disorder is already known or discovered after the first event, so that the drug in question can be avoided thereafter. The

abnormal sensitivity of patients with PORPHY-
RIAS to BARBITURATES is an example. Hereditary biochemical defects of red blood cells are
responsible for many drug-induced haemolytic
anaemias (see under ANAEMIA) and for FAVISM.
Porphyria variegata, the South African variety
of porphyria, is an example of an inborn error
of metabolism which was without serious
symptoms until the advent of barbiturate drugs,
prescription of which is now strongly discour-
aged. If anyone with this metabolic disorder
takes barbiturates, the consequences may be
fatal.

Idoxuridine
An iodine-containing antiviral agent once used
to treat HERPES SIMPLEX involvement of the
cornea of the EYE, its effectiveness is now
doubtful.

Ifosfamide
See CYTOTOXIC.

Iridology
The study of the iris (see EYE). It is an old practice dating back to the days of Aristotle, and has
been revived as a non-conventional treatment
(see COMPLEMENTARY AND ALTERNATIVE MEDI-
CINE (CAM)).

Ileitis
Inflammation of the ileum – the lower part of
the small INTESTINE. It may be caused by
CROHN'S DISEASE, typhoid fever (see ENTERIC
FEVER), TUBERCULOSIS or the bacterium *Yers-
inia enterocolitica*. Ileitis may also accompany
ULCERATIVE COLITIS (see also INFLAMMATORY
BOWEL DISEASE (IBD)).

Patients and their relatives can obtain help
and guidance from the National Association for
Colitis and Crohn's Disease.

Ileo-Caecal
The term applied to the region of the junction
between the small and large intestines in the
right lower corner of the abdomen. The ileo-
caecal valve is a structure which allows the contents of the INTESTINE to pass onwards from the
small to the large intestine, but, in the great
majority of cases, prevents their passage in the
opposite direction.

Ileostomy
The operation by which an artificial opening is
made into the ILEUM and brought through the
abdominal wall to create an artificial opening or
STOMA. It is most often performed as part of the
operation for cancer of the RECTUM, in which

the rectum has usually to be removed. An ileostomy is then performed which acts as an artificial anus, to which a bag is attached to collect
the waste matter. Distressing though this may at
first be, the vast majority of people with an ileostomy learn to lead a fully active and normal
life. Help and advice in adjusting to what can
be described as an 'ileostomy life' can be
obtained from the Ileostomy and Internal
Pouch Support Group.

Ileum
The lower part of the small INTESTINE.

Ileus
Paralysis of the bowel muscle (see INTESTINE,
DISEASES OF).

Ilium
The uppermost of the three bones forming each
side of the PELVIS. (See also BONE.)

Illusions
See HALLUCINATIONS.

Imidazoles
A group of antifungal drugs active against a
wide range of fungi and yeasts (see FUNGAL AND
YEAST INFECTIONS). Some are also effective
against bacteria and HELMINTHS. Econazole,
clotrimazole, ketoconazole, fluconazole and
itraconazole are examples: the drugs are given
by mouth or externally as creams.

Imipramine
A well-established, relatively safe tricyclic antidepressant (see ANTIDEPRESSANT DRUGS) used
to treat DEPRESSION; the drug does, however,
have antimuscarinic and cardiac side-effects. It
is also used to treat ENURESIS by an action distinct from its antidepressant effect.

Immersion Foot
The term applied to a condition which develops
as a result of prolonged immersion of the feet
in cold or cool water. It was a condition
commonly seen during World War II in
shipwrecked sailors and airmen who had
crashed into the sea, spending long periods
there before being rescued. Such prolonged
exposure results in VASOCONSTRICTION of the
smaller arteries in the feet, leading to coldness
and blueness and finally, in severe cases, to
ulceration and GANGRENE. (See also TRENCH
FOOT.)

Immune System
See IMMUNITY.

Age	Disease and mode of administration
3 days	BCG (Bacille Calmette-Guerin) by injection if tuberculosis in family in past 6 months.
2 months	Poliomyelitis (oral); adsorbed diphtheria, whooping-cough (pertussis)[1] and tetanus[2] (triple vaccine given by injection); HiB injection.[3]
3 months	Poliomyelitis (oral); diphtheria, whooping-cough (pertussis)[1] and tetanus[2] (triple vaccine given by injection); HiB injection.[3]
4 months	Poliomyelitis (oral); diphtheria, whooping-cough (pertussis)[1] and tetanus[2] (triple vaccine given by injection); HiB injection.[3]
12–18 months	Measles, mumps, and rubella (German measles)[4] (given together live by injection).
(SCHOOL ENTRY)	
4–5 years	Poliomyelitis (oral); adsorbed diphtheria and tetanus (given together by injection); give MMR vaccine if not already given at 12–18 months.
10–14 females	Rubella (by injection) if they have missed MMR.
10–14	BCG (Bacille Calmette-Guerin) by injection to tuberculin-negative children to prevent tuberculosis.
15–18	Poliomyelitis single booster dose (oral); tetanus (by injection).

[1] Pertussis may be excluded in certain susceptible individuals.

[2] Known as DPT or triple vaccine.

[3] *Haemophilus influenzae* immunisation (type B) is being introduced to be given at same time, but different limb.

[4] Known as MMR vaccine. (Some parents are asking to have their infants immunised with single-constituent vaccines because of controversy over possible side-effects – yet to be confirmed scientifically – of the combined MMR vaccine.)

Recommended immunisation schedules in the United Kingdom

Immunisation

The introduction of antigens (see ANTIGEN) into a body to produce IMMUNITY. The table above gives the immunisation programme recommended by the UK departments of health.

Immunity

The body's defence against foreign substances such as bacteria, viruses and parasites. Immunity also protects against drugs, toxins and cancer cells. It is partly non-specific – that is, it does not depend on previous exposure to the foreign substance. For example, micro-organisms are engulfed and inactivated by polymorphonuclear LEUCOCYTES as a first line of defence before specific immunity has developed.

Acquired immunity depends upon the immune system recognising a substance as foreign the first time it is encountered, storing this information so that it can mount a reaction the next time the substance enters the body. This is the usual outcome of natural infection or prophylactic IMMUNISATION. What happens is that memory of the initiating ANTIGEN persists in selected lymphocytes (see LYMPHOCYTE). Further challenge with the same antigen stimulates an accelerated, more vigorous secondary response by both T- and B-lymphocytes (see

below). Priming the immune system in this manner forms the physiological basis for immunisation programmes.

Foreign substances which can provoke an immune response are termed 'antigens'. They are usually proteins but smaller molecules such as drugs and chemicals can also induce an immune response. Proteins are taken up and processed by specialised cells called 'antigen-presenting cells', strategically sited where microbial infection may enter the body. The complex protein molecules are broken down into short amino-acid chains (peptides – see PEPTIDE) and transported to the cell surface where they are presented by structures called HLA antigens (see HLA SYSTEM).

Foreign peptides presented by human leucocyte antigen (HLA) molecules are recognised by cells called T-lymphocytes. These originate in the bone marrow and migrate to the THYMUS GLAND where they are educated to distinguish between foreign peptides, which elicit a primary immune response, and self-antigens (that is, constituents of the person themselves) which do not. Non-responsiveness to self-antigens is termed 'tolerance' (see AUTOIMMUNITY). Each population or clone of T-cells is uniquely responsive to a single peptide sequence because it expresses a surface molecule ('receptor') which fits only that peptide. The responsive T-cell clone induces a specific response in other T- and B-lymphocyte populations. For example, CYTOTOXIC T-cells penetrate infected tissues and kill cells which express peptides derived from invading micro-organisms, thereby helping to eliminate the infection.

B-lymphocytes secrete ANTIBODIES which are collectively termed IMMUNOGLOBULINS (Ig) – see also GAMMA-GLOBULIN. Each B-cell population (clone) secretes antibody uniquely specific for antigens encountered in the blood, extracellular space, and the LUMEN of organs such as the respiratory passages and gastro-intestinal tract.

Antibodies belong to different Ig classes; IgM antibodies are synthesised initially, followed by smaller and therefore more penetrative IgG molecules. IgA antibodies are adapted to cross the surfaces of mucosal tissues so that they can adhere to organisms in the gut, upper and lower respiratory passages, thereby preventing their attachment to the mucosal surface. IgE antibodies also contribute to mucosal defence but are implicated in many allergic reactions (see ALLERGY).

Antibodies are composed of constant portions, which distinguish antibodies of different class; and variable portions, which confer unique antigen-binding properties on the product of each B-cell clone. In order to match the vast range of antigens that the immune system has to combat, the variable portions are synthesised under the instructions of a large number of encoding GENES whose products are assembled to make the final antibody. The antibody produced by a single B-cell clone is called a monoclonal antibody; these are now synthesised and used for diagnostic tests and in treating certain diseases.

Populations of lymphocytes with different functions, and other cells engaged in immune responses, carry distinctive protein markers. By convention these are classified and enumerated by their 'CD' markers, using monoclonal antibodies specific for each marker.

Immune responses are influenced by cytokines which function as HORMONES acting over a short range to accelerate the activation and proliferation of other cell populations contributing to the immune response. Specific immune responses collaborate with non-specific defence mechanisms. These include the COMPLEMENT SYSTEM, a protein-cascade reaction designed to eliminate antigens neutralised by antibodies and to recruit cell populations which kill micro-organisms.

Immunoassay

Procedures which measure the concentration of any antigenic material (see ANTIGEN) to which an antibody (see ANTIBODIES) can be created. The amount of antigen bound to this antibody is proportional to the parent substance. Enzymes (see ENZYME-LINKED IMMUNOSORBENT ASSAY (ELISA)) or radioactive labels (RADIOIMMUNOASSAY) are used to measure the concentration of antigenic material.

Immunodeficiency

Impaired IMMUNITY resulting from inherited or acquired abnormalities of the immune system. This leads to increased vulnerability to infection. Important inherited examples of immunodeficiency are defects in function of GRANULOCYTES and the COMPLEMENT SYSTEM. Common acquired forms of immunodeficiency are defective function of B-type lymphocytes and hence antibody deficiency in 'common variable hypogammaglobulinaemia', and grossly deficient CD4 T-cell function – malfunctioning T-type lymphocytes – in AIDS, secondary to HIV infection (see AIDS/HIV).

Immunogenicity

The characteristic of a substance that can provoke an immune response (see IMMUNITY). This includes how 'foreign' a substance entering or contacting the body is; route of entry; dose; number and period of exposure to antigen; and the genetic make-up of the host. The characteristics of molecules that determine immunogenicity are:

- Foreignness: molecules recognised as 'self' are generally not immunogenic; the body tolerates these self-molecules. To be immunogenic, molecules must be recognised as non-self or foreign.
- Molecular size: proteins with high molecular weights (over 100,000) are the most effective immunogens; those below 10,000 are weakly immunogenic; and small ones, for example, AMINO ACIDS, are non-immunogenic.
- Chemical complexity: the greater the chemical complexity, the more immunogenic the substance.
- Dosage, route and timing of antigen administration: all these are important factors.

Immunoglobulins

Immunoglobulins are a group of naturally occurring proteins that act as ANTIBODIES. They are structurally related, their differences determining their biological behaviour. Humans have five types of immunoglobulin with different protective functions: IgA, IgD,

IgE, IgG and IgM. In the laboratory these are separated and identified by a chemical process called electrophoresis. Most antibodies have a molecular weight of 160,000.

Certain immunoglobulins can be used in the active or passive immunity of people against infectious diseases such as RABIES and viral HEPATITIS (see also IMMUNITY and GAMMA-GLOBULIN). They are also used in treating certain immunological conditions such as KAWASAKI DISEASE.

Immunologist
A specialist (medically or scientifically qualified) who practises or researches IMMUNOLOGY.

Immunology
The study of immune responses to the environment. Its main clinical applications include improving resistance to microbial infections (see IMMUNITY), combating the effects of impaired immunity (see IMMUNODEFICIENCY), controlling harmful immune reactions (see ALLERGY), and manipulating immune responses (see IMMUNOTHERAPY) to prevent harmful immunological responses such as graft rejection and autoimmune diseases (see AUTOIMMUNITY). The clinical study of disordered immunity now forms the allied discipline of clinical immunology, which is closely linked to the laboratory-based discipline of immunopathology.

Immunosuppressant
A drug that reduces the body's resistance to infection and other foreign agents. It does so by suppressing the activity of the immune system (see IMMUNITY). Examples of such drugs are AZATHIOPRINE, CYCLOPHOSPHAMIDE and CICLOSPORIN A. Immunosuppressants are used to help transplanted organs and tissues to survive the potential immune reaction from the host. They are also used to treat AUTOIMMUNE DISORDERS such as RHEUMATOID ARTHRITIS.

Immunosuppression
The term given to suppression of harmful immune responses (see IMMUNITY), the most obvious application being the prevention of organ rejection by people who receive kidney, heart or bone-marrow transplants (see TRANSPLANTATION). Immunosuppression is also used in certain diseases in a way that is non-specific – that is, it inhibits the entire immune system, not just harmful reactions. CORTICOSTEROIDS are the commonest dugs used in this way, as are METHOTREXATE and AZATHIOPRINE. Tacrolimus, a macrolide (see MACROLIDES) IMMUNOSUPPRESSANT, is used not only for

engrafted patients but also in treating eczema (see DERMATITIS).

There has been a rapid introduction in recent years of monoclonal antibodies which prevent T-cells from proliferating. They can be recognised by the suffix 'mab' (standing for monoclonal antibody) and include rituximab and alemtuzumab. Infliximab, used in CROHN'S DISEASE and RHEUMATOID ARTHRITIS, inhibits tumour necrosis factor alpha.

Immunotherapy
The manipulation of IMMUNITY by immunological (see IMMUNOLOGY) means to reduce harmful reactions or to boost beneficial responses. Severe ALLERGY to wasp or bee stings is often treated by a course of injections with allergen purified from insect venom. There are current attempts to treat autoimmune diseases (see AUTOIMMUNITY) with monoclonal antibodies to the T-cell populations or cytokines implicated in the immunopathogenesis of the disorder.

Strategies are also being evaluated for treating cancer by boosting the patient's own immunity to cancer cells. One approach is immunisation with cancer cells manipulated *in vivo* to increase a T-lymphocyte attack on antigens expressed by tumour cells. Another method is to manipulate the cytokine network into encouraging an immune attack on, or self-destruction ('apoptosis') of, malignant cells.

Immunotherapy is however a developing science, and its place in the routine treatment of immunological and malignant diseases is still evolving.

Impaction
A term applied to a condition in which two things are firmly lodged together. For example, when one piece of bone is driven within another following a fracture, this is known as an impacted fracture; when a tooth is firmly lodged in its socket so that its eruption is prevented, this is known as dental impaction. Intractable constipation is termed faecal impaction.

Imperforate
An adjective meaning lack of an opening. For example, occasionally the ANUS fails to develop properly, resulting in partial or complete obstruction of the opening. Sometimes pubertal girls have an imperforate HYMEN which obstructs the opening to the VAGINA and prevents menstrual flow of blood draining to the exterior.

Impetigo
An infectious skin disease caused usually by

Staphylococcus aureus and less often by *Streptococcus pyogenes*. The itching rash is seen especially on the face but may spread widely. Vesicles and pustules erupt and dry to form yellow-brown scabs. Untreated, the condition may last for weeks. In very young infants, large blisters may form (bullous impetigo).

Treatment Crusts should be gently removed with SALINE. Mild cases respond to frequent application of mupiricin or NEOMYCIN/BACITRACIN ointment; more severe cases should be treated orally or, sometimes, intravenously with FLUCLOXACILLIN or one of the CEPHALOSPORINS. If the patient is allergic to penicillin, ERYTHROMYCIN can be used.

For severe, intractable cases, an oral retinoid drug called isotretinoin (commercially produced as Roaccutane®) can be used. It is given systemically but treatment must be supervised by a consultant dermatologist as serious side-effects, including possible psychiatric disturbance, can occur. The drug is also teratogenic (see TERATOGENESIS), so women who are, or who may become, pregnant must not take isotretinoin. It acts mainly by suppressing SEBUM production in the sebaceous glands and can be very effective. Recurrent bouts of impetigo should raise suspicion of underlying SCABIES or head lice. Bactericidal soaps and instilling an antibiotic into the nostrils may also help.

Implantation
(1) The placing of a substance such as a drug, or an object such as a pacemaker, in a body tissue.
(2) The surgical replacement of injured or unhealthy tissue or organ with healthy tissue or organ (also known as TRANSPLANTATION).
(3) Attachment of the early EMBRYO to the lining of the UTERUS, which occurs around six days after conception; the site where this happens is where the placenta will develop.

Impotence
Inability of the male to perform the sexual act. It may be partial or complete, temporary or permanent. Psychological factors are the most common cause and these include anxiety, ignorance, fear, guilt, weakness of sexual desire or abnormality of such desire. Counselling or sex therapy, preferably with the partner, has a 50-per-cent chance of helping to cure long-term impotence of psychological origin. Among organic causes are lesions (see LESION) of the external genitalia; disturbances of the ENDOCRINE GLANDS, such as diminished activity of the gonads, thyroid gland or pituitary gland; diseases of the central NERVOUS SYSTEM; any

severe disturbance of health, such as DIABETES MELLITUS; and addiction to alcohol.

An oral drug for treating erectile function is sildenafil citrate (Viagra®), the first in a new class of drugs called phosphodiesterase type 5 inhibitors, also including tadalafil (Cialis®) and vardenafil (Levitra®). They work by improving blood flow to the penis. They can be taken an hour before intercourse (up to 12 hours before, in the case of tadalafil). These drugs are not aphrodisiacs, and side-effects include headache, facial flushing and indigestion. There are some suggestions that they may affect retinal function.

Intracavernosal injection or urethral application of alprostadil, a drug which increases local blood supply to the penis, has been used for some years under medical supervision, but success has been variable and oral sildenafil seems to be a more convenient and effective treatment for a man with this disorder.

Impression
In dentistry, a mould (using a rubber or alginate compound) of the teeth and gums from which a plaster-of-Paris model is prepared. This model provides a base on which to construct a denture, bridge or dental inlay. A similar process is used in ORTHODONTICS to make dental appliances to correct abnormalities in the positioning of teeth.

Imprinting
In the context of animal behaviour, this is a quick and irreversible type of learning in which patterns are imprinted on the animal's mind during the first few hours of life. The smell and feel of its mother are one such imprint.

IMR
See INFANT MORTALITY RATE (IMR).

Inanition
Exhaustion in an individual caused by lack of appropriate nutrients in the circulating blood. Starvation, malnutrition or intestinal disorders are among the causes.

Inbreeding
The birth of offspring to parents who are closely related (see CONSANGUINOUS). In traditional rural communities, marriage between cousins was common and this could lead to a higher-than-average number of children with congenital anomalies or learning difficulties. This is now seen in certain ethnic groups who have brought the custom of inbreeding with them to their new homes in the western world.

Incidence

One of the main ways to measure the frequency of a disease in a particular population. The incidence of a disease is the number of new cases that occur during a particular time. PREVALENCE, the other measure, is the total number of cases of disease present at any one time and covers both old and new cases.

Incision

A cut or wound; a term especially applied to surgical openings.

Incisor

The term for the four front TEETH of each jaw.

Inclusion Bodies

Particles found in the CYTOPLASM and NUCLEUS of CELLS, usually a consequence of a viral infection. This phenomenon can be helpful in the diagnosis of such an infection.

Incompatibility

(1) In the pharmacological context, the use of two or more drugs in treatment which together produce adverse consequences for the patient. The *British National Formulary* carries an appendix devoted to drug interactions.
(2) In the haematological context, an adverse reaction in a patient given a blood TRANSFUSION in which the donor blood is incompatible with that of the recipient.

Incompetence

Incompetence is a term applied to the valves of the heart when, as a result of disease in the valves or alterations in size of the chambers of the heart, the valves become unable to close the orifices which they should protect. (See HEART, DISEASES OF.)

Incontinence

Urinary incontinence The International Continence Society defines urinary incontinence as an involuntary loss of URINE that is objectively shown and is a social and hygiene problem. The elderly suffer most from this disorder because the effectiveness of the sphincter muscles surrounding the URETHRA declines with age. Men are less often affected than women; 20 per cent of women over 40 years of age have problems with continence. It is estimated that around three million people are regularly incontinent in the UK, a prevalence of about 40 per 1,000 adults.

Incontinence can be divided broadly into two groups: stress incontinence and incontinence due to an overactive URINARY BLADDER – also called detrusor instability – which affects one-third of incontinent women, prevalence increasing with age. Bladder symptoms do not necessarily correlate with the underlying diagnosis, and accurate diagnosis may require urodynamic studies – examination of urine within, and the passage of urine through and from, the urinary tract. However, such studies are best deferred until conservative treatment has failed or when surgery is planned.

Incontinence causes embarrassment, inconvenience and distress in women, and men are reluctant to seek advice for what remains a social taboo for most people. Sufferers should be encouraged to seek help early and to discuss their anxieties and problems frankly. Often it is a condition which can be managed effectively at primary care centres, and quite simple measures can greatly improve the lives of those affected.

STRESS INCONTINENCE is the most common cause of urinary incontinence in women. This is the involuntary loss of urine during activities that raise the intra-abdominal pressure, such as sneezing, coughing, laughing, exercise or lifting. The condition is caused by injury or weakness of the urethral sphincter muscle; this weakness may be either congenital or the result of childbirth, PROLAPSE of the VAGINA, MENOPAUSE or previous surgery. A CYSTOCOELE may be present. Urinary infection may cause incontinence or aggravate the symptoms of existing incontinence.

The first step is to diagnose and treat infection, if present. Patients benefit from simple advice on incontinence pads and garments, and on fluid intake. Those with a high fluid intake should restrict this to a litre a day, especially if frequency is a problem. Constipation should be treated and smoking stopped. The use of DIURETICS should be reduced if possible, or stopped entirely. Postmenopausal women may benefit from oestrogen-replacement therapy; elderly people with chronic incontinence may need an indwelling urethral catheter.

Pelvic-floor exercises can be successful and the insertion of vaginal cones can be a useful subsidiary treatment, as can electrical stimulation of the pelvic muscles. If these procedures are unsuccessful, then continence surgery may be necessary. The aim of this is to raise the neck of the bladder, support the mid part of the urethra and increase urethral resistance. Several techniques are available.

URGE INCONTINENCE An overactive or unstable bladder results in urge incontinence, also known as detrusor incontinence – the result of uninhibited contractions of the detrusor muscle of the bladder. The bladder contracts (spontaneously or on provocation) during the filling phase while the patient attempts to stop passing any urine. Hyperexcitability of the muscle or a disorder of its nerve supply are likely causes. The symptoms include urgency (acute wish to pass urine), frequency and stress incontinence. Diagnosis can be confirmed with CYSTOMETRY. Bladder training is the first step in treatment, with the aim of reducing the frequency of urination to once every three to four hours. BIOFEEDBACK, using visual, auditory or tactile signals to stop bladder contractions, will assist the bladder training. Drug treatments such as CALCIUM-CHANNEL BLOCKERS, antimuscarinic agents (see ANTIMUSCARINE), TRICYCLIC ANTIDEPRESSANT DRUGS, and oestrogen replacement can be effective. Surgery is rarely used and is best reserved for difficult cases.

OVERFLOW INCONTINENCE Chronic urinary retention with consequent overflow – more common in men than in women. The causes include antispasmodic drugs, continence surgery, obstruction from enlargement and post-prostatectomy problems (in men), PSYCHOSIS, and disease or damage to nerve roots arising from the spinal cord. Urethral dilatation or urethrotomy may be required when obstruction is the cause. Management is intermittent self-catheterisation or a suprapubic catheter and treatment of any underlying cause.

Faecal incontinence is the inability to control bowel movements and may be due to severe CONSTIPATION, especially in the elderly; to local disease; or to injury or disease of the spinal cord or nervous supply to rectum and anal muscles. Those with the symptom require further investigation.

Incoordination

A term applied to irregularity of movements produced either by loss of the sensations by which they are governed, or by defects in the muscles themselves or somewhere in the nervous system.

Incubation

The period elapsing between the time when a person becomes infected by some agent and the first appearance of the symptoms of the disease. Most acute infectious diseases have fairly definite periods of incubation, and it is of great importance that people who have run the risk of infection should know the length of time which must elapse before they can be sure whether or not they are to contract the disease

in question. A person who has been exposed to infection is, during the incubation period, technically known as a contact. By isolating and watching contact cases, medical officers can often successfully check a threatened EPIDEMIC.

It must be noted that diseases are not communicated to others by a person who is incubating an illness. Some diseases, however, such as MEASLES, become infectious as soon as the first symptoms set in after the incubation period is over; others, like SCARLET FEVER and SMALLPOX, are not so infectious then as in their later stages. The incubation period for any given disease is remarkably constant, although in the case of a severe attack the incubation is usually slightly shortened, and if the oncoming attack is a mild one, the period may be lengthened. All, however, may take a few days longer than the time stated to show themselves (see INFECTION), and several – especially WHOOPING-COUGH – may be difficult to recognise in their early stages.

Incubation periods of the more common infectious diseases:

	days
Chickenpox	14–21
Diphtheria	2–5
German measles	14–21
Measles	10–15
Mumps	18–21
Poliomyelitis	3–21
Smallpox	10–16
Typhoid fever	7–21
Whooping-cough	7–10

Index Finger

The forefinger or second digit of the hand.

Index Medicus

A monthly publication produced by the National Library of Medicine in the USA. The publication indexes leading biomedical literature from throughout the world. Indexing is by author and by subject.

Indian Hemp

See CANNABIS.

Indigestion

See DYSPEPSIA.

Indinavir

A protease-inhibitor antiviral drug used in combination with nucleoside reverse transcriptase inhibitors (see REVERSE TRANSCRIPTASE INHIBITOR) to treat HIV infection (see AIDS/HIV). A drug with a range of potentially serious side-effects, its use should be coupled with counselling and monitoring of the effects.

Indispensable Amino Acids

This is the new, preferred term for essential amino acids – amino acids which are essential for the body's normal growth and development, but which the body is unable to produce. Nine essential amino acids exist – HISTIDINE, ISO-LEUCINE, LEUCINE, LYSINE, METHIONINE, PHENYLALANINE, THREONINE, TRYPTOPHAN, and VALINE – and they are present in foods rich in protein: dairy products, eggs, meat, and liver.

Indometacin

Previously indomethacin, this is one of many drugs used in the treatment of GOUT and RHEUMATOID ARTHRITIS. A proprionic-acid derivative, it may help to relieve night pain and morning stiffness. It is also used to treat the congenital abnormality of the heart known as DUCTUS ARTERIOSUS.

Indoramin

An alpha-adrenoreceptor-blocking drug used in the treatment of high blood pressure. It has several side-effects including sleepiness, dizziness, depression and failure to ejaculate. (See ALPHA ADRENERGIC BLOCKERS; ADRENERGIC RECEPTORS.)

Induction

Bringing about a particular event – for example, the induction or starting of labour (see PREG-NANCY AND LABOUR), or the induction of ANAESTHESIA. Newly arrived hospital doctors are given an induction period during their first day or two at work.

Induration

The pathological hardening of a tissue or organ. This may occur when a tissue is infected or when it is invaded by cancer. (See also SCLEROSIS.)

Industrial Diseases

See OCCUPATIONAL HEALTH, MEDICINE AND DISEASES.

Industrial Injuries Benefit

The Industrial Injuries Scheme provides money for people who have suffered injury or illness because of their work. Benefits for employment-related disability (self-employment is excluded) have been altered many times since they were introduced in 1948. There is now a mix of benefits, eligibility for which depends on several factors: the date,

onset and type of disability are among the most important. 'Industrial' includes almost all forms of employment. In addition to accidents, there is a long list of prescribed industrial diseases ranging from BURSITIS, hearing loss, ASTHMA and viral HEPATITIS to unusual ones such as ORF. Psychological as well as physical disablement may attract benefit, which is calculated on a percentage basis according to the extent of disability. The onus is on the individual to claim, and trade unions and representative organisations can advise on procedures. Injured employees should always report details of an accident to their employer and record it in the accident book promptly: even seemingly minor injuries may subsequently lead to some disability. Relevant information leaflets are available – for example, from local benefit agencies, local-authority advice centres and public libraries.

Infant

A baby who is under one year old.

Infant Feeding

The newborn infant may be fed naturally from the breast, or artificially from a bottle.

Breast feeding Unless there is a genuine contraindication, every baby should be breast fed. The nutritional components of human milk are in the ideal proportions to promote the healthy growth of the human newborn. The mother's milk, especially colostrum (the fluid secreted before full lactation is established) contains immune cells and antibodies that increase the baby's resistance to infection. From the mother's point of view, breast feeding helps the womb to return to its normal size and helps her to lose excess body fat gained during pregnancy. Most importantly, breast feeding promotes intimate contact between mother and baby. A final point to be borne in mind, however, is that drugs taken by a mother can be excreted in her milk. These include antibiotics, sedatives, tranquillisers, alcohol, nicotine and high-dose steroids or vitamins. Fortunately this is rarely a cause of trouble. (See also main entry on BREAST FEEDING.)

Artificial feeding Unmodified cows' milk is not a satisfactory food for the human newborn and may cause dangerous metabolic imbalance. If breast feeding is not feasible, one of the many commerciallly available formula milks should be used. Most of these are made from cows' milk which has been modified to reflect the composition of human milk as closely as possible. For the rare infant who develops cows'-milk-protein intolerance, a milk based on soya-bean protein is indicated.

Feeding and weight gain The main guide as to whether an infant is being adequately fed is the weight. During the first days of life a healthy infant loses weight, but should by the end of the second week return to birth weight. From then on, weight gain should be approximately 6oz. (170g) each week.

The timing of feeds reflects social convention rather than natural feeding patterns. Among the most primitive hunter-gatherer tribes of South America, babies are carried next to the breast and allowed to suckle at will. Fortunately for developed society, however, babies can be conditioned to intermittent feedings.

As the timing of breast feeding is flexible – little or no preparation time being required – mothers can choose to feed their babies on demand. Far from spoiling the baby, demand feeding is likely to lead to a contented infant, the only necessary caution being that a crying baby is not always a hungry baby.

In general, a newborn will require feeding every two to four hours and, if well, is unlikely to sleep for more than six hours. After the first months, a few lucky parents will find their infant sleeping through the night.

Weaning Weaning on to solid foods is again a matter of individuality. Most babies will become dissatisfied with a milk-only diet at around six months and develop enthusiasm for cereal-based weaning foods. Also at about this time they enjoy holding objects and transferring them to their mouths – the mouth being an important sense organ in infants. It is logical to include food items that they can hold, as this clearly brings the baby pleasure at this time. Introduction of solids before the age of four months is unusual and best avoided. The usual reason given for early weaning is that the baby appears hungry, but this is unlikely to be the case; crying due to COLIC, for example, is more probable. Some mothers take the baby's desire to suck – say, on their finger – as a sign of hunger when this is, in fact, reflex activity.

Delaying the start of weaning beyond nine months is nutritionally undesirable. As weaning progresses, the infant's diet requires less milk. Once established on a varied solid diet, breast and formula milks can be safely replaced with cows' milk. There is, however, no nutritional contraindication to continued breast feeding until the mother wishes to stop.

It is during weaning that infants realise they can arouse extreme maternal anxiety by refusing to eat. This can lead to force-feeding and battles of will which may culminate in a breakdown of the mother-child relationship. To avoid this, parents must resist the temptation to coax the child to eat. If the child refuses solid food, the meal should be taken away with a minimum of fuss. Children's appetites reflect their individual genetic structure and a well child will eat enough to grow and maintain satisfactory weight gain. If a child is not eating properly, weight gain will be inadequate over a prolonged period and an underlying illness is the most likely cause. Indeed, failure to thrive is the paediatrician's best clue to chronic illness.

Advice on feeding Many sources of conflicting advice are available to new parents. It is impossible to satisfy everyone, and ultimately it is the well-being of the mother and infant and the closeness of their relationship that matter. In general, mothers should be wary of rigid advice. An experienced midwife, health visitor or well-baby-clinic nursing sister are among the most reliable sources of information.

	Protein per cent	Fat per cent	Sugar per cent	Calories per cent
Human milk	1·1	4·2	7·0	70
Cows' milk	3·5	3·9	4·6	66

Composition of human and cows' milk

Infantile Paralysis
An old name for POLIOMYELITIS.

Infantile Spasms
Also known as salaam attacks, these are a rare but serious type of EPILEPSY, usually starting in the first eight months of life. The spasms are short and occur as involuntary flexing of the neck, arms, trunk and legs. They may occur several times a day. If the baby is sitting, it may collapse into a 'salaam' position; more usually there is a simple body jerk, sometimes accompanied by a sudden cry. An electroencephalogram (see ELECTROENCEPHALOGRAPHY (EEG)) shows a picture of totally disorganised electrical activity called hypsarrhythmia. The condition results from any one of many brain injuries, infections or metabolic insults that may have occurred before, during, or in the first few months after birth. Its importance is that in most cases, the baby's development is seriously affected such that they are likely to be left with a profound learning disability. Consequently, prompt diagnosis is important. Treatment is with CORTICOSTEROIDS or with certain anticonvulsants – the hope being that prompt and

aggressive treatment might prevent further brain damage leading to learning disability.

Infantilism

The condition characterised by imperfect sexual development at puberty. It may or may not be associated with small stature, and may be due to lack of development of certain of the ENDO-CRINE GLANDS: for example, the gonads, pituitary gland or adrenal glands. In other cases it may be associated with a generalised disease such as diabetes mellitus, asthma, ulcerative colitis and rheumatoid arthritis (for more information, see under separate entries).

Infant Mortality Rate (IMR)

The number of deaths of infants under one year of age. The IMR in any given year is calculated as the number of deaths in the first year of life in proportion to every 1,000 registered live births in that year. Along with PERINATAL MORTALITY, it is accepted as one of the most important criteria for assessing the health of the community and the standard of the social conditions of a country.

The improvement in the infant mortality rate has occurred mainly in the period from the second month of life. There has been much less improvement in the neonatal mortality rate – that is, the number of infants dying during the first four weeks of life, expressed as a proportion of every 1,000 live births. During the first week of life the main causes of death are asphyxia, prematurity, birth injuries and congenital abnormalities. After the first week the main cause of death is infection.

Social conditions also play an important role in infant mortality. In England and Wales the infant mortality rate in 1930–32 was: Social Class I (professional), 32·7; Social Class III (skilled workers), 57·6; Social Class V (unskilled workers), 77·1. Many factors come into play in producing these social variations, but overcrowding is undoubtedly one of the most important.

1838–9	146	1950–52	30
1851–60	154	1960–62	22
1900–02	142	1970–72	18
1910–12	110	1980–82	12
1920–22	82	1990–92	7
1930–32	67	1996	6·2
1940–42	59	1999	5·8
2000	5.6		

Infant mortality rate in the United Kingdom 1838–2000. Deaths of infants under 1 year age per thousand live births

It is thus evident that for a reduction of the infant mortality rate to the minimum figure, the following conditions must be met. Mothers and potential mothers must be housed adequately in healthy surroundings, particularly with regard to safe water supplies and sewage disposal. The pregnant and nursing mother must be ensured an adequate diet. Effective antenatal supervision must be available to every mother, as well as skilled supervision during labour (see PREGNANCY AND LABOUR). The newborn infant must be adequately nursed and fed and mothers encouraged to breast feed. Environmental and public-health measures must be taken to ensure adequate housing, a clean milk supply and full availability of medical care including such protective measures as IMMUNISATION against diphtheria, measles, poliomyelitis and whooping-cough. (See also PERINATAL MORTALITY.)

Infarction

The changes in an organ when an artery is suddenly blocked, leading to the formation of a dense, wedge-shaped mass of dead tissue in the part of the organ supplied by the artery. It occurs as the result of EMBOLISM or of THROMBOSIS.

Infection

The process by which a disease is transmitted via micro-organisms from one person to another. The micro-organism may be a bacterium (see BACTERIA), a RICKETTSIA, a VIRUS, a protozoon – single-celled animal organism – or a metazoon – multicellular animal organism. Invasion of the body by a metazoon (e.g. by an intestinal worm) is more often known as an infestation.

The skin is an important protection against micro-organisms entering the body tissues. A large measure of protection is afforded by the factors which ensure IMMUNITY against diseases.

Modes of infection The infective material may be transmitted to the person by direct contact with a sick person, when the disease is said to be contagious, although such a distinction is purely artificial. Different diseases are especially infectious at different periods of their course. Protecting people can be difficult, since some diseases are infectious before the patient shows any symptoms (see INCUBATION).

Infection may be conveyed on dust, in drinking-water, in food (particularly milk), in the body's waste products and secretions, or even on clothes and linen which have been in contact with the infected individual (called fomites).

Some people who have recovered from a disease, or who have simply been in contact with an infectious case, harbour the infectious agent. This is particularly the case in typhoid fever (see ENTERIC FEVER), the bacillus continuing to develop in the gall-bladder of some people who have had the disease for years after the symptoms have disappeared. In the case of CHOLERA, which is ENDEMIC in some developing countries with hot climates, 80 per cent or more of the population may harbour the bacillus and spread infection when other circumstances favour this. Similarly in the case of DYSENTERY, people who have completely recovered may still be capable of infecting dust and drinking-water by their stools. DIPHTHERIA and meningococcal MENINGITIS, which is particularly liable to infect children, are other examples.

Flies can infect milk and other food with the organisms causing typhoid fever and food poisoning. Mosquitoes carry the infective agents of MALARIA, DENGUE and YELLOW FEVER, these undergoing part of their development in the body of the mosquito. Fleas convey the germ of plague from rats to humans, and lice are responsible for inoculating TYPHUS FEVER and one form of RELAPSING FEVER by their bite. A tick is responsible for spreading another form of relapsing fever, and kala-azar (LEISHMANIASIS) is spread by the bites of sandflies.

Notifiable diseases Certain of the common and most serious infectious diseases are notifiable in the United Kingdom. A doctor diagnosing someone infected by a notifiable disease must inform the authorities. For the current list of notifiable infectious diseases in the UK, see the main entry for NOTIFIABLE DISEASES.

Prevention is an important aspect of the control of infectious diseases, and various steps can be taken to check the spread of such infections as dysentery, tuberculosis, malaria and others. (See also IMMUNITY; INCUBATION.)

Infectious Mononucleosis
See MONONUCLEOSIS.

Infertility
This is diagnosed when a couple has not achieved a pregnancy after one year of regular unprotected sexual intercourse. Around 15–20 per cent of couples have difficulties in conceiving; in half of these cases the male partner is infertile, while the woman is infertile also in half; but in one-third of infertile couples both

partners are affected. Couples should be investigated together as efficiently and quickly as possible to decrease the distress which is invariably associated with the diagnosis of infertility. In about 10–15 per cent of women suffering from infertility, ovulation is disturbed. Mostly they will have either irregular periods or no periods at all (see MENSTRUATION).

Checking a hormone profile in the woman's blood will help in the diagnosis of ovulatory disorders like polycystic ovaries, an early menopause, anorexia or other endocrine illnesses. Ovulation itself is best assessed by ultrasound scan at mid-cycle or by a blood hormone progesterone level in the second half of the cycle.

The FALLOPIAN TUBES may be damaged or blocked in 20–30 per cent of infertile women. This is usually caused by previous pelvic infection or ENDOMETRIOSIS, where menstrual blood is thought to flow backwards through the fallopian tubes into the pelvis and seed with cells from the lining of the uterus in the pelvis. This process often leads to scarring of the pelvic tissues; 5–10 per cent of infertility is associated with endometriosis.

To assess the Fallopian tubes adequately a procedure called LAPAROSCOPY is performed. An ENDOSCOPE is inserted through the umbilicus and at the same time a dye is pushed through the tubes to assess their patency. The procedure is performed under a general anaesthetic.

In a few cases the mucus around the cervix may be hostile to the partner's sperm and therefore prevent fertilisation.

Defective production is responsible for up to a quarter of infertility. It may result from the failure of the testes (see TESTICLE) to descend in early life, from infections of the testes or previous surgery for testicular torsion. The semen is analysed to assess the numbers of sperm and their motility and to check for abnormal forms.

In a few cases the genetic make-up of one partner does not allow the couple ever to achieve a pregnancy naturally.

In about 25 per cent of couples no obvious cause can be found for their infertility.

Treatment Ovulation may be induced with drugs.

In some cases damaged Fallopian tubes may be repaired by tubal surgery. If the tubes are destroyed beyond repair a pregnancy may be achieved with in vitro fertilisation (IVF) – see under ASSISTED CONCEPTION.

Endometriosis may be treated either with drugs or laser therapy, and pregnancy rates after both forms of treatment are between 40–50 per cent, depending on the severity of the disease.

Few options exist for treating male-factor infertility. These are artificial insemination by husband or donor and more recently in vitro fertilisation. Drug treatment and surgical repair of VARICOCELE have disappointing results.

Following investigations, between 30 and 40 per cent of infertile couples will achieve a pregnancy usually within two years.

Some infertile men cannot repair any errors in the DNA in their sperm, and it has been found that the same DNA repair problem occurs in malignant cells of some patients with cancer. It is possible that these men's infertility might be nature's way of stopping the propagation of genetic defects. With the assisted reproduction technique called intracytoplasmic sperm injection, some men with defective sperm can fertilise an ovum. If a man with such DNA defects fathers a child via this technique, that child could be sterile and might be at increased risk of developing cancer. (See ARTIFICIAL INSEMINATION; ASSISTED CONCEPTION.)

Infestation

A term applied to the occurrence of animal parasites in the intestine, hair or clothing.

Infibulation

The most extensive form of female CIRCUMCISION, involving removal of CLITORIS and both LABIA.

Infiltration

The invasion of tissues or organs by cells or fluid not normally present – for example, local anaesthetic is infiltrated into an area of tissue to produce analgesia in a defined area.

Inflammation

The reaction of the tissues to any injury, which may be the result of trauma, infection or chemicals. Local blood vessels dilate, thus increasing blood flow to the injured site. White blood cells invade the affected tissue, engulfing bacteria or other foreign bodies; related cells consume any dead cells, thus producing PUS after which the site starts to heal. The patient feels pain and the affected tissue becomes hot, red and swollen, with its functioning affected. If the infection is severe it may persist locally – chronic inflammation – or spread elsewhere in the body – systemic infection.

Inflammatory Bowel Disease (IBD)

CROHN'S DISEASE and ULCERATIVE COLITIS are chronic inflammatory diseases characterised by relapsing and remitting episodes over many years. The diseases are similar and are both classified as IBD, but a significant distinction is that Crohn's disease can affect any part of the GASTROINTESTINAL TRACT from mouth to anus, whereas ulcerative colitis affects only the COLON. The incidence of IBD varies widely between countries, being rare in the developing world but much more common in westernised nations, where the incidence of Crohn's disease is around 5–7 per 100,000 (and rising) and that of ulcerative colitis at a broadly stable 10 per 100,000. It is common for both disorders to develop in young adults, but there is a second spike of incidence in people in their 70s. Details about the two disorders are given under the individual entries elsewhere in the dictionary. Inflammatory bowel disease should not be confused with IRRITABLE BOWEL SYNDROME (IBS) which has some of the same symptoms of IBD but a different cause and outcome.

Infliximab

An IMMUNOSUPPRESSANT monoclonal antibody (see ANTIBODIES) designed to inhibit the pro-inflammatory cytokine (see CYTOKINES), tumour necrosis factor alpha. It is used in treating CROHN'S DISEASE and RHEUMATOID ARTHRITIS.

Influenza

Influenza is an acute infectious disease, characterised by a sudden onset, fever and generalised aches and pains. It usually occurs in epidemics and pandemics (see EPIDEMIC; PANDEMIC).

Cause The disease is caused by a VIRUS of the influenza group. There are at least three types of influenza virus, known respectively as A, B and C. One of their most characteristic features is that infection with one type provides no protection against another. Equally important is the ease with which the influenza virus can change its character. It is these two characteristics which explain why one attack of influenza provides little, if any, protection against a subsequent attack, and why it is so difficult to prepare an effective vaccine against the disease.

Epidemics of influenza due to virus A occur in Britain at two- to four-year intervals, and outbreaks of virus B influenza in less frequent cycles. Virus A influenza, for instance, was the prevalent infection in 1949, 1951, 1955 and 1956, whilst virus B influenza was epidemic in 1946, 1950, 1954 and, along with virus A, in 1958–59. The pandemic of 1957, which swept most of the world, although fortunately not in a severe form, was due to a new variant of virus A – the so-called Asian virus – and it has been suggested that it was this variant that was responsible for the pandemics of 1889 and 1918. Since 1957, variants of virus A have been the predominating causes of influenza, accompanied on occasions by virus B.

In 1997 and 2004, outbreaks of Chinese avian influenza caused alarm. The influenza virus had apparently jumped species from birds – probably chickens – to infect some people. Because no vaccine is available, there was a risk that this might start an epidemic.

Symptoms The incubation period of influenza A and B is 2–3 three days, and the disease is characterised by a sudden onset. In most cases this is followed by a short, sharp febrile illness of 2–4 days' duration, associated with headache, prostration, generalised aching, and respiratory symptoms. In many cases the respiratory symptoms are restricted to the upper respiratory tract, and consist of signs of irritation of the nose, pharynx and larynx. There may be nosebleeds, and a dry, hacking cough is often a prominent and troublesome symptom. The fever is usually remittent and the temperature seldom exceeds 39·4 °C (103 °F), tending to fluctuate between 38·3 and 39·4 °C (101 and 103 °F).

The most serious complication is infection of the lungs. This infection is usually due to organisms other than the influenza virus, and is a complication which can have serious results in elderly people.

The very severe form of 'flu which tends to occur during pandemics – and which was so common during the 1918–19 pandemic – is characterised by the rapid onset of bronchopneumonia and severe prostration. Because of the toxic effect on the heart, there is a particularly marked form of CYANOSIS, known as heliotrope cyanosis.

Convalescence following influenza tends to be prolonged. Even after an attack of average severity there tends to be a period of weakness and depression.

Treatment Expert opinion is still divided as to the real value of influenza vaccine in preventing the disease. Part of the trouble is that there is little value in giving any vaccine until it is known which particular virus is causing the infection. As this varies from winter to winter, and as the protection given by vaccine does not exceed one year, it is obviously not worthwhile attempting to vaccinate the whole community. The general rule therefore is that, unless there is any evidence that a particularly virulent type of virus is responsible, only the most vulnerable should be immunised – such as children in boarding schools, elderly people, and people who suffer from chronic bronchitis or asthma, chronic heart disease, renal failure, diabetes mellitus or immunosuppression (see under separate entries). In the face of an epidemic, people in key positions, such as doctors, nurses and those concerned with public safety, transport and other public utilities, should be vaccinated.

For an uncomplicated attack of influenza, treatment is symptomatic: that is, rest in bed, ANALGESICS to relieve the pain, sedatives, and a light diet. A linctus is useful to sooth a troublesome cough. The best analgesics are ASPIRIN or PARACETAMOL. None of the sulphonamides or the known antibiotics has any effect on the influenza virus; on the other hand, should the lungs become infected, antibiotics should be given immediately, because such an infection is usually due to other organisms. If possible, a sample of sputum should be examined to determine which organisms are responsible for the lung infection. The choice of antibiotic then depends upon which antibiotic the organism is most sensitive to.

Information Technology in Medicine

The advent of computing has had widespread effects in all areas of society, with medicine no exception. Computer systems are vital – as they are in any modern enterprise – for the administration of hospitals, general practices and health authorities, supporting payroll, finance, stock ordering and billing, resource and bed management, word-processing correspondence, laboratory-result reporting, appointment and record systems, and management audit.

The imaging systems of COMPUTED TOMOGRAPHY (CT) and magnetic resonance imaging (see MRI) have powerful computer techniques underlying them.

Computerised statistical analysis of study data, population databases and disease registries is now routine, leading to enhanced understanding of the interplay between diseases and the population. And the results of research, available on computerised indexes such as MEDLINE, can be obtained in searches that take only seconds, compared with the hours or days necessary to accomplish the same task with its paper incarnation, *Index Medicus*.

Medical informatics The direct computerisation of those activities which are uniquely medical – history-taking, examination, diagnosis and treatment – has proved an elusive goal, although one hotly pursued by doctors, engineers and scientists working in the discipline of medical informatics. Computer techniques have scored some successes: patients are, for example, more willing to be honest about taboo areas, such as their drug or alcohol consumption, or their sexual proclivities, with a computer than face to face with a clinician; however, the practice of taking a history remains the cornerstone of clinical practice. The examination of the patient is unlikely to be supplanted by technological means in the foreseeable future; visual and tactile recognition systems are still in their infancy. Skilled interpretation of the result by machine rather than the human mind seems equally as remote. Working its way slowly outwards from its starting point in mathematical logic, ARTIFICIAL INTELLIGENCE that in any way mimics its natural counterpart seems a distant prospect. Although there have been successes in computer-supported diagnosis in some specialised areas, such as the diagnosis of abdominal pain, workable systems that could supplant the mind of the generalist are still the dream of the many developers pursuing this goal, rather than a reality available to doctors in their consulting rooms now.

In therapeutics, computerised prescribing systems still require the doctor to make the decision about treatment, but facilitate the process of writing, issuing, and recording the prescription. In so doing, the system can provide automated checks, warning if necessary about allergies, potential drug interactions, or dosing errors. The built-in safety that this process offers is enhanced by the superior legibility of the script that ensues, reducing the potential for error when the medicine is dispensed by the nurse or the pharmacist.

Success in these individual applications continues to drive development, although the process has its critics, who are not slow to point to the lengthier consultations that arise when a computer is present in the consulting room and its distracting effect on communication with the patient.

Underlying these many software applications lies the ubiquitous personal computer – more powerful today than its mainframe predecessor of only 20 years ago – combined with networking technology that enables interconnection and the sharing of data. As in essence the doctor's role involves the acquisition, manipulation and application of information – from the individual patient, and from the body of medical knowledge – great excitement surrounds the development of open systems that allow different software and hardware platforms to interact. Many problems remain to be solved, not least the fact that for such systems to work, the whole organisation, and not just a few specialised individuals, must become computer literate. Such systems must be easy to learn to use, which requires an intuitive interface between user(s) and system(s) that is predictable and logical in its ordering and presentation of information.

Many other issues stand in the way of the development towards computerisation: standard systems of nomenclature for medical concepts have proved surprisingly difficult to develop, but are crucial for successful information-sharing between users. Sharing information between existing legacy systems is a major challenge, often requiring customised software and extensive human intervention to enable the previous investments that an organisation has made in individual systems (e.g. laboratory-result reporting) to be integrated with newer technology. The beginnings of a global solution to this substantial obstacle to networking progress is in sight: the technology that enables the Internet – an international network of telephonically linked personal computers – also enables the establishment of intranets, in which individual servers (computers dedicated to serving information to other computers) act as repositories of 'published' data, which other users on the network may 'browse' as necessary in a client-server environment.

Systems that support this process are still in early stages of development, but the key conceptualisations are in place. Developments over the next 5–10 years will centre on the electronic patient record available to the clinician on an integrated clinical workstation. The clinical workstation – in essence a personal computer networked to the hospital or practice system – will enable the clinician to record clinical data and diagnoses, automate the ordering of investigations and the collection of the results, and facilitate referral and communication between the many professionals and departments involved in any individual patient's care.

Once data is digitised – and that includes text, statistical tables, graphs, illustrations and radiological images, etc. – it may be as freely networked globally as locally. Consultations in which live video and sound transmissions are the bonds of the doctor-patient relationship (the techniques of telemedicine) are already reality, and have proved particularly convenient and cost-effective in linking the patient and the generalist to specialists in remote areas with low population density.

As with written personal medical records,

confidentiality of personal medical information on computers is essential. Computerised data are covered by the Data Protection Act 1984. This stipulates that data must:

● be obtained and processed fairly and lawfully.
● be held only for specified lawful purposes.
● not be used in a manner incompatible with those purposes.
● only be recorded where necessary for these purposes.
● be accurate and up to date.
● not be stored longer than necessary.
● be made available to the patient on request.
● be protected by appropriate security and backup procedures.

As these problems are solved, concerns about privacy and confidentiality arise. While paper records were often only confidential by default, the potential for breaches of security in computerised networks is much graver. External breaches of the system by hackers are one serious concern, but internal breaches by authorised users making unauthorised use of the data are a much greater risk in practice. Governing network security so that clinical users have access on a need-to-know basis is a difficult business: the software tools to enable this – encryption, and anonymisation (ensuring that clinical information about patients is anonymous to prevent confidential information about them leaking out) of data collected for management and research processes – exist in the technical domain but remain a complex conundrum for solution in the real world.

The mushroom growth of websites covering myriad subjects has, of course, included health information. This ranges from clinical details on individual diseases to facts about medical organisations and institutes, patient support groups, etc. Some of this information contains comments and advice from orthodox and unorthodox practitioners. This open access to health information has been of great benefit to patients and health professionals. But web browsers should be aware that not all the medical information, including suggested treatments, has been subject to PEER REVIEW, as is the case with most medical articles in recognised medical journals.

Informed Consent

Patients' rights are a growing concern for doctors and patients. A controversial aspect of their clinical relationship is consent: doctors need signed agreement from patients before carrying out operations or procedures; before entering patients in clinical trials; and before publishing clinical details or photographs of patients for medical education in print or electronic media. Consent is said to be informed when patients are fully aware of the consequences and risks of the procedure in question. For example, doctors and other health professionals should tell patients of the complications of a treatment and the likelihood of its success. They should make sure that the patients understand the information given; patients should be given the opportunity to ask questions and, where appropriate, immediate relatives should be involved in the process. Doctors are often inclined to highlight the benefits of a treatment, while downplaying the risks, but the General Medical Council in the United Kingdom has shown its willingness to discipline doctors who go beyond the consent that they were given by patients.

Although the precise limits will remain difficult to define in some settings, informed consent should be obtained from patients in accordance with guidelines from professional medical organisations. Patients or close relatives should consult the local NHS authorities or help-groups if they are dissatisfied with their doctors' explanations.

Infrared Radiation

The band of electromagnetic radiation which has a longer wavelength than that of the red in the visible spectrum. Infrared radiation is used in the special photographic process essential to THERMOGRAPHY. Its property of transmitting radiant heat has made infrared radiation invaluable in PHYSIOTHERAPY, where it warms tissues, soothes pain and increases the local circulation.

Infundibulum

A funnel-shaped passage. The word is used specifically to describe the hollow conical stalk that links the HYPOTHALAMUS to the posterior lobe of the PITUITARY GLAND.

Infusion

The intravenous or subcutaneous injection of one of a variety of therapeutic solutions, such as saline, glucose, or gum acacia, in the treatment of severe DEHYDRATION, HYPOGLYCAEMIA, or other plasma electrolyte imbalance. Blood infusions may be given in cases of severe ANAEMIA – for example, after heavy bleeding. Infusions may be given in intermittent amounts of around 570 ml (1 pint) at a time, or alternatively by continuous drip-feed over several hours.

Ingestion

(1) The act of taking fluid, food, or medicine

into the stomach. (2) The way in which a phagocytic cell surrounds and absorbs foreign substances such as bacteria in the blood.

Ingrowing Toenail
The sides of the toenail curve downwards, resulting in inflammation of the skin next to the nail which spreads to the base of the nail. The skin and nail base may become painful and badly infected. If antibiotics and local dressing do not cure the condition, surgery to remove part of the nail will be required.

Inguinal Hernia
An extrusion of the abdominal PERITONEUM, sometimes containing a loop of bowel, through natural openings in the region of either groin (see HERNIA).

Inguinal Region
The groin – that area of the body where the lower part of the abdomen meets the upper thigh. The inguinal ligaments extend on each side from the superior spines of the iliac bones to the pubic bone. It is also called Poupart's ligament (see diagram of ABDOMEN).

Inhalants
Substances that can be inhaled into the body through the lungs. They may be delivered in traditional form dissolved in hot water and inhaled in the steam, or as an aerosol – a suspension of very small liquid or solid particles in the air. The latter are now usually delivered by devices in which the aerosol is kept under pressure in a small hand-held cylinder and delivered in required doses by a release mechanism.

Aerosols Asthmatic patients (see ASTHMA) find aerosol devices to be of value in controlling their attacks. They provide an effective and convenient way of applying drugs directly to the bronchi, thus reducing the risks of unwanted effects accompanying SYSTEMIC therapy. BRONCHODILATOR aerosols contain either a beta-sympathomimetic agent or ipratropium bromide, which is an ANTICHOLINERGIC drug.

ISOPRENALINE was the first compound to be widely used as an aerosol. It did however stimulate $beta_1$ receptors in the heart as well as $beta_2$ receptors in the bronchi, and so produced palpitations and even dangerous cardiac arrhythmias. Newer beta-adrenoceptor agonists are specific for the $beta_2$ receptors and thus have a greater safety margin. They include SALBUTAMOL, TERBUTALINE, rimiterol, fenoterol and reproterol. Unwanted effects such as palp-

tations, tremor and restlessness are uncommon with these, more specific preparations. In patients who get insufficient relief from the beta-adrenoreceptor agonist, the drug ipratropium bromide is worth adding. Salmeterol is a longer-acting choice for twice-daily administration: it is not intended for the relief of acute attacks, for which shorter-acting $beta_2$ stimulants such as salbutamol should be used. Salmeterol should be added to existing corticosteroid therapy (see CORTICOSTEROIDS), rather than replacing it.

Patients must be taught carefully and observed while using their inhalers. It is important for them to realise that if the aerosol no longer gives more than slight transient relief, they should not increase the dose but seek medical help.

Inhalation
A method of applying drugs in a finely divided or gaseous state, so that, when breathed in, they may come into contact with the nose, throat and lungs. There are two chief means by which drugs are mingled with the air and so taken in by breathing: these are traditional steam inhalations, and modern aerosol devices which deliver a fine spray direct into the mouth. (See INHALANTS; INHALER.)

Inhaler
A mechanism for administering a drug in the form of a powder or aerosol. mainly used by patients with ASTHMA. Inhalers are basically of two types: aerosol, and dry-powder inhaler. The former delivers the drug as an aerosol spray when the patient presses the top of the canister containing the drug; the latter works by putting a drug capsule in the end of the chamber and, when the patient presses the top, the capsule is pierced and the drug released. A variety of 'spacing devices' are available to use with pressurised (aerosol) inhalers, providing metered doses. The space introduced between the inhaler and the mouth reduces the velocity of the aerosol and thus the impact it has on the oropharynx. More time is therefore allowed for evaporation of the propellant, with a greater concentration of drug particles being inhaled. Inhalers with larger spacing devices and a one-way valve are very effective and particularly useful for children and patients needing higher doses of the drug. (See INHALANTS; NEBULISERS.)

Inheritance
The transfer of characteristics, traits and disorders from parents to children by means of

GENES carried in the CHROMOSOMES of the germ cells. (See GERM CELL; GENETIC CODE; GENETIC DISORDERS.)

Inhibition

Inhibition means arrest or restraint of some process effected by nervous influence. The term is applied to the action of certain inhibitory nerves: for example, the vagus nerve which contains fibres that inhibit or control the action of the heart. The term is also applied generally to the mental processes by which instinctive but undesirable actions are checked by a process of self-control.

Injections

An injection is the introduction of a substance into the body using a syringe and an attached needle. Injections may be given under the skin (subcutaneous), via a vein (intravenous), deep into a muscle (intramuscular), or into the fluid surrounding the spinal cord (intrathecal).

Inner Ear

This comprises three fluid-filled chambers, or labyrinths, situated in the bony temporal area that are concerned with identifying a person's position in space. Each chamber lies in a different plane, and movement of fluid within it is picked up by sensory cells that transmit the information to the brain. Disease or damage to the inner ear upsets the sense of balance and causes vertigo. MOTION TRAVEL SICKNESS is caused by the inner ear being unable to accommodate the changes in position resulting from motion. (See EAR.)

Innervation

The nerve supply to a tissue, organ or part of the body. It carries motor impulses to and sensory impulses away from the part.

Inoculation

The process by which infective material is brought into the system through a small wound in the skin or in a mucous membrane. Many infectious diseases are contracted by accidental inoculation of microbes – as is blood-poisoning (see SEPTICAEMIA). Inoculation is now used as a preventive measure against many infectious diseases. (See also VACCINE.)

Inositol

A sugar compound that is one constituent of some phospholipids (see LIPID) found in cells. It is found in many foods but, although sometimes classified as a VITAMIN, it is not a vital part of the human diet.

Inotropic

Adjective describing anything that affects the force of muscle contraction. It is usually applied to the heart muscle; an inotrope such as DIGOXIN is a drug that improves its contraction. Beta-blocker drugs such as PROPRANOLOL HYDROCHLORIDE have negative inotropic properties.

Inpatient

A person who requires a hospital bed for investigation or treatment.

Inquest

An official inquiry conducted by a CORONER into the cause of an individual's death. The coroner is a judicial officer who, when a death is sudden, unexpected or occurs in suspicious circumstances, considers the results of medical and legal investigation and, sitting with a jury or on his or her own, makes the conclusions public. He/she has wide powers, and, in deaths of uncertain cause, no official death certificate can be issued without his or her approval. A coroner may be legally or medically qualified (or both). In Scotland the comparable officer is the procurator fiscal.

Insanity

See MENTAL ILLNESS.

Insecticides

Substances which kill insects. Since the discovery of the insecticidal properties of DDT (see DICHLORODIPHENYL TRICHLOROETHANE) in 1940, a steady stream of new ones has been introduced. Their combined use has played an outstanding part in international public health campaigns, such as that of the World Health Organisation for the eradication of MALARIA.

Unfortunately, insects are liable to become resistant to insecticides, just as bacteria are liable to become resistant to antibiotics, and it is for this reason that so much research work is being devoted to the discovery of new ones. Researchers are also exploring new methods, such as releasing sexually sterile insects into the natural population.

The useful effects of insecticides must be set against increasing evidence that the indiscriminate use of some of these potent preparations is having an adverse effect – not only upon human beings, but also upon the ecosystems. Some, such as DDT – the use of which is now banned in the UK – are very stable compounds that enter the food chain and may ultimately be lethal to many animals, including birds and fishes.

Insemination

The ejaculation of SEMEN in the VAGINA in the act of sexual intercourse. In ARTIFICIAL INSEMINATION the semen is placed there by the use of an instrument. (See also ASSISTED CONCEPTION.)

Insight

A person's knowledge of him or herself. The description is especially relevant to a person's realisation that he or she has psychological difficulties. Thus, someone with a psychosis (see MENTAL ILLNESS) lacks insight. Insight also refers to an individual's concept of his or her personality and problems.

Insomnia

See SLEEP, DISORDERS OF; HYPNOTICS.

Inspissation

The process of the drying or thickening of fluids or excretions by evaporation.

Institutionalisation

A condition brought about by a prolonged stay in an impersonal institution. The individual becomes apathetic and listless as a result of inadequate stimulation in an uninteresting environment. The condition can occur in mental institutions or long-stay nursing homes; the affected person loses the ability to make any decisions and becomes pathetic and increasingly dependent on others.

Insufflation

Insufflation means the blowing of powder or vapour into a cavity, especially through the air passages, for the treatment of disease.

Insulin

A POLYPEPTIDE hormone (see HORMONES) produced in the PANCREAS by the beta cells of the ISLETS OF LANGERHANS. It plays a key role in the body's regulation of CARBOHYDRATE, FAT, and PROTEIN, and its deficiency leads to DIABETES MELLITUS. Diabetic patients are described as type 1 (insulin dependent), or type 2 (non-insulin dependent), although many of the latter may need insulin later on, in order to maintain good control.

Insulin is extracted mainly from pork pancreas and purified by crystallisation; it may be made biosynthetically by recombinant DNA technology using *Escherichia coli,* or semisynthetically by enzymatic modification of porcine insulin to produce human insulin. The latter is the form now generally used, although some patients find it unsuitable and have to return to porcine insulin.

The hormone acts by enabling the muscles and other tissues requiring sugar for their activity to take up this substance from the blood. All insulin preparations are to a greater or lesser extent immunogenic in humans, but immunological resistance to insulin action is uncommon.

Previously available in three strengths, of 20, 40, and 80 units per millilitre (U/ml), these have now largely been replaced by a standard strength of 100 U/ml (U100). Numerous different insulin preparations are listed; these differ in their speed of onset and duration of action, and hence vary in their suitability for individual patients.

Insulin is inactivated by gastrointestinal enzymes and is therefore generally given by subcutaneous injection, usually into the upper arms, thighs, buttocks, or abdomen. Some insulins are also available in cartridge form, which may be administered by injection devices ('pens'). The absorption may vary from different sites and with strenuous activity. About 25 per cent of diabetics require insulin treatment: most children from the onset, and all patients presenting with ketoacidosis. Insulin is also often needed by those with a rapid onset of symptoms such as weight loss, weakness, and sometimes vomiting, often associated with ketonuria.

The aim of treatment is to maintain good control of blood glucose concentration, while avoiding severe HYPOGLYCAEMIA; this is usually achieved by a regimen of preprandial injections of short-acting insulin (often with a bedtime injection of long-acting insulin). Insulin may also be given by continuous subcutaneous infusion with an infusion pump. This technique has many disadvantages: patients must be well motivated and able to monitor their own blood glucose, with access to expert advice both day and night; it is therefore rarely used.

Hypoglycaemia is a potential hazard for many patients converting from porcine to human insulin, because human insulin may result in them being unaware of classical hypoglycaemic warning symptoms. Drivers must be particularly careful, and individuals may be forbidden to drive if they have frequent or severe hypoglycaemic attacks. For this reason, insurance companies should be warned, and diabetics should – after taking appropriate medical advice – either return to porcine insulin or consider stopping driving.

Insulinase

An ENZYME occurring in body tissues, such as

the kidney and liver, that breaks down INSULIN in the body.

Insulinoma

A tumour in the beta cells in the Islets of Langerhans in the PANCREAS that produces insulin. Symptoms of HYPOGLYCAEMIA occur. Treatment is surgical removal or oral administration of diazoxide.

Insulin Shock

A disorder in which the body produces excess INSULIN, which then reduces the amount of glucose in the blood (HYPOGLYCAEMIA). Treatment is with glucose or GLUCAGON. Untreated, the patient goes into a COMA and dies.

Integument

Another name for skin. The term is also used for a layer or membrane surrounding any of the body's organs.

Intelligence Quotient (IQ)

This is the ratio between the mental age and chronological age multiplied by 100. Thus, if a boy of 10 years of age is found to have a mental age of 12 years, his IQ will be 120. On the other hand, if he is found to have a mental age of 8 years, his IQ will be 80.

The mental age is established by various tests, the most widely used of which are the Stanford-Binet Scale, the Wechsler Adult Intelligence Scale, and the Mill Hill Vocabulary Test.

Average intelligence is represented by an IQ of 100, with a range of 85 to 115. For practical purposes it is taken that the intellectual level reached by the average 15-year-old is indistinguishable from that of an adult.

Intelligence Test

A standardised procedure of mental assessment to determine an individual's intellectual ability. The result is produced as a score termed the INTELLIGENCE QUOTIENT (IQ). The Wechsler Adult Intelligence Scale (WAIS) and one for children, the Wechsler Intelligence Scale for Children (WICS), are commonly used, as is the Stanford-Binet Scale. Assessments are made for educational purposes and to help in the diagnoses of people with possible mental retardation or intellectual deterioration.

Intensive Care Medicine

The origin of this important branch of medicine lies in the effective use of positive-pressure VENTILATION of the lungs to treat respiratory breathing failure in patients affected by POLIO-MYELITIS in an outbreak of this potentially fatal disease in Denmark in 1952. Doctors reduced to 40 per cent, the 90 per cent mortality in patients receiving respiratory support with the traditional cuirass ventilator by using the new technique. They achieved this with a combination of manual positive-pressure ventilation provided through a TRACHEOSTOMY by medical students, and by looking after the patients in a specific area of the hospital, allowing the necessary staffing and equipment resources to be concentrated in one place.

The principle of one-to-one, 24-hours-a-day care for seriously ill patients has been widely adopted and developed for the initial treatment of many patients with life-threatening conditions. Thus, severely injured patients – those with serious medical conditions such as coronary thrombosis or who have undergone major surgery, and individuals suffering from potentially lethal toxic affects of poisons – are treated in an INTENSIVE THERAPY UNIT (ITU). Patients whose respiratory or circulatory systems have failed benefit especially by being intensively treated. Most patients, especially post-operative ones, leave intensive care when their condition has been stabilised, usually after 24 or 48 hours. Some, however, need support for several weeks or even months. Since 1952, intensive medicine has become a valued specialty and a demanding one because of the range of skills needed by the doctors and nurses manning the ITUs.

Intensive Therapy Unit (ITU)

Sometimes called an intensive care unit, this is a hospital unit in which seriously ill patients undergo resuscitation, monitoring and treatment. The units are staffed by doctors and nurses trained in INTENSIVE CARE MEDICINE, and patients receive 24-hour, one-to-one care with continuous monitoring of their condition with highly specialised electronic equipment that assesses vital body functions such as heart rate, respiration, blood pressure, temperature and blood chemistry. The average ITU in Britain has four to six beds, although units in larger hospitals, especially those dealing with tertiary-care referrals – for example, neurosurgical or organ transplant cases – are bigger, but 15 beds is usually the maximum. Annual throughput of patients ranges from fewer than 200 to more than 1,500 patients a year. As well as general ITUs, specialty units are provided for neonatal, paediatric, cardiothoracic and neurological patients in regional centres. The UK has 1–2 per cent of its hospital beds allocated to intensive care, a figure far below the average of 20 per cent provided in the United States. Thus patients undergoing intensive care in the UK are usually more seriously ill than those in the US. This is reflected in the shortage of available ITU beds in Britain, especially in the winter. (See CORONARY CARE UNIT (CCU); HIGH DEPENDENCY UNIT.)

Intercostal

The term applied to the nerves, vessels and muscles that lie between the ribs, as well as to diseases affecting these structures.

Interferon

It has been known for many years that one VIRUS will interfere with the growth of another. In 1957, UK research workers isolated the factor that was responsible for the phenomenon, giving it the name of interferon. There are now known to be three human interferons. They are glycoproteins and are released from cells infected with virus or exposed to stimuli which mimic virus infection. They not only inhibit the growth of viruses; they also inhibit the growth and reduplication of cells, and this is the basis for their investigation as a means of treating cancer. Hitherto the major difficulty has been obtaining sufficient supplies of interferon, but methods have now been evolved which promise to provide adequate amounts of it. The most promising of these is by means of what is known as genetic engineering, or manipulation, whereby a portion of DNA from interferon is inserted into the micro-organism known as *Escherichia coli* (see ESCHERICHIA) which thus becomes a source of almost unlimited amounts of interferon as it can be grown so easily.

Interferon alfa – previously termed leucocyte interferon or lymphoblastoid interferon – has some antitumour effect in some solid tumours and lymphomas. It is also used to treat HEPA-TITIS B and C (chronic variety). Various side-effects include suppression of MYELOBLAST production. Interferon beta – previously termed fibroblast interferon – is used (under restricted conditions in the UK) to treat patients with relapsing, remitting MULTIPLE SCLEROSIS (MS), and interferon beta-16 is licensed for use in patients with the secondary progressive type of this disorder. The use of interferon, which has a range of side-effects, should be recommended by a neurologist.

Interleukins

Interleukins are lymphokines – that is, poly-peptides produced by activated lymphocytes. They are involved in signalling between cells of the immune system (see IMMUNITY) and are released by several cell types, including lympho-cytes. They interact to control the immune response of cells and also participate in HAEMO-POIESIS. There are seven varieties, interleukins 1 to 7. For example, interleukin 1 is produced as a result of inflammation and stimulates the pro-liferation of T and B lymphocytes, enhancing the immune response by stimulating other lymphocytes and activating dormant T cells. Interleukin 2 has anti-cancer effects as it is able to activate T lymphocytes to become killer cells which destroy foreign antigens (see ANTIGEN) such as cancer cells, and this anti-cancer effect is being developed for clinical use. The remaining interleukins have a range of properties in cell growth and differentiation.

Intermediate Care

Described by the UK government as 'a bridge between hospital and home' to speed discharge from acute care and provide recovery and rehabilitation services, this concept was a key element in the *NHS Plan: plan for investment; a plan for reform*, published in 2000. The gov-ernment sees cottage hospitals, private nursing homes, and domiciliary and community set-tings as providing the heart of the proposed intermediate-care sector. Also in the plan, how-ever, is the warning that the NHS would meet the costs only of nursing care for nursing-home residents: personal care would in future be charged for. (In Scotland the NHS funds personal-care costs.) The change in England would alter the principles on which the NHS was founded in 1948 – that all citizens would receive a universal, comprehensive service funded by the government. New care trusts will commission and deliver both primary and community health care as well as social care. The trusts will hold unified, capped budgets and they will define what is NHS care and what is social care. The social-care elements will be subject to the charging policies of local author-ities. Of the 160,000 or so nursing-home resi-dents in England, under 10 per cent have their care fully funded by the NHS. The funding future of this 10 per cent is uncertain, as will be the personal-care funding of 270,000 NHS patients expected to transfer from hospital into intermediate care each year. It is too early to say what effect these changes will have on a vulner-able section of the population. While the prin-ciple of using intermediate care to free expen-sive hospital beds is sensible, the uncertainties over funding and the grey area between the need for nursing and/or residential care will be a worry for elderly people, especially those of limited means. (Legislation to implement the government's planned changes to the NHS was going through Parliament as this text was going to press, so modifications to them are possible.)

Intermittent

A term applied to fevers which continue for a time, subside completely and then return again. The name is also used in connection with a pulse in which occasional heartbeats are not felt, in consequence of irregular action of the heart.

Intermittent Claudication

A condition occurring in middle-aged and elderly people, which is characterised by pain in the legs after walking a certain distance. The pain is relieved by resting for a short time. It is due to arteriosclerosis (see ARTERIES, DISEASES OF) of the arteries to the leg, which results in inadequate blood supply to the muscles. Drugs usually have little effect in easing the pain, but useful preventive measures are to stop smoking, reduce weight (if overweight), and to take as much exercise as possible within the limits imposed by the pain.

Intermittent Self-Catheterisation

A technique in which a patient (of either sex) inserts a disposable catheter (see CATHETERS) through the URETHRA into the bladder to empty it of urine. It is increasingly used to manage patients with chronic retention of urine, or whose bladders do not empty properly – usually the result of neurological disorder affecting the bladder (neuropathic bladder). (See URINARY BLADDER, DISEASES OF.)

Intern

An American term for a doctor-in-training who carries out his or her duties and learns in hospital, usually spending some of his/her time living there. The terms preferred in the UK are house officer or senior house officer (SHO).

International Classification of Disease (ICD)

A World Health Organisation classification of all known diseases and syndromes. The diseases are divided according to system (respiratory, renal, cardiac, etc.) or type (accidents, malignant growth, etc.). Each of them is given a three-digit number to facilitate computerisation. This classification allows mortality and morbidity rates to be compared nationally and regionally. A revised ICD is published every ten years; a similar classification is being developed for impairments, disabilities and handicaps.

Internet

Access to medical information via the Internet is widespread in some populations, often serving more patients than doctors. In addition to the huge variety of information available, patients can share experiences via electronic discussion groups, or obtain e-mail advice on a fee-for-service basis. Some professional organisations and journals provide free access to information, and the Internet can be a useful resource for medical practitioners and researchers. Concerns have arisen about the growth in electronic medical information: some believe that patients who have unlimited access to information via the Internet will be less likely to tolerate health-care rationing or will demand treatments that may be inappropriate in their individual circumstances. Other criticisms relate to the quality and accuracy of the information provided, potential breaches of patient CONFIDENTIALITY, and the risk of increased accusations of medical negligence (see also ETHICS).

Internode

The length of the AXON (of a nerve cell) that is covered with a MYELIN sheath. The nodes of Ranvier, which have no myelin sheath, separate the internodes. (See also NERVE.)

Intersexuality

Intersexuality is a state of indeterminate sexuality of an individual, and may present in many different forms. A characteristic is that only one type of gonad – testis or ovary – is present; in a HERMAPHRODITE both types are present. Intersexuality may be due to a fault in the genetic mechanism of sex determination as early as conception, or to later errors in sexual differentiation of the embryo and fetus, or after birth. Some cases may result from abnormal metabolism of the sex hormones, or may be drug-induced (for example, women given androgens [see ANDROGEN] or PROGESTERONE for repeated miscarriages may give birth to girls with some genital VIRILISATION). Abnormalities of the sex chromosomes may be associated with delayed (or failure of) sexual development, so that the individual shows some of the characteristics (often underdeveloped) of both sexes. Some of the more common presentations of the condition include HYPOGONADISM, CRYPTORCHIDISM, and primary AMENORRHOEA.

Intersexuality inevitably leads to considerable psychological disturbance as the child grows up. It is therefore important to reach an early decision as to the child's sex – or at least, the sex that he or she is to be brought up as. Surgical or hormonal means should then be employed, when appropriate, to develop the attributes of that sex and diminish those of the other, together with psychological counselling.

Interstitial

Interstitial is a term applied to indifferent tissue set among the proper active tissue of an organ. It is generally of a supporting character and formed of fibrous tissue. The term is also applied to the fluid always present in this in a small amount, and to diseases which specially affect this tissue, such as interstitial keratitis.

Interstitial Cells

Also called Leydig cells, these cells are scattered between the SEMINIFEROUS TUBULES of the testis (see TESTICLE). LUTEINISING HORMONE from the anterior PITUITARY GLAND stimulates the interstitial cells to produce androgens, or male hormones.

Intertrigo

Inflammation between two skin surfaces in contact, typically in the toe clefts, axillae, under the breasts or in the anogenital folds. Heat, friction and obesity are aggravating factors. Secondary fungal or bacterial infection with CANDIDA or bacteria is common.

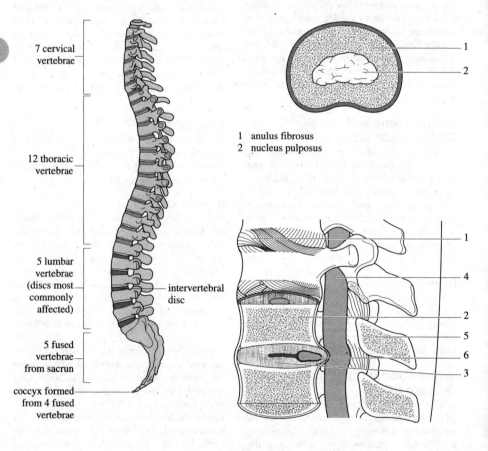

7 cervical vertebrae

12 thoracic vertebrae

5 lumbar vertebrae (discs most commonly affected)

intervertebral disc

5 fused vertebrae from sacrun

coccyx formed from 4 fused vertebrae

1 anulus fibrosus
2 nucleus pulposus

1 intervertebral disc
2 vertebral body
3 anulus fibrosus
4 spinal cord
5 vertebral spine
6 nucleus pulposus (protruding into spinal cord) as a result of 'slipped' disc

Lateral view of prolapsed intervertebral disc.

Interventional Radiology

The use of radiology (see X-RAYS) to enable doctors to carry out diagnostic or treatment procedures under direct radiological vision. This X-ray procedure is used in MINIMALLY INVASIVE SURGERY (MIS) – for example, ANGIOPLASTY, the removal of stones from the kidney (see KIDNEYS, DISEASES OF), and the observation of obstructions in the bile ducts (percutaneous CHOLANGIOGRAPHY). (See also magnetic resonance imaging – MRI.)

Intervention Study

Comparison of outcomes between two or more groups of patients who have been intentionally given different treatments or preventative measures, for example, diets. The subjects in the trial should be randomly allocated to the groups, with patients in one group – called controls – receiving no active treatment. If possible, neither patients nor doctors participating in a study should know which patients are receiving what treatment (double blind study/trial). Furthermore, groups should exchange treatments after a prearranged time (crossover study/trial). (See CLINICAL TRIALS; RANDOMISED CONTROLLED TRIAL.)

Intervertebral Disc

The fibrous disc that acts as a cushion between the bony vertebrae (see SPINAL COLUMN), enabling them to rotate and bend one on another. The disc tends to degenerate with age and may get ruptured and displaced – prolapsed or slipped disc – as a result of sudden strenuous action. Prolapsed disc occurs mainly in the lower back; it is more common in men than in women, and in the 30–40 age group.

Intestine

All the alimentary canal beyond below the stomach. In it, most DIGESTION is carried on, and through its walls all the food material is absorbed into the blood and lymph streams. The length of the intestine in humans is about 8·5–9 metres (28–30 feet), and it takes the form of one continuous tube suspended in loops in the abdominal cavity.

Divisions The intestine is divided into small intestine and large intestine. The former extends from the stomach onwards for 6·5 metres (22 feet) or thereabouts. The large intestine is the second part of the tube, and though shorter (about 1·8 metres [6 feet] long) is much wider than the small intestine. The latter is divided rather arbitrarily into three parts: the duodenum, consisting of the first 25–30 cm (10–12 inches), into which the ducts of the liver and pancreas open; the jejunum, comprising the next 2·4–2·7 metres (8–9 feet); and finally the ileum, which at its lower end opens into the large intestine.

The large intestine begins in the lower part of the abdomen on the right side. The first part is known as the caecum, and into this opens the appendix vermiformis. The appendix is a small tube, closed at one end and about the thickness of a pencil, anything from 2 to 20 cm (average 9 cm) in length, which has much the same structure as the rest of the intestine. (See APPENDICITIS.) The caecum continues into the colon. This is subdivided into: the ascending colon which ascends through the right flank to beneath the liver; the transverse colon which crosses the upper part of the abdomen to the left side; and the descending colon which bends downwards through the left flank into the pelvis where it becomes the sigmoid colon. The last part of the large intestine is known as the rectum, which passes straight down through the back part of the pelvis, to open to the exterior through the anus.

Structure The intestine, both small and large, consists of four coats, which vary slightly in structure and arrangement at different points but are broadly the same throughout the entire length of the bowel. On the inner surface there is a mucous membrane; outside this is a loose submucous coat, in which blood vessels run; next comes a muscular coat in two layers; and finally a tough, thin peritoneal membrane.

MUCOUS COAT The interior of the bowel is completely lined by a single layer of pillar-like cells placed side by side. The surface is increased by countless ridges with deep furrows thickly studded with short hair-like processes called villi. As blood and lymph vessels run up to the end of these villi, the digested food passing slowly down the intestine is brought into close relation with the blood circulation. Between the bases of the villi are little openings, each of which leads into a simple, tubular gland which produces a digestive fluid. In the small and large intestines, many cells are devoted to the production of mucus for lubricating the passage of the food. A large number of minute masses, called lymph follicles, similar in structure to the tonsils are scattered over the inner surface of the intestine. The large intestine is bare both of ridges and of villi.

SUBMUCOUS COAT Loose connective tissue which allows the mucous membrane to play freely over the muscular coat. The blood vessels and lymphatic vessels which absorb the food in the villi pour their contents into a network of large vessels lying in this coat.

MUSCULAR COAT The muscle in the small intestine is arranged in two layers, in the outer of which all the fibres run lengthwise with the bowel, whilst in the inner they pass circularly round it.

PERITONEAL COAT This forms the outer covering for almost the whole intestine except parts of the duodenum and of the large intestine. It is a tough, fibrous membrane, covered upon its outer surface with a smooth layer of cells.

Intestine, Diseases of

The principal signs of trouble which has its origin in the intestine consist of pain somewhere about the abdomen, sometimes vomiting, and irregular bowel movements: constipation, diarrhoea or alternating bouts of these.

Several diseases and conditions are treated under separate headings. (See APPENDICITIS; CHOLERA; COLITIS; CONSTIPATION; CROHN'S DISEASE; DIARRHOEA; DYSENTERY; ENTERIC FEVER; HAEMORRHOIDS; HERNIA; INFLAMMATORY BOWEL DISEASE (IBD); ILEITIS; INTUSSUSCEPTION; IRRITABLE BOWEL SYNDROME (IBS); PERITONITIS; RECTUM, DISEASES OF; ULCERATIVE COLITIS.)

Inflammation of the outer surface is called peritonitis, a serious disease. That of the inner surface is known generally as enteritis, inflammation of special parts receiving the names of colitis, appendicitis, irritable bowel syndrome (IBS) and inflammatory bowel disease (IBD). Enteritis may form the chief symptom of certain infective diseases: for example in typhoid fever (see ENTERIC FEVER), cholera and dysentery. It may be acute, although not connected with any definite organism, when, if severe, it is a very serious condition, particularly in young children. Or it may be chronic, especially as the result of dysentery, and then constitutes a less serious if very troublesome complaint.

Perforation of the bowel may take place as the result either of injury or of disease. Stabs and other wounds which penetrate the abdomen may damage the bowel, and severe blows or crushes may tear it without any external wound. Ulceration, as in typhoid fever, or, more rarely, in TUBERCULOSIS, may cause an opening in the bowel-wall also. Again, when the bowel is greatly distended above an obstruction, faecal material may accumulate and produce

ulcers, which rupture with the ordinary movements of the bowels. Whatever the cause, the symptoms are much the same.

Symptoms The contents of the bowel pass out through the perforation into the peritoneal cavity, and set up a general peritonitis. In consequence, the abdomen is painful, and after a few hours becomes extremely tender to the touch. The abdomen swells, particularly in its upper part, owing to gas having passed also into the cavity. Fever and vomiting develop and the person passes into a state of circulatory collapse or SHOCK. Such a condition may be fatal if not properly treated.

Treatment All food should be withheld and the patient given intravenous fluids to resuscitate them and then to maintain their hydration and electrolyte balance. An operation is urgently necessary, the abdomen being opened in the middle line, the perforated portion of bowel found, the perforation stitched up, and appropriate antibiotics given.

Obstruction means a stoppage to the passage down the intestine of partially digested food. Obstruction may be acute, when it comes on suddenly with intense symptoms; or it may be chronic, when the obstructing cause gradually increases and the bowel becomes slowly more narrow until it closes altogether; or subacute, when obstruction comes and goes until it ends in an acute attack. In chronic cases the symptoms are milder in degree and more prolonged.

Causes Obstruction may be due to causes outside the bowel altogether, for example, the pressure of tumours in neighbouring organs, the twisting around the bowel of bands produced by former peritonitis, or even the twisting of a coil of intestine around itself so as to cause a kink in its wall. Chronic causes of the obstruction may exist in the wall of the bowel itself: for example, a tumour, or the contracting scar of an old ulcer. The condition of INTUSSUSCEPTION, where part of the bowel passes inside of the part beneath it, in the same way as one turns the finger of a glove outside in, causes obstruction and other symptoms. Bowel within a hernia may become obstructed when the hernia strangulates. Finally some body, such as a concretion, or the stone of some large fruit, or even a mass of hardened faeces, may become jammed within the bowel and stop up its passage.

Symptoms There are four chief symptoms: pain, vomiting, constipation and swelling of the abdomen.

Treatment As a rule the surgeon opens the abdomen, finds the obstruction and relieves it or if possible removes it altogether. It may be necessary to form a COLOSTOMY or ILEOSTOMY as a temporary or permanent measure in severe cases.

Tumours are rare in the small intestine and usually benign. They are relatively common in the large intestine and are usually cancerous. The most common site is the rectum. Cancer of the intestine is a disease of older people; it is the second most common cancer (after breast cancer) in women in the United Kingdom, and the third most common (after lung and prostate) in men. Around 25,000 cases of cancer of the large intestine occur in the UK annually, about 65 per cent of which are in the colon. A history of altered bowel habit, in the form of increasing constipation or diarrhoea, or an alternation of these, or of bleeding from the anus, in a middle-aged person is an indication for taking medical advice. If the condition is cancer, then the sooner it is investigated and treated, the better the result.

Intima
The innermost coat lining the arteries and the veins.

Intolerance
An adverse reaction of a patient to a drug or treatment. (See ADVERSE REACTIONS TO DRUGS.)

Intoxication
A term applied to states of poisoning. The poison may be some chemical substance introduced from outside, for example, ALCOHOL; or it may be due to the products of bacterial action, the bacteria either being introduced from outside or developing within the body. The term autointoxication is applied in the latter case.

Intra-
Prefix indicating inside or within. For example, intracellular: within a cell; intra-articular: within a joint.

Intracoronary Artery Stenting
A narrowed or blocked coronary artery (see ARTERIES) can compromise the blood supply to the heart muscle (see HEART, DISEASES OF). A

supportive tube or stent passed into each affected artery can restore the blood supply. The stent has a HEPARIN coating to stop blood clots from forming. Since it was first performed in 1987, intracoronary stents have cut the reblockage rate from one in three patients who have had coronary ANGIOPLASTY to fewer than one in ten in cases where a stent was used with angioplasty.

Intracranial
Intracranial is the term applied to structures, diseases, etc. contained in or rising within the head.

Intracranial Pressure
This is the pressure that is maintained by the brain tissue, intracellular and extracellular fluid, cerebrospinal fluid and blood. An increase in intracranial pressure may occur as a result of inflammation, injury, haemorrhage, or tumour in the brain tissue as well as of some congenital conditions. The pressure is measured by lumbar puncture in which a syringe attached to a mamometer (pressure-measuring device) is inserted into the cerebrospinal fluid surrounding the lower part of the spinal cord. Where continuous pressure monitoring is necessary, an in-dwelling device can be implanted into a cerebral ventricle. Normal pressure is around 10 mm of mercury (Hg), with the acceptable upper limit being 25 mm Hg.

Intracytoplasmic Sperm Injection
Intracytoplasmic sperm injection (ICSI) is the most significant therapeutic advance in male INFERTILITY treatment in the past 30 years. The technique is used when in vitro fertilisation (IVF – see under ASSISTED CONCEPTION) is not possible because the man has very few, motile, normal sperm (see SPERMATOZOON), or when previous attempts at IVF have not produced a fertilised EMBRYO. ICSI requires a single sperm which is injected directly into the cytoplasm of an egg previously retrieved from the woman. Once fertilised, the embryo is transferred to her UTERUS. For men with no sperm in the semen, it may be possible to retrieve sperm by needle aspiration of the EPIDIDYMIS under local anaesthetic (see ANAESTHESIA). Other techniques involve microsurgical retrieval from the epididymis or TESTICLE under a general anaesthetic. Potential complications include scrotal pain, bruising, HAEMATOMA formation and infection. ICSI and surgical sperm-retrieval require extensive training and expertise and is currently available in only a few selected

infertility units. Safety concerns relate to a higher-than-expected rate of abnormalities in the SEX CHROMOSOMES after ICSI, and also the potential risk of transmitting paternal genetic defects in the Y chromosome to sons born after ICSI.

Intrathecal

Intrathecal means within the membranes or meninges which envelop the SPINAL CORD. The intrathecal space, between the arachnoid and the pia mater, contains the CEREBROSPINAL FLUID (see INTRACRANIAL PRESSURE).

Intrauterine Contraceptive Device (IUCD)

A mechanical device, commonly a coil, inserted into the UTERUS to prevent CONCEPTION, probably by interfering with the implantation of the EMBRYO. For many women, IUCDs are an effective and acceptable form of contraception, although only about 10 per cent of women in the UK use them. The devices are of various shapes and made of plastic or copper; most have a string that passes through the cervix and rests in the vagina.

About one-third of women have adverse effects as the result of IUCD use: common ones are backache and heavy menstrual bleeding (see MENSTRUATION). The frequency of unwanted pregnancies is about 2 per 100 women-years of use. (See CONTRACEPTION.)

Intrauterine Insemination

A method of helping CONCEPTION to occur when a man is infertile (see INFERTILITY) because his sperm (see SPERMATOZOON) cannot penetrate either the cervical mucus at the entrance of the UTERUS or the barriers that surround the OVUM. The sperm, often treated chemically beforehand to increase motility, are injected directly into the uterus via the VAGINA.

Intravenous

A term which means inside a vein. An intravenous injection is one that is given into a vein. Blood transfusions are given intravenously, as are other infusions of fluid.

Intravenous Pyelogram (Urogram)

A procedure for getting X-ray pictures of the URINARY TRACT. A radio-opaque medium is injected into a vein and, when it is excreted by the kidneys, the substance can be identified on X-rays. Any abnormalities in structure or foreign bodies such as calculi are outlined by the dye (see KIDNEYS, DISEASES OF).

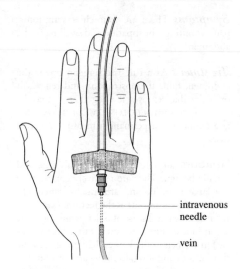

intravenous needle

vein

Position of intravenous needle inserted into vein on back of hand for administration of intravenous fluid or blood transfusion.

Intrinsic Factor

Secreted in the lining of the stomach, this factor is one of the GLYCOPROTEINS, and is essential for the absorption into the bloodstream of vitamin B_{12} (see APPENDIX 5: VITAMINS). Absence of intrinsic factor causes a deficiency of this essential vitamin, which in turn causes PERNICIOUS ANAEMIA.

Intromission

The introduction of one organ or part into another. An example is the insertion of the erect penis into the vagina during copulation.

Introspection

The observation of one's own thoughts or feelings. The term is generally applied to this process when it occurs to an abnormal extent in association with MELANCHOLIA.

Introversion

(1) In physical terms, to turn a hollow structure into itself – for example, a length of the intestine may 'enter' the succeeding portion, also known as INTUSSUSCEPTION.

(2) A psychological term to describe what happens when an individual is more interested in his or her 'inner world' than in what is happening around in the real world. An INTROVERT tends to have few friends and prefers to persist in activities that they have started. Karl Jung (see JUNGIAN ANALYSIS) described introversion as a person's tendency to distance him or herself from others; to have philosophical interests;

and to have reactions that are reserved and defensive.

Introvert

Physically it means turning inside out. Psychologically, the term refers to an individual whose character looks inwards on him or herself and who may also be obsessive and have few friends. (See INTROVERSION.)

Intubation

A procedure consisting in the introduction, through the mouth or nose into the larynx, of a tube designed to keep the air passage open at this point.

Intuition

The immediate understanding of a situation by someone without the customary mental process of reasoning.

Intussusception

A form of obstruction of the bowels in which part of the INTESTINE enters within that part immediately beneath it. This can best be understood by observing what takes place in the fingers of a tightly fitting glove as they turn outside-in when the glove is pulled off the hand. Mostly, the condition affects infants. Often it occurs during the course of a viral infection or a mild attack of gastroenteritis, or it may be that swelling of lymphoid tissue in the gut provokes the event. The point at which it most often occurs is the junction between the small and the large intestines, the former passing within the latter. The symptoms are those of intestinal obstruction in general (see INTESTINE, DISEASES OF – Obstruction), and in addition there is often a discharge of blood-stained mucus from the bowel. Unless the symptoms rapidly subside, when it may be assumed that the bowel has righted itself, treatment consists of either hydrostatic reduction by means of a barium or air ENEMA, or an operation. At operation the intussusception is either reduced or, if this not possible, the obstructed part is cut out and the ends of the intestine then stitched together. If treated adequately and in time, the mortality is now reduced to around 1 per cent. The condition may recur in about 5 per cent of patients.

In Utero

Literally 'in the UTERUS' and used to refer to events occurring to a baby before birth.

Invasion

The entry of bacteria into the body; the spread of cancer into normal, nearby tissues or organs.

In Vitro

A term commonly used in medical research and experimental biology. Literally 'in a glass', it refers to observations made outside the body: for example, on the action of drugs on bacteria. The opposite term is IN VIVO, which refers to observations of processes in the body.

In Vitro Fertilisation (IVF)

Fertilisation of the egg (ovum) outside the body. The fertilised ovum is then incubated until the blastocyst stage develops, when it is implanted into the UTERUS. The procedure was developed in Britain and the first successful in vitro baby, a girl, was born in 1978. IVF is used when a woman has blocked FALLOPIAN TUBES or when the sperm and ovum are unable to fuse in the reproductive tract. Hormone treatment results in the potential mother's producing several mature ova, some of which are removed from the ovary using a LAPAROSCOPE and fertilised with her partner's semen. (See ASSISTED CONCEPTION.)

In Vivo

A Latin term to describe biological events that take place inside the bodies of living organisms.

Involucrum

The sheath of new bone which is formed round a piece of dead bone in, for example, OSTEOMYELITIS.

Involuntary Muscle

Muscle that does not operate under a person's conscious control. Involuntary muscle – also called smooth muscle, because the cells do not contain the striations that occur in VOLUNTARY MUSCLE – is found in blood vessels, the heart, stomach, and intestines. (See PARASYMPATHETIC NERVOUS SYSTEM.)

Involution

The process of change whereby the UTERUS returns to its resting size after parturition (birth). The term is also applied to any retrograde biological change, as in senility (see AGEING).

Iodides

Salts of iodine, those which are especially used in medicine being the iodide of potassium and iodide of sodium. Iodides are excreted in the mucus secretions, as well as in the urine, saliva and sweat, and have an action in liquefying the mucus secretion of the bronchial tree. They are therefore used in EXPECTORANTS. They are also used to assist in providing a supply of iodine in patients with goitre, or in individuals who live in an area where goitre is liable to occur because of a deficiency of IODINE in the drinking water. They may be given in the form of iodised salt. (See THYROID GLAND, DISEASES OF – Goitre.)

Iodine

A non-metallic element which is found largely in seaweed. The body contains about 30 mg, largely concentrated in the THYROID GLAND where it is used to synthesise thyroid hormones. Iodine has a highly irritating action and, when applied to the skin, stains the latter dark brown and causes it to peel off in flakes, while internally it is a violent irritant poison in large doses.

Externally iodine is used as an antiseptic. Its drawback is that it is fixed by protein, which reduces its antiseptic efficiency in open wounds. Its main use in this sphere therefore is for sterilising the unbroken skin, as before an operation. Radioactive iodine is used for diagnosing and treating disease of the thyroid gland.

Ion Atom

An atom (or a collection of atoms) that has an electrical charge. Positive atoms are cations, negative ones are anions. Calcium, hydrogen, potassium and sodium are positive ions. Negative ones include bicarbonate chloride and phosphate. All the substances are critical to the body's physiological activities.

Ion Exchange Resins

Synthetic organic substances, capable of exchanging ions – cationic or anionic – from the contents of the intestine. Originally used in the prevention of OEDEMA, they have been superseded in this role by the modern DIURETICS, and are now used chiefly in the treatment of HYPERKALAEMIA. They are usually taken by mouth or as an ENEMA.

Ionisation

Ionisation means the breaking up of a substance in solution into its constituent.

Ipecacuanha

The root of *Cephaëlis ipecacuanha*, a Brazilian shrub. It contains an alkaloid, emetine, which acts as an irritant when brought into contact with the interior of the stomach, producing vomiting. Formerly used to induce vomiting among young children after poisoning and if still alert, but now of uncertain value, it was used in many traditional expectorant mixtures

(see EXPECTORANTS) given in the treatment of BRONCHITIS. (See POISONS.)

Ipratropium

An ANTICHOLINERGIC, BRONCHODILATOR drug, given by aerosol inhalation to treat ASTHMA, BRONCHITIS and RHINITIS.

IQ

See INTELLIGENCE QUOTIENT (IQ).

Iridectomy

The operation by which a hole is made in the iris of the EYE – as, for example, in the treatment of GLAUCOMA or as part of CATARACT surgery.

Iris

See EYE.

Iritis

See UVEITIS.

Iron

A metal which is an essential constituent of the red blood corpuscles, where it is present in the form of HAEMOGLOBIN. It is also present in muscle as MYOGLOBIN, and in certain respiratory pigments which are essential to the life of many tissues in the body. Iron is absorbed principally in the upper part of the small intestine. It is then stored: mainly in the liver; to a lesser extent in the spleen and kidneys, where it is available, when required, for use in the bone marrow to form the haemoglobin in red blood corpuscles. The daily iron requirement of an adult is 15–20 milligrams. This requirement is increased during pregnancy.

Uses The main use of iron is in the treatment of iron-deficiency anaemias (See ANAEMIA.) Iron preparations sometimes cause irritation of the gastrointestinal tract, and should therefore always be taken after meals. They sometimes produce a tendency towards constipation. Whenever possible, iron preparations should be given by mouth; if PARENTERAL administration is clinically necessary because of malabsorption, a suitable preparation is iron sorbitol injection given intramuscularly. Most patients respond successfully to oral iron preparations.

Irradiation

The use of naturally occurring isotopes, or artificially produced X-rays, in the killing of tumour cells. The amount of radiation is the adsorbed dose; the SI unit is the gray (Gy).

Different tumours seem to be particularly sensitive to radiation; radiotherapy plays an important role in the management of germ-cell tumours (SEMINOMA; TERATOMA) and lymphomas (see LYMPHOMA). Many head and neck tumours, gynaecological cancers, and localised prostate and bladder cancers are curable with radiotherapy. It may be used to reduce the pain – for example, from bone metastases.

Unwanted effects Generalised: lethargy, loss of appetite. Skin: ERYTHEMA, dry desquamation with itching, moist desquamation. Patients should keep the treated area(s) dry and clean and avoid soap, antiseptic mouthwashes, smoking and spicy food if possible. (See ISOTOPE; RADIATION SICKNESS; RADIOTHERAPY).

Irrigation

Irrigation is the method of washing-out wounds, or cavities of the body, like the bladder and bowels. (See DOUCHE; ENEMA.)

Irritable Bowel Syndrome (IBS)

A disorder of the intestinal tract that affects its motility and causes abdominal distension and irregular defaecation. Traditional, but now discarded, names have been spastic or irritable colon. The disease affects around 20 per cent of the general population but in most it is no more than a minor nuisance. The causes are not fully understood, but it is generally believed that symptoms develop in response to psychological factors, changed gastrointestinal motility, or altered visceral sensation. About 50 per cent of patients meet criteria for a psychiatric diagnosis. Anxiety, depression, neurosis, panic attacks, acute disease are among possible triggering factors. Some patients have diarrhoea, others are constipated, and some alternate between the two. Many have increased sensitivity to distension of the intestine. Dietary factors such as intolerance to dairy products and wheat are apparent in certain patients.

Common features of IBS include:
- abdominal distension.
- altered bowel habit.
- colicky lower abdominal pain, eased by defaecation.
- mucous discharge from rectum.
- feelings of incomplete defaecation.

Investigations usually produce normal results. Positive diagnosis in people under 40 is usually straightforward. In older patients, however, barium ENEMA, X-rays and COLONOSCOPY should be done to exclude colorectal cancer.

Reassurance is the initial and often effective treatment. If this fails, treatment should be directed at the major symptoms. Several months of the antidepressant amitriptyline (see ANTIDEPRESSANT DRUGS) may benefit patients with intractable symptoms, given at a dose lower than that used to treat depression. The majority of patients follow a relapsing/remitting course, with episodes provoked by stressful events in their daily lives. (See also INTESTINE, DISEASES OF.)

Irritant

Any substance that produces irritation in a tissue. Examples are: stinging nettles, which cause pain and swelling; certain insect bites or stings which do the same; and anti riot gases such as CS gas, which cause the eyes to water and provoke coughing. Regular, unprotected handling of certain substances – for example, oil – can irritate the skin and cause DERMATITIS. Some people are more sensitive than others to the effect of irritants; sometimes an irritant will produce an allergic reaction (see ALLERGY) and in serious cases ANAPHYLAXIS, which may require medical treatment.

Ischaemia

Bloodlessness of a part of the body, due to contraction, spasm, constriction or blocking (by EMBOLUS or by THROMBUS) of the arteries: for example, of the heart.

Ischaemic Heart Disease

See HEART, DISEASES OF.

Ischaemic Stroke

A STROKE that occurs when the flow of blood to a part of the brain is interrupted by a partial or complete THROMBOSIS of the supplying artery or ARTERIES, or by a clot of blood that has detached itself from elsewhere in the circulatory system – for instance, a deep vein thrombosis (DVT) – and blocked a cerebral artery. Stroke is the second most common cause of death worldwide. Its treatment is difficult and prevention is best targeted at those who are at the highest absolute risk of stroke, because such people are likely to derive the greatest benefit. They generally have a history of occlusive vascular diseases such as previous ischaemic stroke or a transient ischaemic attack (TIA), coronary heart disease (see HEART, DISEASES OF) or PERIPHERAL VASCULAR DISEASE. In the UK strokes affect about 200 people per 100,000 population annually, with the incidence rising sharply after the age of 55. At the age of 70 the incidence is around 15 people per 1,000 of population; at 80 the figure is double that.

About 80 per cent of patients survive an acute stroke and they are at risk of a further episode within a few weeks and months; about 10 per cent in the first year and 5 per cent a year after that. HYPERTENSION, smoking, HYPERLIPIDAEMIA and raised concentration of blood sugar, along with OBESITY, are significant pointers to further strokes and preventive steps to reduce these factors are worthwhile, although the reduction in risk is hard to assess. Even so, the affected person should stop smoking, greatly reduce alcohol intake, check for and have treated diabetes, reduce weight and exercise regularly. In any case, a diet rich in fresh fruit and vegetables and low in fat and salt, exercise and the avoidance of smoking may reduce the risk of having a first stroke.

The evidence is inconclusive that patients with ischaemic stroke should be treated with antihypertensives. Furthermore, neither the starting blood pressure nor the best drug regimen or its starting time are generally agreed. Studies on the most effective methods of preventing and treating stroke are continuing; meanwhile available evidence suggests that an active approach to prevention of primary and secondary hypertension will benefit patients and usually be cost-effective.

Ischiorectal Abscess

An ABSCESS arising in the space between the RECTUM and ischial bone (see ISCHIUM) and often resulting in a FISTULA. It may occur spontaneously or be secondary to an anal fissure, thrombosed HAEMORRHOIDS or other anal disease. The disorder is painful and usually accompanied by fever. Treatment is by a combination of antibiotics and surgery.

Ischium

Ischium is the bone which forms the lower and hinder part of the pelvis. It bears the weight of the body in sitting.

Ishihara's Test

A test for colour vision, introduced by a Japanese doctor, comprising several plates with round dots of different colours and sizes. It is also the name of a type of blood test for SYPHILIS.

Islets of Langerhans

Groups of specialised cells distributed throughout the PANCREAS, that produce three hormones: INSULIN, GLUCAGON, and SOMATOSTATIN.

Iso-Immunisation

The IMMUNISATION of a person by an ANTIGEN they do not have but which is present in other people. For example, a rhesus-negative mother does not carry the rhesus antigen. If she carries a rhesus-positive baby, passage of the rhesus antigen from the baby into the mother's circulation may cause her to be iso-immunised. Her immune system (see IMMUNITY) may then produce ANTIBODIES to the rhesus antigen. When she next becomes pregnant, if the baby is again rhesus positive, the mother will produce large amounts of anti-Rh antibodies which can enter the fetal circulation and cause its blood cells to break up. (See HAEMOLYTIC DISEASE OF THE NEWBORN; BLOOD GROUPS.)

Isolation

This is important when treating patients with serious infection or whose immune systems (see IMMUNITY) are severely compromised by illness or radio- or chemotherapy. The procedure also protects staff caring for infectious patients. (See INCUBATION; INFECTION; QUARANTINE.)

Isoleucine

One of the essential AMINO ACIDS, which are fundamental components of all proteins. It cannot be synthesised by the body and so must be obtained from the diet.

Isometric

Of similar measurement. Isometric exercises are based on the isometric contraction of the muscles. Fibres are provoked into working by pushing or pulling an immovable object, but this technique prevents them from shortening in length. These exercises improve a person's fitness and builds up his or her muscle strength.

Isoniazid

One of the anti-tuberculous drugs. It has the advantages of being relatively non-toxic and of being active when taken by mouth. Unfortunately, like streptomycin, it may render the *Mycobacterium tuberculosis* resistant to its action. This tendency to produce resistance is considerably reduced if it is given in conjunction with RIFAMPICIN and PYRAZINAMIDE.

Isoprenaline

An INOTROPIC sympathomimetic drug which is used as a short-term emergency treatment of heart block or severe BRADYCARDIA. (See HEART, DISEASES OF.)

Isotonic

A term applied to solutions which have the same power of diffusion as one another. An isotonic solution used in medicine is one which can be mixed with body fluids without causing any disturbance. An isotonic saline solution for injection into the blood, so that it may possess the same osmotic pressure (see OSMOSIS) as the blood SERUM, is one of 0·9 per cent strength – that is, containing 9 grams of sodium chloride to 1 litre of water. This is also known as normal or physiological salt solution. An isotonic solution of bicarbonate of soda for injection into the blood is one of 1·35 per cent strength in water. An isotonic solution of glucose for injection into the blood is one of 5 per cent strength in water.

Solutions which are weaker, or stronger, than the fluids of the body with which they are intended to be mixed are known as hypotonic and hypertonic, respectively.

Isotope

This is a form of a chemical element with the same chemical properties as other forms, but which has a different atomic mass. It contains an identical number of positively charged particles called protons, in the nucleus, giving it the same atomic number, but the numbers of neutrons differ. A radioactive isotope, or radionuclide, is one that decays into other isotopes, and in doing so emits alpha, beta or gamma radiation.

Applications of radionuclides to diagnosis The use of radionuclides in diagnosis is based on the fact that it is possible to tag many of the substances normally present in the body with a radioactive label. Certain synthetic radioactive elements, such as technetium, can also be used. Because it is possible to detect minute quantities of radioactive material, only very small doses are needed, making the procedure a safe one. Furthermore the body pool of the material is therefore not appreciably altered, and metabolism is not disturbed. Thus in studies of iodine metabolism the ratio of radioactive atoms administered to stable atoms in the body pool is of the order of 1:1,000 million. By measuring radioactivity in the body, in blood samples, or in the excreta it is possible to gain information about the fate of the labelled substance, and hence of the chemically identical inactive material. Therefore it is theoretically possible to trace the absorption, distribution and excretion of any substance normally present in the body, provided that it can be tagged with a suitable radioactive label.

If the investigation necessitates tracing the path of the material through the body by means of external counting over the body surface, it is obviously essential to use an isotope that emits gamma radiation or positrons. If, however, only measurements on blood sample or excreta are required, it is possible to use pure beta emitters. Whole-body counters measure the total radioactivity in the body, and these are of great value in absorption studies.

Moving images can provide information on body functions such as the movements of the heart, blood flow, bile flow in the liver, and urine in the kidneys. The development of COMPUTED TOMOGRAPHY or CT scanning has replaced radionuclide scanning for some imaging procedures.

Five main groups of diagnostic uses may be defined:

(1) **METABOLIC STUDIES** The use of radioactive materials in metabolic studies is based on the fundamental property that all isotopes of an element are chemically identical. The radioactive isotope is used as a true isotope tracer – that is, when introduced into the body (in whatever form) it behaves in the same way as the inactive element. For example, isotopes of iodine are used to measure thyroid function (see THYROID GLAND), and isotopes of calcium enable kinetic studies of bone formation and destruction to be performed.

(2) **ABSORPTION AND DISTRIBUTION STUDIES** The fate of labelled substances given by mouth can be followed to assess their absorption, utilisation and excretion. In most of these studies the isotope is a true isotope tracer. For example, iron absorption can be measured with radioactive iron; vitamin B_{12} absorption may be investigated with vitamin B_{12} tagged with radioactive cobalt.

(3) **BODY COMPOSITION BY DILUTION STUDIES** By introducing an isotope into a compartment, such as the blood or extracellular space, it is possible to measure the volume of that compartment by determining the dilution of radioactivity when equilibrium has been reached.

(4) **PHYSICAL TRACING STUDIES** In this type of study the isotope is not necessarily used as a true isotopic tracer. In other words, it does not trace the path of the corresponding inactive isotope. For example, xenon-133 is used in measurements of blood flow in muscles, and in lung-function studies; krypton-85 is used to detect intracardiac shunts (abnormal blood flows in the heart). Neither of these elements is normally present in the body. The survival of ERYTHROCYTES may be followed and the organ

of sequestration revealed by labelling them with radioactive chromium.

(5) SCANNING OF ORGANS AND TISSUES Scanning is a technique which is used to determine the distribution of radioactive isotopes within the body or within one particular organ. In the conventional scanner, the radiation detector – which is a scintillation counter – 'sees' only a small cross-sectional area of the body at a time. The activity 'seen' at each point is registered, and a 'map' of the activity seen over the scanned area is recorded. Various methods of presentation have been used, and the recently improved display systems present the information gathered by the scanner more effectively. More recent developments are stationary detectors such as the gamma camera, auto-fluoroscope, and other devices which can view the whole of the area simultaneously. Thus when selective concentration of an isotope in a tissue occurs, it is possible to examine the distribution of that isotope by means of scanning. A toxic nodule in the thyroid may be identified by its selective concentration of iodine-131. Areas of absent function on the radioactive scan ('cold' areas) suggest the presence of tumours, abscesses, and similar lesions. Iodine-131 may be used to localise tumours of the thyroid, and chlormerodrin labelled with mercury-197 to delineate tumours of the kidneys. Of even greater practical application is the localising of brain tumours with human serum albumin labelled with iodine-131 or with radioactive technetium.

Treatment Radioactive isotopes are also used in medical treatment. The overactivity of the thyroid gland in thyrotoxicosis can be treated by the ingestion of radioactive iodine. The ingested iodine is taken up by the thyroid gland where local irradiation of the gland takes place, reducing its activity. Radioactive phosphorus is used in the treatment of polycythemia rubra vera. It is largely taken up in bone as this is the main source of body phosphate, and irradiation of the bone marrow results, controlling the overactivity that is characteristic of polycythaemia rubra vera (see under POLYCYTHAE-MIA). In cobalt teletherapy the isotope cobalt 60 is used to deliver 1·2–1·3 million volt radiation which is equivalent to X-rays generated at a peak voltage of 3–4 million volts. (See RADIOTHERAPY.)

Itch
Itch is a popular name for SCABIES.

Itching
See PRURITUS.

-Itis
A suffix added to the name of an organ to signify any INFLAMMATION of that organ.

ITP
See IDIOPATHIC THROMBOCYTOPENIC PURPURA (ITP).

Itraconazole
A triazole antifungal drug taken orally for oropharyngeal and vulvovaginal CANDIDA, PITYRIASIS versicolor, and tinea corporis and pedis (see under RINGWORM). It is also used for systemic fungal infections such as ASPERGILLOSIS, candidiasis and cryptococcosis where other fungicidal drugs have not worked. Itraconazole is metabolised in the liver so should not be given to patients who have or have had liver disease. The drug can be given as maintenance treatment of AIDS (see AIDS/HIV) patients to prevent resurgence of underlying fungal disease to which they are vulnerable. (See FUNGAL AND YEAST INFECTIONS.)

IUCD (IUD)
Abbreviation for an intrauterine contraceptive device (coil). It acts mechanically to prevent conception, but the coil is not suitable for all women and has a failure rate of 2·3 per cent (see CONTRACEPTION).

IUS
Intrauterine system – a hormonal contraceptive device that is placed in the UTERUS. It is a long-term reversible method of CONTRACEPTION.

IVF
See IN VITRO FERTILISATION (IVF); ASSISTED CONCEPTION.

Ivory
Ivory, or dentine, is the hard material which forms the chief bulk of the TEETH.

J

Jacksonian Epilepsy
See EPILEPSY.

Jaundice
Jaundice is a yellow discoloration of the skin due to the deposition of BILE pigment in its deeper layers. It is the main sign of several disorders of the liver and biliary system. Many babies develop jaundice soon after birth because of the accumulation of BILIRUBIN (yellow bile pigment) in the blood. In most, this is due to liver immaturity and soon disappears, but a serious disorder, HAEMOLYTIC DISEASE OF THE NEWBORN, is a potentially dangerous type of neonatal jaundice that requires treatment.

Types In adults, three types of jaundice occur. They are all the result of disturbance in the mechanism by which HAEMOGLOBIN from the breakdown of ageing red blood cells (erythrocytes) is not properly processed in the liver. Normally the breakdown product of this haemoglobin – bilirubin – is made water-soluble in the liver and excreted via the bile ducts into the small intestine, where it colours the stools dark brown.

HAEMOLYTIC JAUNDICE In this type, the amount of bilirubin produced is too much for the liver to deal with, the excess usually being the result of an abnormal level of haemoglobin from the breakdown of blood cells. This haemolytic anaemia, as it is known, has several causes (see ANAEMIA).

HEPATOCELLULAR JAUNDICE In this disorder, bilirubin builds up in the blood because liver cells have been damaged or have died – usually as a result of a viral infection (there are four types) causing HEPATITIS, or of liver failure.

OBSTRUCTIVE JAUNDICE Also called cholestatic jaundice, this type is characterised by the inability of bile to be discharged from the liver because the bile ducts are blocked as a result of gall-stones (see under GALL-BLADDER, DISEASES OF) or a growth. Sometimes the ducts are absent (atresia) or have been destroyed in the liver as a result of CIRRHOSIS.

Symptoms Yellowness, appearing first in the whites of the eyes and later over the whole skin, is the symptom that attracts notice. Indigestion, nausea, poor appetite and general malaise are other symptoms. The skin may itch, and the faeces are pale because of the absence of bile.

Treatment The essential step is to treat the underlying cause if possible: for instance, gall-stones, if these be the cause of the jaundice. Comprehensive laboratory investigations are usually required, and supportive measures are needed. (See also LIVER, DISEASES OF.).

Jaw
The name applied to the bones that carry the teeth. The two upper jaw-bones, the maxillae, are firmly fixed to the other bones of the face. The lower jaw, the mandible, is shaped somewhat like a horseshoe, and, after the first year of life, consists of a single bone. It forms a hinge-joint with the squamous part of the temporal bone, immediately in front of the ear. Both upper and lower jaw-bones possess deep sockets, known as alveoli, which contain the roots of the teeth. (See DISLOCATIONS; BONE, DISORDERS OF; GUMBOIL; TEETH.)

Jejunum
Part of the small INTESTINE.

Jelly
See GELATIN.

Jenner, Edward
Edward Jenner was an English country practitioner (1749–1823). He had noticed that cowpox, which milkmaids caught from cattle, gave these women immunity from the scourge of SMALLPOX. In 1796 he transformed this observation into the medical technique of VACCINATION, inoculating a country boy with matter from the arm of a milkmaid infected with cowpox. Despite hostility from some doctors, Parliament voted him a grant of £10,000 for a society to promote vaccination and the technique spread worldwide, giving benefit to an immense number of people.

Jerk
A sudden involuntary movement. The term is often used to describe the tendon reflexes.

Joint-Mouse
A popular term for a loose body in a joint. It is found especially in the knee. (See JOINTS, DISEASES OF.)

Joint Replacement
See ARTHROPLASTY.

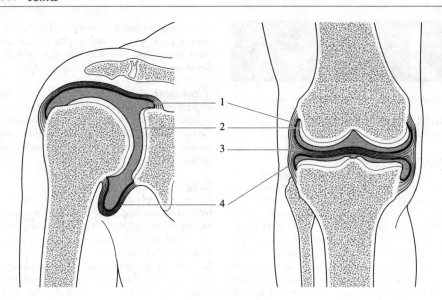

1 synovial membrane
2 articular cartilage
3 articular disc
4 capsule

Diagram of synovial joints. (Left) A right shoulder-joint (simple synovial) from the front. (Right) Right knee-joint (synovial with articular disc) from the front.

Joints

A joint is the articulation point between different parts of the skeleton, whether bone or cartilage. Joints are divided into those which are fixed or relatively fixed (fibrous and cartilaginous joints), and those which allow free movement (synovial joints). In the former, exemplified by the sutures between the bones of the skull, a layer of cartilage or fibrous tissue lies between the bones, binding them firmly together. Amphiarthrodial joints, exemplified by the joints between the vertebral bodies (see SPINAL COLUMN), have a thick disc of fibro-cartilage between the bones. Although the individual joint is capable of very little movement, a series of these gives to the spinal column, as a whole, a flexible character.

All movable joints involve four structures: the bones whose junction forms the joint; a layer of cartilage covering the ends of these, making them smooth; a fibrous sheath, the capsule, thickened at various points into bands or ligaments, which hold the bones together; and, finally, the synovial membrane, which lines the capsule and produces a synovial fluid, lubricating the movements of the joint. In addition, the bones are kept in position at the joints by the various muscles passing over them and by atmospheric pressure. Where the ends of the bones do not quite correspond, a subsidiary disc of fibro-cartilage may help to adapt the ends of the bones more perfectly to each other. Larger cavities may be filled by movable pads of fat under the synovial membrane, giving additional protection to the joint.

Varieties After this main division of joints into those which are fixed and those movable, the movable joints may be further subdivided. In gliding joints, such as the wrist and ankle, the bones have flat surfaces capable of only a limited amount of movement. In hinge joints, such as the elbow and knee, movement takes place around one axis. Ball-and-socket joints, exemplified by the shoulder and hip, allow free movement in any direction. Subsidiary varieties are named according to the shape of the bones which enter the joint.

Joints, Diseases of

'Rheumatism' is the colloquial term for non-specific musculoskeletal symptoms arising in the joints, ligaments, tendons and muscles. 'Arthritis' describes a pathological musculoskeletal disorder. Most common are sprains of ligaments, strains of tendons and muscles,

BURSITIS, TENDINITIS and non-specific back pain (see BACKACHE).

Osteoarthritis (OA) rarely starts before

40, but by the age of 80 affects 80 per cent of the population. There are structural and functional changes in the articular cartilage, as well as changes in the collagenous matrix of tendons and ligaments. OA is not purely 'wear and tear'; various sub-groups have a genetic component. Early OA may be precipitated by localised alteration in anatomy, such as a fracture or infection of a joint. Reactive new bone growth typically occurs, causing sclerosis (hardening) beneath the joint, and osteophytes – outgrowths of bone – are characteristic at the margins of the joint. The most common sites are the first metatarsal (great toe), spinal facet joints, the knee, the base of the thumb and the terminal finger joints (Heberden's nodes).

OA has a slow but variable course, with periods of pain and low-grade inflammation. Acute inflammation, common in the knee, may result from release of pyrophosphate crystals, causing pseudo-gout.

Urate gout results from crystallisation of

URIC ACID in joints, against a background of hyperuricaemia. This high concentration of uric acid in the blood may result from genetic and environmental factors, such as excess dietary purines, alcohol or diuretic drugs.

Inflammatory arthritis is less common

than OA, but potentially much more serious. Several types exist, including:

SPONDYLARTHRITIS This affects younger men, chiefly involving spinal and leg joints. This may lead to inflammation and eventual ossification of the enthesis – that is, where the ligaments and tendons are inserted into the bone around joints. This may be associated with disorders in other parts of the body: skin inflammation (PSORIASIS), bowel and genito-urinary inflammation, sometimes resulting in infection of the organs (such as dysentery). The syndromes most clearly delineated are ankylosing spondylitis (see SPINE AND SPINAL CORD, DISEASES AND INJURIES OF), psoriatic or colitic spondylitis, and REITER'S SYNDROME. The diagnosis is made clinically and radiologically; no association has been found with autoantibodies (see AUTOANTIBODY). A particularly clear gene locus, HLA B27, has been identified in ankylosing spondylitis. Psoriasis can be associated with a characteristic peripheral arthritis.

Systemic autoimmune rheumatic diseases (see AUTOIMMUNE DISORDERS).

RHEUMATOID ARTHRITIS (RA) – see also main entry. The most common of these diseases. Acute inflammation causes lymphoid synovitis, leading to erosion of the cartilage, associated joints and soft tissues. Fibrosis follows, causing deformity. Autoantibodies are common, particularly Rheumatoid Factor. A common complication of RA is Sjögren's syndrome, when inflammation of the mucosal glands may result in a dry mouth and eyes.

SYSTEMIC LUPUS ERYTHEMATOSUS (SLE) and various overlap syndromes occur, such as systemic sclerosis and dermatomyositis. Autoantibodies against nuclear proteins such as DNA lead to deposits of immune complexes and VASCULITIS in various tissues, such as kidney, brain, skin and lungs. This may lead to various symptoms, and sometimes even to organ failure.

Infective arthritis includes:

SEPTIC ARTHRITIS An uncommon but potentially fatal disease if not diagnosed and treated early with approriate antibiotics. Common causes are TUBERCLE bacilli and staphylococci (see STAPHYLOCOCCUS). Particularly at risk are the elderly and the immunologically vulnerable, such as those under treatment for cancer, or on CORTICOSTEROIDS or IMMUNOSUPPRESSANT drugs.

RHEUMATIC FEVER Now rare in western countries. Resulting from an immunological reaction to a streptococcal infection, it is characterised by migratory arthritis, rash and cardiac involvement.

Other infections which may be associated with arthritis include rubella (German measles), parvovirus and LYME DISEASE.

Treatment Septic arthritis is the only type that can be cured using antibiotics, while the principles of treatment for the others are similar: to reduce risk factors (such as hyperuricaemia); to suppress inflammation; to improve function with physiotherapy; and, in the event of joint failure, to perform surgical arthroplasty. NON-STEROIDAL ANTI-INFLAMMATORY DRUGS (NSAIDS) include aspirin, paracetamol and many recently developed ones, such as the proprionic acid derivatives IBUPROFEN and naproxen, along with other drugs that have similar properties such as PIROXICAM. They all carry a risk of toxicity, such as renal dysfunction, or gastrointestinal irritation with haemorrhage. Stronger suppression of inflammation requires corticosteroids and CYTOTOXIC drugs such as azathioprine or cyclophosphamide. Recent research promises more specific and less toxic anti-inflammatory drugs, such as the monoclonal antibodies like infliximab. An important treatment for some osteoarthritic joints is surgical replacement of the joints.

Joule
The unit of energy in the International System of Units. The official abbreviation is J. 4,186·8 J = 1 CALORIE (or kilocalorie). (See also BRITISH THERMAL UNIT (BTU); WEIGHTS AND MEASURES.)

Jugular
Jugular is a general name for any structure in the neck, but is especially applied to three large veins, the anterior, external and internal jugular veins, which convey blood from the head and neck regions to the interior of the chest.

Jumper's Knee
See PATELLAR TENDINITIS.

Jungian Analysis
A school of 'analytical psychology', first described by Carl Gustav Jung in 1913. It introduced the concepts of 'introvert' and 'extrovert' personalities, and developed the theory of the 'collective unconscious' with its archetypes of man's basic psychic nature. In contrast with Freudian analysis (see FREUDIAN THEORY), in Jungian analysis the relationship between therapist and patient is less one-sided because the therapist is more willing to be active and to reveal information about him or herself. (See also PSYCHOANALYSIS.)

Juvenile Idiopathic Arthritis (JIA)
Previously called juvenile rheumatoid arthritis and juvenile chronic arthritis, this is a set of related conditions of unknown cause affecting children. Characteristically, the synovial membrane of a joint or joints becomes inflamed and swollen for at leat six weeks (and often very much longer – even years). About 1 in 10,000 children develop it each year, many of whom have certain HLA genetic markers, thought to be important in determining who gets the illness. Inflammatory CYTOKINES play a big part.

Clinical features There are various types. The oligoarthritic type involves 1–4 joints (usually knee or ankle) which become hot, swollen and painful. One complication is an inflammation of the eyes – UVEITIS. The condition often 'burns out', but may reappear at any time, even years later.

The polyarthritic type is more like RHEUMATOID ARTHRITIS in adults, and the child may have persistent symptoms leading to major joint deformity and crippling.

The systemic type, previously called Still's disease, presents with a high fever and rash, enlarged liver, spleen and lymph nodes, and arthritis – although the latter may be mild. In some children the illness becomes recurrent; in others it dies down only to return as polyarthritis.

Complications These include uveitis, which can lead to loss of vision; a failure to thrive; osteoporosis (see under BONE, DISORDERS OF); joint deformity; and psychosocial difficulties.

Treatment This includes ANTIPYRETICS and ANALGESICS, including NON-STEROIDAL ANTI-INFLAMMATORY DRUGS (NSAIDS), intra-articular steroid injections, anti-tumour necrosis factor drugs and steroids.

Physiotherapy is vital, and children may need to wear splints or other orthotic devices to alleviate deformity and pain. Orthopaedic operative procedures may be necessary.

K

Kala-Azar
Another name for visceral LEISHMANIASIS.

Kanamycin
An antibiotic derived from *Streptomyces kanamyceticus*. It is active against a wide range of organisms, including *Staphylococcus aureus* and *Mycobacterium tuberculosis*.

Kaolin
Kaolin, or china clay, is a smooth white powder consisting of natural white aluminium silicate resulting from the decomposition of minerals containing felspar. It is used as a dusting powder for eczema (see DERMATITIS) and other forms of irritation in the skin. It is also used internally in cases of diarrhoea. Talc, French chalk and Fuller's earth are similar silicates.

Kaolin poultice contains kaolin, boric acid, glycerin and various aromatic substances.

Kaolinosis
Kaolinosis is a form of PNEUMOCONIOSIS caused by the inhaling of clay dust.

Kaposi's Sarcoma
Once a very rare disease in western countries, although more common in Africa, Kaposi's sarcoma is now a feature of AIDS (see AIDS/HIV) – indeed, its increasing occurrence was one of the first pointers to the development of AIDS. It is a condition in which malignant skin tumours develop, originating from the blood vessels. The tumours form purple lumps which customarily start on the feet and ankles, then spread up the legs and develop on the arm and hands. In AIDS the sarcoma appears in the respiratory tract and gut, causing serious bleeding. Radiotherapy normally cures mild cases of Kaposi's sarcoma, but severely affected patients will need anti-cancer drugs to check the tumour's growth.

Kawasaki Disease
Also called mucocutaneous lymph node syndrome, this disorder of unknown origin occurs mainly in children under five and was first described in Japan. It is characterised by high fever, conjunctivitis (see under EYE, DISORDERS OF), skin rashes and swelling of the neck glands. After about two weeks the skin from fingertips and toes may peel. The disease may last for several weeks before spontaneously resolving. It is possible that it is caused by an unusual immune response to INFECTION (see IMMUNITY).

Arteritis is a common complication and can result in the development of coronary artery aneurysms (see ANEURYSM) in up to 60 per cent of those affected. These aneurysms and even myocardial infarction (see HEART, DISEASES OF – Coronary thrombosis) are often detected after the second week of illness. The disease can be hard to diagnose as it mimics many childhood viral illnesses, especially in its early stages. The incidence in the UK is over 3 per 100,000 children under five years of age.

Treatment Because of the danger of coronary artery disease, prompt treatment is important. This is with intravenous IMMUNOGLOBULINS and low-dose aspirin. To be effective, treatment must start in the first week or so of the illness – a time when it is most difficult to diagnose.

Keloid
Hard lumpy nodule of the skin due to overgrowth of fibrous tissue in the dermis. It usually follows surgical or accidental trauma or burns, but, rarely, may complicate acne on the upper trunk. Most commonly seen in the skin over the sternum, shoulders and upper back; coloured people are particularly prone. Injection of corticosteroid into the keloid may cause partial resolution. Excision should be avoided.

Keratin
The substance of which horn and the surface layer of the skin are composed.

Keratinisation
Deposition of KERATIN in cells, in particular those in the skin. The cells become horny and flattened and lose their nuclei, forming hair and nails or hard areas of skin.

Keratitis
See under EYE, DISORDERS OF.

Keratomalacia
Softening of the cornea due to a severe vitamin A deficiency (see EYE, DISORDERS OF).

Keratoplasty
See CORNEAL GRAFT.

Keratosis
Also known as actinic keratosis; a rough, scaly area on exposed skin caused by chronic solar

damage from exposure to sun. The face and backs of the hands are most commonly affected. (See also MELANOMA; PHOTODERMATOSES.) CRYOTHERAPY is effective, but prevention by appropriate clothing and sun-blocking creams is a better strategy.

Kerion
A suppurating form of RINGWORM.

Kernicterus
The staining with BILE of the basal nuclei of the BRAIN, with toxic degeneration of the nerve cells, which sometimes occurs in severe HAEMOLYTIC DISEASE OF THE NEWBORN – especially if prompt treatment by exchange TRANSFUSION has not been carried out. Rare nowadays, the result is a form of CEREBRAL PALSY.

Kernig's Sign
This is found in MENINGITIS. A healthy person's thigh can be bent to a right-angle with the body when the knee is straight; in cases of meningitis the knee cannot be straightened when the thigh is bent this way – not without causing the patient intense pain.

Ketamine
An anaesthetic drug, administered by intravenous or intramuscular injection and used mainly in children. The drug has good analgesic properties when used in subanaesthetic doses. One disadvantage is that when used as an anaesthetic, a high incidence of hallucinations occur. Ketamine is contraindicated in patients with HYPERTENSION.

Ketoconazole
An imidazole (see IMIDAZOLES) antifungal drug available for both oral and topical use. Better absorbed orally than other imidazoles, it also has an anti-androgen effect which may give rise to GYNAECOMASTIA and IMPOTENCE in men. In view of its potential hepatotoxicity it should not be given orally for trivial infections, but reserved instead for SYSTEMIC fungal infections (see FUNGAL AND YEAST INFECTIONS).

Ketogenesis
The production of ketones (see KETONE) in the body; abnormal ketogenesis may result in KETOSIS.

Ketogenic Diet
This contains such an excess of fats that acetone and other KETONE bodies appear in the urine. The diet is sometimes used in the treatment of EPILEPSY and chronic infections of the urinary tract by *Escherichia coli*; butter, cream, eggs and fat meat are allowed, whilst sugar, bread and other carbohydrates are cut out as far as possible.

Ketone
Another name for acetone or dimethyl ketone. The term, ketone bodies, is applied to a group of substances closely allied to acetone, especially beta-hydroxybutyric acid and acetoacetic acid. These are produced in the body from imperfect oxidation of fats and protein foods, and are found in especially large amount in severe cases of DIABETES MELLITUS. Ketonuria is the term applied to the presence of these bodies in the urine.

Ketoprofen
See NON-STEROIDAL ANTI-INFLAMMATORY DRUGS (NSAIDS).

Ketorolac
A non-opioid analgesic (see ANALGESICS) used in the short-term management of moderate to severe acute post-operative pain. It may be given orally or by intramuscular or intravenous injection. Gastrointestinal side-effects are common in elderly people, and there are a range of side-effects from ANAPHYLAXIS to HYPERTENSION, prolonged bleeding time and liver function changes. Contraindications include hypersensitivity to ASPIRIN, ASTHMA, renal impairment and pregnancy (including during labour and delivery).

Ketosis
A condition in which an excessive amount of ketones (see KETONE) are produced by the body and these accumulate in the bloodstream. The affected person becomes drowsy, suffers a headache, breathes deeply, and may lapse into a COMA. The condition results from an unbalanced metabolism of fat, which may occur in DIABETES MELLITUS or starvation.

Keyhole Surgery
See MINIMALLY INVASIVE SURGERY (MIS).

Khat
Tender leaves of a shrub that grows in the Middle East called *Catha edelis*. The leaves are wrapped around betel nuts and chewed: the result is a feeling of EUPHORIA and an ability to tolerate harsh living conditions.

Kidney, Artificial
See DIALYSIS.

Kidneys

These are a pair of glands located in the upper abdomen close to the spine and embedded in fat and loose connective tissue.

Structure Each kidney is about 10 cm long, 6.5 cm wide, 5 cm thick, and weighs around 140 grams.

Adult kidneys have a smooth exterior, enveloped by a tough fibrous coat that is bound to the kidney only by loose fibrous tissue and by a few blood vessels that pass between it and the kidney. The outer margin of the kidney is convex; the inner is concave with a deep depression, known as the hilum, where the vessels enter. The URETER, which conveys URINE to the URINARY BLADDER, is also joined at this point. The ureter is spread out into an expanded, funnel-like end, known as the pelvis, which further divides up into little funnels known as the calyces. A vertical section through a kidney (see diagram) shows two distinct layers: an outer one, about 4 mm thick, known as the cortex; and an inner one, the medulla, lying closer to the hilum. The medulla consists of around a dozen pyramids arranged side by side, with their base on the cortex and their apex projecting into the calyces of the ureter. The apex of each pyramid is studded with tiny holes, which are the openings of the microscopic uriniferous tubes.

In effect, each pyramid, taken together with the portion of cortex lying along its base, is an independent mini-kidney. About 20 small tubes are on the surface of each pyramid; these, if traced up into its substance, repeatedly subdivide so as to form bundles of convoluted tubules, known as medullary rays, passing up towards the cortex. One of these may be traced further back, ending, after a tortuous course, in a small rounded body: the Malpighian corpuscle or glomerulus (see diagram). Each glomerulus and its convoluted tubule is known as a nephron, which constitutes the functional unit of the kidney. Each kidney contains around a million nephrons.

After entering the kidney, the renal artery divides into branches, forming arches where the cortex and medulla join. Small vessels come off these arches and run up through the cortex, giving off small branches in each direction. These end in a tuft of capillaries, enclosed in Bowman's capsule, which forms the end of the uriniferous tubules just described; capillaries with capsule constitute a glomerulus.

After circulating in the glomerulus, the blood leaves by a small vein, which again divides into capillaries on the walls of the uriniferous tubules. From these it is finally collected into the renal veins and then leaves the kidney. This double circulation (first through the glomerulus and then around the tubule) allows a large volume of fluid to be removed from the blood in the glomerulus, the concentrated blood passing on to the uriniferous tubule for removal of parts of its solid contents. Other arteries come straight from the arches and supply the medulla direct; the blood from these passes through another set of capillaries and finally into the renal veins. This circulation is confined purely to the kidney, although small connections by both arteries and veins exist which pass through the capsule and, joining the lumbar vessels, communicate directly with the aorta.

Function The kidneys work to separate fluid and certain solids from the blood. The glomeruli filter from the blood the non-protein portion of the plasma – around 150–200 litres in 24 hours, 99 per cent of which is reabsorbed on passing through the convoluted tubules.

Three main groups of substances are classified according to their extent of uptake by the tubules:

(1) SUBSTANCES ACTIVELY REABSORBED These include amino acids, glucose, sodium, potassium, calcium, magnesium and chlorine (for more information, see under separate entries).

(2) SUBSTANCES DIFFUSING THROUGH THE TUBULAR EPITHELIUM when their concentration in the filtrate exceeds that in the PLASMA, such as UREA, URIC ACID and phosphates.

(3) SUBSTANCES NOT RETURNED TO THE BLOOD from the tubular fluid, such as CREATINE, accumulate in kidney failure, resulting in general 'poisoning' known as URAEMIA.

Kidneys, Diseases of

Diseases affecting the kidneys can be broadly classified into congenital and genetic disorders; autoimmune disorders; malfunctions caused by impaired blood supply; infections; metabolic disorders; and tumours of the kidney. Outside factors may cause functional disturbances – for example, obstruction in the urinary tract preventing normal urinary flow may result in hydronephrosis (see below), and the CRUSH SYNDROME, which releases proteins into the blood as a result of seriously damaged muscles (rhabdomyolysis), can result in impaired kidney function. Another outside factor, medicinal drugs, can also be hazardous to the kidney. Large quantities of ANALGESICS taken over a long time damage the kidneys and acute tubular NECROSIS can result from certain antibiotics.

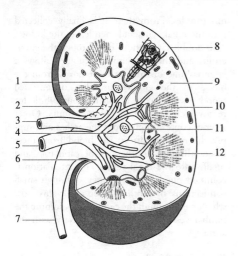

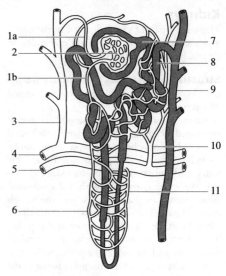

1 calyx minor	7 ureter
2 hilum	8 fibrous capsule
3 renal artery	9 cortex
4 pelvis	10 pyramid
5 renal vein	11 papilla
6 calyx major	12 medulla

Vertical section through the kidney.

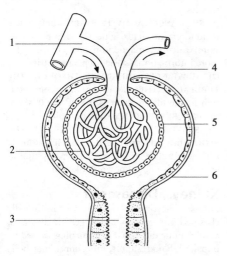

1a	afferent arteriole
1b	efferent arteriole
2	glomerulus
3	interlobular artery
4	arcuate artery
5	arcuate vein
6	descending limb of Henle's loop
7	proximal convoluted tubule
8	distal convoluted tubule
9	collecting tubule
10	uriniferous interlobular vein
11	ascending limb of Henle's loop

Diagram of renal tubules and blood supply of the kidney positioned in the cortex and medulla (see vertical-section diagram).

1 afferent blood vessel	4 efferent blood vessel
2 capillary tuft	5 glomerular capsule
3 tubule	6 capsule

Diagram of glomerulus (Malpighian corpuscle).

Fortunately the body has two kidneys and, as most people can survive on one, there is a good 'functional reserve' of kidney tissue.

Symptoms Many patients with kidney disorders do not have any symptoms, even when the condition is quite advanced. However, others experience loin pain associated with obstruction (renal colic) or due to infection; fevers; swelling (oedema), usually of the legs but occasionally including the face and arms; blood in the urine (haematuria); and excess quantities of urine (polyuria), including at night (nocturia), due to failure of normal mechanisms in the kidney for concentrating urine. Patients with chronic renal failure often have very diffuse symptoms including nausea and vomiting, tiredness due to ANAEMIA, shortness of breath, skin irritation, pins and needles (paraesthesia) due to damage of the peripheral nerves (peripheral neuropathy), and eventually (rarely seen nowadays) clouding of consciousness and death.

Signs of kidney disease include loin tenderness, enlarged kidneys, signs of fluid retention, high blood pressure and, in patients with end-stage renal failure, pallor, pigmentation and a variety of neurological signs including absent reflexes, reduced sensation, and a coarse flapping tremor (asterixis) due to severe disturbance of the body's normal metabolism.

Renal failure Serious kidney disease may lead to impairment or failure of the kidney's ability to filter waste products from the blood and excrete them in the urine – a process that controls the body's water and salt balance and helps to maintain a stable blood pressure. Failure of this process causes URAEMIA – an increase in urea and other metabolic waste products – as well as other metabolic upsets in the blood and tissues, all of which produce varying symptoms. Failure can be sudden or develop more slowly (chronic). In the former, function usually returns to normal once the underlying cause has been treated. Chronic failure, however, usually irreparably reduces or stops normal function.

Acute failure commonly results from physiological shock following a bad injury or major illness. Serious bleeding or burns can reduce blood volume and pressure to the point where blood-supply to the kidney is greatly reduced. Acute myocardial infarction (see HEART, DISEASES OF) or pancreatitis (see PANCREAS, DISORDERS OF) may produce a similar result. A mismatched blood transfusion can produce acute failure. Obstruction to the urine-flow by a stone (calculus) in the urinary tract, a bladder tumour or an enlarged prostate can also cause acute renal failure, as can glomerulonephritis (see below) and the haemolytic-uraemia syndrome.

HYPERTENSION, DIABETES MELLITUS, polycystic kidney disease (see below) or AMYLOIDOSIS are among conditions that cause chronic renal failure. Others include stone, tumour, prostatic enlargement and overuse of analgesic drugs. Chronic failure may eventually lead to end-stage renal failure, a life-threatening situation that will need DIALYSIS or a renal transplant (see TRANSPLANTATION).

Familial renal disorders include autosomal dominant inherited polycystic kidney disease and sex-linked familial nephropathy. Polycystic kidney disease is an important cause of renal failure in the UK. Patients, usually aged 30–50, present with HAEMATURIA, loin or abdominal discomfort or, rarely, urinary-tract infection, hypertension and enlarged kidneys. Diagnosis is based on ultrasound examination of the abdomen. Complications include renal failure, hepatic cysts and, rarely, SUBARACHNOID HAEMORRHAGE. No specific treatment is available. Familial nephropathy occurs more

often in boys than in girls and commonly presents as Alport's syndrome (familial nephritis with nerve DEAFNESS) with PROTEINURIA, haematuria, progressing to renal failure and deafness. The cause of the disease lies in an absence of a specific ANTIGEN in a part of the glomerulus. The treatment is conservative, with most patients eventually requiring dialysis or transplantation.

Acute glomerulonephritis is an immune-complex disorder due to entrapment within glomerular capillaries of ANTIGEN (usually derived from B haemolytic streptococci – see STREPTOCOCCUS) antibody complexes initiating an acute inflammatory response (see IMMUNITY). The disease affects children and young adults, and classically presents with a sore throat followed two weeks later by a fall in urine output (oliguria), haematuria, hypertension and mildly abnormal renal function. The disease is self-limiting with 90 per cent of patients spontaneously recovering. Treatment consists of control of blood pressure, reduced fluid and salt intake, and occasional DIURETICS and ANTIBIOTICS.

Chronic glomerulonephritis is also due to immunological renal problems and is also classified by taking a renal biopsy. It may be subdivided into various histological varieties as determined by renal biopsy. Proteinuria of various degrees is present in all these conditions but the clinical presentations vary, as do their treatments. Some resolve spontaneously; others are treated with steroids or even the cytotoxic drug CYCLOPHOSPHAMIDE or the immunosuppressant cyclosporin. Prognoses are generally satisfactory but some patients may require renal dialysis or kidney transplantation – an operation with a good success rate.

Hydronephrosis A chronic disease in which the kidney becomes greatly distended with fluid. It is caused by obstruction to the flow of urine at the pelvi-ureteric junction (see KIDNEYS – Structure). If the ureter is obstructed, the ureter proximal to the obstruction will dilate and pressure will be transmitted back to the kidney to cause hydronephrosis. Obstruction may occur at the bladder neck or in the urethra itself. Enlargement of the prostate is a common cause of bladder-neck obstruction; this would give rise to hypertrophy of the bladder muscle and both dilatation of the ureter and hydronephrosis. If the obstruction is not relieved, progressive destruction of renal tissue will occur. As a result of the stagnation of the urine, infection is probable and CYSTITIS and PYELONEPHRITIS may occur.

Impaired blood supply may be the outcome of diabetes mellitus and physiological shock, which lowers the blood pressure, also affecting the blood supply. The result can be acute tubular necrosis. POLYARTERITIS NODOSA and SYSTEMIC LUPUS ERYTHEMATOSUS (SLE) may damage the large blood vessels in the kidney. Treatment is of the underlying condition.

Infection of the kidney is called pyelonephritis, a key predisposing factor being obstruction of urine flow through the urinary tract. This causes stagnation and provides a fertile ground for bacterial growth. Acute pyelonephritis is more common in women, especially during pregnancy when bladder infection (CYSTITIS) spreads up the ureters to the kidney. Symptoms are fever, malaise and backache. Antibiotics and high fluid intake are the most effective treatment. Chronic pyelonephritis may start in childhood as a result of congenital deformities that permit urine to flow up from the bladder to the kidney (reflux). Persistent reflux leads to recurrent infections causing permanent damage to the kidney. Specialist investigations are usually required as possible complications include hypertension and kidney failure.

Tumours of the kidney are fortunately rare. Non-malignant ones commonly do not cause symptoms, and even malignant tumours (renal cell carcinoma) may be asymptomatic for many years. As soon as symptoms appear – haematuria, back pain, nausea, malaise, sometimes secondary growths in the lungs, bones or liver, and weight loss – urgent treatment including surgery, radiotherapy and chemotherapy is necessary. This cancer occurs mostly in adults over 40 and has a hereditary element. The prognosis is not good unless diagnosed early. In young children a rare cancer called nephroblastoma (Wilm's tumour) can occur; treatment is with surgery, radiotherapy and chemotherapy. It may grow to a substantial size before being diagnosed.

Cystinuria is an inherited metabolic defect in the renal tubular reabsorption of cystine, ornithine, lysine and arginine. Cystine precipitates in an alkaline urine to form cystine stones. Triple phosphate stones are associated with infection and may develop into a very large branching calculi (staghorn calculi). Stones present as renal or ureteric pain, or as an infec-

tion. Treatment has undergone considerable change with the introduction of MINIMALLY INVASIVE SURGERY (MIS) and the destruction of stone by sound waves (LITHOTRIPSY).

Kinaesthetic Sensations
A term used to describe those sensations which underlie muscle tension and position of joint and muscle. These sensations send impulses along nerves to the brain, and thus inform it of the position of the limb in space and of the relative position to each other of individual muscles and muscle-groups and of joints.

Kinins
Substances present in the body which are powerful VASODILATORS. They also induce pain and are probably involved in the production of the headache of MIGRAINE. In addition, they play a part in the production of ALLERGY and ANAPHYLAXIS.

Kiss of Life
Emergency mouth-to-mouth resuscitation of an unconscious person (see APPENDIX 1: BASIC FIRST AID).

Klebsiella
Gram-negative (see GRAM'S STAIN) bacteria found in the intestinal, respiratory, and urogenital tracts of people and animals. Varieties of the bacteria, which are rod-shaped and non-motile, can cause PNEUMONIA and urinary infections (see URINARY BLADDER, DISEASES OF).

Kleptomania
A psychological disorder in which the person afflicted has an irresistible compulsion to steal things, without necessarily having any need for the object stolen.

Klinefelter's Syndrome
The original syndrome described by Klinefelter consisted of GYNAECOMASTIA, testicular ATROPHY and INFERTILITY. Intelligence was unimpaired. Patients have been described who have associated mental defects and striking tallness of stature, but the only constant feature of the syndrome is testicular atrophy with resulting azoospermia and infertility.

The atrophy of the testis is the result of fibrosis, which begins to appear in childhood and progresses until all the seminiferous tubules are replaced by fibrous tissue. Gynaecomastia, mental retardation and eunuchoidism (see EUNUCH; loss of male secondary sexual characteristics – small penis, loss of body hair and a high-pitched voice) may be present. Most patients with Klinefelter's syndrome have 47 chromosomes instead of the normal 46. The extra chromosome is an X chromosome, so that the sex chromosome constitution is XXY instead of XY. Klinefelter's syndrome is one of the most common chromosome abnormalities and occurs in 1 in 300 of the male population. Patients with this syndrome show that the Y chromosome is strongly sex-determining: thus, a patient who has an XXY chromosome constitution may have the appearance of a normal male, with infertility the only incapacity, while the loss of a Y chromosome leads to the development of a bodily form which is essentially feminine (see TURNER'S SYNDROME).

Klumpke's Paralysis

Injury as a result of the stretching of a baby's brachial plexus during its birth may cause partial paralysis of the arm with atrophy of the muscles of the forearm and hand.

Knee

The joint formed by the FEMUR, TIBIA and patella (knee-cap). It belongs to the class of hinge-joints, although movements are much more complex than the simple motion of a hinge, the condyles of the femur partly rolling, partly sliding over the flat surfaces on the upper end of the tibia, and the acts of straightening and of bending the limb being finished and begun, respectively, by a certain amount of rotation. The cavity of the joint is very intricate: it consists really of three joints fused into one, but separated in part by ligaments and folds of the synovial membrane. The ligaments which bind the bones together are extremely strong, and include the popliteal and the collateral ligaments, a very strong patellar ligament uniting the patella to the front of the tibia, two CRUCIATE LIGAMENTS in the interior of the joint, and two fibro-cartilages which are interposed between the surfaces of tibia and femur at their edge. All these structures give to the knee-joint great strength, so that it is seldom dislocated. The cruciate ligaments, although strong, sometimes rupture or stretch under severe physical stress such as contact sports or athletics. Surgical repair may be required, followed by prolonged physiotherapy.

A troublesome condition often found in the knee – and common among athletes, footballers and other energetic sportspeople – consists of the loosening of one of the fibro-cartilages lying at the head of the tibia, especially of that on the inner side of the joint. The cartilage may either be loosened from its attachment and tend to slip beyond the edges of the bones, or it may become folded on itself. In either case, it tends to cause locking of the joint when sudden movements are made. This causes temporary inability to use the joint until the cartilage is replaced by forcible straightening, and the accident is apt to be followed by an attack of synovitis, which may last some weeks, causing lameness with pain and tenderness especially felt at a point on the inner side of the knee. This condition can be relieved by an operation – sometimes by keyhole surgery (see MINIMALLY INVASIVE SURGERY (MIS)) – to remove the loose portion of the cartilage. Patients whose knees are severely affected by osteoarthritis or rheumatoid arthritis which cause pain and stiffness can now have the joint replaced with an artificial one. (See also ARTHROPLASTY; JOINTS, DISEASES OF.)

Knee Jerk

See REFLEX ACTION.

Knee-Joint Replacement

A surgical operation to replace a diseased – usually osteoarthritic – KNEE with an artificial (metal or plastic) implant which covers the worn cartilage. As much of the original joint as possible is retained. The operations, like hip replacements, are usually done on older people (there is some restriction of movement) and about 90 per cent are successful.

Knock-Knee

Knock-knee, or genu valgum, is a deformity of the lower limbs in such a direction that when the limbs are straightened the legs diverge from one another. As a result, in walking the knees knock against each other. The amount of knock-knee is measured by the distance between the medial malleoli of the ankles, with the inner surfaces of the knee touching and the knee-caps facing forwards. The condition is so common in children between the ages of 2–6 years that it may almost be regarded as a normal phase in childhood. When marked, or persisting into later childhood, it can be corrected by surgery (osteotomy).

Koch's Bacillus

The original name for *Mycobacterium tuberculosis*, which causes TUBERCULOSIS. It stems from the name of the German doctor who first identified the bacillus.

Koilonychia

The term applied to nails that are hollow and depressed like a spoon, a condition sometimes associated with chronic iron deficiency.

Koplik's Spots
Bluish-white spots appearing on the mucous membrane of the mouth in cases of MEASLES about the third day, and forming the first part of the rash in this disease.

Korsakoff's Syndrome
A form of mental disturbance occurring in chronic alcoholism and other toxic states, such as URAEMIA, lead poisoning and cerebral SYPHILIS. Its special features are talkativeness with delusions in regard to time and place – the patient, although clear in other matters, imagining that he or she has recently made journeys.

Krebs Cycle
A series of key cellular chemical reactions starting and ending with oxaloacetic acid. Also called the citric acid or tricarboxylic acid cycle, it produces energy in the form of ADENOSINE TRIPHOSPHATE (ATP) and is the last stage in the biological oxidation of fats, proteins, and carbohydrates. Named after Sir Hans Krebs, a German biochemist working in England in 1900, who won the Nobel Prize for his discovery.

Kuntscher Nail
A surgical nail inserted into the medulla of a fractured bone to fixate it. First introduced by a 20th-century German surgeon.

Kupffer Cells
Star-shaped cells present in the blood-sinuses of the LIVER. They form part of the RETICULO-ENDOTHELIAL SYSTEM and are to a large extent responsible for the breakdown of HAEMO-GLOBIN into the BILE pigments.

Kuru
A slowly progressive, fatal disease due to spongiform degeneration in the central nervous system, particularly the cerebellum (see BRAIN). It is confined to the Fore people in the Eastern Highlands of New Guinea, and causes increasingly severe muscular trembling. Kuru is believed to be due to an infection with a PRION, similar to that causing CREUTZFELDT-JAKOB DISEASE (CJD), acquired from the cannibalistic rite of eating the organs, particularly the brains, of deceased relatives (out of respect). This origin of the disease was suggested by the fact that originally it was a disease of women and children, and it was they who practised this rite. Since the rite was given up, the disease has largely disappeared.

Kveim Test
The characteristic histological test used for the diagnosis of SARCOIDOSIS. The test involves an intradermal injection of sarcoid SPLEEN tissue. If positive, non-caseating granulomata (see GRANULOMA) are seen at the injection site in 4–6 weeks. A positive test is highly specific for sarcoid, but if negative, this would not be excluded.

Kwashiorkor
One of the most important causes of ill health and death among children in the tropics. It is predominantly a deficiency disease due to a diet short of protein; there is also some evidence of a lack of the so-called essential fatty acids. It affects typically the small child weaned from the breast and not yet able to cope with an adult diet, or for whom an adequate amount of first-class protein is not available, and it is mainly found in the less well-developed countries.

The onset of the disease is characterised by loss of appetite, often with diarrhoea and loss of weight. The child is flabby, the skin is dry, and the hair is depigmented, dry, sparse and brittle. At a later stage OEDEMA develops and the liver is often enlarged. In the early stages the condition responds rapidly to a diet containing adequate first-class protein, but in the later stages this must be supplemented by careful nursing, especially as the child is very prone to infection.

Kyphoscoliosis
A combination of SCOLIOSIS and KYPHOSIS in which the spine (see SPINAL COLUMN) is abnormally curved sideways and forwards. The condition may be the result of several diseases affecting the spinal muscles and vertebrae, or it may happen during development for no obvious reason. Although braces may reduce the deformity, an operation may be necessary to correct it.

Kyphosis
The term applied to curvature of the spine in which the concavity of the curve is directed forwards. (See SPINE AND SPINAL CORD, DISEASES AND INJURIES OF.)

Labetalol

Labetalol is an alpha- and beta-adrenoceptor blocker (see ADRENERGIC RECEPTORS) used to treat HYPERTENSION. Beta blockers block the beta-adrenoceptors in the heart, peripheral blood vessels and bronchi. Many drugs belonging to this group are now available, and all are equally effective – but with differences that may make them suitable for a particular patient. Labetalol has the added property of dilating arterioles (small arteries), thus lowering resistance in the small peripheral blood vessels and helping to reduce blood pressure.

Labia

Lips. The labia majora and labia minora are the outer and inner lip-like folds of skin surrounding the entrance to the VAGINA.

Labium

Labium is the Latin word for a lip or lip-shaped organ.

Labour

See PREGNANCY AND LABOUR.

Labyrinth

A convoluted system of structures forming the inner EAR and involved in hearing and balance.

Labyrinthitis

Inflammation of the LABYRINTH of the EAR. Usually caused by bacterial or viral infection, the former often the result of inadequately treated otitis media (see EAR, DISEASES OF – Diseases of the middle ear), or MEASLES. Symptoms are VERTIGO, nausea, vomiting, nystagmus (see EYE, DISORDERS OF), TINNITUS and loss of hearing. Bacterial infection needs treatment with ANTIBIOTICS; viral infection is usually self-limiting. ANTIHISTAMINE DRUGS will help reduce the vertigo. Rarely, surgery may be required to drain the infection in bacteria-based labyrinthitis.

Laceration

A wound to the skin or surface of an organ which results in a cut with irregular edges (cf. an incision produced with a knife, which has smooth, regular edges).

Lacrimal

See EYE – Lacrimal apparatus.

Lacrimal Bones

The smallest bones of the face, one forming part of the bony structure of each orbit containing an EYE.

Lacrimal Nerve

A branch of the ophthalmic nerve supplying the lacrimal gland and conjunctiva of the EYE.

Lacrimation

Crying, or the secretion of an excess quantity of tears.

Lactase

An ENZYME produced by glands in the small INTESTINE which changes lactose (milk sugar) into glucose and galactose during the process of digestion.

Lactation

The period during which an infant is suckled on the mother's breast. (See also BREAST FEEDING; INFANT FEEDING.)

Lacteal

A lymphatic vessel that transmits CHYLE from the INTESTINE. (See also LYMPH.)

Lactic Acid

A colourless, syrupy, sour liquid, which is produced by the action of a bacterium upon lactose, the sugar found in milk. The growth of this organism and consequent formation of lactic acid cause the souring of milk, and the same change takes place to a limited extent when food is long retained in the stomach.

Lactic acid ($CH_3.CHOH.COOH$) is produced in the body during muscular activity, the lactic acid being derived from the breakdown of GLYCOGEN. Muscle fatigue is associated with an accumulation of lactic acid in the muscle. Recovery follows when enough oxygen gets to the muscle, part of the lactic acid being oxidised and most of it then being built up once more into glycogen.

Lactobacillus

A gram-positive (see GRAM'S STAIN), rod-shaped, non-motile bacterium (see BACTERIA). It produces LACTIC ACID by fermenting CARBOHYDRATE. Lactobacilli are found in fermenting animal and plant products, especially dairy products; they also occur in the GASTROINTESTINAL TRACT and the VAGINA. *L. acidophilus* occurs in milk and is a contributory cause to the development of dental caries (see TEETH, DIS-ORDERS OF).

Lactose
The official name for sugar of milk.

Lactose Intolerance
is due to lack in the INTESTINE of the ENZYME known as LACTASE which is responsible for the digestion of lactose, the sugar in milk. The result is that drinking milk or eating milk-containing products is followed by nausea, a sensation of bloating, or distension, in the gut, abdominal pain and diarrhoea. (Similar disturbances after taking milk may also occur in those who do not lack lactase but have an allergy to milk protein). Treatment is by means of a low-lactose diet avoiding fresh or powdered milk and milk puddings. Many can tolerate fermented milk products, as well as the small amounts of milk used in baking and added to margarine and sausages. However, infamts may have to be fed exclusively on a lactose-free formula as even breast milk may produce symptoms.

Lactulose
An osmotic laxative (see OSMOSIS; LAXATIVES), lactulose is a semisynthetic disaccharide – a type of carbohydrate – which is not absorbed from the GASTROINTESTINAL TRACT. It reduces the acidity of FAECES.

Lacuna
A small pit or depression.

Lamblia
See GIARDIASIS.

Lamella
A small disc of glycerin jelly, 3 mm (1/8 inch) in diameter, containing an active drug for application to the eye. It is applied by insertion behind the lower lid.

Laminectomy
An operation in which the arches of one or more vertebrae in the SPINAL COLUMN are removed so as to expose a portion of the SPINAL CORD for removal of a tumour, relief of pressure due to a fracture (see under BONE, DISORDERS OF), or disc protrusion.

Lamotrigine
An antiepileptic drug for the treatment of patients with EPILEPSY, whose condition is characterised by partial seizures.

Lanolin
Derived from wool fat, it is an ingredient of many ointments and creams but may cause allergic contact DERMATITIS.

Lansoprazole
One of the PROTON-PUMP INHIBITORS, it blocks the 'proton pump' ENZYME system of the STOMACH's acid-producing PARIETAL cells. It is used in short-term treatment of PEPTIC ULCER and in combination with antibacterial drugs to eliminate infection with the bacteria HELICOBACTER PYLORI.

Lanugo
Soft fine hair covering the FETUS. It disappears by the ninth month of gestation and is therefore only seen on premature babies.

Laparoscope
An instrument consisting, essentially, of a rigid or flexible cylinder, an eyepiece and a light source, which is inserted through a small incision into the abdominal cavity (which has already been distended with carbon dioxode gas). The laparoscope allows the contents of the abdominal cavity to be examined without performing a LAPAROTOMY. Some operations may be performed using the laparoscope to guide the manipulation of instruments inserted through another small incision – for example, STERILISATION; CHOLECYSTECTOMY. (See also ENDOSCOPE; MINIMALLY INVASIVE SURGERY (MIS).)

Laparoscopy
Also called peritoneoscopy, this is a technique using an instrument called an ENDOSCOPE for viewing the contents of the ABDOMEN. The instrument is inserted via an incision just below the UMBILICUS and air is then pumped into the peritoneal (abdominal) cavity. Visual inspection may help in the diagnosis of cancer, APPENDICITIS, SALPINGITIS, and abnormalities of the LIVER, GALL-BLADDER, OVARIES or GASTROINTESTINAL TRACT. A BIOPSY can be taken of tissue suspected of being abnormal, and operations such as removal of the gall-bladder or appendix may be carried out. (See also MINIMALLY INVASIVE SURGERY (MIS).)

Laparotomy
A general term applied to any operation in which the abdominal cavity is opened (see ABDOMEN). A laparotomy may be exploratory to establish a diagnosis, or carried out as a preliminary to major surgery. Viewing of the peritoneal cavity (see PERITONEUM) through an

ENDOSCOPE is called a LAPAROSCOPY or peritoneoscopy.

Larva

The pre-adult stage in insects and nematodes occurring between the egg and the sexually mature adult.

Larva Migrans

A self-limiting, intensely itching skin eruption caused by nematode (roundworm) larvae, usually of the dog and cat hookworm (see ANCYLOSTOMIASIS). The migrating larvae leave red, raised, irregular tracks in the skin, often on the foot and less frequently elsewhere. The disease is usually acquired by people who take their holidays on tropical beaches. It can be cured by a three-day course of oral ALBENDAZOLE.

Laryngeal Reflex

A 'protective' cough occurring as a result of irritation of the LARYNX – for example, a small particle of food may be accidentally 'inhaled' into the larynx, which reacts with an expulsive cough to prevent the food from entering the lungs.

Laryngectomy

Operation for removal of the LARYNX.

Laryngitis

See LARYNX, DISORDERS OF.

Laryngology

See OTOLARYNGOLOGY.

Laryngoscope

Examination of the LARYNX may be performed indirectly with use of a laryngeal mirror, or directly by use of a laryngoscope – a type of endoscope. The direct examination is usually performed under general anaesthetic.

Laryngo-Tracheo-Bronchitis

Also known as croup – see under LARYNX, DISORDERS OF.

Larynx

The organ of voice which also forms one of the higher parts of the AIR PASSAGES. It is placed high up in the front of the neck and there forms a considerable prominence on the surface (Adam's apple). The vocal cords vibrating in different notes, according to their tenseness and the like, produce the sounds of VOICE AND SPEECH.

Larynx, Disorders of

Obstruction of the larynx is potentially dangerous in adults but can sometimes be life-threatening in infants and children. Stridor – noisy, difficult breathing – is a symptom of obstruction. There are several causes, including congenital abnormalities of the larynx. Others are inflammatory conditions such as acute laryngitis (see below), acute EPIGLOTTITIS and laryngo-tracheo-bronchitis (croup – see below); neurological abnormalities; trauma; and inhalation of foreign bodies.

Laryngitis Inflammation of the mucous membrane of the larynx and vocal chords may be acute or chronic. The cause is usually an infection, most commonly viral, although it may be the result of secondary bacterial infection, voice abuse or irritation by gases or chemicals.

ACUTE LARYNGITIS may accompany any form of upper-respiratory-tract infection. The main symptom is hoarseness and often pain in the throat. The voice becomes husky or it may be lost. Cough, breathing difficulties and sometimes stridor may occur. Acute airway obstruction is unusual following laryngitis but may occasionally occur in infants (see laryngo-tracheo-bronchitis, below).

Treatment Vapour inhalations may be soothing and reduce swelling. Usually all that is needed is rest and analgesics such as paracetamol. Rarely, airway intervention – either ENDOTRACHEAL INTUBATION or TRACHEOSTOMY – may be necessary if severe airway obstruction develops (see APPENDIX 1: BASIC FIRST AID). Affected patients should rest their voice and avoid smoking.

Chronic laryngitis can result from repeated attacks of acute laryngitis; excessive use of the voice – loud and prolonged, singing or shouting; tumours, which may be benign or malignant; or secondary to diseases such as TUBERCULOSIS and SYPHILIS.

Benign tumours or small nodules, such as singer's nodules, may be surgically removed by direct laryngoscopy under general anaesthetic; while cancer of the larynx may be treated either by RADIOTHERAPY or by SURGERY, depending on the extent of the disease. Hoarseness may be the only symptom of vocal-chord disturbance or of laryngeal cancer: any case which has lasted for six weeks should be referred for a specialist opinion.

Laryngectomy clubs are being established

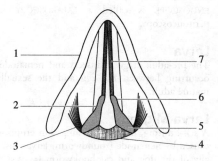

1 thyroid cartilage
2 arytenoid cartilage
3 upper border of cricoid cartilage
4 posterior cricoarytenoid muscles
5 muscular process
6 vocal process

Diagram of the opening of the larynx to show the action of the muscles. A horizontal section has been made at the level of the true vocal cords. The two cords are widely separated by the action of 4.

1 thyroid cartilage	5 muscular process
2 arytenoid cartilage	6 vocal process
3 lateral arytenoid	7 thyroarytenoid
4 arytenoid muscles	

Diagram of the opening of the larynx to show the action of the muscles. The cords are now held together by the action of 3, 4 and 7.

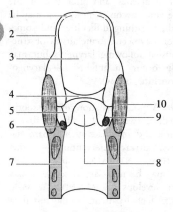

larynx from behind

1 epiglottis
2 aryepiglottic fold
3 tubercle
4 ventricular fold
5 vocal fold
6 interior thyroarytenoid muscle
7 cricothyroid membrane
8 cricothyroid membrane
9 ventricle of larynx
10 thyroid cartilage
11 adipose tissue

Anatomy of the larynx.

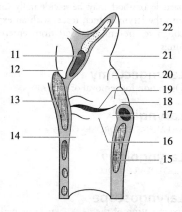

larynx from left side

12 ventricle
13 thyroid cartilage
14 cricothyroid membrane
15 cricoid cartilage
16 vocal cord
17 respiratory glottis
18 false vocal cord
19 arytenoideus muscle
20 corniculate cartilage
21 cuneiform cartilage
22 epiglottis

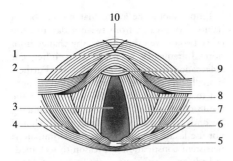

1 epiglottis	6 aryepiglottic fold
2 vallecula	7 vestibular fold
3 trachea	8 vocal fold
4 ventricular fold	9 tubercle of epiglottis
5 cornic cartilage	10 glossoepiglottic fold

A laryngoscopic view of the interior of the larynx.

throughout the country to support patients following laryngectomy. Speech therapists provide speech rehabilitation.

Laryngo-tracheo-bronchitis

Also known as croup. An acute infection of the respiratory tract in infants and young children, usually caused by parainfluenza virus. The onset is variable but the croupy cough and stridulous breathing usually occur a few days after the onset of a viral upper-respiratory-tract infection. A harsh barking cough is typical of the condition. The majority of affected children can be treated with HUMIDIFICATION and a single dose of inhaled corticosteroid (budesonide – see CORTICOSTEROIDS) or a single day's treatment with oral prednisolone. Severe croup can cause serious breathing problems when the child should be referred for urgent specialist assessment, and hospitalisation is preferable in all cases. Rarely, some form of intervention is necessary and this will either be in the form of endotracheal intubation or of a tracheostomy.

Laser

Laser stands for Light Amplification by Stimulated Emission of Radiation. The light produced by a laser is of a single wavelength and all the waves are in phase with each other, allowing a very high level of energy to be projected as a parallel beam or focused on to a small spot.

Various gases, liquids and solids will emit light when they are suitably stimulated. A gassed laser is pumped by the ionising effect of a high-voltage current. This is the same process as that used in a fluorescent tube. Each type of laser has a different effect on biological tissues and this is related to the wavelength of the light

produced. The wavelength determines the degree of energy absorption by different tissues, and because of this, different lasers are needed for different tasks. The argon laser produces light in the visible green wavelength which is selectively absorbed by HAEMOGLOBIN. It heats and coagulates (see COAGULATION) tissues so can be used to seal bleeding blood vessels and to selectively destroy pigmented lesions. The carbon-dioxide laser is the standard laser for cutting tissue: the infra-red beam it produces is strongly absorbed by water and so vaporises cells. Thus, by moving a finely focused beam across the tissue, it is possible to make an incision.

The two main uses of laser in surgery are the endoscopic (see ENDOSCOPE) photocoagulation of bleeding vessels, and the incision of tissue. Lasers have important applications in OPHTHALMOLOGY in the treatment of such disorders as detachment of the retina and the diabetic complications of proliferative retinopathy and of the cornea (see EYE, DISORDERS OF). The destruction of abnormal cells – a sign of pre-malignancy – in the CERVIX UTERI is done using lasers. The beams may also be used to remove scar tissue from the FALLOPIAN TUBES resulting from infection, thus unblocking the tubes and improving the chances of CONCEPTION. Lasers also have several important applications in DERMATOLOGY. They are used in the treatment of pigmented lesions such as LENTIGO, in the obliteration of port-wine stains, in the removal of small, benign tumours such as verrucas, and finally in the removal of tattoos.

Low-intensity laser beams promote tissue healing and reduce inflammation, pain and swelling. Their effect is achieved by stimulating blood and lymph flow and by cutting the production of PROSTAGLANDINS, which provoke inflammation and pain. The beams are used to treat ligament sprains, muscle tears and inflamed joints and tendons.

The three great advantages of lasers are their potency, their speed of action, and the ability to focus on an extremely small area. For these reasons they are widely used, and have allowed great advances to be made in microsurgery, and particularly in FIBREOPTIC ENDOSCOPY.

Lasik

Acronym for laser in-situ keratomileusis, which is a variety of surgery of the EYE used to correct severe myopia (short-sightedness – see REFRACTION; EYE, DISORDERS OF). A thin flap of the cornea is lifted, the area underneath reshaped using an EXCIMER LASER, and the flap is then returned to its place, the altered contour of the cornea improving the patient's sight.

Lassa Fever

First reported in Lassa, in Nigeria, and caused by an arenavirus transmitted by rodents or direct from an infected person. The incubation period is 3–21 days. It is characterised by headache, lethargy and severe muscular pains, and there is often a rash due to bleeding into the skin and mucous membranes. Sore throat is often present. It may carry a high mortality rate, particularly in pregnant women. There is no specific treatment, and all that can be done is supportive nursing.

Lassar's Paste

Officially known as Zinc and Salicylic Acid Paste, BP, this preparation is an old remedy for eczema (see DERMATITIS).

Lassitude

See LETHARGY.

Latanoprost

An analogue of prostaglandin (see PROSTA-GLANDINS), used to treat open-angled GLAU-COMA and raised intra-ocular pressure in the EYE. Delivered as an eye drop, the drug is used in patients who cannot tolerate, or who fail to respond to, other treatments.

Lateral

Referring to the sides of an organ or of the body, or that part furthest from the mid line or median plane.

Latissimus Dorsi

A large, flat, triangular muscle in the back.

Laughing Gas

A popular name for NITROUS OXIDE GAS.

Lavage

The name applied to the washing-out of the stomach, for example to deal with potentially harmful drug ingestion. (See GASTRIC LAVAGE.)

Laxatives

Drugs or other substances used to treat CON-STIPATION. Also called aperients or purgatives, laxatives are classified according to their mode of action. The four main groups are bulk, stimulant, faecal softeners and osmotics. In addition, bowel-cleansing solutions are used before surgery, ENDOSCOPY, or radiological examination of the COLON, to ensure that the bowel is clear of solid matter. However, these are not procedures for treating constipation.

People should be aware that normal bowel habits vary greatly, from twice a day to once every two or even three days. Any change from normal frequency to irregular or infrequent defaecation may signal constipation. Furthermore, before laxatives are prescribed, it is essential to ensure that the constipation is not the result of an underlying condition producing 'secondary' constipation. Individuals should not use laxatives too often or indiscriminately; persistent constipation is a reason to seek medical advice.

Bulk laxatives include bran and most high-fibre foods, such as fruit, vegetables and wholemeal foods. These leave a large indigestible residue that holds water in the gut and produces a large soft stool. Isphaghula husk, methyl cellulose and sterculia are helpful when bran is ineffective. Inorganic salts such as magnesium sulphate (Epsom Salts) have a similar effect.

Stimulant laxatives – for example, bisacodyl, senna and docusate sodium – stimulate PERI-STALSIS, although the action may be accompanied by colicky pains.

Faecal softeners (emollients) There are two groups: surface active agents such as dioctyl sodium and sulphosuccinate which retain water in the stools and are often combined with a stimulant purgative; and liquid paraffin which is chemically inert and is said to act by lubrication.

Osmotic laxatives These substances act by holding fluid in the bowel by OSMOSIS, or by altering the manner in which water is distributed in the FAECES. Magnesium salts are used to produce rapid bowel evacuation, although one of them, magnesium hydroxide, should be used only occasionally. Phosphate or sodium citrate enemas (see ENEMA) can be used for constipation, while the former is used to ensure bowel evacuation before abdominal radiological procedures, endoscopy and surgery.

Lead Poisoning

Lead and lead compounds are used in a variety of products including petrol additives (in the UK, lead-free petrol is now mandatory), piping (lead water pipes were once a common source of poisoning), weights, professional paints, dyes, ceramics, ammunition, homeopathic remedies, and ethnic cosmetic preparations. Lead compounds are toxic by ingestion, by inhalation and, rarely, by skin exposures. Metallic lead, if ingested, is absorbed if it remains in the gut. The absorption is greater in children, who may ingest lead from the paint on old cots – although lead-containing paints are no longer used for items that children may be in contact with.

Acute poisonings are rare. Clinical features include metallic taste, abdominal pain, vomiting, diarrhoea, ANOREXIA, fatigue, muscle weakness and SHOCK. Neurological effects may include headache, drowsiness, CONVULSIONS and COMA. Inhalation results in severe respiratory-tract irritation and systemic symptoms as above.

Chronic poisonings cause gastrointestinal disturbances and constipation. Other effects are ANAEMIA, weakness, pallor, anorexia, insomnia, renal HYPERTENSION and mental fatigue. There may be a bluish 'lead line' on the gums, although this is rarely seen. Neuromuscular dysfunction may result in motor weakness and paralysis of the extensor muscles of the wrist and ankles. ENCEPHALOPATHY and nephropathy are severe effects. Chronic low-level exposures in children are linked with reduced intelligence and behavioural and learning disorders.

Treatment Management of patients who have been poisoned is supportive, with removal from source, gastric decontamination if required, and X-RAYS to monitor the passage of metallic lead through the gut if ingested. It is essential to ensure adequate hydration and renal function. Concentrations of lead in the blood should be monitored; where these are found to be toxic, chelation therapy should be started. Several CHELATING AGENTS are now available, such as DMSA (Meso-2,3-dimercaptosuccinic acid), sodium calcium edetate (see EDTA) and PENICILLAMINE. (See also POISONS.)

Learning Disability

Learning disability, previously called mental handicap, is a problem of markedly low intellectual functioning. In general, people with learning disability want to be seen as themselves, to learn new skills, to choose where to live, to have good health care, to have girlfriends or boyfriends, to make decisions about their lives, and to have enough money to live on. They may live at home with their families, or in small residential units with access to work and leisure and to other people in ordinary communities. Some people with learning disabilities, however, also have a MENTAL ILLNESS. Most can be treated as outpatients, but a few need more intensive inpatient treatment, and a very small minority with disturbed behaviour need secure (i.e. locked) settings.

In the United Kingdom, the 1993 Education Act refers to 'learning difficulties': generalised (severe or moderate), or specific (e.g. DYSLEXIA, dyspraxia [or APRAXIA], language disorder). The 1991 Social Security (Disability Living Allowance) Regulations use the term 'severely mentally impaired' if a person suffers from a state of arrested development or incomplete physical development of the brain which results in severe impairment of intelligence and social functioning. This is distinct from the consequences of DEMENTIA. Though 'mental handicap' is widely used, 'learning disability' is preferred by the Department of Health.

There is a distinction between impairment (a biological deficit), disability (the functional consequence) and handicap (the social consequence).

People with profound learning disability are usually unable to communicate adequately and may be seriously movement-impaired. They are totally dependent on others for care and mobility. Those with moderate disability may achieve basic functional literacy (recognition of name, common signs) and numeracy (some understanding of money) but most have a life-long dependency for aspects of self-care (some fastenings for clothes, preparation of meals, menstrual hygiene, shaving) and need supervision for outdoor mobility.

Children with moderate learning disability develop at between half and three-quarters of the normal rate, and reach the standard of an average child of 8–11 years. They become independent for self-care and public transport unless they have associated disabilities. Most are capable of supervised or sheltered employment. Living independently and raising a family may be possible.

Occurrence Profound learning disability affects about 1 in 1,000; severe learning disability 3 in 1,000; and moderate learning disability requiring special service, 1 per cent. With improved health care, survival of people with profound or severe learning disability is increasing.

Causation Many children with profound or severe learning disability have a diagnosable biological brain disorder. Forty per cent have a chromosome disorder – see CHROMOSOMES (three quarters of whom have DOWN'S (DOWN) SYNDROME); a further 15 per cent have other genetic causes, brain malformations or recognisable syndromes. About 10 per cent suffered brain damage during pregnancy (e.g. from CYTOMEGALOVIRUS (CMV) infection) or from lack of oxygen during labour or delivery. A similar proportion suffer postnatal brain damage from head injury – accidental or otherwise – near-miss cot death or drowning, cardiac arrest, brain infection (ENCEPHALITIS or MENINGITIS), or in association with severe seizure disorders.

Explanations for moderate learning disability include Fragile X or other chromosome abnormalities in a tenth, neurofibromatosis (see VON RECKLINGHAUSEN'S DISEASE), fetal alcohol syndrome and other causes of intra-uterine growth retardation. Genetic counselling should be considered for children with learning disability. Prenatal diagnosis is sometimes possible. In many children, especially those with mild or moderate disability, no known cause may be found.

Medical complications EPILEPSY affects 1 in 20 with moderate, 1 in 3 with severe and 2 in 3 with profound learning disability, although only 1 in 50 with Down's syndrome is affected. One in 5 with severe or profound learning disability has CEREBRAL PALSY.

Psychological and psychiatric needs Over half of those with profound or severe – and many with moderate – learning disability show psychiatric or behavioural problems, especially in early years or adolescence. Symptoms may be atypical and hard to assess. Psychiatric disorders include autistic behaviour (see AUTISM) and SCHIZOPHRENIA. Emotional problems include anxiety, dependence and depression. Behavioural problems include tantrums, hyperactivity, self-injury, passivity, masturbation in public, and resistance to being shaved or helped with menstrual hygiene. There is greater vulnerability to abuse with its behavioural consequences.

Respite and care needs Respite care is arranged with link families for children or staffed family homes for adults where possible. Responsibility for care lies with social services departments which can advise also about benefits.

Education Special educational needs should be met in the least restrictive environment available to allow access to the national curriculum with appropriate modification and support. For older children with learning disability, and for young children with severe or profound learning disability, this may be in a special day or boarding school. Other children can be provided for in mainstream schools with extra classroom support. The 1993 Education Act lays down stages of assessment and support up to a written statement of special educational needs with annual reviews.

Pupils with learning disability are entitled to remain at school until the age of 19, and most with severe or profound learning disability do so. Usually those with moderate learning disability move to further education after the age of 16.

Advice is available from the Mental Health Foundation, the British Institute of Learning Disabilities, MENCAP (Royal Society for Mentally Handicapped Children and Adults), and ENABLE (Scottish Society for the Mentally Handicapped).

Leber's Disease
A hereditary disease in which blindness comes on at about the age of 20.

Lecithin
A very complex fat found in various tissues of the body, but particularly in the brain and nerves, of which it forms a large part. It is also found in large quantities in the yolk of an egg.

Leeches
Animals provided with suckers surrounding the mouth, and living a semi-parasitic life, their food being mainly derived from the blood of other animals. They abstract blood by means of the sucker, which has several large, sharp teeth. Land leeches live in tropical forests and can attach themselves to a person's ankles and lower legs. Aquatic leeches are found in warm water and may attach themselves to swimmers. Their bites are painless, their saliva reducing the clotting properties of blood with hirudin; the result is that the wound continues to bleed after the leech has detached itself or been gently removed (lighted match, alcohol, salt and vinegar are effective removal agents). The medicinal leech, *Hirudo medicinalis*, was formerly employed for the abstraction of small quantities of blood in inflammatory and other conditions. Nowadays it is occasionally used to drain haematomas and to manage healing in certain types of plastic surgery.

Left to Right Shunt
A term used when a hole in the septum (internal wall) of the HEART allows blood to flow from the systemic circulation properly confined to the left side of the heart to the pulmonary circulation, confined to the right. The

shunt is usually detected by hearing a murmur, and the diagnosis confirmed by ECHOCARDIOGRAPHY (see also SEPTAL DEFECT).

Legionnaire's Disease
A form of PNEUMONIA due to a bacterium known as *Legionella pneumophila*, so-called because the first identified outbreak was in a group of US ex-servicemen (members of the American Legion). Inhalation of water aerosols seems the most likely way that people acquire the disease, for example from air-conditioning outlets. Some rubber outlets in showers and taps are able to support the growth of legionnellae so that high concentrations of the organism are released when the tap is first used in the morning. In the presence of the disease, treatment of infected water systems is essential by cleaning, chlorination, heating or a combination of all three.

The pneumonia caused by legionnellae has no distinctive clinical or radiological features, so that the diagnosis is based on an antibody test performed on a blood sample. There is no evidence that the disease is transmitted directly from person to person. The incubation period is 2–10 days; the disease starts with aches and pains followed rapidly by a rise in temperature, shivering attacks, cough and shortness of breath. The X-ray tends to show patchy areas of consolidation in the lungs. Erythromycin and rifampicin are the most useful antibiotics, although rifampicin should never be given alone because of the rapid development of drug resistance.

Leiomyoma
A benign tumour made up of unstriped or involuntary muscle fibres.

Leishmaniasis
A group of infections caused by parasites transmitted to humans by sandflies.

Visceral leishmaniasis (kala-azar) A systemic infection caused by *Leishmania donovani* which occurs in tropical and subtropical Africa, Asia, the Mediterranean littoral (and some islands), and in tropical South America. Onset is frequently insidious; incubation period is 2–6 months. Enlargement of spleen and liver may be gross; fever, anaemia, and generalised lymphadenopathy are usually present. Diagnosis is usually made from a bone-marrow specimen, splenic-aspirate, or liver-biopsy specimen; amastigotes (Leishman-Donovan bodies) of *L. donovani* can be visualised. Several serological tests are of value in diagnosis.

Untreated, the infection is fatal within two years, in approximately 70 per cent of patients. Treatment traditionally involved sodium stibogluconate, but other chemotherapeutic agents (including allupurinol, ketoconazole, and immunotherapy) are now in use, the most recently used being liposomal amphotericin B. Although immunointact persons usually respond satisfactorily, they are likely to relapse if they have HIV infection (see AIDS/HIV).

Cutaneous leishmaniasis This form is caused by infection with *L. tropica*, *L. major*, *L. aethiopica*, and other species. The disease is widely distributed in the Mediterranean region, Middle East, Asia, Africa, Central and South America, and the former Soviet Union. It is characterised by localised cutaneous ulcers – usually situated on exposed areas of the body. Diagnosis is by demonstration of the causative organism in a skin biopsy-specimen; the leishmanin skin test is of value. Most patients respond to sodium stibogluconate (see above); local heat therapy is also used. Paromomycin cream has been successfully applied locally.

Mucocutaneous leishmaniasis This form is caused by *L. braziliensis* and rarely *L. mexicana*. It is present in Central and South America, particularly the Amazon basin, and characterised by highly destructive, ulcerative, granulomatous lesions of the skin and mucous membranes, especially involving the mucocutaneous junctions of the mouth, nasopharynx, genitalia, and rectum. Infection is usually via a superficial skin lesion at the site of a sandfly bite. However, spread is by haematogenous routes (usually after several years) to a mucocutaneous location. Diagnosis and treatment are the same as for cutaneous leishmaniasis.

Lens of the Eye
See EYE.

Lentigo
Lentigines (freckles) are brown MACULES varying in diameter from 1–10 mm or more. Simple lentigines arise in childhood, not necessarily on exposed areas. They may also occur on the lips and are harmless and usually very small. Solar or actinic lentigines are common on the face, neck and backs of the hands in older people and reflect the total cumulative lifetime's exposure to sunlight.

Leproma
A nodule in the skin occurring in LEPROSY.

Leprosy

Also known as Hansen's disease, this is a chronic bacterial infection caused by *Mycobacterium leprae* affecting the skin, mucous membranes, and nerves. Infection is now almost confined to tropical and subtropical countries – mostly in Africa and India. There are two distinct (polarised) clinical forms: tuberculoid and lepromatous. The former usually takes a benign course and frequently burns out, whereas the latter is relentlessly progressive; between these two polar forms lies an intermediate/dimorphous group. Susceptibility may be increased by malnutrition. Nasal secretions (especially in lepromatous disease) are teeming with *M. leprae* and constitute the main source of infection; however, living in close proximity to an infected individual seems necessary for someone to contract the disease. *M. leprae* can also be transmitted in breast milk from an infected mother.

Only a small minority of those exposed to *M. leprae* develop the disease. The incubation period is 3–5 years or longer. The major clinical manifestations involve skin and nerves: the former range from depigmented, often anaesthetic areas, to massive nodules; nerve involvement ranges from localised nerve swelling(s) to extensive areas of anaesthesia. Advanced nerve destruction gives rise to severe deformities: foot-drop, wrist-drop, claw-foot, extensive ulceration of the extremities with loss of fingers and toes, and bone changes. Eye involvement can produce blindness. Laryngeal lesions produce hoarseness and more serious sequelae. The diagnosis is essentially a clinical one; however, skin-smears, histological features and the lepromin skin-test help to confirm the diagnosis and enable the form of disease to be graded.

Although the World Health Organisation had originally hoped to eliminate leprosy worldwide by 2000, that has proved an unrealistic target. The reason is an absence of basic information. Doctors are unable to diagnose the disorder before a patient starts to show symptoms; meanwhile he or she may have already passed on the infection. Doctors do not know exactly how transmission occurs or how it infects humans – nor do they know at what point a carrier of the bacterium may infect others. The incidence of new infections is still more than 650,000 cases a year or about 4.5 cases per 10,000 people in those countries worst affected by the disease.

Treatment Introduction of the sulphone compound, dapsone, revolutionised management of the disease. More recently, rifampicin and clofazimine have been added as first-line drugs for treatment. Second-line drugs include minocycline, ofloxacin and clarithromycin; a number of regimens incorporating several of these compounds (multi-drug regimens – introduced in 1982) are now widely used. A three-drug regime is recommended for multibacillary leprosy and a two-drug one for parcibacillary leprosy. Dapsone resistance is a major problem worldwide, but occurs less commonly when multi-drug regimens are used. Older compounds – ethionamide and prothionamide – are no longer used because they are severely toxic to the liver. Corticosteroids are sometimes required in patients with 'reversal reaction'. Supportive therapy includes physiotherapy; both plastic and orthopaedic surgery may be necessary in advanced stages of the disease. Improvement in socio-economic conditions, and widespread use of BCG vaccination are of value as preventive strategies. Early diagnosis and prompt institution of chemotherapy should prevent long-term complications.

Leptospira

A group, or genus, of spiral micro-organisms, normally found in rodents and other small mammals in which they cause no harm. When transmitted to humans by these animals, either directly or indirectly as through cows, they give rise to various forms of illness (see LEPTOSPIROSIS).

Leptospirosis

The disease caused by infection with LEPTOSPIRA. The three most common members of this group in the United Kingdom are *L. icterohaemorrhagiae*, *L. cani-cola*, and *L. hebdomadis*. It is an occupational hazard of farmers, sewage and abattoir workers, fish cutters and veterinary surgeons, but the infection can also be acquired from bathing in contaminated water. The disease varies in intensity from a mild influenza-like illness to a fatal form of JAUNDICE due to severe liver disease. The kidneys are often involved and there may be MENINGITIS. Penicillin or tetracycline are the usual treatment, but unless they are given early in the disease their effect is limited. The tetracycline antibiotic doxycycline (see TETRACYCLINES) given once weekly during periods of exposure prevents infection.

Spirochaetosis icterohaemorrhagica

Also known as Weil's disease, this is the term applied to infection with the *Leptospira icterohaemorrhagiae* which is transmitted to humans by rats – these animals excreting the organism in their urine, hence the liability of sewage workers to the disease. The condition is characterised by fever, jaundice, enlarged liver, nephritis, and bleeding from mucous membranes.

Lesbian

A female homosexual (see HOMOSEXUALITY); lesbians form about 2 per cent of the female population in the UK. Some engage in active sexual behaviour with another woman, with MASTURBATION, mutual stimulation of the CLITORIS and oral sex being the usual techniques for achieving ORGASM.

Lesion

Lesion meant originally an injury, but is now applied generally to all disease changes in organs and tissues.

Lethal Gene

A gene that produces a GENOTYPE which causes the death of an organism before that organism has reproduced – or which prevents it from reproducing. Lethal genes are usually RECESSIVE, so the organism will die only if both its 'parents' carry the gene. Should only one parent have the lethal gene, its consequences will be masked by the dominant ALLELE passed on by the normal parent.

Lethargy

Lethargy, or lassitude, means a loss of energy. It is a common presenting complaint both to general practitioners and to hospital consultants. It may have a physical cause or a psychological cause; it may be the result of inadequate rest, environmental noise, boredom, insomnia or recent illness. Certain medicinal drugs can cause lethargy, the most common being beta blockers (see BETA-ADRENOCEPTOR-BLOCKING DRUGS) and DIURETICS, and drugs of abuse may also be a cause (see DEPENDENCE). The common psychosocial problems producing lethargy are DEPRESSION and anxiety.

If the patient with lethargy runs a fever, the differential diagnosis is that of a PUO (pyrexia of unknown origin). Many patients with fatigue can establish the onset of the symptom to a febrile illness even though they no longer run a fever. The lethargy that follows some viral infecions, such as HEPATITIS A and glandular fever (see MONONUCLEOSIS) is well recognised; MYALGIC ENCEPHALOMYELITIS (ME) or chronic fatigue syndrome is another disorder associated with lethargy and tiredness. Organic causes of lethargy include ANAEMIA, malnutrition and

hypothyroidism (see THYROID GLAND, DISEASES OF). Some of these patients have a true depressive illness and their presentation and response to treatment is little different from that of sufferers of any other depressive illness, URAEMIA, alcoholism and DIABETES MELLITUS.

Leucine

One of the essential, or indispensable, AMINO ACIDS. They are so-called because they cannot be synthesised, or manufactured, in the body, and are therefore essential constituents of the diet.

Leuco-

Or leuko- – a prefix meaning white.

Leucocytes

The scientific name for white blood cells. Leucocytes contain no HAEMOGLOBIN so are colourless, and have a well-formed NUCLEUS. Healthy people have around 8,000 leucocytes per cubic millimetre of blood. There are three main classes of white cells: granulocytes, lymphocytes and monocytes.

Granulocytes Also known as polymorphonuclear leucocytes ('polys'), these normally constitute 70 per cent of the white blood cells. They are divided into three groups according to the staining reactions of these granules: neutrophils, which stain with neutral dyes and constitute 65–70 per cent of all the white blood cells; eosinophils, which stain with acid dyes (e.g. eosin) and constitute 3–4 per cent of the total white blood cells; and basophils, which stain with basic dyes (e.g. methylene blue) and constitute about 0·5 per cent of the total white blood cells.

Lymphocytes constitute 25–30 per cent of the white blood cells. They have a clear, non-granular cytoplasm and a relatively large nucleus which is only slightly indented. They are divided into two groups: small lymphocytes, which are slightly larger than erythrocytes (about 8 micrometres in diameter); and large lymphocytes, which are about 12 micrometres in diameter.

Monocytes Motile phagocytic cells that circulate in the blood and migrate into the tissues, where they develop into various forms of MACROPHAGE such as tissue macrophages and KUPFFER CELLS.

Site of origin The granulocytes are formed in the red BONE MARROW. The lymphocytes are formed predominantly in LYMPHOID TISSUE. There is some controversy as to the site of origin of monocytes: some say they arise from lymphocytes, whilst others contend that they are derived from histiocytes – i.e. the RETICULO-ENDOTHELIAL SYSTEM.

Function The leucocytes constitute one of the most important of the defence mechanisms against infection. This applies particularly to the neutrophil leucocytes (see LEUCOCYTOSIS). (See also ABSCESS; BLOOD – Composition; INFLAMMATION; PHAGOCYTOSIS; WOUNDS.)

Leucocytosis

A condition in which the polymorphonuclear LEUCOCYTES in the blood are increased in number. It occurs in many different circumstances, and forms a valuable means of diagnosis in certain diseases; however, the condition may occur as a normal reaction in certain conditions (e.g. pregnancy, menstruation, and during muscular exercise). It is usually due to the presence of inflammatory processes (see INFLAMMATION) – the increased number of leucocytes helping to destroy the invading bacteria. Thus, during any acute infective diseases, such as pneumonia, the number is greatly increased. In all suppurative conditions (where PUS is formed) there is also a leucocytosis, and if it seems that an ABSCESS is forming deep in the abdomen, or in some other site where it cannot be readily examined – as, for example, an abscess resulting from APPENDICITIS – the examination of a drop of blood gives a valuable aid in the diagnosis, and may be sufficient, in the absence of other signs, to point out the urgent need of an operation.

Leucoderma

Leucoderma, or leucodermia, is a condition of the skin in which areas of it become white, as the result of various skin diseases.

Leucopenia

A condition in which the number of LEUCOCYTES in the blood is greatly reduced – by, say, ANAEMIA or cancer. It is also a dangerous sign in severe SEPTICAEMIA.

Leucoplakia

See LEUKOPLAKIA.

Leucorrhoea

Discharge of mucus from the VAGINA. It may be whitish or yellowish and is normal in some women, usually increasing before and after MENSTRUATION. It is distinct from abnormal discharges with an offensive smell and yellow or green colouring: these may be caused by micro-organisms or by fungal infection such as *Candida albicans*. Another causative agent is the protozoan parasite, *Trichomonas vaginalis* (see TRICHOMONIASIS). A pessary or tampon that a woman has forgotten to remove will cause a substantial and offensive discharge. Children rarely have vaginal discharge; if they do, it is usually due to an infection or foreign body in the vagina. (See also UTERUS, DISEASES OF.)

Leucotomy

See PSYCHOSURGERY.

Leukaemia

Leukaemia is an umbrella term for several malignant disorders of white blood cells in which they proliferate in a disorganised manner. The disease is also characterised by enlargement of the SPLEEN, changes in the BONE MARROW, and by enlargement of the LYMPH glands all over the body. The condition may be either acute or chronic.

According to the type of cells that predominate, leukaemia may be classified as acute or chronic lymphoblastic leukaemia or myeloid leukaemia. Acute lymphoblastic leukaemia (ALL) is mostly a disease of childhood and is rare after the age of 25. Acute myeloid leukaemia is most common in children and young adults, but may occur at any age. Chronic lymphatic leukaemia occurs at any age between 35 and 80, most commonly in the 60s, and is twice as common in men as in women. Chronic myeloid leukaemia is rare before the age of 25, and most common between the ages of 30 and 65; men and women are equally affected. Around 2,500 patients with acute leukaemia are diagnosed in the United Kingdom, with a similar number annually diagnosed with chronic leukaemia.

Cause Both types of acute leukaemia seem to arise from a MUTATION in a single white cell. The genetically changed cell then goes through an uncontrolled succession of divisions resulting in many millions of abnormal white cells in the blood, bone marrow and other tissues. Possible causes are virus infection, chemical exposure, radiation and genetic background. The cause of chronic lymphocytic leukaemia is not known; the chronic myeloid version may have a genetic background.

Symptoms In acute cases the patient is pale due to anaemia, may have a purpuric rash due

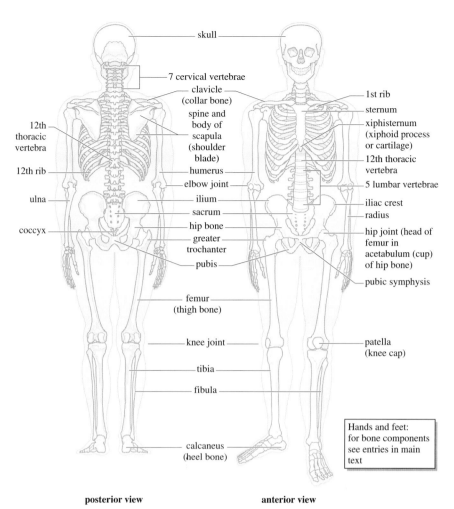

skull

7 cervical vertebrae

clavicle (collar bone)

spine and body of scapula (shoulder blade)

12th thoracic vertebra

12th rib

ulna

coccyx

1st rib

sternum

xiphisternum (xiphoid process or cartilage)

12th thoracic vertebra

5 lumbar vertebrae

iliac crest

radius

hip joint (head of femur in acetabulum (cup) of hip bone)

pubic symphysis

humerus

elbow joint

ilium

sacrum

hip bone

greater trochanter

pubis

femur (thigh bone)

knee joint

patella (knee cap)

tibia

fibula

calcaneus (heel bone)

Hands and feet: for bone components see entries in main text

posterior view   **anterior view**

parietal bone

temporal bone

zygomatic arch

lambdoid suture

external occipital protuberance

occipital bone

external auditory meatus

mastoid process

temporomandibular joint

first and second cervical vertebrae

third to seventh cervical vertebrae

coronal suture

frontal bone

nasal bone

zygomatic bone

anterior nasal spine

maxilla

mental protuberance

body of mandible (jaw)

ramus of mandible

angle of mandible

carotid tubercle of sixth cervical vertebra

first rib

Complete skeleton (top). Right lateral view of skull (bottom).

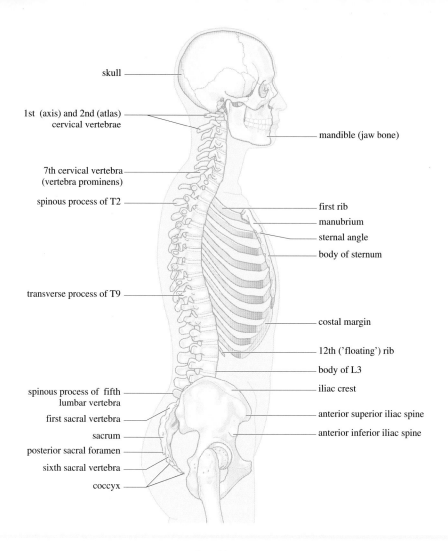

skull

1st (axis) and 2nd (atlas)
cervical vertebrae

mandible (jaw bone)

7th cervical vertebra
(vertebra prominens)

spinous process of T2

first rib

manubrium

sternal angle

body of sternum

transverse process of T9

costal margin

12th ('floating') rib

body of L3

iliac crest

spinous process of fifth
lumbar vertebra

anterior superior iliac spine

first sacral vertebra

anterior inferior iliac spine

sacrum

posterior sacral foramen

sixth sacral vertebra

coccyx

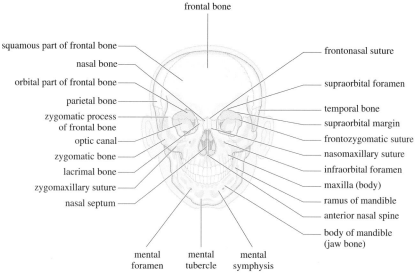

frontal bone

squamous part of frontal bone

frontonasal suture

nasal bone

orbital part of frontal bone

supraorbital foramen

parietal bone

temporal bone

zygomatic process
of frontal bone

supraorbital margin

optic canal

frontozygomatic suture

zygomatic bone

nasomaxillary suture

lacrimal bone

infraorbital foramen

zygomaxillary suture

maxilla (body)

nasal septum

ramus of mandible

anterior nasal spine

body of mandible
(jaw bone)

mental
foramen

mental
tubercle

mental
symphysis

Skull, vertebral column, rib cage and pelvis (top). Skull, frontal view (bottom).

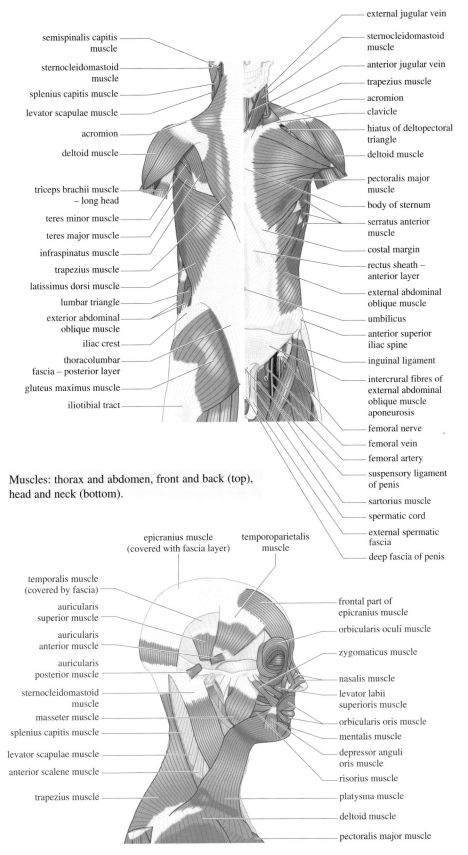

[3]

external jugular vein

sternocleidomastoid muscle

anterior jugular vein

trapezius muscle

acromion

clavicle

hiatus of deltopectoral triangle

deltoid muscle

pectoralis major muscle

body of sternum

serratus anterior muscle

costal margin

rectus sheath – anterior layer

external abdominal oblique muscle

umbilicus

anterior superior iliac spine

inguinal ligament

intercrural fibres of external abdominal oblique muscle aponeurosis

femoral nerve

femoral vein

femoral artery

suspensory ligament of penis

sartorius muscle

spermatic cord

external spermatic fascia

deep fascia of penis

semispinalis capitis muscle

sternocleidomastoid muscle

splenius capitis muscle

levator scapulae muscle

acromion

deltoid muscle

triceps brachii muscle – long head

teres minor muscle

teres major muscle

infraspinatus muscle

trapezius muscle

latissimus dorsi muscle

lumbar triangle

exterior abdominal oblique muscle

iliac crest

thoracolumbar fascia – posterior layer

gluteus maximus muscle

iliotibial tract

Muscles: thorax and abdomen, front and back (top), head and neck (bottom).

epicranius muscle (covered with fascia layer)

temporoparietalis muscle

temporalis muscle (covered by fascia)

auricularis superior muscle

auricularis anterior muscle

auricularis posterior muscle

sternocleidomastoid muscle

masseter muscle

splenius capitis muscle

levator scapulae muscle

anterior scalene muscle

trapezius muscle

frontal part of epicranius muscle

orbicularis oculi muscle

zygomaticus muscle

nasalis muscle

levator labii superioris muscle

orbicularis oris muscle

mentalis muscle

depressor anguli oris muscle

risorius muscle

platysma muscle

deltoid muscle

pectoralis major muscle

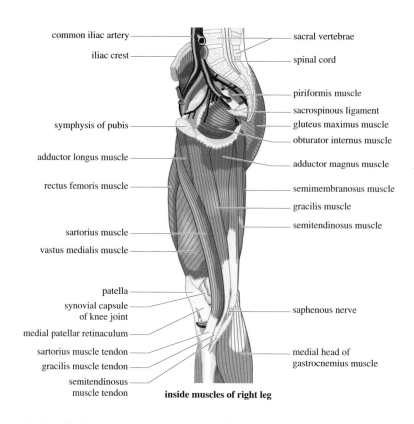

common iliac artery — sacral vertebrae

iliac crest — spinal cord

— piriformis muscle

— sacrospinous ligament

symphysis of pubis — gluteus maximus muscle

— obturator internus muscle

adductor longus muscle — adductor magnus muscle

rectus femoris muscle — semimembranosus muscle

— gracilis muscle

— semitendinosus muscle

sartorius muscle —

vastus medialis muscle —

patella —

synovial capsule of knee joint —

— saphenous nerve

medial patellar retinaculum —

sartorius muscle tendon —

gracilis muscle tendon — medial head of gastrocnemius muscle

semitendinosus muscle tendon —

inside muscles of right leg

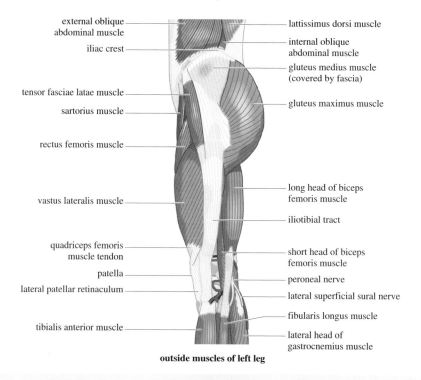

external oblique abdominal muscle — lattissimus dorsi muscle

iliac crest — internal oblique abdominal muscle

— gluteus medius muscle (covered by fascia)

tensor fasciae latae muscle — gluteus maximus muscle

sartorius muscle —

rectus femoris muscle —

— long head of biceps femoris muscle

vastus lateralis muscle — iliotibial tract

quadriceps femoris muscle tendon — short head of biceps femoris muscle

patella — peroneal nerve

lateral patellar retinaculum — lateral superficial sural nerve

— fibularis longus muscle

tibialis anterior muscle — lateral head of gastrocnemius muscle

outside muscles of left leg

Muscles of the legs.

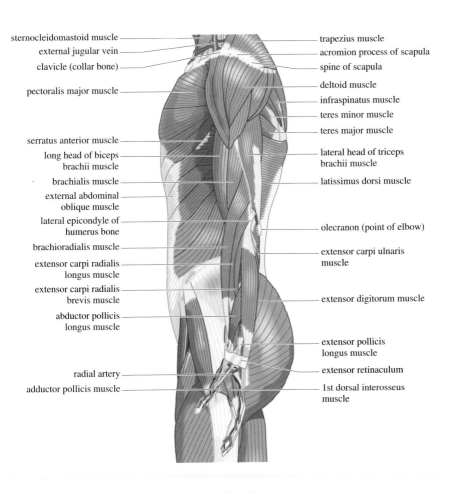

sternocleidomastoid muscle
external jugular vein
clavicle (collar bone)

pectoralis major muscle

serratus anterior muscle
long head of biceps
brachii muscle
brachialis muscle
external abdominal
oblique muscle
lateral epicondyle of
humerus bone
brachioradialis muscle
extensor carpi radialis
longus muscle
extensor carpi radialis
brevis muscle
abductor pollicis
longus muscle

radial artery
adductor pollicis muscle

trapezius muscle
acromion process of scapula
spine of scapula

deltoid muscle
infraspinatus muscle
teres minor muscle
teres major muscle

lateral head of triceps
brachii muscle
latissimus dorsi muscle

olecranon (point of elbow)

extensor carpi ulnaris
muscle

extensor digitorum muscle

extensor pollicis
longus muscle
extensor retinaculum
1st dorsal interosseus
muscle

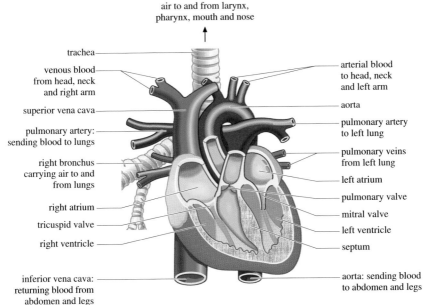

air to and from larynx,
pharynx, mouth and nose

trachea
venous blood
from head, neck
and right arm
superior vena cava

pulmonary artery:
sending blood to lungs

right bronchus
carrying air to and
from lungs
right atrium
tricuspid valve
right ventricle

inferior vena cava:
returning blood from
abdomen and legs

arterial blood
to head, neck
and left arm
aorta
pulmonary artery
to left lung
pulmonary veins
from left lung
left atrium
pulmonary valve
mitral valve
left ventricle
septum

aorta: sending blood
to abdomen and legs

Muscles of shoulder and right arm (top). Interior of heart and attendant blood vessels (bottom).

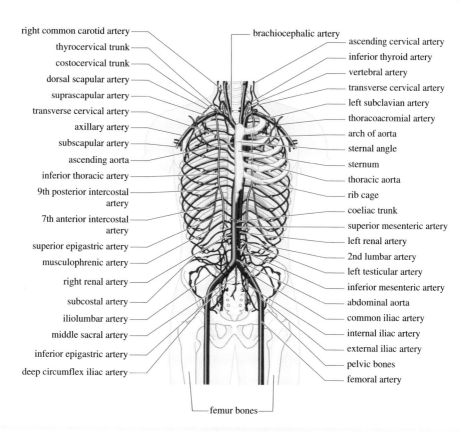

right common carotid artery

thyrocervical trunk

costocervical trunk

dorsal scapular artery

suprascapular artery

transverse cervical artery

axillary artery

subscapular artery

ascending aorta

inferior thoracic artery

9th posterior intercostal artery

7th anterior intercostal artery

superior epigastric artery

musculophrenic artery

right renal artery

subcostal artery

iliolumbar artery

middle sacral artery

inferior epigastric artery

deep circumflex iliac artery

brachiocephalic artery

ascending cervical artery

inferior thyroid artery

vertebral artery

transverse cervical artery

left subclavian artery

thoracoacromial artery

arch of aorta

sternal angle

sternum

thoracic aorta

rib cage

coeliac trunk

superior mesenteric artery

left renal artery

2nd lumbar artery

left testicular artery

inferior mesenteric artery

abdominal aorta

common iliac artery

internal iliac artery

external iliac artery

pelvic bones

femoral artery

femur bones

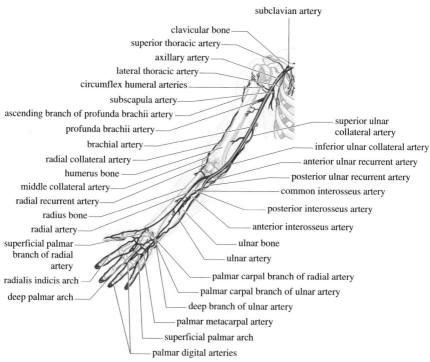

subclavian artery

clavicular bone

superior thoracic artery

axillary artery

lateral thoracic artery

circumflex humeral arteries

subscapula artery

ascending branch of profunda brachii artery

profunda brachii artery

brachial artery

radial collateral artery

humerus bone

middle collateral artery

radial recurrent artery

radius bone

radial artery

superficial palmar branch of radial artery

radialis indicis arch

deep palmar arch

superior ulnar collateral artery

inferior ulnar collateral artery

anterior ulnar recurrent artery

posterior ulnar recurrent artery

common interosseus artery

posterior interosseus artery

anterior interosseus artery

ulnar bone

ulnar artery

palmar carpal branch of radial artery

palmar carpal branch of ulnar artery

deep branch of ulnar artery

palmar metacarpal artery

superficial palmar arch

palmar digital arteries

Arteries: thorax and abdomen (top); right arm, front view (bottom).

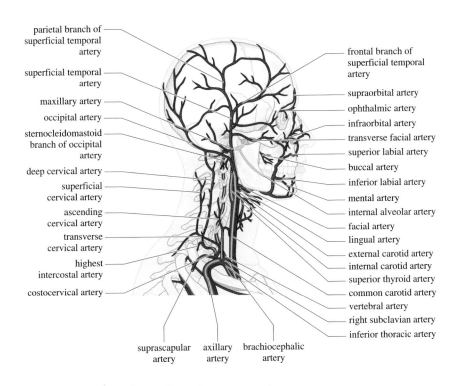

parietal branch of superficial temporal artery
superficial temporal artery
maxillary artery
occipital artery
sternocleidomastoid branch of occipital artery
deep cervical artery
superficial cervical artery
ascending cervical artery
transverse cervical artery
highest intercostal artery
costocervical artery

frontal branch of superficial temporal artery
supraorbital artery
ophthalmic artery
infraorbital artery
transverse facial artery
superior labial artery
buccal artery
inferior labial artery
mental artery
internal alveolar artery
facial artery
lingual artery
external carotid artery
internal carotid artery
superior thyroid artery
common carotid artery
vertebral artery
right subclavian artery
inferior thoracic artery

suprascapular artery
axillary artery
brachiocephalic artery

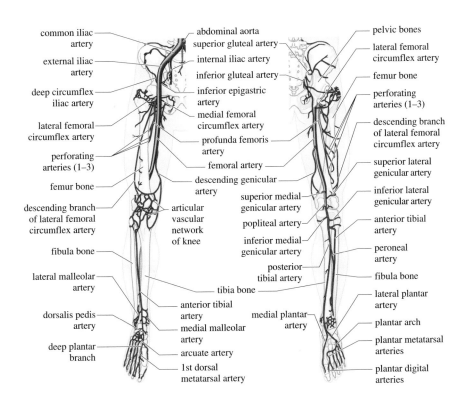

common iliac artery
external iliac artery
deep circumflex iliac artery
lateral femoral circumflex artery
perforating arteries (1–3)
femur bone
descending branch of lateral femoral circumflex artery
fibula bone
lateral malleolar artery
dorsalis pedis artery
deep plantar branch

abdominal aorta
superior gluteal artery
internal iliac artery
inferior gluteal artery
inferior epigastric artery
medial femoral circumflex artery
profunda femoris artery
femoral artery
descending genicular artery
superior medial genicular artery
articular vascular network of knee
popliteal artery
inferior medial genicular artery
posterior tibial artery
tibia bone
anterior tibial artery
medial malleolar artery
arcuate artery
1st dorsal metatarsal artery

medial plantar artery

pelvic bones
lateral femoral circumflex artery
femur bone
perforating arteries (1–3)
descending branch of lateral femoral circumflex artery
superior lateral genicular artery
inferior lateral genicular artery
anterior tibial artery
peroneal artery
fibula bone
lateral plantar artery
plantar arch
plantar metatarsal arteries
plantar digital arteries

Arteries: skull and neck, right side (top);
right leg; anterior view (right), posterior (left)

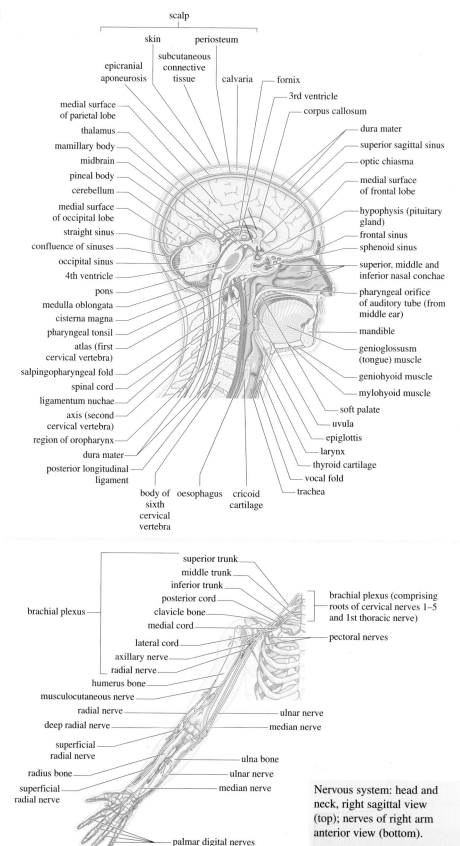

[8]

scalp

skin periosteum

epicranial
aponeurosis
subcutaneous
connective
tissue
calvaria — fornix

— 3rd ventricle

— corpus callosum

medial surface
of parietal lobe
thalamus
mamillary body
midbrain
pineal body
cerebellum
medial surface
of occipital lobe
straight sinus
confluence of sinuses
occipital sinus
4th ventricle
pons
medulla oblongata
cisterna magna
pharyngeal tonsil
atlas (first
cervical vertebra)
salpingopharyngeal fold
spinal cord
ligamentum nuchae
axis (second
cervical vertebra)
region of oropharynx
dura mater
posterior longitudinal
ligament

— dura mater
— superior sagittal sinus
— optic chiasma
— medial surface
of frontal lobe
— hypophysis (pituitary
gland)
— frontal sinus
— sphenoid sinus
— superior, middle and
inferior nasal conchae
— pharyngeal orifice
of auditory tube (from
middle ear)
— mandible
— genioglossum
(tongue) muscle
— geniohyoid muscle
— mylohyoid muscle
— soft palate
— uvula
— epiglottis
— larynx
— thyroid cartilage
— vocal fold
— trachea

body of oesophagus cricoid
sixth cartilage
cervical
vertebra

superior trunk
middle trunk
inferior trunk
posterior cord
clavicle bone
medial cord
lateral cord
axillary nerve
radial nerve
humerus bone
musculocutaneous nerve
radial nerve
deep radial nerve
superficial
radial nerve
radius bone
superficial
radial nerve

brachial plexus

brachial plexus (comprising
roots of cervical nerves 1–5
and 1st thoracic nerve)
pectoral nerves

ulnar nerve
median nerve

ulna bone
ulnar nerve
median nerve

palmar digital nerves

Nervous system: head and
neck, right sagittal view
(top); nerves of right arm
anterior view (bottom).

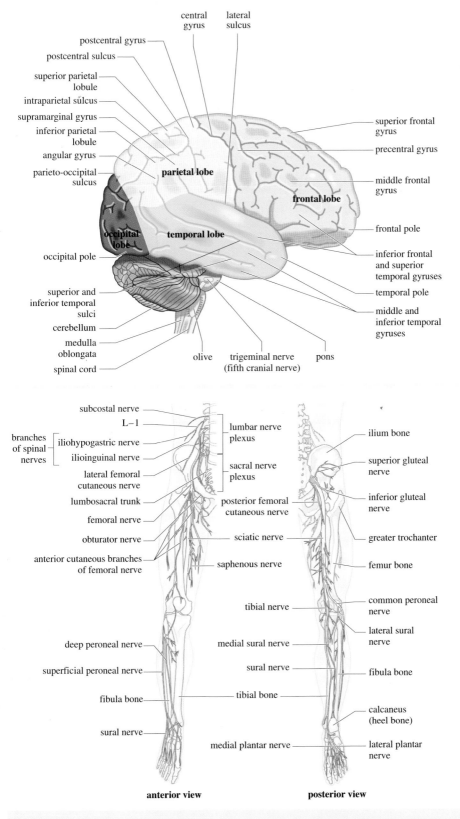

central gyrus
lateral sulcus
postcentral gyrus
postcentral sulcus
superior parietal lobule
intraparietal sulcus
supramarginal gyrus
inferior parietal lobule
angular gyrus
parieto-occipital sulcus
parietal lobe
occipital lobe
occipital pole
superior and inferior temporal sulci
cerebellum
medulla oblongata
spinal cord
temporal lobe
olive
trigeminal nerve (fifth cranial nerve)
pons
superior frontal gyrus
precentral gyrus
middle frontal gyrus
frontal lobe
frontal pole
inferior frontal and superior temporal gyruses
temporal pole
middle and inferior temporal gyruses

subcostal nerve
L–1
branches of spinal nerves
iliohypogastric nerve
ilioinguinal nerve
lateral femoral cutaneous nerve
lumbosacral trunk
femoral nerve
obturator nerve
anterior cutaneous branches of femoral nerve
deep peroneal nerve
superficial peroneal nerve
fibula bone
sural nerve
lumbar nerve plexus
sacral nerve plexus
posterior femoral cutaneous nerve
sciatic nerve
saphenous nerve
tibial nerve
medial sural nerve
sural nerve
tibial bone
medial plantar nerve
ilium bone
superior gluteal nerve
inferior gluteal nerve
greater trochanter
femur bone
common peroneal nerve
lateral sural nerve
fibula bone
calcaneus (heel bone)
lateral plantar nerve

anterior view
posterior view

Nervous system: external, right lateral view of brain (top); nerves of legs (bottom).

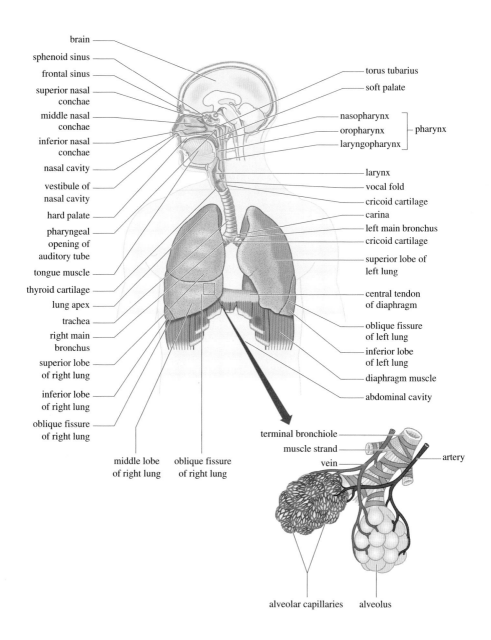

brain
sphenoid sinus
frontal sinus
superior nasal conchae
middle nasal conchae
inferior nasal conchae
nasal cavity
vestibule of nasal cavity
hard palate
pharyngeal opening of auditory tube
tongue muscle
thyroid cartilage
lung apex
trachea
right main bronchus
superior lobe of right lung
inferior lobe of right lung
oblique fissure of right lung

torus tubarius
soft palate
nasopharynx
oropharynx
laryngopharynx
pharynx
larynx
vocal fold
cricoid cartilage
carina
left main bronchus
cricoid cartilage
superior lobe of left lung
central tendon of diaphragm
oblique fissure of left lung
inferior lobe of left lung
diaphragm muscle
abdominal cavity

middle lobe of right lung   oblique fissure of right lung

terminal bronchiole
muscle strand
vein
artery

alveolar capillaries   alveolus

Schematic view of respiratory system with enlarged diagram of alveoli, the site where oxygen is absorbed into the blood and carbon dioxide removed from it.

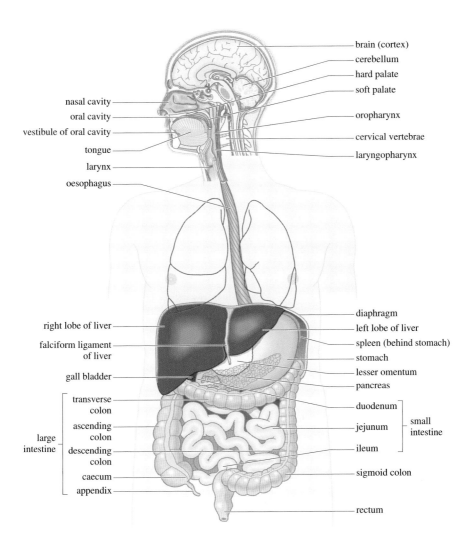

brain (cortex)
cerebellum
hard palate
soft palate
nasal cavity
oral cavity
oropharynx
vestibule of oral cavity
tongue
cervical vertebrae
larynx
laryngopharynx
oesophagus

right lobe of liver
diaphragm
left lobe of liver
falciform ligament of liver
spleen (behind stomach)
stomach
gall bladder
lesser omentum
pancreas
transverse colon
duodenum
ascending colon
jejunum
small intestine
large intestine
descending colon
ileum
caecum
sigmoid colon
appendix
rectum

Gastrointestinal tract from mouth to anus including organs – stomach, liver, pancreas, small and large intestines, essential to the digestion, absorption, metabolism and excretion of food – and partly hidden spleen.

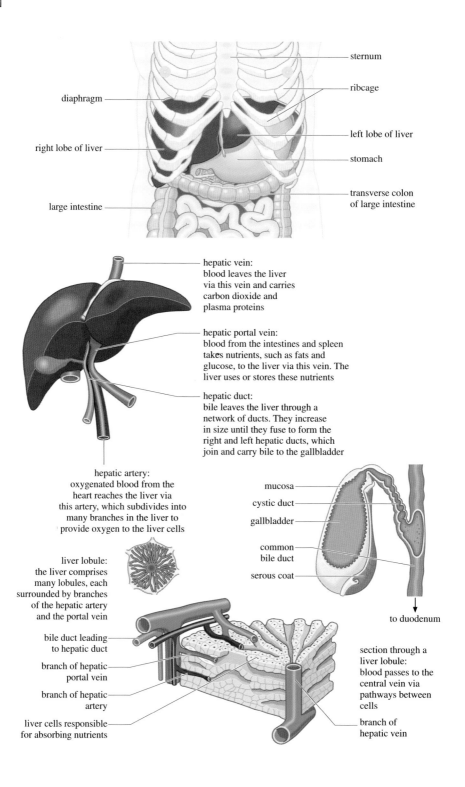

sternum

ribcage

diaphragm

left lobe of liver

right lobe of liver

stomach

transverse colon
of large intestine

large intestine

hepatic vein:
blood leaves the liver
via this vein and carries
carbon dioxide and
plasma proteins

hepatic portal vein:
blood from the intestines and spleen
takes nutrients, such as fats and
glucose, to the liver via this vein. The
liver uses or stores these nutrients

hepatic duct:
bile leaves the liver through a
network of ducts. They increase
in size until they fuse to form the
right and left hepatic ducts, which
join and carry bile to the gallbladder

hepatic artery:
oxygenated blood from the
heart reaches the liver via
this artery, which subdivides into
many branches in the liver to
provide oxygen to the liver cells

mucosa

cystic duct

gallbladder

liver lobule:
the liver comprises
many lobules, each
surrounded by branches
of the hepatic artery
and the portal vein

common
bile duct

serous coat

to duodenum

bile duct leading
to hepatic duct

branch of hepatic
portal vein

branch of hepatic
artery

liver cells responsible
for absorbing nutrients

section through a
liver lobule:
blood passes to the
central vein via
pathways between
cells

branch of
hepatic vein

(From top to bottom) position of liver in abdomen; schematic view of liver's blood circulation;
gall-bladder; section through a liver lobule.

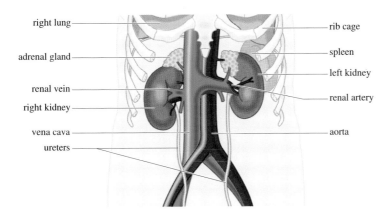

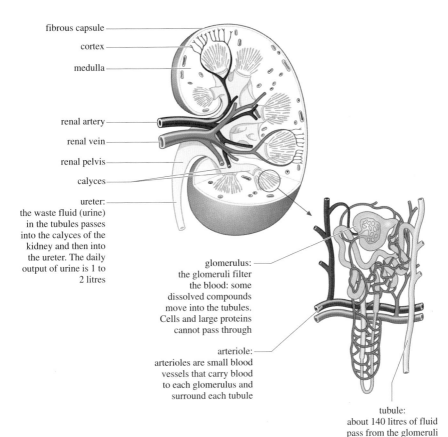

right lung

adrenal gland

renal vein

right kidney

vena cava

ureters

rib cage

spleen

left kidney

renal artery

aorta

fibrous capsule

cortex

medulla

renal artery

renal vein

renal pelvis

calyces

ureter:
the waste fluid (urine)
in the tubules passes
into the calyces of the
kidney and then into
the ureter. The daily
output of urine is 1 to
2 litres

glomerulus:
the glomeruli filter
the blood: some
dissolved compounds
move into the tubules.
Cells and large proteins
cannot pass through

arteriole:
arterioles are small blood
vessels that carry blood
to each glomerulus and
surround each tubule

tubule:
about 140 litres of fluid
pass from the glomeruli
into the tubules each day

Position of kidneys at back of abdomen (top); vertical section of kidney; diagram of the
glomerulus which filters waste from the blood (bottom).

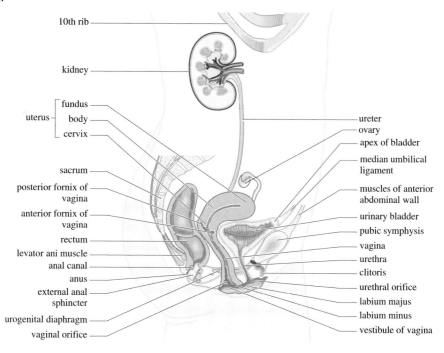

10th rib

kidney

uterus — fundus / body / cervix

ureter
ovary
apex of bladder
median umbilical ligament

sacrum
posterior fornix of vagina
anterior fornix of vagina
rectum
levator ani muscle
anal canal
anus
external anal sphincter
urogenital diaphragm
vaginal orifice

muscles of anterior abdominal wall
urinary bladder
pubic symphysis
vagina
urethra
clitoris
urethral orifice
labium majus
labium minus
vestibule of vagina

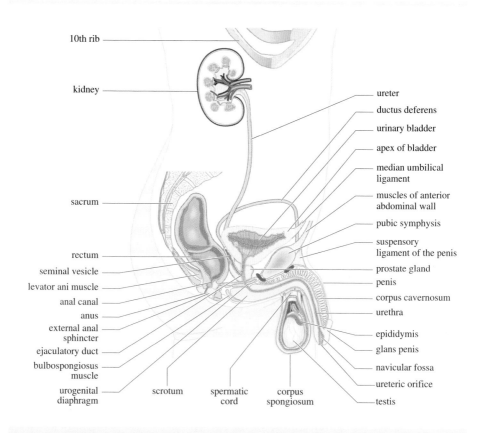

10th rib

kidney

sacrum

rectum
seminal vesicle
levator ani muscle
anal canal
anus
external anal sphincter
ejaculatory duct
bulbospongiosus muscle
urogenital diaphragm

scrotum

spermatic cord

corpus spongiosum

ureter
ductus deferens
urinary bladder
apex of bladder
median umbilical ligament
muscles of anterior abdominal wall
pubic symphysis
suspensory ligament of the penis
prostate gland
penis
corpus cavernosum
urethra
epididymis
glans penis
navicular fossa
ureteric orifice
testis

Female (top) and male urogenital systems.

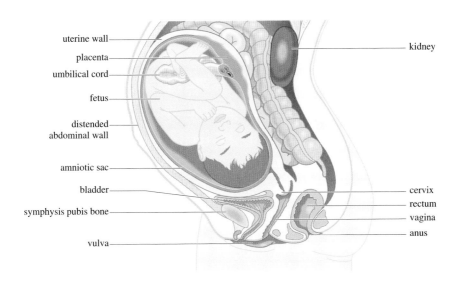

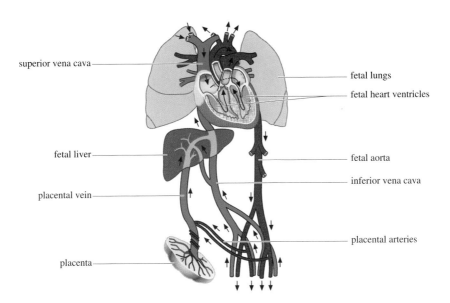

Sagittal section of mother's uterus with near-term baby and diagram of fetal circulation.

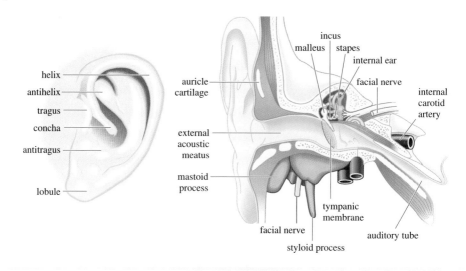

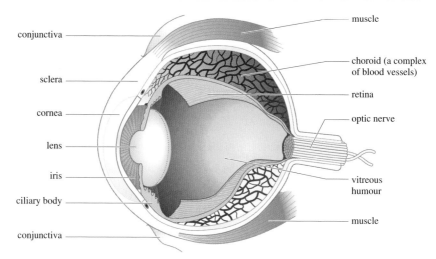

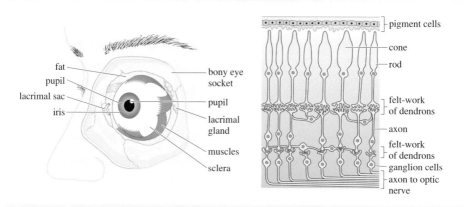

External and internal structures of the ear (top).
Cross-section of eye-ball (middle).
Position of eye in bony socket of the skull (bottom left).
Cross-section of the retina showing cell structures that 'convert' light rays into nervous
impulses that go to the brain along the optic nerve (bottom right).

to lack of platelets, and may have enlarged lymphatic glands and spleen. The temperature is raised, and the condition may be mistaken for an acute infection (or may first become apparent because the patient develops a severe infection due to a lack of normal white blood cells).

In the chronic type of the disease the onset is gradual, and the first symptoms which occasion discomfort are either swelling of the abdomen and shortness of breath, due to painless enlargement of the spleen; or the enlargement of glands in the neck, armpits and elsewhere; or the pallor, palpitation, and other symptoms of anaemia which often accompany leukaemia. Occasional bleeding from the nose, stomach, gums or bowels may occur, and may be severe. Generally, there is a slight fever.

When the blood is examined microscopically, not only is there an enormous increase in the number of white cells, which may be multiplied 30- or 60-fold, but various immature forms are also found. In the lymphatic form of the disease, most white cells resemble lymphocytes, which, in healthy blood, are present only in small numbers. In the myeloid form, myelocytes, or large immature cells from the bone marrow, which are never present in healthy blood, appear in large numbers, and there may also be large numbers of immature, nucleated erythrocytes.

Treatment This varies according to the type of leukaemia and to the particular condition of the patient. Excellent results are being obtained in the control of ALL using blood transfusions, CHEMOTHERAPY, RADIOTHERAPY and bone-marrow TRANSPLANTATION. In the case of acute leukaemia, the drugs now being used include MERCAPTOPURINE, METHOTREXATE and CYCLOPHOSPHAMIDE. Blood transfusion and CORTICOSTEROIDS play an important part in controlling the condition during the period before a response to chemotherapy can be expected. Chemotherapy has almost completely replaced radiotherapy in the treatment of chronic leukaemia. For the myeloid form, BUSULFAN is the most widely used drug, replaced by hydroxyurea, mercaptopurine, or one of the nitrogen mustard (see NITROGEN MUSTARDS) derivatives in the later stages of the disease. For the lymphatic form, the drugs used are CHLORAMBUCIL, CYCLOPHOSPHAMIDE, and the nitrogen mustard derivatives.

Prognosis Although there is still no guaranteed cure, the outlook in both acute and chronic leukaemia has greatly improved – particularly for the acute form of the disease. Between 70 and 80 per cent of children with acute lymphoblastic leukaemia may be cured; between 20 and 50 per cent of those with acute myeloid leukaemia now have much-improved survival rates. Prognosis of patients with chronic lymphocytic leukaemia is often good, depending on early diagnosis.

Leuko-
See LEUCO-.

Leukoplakia
A white plaque on mucous membranes caused by overgrowth of the tissues. It is occasionally a pre-cancerous condition.

Leukotrienes
A group of naturally occurring, slow-reacting substances (SRSS) which have powerful smooth-muscle stimulating properties, particularly on bronchial smooth muscle. Leukotrienes are a metabolic derivative of PROSTAGLANDINS. Leukotriene receptor antagonists, such as montelukast and zafirlukast, are drugs useful in asthma.

Levallorphan Tartrate
An antidote to MORPHINE. It is usually given intravenously.

Levamisole
A drug used to treat ASCARIASIS. Its main advantage seems to be in mass treatment, as one dose may prove effective. It is also being used in the treatment of a group of diseases of obscure origin, including CROHN'S DISEASE and RHEUMATOID ARTHRITIS. The drug is available in the UK with certain restrictions.

Levator
(1) Any muscle that raises the organ or structure into which it is inserted.
(2) A surgical instrument for raising depressed fragments of bone in a fracture, particularly a fracture of the skull.

Levodopa
A drug used in the treatment of PARKINSONISM. It is converted to DOPAMINE in the brain, correcting the deficiency which causes the disorder. Levodopa is often given with carbidopa or benserazide, both dopamine decarboxylase inhibitors, to prevent its conversion to dopamine in the body before it reaches the brain. It may cause nausea, HYPOTENSION or cardiac DYSRHYTHMIA.

Levorphanol

A synthetic derivative of MORPHINE. It is an effective analgesic but, like morphine, is a drug of addiction.

LHRH

Abbreviation for LUTEINISING HORMONE-RELEASING HORMONE (LHRH), which is released by the PITUITARY GLAND.

LHRH Analogue

A synthetically produced agent with the same properties as LUTEINISING HORMONE-RELEASING HORMONE (LHRH).

Libido

The natural desire for sexual intercourse. Lack of desire or diminished libido may occur in any general medical illness as well as in endocrine diseases when there is a lack of production of the sex hormones. The strength or weakness of the sexual drive may be associated with psychiatric diseases; it may also be the result of certain drugs. It must be distinguished from IMPOTENCE, where the desire for intercourse is normal but the performance is defective due to the inability to achieve or maintain an erection.

Librium

See CHLORDIAZEPOXIDE.

Lice

See PEDICULOSIS.

Lichen

Lichen, or lichenification, is a term used to describe a thickening of chronically inflamed skin to give a tree-bark-like appearance.

Lichen simplex (neurodermatitis) is a form of eczema (see DERMATITIS) perpetuated by constant rubbing of the affected skin. Typically, well-defined plaques occur on one or both sides of the nape of the neck, on the ulnar forearm near the elbow, or on the sides of the calves. It is often associated with emotional stress.

Lichen planus is a less common inflammation of the skin characterised by small, shiny, flat-topped violaceous papules which may coalesce to form large plaques. Itching can be intense. Typically seen on the flexor aspects of the wrists, the lower back and on the legs below the knees, it may also affect the mucous membranes of the mouth and lips. The cause is unknown. While in some patients the disorder appears to be nervous or emotional in origin, it can be caused by certain drugs such as

CHLOROQUINE. Severe cases may require oral CORTICOSTEROIDS to control the eruption.

Lidocaine

A local anaesthetic given by injection, previously called lignocaine. It is also used in the treatment of certain disorders of cardiac rhythm known as ventricular arrhythmias which may be particularly dangerous following a coronary thrombosis (see HEART, DISEASES OF).

Life Expectancy

The number of years an individual can expect to live. Life expectancy at birth in most western countries is over 75 years for women (nearly 80 in the UK in 1998) and over 70 for men (over 74 in the UK in 1998) – a figure that has been steadily rising as living standards have improved. The longer a person lives, the greater is his or her life expectancy.

Lifestyle Medicines

Drugs used for non-health problems or for disorders that are in the grey area between a genuine health need and a desire to change a 'lifestyle failing' by the use of medication. Examples are: SILDENAFIL CITRATE, which is prescribed for men unable to achieve penile erection (erectile dysfunction); and ORLISTAT, a drug used to combat OBESITY.

Ligaments

Strong bands of fibrous tissue which serve to bind together the bones entering into a joint. In some cases they are cord-like; in others, flattened bands – whilst most joints are surrounded by a fibrous capsule or capsular ligament. (See JOINTS.)

Ligation

Tying-off – for example, of a blood vessel – by completely encircling it with a tight band, usually of catgut or some other suture material.

Ligature

A cord or thread used to tie around arteries in order to stop the circulation through them, or to prevent escape of blood from their cut ends. Ligatures are generally made of catgut or silk, and are tied with a reef-knot.

Light Reflex

Pupillary constriction in the EYE in response to light. The direct light reflex involves pupillary constriction in the eye into which a light is shone; the consensual light reflex is the pupillary constriction that occurs in the other eye. The afferent or inward pathway of the reflex is via the optic nerve, and the efferent or outward pathway is via the occulomotor nerve.

Limbic System

A circular, complex system of NERVE pathways in the middle of the BRAIN. This connected cluster of neuronal nuclei is involved in the working of the AUTONOMIC NERVOUS SYSTEM, helping to control the expression of instinct and mood in activities of the motor systems and the ENDOCRINE GLANDS of the body. The brain regions involved include the amygdala (an almond-shaped basal ganglion deep in each cerebral hemisphere), and the HYPO-THALAMUS. If the limbic system is impaired by injury or disease, the person may suffer abnormal emotional responses such as unprovoked rage, unreasonable fear and anxiety, depression, greater-than-normal sexual interest, and crying or laughing for no good reason.

Limb Lengthening

An orthopaedic procedure in which the length of a limb, usually a leg, is increased. The bone is surgically divided and slowly stretched in a special frame. The operation is usually done on people with unequal leg lengths as a result of injury or from PARALYSIS in childhood. Exceptionally, it may be done in both legs to help people of short stature.

Limbs, Artificial

See PROSTHESIS.

Lime-Juice

A yellow liquid obtained by squeezing lime-fruit, *Citrus limetta*. In common with lemon-juice, it is a rich source of vitamin C (16·8–62·5 mg per 100 ml) and contains a large quantity of citric acid. It is used as a refreshing drink and as a preventive of, and remedy for, SCURVY. Lime-juice which has been boiled, or preserved for a prolonged period, loses its anti-scorbutic properties.

Linctus

A term applied to any thick, syrupy medicine. Most of these are remedies for excessive coughing.

Lindane

An insecticide used in SCABIES and lice infestations (see PEDICULOSIS); however, head lice are now often resistant. Used excessively, lindane may be neurotoxic (damage the nervous system).

Linea Alba

The line of fibrous tissue stretching down the mid line of the belly from the lower end of the sternum to the pubic bone (see PUBIS). The linea alba gives attachment to the muscles of the wall of the stomach.

Linea Nigra

During pregnancy, the LINEA ALBA becomes pigmented and appears as a dark line down the middle of the belly, and is called the linea nigra.

Linear Accelerator

See RADIOTHERAPY.

Lingual

Referring or related to the TONGUE: for example, the lingual nerve supplies sensation to the tongue.

Liniments

Liniments, or EMBROCATIONS, are oily mixtures intended for external application by rubbing. Their chief use is in the production of pain relief, particularly in rheumatic conditions. They may be highly toxic if taken orally.

Linkage

A description that in GENETICS means circumstances in which two or more GENES lie near each other on a chromosome (see CHROMO-SOMES) and so may well be inherited together.

Linoleic Acid

An unsaturated fatty acid occurring widely in the glycerides of plants. It is an essential nutrient for mammals, including humans.

Lint

This was originally made of teased-out linen; now it consists of a loose cotton fabric, one side of which is fluffy, the other being smooth and applied next to the skin when the surface is broken. Marine lint consists of tow impregnated with tar, and is used where large quantities of some absorbent and deodorising dressing are required. Cotton lint is impregnated with various substances, the most common being boracic lint. Lint containing perchloride of iron (15 per cent) is valuable as a styptic (see STYPTICS).

Liothyronine Acid

A preparation based on the thyroid (see THY-ROID GLAND) hormone triiodothyronine, which is prescribed to replace the lack of natural thyroid hormone (hypothyroidism). The drug is also used to treat goitre and cancer of the thyroid gland. (See THYROID GLAND, DISEASES OF.)

Lipaemia

The presence of an excessive amount of FAT in the blood.

Lipase

An ENZYME widely distributed in plants, and present also in the liver and gastric and pancreatic juices, which breaks down fats to the constituent fatty acids and glycerol.

Lipid

A substance which is insoluble in water, but soluble in fat solvents such as alcohol and ether. The main lipid groups are the triglycerides, phospholipids, and glycolipids. They play an important role in nutrition, health (particularly in the functioning of the cell membranes, and the immune response), and disease (notably cardiovascular disease). There is a strong correlation between the concentration of CHOLESTEROL in the blood (transported as lipoproteins) and the risk of developing ATHEROMA and coronary heart disease (see HEART, DISEASES OF). Lipoproteins are classified by their density and mobility, the chief groups being low-density (LDL) and high-density (HDL). High SERUM concentrations of LDL increase the risk of cardiovascular disease, while HDL is thought to protect the vessel wall by removing cholesterol, and has an inverse relationship to risk. The various serum lipid abnormalities have been classified into five groups, according to the cause and particular lipoprotein raised. Most important are type II (increased LDL, genetically determined) and type IV (increased VLDL, associated with obesity, diabetes, and excess alcohol). Various lipid-lowering drugs are available, but any drug treatment must be combined with a strict diet, reduction of blood pressure, and cessation of smoking.

Lipidosis

Any disorder of LIPID metabolism in body cells. Some hereditary disorders cause deposition of lipids within the brain.

Lipid-Regulating Drugs

These drugs reduce the amount of low-density LIPOPROTEINS, which transport CHOLESTEROL and triglycerides (see TRIGLYCERIDE) in the blood, or raise the concentration of high-density lipoproteins. The aim is to reduce the progression of ATHEROSCLEROSIS and therefore help prevent coronary heart disease (see HEART,

DISEASES OF). These drugs should be combined with reducing other risk factors for raised lipid concentrations, such as a high-fat diet, smoking and obesity. Lipid-regulating drugs include STATINS, fibrates, anion-exchange resins, and NICOTINIC ACID, which may be used singly or in combination under careful medical supervision (see HYPERLIPIDAEMIA).

Lipodystrophy

A congenital maldistribution of FAT tissue. Subcutaneous fat is totally absent from a portion of the body and hypertrophied in the remainder. Another form of lipodystrophy occurs at the site of INSULIN injections, but is much less frequently seen nowadays; the new, synthetic preparations of insulin are pure and unlikely to cause this reaction, which was not uncommon with the older preparations. Occasionally the converse occurs at the site of insulin injections, where the lipogenic action of insulin stimulates the fat cells to hypertrophy. This can also be disfiguring and usually results from using the same site for injections too frequently.

Lipoid Factor

An agent involved in the clotting mechanism of the blood. It helps in the activation of THROMBOPLASTIN in the blood PLASMA (see COAGULATION).

Lipolysis

The enzymatic breaking-down of FAT.

Lipoma

A TUMOUR mainly composed of FAT. Such tumours arise in almost any part of the body, developing in fibrous tissues – particularly in that beneath the skin. They are benign in nature, and seldom give any trouble beyond that connected with their size and position. If large, they can be excised.

Lipoproteins

Compounds containing lipids and proteins (see LIPID; PROTEIN). Most lipids in blood PLASMA are present in this form and are characterised according to their densities: very low (VLDL), intermediate (IDL), low (LD), high (HDL) and very high (VHDL). Concentrations of lipoproteins are key factors in assessing the risk of cardiovascular disease (see HEART, DISEASES OF).

Liposarcoma

A rare malignant TUMOUR of adipose or fatty tissue. It occurs most frequently in the thighs, buttocks or retro-peritoneum. The four main types are: well differentiated; myxoid; round cell; and pleomorphic (variety of forms).

Liposomes

These are essentially tiny oil droplets consisting of layers of fatty material, known as phospholipid, separated by aqueous compartments. Drugs can be incorporated into the liposomes, which are then injected into the bloodstream or into the muscles, or given by mouth. Using this method of giving drugs, it is possible to protect them from being broken down in the body before they reach the part of the body where their curative effect is required: for example, in the liver or in a tumour.

Liposuction

A surgical procedure, also called suction lipectomy, for extracting unwanted accumulations of subcutaneous FAT with the use of a powerful suction tube passed through the skin at different sites. Widely used in cosmetic surgery to improve the contour of the body, particularly that of women, the technique can have unwanted side-effects.

Lips

These form a pair of 'curtains' before the mouth, each composed of a layer of skin and of mucous membrane, between which lies a considerable amount of fat and of muscle fibres.

Fissures coming on in cold weather are often difficult to get rid of. Peeling and cracking of the vermilion of the lips is common in those exposed for long periods to wind and sunlight. Treatment consists of the application of aqueous cream. If the main cause is excessive exposure to sunlight – in which case the lower lip is mainly affected – a protective cream should be applied.

Herpes in the form of 'cold sores' often develops on the lip as a result of a cold or other feverish condition, but quickly passes off (see HERPES SIMPLEX).

Ulcers may form on the inner surface of the lip, usually in consequence of bad teeth or of DYSPEPSIA.

Small cysts sometimes form on the inner surface of the lip, and are seen as little bluish swellings filled with mucus; they are of no importance.

Hare-lip is a deformity sometimes present at birth (see PALATE, MALFORMATIONS OF).

Cancer of the lip sometimes occurs – almost always in men, and usually on the lower lip. (See also MOUTH, DISEASES OF.)

Liquor

See SOLUTION.

Liquorice

The root of *Glycyrrhiza glabra*, a plant of southern Europe and Asia. It is a mild expectorant (see EXPECTORANTS), but is mainly used to cover the taste of disagreeable and more powerful drugs. Solid and liquid extracts are made from it, but the most commonly used preparation is compound liquorice powder, which contains also senna and sulphur.

Listeriosis

A rare disease, although the causal organism, *Listeria monocytogenes*, is widely distributed in soil, silage, water, and various animals, with consequent risk of food contamination – for example, from unpasteurised soft cheese. Neonates are mainly affected – often as a result of a mild or inapparent infection in the pregnant mother. The disease presents in two main forms: MENINGOENCEPHALITIS, or SEPTICAEMIA with enlarged LYMPH glands. Elderly adults occasionally develop the first form, while younger adults are more likely to develop a mild or even inapparent form. The disease is treated with ANTIBIOTICS such as ampicillin (see PENICILLIN) or CHLORAMPHENICOL.

Lithiasis

A general name applied to the formation of CALCULI and concretions in tissues or organs: for example, cholelithiasis means the formation of calculi in the GALL-BLADDER.

Lithium Carbonate

A drug widely used in the PROPHYLAXIS treatment of certain forms of MENTAL ILLNESS. The drug should be given only on specialist advice. The major indication for its use is acute MANIA; it induces improvement or remission in over 70 per cent of such patients. In addition, it is effective in the treatment of manic-depressive patients (see MANIC DEPRESSION), preventing both the manic and the depressive episodes. There is also evidence that it lessens aggression in prisoners who behave antisocially and in patients with learning difficulties who mutilate themselves and have temper tantrums.

Because of its possible toxic effects – including kidney damage – lithium must only be administered under medical supervision and with monitoring of the blood levels, as the gap between therapeutic and toxic concentrations is narrow. Due to the risk of its damaging the unborn child, it should not be prescribed, unless absolutely necessary, during pregnancy – particularly not in the first three months. Mothers should not take it while breast feeding, as it is excreted in the milk in high concentrations. The drug should not be taken with DIURETICS.

Litholapaxy

Litholapaxy is the term applied to the operation in which a stone in the URINARY BLADDER is crushed by an instrument introduced along the URETHRA, and the fragments washed out through a catheter (see CATHETERS).

Lithotomy

The operation of cutting for stone in the bladder. The operation is of great historic interest, because more has probably been written about it in early times than about any other type of surgery – and because, for a long time, it formed almost the only operation in which the surgeon dared to attack diseases of the internal organs.

Lithotripsy

Extracorporeal shock-wave lithotripsy (ESWL) causes disintegration of renal and biliary stones (see CALCULI) without physical contact, and is therefore an attractive procedure for patients and surgeons alike.

Shock waves generated outside the body can be accurately focused with a reflector whilst the patient is suspended in water, to facilitate transmission of the waves. These are focused on the calculus. The resultant fine fragments are passed spontaneously in the urine with minimal, if any, discomfort. The procedure has been shown to be safe, short and effective, and is most acceptable to patients.

Litigation

See MEDICAL LITIGATION.

Litmus

Litmus, which is prepared from several lichens, is a vegetable dye-substance, which on contact with alkaline fluids becomes blue, and on contact with acid fluids, red. Slips of paper, impregnated with litmus, form a valuable test for the acidity of the secretions and discharges.

Litre

A unit measurement of volume. One litre (l) is equivalent to the volume occupied by one kilo-gram of pure water at 4 °C and 760 mm Hg pressure. For day-to-day measurement, 1 litre is taken as being equal to 1,000 cubic centimetres (cm^3).

Little's Disease

A form of CEREBRAL PALSY.

Liver

The liver is the largest gland in the body, serving numerous functions, chiefly involving various aspects of METABOLISM.

Form The liver is divided into four lobes, the greatest part being the right lobe, with a small left lobe, while the quadrate and caudate lobes are two small divisions on the back and under-surface. Around the middle of the under-surface, towards the back, a transverse fissure (the porta hepatis) is placed, by which the hepatic artery and portal vein carry blood into the liver, and the right and left hepatic ducts emerge, carrying off the BILE formed in the liver to the GALL-BLADDER attached under the right lobe, where it is stored.

Position Occupying the right-hand upper part of the abdominal cavity, the liver is separated from the right lung by the DIAPHRAGM and the pleural membrane (see PLEURA). It rests on various abdominal organs, chiefly the right of the two KIDNEYS, the suprarenal gland (see ADRENAL GLANDS), the large INTESTINE, the DUODENUM and the STOMACH.

Vessels The blood supply differs from that of the rest of the body, in that the blood collected from the stomach and bowels into the PORTAL VEIN does not pass directly to the heart, but is first distributed to the liver, where it breaks up into capillary vessels. As a result, some harmful substances are filtered from the bloodstream and destroyed, while various constituents of the food are stored in the liver for use in the body's metabolic processes. The liver also receives the large hepatic artery from the coeliac axis. After circulating through capillaries, the blood from both sources is collected into the hepatic veins, which pass directly from the back surface of the liver into the inferior vena cava.

Minute structure The liver is enveloped in a capsule of fibrous tissue – Glisson's capsule – from which strands run along the vessels and penetrate deep into the organ, binding it together. Subdivisions of the hepatic artery, portal vein, and bile duct lie alongside each other, finally forming the interlobular vessels,

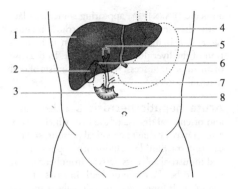

1 liver
2 gall-bladder
3 ampulla of Vater (leading into duodenum)
4 outline of stomach
5 hepatic ducts
6 bile duct
7 common bile duct
8 section of duodenum

Postions of liver, gall-bladder and connecting bile ducts.

which lie between the lobules of which the whole gland is built up. Each is about the size of a pin's head and forms a complete secreting unit; the liver is built up of hundreds of thousands of such lobules. These contain small vessels, capillaries, or sinusoids, lined with stellate KUPFFER CELLS, which run into the centre of the lobule, where they empty into a small central vein. These lobular veins ultimately empty into the hepatic veins. Between these capillaries lie rows of large liver cells in which metabolic activity occurs. Fine bile capillaries collect the bile from the cells and discharge it into the bile ducts lying along the margins of the lobules. Liver cells are among the largest in the body, each containing one or two large round nuclei. The cells frequently contain droplets of fat or granules of GLYCOGEN – that is, animal starch.

Functions The liver is, in effect, a large chemical factory and the heat this produces contributes to the general warming of the body. The liver secretes bile, the chief constituents of which are the bile salts (sodium glycocholate and taurocholate), the bile pigments (BILIRUBIN and biliverdin), CHOLESTEROL, and LECITHIN. These bile salts are collected and formed in the liver and are eventually converted into the bile acids. The bile pigments are the iron-free and globin-free remnant of HAEMOGLOBIN, formed in the Kupffer cells of the liver. (They can also be formed in the spleen, lymph glands, bone marrow and connective tissues.) Bile therefore

serves several purposes: it excretes pigment, the breakdown products of old red blood cells; the bile salts increase fat absorption and activate pancreatic lipase, thus aiding the digestion of fat; and bile is also necessary for the absorption of vitamins D and E.

The other important functions of the liver are as follows:

● In the EMBRYO it forms red blood cells, while the adult liver stores vitamin B_{12}, necessary for the proper functioning of the bone marrow in the manufacture of red cells.

● It manufactures FIBRINOGEN, ALBUMINS and GLOBULIN from the blood.

● It stores IRON and copper, necessary for the manufacture of red cells.

● It produces HEPARIN, and – with the aid of vitamin K – PROTHROMBIN.

● Its Kupffer cells form an important part of the RETICULO-ENDOTHELIAL SYSTEM, which breaks down red cells and probably manufactures ANTIBODIES.

● Noxious products made in the intestine and absorbed into the blood are detoxicated in the liver.

● It stores carbohydrate in the form of glycogen, maintaining a two-way process: glucose ⇆ glycogen.

● CAROTENE, a plant pigment, is converted to vitamin A, and B vitamins are stored.

● It splits up AMINO ACIDS and manufactures UREA and uric acids.

● It plays an essential role in the storage and metabolism of FAT.

Liver, Diseases of

The LIVER may be extensively diseased without any obviously serious symptoms, unless the circulation through it is impeded, the outflow of BILE checked, or neighbouring organs implicated. JAUNDICE is a symptom of several liver disorders, and is discussed under its separate heading. ASCITES, which may be caused by interference with the circulation through the portal vein of the liver, as well as by other reasons, is also considered separately. The presence of gallstones is a complication of some diseases connected with the liver, and is treated under GALLBLADDER, DISEASES OF. For hydatid cyst of the liver, see TAENIASIS. Liver diseases in a tropical environment are dealt with later in this section.

Inflammation of the liver, or HEPATITIS, may occur as part of a generalised infection or may be a localised condition. Infectious hepatitis, which is the result of infection with a virus, is one of the most common forms. Many different viruses can cause hepatitis, including that responsible for glandular fever (see MONO-NUCLEOSIS). Certain spirochaetes may also be the cause, particularly that responsible for LEPTOSPIROSIS, as can many drugs. Hepatitis may also occur if there is obstruction of the BILE DUCT, as by a gall-stone.

Cirrhosis of the liver A disorder caused by chronic damage to liver cells. The liver develops areas of fibrosis or scarring; in response, the remaining normal liver cells increase and form regeneration nodules. Those islands of normality, however, suffer from inadequate blood supply, thus adversely affecting liver function. Alcohol is the most common cause of cirrhosis in the United Kingdom and the USA, and the incidence of the disorder among women in the UK has recently risen sharply as a consequence of greater consumption of alcohol by young women in the latter decades of the 20th century. In Africa and many parts of Asia, infection with hepatitis B virus is a common cause. Certain drugs – for example, PARACETAMOL – may damage the liver if taken in excess. Unusual causes of cirrhosis include defects of the bile ducts, HAEMOCHROMATOSIS (raised iron absorption from the gut), CYSTIC FIBROSIS, cardiac cirrhosis (the result of heart failure causing circulatory congestion in the liver), and WILSON'S DISEASE (raised copper absorption).

Symptoms Some people with cirrhosis have no signs or symptoms and the disease may be diagnosed at a routine medical examination. Others may develop jaundice, OEDEMA (including ascites – fluid in the abdomen), fever, confusion, HAEMATEMESIS (vomiting blood), loss of appetite and lethargy. On examination, cirrhotic patients often have an enlarged liver and/or SPLEEN, and HYPERTENSION. Liver function tests, cholangiography (X-ray examination of the bile ducts) and biopsy of liver tissue will help to reach a diagnosis.

Treatment Nothing can be done to repair a cirrhosed organ, but the cause, if known, must be removed and further advance of the process thus prevented. In the case of the liver, a high-protein, high-carbohydrate, low-fat diet is given, supplemented by liver extract and vitamins B and K. The consumption of alcohol should be banned. In patients with liver failure and a poor prognosis, liver TRANSPLANTATION is worthwhile but only after careful consideration.

Abscess of the liver When an ABSCESS develops in the liver, it is usually a result of

amoebic DYSENTERY, appearing sometimes late in the disease – even after the diarrhoea is cured (see below). It may also follow upon inflammation of the liver due to other causes. In the case of an amoebic abscess, treatment consists of oral metronidazole.

Acute hepatic necrosis is a destructive and often fatal disease of the liver which is very rare. It may be due to chemical poisons, such as carbontetrachloride, chloroform, phosphorus and industrial solvents derived from benzene. It may also be the cause of death in cases of poisoning with fungi. Very occasionally, it may be a complication of acute infectious hepatitis.

Cancer of the liver is not uncommon, although it is rare for the disease to begin in the liver – the involvement of this organ being usually secondary to disease situated somewhere in the stomach or bowels. Cancer originating in the liver is more common in Asia and Africa. It usually arises in a fibrotic (or cirrhotic) liver and in carriers of the hepatitis B virus. There is great emaciation, which increases as the disease progresses. The liver is much enlarged, and its margin and surface are rough, being studded with hard cancer masses of varying size, which can often be felt through the abdominal wall. Pain may be present. Jaundice and oedema often appear.

Liver disease in the tropics
ACUTE LIVER DISEASE The hepatitis viruses (A–F) are of paramount importance. Hepatitis E (HEV) often produces acute hepatic failure in pregnant women; extensive epidemics – transmitted by contaminated drinking-water supplies – have been documented. HBV, especially in association with HDV, also causes acute liver failure in infected patients in several tropical countries: however, the major importance of HBV is that the infection leads to chronic liver disease (see below). Other hepatotoxic viruses include the EPSTEIN BARR VIRUS, CYTO-MEGALOVIRUS (CMV), the flavivirus causing YELLOW FEVER, Marburg/Ebola viruses, etc. Acute liver disease also occurs in the presence of several acute bacterial infections, including *Salmonella typhi*, brucellosis, leptospirosis, syphilis, etc. The complex type of jaundice associated with acute systemic bacterial infection – especially pneumococcal PNEUMONIA and pyomiositis – assumes a major importance in many tropical countries, especially those in Africa and in Papua New Guinea. Of protozoan infections, plasmodium *falciparum* malaria, LEISHMANIASIS, and TOXOPLASMOSIS should be

considered. *Ascaris lumbricoides* (the roundworm) can produce obstruction to the biliary system.

CHRONIC LIVER DISEASE Long-term disease is dominated by sequelae of HBV and HCV infections (often acquired during the neonatal period), both of which can cause chronic active hepatitis, cirrhosis, and hepatocellular carcinoma ('hepatoma') – one of the world's most common malignancies. Chronic liver disease is also caused by SCHISTOSOMIASIS (usually *Schistosoma mansoni* and *S. japonicum*), and acute and chronic alcohol ingestion. Furthermore, many local herbal remedies and also orthodox chemotherapeutic compounds (e.g. those used in tuberculosis and leprosy) can result in chronic liver disease. HAEMOSIDEROSIS is a major problem in southern Africa. Hepatocytes contain excessive iron – derived primarily from an excessive intake, often present in locally brewed beer; however, a genetic predisposition seems likely. Indian childhood cirrhosis – associated with an excess of copper – is a major problem in India and surrounding countries. Epidemiological evidence shows that much of the copper is derived from copper vessels used to store milk after weaning. Veno-occlusive disease was first described in Jamaica and is caused by pyrrolyzidine alkaloids (present in bush-tea). Several HIV-associated 'opportunistic' infections can give rise to hepatic disease (see AIDS/HIV).

A localised (focal) form of liver disease in all tropical/subtropical countries results from invasive *Entamoeba histolytica* infection (amoebic liver 'abscess'); serology and imaging techniques assist in diagnosis. Hydatidosis also causes localised liver disease; one or more cysts usually involve the right lobe of the liver. Serological tests and imaging techniques are of value in diagnosis. Whilst surgery formerly constituted the sole method of management, prolonged courses of albendazole and/or praziquantel have now been shown to be effective; however, surgical intervention is still required in some cases.

Hepato-biliary disease is also a problem in many tropical/subtropical countries. In southeast Asia, *Clonorchis sinensis* and *Opisthorchis viverini* infections cause chronic biliary-tract infection, complicated by adenocarcinoma of the biliary system. Praziquantel is effective chemotherapy before advanced disease ensues. *Fasciola hepatica* (the liver fluke) is a further hepato-biliary helminthic infection; treatment is with bithionol or triclabendazole, praziquantel being relatively ineffective.

Liver Fluke
Fasciola hepatica is a parasite infesting sheep and occasionally invading the bile ducts and liver of humans (see FASCIOLIASIS).

Liver Spots
A misnomer applied to the brown MACULES often seen on the backs of the hands of those chronically exposed to sunlight (see LENTIGO). They have no connection with any liver disorder.

Living Will
Also known as an advance directive or advance statement about medical treatment. This is a means of exercising choice in advance for patients who suspect that they will suffer mental impairment and become unable to speak for themselves. Advance statements can have legal force if made by an informed and competent adult, clearly refusing some or all future medical treatment once that individual has irrevocably lost mental capacity. Some statements intend to give other instructions, such as requesting certain treatments: these can be helpful in clarifying the patients's wishes, but only a clear refusal of treatment is legally binding in most of the UK. (In Scotland, patients have some legal powers to use an advance statement to nominate another person to act as a proxy decision-maker.)

As there is no statute defining the scope and limits of advance statements in the UK, their legal status depends principally on case precedents. As well as written documents, competent patients can make equally valid advance oral refusals which should be recorded in the medical notes. Some health professionals or health facilities may have a conscientious objection (see ETHICS) to the concept of withdrawing life-prolonging treatment from incompetent patients, even at the patient's advance request. Such objections need to be made known to patients well in advance of a living will becoming eligible for implementation, so that the patient can make other arrangements. The British Medical Association has issued a code of practice on the subject; this provides widely approved guidance on various facets of drafting, storing, witnessing and implementing advance statements. It is also dealt with in the GMC document on withdrawing treatment.

Loa
See LOIASIS.

Lobe
The term applied to the larger divisions of

various organs, such as to the four lobes of the LIVER, the three lobes of the right and the two lobes of the left lung, which are separated by fissures from one another (see LUNGS), and to the lobes or superficial areas into which the BRAIN is divided. The term lobar is applied to structures which are connected with lobes of organs, or to diseases which have a tendency to be limited by the boundaries of lobes, such as lobar PNEUMONIA.

Lobectomy

The operation of cutting out a lobe of the lung in such diseases as abscess of the lung and bronchiectasis and carcinoma (see LUNGS, DISEASES OF).

Lobotomy

Lobotomy is the cutting of a lobe of the BRAIN. (See also PSYCHOSURGERY.)

Lobule

The term applied to a division of an organ smaller than a lobe: for example, the lobules of the lung are of the size of millet seeds (see LUNGS); those of the LIVER, slightly larger. Lobules form the smallest subdivisions or units of an organ, each lobule being similar to the others, of which there may be perhaps several hundred thousand in the organ.

Local Anaesthesia

Loss of sensation produced in a part of the body to stop pain while a person is examined, investigated or treated (see also ANAESTHESIA). The anaesthesia is effected by giving drugs in a local area temporarily to stop the action of pain-carrying nerve fibres. To anaesthetise a large area, a nerve block is done. Various drugs are used, depending on the depth and length of local anaesthesia required.

Lochia

Lochia is the discharge which takes place during the first week or two after childbirth. During the first four days it consists chiefly of blood; after the fifth day the colour should become paler, and after the first week the quantity should diminish. If the discharge becomes smelly, it may indicate an infection and immediate investigation and treament are necessary. (See also PUERPERIUM.)

Locked-In Syndrome

This describes a condition in which a patient is awake and retains the power of sense perception, but is unable to communicate except by limited eye movements because the motor nervous system is paralysed. Several diseases can cause this syndrome, which results from interruption of some of the nerve tracts between the mid brain and the pons (see BRAIN). Sometimes the syndrome is caused by severe damage to muscles or the nerves enervating them. Locked-in syndrome may sometimes be confused with a PERSISTENT VEGETATIVE STATE (PVS).

Lockjaw

A painful spasm of the JAW muscles, making it hard to open the mouth. It is a prominent symptom of TETANUS and was once the popular name for this condition.

Locomotor Ataxia

The uncoordinated movements and unsteady lurching gait that occurs in the tertiary stage of untreated SYPHILIS.

Locum Tenens

A doctor who stands in for another.

Lofexidine

An opioid antagonist drug used to modify the symptoms of addicted patients undergoing opioid-withdrawal treatment.

Logorrhoea

Logorrhoea is the technical term for garrulousness ('chatterbox') – a feature which may be exaggerated in certain states of mental instability.

Loiasis

Loiasis is the disease caused by the filarial worm *Loa loa*, a thread-like worm which differs from *W. bancrofti* in that it is shorter and thicker, and is found in the bloodstream during the day, not at night. It is transmitted by the mango fly, *Chrysops dimidiata*, but other flies of this genus can also transmit it. It is confined to West and Central Africa. The characteristic feature of the disease is the appearance of fugitive swellings which may arise anywhere in the body in the course of the worm's migration through it: these are known as Calabar swellings. The worm is often found in the eye, hence the old name of the worm in Africa – the eye worm. Diethylcarbamazine is the treatment for this form of FILARIASIS.

Loin

The name applied to the part of the back between the lower ribs and the pelvis. (For pain in the loins, see BACKACHE; LUMBAGO.)

Long-Sight

Also known as hypermetropia: see under EYE, DISORDERS OF – Errors of refraction.

Loop Diuretics

Drugs used in pulmonary oedema (excess fluid in the lungs) caused by failure of the left VEN-TRICLE of the HEART. DIURETICS cause an increase in excretion of URINE, thus reducing the amount of fluid in the body. Intravenous administration of loop diuretics relieves patients' breathlessness. They work by inhibiting resorption of fluid in the renal tubule loops of the KIDNEYS. Frusemide and bumetanide are commonly used loop diuretic drugs that act quickly and last for six hours so that they can be given twice in 24 hours without disturbing the patient's sleep.

Loperamide

A drug that reduces the motility of the GASTRO-INTESTINAL TRACT. It is of limited use as an adjunct to fluid replacement in diarrhoea in adults, and is sometimes used in chronic non-infective diarrhoea in children.

Lorazepam

A benzodiazepine tranquilliser (see BENZO-DIAZEPINES), shown to be of limited use in the short-term treatment of anxiety or insomnia, in STATUS EPILEPTICUS, or for perioperative use. Its use is not recommended for children. As with other benzodiazepines, the smallest possible dose should be given for the shortest possible time, as DEPENDENCE is a well-recognised danger.

Lordosis

An unnatural curvature of the spine forwards. It occurs chiefly in the lumbar region, where the natural curve is forwards, as the result of muscular weakness, spinal disease, etc. (See SPINAL COLUMN.)

Lotions

Fluid preparations intended for bringing into contact with, or for washing, the external surface of the body. Lotions are generally of a watery or alcoholic composition, and many of them are known as 'liquors'. Those external applications which are of an oily nature, and intended to be rubbed into the surface, are known as liniments.

Louse

See PEDICULOSIS.

Lozenges

These are small tablets containing drugs mixed with sugar, gum, glycerin-jelly or fruit-paste. They are used in various affections of the mouth and throat, being sucked and slowly dissolved by the saliva, which brings the drugs they contain into contact with the affected surface. Some of the substances used in lozenges are benzalkonium (disinfectant), benzocaine (analgesic), betamethasone (corticosteroid), bismuth (disinfectant), formaldehyde (disinfectant), hydrocortisone (corticosteroid), liquorice, and penicillin (antibiotic).

LSD

See LYSERGIC ACID DIETHYLAMIDE (LSD).

Lucid Interval

A temporary restoration of consciousness after a person has been rendered unconscious from a blow to the head. The victim subsequently relapses into COMA. This is a sign of raised INTRACRANIAL PRESSURE from arterial bleeding and indicates that surgery may be required to control the intracranial haemorrhage. (See also GLASGOW COMA SCALE.)

Ludwig's Angina

An uncommon bacterial infection affecting the floor of the mouth. It can spread to the throat and become life-threatening. Usually caused by infected gums or teeth, it causes pain, fever and swelling, resulting in difficulty in opening the mouth or swallowing. Urgent treatment with ANTIBIOTICS is called for, otherwise the patient may need a TRACHEOSTOMY to relieve breathing problems.

Lugol's Solution

A compound solution of iodine and potassium iodide used in the preoperative preparation of patients with thyrotoxicosis (see THYROID GLAND, DISEASES OF). The solution is taken orally.

Lumbago

Pain in the lower (lumbar) region of the back. It may be muscular, skeletal or neurological in origin. A severe form associated with SCIATICA may be due to a prolapsed INTERVERTEBRAL DISC. Less severe forms may be caused by OSTEOARTHRITIS of the spine, a trapped nerve, inflammation of connective tissue, or may follow an old injury.

The treatment will depend upon the cause, but mild lumbago will usually respond to NON-STEROIDAL ANTI-INFLAMMATORY DRUGS (NSAIDS) and the application of warmth. Sufferers should remember to bend their knees rather than their backs when lifting objects.

Moderate activity rather than bed rest is recommended for most patients.

Lumbar

A term used to denote structures in, or diseases affecting, the region of the loins (see LOIN) – as, for example, the lumbar vertebrae, lumbar abscess.

Lumbar Puncture

A procedure for removing CEREBROSPINAL FLUID (CSF) from the spinal canal in the LUMBAR region in order: (1) to diagnose disease of the nervous system; (2) to introduce medicaments – spinal anaesthetics or drugs. A hollow needle is inserted into the lower section of the space around the SPINAL CORD (see diagram) and the cerebrospinal fluid withdrawn. The

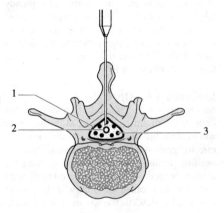

1 dura mater
2 filum terminale
3 cauda equina

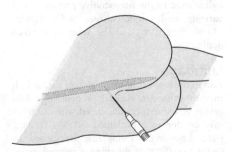

The patient lies on his/her left side with the back on the edge of the bed and the hips and knees flexed as shown in this diagram. The needle is inserted through the skin between the processes of the third and fourth lumbar vertebrae. The needle is then passed through the spinal ligaments and the dura into the subarachnoid space which contains the spinal fluid. A sample of fluid is slowly withdrawn.

procedure should not be done too rapidly or the subject may develop a severe headache. Examination of the cerebrospinal fluid helps in the diagnosis and investigation of disorders of the brain and spinal cord – for example, MENINGITIS and SUBARACHNOID HAEMORRHAGE. When using the procedure to inject drugs into the CSF, the operator must take care to inject only those agents specifically produced for CSF injection. Deaths have occurred because the wrong drug has been injected, and there have been demands for specialised equipment and strict procedures that will prevent such tragedies.

Lumbar Sympathectomy

Destruction of the LUMBAR chain of sympathetic nerves (see NERVOUS SYSTEM) by means of surgery, DIATHERMY or injection of chemicals (phenol or alcohol). The technique is used to improve the blood flow to the leg in patients with peripheral vascular disease, and to treat some types of chronic leg pain. It has only limited success.

Lumbar Vertebra

There are five lumbar vertebrae in the lower SPINAL COLUMN between the thoracic vertebrae and the sacrum.

Lumbricus

Lumbricus is a name sometimes applied to the roundworm, or *Ascaris lumbricoides.* (See ASCARIASIS.)

Lumen

(1) The space enclosed by a tubular structure or hollow organ (e.g. the gastrointestinal tract or urinary bladder).
(2) The SI unit of luminous flux (1 lumen [1m] = the amount of light emitted per second in a unit solid angle of 1 steradian by a 1-candela point source).

Lumpectomy

An operation for suspected breast cancer (see BREASTS, DISEASES OF), in which the tumour is removed from the breast rather than with it (see MASTECTOMY).

Lunatic

An out-of-date and now derogatory term applied to people of disordered mind, because lunacy was supposed at one time to be largely influenced by the moon. (See MENTAL ILLNESS.)

Lung Volumes

The volume of air within the LUNGS changes with the respiratory cycle (see RESPIRATION). The volumes defined in the following table can be measured, and may be useful indicators of some pulmonary diseases.

Normal values for a 60 kg man are (in ml):

TLC	5,000–6,000
TV	400–600
IRV	3,300–3,750
ERV	950–1,200
RV	1,200–1,700
VC	3,400–4,800
FRC	2,300–2,600

Total lung capacity (TLC) The volume of air that can be held in the lungs at maximum inspiration.

Tidal volume (TV) The volume of air taken into and expelled from the lungs with each breath.

Inspiratory reserve volume (IRV) The volume of air that can still be inspired at the end of a normal quiet inspiration.

Expiratory reserve volume (ERV) The volume of air that can still be expired at the end of a normal quiet expiration.

Residual volume (RV) The volume of air remaining in the lungs after a maximal expiration.

Vital capacity (VC) The maximum amount of air that can be expired after a maximal inspiration.

Functional residual capacity (FRC) The volume of air left in the lungs at the end of a normal quiet expiration.

Lungs

Positioned in the chest, the lungs serve primarily as respiratory organs (see RESPIRATION), also acting as a filter for the blood.

Form and position Each lung is a sponge-like cone, pink in children and grey in adults. Its apex projects into the neck, with the base resting on the DIAPHRAGM. Each lung is enveloped by a closed cavity, the pleural cavity, consisting of two layers of pleural membrane separated by a thin layer of fluid. In healthy states this allows expansion and retraction as breathing occurs.

Heart/lung connections The HEART lies in contact with the two lungs, so that changes in lung volume inevitably affect the pumping action of the heart. Furthermore, both lungs are connected by blood vessels to the heart. The pulmonary artery passes from the right ventricle and divides into two branches, one of which runs straight outwards to each lung, entering its substance along with the bronchial tube at the hilum or root of the lung. From this point also emerge the pulmonary veins, which carry the blood oxygenated in the lungs back to the left atrium.

Fine structure of lungs Each main bronchial tube, entering the lung at the root, divides into branches. These subdivide again and again, to be distributed all through the substance of the lung until the finest tubes, known as respiratory bronchioles, have a width of only 0·25 mm (1/100 inch). All these tubes consist of a mucous membrane surrounded by a fibrous sheath. The surface of the mucous membrane comprises columnar cells provided with cilia (hair-like structures) which sweep mucus and unwanted matter such as bacteria to the exterior.

The smallest divisions of the bronchial tubes, or bronchioles, divide into a number of tortuous tubes known as alveolar ducts terminating eventually in minute sacs, known as alveoli, of which there are around 300 million.

The branches of the pulmonary artery accompany the bronchial tubes to the furthest recesses of the lung, dividing like the latter into finer and finer branches, and ending in a dense network of capillaries. The air in the air-vesicles is separated therefore from the blood only by two delicate membranes: the wall of the air-vesicle, and the capillary wall, through which exchange of gases (oxygen and carbon dioxide) readily takes place. The essential oxygenated blood from the capillaries is collected by the pulmonary veins, which also accompany the bronchi to the root of the lung.

The lungs also contain an important system of lymph vessels, which start in spaces situated between the air-vesicles and eventually leave the lung along with the blood vessels, and are connected with a chain of bronchial glands lying near the end of the TRACHEA.

Lungs, Diseases of

Various conditions affecting the LUNGS are dealt with under the following headings: ASTHMA; BRONCHIECTASIS; CHEST, DEFORMITIES OF; CHRONIC OBSTRUCTIVE PULMONARY DISEASE (COPD); COLD, COMMON; EMPHYSEMA; EXPECTORATION; HAEMOPTYSIS; HAEMORRHAGE; OCCUPATIONAL HEALTH, MEDICINE

AND DISEASES; PLEURISY; PNEUMONIA; PULMONARY EMBOLISM; TUBERCULOSIS.

Inflammation of the lungs is generally
known as PNEUMONIA, when it is due to infection; as ALVEOLITIS when the inflammation is immunological; and as PNEUMONITIS when it is due to physical or chemical agents.

Abscess of the lung consists of a collection of PUS within the lung tissue. Causes include inadequate treatment of pneumonia, inhalation of vomit, obstruction of the bronchial tubes by tumours and foreign bodies, pulmonary emboli (see EMBOLISM) and septic emboli. The patient becomes generally unwell with cough and fever. BRONCHOSCOPY is frequently performed to detect any obstruction to the bronchi. Treatment is with a prolonged course of antibiotics. Rarely, surgery is necessary.

Pulmonary oedema is the accumulation of fluid in the pulmonary tissues and air spaces. This may be caused by cardiac disease (heart failure or disease of heart valves – see below, and HEART, DISEASES OF) or by an increase in the permeability of the pulmonary capillaries allowing leakage of fluid into the lung tissue (see ACUTE RESPIRATORY DISTRESS SYNDROME (ARDS)).

Heart failure (left ventricular failure) can be caused by a weakness in the pumping action of the HEART leading to an increase in back pressure which forces fluid out of the blood vessels into the lung tissue. Causes include heart attacks and HYPERTENSION (high blood pressure). Narrowed or leaking heart valves hinder the flow of blood through the heart; again, this produces an increase in back pressure which raises the capillary pressure in the pulmonary vessels and causes flooding of fluid into the interstitial spaces and alveoli. Accumulation of fluid in lung tissue produces breathlessness. Treatments include DIURETICS and other drugs to aid the pumping action of the heart. Surgical valve replacement may help when heart failure is due to valvular heart disease.

Acute respiratory distress syndrome Formerly known as adult respiratory distress syndrome (ARDS), this produces pulmonary congestion because of leakage of fluid through pulmonary capillaries. It complicates a variety of illnesses such as sepsis, trauma, aspiration of gastric contents and diffuse pneumonia. Treatment involves treating the cause and supporting the patient by providing oxygen.

Collapse of the lung may occur due to blockage of a bronchial tube by tumour, foreign body or a plug of mucus which may occur in bronchitis or pneumonia. Air beyond the blockage is absorbed into the circulation, causing the affected area of lung to collapse. Collapse may also occur when air is allowed into the pleural space – the space between the lining of the lung and the lining of the inside of the chest wall. This is called a pneumothorax and may occur following trauma, or spontaneously – for example, when there is a rupture of a subpleural air pocket (such as a cyst) allowing a communication between the airways and the pleural space. Lung collapse by compression may occur when fluid collects in the pleural space (pleural effusion): when this fluid is blood, it is known as a haemothorax; if it is due to pus it is known as an empyema. Collections of air, blood, pus or other fluid can be removed from the pleural space by insertion of a chest drain, thus allowing the lung to re-expand.

Tumours of the lung are the most common cause of cancer in men and, along with breast cancer, are a major cause of cancer in women. Several types of lung cancer occur, the most common being squamous cell carcinoma, small- (or oat-) cell carcinoma, adenocarcinoma, and large-cell carcinoma. All but the adenocarcinoma have a strong link with smoking. Each type has a different pattern of growth and responds differently to treatment. More than 30,000 men and women die of cancer of the trachea, bronchus and lung annually in England and Wales.

The most common presenting symptom is cough; others include haemoptysis (coughing up blood), breathlessness, chest pain, wheezing and weight loss. As well as spreading locally in the lung – the rate of spread varies – lung cancer commonly spawns secondary growths in the liver, bones or brain. Diagnosis is confirmed by X-rays and bronchoscopy with biopsy.

Treatment Treatment for the two main categories of lung cancer – small-cell and non-small-cell cancer – is different. Surgery is the only curative treatment for the latter and should be considered in all cases, even though fewer than half undergoing surgery will survive five years. In those patients unsuitable for surgery, radical RADIOTHERAPY should be considered. For other patients the aim should be the control of symptoms and the maintenance of quality of life, with palliative radiotherapy one of the options.

Small-cell lung cancer progresses rapidly, and untreated patients survive for only a few months. Because the disease is often widespread by the time of diagnosis, surgery is rarely an option. All patients should be considered for CHEMOTHERAPY which improves symptoms and prolongs survival.

Wounds of the lung may cause damage to the lung and, by admitting air into the pleural cavity, cause the lung to collapse with air in the pleural space (pneumothorax). This may require the insertion of a chest drain to remove the air from the pleural space and allow the lung to re-expand. The lung may be wounded by the end of a fractured rib or by some sharp object such as a knife pushed between the ribs.

Lupus

This is the Latin word for wolf, and a term applied to certain chronic skin diseases which can destroy skin, underlying cartilage and even bone to cause serious deformity if uncontrolled.

Lupus vulgaris is a form of TUBERCULOSIS of the skin. It typically begins in childhood and may spread slowly for decades if untreated. The face and neck are the usual sites. In untreated disease, large, well-demarcated areas may be affected with redness, scaling and thickening. If the affected skin is blanched by pressure, yellow-brown foci may be observed – the so-called apple-jelly nodules. The disease causes extensive scarring as it spreads and may destroy cartilage in its path – for example, on the nose or ear – causing gross deformity. The disease was common in the UK up to 50 years ago, but is now rare. It is treated with a combination of tuberculostatic drugs.

Lupus erythematosus is an autoimmune disease which can affect skin or internal organs.

Discoid lupus erythematosus (DLE) In this disease, only the skin is affected. Sharply defined red, scaly and eventually atrophic patches appear on the face, especially on the nose and cheeks. ALOPECIA with scarring is seen if the scalp is affected. The condition is aggravated by sunlight. Topical CORTICOSTEROIDS are helpful.

Systemic lupus erythematosus (SLE) See separate dictionary entry.

Luteinising Hormone

A hormone secreted by the anterior PITUITARY GLAND which stimulates OVULATION, maturation of the CORPUS LUTEUM, and the synthesis of progesterone by the ovary (see OVARIES) and testosterone by the testis (see TESTICLE).

Luteinising Hormone-Releasing Hormone (LHRH)

A natural hormone released by the HYPO-THALAMUS gland in the BRAIN. It stimulates the release of GONADOTROPHINS from the PITUIT-ARY GLAND; these control the production of the sex hormones (see ANDROGEN; OESTROGENS).

Lux

The unit of illumination. The abbreviation is lx.

Luxation

Another word for dislocation (see DISLOCATIONS).

Lycanthropy

Morbid delusion that one is a wolf.

Lying-In

See PREGNANCY AND LABOUR.

Lyme Disease

This comprises ARTHRITIS associated with skin rashes, fever and sometimes ENCEPHALITIS or carditis (inflammation of the heart). It is caused by a SPIROCHAETE which is transmitted by tick bite. Treatment is with antibiotics.

Lymph

Lymph is the fluid which circulates in the lymphatic vessels of the body. It is a colourless fluid, like blood PLASMA in composition, only rather more watery. It contains salts similar to those of blood plasma, and the same proteins, although in smaller amount: FIBRINOGEN, serum albumin (see ALBUMINS), and serum GLOBULIN. It also contains lymphocytes (white blood cells), derived from the glands. In some lymphatic vessels, the lymph contains, after meals, a great amount of FAT in the form of a fine milky emulsion. These are the vessels which absorb fat from the food passing down the INTESTINE, and convey it to the thoracic duct; they are called lacteals because their contents look milky (see CHYLE).

The lymph is derived, initially, from the blood, the watery constituents of which exude through the walls of the CAPILLARIES into the tissues, conveying material for the nourishment of the tissues and absorbing waste products.

The spaces in the tissues communicate with lymph capillaries, which have a structure similar to that of the capillaries of the blood-vessel system, being composed of delicate flat cells joined edge to edge. These unite to form fine vessels, resembling minute veins in structure, called lymphatics, which ramify throughout the body, passing through lymphatic glands and ultimately discharging their contents into the jugular veins in the root of the neck. Other lymph vessels commence in great numbers as minute openings on the surface of the PLEURA and PERITONEUM, and act as drains for these otherwise closed cavities. When fluid is effused into these cavities – as in a pleural effusion, for example – its absorption takes place through the lymphatic vessels. The course of these vessels is described under the entry on GLAND.

Lymph circulates partly by reason of the pressure at which it is driven through the walls of the blood capillaries, but mainly in consequence of incidental forces. The lymph capillaries and vessels are copiously provided with valves, which prevent any back flow of lymph, and every time these vessels are squeezed (as by the contraction of a muscle, or movement of a limb) the lymph is pumped along.

The term lymph is also applied to the serous fluid contained in the vesicles which develop as the result of vaccination, and used for the purpose of vaccinating other individuals.

Lymphadenectomy
Surgical removal of the LYMPH NODES. The procedure is usually carried out when cancer has infiltrated the nodes in the lymphatic drainage zone of an organ or tissue invaded by a malignant growth. RADIOTHERAPY or CHEMOTHERAPY may be given if laboratory tests show that the type or extent of spread of the cancer cells merits this.

Lymphadenitis
Inflammation of lymphatic glands (see LYMPHATICS; GLAND).

Lymphadenoma
Another name for Hodgkin's disease. (See LYMPHOMA.)

Lymphadenopathy
Medical description of swollen lymph glands (see GLAND). One cause is HIV infection (see AIDS/HIV); another is spread of malignant cells from a tumour in the catchment area of lymphatic drainage.

Lymphangiectasis
Lymphangiectasis means an abnormal dilatation of the lymph vessels, as in FILARIASIS.

Lymphangiography
A procedure whereby the LYMPHATICS and lymphatic glands can be rendered visible on X-ray films by means of the injection of radio-opaque substances. It has now been replaced largely by magnetic resonance imaging (MRI).

Lymphangioma
An uncommon, non-malignant tumour occurring in the skin or the tongue. It comprises an abnormal collection of lymph vessels and tends to be present from birth. Sometimes it disappears spontaneously, but it may need surgical removal.

Lymphangitis
Inflammation situated in the lymphatic vessels.

Lymphatics
Vessels which convey the LYMPH. (For an account of their arrangement, see GLAND.)

Lymph Nodes
Swellings which occur at various points in the lymphatic system through which LYMPH drains. They consist of a cortex, medulla and lymph sinuses and have two main functions: (1) the interception and removal of abnormal or foreign material from the lymph; (2) the production of immune responses (see IMMUNITY). The lymph nodes become enlarged when the area of the body which they drain is the site of infection or as a manifestation of some systemic diseases. Occasionally they are the site of primary or metastatic malignant disease.

Lymphocyte
A variety of white blood cell produced in the LYMPHOID TISSUE and lymphatic glands (see LYMPHATICS; GLAND) of the body. It contains a simple, rounded nucleus surrounded by protoplasm generally described as non-granular. Two varieties of lymphocyte are described, small and large, and together they form over 20 per cent of the white cells of the blood. They play an important part in the production of ANTIBODIES, and in the rejection of transplanted organs such as the heart (see TRANSPLANTATION). This they do in two different ways: what are known as B-lymphocytes produce antibodies, while T-lymphocytes attack and destroy antigens (see ANTIGEN) directly. The latter are known as T-lymphocytes because they are produced by the THYMUS GLAND. Their numbers are increased in TUBERCULOSIS and certain other diseases. Such an increase is known as LYMPHOCYTOSIS.

Lymphocytosis

An increase in the number of lymphocytes in the blood (see LYMPHOCYTE) – for example, in response to viral infection or in chronic lymphocytic LEUKAEMIA.

Lymphoedema

Swelling of a part or organ due to obstruction to the LYMPH vessels draining it.

Lymphogranuloma Inguinale

A venereal disease in which the chief characteristic is enlargement of glands in the groin – the infecting agent being a virus.

Lymphoid Tissue

Tissue involved in the formation of LYMPH, lymphocytes (see LYMPHOCYTE), and ANTIBODIES. It consists of the LYMPH NODES, THYMUS GLAND, TONSILS and SPLEEN.

Lymphokines

Lymphokines are polypeptides that are produced by lymphocytes (see LYMPHOCYTE) as part of their immune response to an ANTIGEN; their function is to communicate with other cells of the immune system (see IMMUNITY). Some lymphokines stimulate B-cells to differentiate into antibody-producing plasma cells; others stimulate T-lymphocytes to proliferate; other lymphokines become interferons (see INTERFERON).

Lymphoma

A malignant tumour of the LYMPH NODES divided histologically and clinically into two types: Hodgkin's disease, and non-Hodgkin's lymphoma. Hodgkin's disease or lymphadenoma was named after Thomas Hodgkin (1798–1866), a Guy's Hospital pathologist, who first described the condition.

Hodgkin's disease The incidence is around four new cases per 100,000 population annually, with slightly more men than women contracting it. The first incidence peak is in age group 20–35 and the second in age group 50–70. The cause of Hodgkin's is not known, although it is more common in patients from small families and well-educated backgrounds. The disease is three times more likely to occur in people who have had glandular fever (see MONONUCLEOSIS) but no link with the EPSTEIN BARR VIRUS has been established (see Burkitt's lymphoma, below)

The disease is characterised histologically by the presence of large malignant lymphoid cells (Reed-Sternberg cells) in the lymph glands.

Clinically the lymph glands are enlarged, rubbery but painless; usually those in the neck or just above the CLAVICLE are affected. Spread is to adjacent lymph glands and in young people a mass of enlarged glands may develop in the MEDIASTINUM. The SPLEEN is affected in about one-third of patients with the disorder. Treatment is either with RADIOTHERAPY, CHEMOTHERAPY or both, depending on when the disease is diagnosed and the nature of the abnormal lymph cells. Cure rates are good, especially if the lymphoma is diagnosed early.

Non-Hodgkin's lymphoma (NHL) This varies in its malignancy depending on the nature and activity of the abnormal lymph cells. The disease is hard to classify histologically, so various classification systems have been evolved. High- and low-grade categories are recognised according to the rate of proliferation of abnormal lymph cells. No single causative factor has been identified, although viral and bacterial infections have been linked to NHL, and genetic and immunological factors may be implicated. The incidence is higher than that of Hodgkin's disease, at 12 new cases per 100,000 population a year, and the median age of diagnosis is 65–70 years. Suppression of the immune system that ocurs in people with HIV infection has been linked with a marked rise in the incidence of non-Hodgkin's lymphoma and Hodgkin's disease.

Most patients have painless swelling of one or more groups of lymph nodes in the neck or groin, and the liver and spleen may enlarge. As other organs can also be affected, patients may present with a wide range of symptoms, including fever, itching and weight loss. If NHL occurs in a single group of lymph nodes, radiotherapy is the treatment of choice; more extensive infiltration of glands will require chemotherapy – and sometimes both types of treatment will be necessary. If these treatments fail, BONE MARROW TRANSPLANT may be carried out. Prognosis is good for low-grade NHL (75 per cent of patients survive five years or more); in more severe types the survival rate is 40–50 per cent for two years.

Another variety of lymphoma is found in children in Africa, sometimes called after Burkitt, the Irish surgeon who first identified it. Burkitt's lymphoma is a rapidly growing malignant tumour occurring in varying sites, and the Epstein Barr virus has a role in its origin and growth. A non-African variety of Burkitt's lymphoma is now also recognised. CYTOTOXIC drug therapy is effective.

Lymphosarcoma

A traditional term for non-Hodgkin's lymphoma (see LYMPHOMA).

Lysergic Acid Diethylamide (LSD)

Lysergic acid diethylamide belongs to the ergot group of ALKALOIDS. It has various effects on the brain, notably analgesic and hallucinogenic, thought to be due to its antagonism of 5-hydroxytryptamine (5-HT). In small doses it induces psychic states, in which the individual may become aware of repressed memories. For this reason it may help in the treatment of certain anxiety states, if used under skilled supervision. LSD rapidly induces TOLERANCE, however, and psychological DEPENDENCE may occur, although not physical dependence. Serious side-effects include psychotic reactions, with an increased risk of suicide.

Lysine

An essential amino acid (see AMINO ACIDS; INDISPENSABLE AMINO ACIDS), lysine was first isolated in 1889 from casein, the principal protein of milk. Like other essential amino acids, it ensures optimum growth in infants and balanced nitrogen metabolism in adults.

Lysis

The gradual ending of a fever, and the opposite of CRISIS, which signifies the sudden ending of a fever. It is also used to describe the process of dissolution of a blood clot, or the destruction of CELLS as a result of damage to or rupture of the PLASMA membrane, thus allowing the cell contents to escape.

Lysol

A brown, clear, oily fluid with antiseptic properties, made from coal-tar and containing 50 per cent CRESOL. When mixed with water it forms a clear soapy fluid.

Lysol Poisoning

When LYSOL is swallowed it burns the mouth and throat. Brown discoloration of the affected tissues, accompanied by the characteristic smell of lysol on the breath, is typical.

Treatment This is urgent. If the skin has been contaminated with the lysol, it must be washed with water, and any lysol-contaminated clothing must be taken off. Do not make the victim vomit if he or she has swallowed a corrosive substance such as lysol or phenol. Call an ambulance and say what the victim has taken. See APPENDIX 1: BASIC FIRST AID.

Lysozyme

An ENZYME present in tears and egg white, lysozyme catalyses the destruction of some bacteria by damaging their walls.

Lyssa

Lyssa is another term for RABIES.

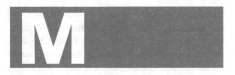

M

Maceration
Maceration is the softening of a solid by soaking in fluid.

Macr-/Macro-
Prefix denoting large-sized cell – for example, a MACROPHAGE is a large PHAGOCYTE.

Macrocyte
Macrocyte is an unusually large red blood cell (see ERYTHROCYTES) especially characteristic of the blood in PERNICIOUS ANAEMIA.

Macrocytosis
This condition is particularly associated with PERNICIOUS ANAEMIA but can also be caused by a number of other things, such as alcohol, pregnancy, myxoedema (see THYROID GLAND, DISEASES OF – Hypothyroidism) and MYELO-MATOSIS, and also by vitamin B_{12} deficiency: this occurs sometimes in vegans (see VEGANISM) as well as in patients with CROHN'S DISEASE.

Macroglossia
An abnormally large TONGUE.

Macrolides
A group of ANTIBIOTICS. The original macrolide, ERYTHROMYCIN, was discovered in the early 1950s and used successfully as an alternative to PENICILLIN. The name 'macrolide' derives from the molecular structure of this group, three others of which are clarithromycin, azithromycin and spiramycin. Macrolides check PROTEIN synthesis in BACTERIA and the latest ones are, like erythromycin, active against several bacterial species including gram-positive COCCI and rods. In addition, they act against *Haemophilus influenzae*. Clarithromycin is potent against *Helicobacter pylori*; azithromycin is effective against infections caused by *Legionella* spp. (see LEGIONNAIRE'S DISEASE) and GONOCOCCI. Spiramycin is a restricted-use macrolide prescribed for pregnant patients with TOXOPLASMOSIS.

Macrophage
A large PHAGOCYTE that forms part of the RETICULO-ENDOTHELIAL SYSTEM. It is found in many organs and tissues, including connective tissue, bone marrow, lymph nodes, spleen, liver and central nervous system. Free macrophages move between cells and, using their scavenger properties, collect at infection sites to remove foreign bodies, including bacteria. Fixed macrophages are found in connective tissue.

Macropsia
Condition in which objects appear larger than normal. It can be due to disease of the MACULA – see also EYE.

Macula
A spot or area of tissue that is different from the surrounding tissue. An example is the macula letea, the yellow spot in the retina of the EYE.

Macules
Areas of small, flat or slightly raised skin discoloration which may occur in a wide range of conditions such as many viral infections, eczema (DERMATITIS), PSORIASIS, SYPHILIS and after burns (see BURNS AND SCALDS), as well as in pregnancy.

Maculopapular
A skin rash that is made up of macules (discoloration of the skin) and papules (raised abnormalities of the skin).

Madura Foot
Tropical infection of the foot by deeply invasive fungi which cause chronic swelling and suppuration with multiple discharging sinuses. Antibiotics are of limited value and advanced disease may require amputation of the affected foot.

Magnesium
Magnesium is a light metallic element; it is one of the essential mineral elements of the body, without which the body cannot function properly. The adult body contains around 25 grams of magnesium, the greater part of which is in the bones. More than two-thirds of our daily supply comes from cereals and vegetables; as most other foods also contain useful amounts, there is seldom any difficulty in maintaining an adequate amount in the body. Magnesium is also an essential constituent of several vital enzymes (see ENZYME). Deficiency leads to muscular weakness and interferes with the efficient working of the heart. The salts of magnesium used as drugs are the hydroxide of magnesium, the oxide of magnesium – generally known as 'magnesia' – and the carbonate of magnesium, all of which have an antacid action; also the sulphate of magnesium known as 'Epsom salts', which acts as a purgative.

Uses Compounds of magnesia are used to correct hyperacidity of the stomach and as a laxative (see LAXATIVES).

Magnesium Trisilicate
A white powder with mild antacid properties (see ANTACIDS) and a prolonged action, it is used for treating peptic ulceration – commonly combined with quickly acting antacids. It has a mild laxative effect (see LAXATIVES).

Magnetic Resonance Imaging (MRI)
See MRI.

Malabsorption Syndrome
This term includes a multiplicity of diseases, all of which are characterised by faulty absorption from the INTESTINE of essential foodstuffs such as fat, vitamins and mineral salts. Among the conditions in this syndrome are COELIAC DISEASE, SPRUE, CYSTIC FIBROSIS and pancreatitis (see PANCREAS, DISORDERS OF). Surgical removal of the small intestine also causes the syndrome. Symptoms include ANAEMIA, diarrhoea, OEDEMA, vitamin deficiencies, weight loss and, in severe cases, MALNUTRITION.

Malacia
Malacia is a term applied to softening of a part or tissue in disease: for example, OSTEOMALACIA or softening of the bones.

Malaise
A vague feeling of feverishness, listlessness and languor, malaise sometimes precedes the onset of serious acute diseases, but more commonly accompanies passing illnesses such as DYSPEPSIA, chills and colds.

Malar
Anything relating to the cheek. For example, the malar (zygomatic) bone is also known as the cheek bone, and a malar flush is reddening of the cheeks.

Malaria
A parasitic disease caused by four species of PLASMODIUM: *P. falciparum, P. vivax, P. ovale,* and *P. malariae.* Clinically, malaria is characterised by recurrent episodes of high fever, sometimes associated with RIGOR; enlargement of the SPLEEN is common. *P. falciparum* infection can also be associated with several serious – often fatal – complications (see below): although other species cause chronic disease, death is unusual.

During a bite by the female mosquito, one or more sporozoites – a stage in the life-cycle of the parasite – are injected into the human circulation; these are taken up by the hepatocytes (liver cells). Following division, merozoites (minute particles resulting from the division) are liberated into the bloodstream where they invade red blood cells. These in turn divide, releasing further merozoites. As merozoites are periodically liberated into the bloodstream, they cause the characteristic fevers, rigors, etc.

Malaria occurs in many tropical and subtropical countries; *P. falciparum* is, however, confined very largely to Africa, Asia and South America. Malaria is present in increasingly large areas; in addition, the parasites are developing resistance to various preventative and treatment drugs. The disease constitutes a significant problem for travellers, who must obtain sound advice on chemoprophylaxis before embarking on tropical trips – especially to a rural area where intense transmission can occur. Transmission has also been recorded at airports, and following blood transfusion.

The World Health Organisation (WHO) has listed malaria as one of Europe's top ten infectious diseases. In 1992, 20,000 cases were reported: this had risen to more than 200,000 by the late 1990s. The resurgence of malaria has been worldwide, in part the result of the development of resistant strains of the disease, and in part because many countries have failed (or been unable) to implement environmental measures to eliminate mosquitoes. Nearly 40 years ago the WHO forecast that by 1980 only four million people would be affected worldwide; now, at the beginning of the 21st century, around 500 million people a year are contracting malaria with about 3,000 people a day dying from the infection – as many as 70 per cent of them children under the age of five, according to WHO figures. The apparently steady advance of global warming means that countries with temperate climates may well warm up sufficiently to enable malaria to become established as an ENDEMIC disease. In any case, the great increase in international air travel has exposed many more people to the risk of malaria, and infected individuals may not exhibit symptoms until they are back home. Doctors seeing a recent traveller with unexplained pyrexia and illness should consider the possibility of malarial infection.

Diagnosis is by demonstration of trophozoites – a stage in the parasite's life-cycle that takes place in red blood cells – in thick/thin blood-films of peripheral blood. Serological tests are of value in deciding whether an individual has had a past infection, but are of no value in acute disease.

P. vivax and P. ovale infections cause less
severe disease than *P. falciparum* (see below), although overall there are many clinical similarities; acute complications are unusual, but chronic ANAEMIA is often present. Primaquine is necessary to eliminate the exoerythrocytic cycle in the hepatocyte (liver cell).

P. falciparum Complications of *P. falciparum* infection include cerebral involvement
(see BRAIN – Cerebrum), due to adhesion of immature trophozoites on to the cerebral vascular endothelium; these lead to a high death rate when inadequately treated. Renal involvement (frequently resulting from HAEMOGLOBINURIA), PULMONARY OEDEMA, HYPOTENSION, HYPOGLYCAEMIA, and complications in pregnancy are also important. In complicated disease, HAEMODIALYSIS and exchange TRANSFUSION have been used. No adequate controlled trial using the latter regimen has been carried out, however, and possible benefits must be weighed against numerous potential side-effects – for instance, the introduction of a wide range of infections, overload of the circulatory system with infused fluids, and other complications.

P. malariae usually produces a chronic infection, and chronic renal disease (nephrotic syndrome) is an occasional sequel, especially in
tropical Africa.

Gross SPLENOMEGALY (hyper-reactive malarious splenomegaly, or tropical splenomegaly syndrome) can complicate all four human *Plasmodium* spp. infections. The syndrome responds to long-term malarial chemoprophylaxis. BURKITT'S LYMPHOMA is found in geographical areas where malaria infection is endemic; the EPSTEIN BARR VIRUS is aetiologically involved.

Prophylaxis Malaria specialists in the United Kingdom have produced guidance for residents travelling to endemic areas for short stays. Drug choice takes account of:
- risk of exposure to malaria;
- extent of drug resistance;
- efficacy of recommended drugs and their side-effects;
- criteria relevant to the individual (e.g. age, pregnancy, kidney or liver impairment).

Personal protection against being bitten by mosquitoes is essential. Permethrin-impregnated nets are an effective barrier, while skin barrier protection and vaporised insecticides are helpful. Lotions, sprays or roll-on applicators all containing diethyltoluamide (DEET) are safe and work when put on the skin. Their effect, however, lasts only for a few hours. Long sleeves and trousers should be worn after dark.

Drug prophylaxis should be started at least a week before travelling into countries where malaria is endemic (two or three weeks in the case of mefloquine). Drug treatment should be continued for at least four weeks after leaving endemic areas. Even if all recommended antimalarial programmes are followed, it is possible that malaria may occur any time up to three months afterwards. Medical advice should be sought if any illness develops. Chloroquine can be used as a prophylactic drug where the risk of resistant falciparum malaria is low; otherwise, mefloquine or proguanil hydrochloride should be used. Travellers to malaria-infested areas should seek expert advice on appropriate prophylactic treatment well before departing.

Treatment Various chemoprophylactic regimes are widely used. Those commmonly prescribed include: chloroquine + paludrine, mefloquine, and Maloprim (trimethoprim + dapsone); Fansidar (trimethoprim + sulphamethoxazole) has been shown to have significant side-effects, especially when used in conjunction with chloroquine, and is now rarely used. No chemotherapeutic regimen is totally effective, so other preventive measures are again being used. These include people avoiding mosquito bites, covering exposed areas of the body between dusk and dawn, and using mosquito repellents.

Chemotherapy was for many years dominated by the synthetic agent chloroquine. However, with the widespread emergence of chloroquine-resistance, quinine is again being widely used. It is given intravenously in severe infections; the oral route is used subsequently and in minor cases. Other agents currently in use include mefloquine, halofantrine, doxycycline, and the artemesinin alkaloids ('qinghaosu').

Researchers are working on vaccines against malaria.

Malathion
Organophosphorus insecticide which is a preferred scabicide and pediculocide; applied externally; resistance is rare.

Maldescended Testis
See under TESTICLE, DISEASES OF.

Malformation
See DEFORMITIES.

Malignant
A term applied in several ways to serious disorders. A TUMOUR is called malignant when it grows rapidly, tending to infiltrate surrounding healthy tissues and to spread to distant parts of the body, leading eventually to death (see CANCER). The term is also applied to types of disease which are much more serious than the usual form – for example, MALIGNANT HYPERTENSION. Malignant pustule is another name for ANTHRAX.

Malignant Hyperpyrexia
See MALIGNANT HYPERTHERMIA.

Malignant Hypertension
Malignant hypertension has nothing to do with cancer; it derives its name from the fact that, if untreated, it runs a rapidly fatal course. (See HYPERTENSION.)

Malignant Hyperthermia
This disorder is a rare complication of general ANAESTHESIA caused, it is believed, by a combination of an inhalation anaesthetic (usually HALOTHANE) and a muscle-relaxant drug (usually succinycholine). A life-endangering rise in temperature occurs, with muscular rigidity the first sign. TACHYCARDIA, ACIDOSIS and SHOCK usually ensue. About 1:20,000 patients having general anaesthesia suffer from this disorder, which progresses rapidly and is often fatal. Surgery and anaesthesia must be stopped immediately and appropriate corrective measures taken, including the intravenous administration of DANTROLENE. It is a dominantly inherited genetic condition; therefore, when a case is identified it is most important that relatives are screened.

Malignant Lymphoma
See LYMPHOMA.

Malignant Melanoma
See MELANOMA.

Malingering
Malingering is a term applied to the feigning of illness. In the great majority of cases, a person who feigns illness has a certain amount of disability, but exaggerates the illness or discomfort for some ulterior motive – for example, to take time off work or to obtain compensation.

Malleolus
Name of either of the two bony prominences at the ANKLE.

Mallet Finger
Deformation of a finger due to sudden forced flexion of the terminal joint, leading to rupture of the tendon. As a result the individual is unable to extend the terminal part of the finger, which remains bent forwards. The middle, ring and little fingers are most commonly involved. Treatment is by splinting the finger. The end result is satisfactory provided that the patient has sufficient patience.

Mallet Toe
The condition in which it is not possible to extend the terminal part of the toe. It is usually due to muscular imbalance but may be caused by congenital absence of the extensor muscle. A callosity (see CALLOSITIES) often forms on the toe, which may be painful. Should this be troublesome, treatment consists of removal of the terminal phalanx.

Malleus
The hammer-shaped lateral bone of the group of three that form the sound-transmitting ossicles in the middle ear. (See EAR.)

Malnutrition
The condition arising from an inadequate or unbalanced DIET. The causes may be a lack of one or more essential nutrients, or inadequate absorption from the intestinal tracts. A diet that is deficient in CARBOHYDRATE usually contains inadequate PROTEIN, and this type of malnutrition occurs widely in Africa and Asia as a result of poverty, famine or war.

Maloprim
A combination of PYRIMETHAMINE and DAPSONE which is used for the prevention of MALARIA in limited circumstances. It has the advantage of only needing to be taken once weekly. It should not be taken by anyone hypersensitive to sulphonamides, and should not be used for the treatment of an acute attack.

Malpractice
An American term implying improper or inadequate medical treatment that fails to match the standards of skill and care reasonably expected from a qualified health-care practitioner – usually a doctor or dentist. Litigation against health professionals for malpractice has been running at substantial levels in the USA for some years. During the past decade the

number of cases has been rising sharply in the United Kingdom, where the more usual term is 'clinical negligence'. The increase is assumed to be partly because of failings in the NHS, and partly because patients have more understanding of health care, accompanied by higher expectations of treatment outcomes.

Patients concerned that they or their relatives might have been subject to negligence which has caused harm should consult a solicitor experienced in the field of clinical negligence. www.avma.org.uk

Malpresentation
A situation during childbirth in which a baby is not in the customary head-first position before delivery. The result is usually a complicated labour in which a caesarean operation may be necessary to effect the birth. (See PREGNANCY AND LABOUR.)

Malta Fever
See BRUCELLOSIS.

Mammary Gland
See BREASTS.

Mammography
The special technique whereby X-rays are used to show the structure of the breast or any abnormalities in it (see BREASTS; BREASTS, DISEASES OF). It is an effective way of distinguishing benign from malignant tumours, and can detect tumours that are not palpable. In a multi-centre study in the USA, called the Breast Cancer Detection Demonstration Project and involving nearly 300,000 women in the 40–49 age group, 35 per cent of the tumours found were detected by mammography alone, 13 per cent by physical examination, and 50 per cent by both methods combined. The optimum frequency of screening is debatable: the American College of Radiologists recommends a baseline mammogram at the age of 40 years, with subsequent mammography at one- to two-year intervals up to the age of 50; thereafter, annual mammography is recommended. In the United Kingdom a less intensive screening programme is in place, with women over 50 being screened every three years. As breast cancer is the commonest malignancy in western women and is increasing in frequency, the importance of screening for this form of cancer is obvious.

Mammoplasty
A surgical operation to reconstruct a breast (see BREASTS) after part or all of it has been removed

to treat breast cancer; to enlarge small breasts; or to reduce the size of overlarge breasts. The routine method for breast enlargement used to be the insertion of silicone (see SILICONES) implants under the skin; controversy about the long-term safety of silicone, however, has restricted their use mainly to women needing reconstruction of their breasts after cancer surgery. Side-effects have included hardening of breast tissue, leaking of implants and development of scar tissue. (See also MASTECTOMY.)

Managed Health Care
This process aims to reduce the costs of health care while maintaining its quality. The concept originated in the United States but has attracted interest in the United Kingdom and Europe, where the spiralling costs of health care have been causing widespread concern. Managed care works through changing clinical practice, but it is not a discrete entity: the American I. J. Iglehart has defined it as 'a variety of methods of financing and organising the delivery of comprehensive health care in which an attempt is made to control costs by controlling the provision of services'. Managed care has three facets: health policy; how that policy is managed; and how individuals needing health care are dealt with. The process and its applications are still evolving and it is likely that different health-care systems will adapt it to suit their own particular circumstances.

Mandelic Acid
Also known as mandelamine, a non-toxic keto-acid used in the treatment of infections of the urinary tract, especially those due to the *Escherichia coli* and the *Streptococcus faecalis* or *Enterococcus*. It is administered in doses of 3 grams several times daily. As it is only effective in an acid urine, ammonium chloride must be taken at the same time.

Mandible
The bone of the lower JAW.

Manganese
A metal, oxides of which are found abundantly in nature. Permanganate of potassium is a well-known disinfectant. The body requires small amounts of the metal for normal growth and development. (See also TRACE ELEMENTS.)

Mania
A form of mental disorder characterised by great excitement. (See MENTAL ILLNESS.)

Manic Depression

Manic depression, or CYCLOTHYMIA, is a form of MENTAL ILLNESS characterised by alternate attacks of mania and depression.

Manipulation

The passive movement (frequently forceful) of bones, joints, or soft tissues, carried out by orthopaedic surgeons, physiotherapists (see PHYSIOTHERAPY), osteopaths (see OSTEOPATHY) and chiropractors (see CHIROPRACTOR) as an important part of treatment – often highly effective. It may be used for three chief reasons: correction of deformity (mainly the reduction of fractures and dislocations, or to overcome deformities such as congenital club-foot – see TALIPES); treatment of joint stiffness (particularly after an acute limb injury, or FROZEN SHOULDER); and relief of chronic pain (particularly when due to chronic strain, notably of the spinal joints – see PROLAPSED INTERVERTEBRAL DISC). Depending on the particular injury or deformity being treated, and the estimated force required, manipulation may be used with or without ANAESTHESIA. Careful clinical and radiological examination, together with other appropriate investigations, should always be carried out before starting treatment, to reduce the risk of harm, or disasters such as fractures or the massive displacement of an intervertebral disc.

Mannitol

An osmotic diuretic (see DIURETICS) given by a slow intravenous infusion to reduce OEDEMA of the BRAIN or raised intraocular pressure in GLAUCOMA.

Manometer

An instrument for measuring the pressure or tension of liquids or gases. (See BLOOD PRESSURE.)

Mantoux Test

A test for TUBERCULOSIS. It consists in injecting into the superficial layers of the skin (i.e. intradermally) a very small quantity of old TUBERCULIN which contains a protein ANTIGEN to TB. A positive reaction of the skin – swelling and redness – shows that the person so reacting has been infected at some time in the past with *Mycobacterium tuberculosis*. However, it does not mean that such a person is suffering from active tuberculosis.

Manubrium

The uppermost part of the STERNUM or breastbone.

MAOIs

See MONOAMINE OXIDASE INHIBITORS (MAOIS).

Marasmus

Progressive wasting, especially in young children, when there is no ascertainable cause. It is generally associated with defective feeding. (See also ATROPHY; INFANT FEEDING.)

Marburg Disease

This is also known as green monkey disease, or vervet monkey disease, because the first recorded human cases acquired their infection from monkeys of this genus. It is a highly dangerous viral infection with a high mortality rate. The incubation period is 4–9 days. The onset is sudden with marked nausea and severe headache; this is followed by rising temperature, diarrhoea, and vomiting. Towards the end of the first week a rash appears which persists for a week and is accompanied by internal bleeding. In those who recover, convalescence is slow and prolonged. Apart from laboratory infections acquired through working with vervet monkeys, all the cases so far reported have occurred in Africa.

March Fracture

A curious condition in which a fracture occurs of the second (rarely, the third) metatarsal bone in the foot without any obvious cause. The usual story is that a pain suddenly developed in the foot while walking or marching (hence the name), and that it has persisted ever since. The only treatment needed is immobilisation of the foot and rest, and the fracture heals satisfactorily. (For more information on fractures, see BONE, DISORDERS OF – Bone fractures.)

March Haemoglobinuria

A complication of walking and running over long distances. It is due to damage to red blood cells in the blood vessels of the soles of the feet. This results in HAEMOGLOBIN being released into the bloodstream, which is then voided in the URINE – the condition known as HAEMOGLOBINURIA. No treatment is required.

Marfan's Syndrome

An inherited disorder affecting about one person in 50,000 in which the CONNECTIVE TISSUE is abnormal. The result is defects of the heart valves, the arteries arising from the heart, the skeleton and the eyes. The victims are unusually tall and thin with a particular facial appearance (the US President Abraham Lincoln was said to have Marfan's) and deformities of the chest and spine. They have spider-like fingers and toes and their joints and ligaments are weak. Orthopaedic intervention may help, as will drugs to control the heart problems. As affected individuals have a 50 per cent chance of passing on the disease to their children, they should receive genetic counselling.

Marijuana

Another term for CANNABIS, hemp, or hashish. (See also DEPENDENCE.)

Marriage Guidance

See RELATE MARRIAGE GUIDANCE.

Marrow

See BONE MARROW.

Marsh Fever

See MALARIA.

Mask

A device that covers the nose and mouth to enable inhalation anaesthetics (see ANAES-THESIA) or other gases such as oxygen to be administered. It is also a covering for the nose and mouth to ensure that antiseptic conditions are maintained during surgery, when dressing a wound or nursing a patient in conditions of isolation. The term is also applied to the expressionless appearance that occurs in certain disorders – for example, in PARKINSONISM.

Masochism

A condition in which a person gets pleasure from physical or emotional pain inflicted by others or themselves. The term is often used in the context of achieving sexual excitement through inflicted pain. Masochism may be a conscious or subconscious activity.

Massage

A method of treatment in which the operator uses his or her hands, or occasionally other appliances, to rub the skin and deeper tissues of the person under treatment. It is often combined with (a) passive movements, in which the masseur/masseuse moves the limbs in various ways, the person treated making no effort; or (b) active movements, which are performed with the combined assistance of masseur/masseuse and patient. Massage is also often combined with baths and gymnastics in order to strengthen various muscles. It helps to improve circulation, prevent adhesions in injured tissues, relax muscular spasm, improve muscle tone and reduce any oedema. (See also CARDIAC MASSAGE.)

Massage for medical conditions is best done by trained practitioners. A complete list of members of the Chartered Society of Physiotherapy can be obtained on application to the Secretary of the Society.

Masseter

An important muscle of MASTICATION that extends from the zygomatic arch in the cheek to the mandible or jawbone. It acts by closing the jaw.

Mass Hysteria

See HYSTERIA.

Mass Miniature Radiography

A method of obtaining X-ray photographs of the chests of large numbers of people. It has been used on a large scale as a means of screening the population for pulmonary TUBERCU-LOSIS. It is no longer used in the United Kingdom.

Mastalgia

The term applied to pain in the breast (see BREASTS; BREASTS, DISEASES OF).

Mast Cells

Round or oval cells found predominantly in the loose CONNECTIVE TISSUE. They contain HISTAMINE and HEPARIN, and carry immunoglobulin E, the antibody which plays a predominant part in allergic reactions (see ANTIBODIES; ALLERGY). Although known to play a part in inflammatory reactions, allergy, and hypersensitivity, their precise function in health and disease is still not quite clear.

Mastectomy

A surgical operation to remove part or all of the breast (see BREASTS). It is usually done to treat cancer, when it is commonly followed by CHEMOTHERAPY or RADIOTHERAPY (see BREASTS, DISEASES OF). There are four types of mastectomy: lumpectomy, quandrantectomy, subcutaneous mastectomy and total mastectomy. The choice of operation depends upon several factors, including the site and nature of the tumour and the patient's age and health. Traditionally, radical mastectomy was used to treat breast cancer; in the past three decades, however, surgeons and oncologists have become more selective in their treatment of the disease, bringing the patient into the decision-making on the best course of action. Lumpectomy is done where there is a discrete lump less than 2 cm in diameter with no evidence of glandular spread. A small lump (2–5 cm) with limited spread to the glands may be removed by quadrantectomy or subcutaneous mastectomy (which preserves the nipple and much of the skin, so producing a better cosmetic effect). Lumps bigger than 5 cm and fixed to the underlying tissues require total mastectomy in which the breast tissue, skin and some fat are dissected down to the chest muscles and removed. In addition, the tail of the breast tissue and regional lymph glands are removed. In all types of mastectomy, surgeons endeavour to produce as good a cosmetic result as possible, subject to the adequate removal of suspect tissue and glands.

Breast reconstructive surgery (MAM-MOPLASTY) may be done at the same time as the mastectomy – the preferred option – or, if that is not feasible, at a later date. Where the whole breast has been excised, some form of artificial breast (prosthesis) will be provided. This may be an external prosthesis fitted into a specially made brassiere, or an internal implant – perhaps a silicone bag, though there has been controversy over the safety of this device. Reconstructive techniques involving the transfer of skin and muscle from nearby areas are also being developed. Post-operatively, patients can obtain advice from Breast Cancer Care.

Mastication

The act whereby, as a result of movements of the lower jaw, lips, tongue, and cheek, food is reduced to a condition in which it is ready to be acted on by the gastric juices in the process of DIGESTION. Adequate mastication before swallowing is an essential part of the digestive process.

Mastitis

The term applied to inflammation of the breast (see BREASTS, DISEASES OF).

Mastocytosis

A rare condition in which the primary abnormality is of MAST CELLS – a type of cell responsible for the storage and release of agents such as HISTAMINE, important in allergic states. Patients may present with an urticarial rash (*urticaria pigmentosa*) but may have symptoms referable to any part of the body, related to collections of active mast cells in these areas.

Mastoid Process

The large process of the temporal bone of the SKULL which can be felt immediately behind the ear. It contains numerous cavities, one of which – the mastoid antrum – communicates with the middle ear, and is liable to suppurate when the middle ear is diseased. (See under EAR, DISEASES OF.)

Masturbation

The production of an ORGASM by self-manipulation of the PENIS or CLITORIS.

Mat Burn

A combination of a burn and an abrasion which occurs in wrestlers when the skin over the bony points is rubbed against the unyielding canvas mat.

Materia Medica

The branch of medical study which deals with the sources, preparations and uses of drugs. (See MEDICINES.)

Maxilla

The name applied to the upper jawbones, which bear the teeth.

ME

See MYALGIC ENCEPHALOMYELITIS (ME).

Mean

A statistical term meaning the value obtained when you add up the total of a set of observations and divide the result by the number of observations. It can give a false impression if there are a few outliers – individual results well beyond the range of the remainder.

Measles

Measles, formerly known as morbilli, is an acute infectious disease occurring mostly in children and caused by an RNA paramyxovirus.

Epidemiology There has been a dramatic fall in the number of sufferers from 1986, when more than 80,000 cases were reported. This is due to the introduction in 1988 of the measles, mumps and rubella vaccine (MMR VACCINE – see also IMMUNISATION); 1990, when the proportion of children immunised reached 90 per cent, was the first year in which no deaths from measles were reported. Even so, fears of side-effects of the vaccine against measles – including scientifically unproven and discredited claims of a link with AUTISM – mean that some children in the UK are not being immunised, and since 2002 local outbreaks of measles have been reported in a few areas of the UK. Side-effects are, however, rare and the government is campaigning to raise the rate of immunisation, with GPs being set targets for their practices.

There are few diseases as infectious as measles, and its rapid spread in epidemics is no doubt due to the fact that this viral infection is most potent in the earlier stages. Hence the difficulty of timely isolation, and the readiness with which the disease is spread, which is mostly by infected droplets. In developing countries measles results in the death of more than a million children annually.

Symptoms The incubation period, during which the child is well, lasts 7–21 days. Initial symptoms are CATARRH, conjunctivitis (see EYE, DISORDERS OF), fever and a feeling of wretchedness. Then Koplik spots – a classic sign of measles – appear on the roof of the mouth and lining of the cheeks. The macular body rash, typical of measles, appears 3–5 days later. Common complications include otitis media (see under EAR, DISEASES OF) and PNEUMONIA. Measles ENCEPHALITIS can cause permanent brain damage. A rare event is a gradual dementing disease (see DEMENTIA) called subacute sclerosing panenecephalitis (SSPE).

Treatment Isolation of the patient and treatment of any secondary bacterial infection, such as pneumonia or otitis, with antibiotics. Children usually run a high temperature which can be relieved with cool sponging and antipyretic drugs. Calamine lotion may alleviate any itching.

Measures
See APPENDIX 6: MEASUREMENTS IN MEDICINE.

Meat
See PROTEIN.

Meatus
A term applied to any passage or opening: for example, external auditory meatus – the passage from the surface to the drum of the EAR.

Mebendazole
An anthelmintic drug (see ANTHELMINTICS) used to treat threadworms (see ENTEROBIASIS). It is the drug of choice, except for in children aged two years or younger. A single dose is usually effective, but reinfection is common and a second treatment may be given after three weeks.

Mebeverine
A direct relaxant of the smooth muscle in the INTESTINE, it may relieve pain in patients with IRRITABLE BOWEL SYNDROME (IBS) or DIVERTICULAR DISEASE. Adverse effects are rare.

Meckel's Diverticulum
A hollow pouch sometimes found attached to the small INTESTINE. It is placed on the small intestine about 90–120 cm (3–4 feet) from its junction with the large intestine, is several centimetres long, and ends blindly. It is lined with cells similar to those which line the stomach, and so may produce acid. This leads to occasional illness – Meckel's diverticulitis with ulceration, which causes abdominal pain and fever (sometimes referred to as 'left-sided appendicitis'). Perforation may result in PERITONITIS and, rarely, may be the lead point of an INTUSSUSCEPTION.

Meconium
The brown, semi-fluid material which collects in the bowels of a FETUS before birth, and which should be discharged either at the time of birth or shortly afterwards. It consists partly of BILE secreted by the liver before birth; partly of debris from the mucous membrane of the intestines.

Media
The middle layer of an organ or tissue, but more usually applied to the wall of an artery or vein, where the media comprises layers of elastic and smooth muscle fibres.

Medial
Near the middle of tissue, organ or body.

Medial Tibial Syndrome
The term applied by athletes to a condition characterised by pain over the inner border of the shin, which occurs in most runners and sometimes in joggers. The syndrome, also known as shin splints, is due to muscular swelling resulting in inadequate blood supply in the muscle: hence the pain. The disorder may be the result of compartment syndrome (build-up of pressure in the muscles), TENDINITIS, muscle or bone inflammation, or damage to the muscle. It usually disappears within a few weeks, responding to rest and PHYSIOTHERAPY, with or without injections. In some cases, however, it becomes chronic and so severe that it occurs even at rest. If the cause is the compartment syndrome, relief is usually obtained by a simple operation to relieve the pressure in the affected muscles.

Median
A statistical term which is the central value of a set of values placed in order of size. The median divides the set into two halves.

Mediastinum

Mediastinum is the space in the chest which lies between the two lungs. It contains the heart and great vessels, the gullet, the lower part of the windpipe, the thoracic duct and the phrenic nerves, as well as numerous structures of less importance.

Medicaid

A joint state and federal health insurance scheme in the United States that provides cover for poorer people in the population.

Medical Audit

A systematic review of the procedures involved in the diagnosis, care and treatment of patients. Such a review includes the input of associated resources – for example, social-services care and funding – and an assessment of the outcome and quality of life for the patient(s). If the review is undertaken by health-care professionals, the process is called CLINICAL AUDIT.

Medical Defence Organisations

These are UK bodies that provide doctors with advice and, where appropriate, financial support in defending claims for medical negligence in their clinical practice. They also advise doctors on all legal aspects of their work, including patients' complaints, and provide representation for members called to account by the GENERAL MEDICAL COUNCIL (GMC) or other regulatory body. The sharp rise in claims for medical negligence in the NHS in the 1980s persuaded the UK Health Departments to introduce a risk-pooling system called the Clinical Negligence Scheme for Trusts, and the defence societies liaise with this scheme when advising their doctor members on responding to claims of negligence (see MEDICAL LITIGATION; MEDICAL NEGLIGENCE).

Medical Devices Agency

An executive agency of the Department of Health in the UK. Set up in 1994, it is responsible for regulating and advising on the sale or use of any product, other than a medicine, used in the health-care environment for the diagnosis, prevention, monitoring or treatment of illness or disease. Equipment ranges from pacemakers (see CARDIAC PACEMAKER) to prostheses (see PROSTHESIS), and from syringes to magnetic resonance imaging (see (MRI).

Medical Education

This term is used to define the process of learning and knowledge-acquisition in the study of medicine. It also encompasses the expertise required to develop education and training for students and learners in all aspects of medical health care. Studies for undergraduate students, postgraduate students and individual health-care practitioners, from the initial stages to the ongoing development of a career in medicine or associated health fields, are also included in medical education. The word 'pedagogy' is sometimes applied to this process.

A range of research investigations has developed within medical education. These apply to course monitoring, audit, development and validation, assessment methodologies and the application of educationally appropriate principles at undergraduate and postgraduate levels. Research is undertaken by medical educationalists whose backgrounds include teaching, social sciences and medicine and related health-care specialties, and who will hold a medical or general educational diploma, degree or other appropriate postgraduate qualification.

Development and validation for all courses are an important part of continuing accreditation processes. The relatively conservative courses at both undergraduate and postgraduate levels, including diplomas and postgraduate qualifications awarded by the specialist medical royal colleges (responsible for standards of specialist education) and universities, have undergone a range of reassessment and redefinition driven by the changing needs of the individual practitioner in the last decade. The stimuli to change aspects of medical training have come from the government through the former Chief Medical Officer, Sir Kenneth Calman, and the introduction of new approaches to specialist training (the Calman programme), from the GENERAL MEDICAL COUNCIL (GMC) and its document *Tomorrow's Doctors*, as well as from the profession itself through the activities of the British Medical Association and the medical royal colleges. The evolving expectations of the public in their perception of the requirements of a doctor, and changes in education of other groups of health professionals, have also led to pressures for changes.

Consequently, many new departments and units devoted to medical education within university medical schools, royal colleges and elsewhere within higher education have been established. These developments have built upon practice developed elsewhere in the world, particularly in North America, Australia and some European countries. Undergraduate education has seen application of new educational methods, including Problem-Based Learning (PBL) in Liverpool, Glasgow and Manchester; clinical and communications skills teaching; early patient contact; and the extensive adoption of Internet (World Wide Web) support and Computer-Aided Learning (CAL). In postgraduate education – driven by European directives and practices, changes in specialist training and the needs of community medicine – new courses have developed around the membership and fellowship examinations for the royal colleges. Examples of these changes driven by medical education expertise include the STEP course for the Royal College of Surgeons of England, and distance-learning courses for diplomas in primary care and rheumatology, as well as examples of good practice as adopted by the Royal College of General Practitioners.

Continuing Professional Development (CPD) and Continuing Medical Education (CME) are also important aspects of medical education now being developed in the United Kingdom, and are evolving to meet the needs of individuals at all stages of their careers.

Bodies closely involved in medical educational developments and their review include the General Medical Council, SCOPME (the Standing Committee on Postgraduate Medical Education), all the medical royal colleges and medical schools, and the British Medical Association through its Board of Medical Education. The National Health Service (NHS) is also involved in education and is a key to facilitation of CPD/CME as the major employer of doctors within the United Kingdom.

Several learned societies embrace medical education at all levels. These include ASME (the Association for the Study of Medical Education), MADEN (the Medical and Dental Education Network) and AMEE (the Association for Medical Education in Europe). Specialist journals are devoted to research reports relating to medical educational developments (e.g. *Academic Medicine, Health Care Education, Medical Education*). The more general medical journals (e.g. *British Medical Journal, New England Journal of Medicine, The Lancet, Annals of the Royal College of Surgeons*) also carry articles on educational matters. Finally, the World Wide Web (WWW) is a valuable source of information relating to courses and course development and other aspects of modern medical education.

The UK government, which controls the number of students entering medical training, has recently increased the quota to take account of increasing demands for trained staff from the NHS. More than 5,700 students – 3,300 women and 2,400 men – are now entering UK medical schools annually with nearly 28,600 at medical school in any one year, and an attrition

rate of about 8–10 per cent. This loss may in part be due to the changes in university-funding arrangements. Students now pay all or part of their tuition fees, and this can result in medical graduates owing several thousand pounds when they qualify at the end of their five-year basic qualification course. Doctors wishing to specialise need to do up to five years (sometimes more) of salaried 'hands-on' training in house or registrar (intern) posts.

Though it may be a commonly held belief that most students enter medicine for humanitarian reasons rather than for the financial rewards of a successful medical career, in developed nations the prospect of status and rewards is probably one incentive. However, the cost to students of medical education along with the widespread publicity in Britain about an under-resourced, seriously overstretched health service, with staff working long hours and dealing with a rising number of disgruntled patients, may be affecting recruitment, since the number of applicants for medical school has dropped in the past year or so. Although there is still competition for places, planners need to bear this falling trend in mind.

Another factor to be considered for the future is the nature of the medical curriculum. In Britain and western Europe, the age structure of a probably declining population will become top-heavy with senior citizens. In the financial interests of the countries affected, and in the personal interests of an ageing population, it would seem sensible to raise the profile of preventive medicine – traditionally rather a Cinderella subject – in medical education, thus enabling people to live healthier as well as longer lives. While learning about treatments is essential, the increasing specialisation and sub-specialisation of medicine in order to provide expensive, high-technology care to a population, many of whom are suffering from preventable illnesses originating in part from self-indulgent lifestyles, seems insupportable economically, unsatisfactory for patients awaiting treatment, and not necessarily professionally fulfilling for health-care staff. To change the mix of medical education would be a difficult long-term task but should be worthwhile for providers and recipients of medical care.

Medical Informatics

See INFORMATION TECHNOLOGY IN MEDICINE.

Medical Litigation

Legal action taken by an individual or group of individuals, usually patients, against hospitals, health-service providers or health professionals in respect of alleged inadequacies in the provision of health care.

In the hospital service, claims for clinical negligence have risen enormously since the 1970s. In 1975 the NHS spent about £1m a year on legal claims; by 2004 the NHS faced over £2 billion in outstanding claims. In 1995 a risk-pooling Clinical Negligence Scheme for Trusts (CNST) was set up in England, and is administered by the NHS Litigation Authority. NHS trusts are expected to follow a set of risk-management standards, the first being that each trust should have a written risk-management strategy with an explicit commitment to managing clinical risk (see RISK MANAGEMENT).

Medical Negligence

Under the strict legal definition, negligence must involve proving a clearly established duty of care which has been breached in a way that has resulted in injury or harm to the recipient of care. There does not need to be any malicious intention. Whether or not a particular injury can be attributed to medical negligence, or must simply be accepted as a reasonable risk of the particular treatment, depends upon an assessment of whether the doctor has fallen below the standard expected of practitioners in the particular specialty. A defence to such a claim is that a respected body of practitioners would have acted in the same way (even though the majority might not) and in doing so would have acted logically.

Medical Oncology

See ONCOLOGY.

Medical Record

The information recorded and kept – on paper or electronically – by health professionals about an individual's illness(es). The information is normally confidential to those responsible for caring for the patient – and to the patient, if he or she should wish to see it. (See CONFIDENTIALITY.)

Medical Research Council

A statutory body in the United Kingdom that promotes the balanced development of medical and related biological research and aims to advance knowledge that will lead to improved health care. It employs its own research staff in more than 40 research establishments. These include the National Institute for Medical Research, the Laboratory of Molecular Biology, and the Clinical Sciences Centre. Grants are provided so that individual scientists can do research which complements the research activities of hospitals and universities. There are several medical charities and foundations – for example, the Imperial Cancer Research Fund, the British Heart Foundation, the Nuffield Laboratories and the Wellcome Trust which fund and foster medical research.

Medicare

A health insurance scheme in the United States, managed by the federal government, that provides cover for Americans over the age of 65 who have certain disabilities.

Medicated

Description of a substance that contains a medicinal drug, commonly applied to items such as sweets and soaps.

Medicine

(1) The skills and science used by trained practitioners to prevent, diagnose, treat and research disease and its related factors.

(2) A drug used to treat an individual with an illness or injury (see MEDICINES).

(3) The diagnosis and treatment of those diseases not normally requiring surgical intervention.

Defensive medicine Diagnostic or treatment procedures undertaken by practitioners in which they aim to reduce the likelihood of legal action by patients. This may result in requests for investigations that, arguably, are to provide legal cover for the doctor rather than more certain clinical diagnosis for the patient.

Medicine of Ageing

Diseases developing during a person's lifetime may be the result of his or her lifestyle, environment, genetic factors and natural AGEING factors.

Lifestyle While this may change as people grow older – for instance, physical activity is commonly reduced – some lifestyle factors are unchanged: for example, cigarette smoking, commonly started in adolescence, may be continued as an adult, resulting in smoker's cough and eventually chronic BRONCHITIS and EMPHYSEMA; widespread ATHEROSCLEROSIS causing heart attacks and STROKE; osteoporosis (see BONE, DISORDERS OF) producing bony fractures; and cancer affecting the lungs and bladder.

Genetic factors can cause sickle cell disease (see ANAEMIA), HUNTINGTON'S CHOREA and polycystic disease of the kidney.

Ageing process This is associated with the MENOPAUSE in women and, in both sexes, with a reduction in the body's tissue elasticity and often a deterioration in mental and physical capabilities. When compared with illnesses described in much younger people, similar illnesses in old age present in an atypical manner – for example, confusion and changed behaviour due to otherwise asymptomatic heart failure, causing a reduced supply of oxygen to the brain. Social adversity in old age may result from the combined effects of reduced body reserve, atypical presentation of illness, multiple disorders and POLYPHARMACY.

Age-related change in the presentation of illnesses This was first recognised by the specialty of geriatric medicine (also called the medicine of ageing) which is concerned with the medical and social management of advanced age. The aim is to assess, treat and rehabilitate such patients. The number of institutional beds has been steadily cut, while availability of day-treatment centres and respite facilities has been boosted – although still inadequate to cope with the growing number of people over 65.

These developments, along with day social centres, provide relatives and carers with a break from the often demanding task of looking after the frail or ill elderly. As the proportion of elderly people in the population rises, along with the cost of hospital inpatient care, close co-operation between hospitals, COMMUNITY CARE services and primary care trusts (see under GENERAL PRACTITIONER (GP)) becomes increasingly important if senior citizens are not to suffer from the consequences of the tight operating budgets of the various medical and social agencies with responsibilities for the care of the elderly. Private or voluntary nursing and residential homes have expanded in the past 15 years and now care for many elderly people who previously would have been occupying NHS facilities. This trend has been accelerated by a tightening of the benefit rules for funding such care. Local authorities are now responsible for assessing the needs of elderly people in the community and deciding whether they are eligible for financial support (in full or in part) for nursing-home care.

With a substantial proportion of hospital inpatients in the United Kingdom being over 60, it is sometimes argued that all health professionals should be skilled in the care of the elderly; thus the need for doctors and nurses trained in the specialty of geriatrics is diminishing. Even so, as more people are reaching their 80s, there seems to be a reasonable case for training staff in the type of care these individuals need and to facilitate research into illness at this stage of life.

Medicines

Medicines are drugs made stable, palatable and acceptable for administration. In Britain, the Medicines Act 1968 controls the making, advertising and selling of substances used for 'medicinal purposes', which means diagnosing, preventing or treating disease, or altering a function of the body. Permission to market a medicine has to be obtained from the government through the MEDICINES CONTROL AGENCY, or from the European Commission through the European Medicines Evaluation Agency. It takes the form of a Marketing Authorisation (formerly called a Product Licence), and the uses to which the medicine can be put are laid out in the Summary of Product Characteristics (which used to be called the Product Data Sheet).

There are three main categories of licensed medicinal product. Drugs in small quantities can, if they are perceived to be safe, be licensed for general sale (GSL – general sales list), and may then be sold in any retail shop. P (pharmacy-only) medicines can be sold from a registered pharmacy by or under the supervision of a pharmacist (see PHARMACISTS); no prescription is needed. P and GSL medicines are together known as OTCs – that is, 'over-the-counter medicines'. POM (prescription-only medicines) can only be obtained from a registered pharmacy on the prescription of a doctor or dentist. As more information is gathered on the safety of drugs, and more emphasis put on individual responsibility for health, there is a trend towards allowing drugs that were once POM to be more widely available as P medicines. Examples include HYDROCORTISONE 1 per cent cream for skin rashes, CIMETIDINE for indigestion, and ACICLOVIR for cold sores. Care is needed to avoid taking a P medicine that might alter the actions of another medicine taken with it, or that might be unsuitable for other reasons. Patients should read the patient-information leaflet, and seek the pharmacist's advice if they have any doubt about the information. They should tell their pharmacist or doctor if the medicine results in any unexpected effects.

Potentially dangerous drugs are preparations referred to under the Misuse of Drugs Act 1971 and subsequent regulations approved in 1985. Described as CONTROLLED DRUGS, these include such preparations as COCAINE, MORPHINE, DIAMORPHINE, LSD (see LYSERGIC ACID

M

DIETHYLAMIDE (LSD)), PETHIDINE HYDRO-
CHLORIDE, AMPHETAMINES, BARBITURATES and
most BENZODIAZEPINES.

Naming of drugs A European Community
Directive (92/27/EEC) requires the use of the
Recommended International Non-proprietary
Name (rINN) for medicinal substances. For
most of these the British Approved Name
(BAN) and rINN were identical; where the two
were different, the BAN has been modified in
line with the rINN. Doctors and other authorised subscribers are advised to write titles of
drugs and preparations in full because unofficial
abbreviations may be misinterpreted. Where a
drug or preparation has a non-proprietary (generic) title, this should be used in prescribing
unless there is a genuine problem over the bio-
availability properties of a proprietary drug and
its generic equivalent.

Where proprietary – commercially registered
– names exist, they may in general be used only
for products supplied by the trademark owners.
Countries outside the European Union have
their own regulations for the naming of
medicines.

Methods of administration The ways in
which drugs are given are increasingly ingenious. Most are still given by mouth; some oral
preparations ('slow release' or 'controlled
release' preparations) are designed to release
their contents slowly into the gut, to maintain
the action of the drug.

Buccal preparations are allowed to dissolve in
the mouth, and sublingual ones are dissolved
under the tongue. The other end of the gastrointestinal tract can also absorb drugs: suppositories inserted in the rectum can be used for
their local actions – for example, as laxatives –
or to allow absorption when taking the drug by
mouth is difficult or impossible – for example,
during a convulsion, or when vomiting.

Small amounts of drug can be absorbed
through the intact skin, and for very potent
drugs like OESTROGENS (female sex hormones)
or the anti-anginal drug GLYCERYL TRINITRATE,
a drug-releasing 'patch' can be used. Drugs can
be inhaled into the lungs as a fine powder to
treat or prevent ASTHMA attacks. They can also
be dispersed ('nebulised') as a fine mist which
can be administered with compressed air or
oxygen. Spraying a drug into the nostril, so that
it can be absorbed through the lining of the
nose into the bloodstream, can avoid destruction of the drug in the stomach. This route is
used for a small number of drugs like antidiuretic hormone (see VASOPRESSIN).

Injection remains an important route of
administering drugs both locally (for example,
into joints or into the eyeball), and into the
bloodstream. For this latter purpose, drugs can
be given under the skin – that is, subcutaneously (s.c. – also called hypodermic injection);
into muscle – intramuscularly (i.m.); or into a
vein – intravenously (i.v.). Oily or crystalline
preparations of drugs injected subcutaneously
form a 'depot' from which they are absorbed
only slowly into the blood. The action of drugs
such as TESTOSTERONE and INSULIN can be prolonged by using such preparations, which also
allow contraceptive 'implants' that work for
some months (see CONTRACEPTION).

Safe disposal of unwanted medicines
Unwanted medicines are a form of 'controlled waste' under the Environmental Protection Act 1990 and must be disposed of in an
appropriate way. The best thing is to take any
extra or unwanted medicines to a registered
pharmacy. Syringes and needles (used by diabetic patients, for example) pose problems:
devices exist to cut off and retain the needle,
and some local authorities in the United Kingdom arrange for collection and safe disposal.
There are also local 'needle exchange' schemes
for intravenous drug abusers.

Safe use of medicines All medicines can
have unwanted effects ('side-effects' or, more
strictly, adverse effects) that are unpleasant and
sometimes harmful. It is best not to take any
medicine, prescribed or otherwise, unless there
is a clear reason for doing so; the possible
adverse effects of treatment, and the risk of their
occurring, have to be set against any likely
benefit. Remember too that one treatment can
affect another already being taken. Many
adverse events depend upon the recommended
dose being exceeded. Some people – for
example, those with allergies (see ALLERGY) to a
particular group of drugs, or those with kidney
or liver disease – are more likely to suffer
adverse effects than otherwise healthy people.

When an individual begins a course of
treatment, he or she should take it as instructed.
With ANTIBIOTICS treatments especially, it is
important to take the whole course of tablets
prescribed, because brief exposure of bacteria to
an antibiotic can make them resistant to treatment. Most drugs can be stopped at once, but
some treatments can cause unpleasant, and
occasionally dangerous, symptoms if stopped
abruptly. Sleeping tablets, anti-EPILEPSY treatment, and medicines used to treat ANGINA PEC-
TORIS are among the agents which can cause

such 'withdrawal symptoms'. CORTICO-STEROIDS are a particularly important group of medicines in this respect, because prolonged courses of treatment with high doses can suppress the ability of the body to respond to severe stresses (such as surgical operations) for many months or even years.

Medicines Commission
A government-appointed expert advisory body on the use of MEDICINES in the UK.

Medicines Control Agency
An executive agency of the Department of Health with the prime function of safeguarding the public health. It ensures that branded and non-branded MEDICINES on the UK market meet appropriate standards of safety, quality and efficacy. The agency applies the strict standards set by the UK Medicines Act (1968) and relevant European Community legislation.

Medicolegal
A term that relates to the practice of medicine and law (see FORENSIC MEDICINE; MEDICAL LITIGATION; MEDICAL NEGLIGENCE).

Medlars
Medical Literature Analysis and Retrieval System – a computerised index system produced by the US National Library of Medicine.

Medline
A computer-based telephone line linkage to MEDLARS for rapid transmission of medical information held by that library. Information can be accessed worldwide. Information is also available via the web.

Medroxyprogesterone
A PROGESTERONE (female sex hormone) preparation which is given intramuscularly in long-acting form as a PROGESTOGEN-only contraception; however, it should be given only with counselling and full details of its action. The drug is also used as second- or third-line treatment for patients with breast cancer and also in carcinoma of the kidney. Progestogens have been proposed for lessening premenstrual symptoms, but proof of their value in this role is not convincing.

Medulla
The inside part of an organ or tissue that is distinct from the outer part – for example, the marrow in the centre of a long bone, or the inner portion of the kidneys or adrenal glands.

Medulla Oblongata
The hindmost part of the BRAIN, continuing into the SPINAL CORD. In it are situated several of the nerve centres which are most essential to life, such as those governing breathing, the action of the heart and swallowing.

Mefenamic Acid
One of the NON-STEROIDAL ANTI-INFLAMMATORY DRUGS (NSAIDS) that is an analgesic (see ANALGESICS) for mild to moderate pain in RHEUMATOID ARTHRITIS, OSTEOARTHRITIS and other musculoskeletal disorders. Also used for DYSMENNORRHOEA and MENORRHAGIA. It must be used with care as it has several side-effects, in particular diarrhoea and occasional haemolytic ANAEMIA. It must not be used in patients with INFLAMMATORY BOWEL DISEASE (IBD).

Megacolon
A greatly enlarged colon that may be present at birth or develop later. It can occur in all age groups and the condition is typified by severe chronic constipation. Megacolon is caused by obstruction of the colon which may be due to faulty innervation, or to psychological factors. Other causes are HIRSCHSPRUNG'S DISEASE or ULCERATIVE COLITIS. In old people the persistent use of powerful laxative drugs may cause the condition.

Megalomania
A delusion of grandeur or an insane belief in a person's own extreme greatness, goodness, or power.

Mega-/Megalo-
Prefixes denoting largeness.

Meibomian Glands
Numerous glands within the tarsal plates of the eyelids. Their secretions form part of the tears. (See EYE.)

Meiosis
Meiosis, or reduction division, is the form of cell division that only occurs in the gonads (see GONAD) – that is, the testis (see TESTICLE) and the ovary (see OVARIES) – giving rise to the germ cells (gametes) of the sperms (see SPERMATOZOON) and the ova (see OVUM).

Two types of sperm cells are produced: one contains 22 autosomes and a Y sex chromosome (see SEX CHROMOSOMES); the other, 22 autosomes and an X sex chromosome. All the ova, however, produced by normal meiosis have 22 autosomes and an X sex chromosome.

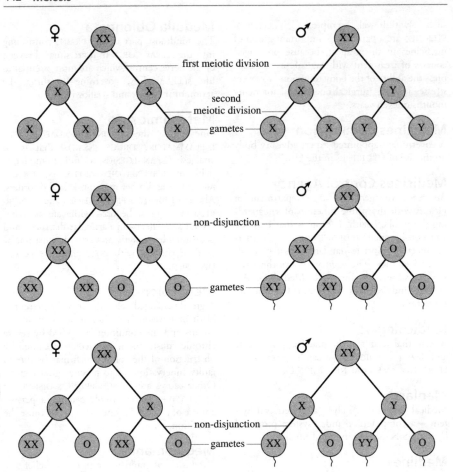

The formation of gametes. Top, normal meiosis. Centre, non-disjunction at first meiotic division. Bottom, non-disjunction at second meiotic division.

Two divisions of the NUCLEUS occur (see also CELLS) and only one division of the chromosomes, so that the number of chromosomes in the ova and sperms is half that of the somatic cells. Each chromosome pair divides so that the gametes receive only one member of each pair. The number of chromosomes is restored to full complement at fertilisation so that the zygote has a complete set, each chromosome from the nucleus of the sperm pairing up with its corresponding partner from the ovum.

The first stage of meiosis involves the pairing of homologous chromosomes which join together and synapse lengthwise. The chromosomes then become doubled by splitting along their length and the chromatids so formed are held together by centromeres. As the homologous chromosomes – one of which has come from the mother, and the other from the father – are lying together, genetic interchange can take place between the chromatids and in this way new combinations of GENES arise. All four chromatids are closely interwoven and recombination may take place between any maternal or any paternal chromatids. This process is known as crossing over or recombination. After this period of interchange, homologous chromosomes move apart, one to each pole of the nucleus. The cell then divides and the nucleus of each new cell now contains 23 and not 46 chromosomes. The second meiotic division then occurs, the centromeres divide and the chromatids move apart to opposite poles of the nucleus so there are still 23 chromosomes in each of the daughter nuclei so formed. The cell divides again so that there are four gametes, each containing a half number (haploid) set of chromosomes. However, owing to the recombination or crossing over, the genetic material is not identical with either parent or with other spermatozoa.

Melaena

Blood in the FAECES in which dark, tarry masses are passed from the bowel. It is due to bleeding from the stomach or from the higher part of the bowel, the blood undergoing chemical changes under the action of the secretions, and being finally converted in large part into sulphide of iron. It is a serious symptom meriting medical investigation. It can indicate peptic ulcer or carcinoma of the stomach.

Melancholia

A term used in the past for illness characterised by great mental and physical DEPRESSION. (See MENTAL ILLNESS.)

Melanin

Pigment which confers colour on the SKIN, hair and EYE. It is produced by cells called melanocytes interspersed along the basal layer of the EPIDERMIS. The maturation of the epidermis into stratum corneum cells packed with melanin granules confers an ultraviolet light barrier which protects the skin against the harmful effects resulting from continued solar exposure. The races do not differ in the number of melanocytes in their skin, only in the rate and quantity of melanin production. Exposure to bright sunlight stimulates melanin production and distribution causing 'suntan'. A hormone from the PITUITARY GLAND may stimulate melanin production on the face in pregnancy (see CHLOASMA).

Melanocyte

Clear branching cell in the epidermis of the SKIN that produces tyrosinase (an ENZYME) and MELANIN.

Melanoma

A malignant tumour arising from melanocytes (see MELANOCYTE). It may start in an existing MOLE or arise *de novo*. Increasing exposure to sunlight of white populations in the 20th century has resulted in an alarming increase in the incidence of this cancer. It is mainly seen in those over 40 years, especially on the legs in women and on the back in men. An enlarging pigmented macule or nodule with irregular contour, profile or colour distribution is always suspect.

Treatment is excision with a margin of normal tissue. The specimen must be examined histologically, and prognosis depends on the depth of invasion. Very superficial melanomas carry an excellent outlook once removed, but deeper tumours may spread to regional lymph glands and beyond with fatal results. Public-awareness campaigns have led to the earlier presentation of melanomas in recent years, with corresponding benefit. (See also SUNBURN.)

Melatonin

A hormone that plays a key role in the body's diurnal (night and day) rhythms. Produced by the PINEAL GLAND and derived from SEROTONIN, it acts on receptors in an area of the brain above the OPTIC CHIASMA, synchronising them to the diurnal rhythm. Melatonin is under investigation as a possible agent to treat insomnia in the elderly, in shift workers and in those with severe learning disability (mental handicap). It may also help people with SEASONAL AFFECTIVE DISORDER SYNDROME (SADS) and those who suffer from jet lag.

Melphalan

One of the ALKYLATING AGENTS, melphalan is used to treat certain forms of malignant disease including breast tumours (see BREASTS, DISEASES OF), MELANOMA and Hodgkin's LYMPHOMA. It can be given orally or by injection. (See CYTOTOXIC.)

Membranes

See BRAIN; CROUP; DIPHTHERIA; labour (under PREGNANCY AND LABOUR).

Memory

The capacity to remember. It is a complex process and probably occurs in many areas of the BRAIN including the LIMBIC SYSTEM and the temporal lobes. There are three main steps: registration, storage, and recall.

During registration, information from the sense organs and the cerebral cortex is put into codes for storage in the short-term memory system. The codes are usually acoustic (based on the sounds and words that would be used to describe the information) but may use any of the five senses. This system can take only a few chunks of information at a time: for example, only about seven longish numbers can be retained and recalled at once – the next new number displaces an earlier one that is then forgotten. And if a subject is asked to describe a person just met, he or she will recall only seven or so facts about that person. This depends on attention span and can be improved by concentration and rehearsal – for example, by reciting the list of things that must be remembered.

Material needing storage for several minutes

stays in the short-term memory. More valuable information goes to the long-term memory where it can be kept for any period from a few minutes to a lifetime. Storage is more reliable if the information is in meaningful codes – it is much easier to remember people's names if their faces and personalities are memorable too. Using techniques such as mnemonics takes this into account.

The final stage is retrieval. Recognising and recalling the required information involves searching the memory. In the short-term memory, this takes about 40-thousandths of a second per item – a rate that is surprisingly consistent, even in people with disorders such as SCHIZOPHRENIA.

Most kinds of forgetting or AMNESIA occur during retrieval. Benign forgetfulness is usually caused by interference from similar items because the required information was not clearly coded and well organised. Retrieval can be improved by recreating the context in which the information was registered. This is why the police reconstruct scenes of crimes, and why revision for exams is more effective if facts are learnt in the form of answers to mock questions.

Loss of memory or amnesia mainly affects long-term memory (information which is stored indefinitely) rather than short-term memory which is measured in minutes. Short-term memory may, however, be affected by unconsciousness caused by trauma. Drivers involved in an accident may be unable to recall the event or the period leading up to it. The cause of amnesia is disease of or damage to the parts of the brain responsible for memory. Degenerative disorders such as ALZHEIMER'S DISEASE, brain tumours, infections (for example, ENCEPHALITIS), STROKE, SUBARACH-NOID HAEMORRHAGE and alcoholism all cause memory loss. Some psychiatric illnesses feature loss of memory and AGEING is usually accompanied by some memory loss, although the age of onset and severity vary greatly.

Menarche

The start of MENSTRUATION. The average age at which it occurs in British females is 12·5 years – a year or two after the first physical indications of PUBERTY start. There is considerable racial and geographical variation.

Mendelism

The term applied to a law enunciated by G. J. Mendel that the offspring is not intermediate in type between its parents, but that the type of one or other parent is predominant. Character-istics are classed as either dominant or recessive. The offspring of the first generation tend to inherit the dominant characteristics, whilst the recessive characteristics remain latent and appear in some of the offspring of the second generation. If individuals possessing recessive characters unite, recessive characters then become dominant characters in succeeding generations. (See GENETICS.)

Mendelson Syndrome

Inhalation of regurgitated stomach contents, usually as a complication of general ANAES-THESIA. It may cause death from ANOXIA or result in extensive lung damage.

Menière's Disease

Named after the Frenchman, Prosper Menière, who first described it in 1861, the disease is characterised by TINNITUS, deafness and intermittent attacks of VERTIGO. The first manifestation is usually deafness on one side; then – as a rule, many months later – there is a sudden attack, without any warning, of intense vertigo. The acute giddiness usually lasts for two or three hours with some unsteadiness persisting for a few days. The time interval between attacks varies from a week to a few months. When they do recur, they tend to do so in clusters. The tinnitus, which tends to be low-pitched, comes on at about the same time as the deafness; it is often described as being like rushing water or escaping steam. The deafness becomes gradually worse until it is complete. The condition is due to excessive fluid in the labyrinth of the ears (see EAR). The cause of this accumulation is not known, although it has been suggested that it might be a form of ALLERGY, or might be due to spasm of small blood vessels. The disorder is diagnosed from AUDIOMETRY, the CALORIC TEST and other investigations.

Treatment Acute vertigo symptoms can sometimes be alleviated with drugs such as CYCLIZINE HYDROCHLORIDE and NICOTINIC ACID, but the disorder is notoriously difficult to treat and no certain cure is available. Surgical decompression of the fluid in the ear's balancing mechanism may relieve vertigo and prevent the disease from worsening. The vestibular nerve to the ear can also be cut to relieve vertigo while preserving hearing.

Meninges

The membranes surrounding the BRAIN and SPINAL CORD. The membranes include the

DURA MATER, a tough, fibrous membrane closely applied to the inside of the skull; the ARACHNOID MEMBRANE, a more delicate membrane, enveloping the brain but separated from its irregular surface by spaces containing fluid; and the pia mater, a delicate network of fibres containing blood vessels and uniting the arachnoid to the brain. The latter two are sometimes referred to as the pia-arachnoid.

These membranes bear the blood vessels which nourish the surface of the brain and the interior of the skull. Meningeal haemorrhage from these vessels forms one of the chief dangers arising from fracture of the skull.

Meningism

A condition with symptoms and signs closely resembling those of MENINGITIS. Most commonly occurring in children, it is usually a symptom of chest infection or of inflammation in the upper respiratory tract. Given the serious implications of meningitis, medical advice should be sought. Examination of the CEREBROSPINAL FLUID may be necessary: in meningism the fluid is normal.

Meningitis

Inflammation affecting the membranes of the BRAIN or SPINAL CORD, or usually both. Meningitis may be caused by BACTERIA, viruses (see VIRUS), fungi, malignant cells or blood (after SUBARACHNOID HAEMORRHAGE). The term is, however, usually restricted to inflammation due to a bacterium or virus. Viral meningitis is normally a mild, self-limiting infection of a few days' duration; it is the most common cause of meningitis but usually results in complete recovery and requires no specific treatment. Usually a less serious infection than the bacterial variety, it does, however, rarely cause associated ENCEPHALITIS, which is a potentially dangerous illness. A range of viruses can cause meningitis, including: ENTEROVIRUSES; those causing MUMPS, INFLUENZA and HERPES SIMPLEX; and HIV.

Bacterial meningitis is life-threatening: in the United Kingdom, 5–10 per cent of children who contract the disease may die. Most cases of acute bacterial meningitis in the UK are caused by two bacteria: *Neisseria meningitidis* (meningococcus), and *Streptococcus pneumoniae* (pneumococcus); other bacteria include *Haemophilus influenzae* (a common cause until virtually wiped out by immunisation), *Escherichia coli*, *Mycobacterium tuberculosis* (see TUBERCULOSIS), *Treponema pallidum* (see SYPHILIS) and *Staphylococci* spp. Of the bacterial infections, meningococcal group B is the type that causes a large number of cases in the UK, while group A is less common.

Bacterial meningitis may occur by spread from nearby infected foci such as the nasopharynx, middle ear, mastoid and sinuses (see EAR, DISEASES OF). Direct infection may be the result of penetrating injuries of the skull from accidents or gunshot wounds. Meningitis may also be a complication of neurosurgery despite careful aseptic precautions. Immuno-compromised patients – those with AIDS or on CYTOTOXIC drugs – are vulnerable to infections.

Spread to contacts may occur in schools and similar communities. Many people harbour the meningococcus without developing meningitis. In recent years small clusters of cases, mainly in schoolchildren and young people at college, have occurred in Britain.

Symptoms include malaise accompanied by fever, severe headache, PHOTOPHOBIA, vomiting, irritability, rigors, drowsiness and neurological disturbances. Neck stiffness and a positive KERNIG'S SIGN appearing within a few hours of infection are key diagnostic signs. Meningococcal and pneumococcal meningitis may co-exist with SEPTICAEMIA, a much more serious condition in terms of death rate or organ damage and which constitutes a grave emergency demanding rapid treatment.

Diagnosis and treatment are urgent and, if bacterial meningitis is suspected, antibiotic treatment should be started even before laboratory confirmation of the infection. Analysis of the CEREBROSPINAL FLUID (CSF) by means of a LUMBAR PUNCTURE is an essential step in diagnosis, except in patients for whom the test would be dangerous as they have signs of raised intracranial pressure. The CSF is clear or turbid in viral meningitis, turbid or viscous in tuberculous infection and turbulent or purulent when meningococci or staphylococci are the infective agents. Cell counts and biochemical make-up of the CSF are other diagnostic pointers. Serological tests are done to identify possible syphilitic infection, which is now rare in Britain.

Patients with suspected meningitis should be admitted to hospital quickly. General practitioners are encouraged to give a dose of intramuscular penicillin before sending the child to hospital. Treatment in hospital is usually with a cephalosporin, such as ceftazidime or ceftriaxone. Once the sensitivity of the organism is known as a result of laboratory studies on CSF and blood, this may be changed to penicillin or, in the case of *H. influenzae*, to amoxicillin. Local infections such as SINUSITIS or middle-ear infection require treatment, and appropriate surgery for skull fractures or meningeal tears should be carried out as necessary. Tuberculous meningitis is treated for at least nine months with anti-tuberculous drugs (see TUBERCULOSIS). If bacterial meningitis causes CONVULSIONS, these can be controlled with diazepam (see TRANQUILLISERS; BENZODIAZEPINES) and ANALGESICS will be required for the severe headache.

Coexisting septicaemia may require full intensive care with close attention to intravenous fluid and electrolyte balance, control of blood clotting and blood pressure.

Treatment of close contacts such as family, school friends, medical and nursing staff is recommended if the patient has *H. influenzae* or *N. meningitidis*. RIFAMPICIN provides effective prophylaxis. Contacts of patients with pneumococcal infection do not need preventive treatment. Vaccines for meningococcal meningitis may be given to family members in small epidemics and to any contacts who are especially at risk such as infants, the elderly and immuno-compromised individuals.

The outlook for a patient with bacterial meningitis depends upon age – the young and old are vulnerable; speed of onset – sudden onset worsens the prognosis; and how quickly treatment is started – hence the urgency of diagnosis and admission to hospital. Recent research has shown that children who suffer meningitis in their first year of life are ten times more likely to develop moderate or severe disability by the age of five than contemporaries who have not been infected. (See *British Medical Journal*, 8 September 2001, page 523.)

Prevention One type of bacterial meningitis, that caused by *Haemophilus*, has been largely controlled by IMMUNISATION; meningococcal C vaccine has largely prevented this type of the disease in the UK. So far, no vaccine against group B has been developed, but research continues. Information on meningitis can be obtained from the Meningitis Trust and the Meningitis Research Foundation.

Meningocele
Meningocele is a protusion of the MENINGES of the brain through a defect in the skull. (See SPINA BIFIDA.)

Meningococcus
See NEISSERIACEAE.

Meningoencephalitis
Meningoencephalitis is the term applied to infection of the membranes, or MENINGES, of the brain and the underlying brain matter. In practically all cases of MENINGITIS there is some involvement of the underlying brain, and it is when this involvement is considerable that the term, meningoencephalitis, is used. One form that has attracted attention in recent years is that caused by amoebae (see AMOEBA), particularly that known as *Naegleria fowleri*, in which the infection is acquired through bathing in contaminated water. Effective chlorination of swimming baths kills this micro-organism.

Meningomyelocele
A protrusion of the MENINGES of the spinal cord through a defect in the spine. (See SPINA BIFIDA.)

Meniscus
A crescentic fibro-cartilage in a joint, such as the cartilages in the knee-joint.

Menopause
This is the term applied to the cessation of MENSTRUATION at the end of reproductive life. Usually it occurs between the ages of 45 and 50, although it may occur before the age of 30 or after the age of 50. It can be a psychologically disturbing experience which is quite often accompanied by physical manifestations. These include hot flushes, tiredness, irritability, lack of concentration, palpitations, aching joints and vaginal irritation. There may also be loss of libido (sex drive). Most women can and do live happy, active lives through the menopause, the length of which varies considerably.

One of the major problems of the menopause which does not give rise to symptoms until many years later is osteoporosis (see BONE, DISORDERS OF). After the menopause, 1 per cent of the bone is lost per annum to the end of life. This is a factor in the frequency of fractures of the femur in elderly women as a result of osetoporosis, but it can be prevented by hormone replacement therapy (see below).

Hormone replacement therapy (HRT) This term has become synonymous with the scientifically correct term 'OESTROGENS replacement therapy' to signify the treatment of menopausal symptoms and signs with oestrogens, now usually combined with PROGESTOGEN. Oestrogen and combined treatment relieve the short-term symptoms such as hot flushes, sweats and vaginal dryness. Atrophic vaginitis and vulvitis (shrinking of the tissues of VULVA and VAGINA due to fall in natural oestrogen levels) also usually respond to treatment with oestrogens.

Cyclical therapy is necessary to avoid abnormal bleeding in women who have reached the menopause. If oestrogens are given alone, there is an increased risk of endometrial hyperplasia (overgrowth of the ENDOMETRIUM) which may lead to endometrial cancer, so these are restricted to women who have had a hysterectomy and are no longer at risk. Other women can be given oestrogen-progestogen combinations.

There is good evidence that oestrogen alone or in combination can prevent the bone-loss associated with the menopause by reducing the demineralisation of bone which normally occurs after the menopause; and, if it is started early and continued for years, it may prevent the development of osteoporosis. Oestrogen is far more effective than calcium supplements and has been shown greatly to reduce fractures affecting the spine, wrists and legs after the age of 50.

However, HRT is no longer licensed for first-line treatment to prevent osteoporosis, as increased risk of stroke, breast cancer and coronary heart disease cannot justify treatment for long periods – unless the woman has severe menopausal symptoms. HRT is recommended for short-term use only in menopausal women whose lives are inconvenienced by vasomotor instability (severe flushes, etc.) or vaginal atrophy, although the latter may respond to local oestrogen treatment – creams or pessaries. In terms of oestrogenic activity, natural oestrogen such as oestradiol, oestrone and oestriol are more appropriate for HRT than synthetic oestrogens like ethinyloestradiol, mestranol and diethylstilboestrol.

Many experts believe that controversy surrounding the risks and benefits of HRT have been settled by a large randomised trial (the Women's Health Initiative), published in 2003, which showed that combined treatment increases the risk of breast tumours, stroke and coronary heart disease (in the first year). Oestrogen alone (given to women who have had a hysterectomy) also increases the risk of stroke. Five years of combined treatment may double the risk of breast cancer, and the heart-disease risk is nearly doubled during the first year of use. This is in spite of the beneficial effects of HRT on blood lipids. However, there are others who consider that different dose combinations of different hormones may one day prove beneficial, so research continues.

HRT can also provoke minor adverse effects such as breast tenderness, fluid retention, leg cramps and nausea. The risk of abnormal blood clotting means that HRT is not normally recommended for women who smoke heavily or have had THROMBOSIS, severe HYPERTENSION, stroke or liver disease. HRT has, however, brought symptomatic benefits to many menopausal women, who can then justify taking the other increased risks – only fully understood since the large trial results were published.

As the evidence stands at present, careful consideration of each woman's medical history and the severity of her menopausal symptoms is necessary in deciding what combination of drugs should be given and for how long. In general, the indications should be severe menopausal symptoms that can be controlled by the lowest dose for the shortest time. Using HRT to alleviate mild symptoms, or to prevent future bone loss, is probably of insufficient benefit to counter the other risks described above.

Menorrhagia

Menorrhagia means an over-abundance of the menstrual discharge. (See MENSTRUATION, DISORDERS OF.)

Menstruation

A periodic change occurring in (female) human beings and the higher apes, consisting chiefly in a flow of blood from the cavity of the womb (UTERUS) and associated with various slight constitutional disturbances. It begins between the ages of 12 and 15, as a rule – although its onset may be delayed until as late as 20, or it may begin as early as ten or 11. Along with its first appearance, the body develops the secondary sex characteristics: for example, enlargement of the BREASTS, and characteristic hair distribution. The duration of each menstrual period varies in different persons from 2–8 days. It recurs in the great majority of cases with regularity, most commonly at intervals of 28 or 30 days, less often with intervals of 21 or 27 days, and ceasing only during pregnancy and lactation, until the age of 45 or 50 arrives, when it stops altogether – as a rule ceasing early if it has begun early, and vice versa. The final stoppage is known as the MENOPAUSE or the CLIMACTERIC.

Menstruation depends upon a functioning ovary (see OVARIES) and this upon a healthy PITUITARY GLAND. The regular rhythm may depend upon a centre in the HYPOTHALAMUS, which is in close connection with the pituitary. After menstruation, the denuded uterine ENDOMETRIUM is regenerated under the influence of the follicular hormone, oestradiol. The epithelium of the endometrium proliferates, and about a fortnight after the beginning of menstruation great development of the endometrial glands takes place under the influence of progesterone, the hormone secreted by the CORPUS LUTEUM. These changes are made for the reception of the fertilised OVUM. In the absence of fertilisation the uterine endometrium breaks down in the subsequent menstrual discharge.

Disorders of menstruation In most healthy women, menstruation proceeds regularly for 30 years or more, with the exceptions connected with childbirth. In many women, however, menstruation may be absent, excessive or painful. The term amenorrhoea is applied to the condition of absent menstruation; the terms menorrhagia and metrorrhagia describe excessive menstrual loss – the former if the excess occurs at the regular periods, and the latter if it is irregular. Dysmenorrhoea is the name given to painful menstruation.

AMENORRHOEA If menstruation has never occurred, the amenorrhoea is termed primary; if it ceases after having once become established it is known as secondary amenorrhoea. The only value of these terms is that some patients with either chromosomal abnormalities (see CHROMOSOMES) or malformations of the genital tract fall into the primary category. Otherwise, the age of onset of symptoms is more important.

The causes of amenorrhoea are numerous and treatment requires dealing with the primary cause. The commonest cause is pregnancy; psychological stress or eating disorders can cause amenorrhoea, as can poor nutrition or loss of weight by dieting, and any serious underlying disease such as TUBERCULOSIS or MALARIA. The excess secretion of PROLACTIN, whether this is the result of a micro-adenoma of the pituitary gland or whether it is drug induced, will cause amenorrhoea and possibly GALACTORRHOEA as well. Malfunction of the pituitary gland will result in a failure to produce the gonadotrophic hormones (see GONADOTROPHINS) with consequent amenorrhoea. Excessive production of cortisol, as in CUSHING'S SYNDROME, or of androgens (see ANDROGEN) – as in the adreno-genital syndrome or the polycystic ovary syndrome – will result in amenorrhoea. Amenorrhoea occasionally follows use of the oral contraceptive pill and may be associated with both hypothyroidism (see under THYROID GLAND, DISEASES OF) and OBESITY.

Patients should be reassured that amenorrhoea can often be successfully treated and does not necessarily affect their ability to have normal sexual relations and to conceive. When weight loss is the cause of amenorrhoea, restoration of body weight alone can result in spontaneous menstruation (see also EATING DISORDERS – Anorexia nervosa). Patients with raised concentration of serum gonadotrophin hormones have primary ovarian failure, and this is not amenable to treatment. Cyclical oestrogen/progestogen therapy will usually establish withdrawal bleeding. If the amenorrhoea is due to mild pituitary failure, menstruation may return after treatment with clomiphene, a non-steroidal agent which competes for oestrogen receptors in the hypothalamus. The patients who are most likely to respond to clomiphene are those who have some evidence of endogenous oestrogen and gonadotrophin production.

IRREGULAR MENSTRUATION This is a change from the normal monthly cycle of menstruation, the duration of bleeding or the amount of blood lost (see menorrhagia, below). Such changes may be the result of an upset in the balance of oestrogen and progesterone hormones which between them control the cycle. Cycles may be irregular after the MENARCHE and before the menopause. Unsuspected pregnancy may manifest itself as an 'irregularity', as can an early miscarriage (see ABORTION). Disorders of the uterus, ovaries or organs in the pelvic cavity can also cause irregular menstruation. Women with the condition should seek medical advice.

MENORRHAGIA Abnormal bleeding from the uterus during menstruation. A woman loses on average about 60 ml of blood during her period; in menorrhagia this can rise to 100 ml. Some women have this problem occasionally, some quite frequently and others never. One cause is an imbalance of progesterone and oestrogen hormones which between them control menstruation: the result is an abnormal increase in the lining (endometrium) of the uterus, which increases the amount of 'bleeding' tissue. Other causes include fibroids, polyps, pelvic infection or an intrauterine contraceptive device (IUD – see under CONTRACEPTION). Sometimes no physical reason for menorrhagia can be identified.

Treatment of the disorder will depend on how severe the loss of blood is (some women will become anaemic – see ANAEMIA – and require iron-replacement therapy); the woman's age; the cause of heavy bleeding; and whether or not she wants children. An increase in menstrual bleeding may occur in the months before the menopause, in which case time may produce a cure. Medical or surgical treatments are available. Non-steroidal anti-inflammatory drugs may help, as may tranexamic acid, which prevents the breakdown of blood clots in the circulation (FIBRINOLYSIS): this drug can be helpful if an IUD is causing bleeding. Hormones such as dydrogesterone (by mouth) may cure the condition, as may an IUD that releases small quantities of a PROGESTOGEN into the lining of the womb.

Traditionally, surgical intervention was either dilatation and curettage of the womb lining (D & C) or removal of the whole uterus (HYSTERECTOMY). Most surgery is now done using minimally invasive techniques. These do not require the abdomen to be cut open, as an ENDOSCOPE is passed via the vagina into the uterus. Using DIATHERMY or a laser, the surgeon then removes the whole lining of the womb.

DYSMENORRHOEA This varies from discomfort to serious pain, and sometimes includes vomiting and general malaise. Anaemia is sometimes a cause of painful menstruation as well as of stoppage of this function.

Inflammation of the uterus, ovaries or FALLOPIAN TUBES is a common cause of dysmenorrhoea which comes on for the first time late in life, especially when the trouble follows the birth of a child. In this case the pain exists more or less at all times, but is aggravated at the periods. Treatment with analgesics and remedying the underlying cause is called for.

Many cases of dysmenorrhoea appear with the beginning of menstrual life, and accompany every period. It has been estimated that 5–10 per cent of girls in their late teens or early 20s are severely incapacitated by dysmenorrhoea for several hours each month. Various causes have been suggested for the pain, one being an excessive production of PROSTAGLANDINS. There may be a psychological factor in some sufferers and, whether this is the result of inadequate sex instruction, fear, family, school or work problems, it is important to offer advice and support, which in itself may resolve the dysmenorrhoea. Symptomatic relief is of value.

Mental Handicap
See LEARNING DISABILITY.

Mental Illness
Defined simply, this is a disorder of the brain's processes that makes the sufferer feel or seem ill, and may prevent that person from coping with daily life. Psychiatrists – doctors specialising in diagnosing and treating mental illness – have, however, come up with a range of much more complicated definitions over the years.

Psychiatrists like to categorise mental illnesses because mental signs and symptoms do occur together in clusters or syndromes, each tending to respond to certain treatments. The idea that illnesses can be diagnosed simply by recognising their symptom patterns may not seem very scientific in these days of high technology. For most common mental illnesses, however, this is the only method of diagnosis; whatever is going wrong in the brain is usually too poorly understood and too subtle to show up in laboratory tests or computed tomography scans of the brain. And symptom-based definitions of mental illnesses are, generally, a lot more meaningful than the vague lay term 'nervous breakdown', which is used to cover an attack of anything from AGORAPHOBIA to total inability to function.

There is still a lot to learn about the workings of the brain, but psychiatry has developed plenty of practical knowledge about the probable causes of mental illness, ways of relieving symptoms, and ways of aiding recovery. Most experts now believe that mental illnesses generally arise from different combinations of inherited risk and psychological STRESS, sometimes with additional environmental exposure – for example, viruses, drugs or ALCOHOL.

The range of common mental illnesses includes anxiety states, PHOBIA, DEPRESSION, alcohol and drug problems, the EATING DISORDERS anorexia and bulimia nervosa, MANIC DEPRESSION, SCHIZOPHRENIA, DEMENTIA, and a group of problems related to coping with life that psychiatrists call personality disorders.

Of these mental illnesses, dementia is the best understood. It is an irreversible and fatal form of mental deterioration (starting with forgetfulness and eventually leading to severe failure of all the brain's functions), caused by rapid death of brain cells and consequent brain shrinkage. Schizophrenia is another serious mental illness which disrupts thought-processes, speech, emotions and perception (how the brain handles signals from the five senses). Manic depression, in which prolonged 'highs' of extremely elevated mood and overexcitement alternate with abject misery, has similar effects on the mental processes. In both schizophrenia and manic depression the sufferer loses touch with reality, develops unshakeable but completely unrealistic ideas (delusions), and hallucinates (vividly experiences sensations that are not real, e.g. hears voices when there is nobody there). This triad of symptoms is called psychosis and it is what lay people, through fear and lack of understanding, sometimes call lunacy, madness or insanity.

The other mental illnesses mentioned above are sometimes called neuroses. But the term has become derogatory in ordinary lay language;

indeed, many people assume that neuroses are mild disorders that only affect weak people who cannot 'pull themselves together', while psychoses are always severe. In reality, psychoses can be brief and reversible and neuroses can cause lifelong disability.

However defined and categorised, mental illness is a big public-health problem. In the UK, up to one in five women and around one in seven men have had mental illness. About half a million people in Britain suffer from schizophrenia: it is three times commoner than cancer. And at any one time, up to a tenth of the adult population is ill with depression.

Treatment settings Most people with mental-health problems get the help they need from their own family doctor(s), without ever seeing a psychiatrist. General practictitioners in Britain treat nine out of ten recognised mental-health problems and see around 12 million adults with mental illness each year. Even for the one in ten of these patients referred to psychiatrists, general practitioners usually handle those problems that continue or recur.

Psychiatrists, psychiatric nurses, social workers, psychologists, counsellors and therapists often see patients at local doctors' surgeries and will do home visits if necessary. Community mental-health centres – like general-practice health centres but catering solely for mental-health problems – offer another short-cut to psychiatric help. The more traditional, and still more common, route to a psychiatrist for many people, however, is from the general practitioner to a hospital outpatient department.

Specialist psychiatric help In many ways, a visit to a psychiatrist is much like any trip to a hospital doctor – and, indeed, psychiatric clinics are often based in the outpatient departments of general hospitals. First appointments with psychiatrists can last an hour or more because the psychiatrist – and sometimes other members of the team such as nurses, doctors in training, and social workers – need to ask lots of questions and record the whole consultation in a set of confidential case notes.

Psychiatric assessment usually includes an interview and an examination, and is sometimes backed up by a range of tests. The interview begins with the patient's history – the personal story that explains how and, to some extent, why help is needed now. Mental-health problems almost invariably develop from a mixture of causes – emotional, social, physical and familial – and it helps psychiatrists to know

what the people they see are normally like and what kind of lives they have led. These questions may seem unnecessarily intrusive, but they allow psychiatrists to understand patients' problems and decide on the best way to help them.

The next stage in assessment is the mental-state examination. This is how psychiatrists examine minds, or at least their current state. Mental-state examination entails asking more questions and using careful observation to assess feelings, thoughts and mental symptoms, as well as the way the mind is working (for example, in terms of memory and concentration). During first consultations psychiatrists usually make diagnoses and explain them. The boundary between a life problem that will clear up spontaneously and a mental illness that needs treatment is sometimes quite blurred; one consultation may be enough to put the problem in perspective and help to solve it.

Further assessment in the clinic may be needed, or some additional tests. Simple blood tests can be done in outpatient clinics but other investigations will mean referral to another department, usually on another day.

Further assessment and tests

PSYCHOLOGICAL TESTS Psychologists work in or alongside the psychiatric team, helping in both assessment and treatment. The range of psychological tests studies memory, intelligence, personality, perception and capability for abstract thinking.

PHYSICAL TESTS Blood tests and brain scans may be useful to rule out a physical illness causing psychological symptoms.

SOCIAL ASSESSMENT Many patients have social difficulties that can be teased out and helped by a psychiatric social worker. 'Approved social workers' have special training in the use of the Mental Health Act, the law that authorises compulsory admissions to psychiatric hospitals and compulsory psychiatric treatments. These social workers also know about all the mental-health services offered by local councils and voluntary organisations, and can refer clients to them. The role of some social workers has been widened greatly in recent years by the expansion of community care.

OCCUPATIONAL THERAPY ASSESSMENT Mental-health problems causing practical disabilities – for instance, inability to work, cook or look after oneself – can be assessed and helped by occupational therapists.

Treatment The aims of psychiatric treatment are to help sufferers shake off, or at least cope with, symptoms and to gain or regain an acceptable quality of life. A range of psychological and physical treatments is available.

COUNSELLING This is a widely used 'talking cure', particularly in general practice. Counsellors listen to their clients, help them to explore feelings, and help them to find personal and practical solutions to their problems. Counsellors do not probe into clients' pasts or analyse them.

PSYCHOTHERAPY This is the best known 'talking cure'. The term psychotherapy is a generalisation covering many different concepts. They all started, however, with Sigmund Freud (see FREUDIAN THEORY), the father of modern psychotherapy. Freud was a doctor who discovered that, as well as the conscious thoughts that guide our feelings and actions, there are powerful psychological forces of which we are not usually aware. Applying his theories to his patients' freely expressed thoughts, Freud was able to cure many illnesses, some of which had been presumed completely physical. This was the beginning of individual analytical psychotherapy, or PSYCHOANALYSIS. Although Freud's principles underpin all subsequent theories about the psyche, many different schools of thought have emerged and influenced psychotherapists (see ADLER; JUNGIAN ANALYSIS; PSYCHOTHERAPY).

BEHAVIOUR THERAPY This springs from theories of human behaviour, many of which are based on studies of animals. The therapists, mostly psychologists, help people to look at problematic patterns of behaviour and thought, and to change them. Cognitive therapy is very effective, particularly in depression and eating disorders.

PHYSICAL TREATMENTS The most widely used physical treatments in psychiatry are drugs. Tranquillising and anxiety-reducing BENZO-DIAZEPINES like diazepam, well known by its trade name of Valium, were prescribed widely in the 1960s and 70s because they seemed an effective and safe substitute for barbiturates. Benzodiazepines are, however, addictive and are now recommended only for short-term relief of anxiety that is severe, disabling, or unacceptably distressing. They are also used for short-term treatment of patients drying out from alcohol.

ANTIDEPRESSANT DRUGS like amitriptyline and fluoxetine are given to lift depressed mood and to relieve the physical symptoms that sometimes occur in depression, such as insomnia and poor appetite. The side-effects of antidepressants are mostly relatively mild, when recom-mended doses are not exceeded – although one group, the monoamine oxidase inhibitors, can lead to sudden and dangerous high blood pressure if taken with certain foods.

Manic depression virtually always has to be treated with mood-stabilising drugs. Lithium carbonate is used in acute mania to lower mood and stop psychotic symptoms; it can also be used in severe depression. However lithium's main use is to prevent relapse in manic depression. Long-term unwanted effects may include kidney and thyroid problems, and short-term problems in the nervous system and kidney may occur if the blood concentration of lithium is too high – therefore it must be monitored by regular blood tests. Carbamazepine, a treatment for EPILEPSY, has also been found to stabilise mood, and also necessitates blood tests.

Antipsychotic drugs, also called neuroleptics, and major tranquillisers are the only effective treatments for relieving serious mental illnesses with hallucinations and delusions. They are used mainly in schizophrenia and include the short-acting drugs chlorpromazine and clozapine as well as the long-lasting injections given once every few weeks like fluphenazine decanoate. In the long term, however, some of the older antipsychotic drugs can cause a brain problem called TARDIVE DYSKINESIA that affects control of movement and is not always reversible. And the antipsychotic drugs' short-term side-effects such as shaking and stiffness sometimes have to be counteracted by other drugs called anticholinergic drugs such as procyclidine and benzhexol. Newer antipsychotic drugs such as clozapine do not cause tardive dyskinesia, but clozapine cannot be given as a long-lasting injection and its concentration in the body has to be monitored by regular blood tests to avoid toxicity.

OTHER PHYSICAL TREATMENTS The other two physical treatments used in psychiatry are particularly controversial: electroconvulsive therapy (ECT) and psychosurgery. In ECT, which can be life-saving for patients who have severe life-threatening depression, a small electric current is passed through the brain to induce a fit or seizure. Before the treatment the patient is anaesthetised and given a muscle-relaxing injection that reduces the magnitude of the fit to a slight twitching or shaking. Scientists do not really understand how ECT works, but it does, for carefully selected patients. Psychosurgery – operating on the brain to alleviate psychiatric illness or difficult personality traits – is extremely uncommon these days. Stereo-tactic surgery, in which small cuts are made in specific brain fibres under X-ray guidance, has superseded the more generalised lobotomies of old. The Mental Health Act 1983 ensures that psychosurgery is performed only when the patient has given fully informed consent and a second medical opinion has agreed that it is necessary. For all other psychiatric treatments (except another rare treatment, hormone implantation for reducing the sex drive of sex offenders), either consent or a second opinion is needed – not both.

TREATMENT IN HOSPITAL Psychiatric wards do not look like medical or surgical wards and staff may not wear uniforms. Patients do not need to be in their beds during the day, so the beds are in separate dormitories. The main part of most wards is a living space with a day room, an activity and television room, quiet rooms, a dining room, and a kitchen. Ward life usually has a certain routine. The day often starts with a community meeting at which patients and nurses discuss issues that affect the whole ward. Patients may go to the occupational therapy department during the day, but there may also be some therapy groups on the ward, such as relaxation training. Patients' symptoms and problems are assessed continuously during a stay in hospital. When patients seem well enough they are allowed home for trial periods; then discharge can be arranged. Patients are usually followed up in the outpatient clinic at least once.

TREATING PATIENTS WITH ACUTE PSYCHIATRIC ILLNESS Psychiatric emergencies – patients with acute psychiatric illness – may develop from psychological, physical, or practical crises. Any of these crises may need quick professional intervention. Relatives and friends often have to get this urgent help because the sufferer is not fit enough to do it or, if psychotic, does not recognise the need. First, they should ring the person's general practitioner. If the general practitioner is not available and help is needed very urgently, relatives or friends should phone the local social-services department and ask for the duty social worker (on 24-hour call). In a dire emergency, the police will know what to do.

Any disturbed adult who threatens his or her own or others' health and safety and refuses psychiatric help may be moved and detained by law. The Mental Health Act of 1983 authorises emergency assessment and treatment of any person with apparent psychiatric problems that fulfil these criteria.

Although admission to hospital may be the best solution, there are other ways that psychiatric services can respond to emergencies. In some districts there are 'crisis intervention' teams of psychiatrists, nurses, and social work-

ers who can visit patients urgently at home (at a GP's request) and, sometimes, avert unnecessary admission. And research has shown that home treatment for a range of acute psychiatric problems can be effective.

LONG-TERM TREATMENT AND COMMUNITY CARE Long-term treatment is often provided by GPs with support and guidance from psychiatric teams. That is fine for people whose problems allow them to look after themselves, and for those with plenty of support from family and friends. But some people need much more intensive long-term treatment and many need help with running their daily lives.

Since the 1950s, successive governments have closed the old psychiatric hospitals and have tried to provide as much care as possible outside hospital – in 'the community'. Community care is effective as long as everyone who needs inpatient care, or residential care, can have it. But demand exceeds supply. Research has shown that some homeless people have long-term mental illnesses and have somehow lost touch with psychiatric services. Many more have developed more general long-term health problems, particularly related to alcohol, without ever getting help.

The NHS and Community Care Act 1990, in force since 1993, established a new breed of professionals called care managers to assess people whose long-term illnesses and disabilities make them unable to cope completely independently with life. Care managers are given budgets by local councils to assess people's needs and to arrange for them tailor-made packages of care, including services like home helps and day centres. But co-ordination between health and social services has sometimes failed – and resources are limited – and the government decided in 1997 to tighten up arrangements and pool community-care budgets.

Since 1992 psychiatrists have had to ensure that people with severe mental illnesses have full programmes of care set up before discharge from hospital, to be overseen by named key workers. And since 1996 psychiatrists have used a new power called Supervised Discharge to ensure that the most vulnerable patients cannot lose touch with mental-health services. There is not, however, any law that allows compulsory treatment in the community.

There is ample evidence that community care can work and that it need not cost more than hospital care. Critics argue, however, that even one tragedy resulting from inadequate care, perhaps a suicide or even a homicide, should reverse the march to community care. And, according to the National Schizophrenia

Fellowship, many of the 10–15 homicides a year carried out by people with severe mental illnesses result from inadequate community care.

Further information can be obtained from the Mental Health Act Commission, and from MIND, the National Association for Mental Health. MIND also acts as a campaigning and advice organisation on all aspects of mental health.

Mental health problems in children
Emotional and behavioural problems are common in children and adolescents, affecting up to one-fifth at any one time. But these problems are often not clear-cut, and they may come and go as the child develops and meets new challenges in life. If a child or teenager has an emotional problem that persists for weeks rather than days and is associated with disturbed behaviour, he or she may have a recognisable mental health disorder.

Anxiety, phobias and depression are fairly common. For instance, surveys show that up to 2.5 per cent of children and 8 per cent of adolescents are depressed at any one time, and by the age of 18 a quarter will have been depressed at least once. Problems such as OBSESSIVE COMPULSIVE DISORDER, ATTENTION DEFICIT DISORDER (HYPERACTIVITY SYNDROME), AUTISM, ASPERGER'S SYNDROME and SCHIZOPHRENIA are rare.

Mental-health problems may not be obvious at first, because children often express distress through irritability, poor concentration, difficult behaviour, or physical symptoms. Physical symptoms of distress, such as unexplained headache and stomach ache, may persuade parents to keep children at home on school days. This may be appropriate occasionally, but regularly avoiding school can lead to a persistent phobia called school refusal.

If a parent, teacher or other person is worried that a child or teenager may have a mental-health problem, the first thing to do is to ask the child gently if he or she is worried about anything. Listening, reassuring and helping the child to solve any specific problems may well be enough to help the child feel settled again. Serious problems such as bullying and child abuse need urgent professional involvement.

Children with emotional problems will usually feel most comfortable talking to their parents, while adolescents may prefer to talk to friends, counsellors, or other mentors. If this doesn't work, and if the symptoms persist for weeks rather than days, it may be necessary to seek additional help through school or the family's general practitioner. This may lead to the child and family being assessed and helped by a psychologist, or, less commonly, by a child psychiatrist. Again, listening and counselling will be the main forms of help offered. For outright depression, COGNITIVE BEHAVIOUR THERAPY and, rarely, antidepressant drugs may be used.

Mepacrine Hydrochloride
A synthetic acridine product used in the treatment of MALARIA. It came to the fore during World War II, when supplies of quinine were short, and proved of great value both as a prophylactic and in the treatment of malaria. It is now used only to treat infestation with tapeworms (see TAENIASIS).

Meralgia Paraesthetica
A condition characterised by pain and PARAESTHESIA on the front and outer aspect of the thigh. It is more common in men than in women, and the victims are usually middle-aged, overweight and out of condition. It is due to compression of the lateral cutaneous nerve of the thigh, and exacerbated by an uncomfortable driving position when motoring long distances. Reduction in weight, improvement in general fitness and correction of faulty posture usually bring relief. If these fail, surgical decompression of the nerve may help.

Mercaptopurine
One of the antimetabolite group of drugs (see ANTIMETABOLITES), which includes methotrexate, fluorouracil and thioguanine. These drugs are incorporated into new nuclear material in the cell or combine irreversibly with vital cellular enzymes, preventing normal cellular metabolism and division. Mercaptopurine is used mainly for the maintenance treatment of acute LEUKAEMIA, though it is increasingly proving valuable in the treatment of CROHN'S DISEASE. As with all CYTOTOXIC drugs, dosage must be carefully controlled; in particular it must be reduced if used concurrently with allopurinol. Side-effects include gastrointestinal upsets (including ulceration), and bone-marrow depression.

Mercury
Mercury is a heavy fluid metal which, with its salts, has been used in medicine for many centuries.

Uses In the past, mercuric salts were used as ANTISEPTICS, anti-parasitic agents and fungicides. Mercury has been widely used in dental amalgams for filling teeth. Because of their toxicity, mercury compounds must not be taken internally.

Mercury has traditionally been used in thermometers for recording body temperature, and in sphygmomanometers for measuring a person's BLOOD PRESSURE. These instruments have been largely replaced in the UK by electronic devices that do not require mercury.

Mesalazine
An aminosalicylate drug used for the treatment of mild to moderate ULCERATIVE COLITIS and the maintenance of remission. It should be used with caution by pregnant women.

Mescaline
Derived from the Mexican peyote cactus, *Anhalonium lewinii*, this is a hallucinogen used for many centuries by Indian tribes in Mexico as an intoxicant to produce ecstatic states for religious celebrations. In recent times its ability to produce temporary psychotic symptoms has been used to investigate the mechanism of PSYCHOSIS. Mescaline has similar effects to those of LSD: changes in mood and thought, illusions, self-absorption and an altered perception of time. Experience of the drug may subsequently provoke panic attacks, deliberate self-injury, real psychosis and sometimes addiction (see DEPENDENCE).

Mesencephalon
The small section of brain stem – excluding the pons and medulla – linking the hindbrain to the forebrain. (See BRAIN.)

Mesentery
Mesentery is the double layer of peritoneal membrane which supports the small INTESTINE. It is of a fan shape, and its shorter edge is attached to the back wall of the abdomen for a distance of about 15 cm (6 inches), while the small intestine lies within its longer edge, for a length of over 6 metres (20 feet). The terms mesocolon, mesorectum, etc., are applied to similar folds of PERITONEUM that support parts of the colon, rectum, etc.

Mesmerism
See HYPNOTISM.

Mesocolon
The double fold of PERITONEUM by which the large INTESTINE is suspended from the back wall of the abdomen.

Mesoderm
The middle layer of the three germ layers of the EMBRYO during its early development. It develops into cartilage, bone, blood, muscle, kidneys, testes and connective tissue.

Mesothelioma
A malignant tumour of the PLEURA, the membrane lining the chest cavity. The condition is more common in people exposed to asbestos dust. It may be asymptomatic or cause pain, cough, and breathing troubles. Surgery or radiotherapy may be effective but often the disease has spread too far before it is discovered. Mesothelioma incurred as a result of contact with asbestos at work may attract industrial COMPENSATION.

Meta-Analysis
A development of systematic reviews of randomised, controlled trials in particular fields of health care. If this re-evaluation of the findings of primary research also includes the aggregation of data from all the re-evaluated studies and a re-analysis of them, the procedure is described as meta-analysis. The technique has been used increasingly in medicine in recent years, and the COCHRANE COLLABORATION has been in the forefront of systematically reviewing and storing clinical and research data to provide a reliable information base on which to take forward the practice of EVIDENCE-BASED MEDICINE. Bias in medical research – because, say, of an inadequately planned statistical base or only small numbers in a trial – is not uncommon, and meta-analysis of a group of broadly similar trials can provide more reliable data and reduce the risk of erroneous conclusions.

Metabolic Disorders
A collection of disorders in which some part of the body's internal chemistry (see METABOLISM; CATABOLISM) is disrupted. Some of these disorders arise from inherited deficiencies in which a specific ENZYME is absent or abnormal, or does not function properly. Other metabolic disorders occur because of malfunctions in the endocrine system (see ENDOCRINE GLANDS). There may be over- or underproduction of a hormone involved in the control of metabolic activities: a prime example is DIABETES MELLITUS – a disorder of sugar metabolism; others include CUSHING'S SYNDROME; hypothyroidism and hyperthyroidism (see THYROID GLAND, DISEASES OF); and insulinoma (an insulin-producing tumour of the pancreas). The bones can be affected by metabolic disorders such as osteoporosis, osteomalacia (rickets) and

Paget's disease (see under BONE, DISORDERS OF). PORPHYRIAS, HYPERLIPIDAEMIA, HYPERCAL-CAEMIA and gout are other examples of disordered metabolism.

There are also more than 200 identified disorders described as inborn errors of metabolism. Some cause few problems; others are serious threats to an individual's life. Individual disorders are, fortunately, rare – probably one child in 10,000 or 100,000; overall these inborn errors affect around one child in 1,000. Examples include GALACTOSAEMIA, PHENYL-KETONURIA, porphyrias, TAY SACHS DISEASE and varieties of mucopolysaccharidosis, HOMOCYSTINURIA and hereditary fructose (a type of sugar) intolerance.

Metabolism
This means tissue change, and includes all the physical and chemical processes by which the living body is maintained – as well as those by which the energy is made available for various forms of work. The constructive, chemical and physical, processes by which food materials are adapted for the use of the body are collectively known as ANABOLISM. The destructive processes by which energy is produced with the breaking-down of tissues into waste products is known as CATABOLISM. Basal metabolism is the term applied to the energy changes necessary for essential processes such as the beating of the heart, respiration, and maintenance of body warmth. This can be estimated, when a person is placed in a state of complete rest, by measuring the amounts of oxygen and carbon dioxide exchanged during breathing under certain standard conditions. (See also CALORIE.)

Metabolites
A biochemical compound that is involved in the mechanism of the body's METABOLISM. The compounds are either produced during metabolism or are in the food eaten by an individual.

Metacarpal Bones
The five long bones which occupy the HAND between the carpal bones at the wrist and the phalanges of the fingers. The large rounded 'knuckles' at the root of the fingers are formed by the heads of these bones.

Metamyelocyte
An immature granulocyte (white blood cell) usually found in the bone marrow's blood-making tissue. It can, however, appear in the blood in a range of diseases, including infection.

Metaphysis
The extremity of a long bone where it joins the epiphysis (see BONE – Growth of bones).

Metaplasia
The term applied to a change of one kind of tissue into another. Although not usually harmful, it may be pre-cancerous if occurring in the cervix (neck of the womb or UTERUS), URINARY BLADDER, or lining of the airways (bronchi).

Metastasis
Metastasis, and metastatic, are terms applied to the process by which malignant disease spreads to distant parts of the body, and also to the secondary tumours resulting from this process. For example, a cancer of the breast may produce metastatic growths in the glands of the armpit; cancer of the stomach may be followed by metastases in the liver. Metastases are colloquially known as secondaries and their spread occurs through the bloodstream, lymphatic system and across the body cavities. Highly malignant tumours – for example, melanomas – are especially prone to spread far and fast. (See CANCER.)

Metastatic
See METASTASIS.

Metatarsal Bones
The five bones in the foot which correspond to the METACARPAL BONES in the hand, lying between the tarsal bones, at the ankle, and the toes.

Metatarsalgia
Pain affecting the metatarsal region of the foot. It is common in adolescents, and associated with FLAT-FOOT; in adults it may be a manifestation of RHEUMATOID ARTHRITIS. Morton's metatarsalgia is a form associated usually with the nerve to the second toe cleft, often induced by the compression of tight shoes.

Metatarsus
Metatarsus is the group name of the five metatarsal bones in the foot. Metatarsus varus is the condition characterised by deviation of the forefoot towards the other foot. It is a common condition in newborn babes and almost always corrects itself spontaneously. Only in the rare cases in which it is due to some deformity of the bones or muscles of the foot is any treatment required.

Meteorism
Also known as tympanites, this is a distension

of the ABDOMEN from excess gas or air in the INTESTINE or peritoneal cavity. On percussion the abdomen sounds resonant, like a drum. Causes include obstruction of the intestines, aerophagy (the swallowing of air), and IRRITABLE BOWEL SYNDROME (IBS). Treatment is of the underlying condition. (See also FLATULENCE.)

Metformin

One of the BIGUANIDES, metformin lowers the blood sugar by increasing cellular uptake of glucose. It is active when taken by mouth and is used to treat some patients with DIABETES MELLITUS, usually in addition to another hypoglycaemic drug.

Methadone Hydrochloride

Also known as Physeptone®, this is a synthetic drug structurally similar to MORPHINE, one of many opioid drugs used to treat severe pain. Methadone is, however, less sedating and has a longer half-life. Furthermore, it is more reliable when taken orally. Although vomiting is common, this is generally less severe than with morphine.

Methadone is valuable as a suppressant for non-productive cough, acting on the medullary 'cough centre' in the central nervous system. It is also helpful in weaning addicts off morphine and heroin, having a slower onset of DEPENDENCE and a less severe withdrawal syndrome. When used for prolonged periods, methadone should not be given more often than twice daily, to avoid the risks of accumulation and opioid overdosage.

Methaemoglobin

A derivative of HAEMOGLOBIN in which the iron has been oxidised from ferrous to ferric form. It does not combine with oxygen and therefore plays no part in oxygen transport. Normal concentration of methaemoglobin in red blood cells is less than 1 per cent of the total haemoglobin. When a large concentration of the haemoglobin is in the form of methaemoglobin, the patient will suffer from HYPOXIA and will be cyanosed (see CYANOSIS). Most cases of METHAEMOGLOBINAEMIA are due to chemical agents.

Methaemoglobinaemia

Methaemoglobinaemia is a condition due to the presence in the blood of METHAEMOGLOBIN. It is characterised by CYANOSIS which turns the skin and lips a blue colour, shortness of breath, headache, fatigue and sickness. There are two main forms: a hereditary form and a toxic form. The latter is caused by certain drugs, including acetanilide, phenacetin, the sulphonamides and benzocaine. The treatment of the toxic form is the withdrawal of the causative drug. In the more severe cases the administration of methylene blue or ascorbic acid may also be needed, and these are the drugs used in the hereditary form.

Methane

An odourless, colourless, highly flammable gas. It occurs naturally in gas from coal mines and oil wells, where it is a hazard because of its explosive properties. 'Natural' gas supplied to homes and industries is almost 100 per cent methane. Unlike coal gas, it is not poisonous unless present in large amounts, when it may displace oxygen and thus asphyxiate (suffocate) anyone exposed to it. Decomposition of organic matter produces methane.

Methanol

A variety of ALCOHOL used as a solvent to remove paint or as a constituent of some antifreeze fluids. It is poisonous: sometimes people drink it as a substitute for ethyl (ordinary) alcohol. Symptoms appear up to 24 hours after imbibing methanol and include nausea, vomiting, dizziness, headache and sometimes unconsciousness. Treatment is to induce vomiting (in conscious victims) and to do a stomach washout (see GASTRIC LAVAGE), but such steps must be taken within two hours of ingestion. Hospital treatment is usually required, when intravenous infusion of sodium bicarbonate (and sometimes ethanol, which slows up breakdown of methanol by the liver) is administered.

Methicillin-Resistant Staphylococcus Aureus (MRSA)

Most staphylococci (see STAPHYLOCOCCUS) have now evolved resistance to benzylpenicillin (see PENICILLIN) because of their ability to produce PENICILLINASE. Cloxacillin and flucloxacillin are antibiotics still effective against most staphylococci; at one time methicillin was used to combat resistant strains, but in hospital environments bacteria acquired immunity to this powerful drug (now withdrawn from use) and to cloxacillin. RIFAMPICIN, VANCOMYCIN, TEICOPLANIN and temocillin are still active against most penicillinase-producing gram-negative bacteria (see GRAM'S STAIN). There is, however, a growing threat to health because of the rise in the number of antibiotic-resistant bacteria, particularly in hospitals. The bacteria themselves are not more virulent than others, but the difficulty in treating them with a safe and effective antibiotic mean that they are more dangerous. It is likely that lapses in normal hygienic practice – such as frequent hand-washing – has resulted in an increase in MRSA disease.

Methionine

Methionine is an essential amino acid (see AMINO ACIDS; INDISPENSABLE AMINO ACIDS) that contains sulphur; it is necessary for normal growth in infants and to maintain nitrogen balance in adults.

Methotrexate

One of the ANTIMETABOLITES used to treat certain forms of malignant disease. Acting to inhibit the ENZYME dihydrofolate reductase, which is essential for purine and pyrimidine synthesis, it is given orally, intravenously, intramuscularly or intrathecally. Methotrexate is used as maintenance therapy for childhood acute lymphoblastic LEUKAEMIA, while other uses include CHORIOCARCINOMA, non-Hodgkin's LYMPHOMA, and various solid tumours. Intrathecally, it is used in the prophylaxis of childhood acute lymphoblastic leukaemia, and as treatment for established meningeal cancer or lymphoma.

Side-effects include suppression of myelocytes in bone marrow, inflammation of mucous membranes, and, rarely, PNEUMONITIS. It should be avoided whenever significant renal impairment is present, while significant pleural effusion or ascites is also a contraindication. Blood counts should be carefully monitored whenever intrathecal methotrexate is given. Oral or parenteral folinic acid helps to prevent, or to speed recovery from, myelosuppression or mucositis.

Methotrexate is used in dermatology, where it may be indicated for cases of severe uncontrolled PSORIASIS unresponsive to conventional therapy; it may also be indicated for severe active RHEUMATOID ARTHRITIS. Because of its potentially severe haematological, pulmonary, gastrointestinal, and other toxicities it should be used only by specialists and appropriate renal and liver function tests carried out before and during treatment. It should be avoided in pregnancy, and conception should be avoided for at least six months after stopping, as should breast feeding. Concurrent administration of aspirin or other NON-STEROIDAL ANTI-INFLAMMATORY DRUGS (NSAIDS) reduces methotrexate excretion, increasing its toxicity, and should therefore be avoided whenever possible.

Methyl

Methyl is an organic radical whose chemical formula is CH_3, and which forms the centre of a wide group of substances known as the methyl group. For example, methyl alcohol is obtained as a by-product in the manufacture of beet-sugar, or by distillation of wood; methyl salicylate is the active constituent in oil of wintergreen; methyl hydride is better known as marsh gas.

Methyl alcohol, or wood spirit (see METHANOL), is distilled from wood and is thus a cheap form of alcohol. It has actions similar to, but much more toxic than, those of ethyl alcohol. It has a specially pronounced action on the nervous system, and in large doses is apt to cause neuritis, especially of the optic nerves, leading to blindness, partial or complete.

Methylbenzene

See TOLUENE.

Methylcellulose

A COLLOID which absorbs water to swell to about 25 times its original volume. It is used in the treatment of CONSTIPATION and also in the management of OBESITY. The rationale for its use in obesity is that by swelling up in the stomach, it reduces the appetite.

Methyldopa

A centrally acting anti-hypertensive (see HYPERTENSION) drug often used in conjunction with a diuretic (see DIURETICS). It can be effective in controlling high blood pressure in pregnancy. The drug is also safe to use in patients with ASTHMA or heart failure.

Methylene Blue

Methylene blue, or methylthionin chloride, is used in a dose of 75–100 mg, as a 1-per-cent intravenous injection, in the treatment of METHAEMOGLOBINAEMIA, which may occur following high doses of local anaesthetics such as prilocaine.

Methylphenidate

A drug that stimulates the CENTRAL NERVOUS SYSTEM. Its action is similar to DEXAMPHETAMINE. A controlled drug, one of its trade names is Ritalin® and it is (controversially) used in the treatment of ATTENTION DEFICIT DISORDER (HYPERACTIVITY SYNDROME) in children, in conjunction with behavioural treatment and family support. Because of the potential for side-effects, its administration should be under specialist supervision.

Methylprednisolone

A mineralcorticoid drug (see CORTICO-STEROIDS) with an action comparable to that of PREDNISOLONE, but effective at a somewhat lower dose.

Methyl Salicylate

Also called oil of Wintergreen, the liquid has analgesic (see ANALGESICS) and counter-irritant properties. Rubbed into the skin, the oil helps to relieve pain in LUMBAGO, SCIATICA and 'rheumatic conditions'.

Methysergide

A drug used to prevent attacks of MIGRAINE. The drug requires hospital supervision, as it has to be used with care because of the toxic effects it sometimes produces – for example, nausea, drowsiness and retroperitoneal FIBROSIS.

Metoclopramide

This drug antagonises the actions of DOPA-MINE. Given orally, intramuscularly, or intravenously, it is used to treat nausea and vomiting, particularly in gastrointestinal disorders, or when associated with cytotoxics or radiotherapy. It is useful in the early treatment of MIGRAINE.

Caution is indicated in prescribing metoclopramide for elderly and young patients, and whenever hepatic or renal impairment is present, and it should be avoided in pregnancy or cases of PORPHYRIAS. Adverse effects include extrapyramidal effects (see under EXTRAPYRAMIDAL SYSTEM) and HYPERPROLACTINAEMIA with occasional TARDIVE DYSKINESIA on prolonged administration. There have also been occasional reports of drowsiness, restlessness, diarrhoea, depression and neuroleptic malignant syndrome, with rare cardiac conduction abnormalities following intravenous administration.

Metolazone

A thiazide-type diuretic (see THIAZIDES; DIURETICS) which is particularly effective when combined with a loop diuretic (see LOOP DIURETICS), when it produces profound diuresis. The drug is also useful for treating kidney stones (see under KIDNEYS, DISEASES OF).

Metoprolol

A beta-adrenergic-receptor blocking agent. (See ADRENERGIC RECEPTORS.)

Metre

The basic unit of length in the modern version of the metric system, known as the International System of Units (SI). It is equivalent to 39·37 inches.

Metritis

Inflammation of the uterus (see UTERUS, DISEASES OF).

Metronidazole

An antimicrobial drug particularly active against anaerobic (see ANAEROBE) bacteria and PROTOZOA. Given by mouth, by rectum or intravenously, it is used to treat infections of the urinary, genital, and digestive systems – for example, TRICHOMONIASIS, amoebiasis (see DYSENTERY), GIARDIASIS, and acute ulcerative GINGIVITIS, and is a useful treatment for dental abscesses. Topically, it is used in the management of ROSACEA and it reduces the odour produced by anaerobic bacteria in fungating tumours.

It may cause a DISULFIRAM-like reaction with alcohol; caution is similarly indicated in patients with impaired liver function or hepatic encephalopathy, and who are pregnant or breast feeding. Rare side-effects include nausea, vomiting, unpleasant taste, furred tongue and gastrointestinal disturbances; rashes, URTICARIA, and angio-oedema (see under URTICARIA); drowsiness, headache, dizziness, ATAXIA and ANAPHYLAXIS.

Metropathia Haemorrhagica

A disorder characterised by irregular bouts of uterine (see UTERUS) bleeding – without previous OVULATION – due to excessive oestrogenic activity. It is associated with endometrial hyperplasia and cysts of the ovary.

Metrorrhagia

Uterine (see UTERUS) bleeding otherwise than at the proper period (see MENSTRUATION). It is usually due to a uterine lesion and should be investigated.

Metyrapone

Metyrapone is a drug that inhibits the production of CORTISOL in the adrenal cortex, which results in an increase in ACTH production and (completing the feedback control cycle) thus greater synthesis of the chemical precursors of cortisol. Metyrapone is used to treat patients with CUSHING'S SYNDROME (a condition caused by excess amounts of corticosteroid hormones in the body) where surgery is not possible.

Miconazole

One of the IMIDAZOLES group of antifungals which includes clotrimazole and ketoconazole. Active against a wide range of fungi and yeasts, their main indications are vaginal candidiasis and dermatophyte skin infections. Miconazole is used as a cream or ointment; it may also be given orally (for oral or gastrointestinal infections), or parenterally (for systemic infections such as aspergillosis or candidiasis). (See MYCOSIS.)

Microangiopathy
Disease of the CAPILLARIES.

Microbe
See BACTERIA; MICROBIOLOGY.

Microbicides
Gels or creams, currently under investigation, designed to reduce the risk of anal or vaginal transmission of viruses such as HIV (see also AIDS/HIV). The aim is to kill or to inactivate the virus, creating a barrier to mucosal cells or preventing the infection from taking hold after it has entered the body. Large-scale trials were launched in Africa in 2004, using dextrin sulphate and PRO-2000 gel.

Microbiology
The study of all aspects of micro-organisms (microbes) – that is, organisms which individually are generally too small to be visible other than by microscopy. The term is applicable to viruses (see VIRUS), BACTERIA, and microscopic forms of fungi, algae, and PROTOZOA.

Among the smallest and simplest micro-organisms are the viruses. First described as filterable agents, and ranging in size from 20–30 nm to 300 nm, they may be directly visualised only by electron microscopy. They consist of a core of deoxyribonucleic or ribonucleic acid (DNA or RNA) within a protective protein coat, or capsid, whose subunits confer a geometric symmetry. Thus viruses are usually cubical (icosahedral) or helical; the larger viruses (pox-, herpes-, myxo-viruses) may also have an outer envelope. Their minimal structure dictates that viruses are all obligate parasites, relying on living cells to provide essential components for their replication. Apart from animal and plant cells, viruses may infect and replicate in bacteria (bacteriophages) or fungi (mycophages), which are damaged in the process.

Bacteria are larger (0·01–5,000 μm) and more complex. They have a subcellular organisation which generally includes DNA and RNA, a cell membrane, organelles such as ribosomes, and a complex and chemically variable cell envelope – but, unlike EUKARYOTES, no nucleus. Rickettsiae, chlamydia, and mycoplasmas, once thought of as viruses because of their small size and absence of a cell wall (mycoplasma) or major wall component (chlamydia), are now acknowledged as bacteria; rickettsiae and chlamydia are intracellular parasites of medical importance. Bacteria may also possess additional surface structures, such as capsules and organs of locomotion (flagella) and attachment (fimbriae and stalks). Individual bacterial cells may be spheres (cocci); straight (bacilli), curved (vibrio), or flexuous (spirilla) rods; or oval cells (coccobacilli). On examination by light microscopy, bacteria may be visible in characteristic configurations (as pairs of cocci [diplococci], or chains [streptococci], or clusters); actinomycete bacteria grow as filaments with externally produced spores. Bacteria grow essentially by increasing in cell size and dividing by fission, a process which in ideal laboratory conditions some bacteria may achieve about once every 20 minutes. Under natural conditions, growth is usually much slower.

Eukaryotic micro-organisms comprise fungi, algae, and protozoa. These organisms are larger, and they have in common a well-developed internal compartmentation into subcellular organelles; they also have a nucleus. Algae additionally have chloroplasts, which contain photosynthetic pigments; fungi lack chloroplasts; and protozoa lack both a cell wall and chloroplasts but may have a contractile vacuole to regulate water uptake and, in some, structures for capturing and ingesting food. Fungi grow either as discrete cells (yeasts), multiplying by budding, fission, or conjugation, or as thin filaments (hyphae) which bear spores, although some may show both morphological forms during their life-cycle. Algae and protozoa generally grow as individual cells or colonies of individuals and multiply by fission.

Micro-organisms of medical importance include representatives of the five major microbial groups that obtain their essential nutrients at the expense of their hosts. Many bacteria and most fungi, however, are saprophytes (see SAPROPHYTE), being major contributors to the natural cycling of carbon in the environment and to biodeterioration; others are of ecological and economic importance because of the diseases they cause in agricultural or horticultural crops or because of their beneficial relationships with higher organisms. Additionally, they may be of industrial or biotechnological importance. Fungal diseases of humans tend to be most important in tropical environments and in immuno-compromised subjects.

Pathogenic (that is, disease-causing) micro-organisms have special characteristics, or virulence factors, that enable them to colonise their hosts and overcome or evade physical, biochemical, and immunological host defences. For example, the presence of capsules, as in the bacteria that cause anthrax (*Bacillus anthracis*), one form of pneumonia (*Streptococcus pneumoniae*), scarlet fever (*S. pyogenes*), bacterial meningitis (*Neisseria meningitidis, Haemophilus influenzae*) is directly related to the ability to cause disease because of their antiphagocytic properties. Fimbriae are related to virulence, enabling tissue attachment – for example, in gonorrhoea (*N. gonorrhoeae*) and cholera (*Vibrio cholerae*). Many bacteria excrete extracellular virulence factors; these include enzymes and other agents that impair the host's physiological and immunological functions. Some bacteria produce powerful toxins (excreted exotoxins or endogenous endotoxins), which may cause local tissue destruction and allow colonisation by the pathogen or whose specific action may explain the disease mechanism. In *Staphylococcus aureus*, exfoliative toxin produces the staphylococcal scalded-skin syndrome, TSS toxin-1 toxic-shock syndrome, and enterotoxin food poisoning. The pertussis exotoxin of *Bordetella pertussis*, the cause of whooping cough, blocks immunological defences and mediates attachment to tracheal cells, and the exotoxin produced by *Corynebacterium diphtheriae* causes local damage resulting in a pronounced exudate in the trachea.

Viruses cause disease by cellular destruction arising from their intracellular parasitic existence. Attachment to particular cells is often mediated by specific viral surface proteins; mechanisms for evading immunological defences include latency, change in viral antigenic structure, or incapacitation of the immune system – for example, destruction of CD 4 lymphocytes by the human immunodeficiency virus.

Microcephaly
Abnormal smallness of the head, usually associated with LEARNING DISABILITY. It may occur as a result of infection of the fetus by, for example, RUBELLA (German measles) or from hypoxic damage to the brain before or during birth.

Micrococcus
A spherical gram-positive bacterium (see BACTERIA; GRAM'S STAIN). It occurs in colonies and is usually harmless in humans. However, micrococcus can become pathogenic and cause abscesses (see ABSCESS), ARTHRITIS, ENDOCARDITIS or MENINGITIS.

Microcyte
A small red blood cell.

Microdissection
The technique of dissecting very small structures under a microscope. Miniature surgical instruments are manipulated via geared connections that convert the coarse movements of the surgeon's fingers into miniscule movements, making it possible to dissect and separate even individual CHROMOSOMES.

Microfilaria
The mobile embryo of certain parasitic nematode worms which are found in the blood or lymph of patients infected with filarial worms. The microfilariae develop into larvae in the body of a blood-sucking insect, for example, a mosquito.

Microgram
Microgram is the 1/1,000th part of a milligram. The abreviation for it is μg. (See APPENDIX 6: MEASUREMENTS IN MEDICINE.)

Micrometre
The 1/1,000th part of a millimetre. The abbreviation for it is μm. (See APPENDIX 6: MEASUREMENTS IN MEDICINE.)

Micro-Organism
A very small, single-celled living organism that cannot usually be seen by the naked eye. The most important micro-organisms in medicine are those that cause disease. This 'pathogenic' group, however, forms only a small proportion of the enormous number of known micro-organisms. The main pathogenic ones are BACTERIA. Others are fungi and RICKETTSIA. Though not true cells, viruses (see VIRUS) are usually classified as micro-organisms. (See also MICROBIOLOGY.)

Micropsia
Condition in which objects appear smaller than normal. It can be due to disease of the macula of the EYE.

Microscope
An optical instrument comprising adjustable magnifying lenses that greatly enlarge a small object under study – for example, an insect, blood cells, or bacteria. Some microscopes use electron beams to magnify minute objects such as chromosomes, crystals, or even large molecules. Optical microscopes are also used for MICROSURGERY when the area being operated on is otherwise inaccessible: for example, in eye

and inner ear surgery; for the removal of tumours from the brain or spinal cord; and for resuturing damaged blood vessels and nerves.

Microsporum

One of the three genera of dermatophytes (fungi) which cause tinea (see RINGWORM). Microsporum of human or animal origin is an important cause of tinea capitis, or ringworm of the scalp.

Microsurgery

The conduct of very intricate surgical operations using specially refined operating microscopes (see MICROSCOPE) and miniaturised precision instruments – for example, forceps, scalpels, scissors, etc. Microsurgery is used in previously inaccessible areas of the brain, eye, inner ear and spinal cord, as well as in the suturing of severed nerves and small blood vessels following traumatic injuries to the limbs or fingers. The technique is also used to reverse VASECTOMY.

Microtome

A laboratory instrument for cutting sections of biological tissues for study under a MICROSCOPE. It is widely used in biological and PATHOLOGY laboratories.

Microwaves

Non-ionising electro-magnetic radiations in the frequency range of 30–300,000 megahertz. They are emitted from electronic devices, such as heaters, some domestic ovens, television receivers, radar units and DIATHERMY units. There is no scientific evidence to justify the claims that they are harmful to humans, or that they produce any harmful effect in the GENES. The only known necessary precaution is the protection of the eyes in those using them in industry, as there is some evidence that prolonged exposure to them in this may induce cataract (see EYE, DISORDERS OF).

Micturition

The act of URINATION (see also URINARY BLADDER; URINE).

Middle Ear

That portion of the EAR lying between the TYMPANIC MEMBRANE and the INNER EAR. It contains the ossicles, the three small bones that transmit sound.

Midges

See BITES AND STINGS.

Mid-Life Crisis

A colloquial description of the feelings of anxiety and distress experienced by some individuals in early middle age. They realise that by 45 years of age they are no longer young, and men in particular try to turn the clock back by changing jobs, dressing trendily, taking up energetic or unusual sports or engaging in extramarital liaisons. Sometimes those in mid-life crises develop mild or even serious DEPRESSION. The feelings of anxiety and insecurity usually disappear with time but some people may benefit from counselling.

Midwife

A member of the profession which provides care and advice during pregnancy, supervises the mother's labour and delivery, and looks after her and the baby after birth (see also PREGNANCY AND LABOUR). Should a pregnancy or labour develop complications, the midwife will seek medical advice. Most midwives are registered general nurses who have also done an 18-month course in midwifery. Trained midwives are registered with the UK Central Council for Nursing Midwifery and Health Visiting and work in hospitals or a domiciliary setting. Midwives practise in hospitals, health units or in a domiciliary (home) setting.

Midwifery

See MIDWIFE; PREGNANCY AND LABOUR.

Migraine

The word migraine derives from HEMICRANIA, the Greek for half a skull, and is a common condition characterised by recurring intense headaches. It is much more usual in women than in men and affects around 10 per cent of the population. It has been defined as 'episodic headache accompanied by visual or gastrointestinal disturbances, or both, attacks lasting hours with total freedom between episodes'.

It usually begins at puberty – although young children can be affected – and tends to stop in middle age: in women, for example, attacks often cease after MENOPAUSE. It frequently disappears during pregnancy. The disorder tends to run in families. In susceptible individuals, attacks may be provoked by a wide variety of causes including: anxiety, emotion, depression, shock, and excitement; physical and mental fatigue; prolonged focusing on computer, television or cinema screens; noise, especially loud and high-pitched sounds; certain foods – such as chocolate, cheese, citrus fruits, pastry; alcohol; prolonged lack of food; irregular meals; menstruation and the pre-menstrual period.

Anything that can provoke a headache in the ordinary individual can probably precipitate an attack in a migrainous subject. It seems as if there is an inherited predispostion that triggers a mechanism whereby in the migrainous subject, the headache and the associated sickness persist for hours, a whole day or even longer.

The precise cause is not known, but the generally accepted view is that in susceptible individuals, one or other of these causes produces spasm or constriction of the blood vessels of the brain. This in turn is followed by dilatation of these blood vessels which also become more permeable and so allow fluid to pass out into the surrounding tissues. This combination of dilatation and outpouring of fluid is held to be responsible for the headache.

Two types of migraine have been recognised: classical and common. The former is relatively rare and the headache is preceded by a slowly extending area of blindness in one or both eyes, usually accompanied by intermittent 'lights'. The phenomenon lasts for up to 30 minutes and is followed by a bad, often unilateral headache with nausea, sometimes vomiting and sensitivity to light. Occasionally, passing neurological symptoms such as weakness in a limb may accompany the attack. The common variety has similar but less severe symptoms. It consists of an intense headache, usually situated over one or other eye. The headache is usually preceded by a feeling of sickness and disturbance of sight. In 15–20 per cent of cases this disturbance of sight takes the form of bright lights: the so-called AURA of migraine. The majority of attacks are accompanied by vomiting. The duration of the headache varies, but in the more severe cases the victim is usually confined to bed for 24 hours.

Treatment consists, in the first place, of trying to avoid any precipitating factor. Patients must find out which drug, or drugs, give them most relief, and they must always carry these about with them wherever they go. This is because it is a not uncommon experience to be aware of an attack coming on and to find that there is a critical quarter of an hour or so during which the tablets are effective. If not taken within this period, they may be ineffective and the unfortunate victim finds him or herself prostrate with headache and vomiting. In addition, sufferers should immediately lie down; at this stage a few hours' rest may prevent the development of a full attack.

When an attack is fully developed, rest in bed in a quiet, darkened room is essential; any loud noise or bright light intensifies the headache or sickness. The less food that is taken during an attack the better, provided that the individual drinks as much fluid as he or she wants. Group therapy, in which groups of around ten migrainous subjects learn how to relax, is often of help in more severe cases, whilst in others the injection of a local anaesthetic into tender spots in the scalp reduces the number of attacks. Drug treatment can be effective and those afflicted by migraine may find a particular drug or combination of drugs more suitable than others. ANALGESICS such as PARACETAMOL, aspirin and CODEINE phosphate sometimes help. A combination of buclizine hydrochloride and analgesics, taken when the visual aura occurs, prevents or diminishes the severity of an attack in some people. A commonly used remedy for the condition is ergotamine tartrate, which causes the dilated blood vessels to contract, but this must only be taken under medical supervision. In many cases METOCLOPRAMIDE (an antiemetic), followed ten minutes later by three tablets of either aspirin or paracetamol, is effective if taken early in an attack. In milder attacks, aspirin, with or without codeine and paracetamol, may be of value. SUMATRIPTAN (5-hydroxytryptamine [5HT$_1$] AGONIST – also known as a SEROTONIN agonist) is of value for acute attacks. It is used orally or by subcutaneous injection, but should not be used for patients with ischaemic heart disease. Naratriptan is another 5HT$_1$ agonist that is an effective treatment for acute attacks; others are almotriptan, rizatriptan and zolmitriptan. Some patients find beta blockers such as propranolol a valuable prophylactic.

People with migraine and their relatives can obtain help and guidance from the Migraine Action Association.

Milia
These are small keratin cysts appearing as white papules on the cheek and eyelids.

Miliaria
Also known as prickly heat. An intensely itchy vesicular and erythematous rash induced by intense heat and humidity. It is caused by a disturbance of sweat-gland function.

Miliary
A term, expressing size, applied to various disease products which are about the size of millet seeds: for example, miliary aneurysms, miliary tuberculosis.

Milium
Milium is a pinhead white cyst of the skin of

the face containing corneal cells. It can be removed on the point of a sterile needle.

Milk

The natural food of all mammalia for a considerable period following their birth. It is practically the only form of animal food in which protein, fat, carbohydrate and salt are all represented in sufficient amount, and it therefore contains all the constituents of a standard diet. Milk is important in human nutrition because it contains first-class animal protein of high biological value; because it is exceptionally rich in calcium; and because it is a good source of vitamin A, thiamine and riboflavine. It also contains a variable amount of ascorbic acid (vitamin C) and of vitamin D – the amount of the latter being higher during the summer months than during the winter months. Raw milk yields 67 Calories (see CALORIE) per 100 millilitres, in which are present (in grams) 87·6 of water, 3·3 of protein, 3·6 of fat, 4·7 of carbohydrate, and 0·12 of calcium. Heat has no effect on the vitamin A or D content of milk, or on the riboflavine content, but it causes a considerable reduction in the vitamin C and thiamine content.

Preparation of milk Milk may be prepared for food in various ways. Boiling destroys the bacteria, especially any *Mycobacteria tuberculosis* which the milk may contain. It also partly destroys vitamin C and thiamine, as does pasteurisation. Curdling of milk is effected by adding rennet, which carries out the initial stage of digestion and thus renders milk more suitable for people who could not otherwise tolerate it. Souring of milk is practised in many countries before milk is considered suitable for food; it is carried out by adding certain organisms such as the LACTIC ACID bacillus, the Bulgarian bacillus, and setting the milk in a warm place for several hours. Sterilisation, which prevents fermentation and decomposition, is usually carried out by raising the milk to boiling temperature (100 °C) for 15 minutes and then hermetically sealing it. Condensed, unsweetened milk – usually known as evaporated milk – is concentrated *in vacuo* at low temperature; the milk is then placed in tins, which are sealed, and is sterilised by heat at a temperature of 105 °C. This destroys 60 per cent of the vitamin C and 30–50 per cent of the thiamine. Sweetened condensed milk is not exposed to such a high temperature. The sugar, which prevents the growth of micro-organisms, is added before the condensing, and finally reaches a concentration of about 40 per cent.

Dried milk is prepared by evaporating all the fluid so that the milk is reduced to the form of powder. Humanised milk is cow's milk treated to render it closely similar to human milk.

Milk Teeth

The temporary teeth of children. (For the time of their appearance, see under TEETH.)

Millilitre

Millilitre is the 1,000th part of 1 litre. It is practically the equivalent of a cubic centimetre (1 cm^3 = 0·999973 ml); ml is the usual abbreviation.

Mind

(1) The seat of consciousness of the human BRAIN. The mind understands, reasons and initiates action and is also the source of emotions. This is a simplistic definition for a concept that has been and continues to be the subject of vigorous debate among theologians, philosophers, biologists, psychologists, psychiatrists and other doctors, their arguments being too complex for inclusion in a dictionary's definition.
(2) MIND: The National Association for Mental Health, a voluntary charitable body that works in the interests of those with MENTAL ILLNESS, advising, educating and campaigning for and supporting them.

Mineralcorticoid

See CORTICOSTEROIDS.

Minim

A 'pre-metric' unit of measurement of volume. It is about one-60th part of a fluid drachm and is used in pharmacy.

Minimum Lethal Dose (MLD)

See MLD.

Minimally Invasive Surgery (MIS)

More popularly called 'keyhole surgery', MIS is surgical intervention, whether diagnostic or curative, that causes patients the least possible physical trauma. It has revolutionised surgery, growing from a technique used by gynaecologists, urologists and innovative general surgeons to one regularly used in general surgery, GYNAECOLOGY, UROLOGY, thoracic surgery, orthopaedic surgery (see ORTHOPAEDICS) and OTORHINOLARYNGOLOGY.

MIS is commonly carried out by means of an operating laparoscope (a type of ENDOSCOPE) that is slipped through a small incision in the skin. MIS now accounts for around 50 per cent

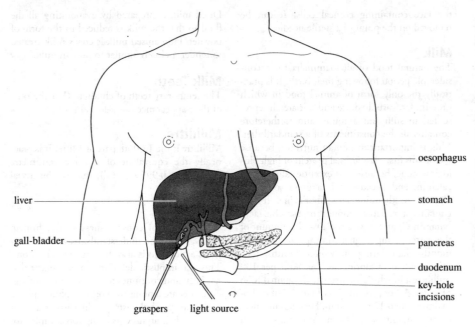

Removal of stones from gall-bladder using the technique of minimally invasive surgery.

of all operations carried out in the UK. A small attachment on the end of the laparoscope provides an image that can be magnified on a screen, leaving the surgeon's hands free to operate while his assistant operates the laparoscope. Halogen bulbs, fibreoptic cables and rod lenses have all contributed to the technical advancement of laparoscopes. Operations done in this manner include extracorporeal shock-wave LITHOTRIPSY for stones in the gall-bladder, biliary ducts and urinary system; removal of the gall-bladder; appendicectomy; removal of the spleen and adrenal glands; and thoracic sympathectomy. MIS is also used to remove cartilage or loose pieces of bone in the knee-joint.

This method of surgery usually means that patients can be treated on a day or overnight basis, allowing them to resume normal activities more quickly than with conventional surgery. It is safer and lessens the trauma and shock for patients needing surgery. MIS is also more cost effective, allowing hospitals to treat more patients in a year. Surgeons undertake special training in the use of MIS, a highly skilled technique, before they are permitted to use the procedures on patients. The use of MIS for hernia repair, colon surgery and repairs of duodenal perforations is under evaluation and its advantages will be enhanced by the development of robotic surgical techniques.

Minocycline

One of the tetracycline broad-spectrum antibiotic drugs (see TETRACYCLINES). Minocycline has a broader spectrum than the others and is effective against *Neisseria meningitidis*, which causes bacterial MENINGITIS. It should not be prescribed for patients with kidney disease.

Minoxidil

A vasodilator drug taken orally to treat people with serious HYPERTENSION. Minoxidil is also used as a lotion to treat male-pattern baldness (in both sexes). The drug can cause fluid retention, weight gain and excessive growth of the hair.

Miosis

Condition of constriction (reduction in size) of the pupil (see EYE). It may be the result of disease affecting the AUTONOMIC NERVOUS SYSTEM. Bright light causes miosis and some drugs – for example, PILOCARPINE or OPIUM – have the same effect.

Miscarriage

See ABORTION.

Misoprostol

A PROSTAGLANDIN analogue used to treat duodenal and gastric ulcers, and those induced by NON-STEROIDAL ANTI-INFLAMMATORY DRUGS

(NSAIDS). It should not be taken by pregnant or breast-feeding women.

Misuse of Drugs

See also MEDICINES. Government legislation covers the manufacture, sale and prescription of drugs in the UK. As well as stating which drugs may be sold over the counter (OTC) without a doctor's or dentist's prescription, and those which can be obtained only with such a prescription, government regulations determine the extent of availability of many substances which are liable to be abused – see Misuse of Drugs Act 1971 (below). The Misuse of Drugs Regulations 1985 define those individuals who in their professional capacity are authorised to supply and possess controlled drugs: see the schedules of drugs listed below under the 1985 regulations.

Misuse of Drugs Act 1971 This legislation forbids activities relating to the manufacture, sale and possession of particular (controlled) drugs. These are classified into three grades according to their dangers if misused. Any offences concerning class A drugs, potentially the most damaging when abused, carry the toughest penalties, while classes B and C attract lesser penalties if abused.

- Class A includes: cocaine, dextromoramide, diamorphine (heroin), lysergic acid (LSD), methadone, morphine, opium, pethidine, phencyclidine acid and injectable preparations of class B drugs.
- Class B includes: oral amphetamines, barbiturates, codeine, glutethimide, marijuana (cannabis), pentazocine and pholcodine.
- Class C includes: drugs related to the amphetamines, anabolic and androgenic steroids, many benzodiazepines, buprenorphine, diethyl propion, human chorionic gonadotrophin (HCG), mazindol, meprobamate, pemoline, phenbuterol, and somatropin.

Misuse of Drugs Regulations 1985 These regulations define those people who are authorised in their professional capacity to supply and possess controlled drugs. They also describe the requirements for legally undertaking these activities, such as storage of the drugs and limits on their prescription.

Drugs are divided into five schedules and some examples follow.

- I: Almost all are prohibited except in accordance with Home Office authority: marijuana (cannabis), LSD.
- II: High potential for abuse but have accepted medical uses: amphetamines, cocaine.
- III: Lower potential for abuse: barbiturates, meprobamate, temazepam.
- IV: Lower potential for abuse than I to III. Minimal control: benzodiazepines.
- V: Low potential for abuse: generally compound preparations containing small amounts of opioids: kaolin and morphine (antidiarrhoeal medicine), codeine linctus (cough suppressant).

(See also CONTROLLED DRUGS.)

Mites

A mite is an arthropod belonging to a group of insects called ACARINA. It may be parasitic or free-living. Most mites are less than 1 mm long and medically significant ones include those that cause DERMATITIS (dermatophagoides) and the harvest mite, which transmits scrub typhus (see under TYPHUS FEVER).

Mitochondria

The rod-like bodies in the CELLS of the body which contain the enzymes (see ENZYME) necessary for the activity of the cell. They have been described as the 'power plant of the cell'

Mitosis

The process of cell division for somatic cells and for the ovum after fertilisation. Each chromosome becomes doubled by splitting lengthwise and forming two chromatids which remain held together by the centromere. These chromatids are exact copies of the original chromosomes and contain duplicates of all the genes they bear. When cell division takes place, the pull of the spindle splits the centromere and each double chromatid separates, one passing to one pole of the nucleus and the other to the opposite pole. The nucleus and the cell itself then also divide, forming two new daughter cells containing precisely the same 23 pairs of chromosomes and carrying exactly the same complement of genes as did the mother cell. (See CHROMOSOMES; FERTILISATION; GENES; HEREDITY.)

Mitral Incompetence

A defect in the MITRAL VALVE of the HEART which allows blood to leak from the left VENTRICLE into the left ATRIUM. It is also known as mitral regurgitation; incompetence may occur along with MITRAL STENOSIS. The left ventricle has to work harder to compensate for the faulty valve, so it enlarges, but eventually the ventricle cannot cope with the extra load and left-sided heart failure may develop. A common cause of mitral incompetence is RHEUMATIC FEVER or damage following a heart attack. The condition is treated with drugs to help the heart, but in severe cases heart surgery may be required.

Mitral Stenosis

Narrowing of the opening between the left ATRIUM and left VENTRICLE of the HEART as a result of rigidity of, and adhesion between, the cusps of the MITRAL VALVE. It is due, almost invariably, to the infection RHEUMATIC FEVER. The atrium has to work harder to force blood through the narrowed channel. The effects are similar to those of MITRAL INCOMPETENCE. Shortness of breath and palpitations and irregular beating (fibrillation) of the atrium are common consequences in adults. Drug treatment with DIGOXIN and DIURETICS helps, but surgery to dilate or replace the faulty valve may be necessary.

Mitral Valve

The mitral valve, so-called because of its resemblance to a bishop's mitre, is the valve which guards the opening between the ATRIUM and VENTRICLE on the left side of the HEART.

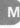

MLD

The minimal lethal dose or smallest amount of a toxic compound needed to cause death.

MMR Vaccine

A combined vaccine offering protection against MEASLES, MUMPS and RUBELLA (German measles), it was introduced in the UK in 1988 and has now replaced the measles vaccine. The combined vaccine is offered to all infants in their second year; health authorities have an obligation to ensure that all children have received the vaccine by school entry – it should be given with the pre-school booster doses against DIPHTHERIA, TETANUS and POLIOMYELITIS, if not earlier – unless there is a valid contra-indication (such as partial immunosuppression), parental refusal, or evidence of previous infection. MMR vaccine may also be used in the control of measles outbreaks, if offered to susceptible children within three days of exposure to infection. The vaccine is effective and generally safe, though minor symptoms such as malaise, fever and rash may occur 5–10 days after immunisation. The incidence of all three diseases has dropped substantially since MMR was introduced in the UK and USA.

A researcher has suggested a link between the vaccine and AUTISM, but massive studies of children with and without this condition in several countries have failed to find any evidence to back the claim. Nonetheless, the publicity war has been largely lost by the UK health departments so that vaccine rates have dropped to a worryingly low level.

(See IMMUNISATION.)

MND

See MOTOR NEURONE DISEASE (MND).

Moclobemide

A reversible monoamine oxidase inhibitor (see MONOAMINE OXIDASE INHIBITORS (MAOIS)), this drug is used as second-line treatment for patients with severe DEPRESSION. As with all MAOIs, those taking moclobemide should avoid too much tyramine-rich food – mature cheese, yeast extracts, fermented soya-bean products – and they should not take the drug with another antidepressant (see ANTIDEPRESSANT DRUGS).

Mode

A statistical term which is the most frequently occurring value of a set of observations. If the results are plotted as a graph, the mode is the peak of the curve which results.

Molar Teeth

The last three TEETH on each side of the JAW.

Mole

(1) A term used to describe the common pigmented spots which occur on human SKIN. It arises from a collection of abnormal melanocytes (see MELANOCYTE) in the dermis adjacent to the epidermodermal junction. Moles are usually not present at birth, and appear in childhood or adolescence. Most moles are less than 5 mm in diameter and are macular at first, becoming raised later. Rarely, moles are present at birth and may occasionally be massive. There is a substantial risk of future malignancy (see MALIGNANT) in massive congenital moles and prophylactic surgical removal is advised if feasible. All humans have moles, but their number varies from ten or fewer to 100 or more. The members of some families are genetically predisposed to large numbers of moles, some of which may be large and irregular in shape and colour. This 'atypical mole syndrome' is associated with an increased risk of future malignant MELANOMA.

(2) An internationally agreed unit (see SI UNITS) for measuring the quantity of a substance at molecular level.

Molecular Biology

The study of molecules (see MOLECULE) that are part of the structure of living organisms.

Molecule

The smallest possible amount of a substance comprising two or more linked atoms which retains the chemical characteristics of that substance. Molecules vary greatly in their size and complexity, ranging from oxygen (two linked oxygen atoms) and water (two hydrogen atoms and one oxygen) to large complex molecules such as deoxyribonucleic acid (DNA) comprising thousands of atoms of carbon, hydrogen, oxygen, nitrogen and phosphorus that form the double-helix structure which helps to form GENES, the basic building blocks of the hereditary material of living things.

Molluscum Contagiosum

Common papular eruption of the skin caused by a virus. Most common in children, it is highly contagious and often transmitted in swimming pools and sauna baths. Mollusca are often multiple and persistent in children with atopic eczema (see DERMATITIS), and epidemics may occur in boarding schools. The typical molluscum is 2–3 mm in diameter, skin-coloured and translucent, with a dimpled centre. The armpits and adjacent chest, upper inner thighs and genital areas are common sites in young children. In adults the infection is usually transmitted sexually and affects the pubic area and lower belly. Mollusca eventually disappear spontaneously, but cure can be expedited by curettage (removal with a CURETTE) under surface anaesthesia.

Mongolian Blue Spots

Irregularly shaped areas of bluish-black pigmentation found occasionally on the buttocks, lower back or upper arms in newborn infants of African, Chinese and Japanese parentage, and sometimes in the babies of black-haired Europeans. They measure from one to several centimetres in diameter, and usually disappear in a few months. They are commonly mistaken for bruises.

Mongolism

See DOWN'S (DOWN) SYNDROME.

Moniliasis

The infection caused by monilia, the genus of fungi now known as *Candida albicans* (see CANDIDA). The infection may occur in the mouth – where it is known as thrush – lungs, intestine, vagina, skin, or nails.

Monoamine Oxidase Inhibitors (MAOIs)

These are drugs that destroy, or prevent the action of, monoamine oxidase (MAO). Monoamines, which include NORADRENALINE and tyramine, play an important part in the metabolism of the BRAIN, and there is some evidence that excitement is due to an accumulation of monoamines in the brain. MAO is a naturally occurring ENZYME which is concerned in the breakdown of monoamines. MAOIs were among the earliest ANTIDEPRESSANT DRUGS used, but they are now used much less than tricyclic and related antidepressants, or SELECTIVE SEROTONIN-REUPTAKE INHIBITORS (SSRIS) and related antidepressants, because of the dangers of dietary or drug interactions – and because MAOIs are less effective than these two groups.

An excessive accumulation of monoamines can induce a dangerous reaction characterised by high blood pressure, palpitations, sweating and a feeling of suffocation. Hence the care with which MAOI drugs are administered. What is equally important, however, is that in no circumstances should a patient receiving any MAOI drug eat cheese, yeast preparations such as Marmite, tinned fish, or high game. The reason for this ban is that all these foodstuffs contain large amounts of tyramine which increases the amount of certain monoamines such as noradrenaline in the body. (See MENTAL ILLNESS.)

There are also certain drugs, such as AMPHETAMINES and PETHIDINE HYDROCHLORIDE, which must not be taken by a patient who is receiving an MAOI drug. The MAOIs of choice are phenelzine or isocarboxazid because their stimulant effects are less than those of other MAOIs, making them safer.

Monoclonal Antibodies

An artificially prepared antibody (see ANTIBODIES) obtained from cell clones – a genetically identical group of cells – and comprising a single type of immunoglobulin. It neutralises only one specific ANTIGEN. The antibodies are prepared by linking antibody-forming lymphocytes (see LYMPHOCYTE) from the spleen of mice with myeloma cells from mice. Monoclonal antibodies are used in the development of new vaccines and in the study of human cells, hormones, and micro-organisms. Research is under way for their use in the treatment of some forms of cancer. (See IMMUNOLOGY.)

Monocyte

A type of white blood cell which has a single

kidney-shaped nucleus. Present in the tissues and lymphatic system as well as in the circulation, it ingests foreign particles such as tissue debris and bacteria. Monocytes are about 20 μm in diameter and 1 mm³ of blood contains around 7,500 of them, many times fewer than the five million erythrocytes (red blood cells).

Monomania
Monomania is a form of MENTAL ILLNESS, in which the affected person has delusion (see DELUSIONS) upon one subject, although he or she can converse rationally and is a responsible individual upon other matters.

Mononucleosis
An acute viral infection in which the patient develops a sore throat, swollen lymph glands and fever. Also known as glandular fever, infectious mononucleosis is caused by members of the herpes group of viruses – the EPSTEIN BARR VIRUS and CYTOMEGALOVIRUS (CMV). The disease is more common among adolescents aged 15–17, an age when their immune defence mechanisms are not fully developed. In the UK many thousands of teenagers catch the disease every year, and kissing is believed to be the method of transmission among many of them. The blood contains many atypical lymphocytes (see LYMPHOCYTE) and the diagnosis is confirmed with the heterophil antibodies test. Patients normally recover within six weeks without treatment, but they may feel tired and depressed for several months afterwards. Some cases of MYALGIC ENCEPHALOMYELITIS (ME) and other chronic fatigue syndromes occur after infection with this virus.

Monoplegia
PARALYSIS of a single limb or part.

Monorchism
The absence of one testis, usually the result of the failure of one TESTICLE to drop down into the SCROTUM before birth. Monorchism is sometimes used to describe the condition when one testicle has been destroyed by disease or injury, or has been surgically removed – when, for example, the man has developed cancer of the testicle.

Monosaccharide
A sugar having six carbon atoms in the molecule, such as glucose, galactose, and laevulose.

Monospot
A screening test, performed on blood, which indicates the likelihood of infection with

EPSTEIN BARR VIRUS, which causes MONONUCLEOSIS.

Monozygotic Twins
Twins who develop from a single OVUM fertilised by a single SPERMATOZOON. Also known as identical or uniovular twins (see MULTIPLE BIRTHS).

Morbid Anatomy
The study of the structural changes that diseases cause in the body, in particular those which can be seen with the naked eye at POST-MORTEM EXAMINATION.

Morbidity
The condition of being diseased. The morbidity rate is the number of cases of disease occurring within a particular number of the population.

Morbilli
Another name for MEASLES.

Morbus
Morbus, the Latin word for disease, is used in such terms as morbus cordis (heart disease), morbus coxae (hip-joint disease).

Moribund
In a state of dying.

Morning-After Pill
See CONTRACEPTION.

Moron
An out-of-date term previously used to describe individuals with mild learning difficulties, but which is now offensive.

Moro Reflex
A primitive REFLEX ACTION occurring in newly born infants in response to a sudden movement or noise. Also known as the startle reflex, the baby will throw its arms and legs wide and stiffen its body. This is followed by flexion of the arms and legs. The reflex disappears by four months; its persistence suggests a possible neurological condition such as CEREBRAL PALSY.

Morphine
Morphine is the name of the chief alkaloid (see ALKALOIDS) upon which the action of OPIUM depends. A traditional and invaluable opioid analgesic (see ANALGESICS) used to control severe pain, it is the standard against which other opioid analgesics are measured. Used widely in patients with post-operative pain or

those in PALLIATIVE care who have severe pain, it produces a sense of EUPHORIA. A serious side-effect is that morphine can cause nausea and vomiting. The drug may also cause DEPEND-ENCE. Morphine is a Class A controlled drug and is classifed in Schedule II of the Misuse of Drugs Regulations 1985 (see CONTROLLED DRUGS; MEDICINES; MISUSE OF DRUGS).

Morphoea

A form of circumscribed SCLERODERMA.

Mortality

See DEATH, CAUSES OF; DEATH RATE; INFANT MORTALITY RATE (IMR).

Mortification

Mortification is another name for GANGRENE.

Mosaicism

If non-dysjunction occurs after the formation of a ZYGOTE – that is, during a mitotic cell division and not a meiotic cell division (see MITOSIS; MEIOSIS) – some of the cells will have one chromosome constitution and others another. The term mosaicism describes a condition in which a substantial minority of cells in an individual's body differ from the majority in their chromosome content. How substantial this minority is will depend upon how early during cleavage the zygote undergoes non-dysjunction. Mosaicism can cause disorders such as DOWN'S (DOWN) SYNDROME and TURNER'S SYNDROME. The proportion and type of abnormal cells affect the physical appearance of the affected individual. This may range from normal to the features typical of people with a chromosomal-abnormality syndrome.

Mosquitoes

See ANOPHELES; BITES AND STINGS; MALARIA.

Motilin

Motilin is a hormone (see HORMONES) formed in the DUODENUM and the JEJUNUM which plays a part in controlling the movements of the stomach and the gut.

Motion

Waste products evacuated in a bowel movement, also called faeces or stool.

Motion (Travel) Sickness

A characteristic set of symptoms experienced by many people when subjected to the constant changes of position caused, for example, by the pitching and rolling motion of a vessel at sea.

Depression, giddiness, nausea and vomiting are the most prominent.

Causes Although the vast majority of people appear to be liable to this ailment at sea, they do not all suffer alike. Many endure acute distress, whilst others are simply conscious of transient feelings of nausea and discomfort. A smaller proportion of people suffer from air and car sickness. The symptoms are a result of over-stimulation of the organs of balance in the inner EAR by continuous changes in the body's position. The movements of the horizon worsen this situation.

Symptoms The symptoms generally show themselves soon after the journey has started, by the onset of giddiness and discomfort in the head, together with a sense of nausea and sinking at the stomach, which soon develops into intense sickness and vomiting. Most people recover quickly when the motion stops.

Treatment Innumerable preventives and remedies have been proposed. Cinnarizine 30 mg orally is useful 2 hours before travel, then 15 mg every 8 hours during the journey if necessary. Dimenhydrinate and promethazine are also commonly taken for motion sickness.

Motor

A term usually applied to nerves, used to describe anything that results in movement. Motor nerves stimulate muscles to contract, producing movement. (See also SENSORY.)

Motor Neurone Disease (MND)

A group of disorders of unknown origin. Certain cells in the neurological system's MOTOR nerves degenerate and die. Upper and lower motor neurones may be affected but sensory cells retain their normal functions. Three types of MND are identified: amyotrophic lateral sclerosis (AML – 50 per cent of patients); progressive muscular atrophy (25 per cent), in which the prognosis is better than for AML; and bulbar palsy (25 per cent). Men are affected more than women, and the disorder affects about seven people in every 100,000. Those affected develop progressive weakness and wasting of their muscles. The diagnosis is confirmed with various tests including the measurement of electrical activity in muscles, electromyography, muscle BIOPSY, blood tests and X-ray examination of the spine. There is no medical treatment: patients need physical and psychological support with aids to help them overcome disabilities. The Motor Neurone Disease

Association provides excellent advice and help for sufferers and their relatives. (See APPENDIX 2: ADDRESSES: SOURCES OF INFORMATION, ADVICE, SUPPORT AND SELF-HELP.)

Mountain Sickness
See ALTITUDE SICKNESS.

Mouth, Diseases of
The mucous membrane of the mouth can indicate the health of the individual and internal organs. For example, pallor or pigmentation may indicate ANAEMIA, JAUNDICE or ADDISON'S DISEASE.

Thrush is characterised by the presence of white patches on the mucous membrane which bleeds if the patch is gently removed. It is caused by the growth of a parasitic mould known as *Candida albicans*. Antifungal agents usually suppress the growth of candida. Candidal infiltration of the mucosa is often found in cancerous lesions.

Leukoplakia literally means a white patch. In the mouth it is often due to an area of thickened cells from the horny layer of the epithelium. It appears as a white patch of varying density and is often grooved by dense fissures. There are many causes, most of them of minor importance. It may be associated with smoking, SYPHILIS, chronic SEPSIS or trauma from a sharp tooth. Cancer must be excluded.

Stomatitis (inflammation of the mouth) arises from the same causes as inflammation elsewhere, but among the main causes are the cutting of teeth in children, sharp or broken teeth, excess alcohol, tobacco smoking and general ill-health. The mucous membrane becomes red, swollen and tender and ulcers may appear. Treatment consists mainly of preventing secondary infection supervening before the stomatitis has resolved. Antiseptic mouthwashes are usually sufficient.

Gingivitis (see TEETH, DISEASES OF) is inflammation of the gum where it touches the tooth. It is caused by poor oral hygiene and is often associated with the production of calculus or tartar on the teeth. If it is neglected it will proceed to periodontal disease.

Ulcers of the mouth These are usually small and arise from a variety of causes. Aphthous ulcers are the most common; they last about ten days and usually heal without scarring. They may be associated with STRESS or DYSPEPSIA. There is no ideal treatment.

Herpetic ulcers (see HERPES SIMPLEX) are similar but usually there are many ulcers and the patient appears feverish and unwell. This condition is more common in children.

Calculus (*a*) Salivary: a calculus (stone) may develop in one of the major salivary-gland ducts. This may result in a blockage which will cause the gland to swell and be painful. It usually swells before a meal and then slowly subsides. The stone may be passed but often has to be removed in a minor operation. If the gland behind the calculus becomes infected, then an ABSCESS forms and, if this persists, the removal of the gland may be indicated. (*b*) Dental, also called TARTAR: this is a calcified material which adheres to the teeth; it often starts as the soft debris found on teeth which have not been well cleaned and is called plaque. If not removed, it will gradually destroy the periodontal membrane and result in the loss of the tooth. (See TEETH, DISORDERS OF.)

Ranula This is a cyst-like swelling found in the floor of the mouth. It is often caused by mild trauma to the salivary glands with the result that saliva collects in the cyst instead of discharging into the mouth. Surgery may be required.

Mumps is an acute infective disorder of the major salivary glands. It causes painful enlargement of the glands which lasts for about two weeks. (See also main entry for MUMPS.)

Tumours may occur in all parts of the mouth, and may be BENIGN or MALIGNANT. Benign tumours are common and may follow mild trauma or be an exaggerated response to irritation. Polyps are found in the cheeks and on the tongue and become a nuisance as they may be bitten frequently. They are easily excised.

A MUCOCOELE is found mainly in the lower lip.

An exostosis or bone outgrowth is often found in the mid line of the palate and on the inside of the mandible (bone of the lower jaw). This only requires removal if it becomes unduly large or pointed and easily ulcerated.

Malignant tumours within the mouth are often large before they are noticed, whereas those on the lips are usually seen early and are more easily treated. The cancer may arise from any of the tissues found in the mouth including epithelium, bone, salivary tissue and tooth-forming tissue remnants. Oral cancers represent about 5 per cent of all reported malignancies, and in England and Wales around 3,300 people are diagnosed annually as having cancer of the mouth and PHARYNX.

Cancer of the mouth is less common below the age of 40 years and is more common in men. It is often associated with chronic irritation from a broken tooth or ill-fitting denture. It is also more common in those who smoke and those who chew betel leaves. Leukoplakia (see above) may be a precursor of cancer. Spread of the cancer is by way of the lymph nodes in the neck. Early treatment by surgery, radiotherapy or chemotherapy will often be effective, except for the posterior of the tongue where the prognosis is very poor. Although surgery may be extensive and potentially mutilating, recent advances in repairing defects and grafting tissues from elsewhere have made treatment more acceptable to the patient.

Mouth-To-Mouth Respiration
See APPENDIX 1: BASIC FIRST AID.

MRI
MRI, or magnetic resonance imaging, is a non-invasive method of imaging the body and its organs. It may also be used to study tissue metabolism. The body is placed in a magnetic field which causes certain atomic nuclei to align in the direction of the field. Pulses of radio-frequency radiation are then applied; interpretation of the frequencies absorbed and re-emitted allows an image in any body plane to be built up. Different tissues – for example, fat and water – can be separately identified and, if the resonance signal for the fat is suppressed, then only the signal from any abnormalities in the fat can be identified. Many diseases result in a rise in the water content of tissues,so MRI is a valuable test for identifying disease, and the operating radiologist is skilled in interpreting the meaning of altered signals.

MRSA
See METHICILLIN-RESISTANT STAPHYLOCOCCUS AUREUS (MRSA).

Mucilage
This is prepared from acacia or tragacanth gum, and is used as an ingredient of mixtures containing solid particles in order to keep the latter from settling, and also as a demulcent.

Mucocoele
An abnormally dilated cavity in the body due to the accumulation of MUCUS; such a 'cyst' may

therefore form wherever there is mucous membrane.

Mucocutaneous Lymph Node Syndrome
See KAWASAKI DISEASE.

Mucolytic
The term used to describe the property of destroying, or lessening the tenacity of, MUCUS. It is most commonly used to describe drugs which have this property and are therefore used in the treatment of BRONCHITIS. The inhalation of steam, for example, has a mucolytic action.

Mucopolysaccaridhosis
A collection of familial metabolic disorders, the best known of which is Hurler's syndrome (see GARGOYLISM). Others include Hunter's, Maroteaux-Lamy and Scheie's syndromes. The disorders, which result from a faulty gene-producing abnormality in a specific ENZYME, affect one child in 10,000. Those affected usually die before reaching adulthood.

Mucosa
A term for MUCOUS MEMBRANE.

Mucous Membrane
The general name given to the membrane which lines many of the hollow organs of the body. These membranes vary widely in structure in different sites, but all have the common character of being lubricated by MUCUS – derived in some cases from isolated cells on the surface of the membrane, but more generally from definite glands placed beneath the membrane, and opening here and there through it by ducts. The air passages, the gastrointestinal tract and the ducts of glands which open into it, and also the urinary passages, are all lined by mucous membrane.

Mucoviscidosis
See CYSTIC FIBROSIS.

Mucus
The general name for the slimy secretion derived from mucous membranes. It is mainly composed of a substance called mucin, which varies according to the particular mucous membrane from which it is derived, and it contains other substances, such as cells cast off from the surface of the membrane, enzymes, and dust particles. Mucin has the following characteristics: it is viscid, clear and tenacious; when dissolved in water it can be precipitated by addition of acetic acid; and when not in solution

already, it is dissolved by weak alkalis, such as lime-water.

Under normal conditions the surface of a mucous membrane is lubricated by only a small quantity of mucus; the appearance of large quantities is a sign of inflammation.

Mullerian Ducts

The Mullerian and the Wolffian ducts are separate sets of primordia that transiently co-exist in embryos of both sexes (see EMBRYO). In female embryos the Mullerian ducts grow and fuse in the mid line, producing the FALLOPIAN TUBES, the UTERUS and the upper third of the VAGINA, whereas the Wolffian ducts regress. In the male the Wolffian ducts give rise to the VAS DEFERENS, the seminal vesicles and the EPI-DIDYMIS, and the Mullerian ducts disappear. This phase of development requires a functioning testis (see TESTICLE) from which an inducer substance diffuses locally over the primordia to bring about the suppression of the Mullerian duct and the development of the Wolffian duct. In the absence of this substance, development proceeds along female lines regardless of the genetic sex.

Multigravida

A pregnant woman who has had more than one pregnancy.

Multipara

A woman who has borne several children.

Multiple Births

Twins occur about once in 80 pregnancies, triplets once in 6,000, and quadruplets about once in 500,000. Quintuplets are exceedingly rare. Such is the natural state of affairs.

In recent years, however, the position has been altered by the introduction of the so-called fertility drugs, such as CLOMIPHENE, and human menopausal gonadotrophin which, through the medium of the PITUITARY GLAND, stimulate the production of ova (see OVUM). Their wide use in the treatment of INFERTILITY has resulted in an increase in the number of multiple births, a recognised hazard of giving too large a dose.

Twins may be binovular or uniovular. Binovular, or fraternal, twins are the result of the mother's releasing two ova within a few days of each other and both being fertilised by separate spermatozoa (see SPERMATOZOON). They both develop separately in the mother's womb and are no more alike than is usual with members of the same family. They are three times as common as uniovular, or identical, twins, who are

developed from a single ovum fertilised by a single spermatozoon, but which has split early in development. This is why they are usually so remarkably alike in looks and mental characteristics. Unlike binovular twins, who may be of the same or different sex, they are always of the same sex.

So far as fraternal, or binovular, twins are concerned, multiple pregnancy may be an inherited tendency; it certainly occurs more often in certain families, but this may be partly due to chance. A woman who has already given birth to twins is ten times more likely to have another multiple pregnancy than one who has not previously had twins. The statistical chance of a third pair of twins is 1:512,000. Identical twins do not run in families.

The relative proportion of twins of each type varies in different races. Identical twins have much the same frequency all over the world: around 3 per 1,000 maternities. Fraternal twins are rare in Mongolian races: less than 3 per 1,000 maternities. In Caucasians they occur two or three times as often as identical twins: between 7 (Spain and Portugal) and 10 (Czech and Slovak Republics and Greece) per 1,000 maternities. They are more common in Afro-Caribbeans, reaching 30 per 1,000 maternities in certain West African populations.

Rarely, uniovular twins may not develop as separate individuals, being physically joined in some way. They are called conjoined or (traditionally) Siamese twins. Depending on the extent of common structures shared by the infants – this ranges from a common umbilical cord to twins with conjoined heads or a common liver – the infants may be successfully separated by surgery. (See CONJOINED TWINS.)

Parents of twins, triplets, etc. can obtain advice and help from the Twins and Multiple Births Association (TAMBA).

Multiple Personality Disorder

The individual with this psychiatric disorder has two or more different personalities, often contrasting. The dominant personality at the time determines the behaviour and attitude of the individual, who customarily seems not to know about the other personality – or personalities. The switch from one personality to another is abrupt and the mental condition of the differing personalities is usually normal. It is possible that child abuse is a factor in the disorder, which is treated by psychotherapy. The classic multiple personality was the fictional form of Dr Jekyll and Mr Hyde.

Multiple Sclerosis (MS)

Multiple sclerosis is a progressive disease of the

BRAIN and SPINAL CORD, which, although slow in its onset, in time may produce marked symptoms such as PARALYSIS and tremors (see TREMOR), and may ultimately result in a severely disabled invalid. The disorder consists of hardened patches, from the size of a pin-head to that of a pea or larger, scattered here and there irregularly through the brain and spinal cord. Each patch is made up of a mass of the CONNECTIVE TISSUE (neuroglia), which should be present only in sufficient amount to bind the nerve-cells and fibres together. In the earliest stage, the insulating sheaths (MYELIN) of the nerve-fibres in the hardened patches break up, are absorbed, and leave the nerve-fibres bare, the connective tissue being later formed between these.

Cause Although this is one of the most common diseases of the central nervous system in Europe – there are around 50,000 affected individuals in Britain alone – the cause is still not known. The disease comes on in young people (onset being rare after the age of 40), apparently without previous illness. The ratio of women-to-men victims is 3:2. It is more common in first and second children than in those later in birth order, and in small rather than big families. There may be a hereditary factor for MS, which could be an autoimmune disorder: the body's defence system attacks the myelin in the central nervous system as if it were a 'foreign' tissue.

Symptoms These depend greatly upon the part of the brain and cord affected by the sclerotic patches. Temporary paralysis of a limb, or of an eye muscle, causing double vision, and tremors upon exertion, first in the affected parts, and later in all parts of the body, are early symptoms. Stiffness of the lower limbs causing the toes to catch on small irregularities in the ground and trip the person in walking, is often an annoying symptom and one of the first to be noticed. Great activity is shown in the reflex movements obtained by striking the tendons and by stroking the soles of the feet. The latter reflex shows a characteristic sign (Babinski sign) in which the great toe bends upwards and the other toes spread apart as the sole is stroked, instead of the toes collectively bending downwards as in the normal person. Tremor of the eye movements (nystagmus) is usually found. Trembling handwriting, interference with the functions of the bladder, giddiness, and a peculiar 'staccato' or 'scanning' speech are common symptoms at a later stage. Numbness and tingling in the extremities occur commonly, particularly in the early stages of the disease. As the disease progresses, the paralyses, which were transitory at first, now become confirmed, often with great rigidity in the limbs. In many patients the disease progresses very slowly.

People with multiple sclerosis, and their relatives, can obtain help and guidance from the Multiple Sclerosis Society. Another helpful organisation is the Multiple Sclerosis Resources Centre. Those with sexual or marital problems arising out of the illness can obtain information from SPOD (Association to Aid the Sexual and Personal Relationships of People with a Disability). (See APPENDIX 2: ADDRESSES: SOURCES OF INFORMATION, ADVICE, SUPPORT AND SELF-HELP.)

Treatment is difficult, because the most that can be done is to lead a life as free from strain as possible, to check the progress of the disease. The use of INTERFERON beta seems to slow the progress of MS and this drug is licensed for use in the UK for patients with relapsing, remitting MS over two years, provided they can walk unaided – a controversial restriction on this (expensive) treatment. CORTICOSTEROIDS may be of help to some patients.

The NATIONAL INSTITUTE FOR CLINICAL EXCELLENCE (NICE) ruled in 2001 that the use of the drugs interferon beta and glatiramer acetate for patients with multiple sclerosis was not cost-effective but recommended that the Department of Health, the National Assembly for Wales and the drug manufacturers should consider ways of making the drugs available in a cost-effective way. Subsequently the government said that it would consider funding a 'risk-sharing' scheme in which supply of drugs to patients would be funded only if treatment trials in individuals with MS showed that they were effective.

The Department of Health has asked NICE to assess two CANNABIS derivatives as possible treatments for multiple sclerosis and the relief of post-operative pain. Trials of an under-the-tongue spray and a tablet could, if successsful, lead to the two drugs being available around 2005.

It is important to keep the nerves and muscles functioning, and therefore the patient should remain at work as long as he or she is capable of doing it, and in any case should exercise regularly.

Mumps

Mumps, also known as epidemic parotitis, is an infectious disease characterised by inflammatory swelling of the PAROTID GLAND and other

SALIVARY GLANDS – often occurring as an EPIDEMIC and affecting mostly young people. Its name comes from the old verb, 'mump', meaning to mope or assume a disconsolate appearance – an apt description of the victim of the disease at its height.

Causes Mumps is due to infection with a virus and is highly infectious from person to person. It is predominantly a disease of childhood and early adult life, but it can occur at any age. Epidemics usually occur in the winter and spring. It is infectious for two or three days before the swelling of the glands appears. A vaccine is now available that gives a high degree of protection against the disease, the incidence of which is falling sharply. The vaccine is combined with those for MEASLES and RUBELLA – see MMR VACCINE; IMMUNISATION.

Symptoms There is an incubation period of 2–3 weeks after infection before the glands begin to swell. The gland first affected is generally the parotid, situated in front of and below the ear. The swelling usually spreads to the submaxillary and sublingual glands lying beneath the jaw. The patient is feverish and the gland is tender. The swelling disappears after about five days. In 15–30 per cent of males, inflammation of the testicles (orchitis) develops. This usually occurs during the second week of the illness, but may not occur until 2–3 weeks later; it may result in partial ATROPHY of the testicles, but practically never in INFERTILITY. In a much smaller proportion of females with mumps, inflammation of the OVARIES or BREASTS may occur. Inflammation of the PANCREAS, accompanied by tenderness in the upper part of the abdomen and digestive disturbances, sometimes results, and MENINGITIS is also an occasional complication. The various complications are found much more often when the disease affects adults than when it occurs in childhood.

Treatment There is no specific treatment but ANALGESICS and plenty of fluid should be available. The child may need to be in bed for a few days and should not return to school until the symptoms have settled. Adults with orchitis may need strong painkillers, and CORTICOSTEROIDS may be required to reduce the painful swelling.

Munchausen's Syndrome

Munchausen's syndrome, also known as 'hospital addiction' syndrome, is a disorder in which the patient presents repeatedly to hospitals with symptoms and signs (often simulated) suggestive of serious physical illness. More common among men than women, it differs from MALINGERING in that no obvious reward results from the imagined or simulated symptoms. Patients may simulate signs and symptoms in a bizarre way – for instance, by swallowing blood or inserting needles into the chest. Abdominal symptoms are particularly common. They often have a history of multiple hospital admissions and operations, and show extensive pathological lying and lack of personal rapport. Although the cause is unclear, it is thought to be a form of hysterical behaviour in a severely disordered personality. Patients are often masochistic, attention-seeking, and constantly trying to obtain ANALGESICS. Occasionally there may be a degree of treatable DEPRESSION, but on the whole management is very difficult as patients often abscond from psychiatric treatment.

A variation of the syndrome – Munchausen's syndrome by proxy, better termed 'fabricated and induced illness' – has been identified, in which the persons affected inflict damage upon others, usually children (or even animals) in their care. Factitious illness refers to simulating symptoms, such as stating that the child has blood in its urine when it is actually the parent's blood. Induced illness includes such events as injecting dirty water into a baby's muscles, dropping mild caustic into their eyes, adding salt to a baby's milk or diluting it 50–50 with water, and so on. Much debate has ensued about the suggestion that some sudden infant deaths are due to smothering rather than natural causes, as a type of induced illness. As a consequence of two successful appeals against conviction for murder in 2004, the UK attorney general ordered a review of all criminal and family court cases in which disputed medical evidence had formed the basis of the decision. Paediatricians are concerned that one result is likely to be an increase in undetected child abuse.

Murmur

The uneven, rustling sound heard by AUSCULTATION over the HEART and various blood vessels in abnormal conditons. For example, murmurs heard when the stethoscope is applied over the heart are highly characteristic of valvular disease of this organ.

Muscarine

The poisonous principle found in some toadstools (see FUNGUS POISONING). It is a cholinergic substance with pharmacological properties resembling those of ACETYLCHOLINE, a chemical neurotransmitter released at the junctions (synapses) of parasympathetic nerves and at the junctions where nerves enter muscles.

Muscle

Muscular tissue is divided, according to its function, into three main groups: voluntary muscle, involuntary muscle, and skeletal muscle – of which the first is under control of the will, whilst the latter two discharge their functions independently. The term 'striped muscle' is often given to voluntary muscle, because under the microscope all the voluntary muscles show a striped appearance, whilst involuntary muscle is, in the main, unstriped or plain. Heart muscle is partially striped, while certain muscles of the throat, and two small muscles inside the ear, not controllable by willpower, are also striped.

Structure of muscle Skeletal or voluntary muscle forms the bulk of the body's musculature and contains more than 600 such muscles. They are classified according to their methods of action. A flexor muscle closes a joint, an extensor opens it; an abductor moves a body part outwards, an adductor moves it in; a depressor lowers a body part and an elevator raises it; while a constrictor (sphincter) muscle surrounds an orifice, closing and opening it. Each muscle is enclosed in a sheath of fibrous tissue, known as fascia or epimysium, and, from this, partitions of fibrous tissue, known as perimysium, run into the substance of the muscle, dividing it up into small bundles. Each of these bundles consists in turn of a collection of fibres, which form the units of the muscle. Each fibre is about 50 micrometres in thickness and ranges in length from a few millimetres to 300 millimetres. If the fibre is cut across and examined under a high-powered microscope, it is seen to be further divided into fibrils. Each fibre is enclosed in an elastic sheath of its own, which allows it to lengthen and shorten, and is known as the sarcolemma. Within the sarcolemma lie numerous nuclei belonging to the muscle fibre, which was originally developed from a simple cell. To the sarcolemma, at either end, is attached a minute bundle of connective-tissue fibres which unites the muscle fibre to its neighbours, or to one of the connective-tissue partitions in the muscle, and by means of these connections the fibre affects muscle contraction. Between the muscle fibres, and enveloped in a sheath of connective tissue, lie here and there special structures known as muscle-spindles. Each of these contains thin muscle

fibres, numerous nuclei, and the endings of sensory nerves. (See TOUCH.) The heart muscle comprises short fibres which communicate with their neighbours via short branches and have no sarcolemma.

Plain or unstriped muscle is found in the following positions: the inner and middle coats of the STOMACH and INTESTINE; the ureters (see URETER) and URINARY BLADDER; the TRACHEA and bronchial tubes; the ducts of glands; the GALL-BLADDER; the UTERUS and FALLOPIAN TUBES; the middle coat of the blood and lymph vessels; the iris and ciliary muscle of the EYE; the dartos muscle of the SCROTUM; and in association with the various glands and hairs in the SKIN. The fibres are very much smaller than those of striped muscle, although they vary greatly in size. Each has one or more oval nuclei and a delicate sheath of sarcolemma enveloping it. The fibres are grouped in bundles, much as are the striped fibres, but they adhere to one another by cement material, not by the tendon bundles found in voluntary muscle.

Development of muscle All the muscles of the developing individual arise from the central layer (mesoderm) of the EMBRYO, each fibre taking origin from a single cell. Later on in life, muscles have the power both of increasing in size – as the result of use, for example, in athletes – and also of healing, after parts of them have been destroyed by injury. An example of the great extent to which unstriped muscle can develop to meet the demands made on it is the uterus, whose muscular wall develops so much during pregnancy that the organ increases from the weight of 30–40 g (1–1½ oz.) to a weight of around 1 kg (2 lb.), decreasing again to its former small size in the course of a month after childbirth.

Physiology of contraction A muscle is an elaborate chemico-physical system for producing heat and mechanical work. The total energy liberated by a contracting muscle can be exactly measured. From 25–30 per cent of the total energy expended is used in mechanical work. The heat of contracting muscle makes an important contribution to the maintenance of the heat of the body. (See also MYOGLOBIN.)

The energy of muscular contraction is derived from a complicated series of chemical reactions. Complex substances are broken down and built up again, supplying each other with energy for this purpose. The first reaction is the breakdown of adenyl-pyrophosphate into phosphoric acid and adenylic acid (derived from nucleic acid); this supplies the immediate energy for contraction. Next phosphocreatine breaks down into creatine and phosphoric acid, giving energy for the resynthesis of adenyl-pyrophosphate. Creatine is a normal nitrogen-ous constituent of muscle. Then glycogen through the intermediary stage of sugar bound to phosphate breaks down into lactic acid to supply energy for the resynthesis of phospho-creatine. Finally part of the lactic acid is oxi-dised to supply energy for building up the rest of the lactic acid into glycogen again. If there is not enough oxygen, lactic acid accumulates and fatigue results.

All of the chemical changes are mediated by the action of several enzymes (see ENZYME).

Involuntary muscle has several peculiarities of contraction. In the heart, rhythmicality is an important feature – one beat appearing to be, in a sense, the cause of the next beat. Tonus is a character of all muscle, but particularly of unstriped muscle in some localities, as in the walls of arteries.

Fatigue occurs when a muscle is made to act for some time and is due to the accumulation of waste products, especially sarcolactic acid (see LACTIC ACID). These substances affect the end-plates of the nerve controlling the muscle, and so prevent destructive overaction of the muscle. As they are rapidly swept away by the blood, the muscle, after a rest (and particularly if the rest is accompanied by massage or by gentle contrac-tions to quicken the circulation) recovers rap-idly from the fatigue. Muscular activity over the whole body causes prolonged fatigue which is remedied by rest to allow for metabolic balance to be re-established.

Muscle Relaxants

These drugs produce partial or complete par-alysis of skeletal muscle (see under MUSCLE – Structure of muscle). Drugs in clinical use are all reversible and are used to help insert a breathing tube into the TRACHEA (endotracheal tube) during general ANAESTHESIA and ARTI-FICIAL VENTILATION OF THE LUNGS. They may be broadly divided into depolarising and non-depolarising muscle relaxants. Depolarising muscle relaxants act by binding to acetylcholine receptors at the motor end-plate where nerves are attached to muscle cells, and producing a more prolonged depolarisation than acetyl-choline, which results in initial muscle fascicu-lation (overactivity) and then flaccid paralysis of the muscle. The only commonly used depolar-ising drug is succinylcholine which has a rapid

onset of action and lasts approximately three minutes. Non-depolarising muscle relaxants bind to the acetylcholine receptors, preventing acetylcholine from gaining access to them. They have a slower onset time and longer dur-ation than depolarisers, although this varies widely between different drugs. They are com-petitive antagonists and they may be reversed by increasing the concentration of acetylcholine at the motor end-plate using an anticholinesterase agent such as neostigmine. These drugs are broken down in the liver and excreted through the kidney, and their action will be prolonged in liver and renal failure. Other uses include the relief of skeletal muscle spasms in TETANUS, PARKINSONISM and spastic disorders. The drugs dantrolene and diazepam are used in these circumstances.

Muscles, Disorders of

Compression syndrome The tense, pain-ful state of muscles induced by excessive accumulation of INTERSTITIAL fluid in them, following unusual exercise. This condition is more liable to occur in the muscles at the front of the shin, because they lie within a tight fascial membrane: here the syndrome is known as the anterior tibial syndrome ('shin splints'). Prevention consists of always keeping fit and in training for the amount of exercise to be under-taken. Equally important is what is known in sporting circles as 'warming down': i.e., at the end of training or a game, exercise should be gradually tailed off. Treatment consists of eleva-tion of the affected limb, compression of it by compression bandages, with ample exercise of the limb within the bandage, and massage. In more severe cases DIURETICS may be given. Occasionally surgical decompression may be necessary.

Cramp Painful spasm of a muscle usually caused by excessive and prolonged contraction of the muscle fibres. Cramps are common, especially among sportsmen and women, nor-mally lasting a short time. The condition usu-ally occurs during or immediately following exercise as a result of a build-up of LACTIC ACID and other chemical by-products in the muscles – caused by the muscular efforts. Cramps may occur more frequently, especially at night, in people with poor circulation, when the blood is unable to remove the lactic acid from the muscles quickly enough.

Repetitive movements such as writing (writer's cramp) or operating a keyboard can cause cramp. Resting muscles may suffer cramp if a person sits or lies in an awkward position which limits local blood supply to them. Profuse sweating as a result of fever or hot weather can also cause cramp in resting muscle, because the victim has lost sodium salts in the sweat; this disturbs the biochemical balance in muscle tissue.

Treatment is to massage and stretch the affected muscle – for example, cramp in the calf muscle may be relieved by pulling the toes on the affected leg towards the knee. Persistent night cramps sometimes respond to treatment with a drug containing CALCIUM or QUININE. If cramp persists for an hour or more, the person should seek medical advice, as there may be a serious cause such as a blood clot impeding the blood supply to the area affected.

Dystrophy See myopathy below.

Inflammation (myositis) of various types may occur. As the result of injury, an ABSCESS may develop, although wounds affecting muscle generally heal well. A growth due to SYPHILIS, known as a gumma, sometimes forms a hard, almost painless swelling in a muscle. Rheumatism is a vague term traditionally used to define intermittent and often migratory discomfort, stiffness or pain in muscles and joints with no obvious cause. The most common form of myositis is the result of immunological damage as a result of autoimmune disease. Because it affects many muscles it is called POLYMYOSITIS.

Myasthenia (see MYASTHENIA GRAVIS) is muscle weakness due to a defect of neuromuscular conduction.

Myopathy is a term applied to an acquired or developmental defect in certain muscles. It is not a neurological disease, and should be distinguished from neuropathic conditions (see NEUROPATHY) such as MOTOR NEURONE DISEASE (MND), which tend to affect the distal limb muscles. The main subdivisions are genetically determined, congenital, metabolic, drug-induced, and myopathy (often inflammatory) secondary to a distant carcinoma. Progressive muscular dystrophy is characterised by symmetrical wasting and weakness, the muscle fibres being largely replaced by fatty and fibrous tissue, with no sensory loss. Inheritance may take several forms, thus affecting the sex and age of victims.

The commonest type is DUCHENNE MUSCULAR DYSTROPHY, which is inherited as a sex-linked disorder. It nearly always occurs in boys.

Symptoms There are three chief types of myopathy. The commonest, known as pseudo-hypertrophic muscular dystrophy, affects particularly the upper part of the lower limbs of children. The muscles of the buttocks, thighs and calves seem excessively well developed, but nevertheless the child is clumsy, weak on his legs, and has difficulty in picking himself up when he falls. In another form of the disease, which begins a little later, as a rule at about the age of 14, the muscles of the upper arm are first affected, and those of the spine and lower limbs become weak later on. In a third type, which begins at about this age, the muscles of the face, along with certain of the shoulder and upper arm muscles, show the first signs of wasting. All the forms have this in common: that the affected muscles grow weaker until their power to contract is quite lost. In the first form, the patients seldom reach the age of 20, falling victims to some disease which, to ordinary people, would not be serious. In the other forms the wasting, after progressing to a certain extent, often remains stationary for the rest of life. Myopathy may also be acquired when it is the result of disease such as thyrotoxicosis (see under THYROID GLAND, DISEASES OF), osteomalacia (see under BONE, DISORDERS OF) and CUSHING'S DISEASE, and the myopathy resolves when the primary disease is treated.

Treatment Some myopathies may be the result of inflammation or arise from an endocrine or metabolic abnormality. Treatment of these is the treatment of the cause, with supportive physiotherapy and any necessary physical aids while the patient is recovering. Treatment for the hereditary myopathies is supportive since, at present, there is no cure – although developments in gene research raise the possibility of future treatment. Physiotherapy, physical aids, counselling and support groups may all be helpful in caring for these patients.

The education and management of these children raise many difficulties. Much help in dealing with these problems can be obtained from Muscular Dystrophy Campaign.

Myositis ossificans, or deposition of bone in muscles, may be congenital or acquired. The congenital form, which is rare, first manifests itself as painful swellings in the muscles. These gradually harden and extend until the child is

M

encased in a rigid sheet. There is no effective treatment and the outcome is fatal.

The acquired form is a result of a direct blow on muscle, most commonly on the front of the thigh. The condition should be suspected whenever there is severe pain and swelling following a direct blow over muscle. The diagnosis is confirmed by hardening of the swelling. Treatment consists of short-wave DIATHERMY with gentle active movements. Recovery is usually complete.

Pain, quite apart from any inflammation or injury, may be experienced on exertion. This type of pain, known as MYALGIA, tends to occur in unfit individuals and is relieved by rest and physiotherapy. .

Parasites sometimes lodge in the muscles, the most common being *Trichinella spiralis*, producing the disease known as TRICHINOSIS (trichiniasis).

Rupture of a muscle may occur, without any external wound, as the result of a spasmodic effort. It may tear the muscle right across – as sometimes happens to the feeble plantaris muscle in running and leaping – or part of the muscle may be driven through its fibrous envelope, forming a HERNIA of the muscle. The severe pain experienced in many cases of LUMBAGO is due to tearing of one of the muscles in the back. These conditions are usually relieved by rest and massage. Partial muscle tears, such as occur in sport, require more energetic treatment: in the early stages this consists of the application of an ice or cold-water pack, firm compression, elevation of the affected limb, rest for a day or so and then gradual mobilisation (see SPORTS MEDICINE).

Tumours occur occasionally, the most common being fibroid, fatty, and sarcomatous growths.

Wasting of muscles sometimes occurs as a symptom of disease in other organs: for example, damage to the nervous system, as in poliomyelitis or in the disease known as progressive muscular atrophy. (See PARALYSIS.)

Muscular Dystrophy
See MUSCLES, DISORDERS OF – Myopathy.

Musculoskeletal
An adjective that relates to muscle and/or bone. The musculoskeletal system comprises the bones of the skeleton and all the muscles attached to them.

Mushroom Poisoning
See FUNGUS POISONING.

Mutagen
A chemical or physical agent that has the property of increasing the rate of MUTATION among CELLS. A mutagen does not usually increase the range of mutations. Chemicals, ionising radiation, and viruses may act as mutagens.

Mutation
A change occurring in the genetic material (DNA) in the CHROMOSOMES of a cell. It is caused by a fault in the replication of a cell's genetic material when it divides to form two daughter cells. Mutations may occur in somatic cells which may result in a local growth of the new type of cells. These may be destroyed by the body's defence mechanism or they may develop into a tumour. If mutation occurs in a germ cell or gamete – the organism's sex cells – the outcome may be a changed inherited characteristic in succeeding generations. Mutations occur rarely, but a small steady number are caused by background radiation in the environment. They are also caused by mutagens (see MUTAGEN). (See also GENETIC DISORDERS.)

Mutism
See under VOICE AND SPEECH.

Myalgia
Pain in a muscle. (See MUSCLES, DISORDERS OF; BORNHOLM DISEASE; LUMBAGO.)

Myalgic Encephalomyelitis (ME)
A syndrome in which various combinations of extreme fatiguability, muscle pain, lack of concentration, panic attacks, memory loss and depression occur. Its existence and causes have been the subject of controversy reflected in the variety of names given to the syndrome: CHRONIC FATIGUE SYNDROME (CFS), post-viral fatigue syndrome, Royal Free disease, epidemic neuromyasthenia and Icelandic disease. ME often follows virus infections of the upper respiratory tract or gut, but it is not clear whether this is an association or cause-and-effect. It may occur in epidemics or as individual cases. Physical examination shows no evidence of diagnosable disease and there is no diagnostic test – diagnosis usually being made by excluding other possible disorders. The suf-

ferer usually recovers in time, although sometimes recovery may take many months or even years. The most severely affected may be bedridden and may need tube-feeding. There is no specific curative treatment, but symptomatic treatment such as resting in the early stages may help. Some experts believe that the illness has a psychological element, and sufferers have been treated with COGNITIVE BEHAVIOUR THERAPY. In 1998 the Chief Medical Officer set up a multidisciplinary working group, including patients, to consider possible cures and treatments for ME/CFS. The report (2002) concluded that the disorder should be recognised as chronic and treatable, but there was no clear agreement on cause(s) and treatment(s). Meanwhile research continues, including a programme by the Centre of Disease Control in Atlanta, USA. Sufferers may find it helpful to consult the ME Association.

Myasthenia Gravis

A serious disorder in which the chief symptoms are muscular weakness and a special tendency for fatigue to come on rapidly when efforts are made. The prevalence is around 1 in 30,000. Two-thirds of the patients are women, in whom it develops in early adult life. In men it tends to develop later in life.

It is a classical example of an autoimmune disease (see AUTOIMMUNITY). The body develops ANTIBODIES which interfere with the working of the nerve endings in muscle that are acted on by ACETYLCHOLINE. It is acetylcholine that transmits the nerve impulses to muscles: if this transmission cannot be effected, as in myasthenia gravis, then the muscles are unable to contract. Not only the voluntary muscles, but those connected with the acts of swallowing, breathing, and the like, become progressively weaker. Rest and avoidance of undue exertion are necessary, and regular doses of neostigmine bromide, or pyridostigmine, at intervals enable the muscles to be used and in some cases have a curative effect. These drugs act by inhibiting the action of cholinesterase – an ENZYME produced in the body which destroys any excess of acetylcholine. In this way they increase the amount of available acetylcholine which compensates for the deleterious effect of antibodies on the nerve endings.

The THYMUS GLAND plays the major part in the cause of myasthenia gravis, possibly by being the source of the original acetylcholine receptors to which the antibodies are being formed. Thymectomy (removal of the thymus) is often used in the management of patients with myasthenia gravis. The incidence of remission following thymectomy increases with the number of years after the operation. Complete remission or substantial improvement can be expected in 80 per cent of patients.

The other important aspect in the management of patients with myasthenia gravis is IMMUNOSUPPRESSION. Drugs are now available that suppress antibody production and so reduce the concentration of antibodies to the acetylcholine receptor. The problem is that they not only suppress abnormal antibody production, but also suppress normal antibody production. The main groups of immunosuppressive drugs used in myasthenia gravis are the CORTICOSTEROIDS and AZATHIOPRINE. Improvement following steroids may take several weeks and an initial deterioration is often found during the first week or ten days of treatment. Azathioprine is also effective in producing clinical improvement and reducing the antibodies to acetylcholine receptors. These effects occur more slowly than with steroids, and the mean time for an azathioprine remission is nine months.

The Myasthenia Gravis Association, which provides advice and help to sufferers, was created and is supported by myasthenics, their families and friends.

Mycobacterium

A gram-positive (see GRAM'S STAIN) rod-like genus of aerobic BACTERIA, some species of which are harmful to humans and animals. For example, *M. tuberculosis* (Koch's bacillus) and *M. leprae* cause, respectively, TUBERCULOSIS and LEPROSY.

Mycoplasma

A genus of micro-organisms which differ from bacteria in that they lack a rigid cell wall. They are responsible for widespread epidemics in cattle and poultry. For a long time the only member of the genus known to cause disease in humans was *Mycoplasma pneumoniae* which is responsible for the form of PNEUMONIA known as primary atypical pneumonia – particularly common in children, for whom it is the single most common cause of the diseaase when contracted out of hospital. Another, *Mycoplasma genitalium*, has now been isolated which is responsible for certain cases of non-gonococcal urethritis. Mycoplasma infections respond to TETRACYCLINES.

Mycosis

The general term applied to diseases due to the growth of fungi in the body. Among some of the simplest and commonest mycoses are

RINGWORM, FAVUS, and thrush (CANDIDA). The MADURA FOOT of India, ACTINOMYCOSIS, and occasional cases of PNEUMONIA and suppurative ear disease are also due to the growth of moulds in the bodily tissues. Other forms of mycosis include ASPERGILLOSIS, candidiasis (see CANDIDA), CRYPTOCOCCOSIS and HISTOPLASMOSIS.

Mycosis Fungoides

An old term for a chronic eruption of the skin characterised by erythematous (see ERYTHEMA) itching plaques (raised patches on the skin resulting from the merging or enlargement of papules – see PAPULE), which, if left untreated, eventually form tumours and ulcers. The disease is now known to be a form of cancer of lymphocytes (see LYMPHOCYTE) called T-cell LYMPHOMA. It may be responsive to PHOTO-CHEMOTHERAPY in its early stages and to RADIOTHERAPY when more advanced.

Mydriasis

Dilation or widening of the pupil of the EYE. Occurring naturally when it is dark, or when someone is emotionally aroused, mydriasis can also result from the administration of ATROPINE eye drops. Alcohol consumption also has a mydriatic effect.

Myectomy

Removal of all or part of a muscle by surgery. It may be used to correct a SQUINT (caused by unbalanced eye muscles) or to remove a FIBROID from the muscular wall of the UTERUS.

Myelin

A substance made up of protein and phospholipid that forms the sheath surrounding the axons of some neurons (see NEURON(E)). These are described as myelinated or medullated nerve fibres, and electric impulses pass along them faster than along non-myelinated nerves. Myelin is produced by Schwann cells which occur at intervals along the nerve fibre. (See MULTIPLE SCLEROSIS (MS).)

Myelitis

Myelitis is inflammation of the SPINAL CORD.

Myeloblast

Present in the blood-producing tissue in the BONE MARROW, this is a cell with a large nucleus and scanty cytoplasm. It is the precursor cell of a granulocyte (see GRANULOCYTES). Myeloblasts sometimes appear in the blood of patients with various diseases including acute myeloblastic LEUKAEMIA.

Myelocyte

The name given to one of the cells of BONE MARROW from which the granular white cells of the blood are produced. They are found in the blood in certain forms of LEUKAEMIA.

Myelography

The injection of a radio-opaque substance into the central canal of the SPINAL CORD in order to assist in the diagnosis of diseases of the spinal cord or spine using X-ray examination. Because of the high risk of causing damage to the spinal cord (arachnoiditis), it has been largely superceded by MRI.

Myeloid

An adjective that relates to the granulocyte (see GRANULOCYTES) precursor cell in the BONE MARROW. For example, myeloid LEUKAEMIA, which arises from abnormal growth in the blood-forming tissue of the bone marrow.

Myeloma

See MYELOMATOSIS.

Myelomatosis

A MALIGNANT disorder of PLASMA cells, derived from B-lymphocytes (see LYMPHOCYTE). In most patients the BONE MARROW is heavily infiltrated with atypical, monoclonal plasma cells, which gradually replace the normal cell lines, inducing ANAEMIA, LEUCOPENIA, and THROMBOCYTOPENIA. Bone absorption occurs, producing diffuse osteoporosis (see under BONE, DISORDERS OF). In some cases only part of the immunoglobulin molecule is produced by the tumour cells, appearing in the urine as Bence Jones PROTEINURIA.

The disease is rare under the age of 30, frequency increasing with age to peak between 60 and 70 years. There may be a long preclinical phase, sometimes as long as 25 years. When symptoms do occur, they tend to reflect bone involvement, reduced immune function, renal failure, anaemia or hyperviscosity of the blood. Vertebral collapse is common, with nerve root pressure and reduced stature. The disease is eventually fatal, infection being a common cause of death. Local skeletal problems should be treated with RADIOTHERAPY, and the general disease with CHEMOTHERAPY – chiefly the ALKYLATING AGENTS melphalan or cyclophosphamide. Red-blood-cell TRANSFUSION is usually required, together with plasmapheresis (see PLASMA EXCHANGE), and orthopaedic surgery may be necessary following fractures.

Myelosuppression

A fall in the production of blood cells in the BONE MARROW. This fall often occurs after CHEMOTHERAPY for cancer. ANAEMIA, infection and abnormal bleeding are symptomatic of myelosuppression.

Myiasis

Infestation of the SKIN, deeper tissues or the INTESTINE by larvae of the tropical tumbu fly.

Myocardial Infarction

See HEART, DISEASES OF – Coronary thrombosis.

Myocarditis

Inflammation of the muscular wall of the HEART.

Myocardium

Myocardium is the muscular substance of the HEART. (See also MUSCLE.)

Myoclonus

A brief, twitching muscular contraction which may involve only a single muscle or many muscles (see MUSCLE). It may be too slight to cause movement of the affected limb, or so violent as to throw the victim to the floor. The cause is not known, but in some cases may be a form of EPILEPSY. A single myoclonic jerk in the upper limbs occasionally occurs in minor motor epilepsy (petit mal). The myoclonic jerks which many people experience on falling asleep are a perfectly normal phenomenon.

Myoglobin

The protein which gives MUSCLE its red colour. It has the property of combining loosely and reversibly with OXYGEN; this means that it is the vehicle whereby muscle extracts oxygen from the HAEMOGLOBIN in the blood circulating through it, and then releases the oxygen for use in muscle METABOLISM.

Myoglobinuria

The occurrence of MYOGLOBIN in the URINE. This is the oxygen-binding pigment in muscle and mild myoglobinuria may occur during exercise. Severe myoglobinuria will result from serious injuries, particularly crushing injuries, to muscles.

Myoma

The term applied to a TUMOUR, almost invariably of a simple nature, which consists mainly of muscle fibres (see MUSCLE – Structure of muscle). These muscle tumours often occur in the UTERUS.

Myomectomy

Removal by surgery of fibroids (see FIBROID) from the muscular wall of the UTERUS.

Myometrium

The muscular coat of the UTERUS.

Myopathy

See under MUSCLES, DISORDERS OF.

Myopia

Sort-sightedness (see under EYE, DISORDERS OF – Errors of refraction).

Myositis

Inflammation of a muscle. (See also MUSCLES, DISORDERS OF – Inflammation (myositis)).

Myositis Ossificans

See under MUSCLES, DISORDERS OF.

Myotonia

A condition in which the muscles (see MUSCLE), though possessed of normal power, contract only very slowly. The stiffness disappears as the muscles are used.

Myringoplasty

The sealing by a surgical tissue-graft of a hole or perforation in the drum (tympanum) which separates the middle and outer sections of the EAR. It is aimed at improving the subject's hearing (see DEAFNESS); sometimes the operation is done to stop persistent DISCHARGE.

Myringotomy

An operation to cut open the drum of the EAR to provide drainage for an infection of the middle ear. It is now done mainly in children with persistent glue ear (see under EAR, DISEASES OF – Diseases of the middle ear).

Myrrh

Myrrh is a gum-resin obtained from *Commiphora molmol*, an Arabian myrtle tree. It stimulates the function of MUCOUS MEMBRANE with which it is brought in contact or by which it is excreted. Tincture of myrrh is used for a gargle in sore throat, as a toothwash when the gums are inflamed, and as an ingredient of cough mixtures.

Myxoedema
See under THYROID GLAND, DISEASES OF –
Hypothyroidism.

Myxoma
A benign TUMOUR comprising gelatinous CON-
NECTIVE TISSUE, most commonly occurring
beneath the SKIN – although the condition may
develop in the ABDOMEN, URINARY BLADDER,
BONE and, rarely, the HEART. Treatment
involves surgery, which is usually successful.

Myxoviruses
These include the INFLUENZA viruses A, B and
C; and the PARAINFLUENZA VIRUSES, types 1 to
3. Myxoviruses, which are one of a group of
RNA-containing viruses, have an affinity for
protein receptors in red blood cells.

Nabilone

A CANNABIS-related drug given by mouth and licensed for use in treating severe nausea and vomiting, particularly when they result from treatment with anticancer drugs.

Naevus

A congenitally determined tissue abnormality. In the SKIN, naevi of blood vessels are best known, but a MOLE is a MELANOCYTE naevus, and warty streaked and linear naevi of the epidermis occasionally occur. There are several patterns of vascular naevi:

Naevus simplex Also known as 'salmon patch'. About one-third of white children are born with macular pink areas of ERYTHEMA on the nape, brow or eyelids which usually disappear after a few months, but patches on the nape may persist.

Naevus flammeus Also known as 'port-wine stain' and present at birth. It is unilateral, usually on the face, and may be extensive. It tends to darken with age and is permanent. Laser treatment is effective.

Strawberry naevus (cavernous haemangioma) is usually not present at birth but appears within a few weeks and grows rapidly, reaching a peak in size after 6–12 months, when the lobulated red nodule may resemble a ripe strawberry. Untreated, the naevus disappears spontaneously over several years. It may occur anywhere and may be very troublesome when occurring around an eye or on the 'nappy' area. If possible it should be left alone, but where it is causing problems other than simply cosmetic ones it is best treated by an expert. This may involve medical treatment with steroids or interferon or laser therapy.

Spider naevus is due to a dilated ARTERIOLE causing a minute red papule in the skin, the small branching vessels resembling spider legs. A few spider naevi are common in young people, but multiple naevi are common in pregnancy and may also be a warning sign of chronic liver disease.

NAI
See NON-ACCIDENTAL INJURY (NAI).

Nail
See SKIN.

Nail-Biting

A common practice in schoolchildren, most of whom gradually give it up as they approach adolescence. Too much significance should therefore not be attached to it; in itself it does no harm, and punishment or restraining devices are not needed. It is a manifestation of tension or insecurity, the cause of which should be removed. In some people the habit is carried into adulthood.

Nails, Diseases of

Disease may affect the nail fold, nail plate or nail bed (see SKIN – Nail). Inflammation of the nail fold is called paronychia: acute paronychia is usually caused by a minor injury allowing in bacteria, which set up infection; chronic paronychia is often an occupational hazard, due to constant exposure of the hands to water – for example, in the catering industry, agriculture and housework – but may also be caused by impaired circulation in the fingers. Often, ANTIBIOTICS are sufficient for treatment, but sometimes surgical incision is needed.

PSORIASIS is a common cause of disease of the nail plate, as are eczema (see DERMATITIS) and fungal infection (see FUNGAL AND YEAST INFECTIONS). Deformity of the nail may point to systemic disease, as in CLUBBING, or the spoon-shaped concave nails (koilonychia) of severe iron deficiency. Acute toxic illnesses may temporarily disturb nail growth causing horizontal ridges (Beau's lines) which grow out slowly.

Onycholysis is separation of the nail plate from its bed. It may be due to psoriasis of the nail bed and trauma, or may occur spontaneously. Gross thickening of nails is common in the toes, caused by psoriasis or fungal infection.

Nalidixic Acid

An antibiotic drug, active against gram-negative (see GRAM'S STAIN) micro-organisms, used to treat and prevent infections of the URINARY TRACT.

Nalorphine

Nalorphine reduces or abolishes most of the actions of MORPHINE and similarly acting NARCOTICS, such as PETHIDINE HYDROCHLORIDE. It was used as an antidote in the treatment of overdosage with these drugs but has now been superseded by NALOXONE.

Naloxone

An effective drug in the treatment of opioid poisoning. It blocks the effects of most opiates; given intravenously, it acts within 2–3 minutes. The drug is also given to newborn babies whose breathing has been depressed by narcotic drugs given to their mothers to relieve pain during childbirth.

Naltrexone

A drug that is an ANTAGONIST to narcotic substances (see NARCOTICS). Given orally, it is used in the maintenance treatment of HEROIN – and other opiate-dependent people.

Nandrolone

One of the ANABOLIC STEROIDS, with the property of building PROTEIN. It is of little value in medical care, although is licensed for use in aplastic ANAEMIA; it has also been used in the past to treat osteoporosis in women (see under BONE, DISORDERS OF), but is no longer recommended for this purpose. Its use as a bodybuilder by some athletes and others has caused controversy: those found using it are barred from most recognised athletic events. Nandrolone should never be taken by pregnant women or by people with liver disease or prostate cancer. Side-effects include ACNE; VIRILISATION with high doses including voice changes, cessation of periods, and inhibition of sperm production; and liver tumours after prolonged use.

Nanometre

A nanometre is a millionth of a millimetre. The approved abbreviation is nm. (See APPENDIX 6: MEASUREMENTS IN MEDICINE.)

Nappy Rash

A common form of irritant contact DERMATITIS in the nappy area in babies under one year old. Wetting of the skin by urine, abrasion, and chemical changes due to faecal contamination all play a part. Good hygiene and use of disposable absorbent nappies have much reduced its incidence. An ointment containing a barrier, such as titanium dioxide, may help; other medications such as mild CORTICOSTEROIDS or antibiotics should be used very cautiously and only under the guidance of a doctor, as harmful effects may result – especially from overuse.

Naproxen

See under NON-STEROIDAL ANTI-INFLAMMATORY DRUGS (NSAIDS).

Narcissism

An abnormal mental state characterised by excessive admiration of one's self. In Greek mythology, Narcissus so loved staring at his own reflection in water that he eventually fell in and drowned.

Narcolepsy

A condition in which uncontrollable episodes of sleep occur two or three times a day. It starts at any age and persists for life. The attacks, which usually last for 10–15 minutes, come on suddenly at times normally conducive to sleep, such as after a meal, or sitting in a bus, but they may occur when walking in the street. In due course, usually after some years, they are associated with cataplectic attacks (see CATAPLEXY), when for a few seconds there is sudden muscular weakness affecting the whole body. The cataplectic attacks can be controlled by the TRICYCLIC ANTIDEPRESSANT DRUGS, imipramine or clomipramine.

Familial narcolepsy is well recognised, and recently a near-100-per-cent association between narcolepsy and the histocompatability antigen HLA-DR2 (see HLA SYSTEM) has been discovered, which suggests that narcolepsy is an immunorelated disease. The Narcolepsy Association (UK) has been founded to help patients with this strange disorder.

Narcosis

A condition of stupor (see under UNCONSCIOUSNESS), resembling sleep, that is usually caused by a drug. It may also occur as a result of liver or kidney failure which causes URAEMIA. The affected person has significantly reduced awareness and is hard to arouse. Treatment is of the underlying cause and the normal precautions for caring for an unconscious or semiconscious subject should be taken. (See APPENDIX 1: BASIC FIRST AID.).

Narcotics

Substances that induce stupor and eventually UNCONSCIOUSNESS. Used in the relief of severe pain, people can become first tolerant of them – so requiring larger doses – and then dependent (see also ANALGESICS; HYPNOTICS; TOLERANCE; DEPENDENCE).

Nasal Congestion

The nose and nasal sinuses (see SINUS) produce up to a litre of MUCUS in 24 hours, most of which enters the stomach via the NASOPHARYNX. Changes in the nasal lining mucosa occur in response to changes in humidity and atmospheric temperature; these may cause severe congestion, as might an allergic reaction or nasal polyp.

Treatment Topical nasal decongestants include sodium chloride drops and corticosteroid nasal drops (for polyps). For common-cold-induced congestion, vapour inhalants, decongestant sprays and nasal drops, including EPHEDRINE drops, are helpful. Overuse of decongestants, however, can produce a rebound congestion, requiring more treatment and further congestion, a tiresome vicious circle. Allergic RHINITIS (inflammation of the nasal mucosa) usually responds to ipratropium bromide spray.

Systemic nasal decongestants given by mouth are not always as effective as topical administrations but they do not cause rebound congestion. Pseudoephedrine hydrochoride is available over the counter, and most common-cold medicines contain anticongestant substances.

Nasogastric Tube

A small-bore plastic or rubber tube passed into the stomach through the nose, pharynx and then the oesophagus. It is used either to aspirate gas and liquid from the stomach or to pass food or drugs into it.

Nasolacrimal Duct

A duct that goes through the nasolacrimal canal in the palatine bone of the SKULL. The duct drains the tears from the lacrimal (tear) glands into the NOSE.

Nasopharynx

Nasopharynx is the upper part of the throat, lying behind the nasal cavity. (See NOSE.)

National Blood Authority

This body manages regional TRANSFUSION centres. Among its aims are the maintenance and promotion of blood and blood products based on a system of voluntary donors; implementing a cost-effective national strategy for ensuring adequate supplies of blood and its products to meet national needs; and ensuring high standards of safety and quality.

National Care Standards Commission

This was set up under the CARE STANDARDS ACT 2000 as an independent regulator in respect of homes for the elderly, the disabled and children in the state and private sectors in the UK.

National Electronic Library for Health

This National Health Service initiative went online in November 2000. It aims to provide health professionals with easy and fast access to best current knowledge from medical journals, professional group guidelines, etc. Unbiased data can be accessed by both clinicians and the public.

National Health Service (NHS)

The United Kingdom's National Health Service was created by Act of Parliament and inaugurated on 5 July 1948. Its original aim was to provide a comprehensive system of health care to everyone, free at the point of delivery. Scotland had its own, similar legislation, as did Northern Ireland. The service is funded by National Insurance contributions and from general taxation, with a small amount from patient charges. The structure, functioning and financing of the NHS have been – and still are – undergoing substantial changes.

National Infection Control and Health Protection Agency

A National Health Service body intended to combat the increasing threat from infectious diseases and biological, chemical and radiological hazards. Covering England, the agency includes the Public Health Laboratory Service, the National Radiological Protection Board, the Centre for Applied Microbiology and Research, and the National Focus Group for Chemical Incidents.

National Institute for Clinical Excellence (NICE)

This special health authority in the National Health Service, launched in 1999, prepares formal advice for all managers and health professionals working in the service in England and Wales on the clinical- and cost-effectiveness of new and existing technologies. This includes diagnostic tests, medicines and surgical procedures. The institute also gives advice on best practice in the use of existing treatments.

NICE – its Scottish equivalent is the Scottish Health Technology Assessment Centre – has three main functions:

- appraisal of new and existing technologies.
- development of clinical guidelines.
- promotion of clinical audit and confidential inquiries. Central to its task is public concern about 'postcode prescribing' – that is, different availability of health care according to geography.

In 2003 the World Health Organisation appraised NICE. Amongst its recomendations were that there should be greater consistency in the methods used for appraisal and the way in which results and decisions were reported. WHO was concerned about the need for transparency about the conflict between NICE's use of manufacturers' commercial evidence in confidence, and believed there should be greater definition of justification for 'threshold' levels for cost-effectiveness in the Centre's judgement of what represents value for money.

In all, WHO was congratulatory – but questions remain about the practical value and imlementation of NICE guidelines.

National Listening Library

National Listening Library is a charity which produces recorded books for handicapped people who cannot read, with the exception of the blind who have their own separate organisation, the Royal National Institute for the Blind. (See also CALIBRE.)

Natriuresis

The excretion of SODIUM in the URINE, particularly if the amount excreted is more than normal. An agent that causes this sodium excretion – usually a diuretic (see DIURETICS) – is termed a natriuretic.

Nausea

The sensation that VOMITING is about to occur; however, nausea does not always lead to vomiting.

Navel

Navel, or UMBILICUS, is the scar on the abdomen marking the point where the umbilical cord joined the body in embryonic life. (See PLACENTA.)

Near Sight

Myopia. See under EYE, DISORDERS OF – Errors of refraction.

Nebula

The term applied to a slight opacity on the cornea (see EYE) producing a haze in the field of vision, and also to any oily preparation to be sprayed from a nebuliser – an apparatus for splitting up a fluid into fine droplets.

Nebulisers

A nebuliser makes an aerosol (see under INHALANTS) by blowing air or oxygen through a solution of a drug. Many inhaled drugs such as SALBUTAMOL, ipratropium and beclomethasone can be given in this way. It has the advantage over a metered dose inhaler (MDI) that no special effort is required to coordinate breathing, and a nebuliser allows a much greater volume of the drug to be delivered to where it is needed (the airways) compared with that of MDIs. The use of higher doses of bronchodilator drugs made possible by the nebuliser means that the risk of unwanted side-effects is also increased. Fortunately the safety profile of anti-asthmatic drugs such as salbutamol is extremely high and overdose is generally well-tolerated.

Necator Americanus

A hookworm, closely resembling but smaller than the *Ancylostoma duodenale.* (See ANCYLOSTOMIASIS.)

Necropsy

A traditional term for an autopsy or POST-MORTEM EXAMINATION.

Necrosis

Death of a limited portion of tissue, the term being most commonly applied to bones when, as the result of disease or injury, a fragment dies and separates. (See BONE, DISEASES OF.)

Necrotising Fasciitis

Also known as CELLULITIS. A potentially lethal infection caused by the gram-positive (see GRAM'S STAIN) bacterium *Streptococcus pyogenes* which has the property of producing dangerous exotoxins. The infection, which starts in the layer of FASCIA under the SKIN, may spread very rapidly, destroying tissue as it spreads. Urgent antibiotic treatment may check the infection, and surgery is sometimes required, but even with treatment patients may die (see STREPTOCOCCUS).

Needle-Stick Injury

Accidental perforation of the skin by an injection needle, commonly of the hand or finger and usually by a nurse or doctor administering a therapeutic injection. The term also refers to accidental injuries from injection needles discarded by drug abusers. Dangerous infections such as viral HEPATITIS or HIV may be acquired from needle-stick injuries, and there are strict procedures about the disposal of used syringes and needles in medical settings.

Needling

An operation performed in the treatment of cataracts (see under EYE, DISORDERS OF), in which the anterior lens capsule of the EYE is torn open with a needle, allowing the aqueous fluid to dissolve the opaque soft lens matter, which is gradually washed away into the bloodstream. This 'extra-capsular extraction' may need to be repeated several times before all the opaque lens matter disperses. Although a relatively simple procedure, it is unsuitable for patients over the age of 35 (when the nucleus of the lens becomes increasingly hard), and CRYO-SURGERY and LASER therapy have become the preferred methods of treatment.

Needling is also used for certain minor dermatological procedures, such as removal of small facial cysts and scabies mites.

Nefopam Hydrochloride

A non-opioid analgesic drug (see ANALGESICS) of use in the relief of pain that fails to respond to other non-opioid analgesics. It causes little depression of respiration but side-effects may be a problem.

Negativism

Negativism means a morbid tendency in a person to do the opposite of what he or she is desired or directed to do. It is especially characteristic of those suffering from SCHIZOPHRENIA, but is not uncommon in non-psychotic persons.

Negligence

See MEDICAL NEGLIGENCE.

Neisseriaceae

A family of bacteria of which three varieties cause disease. *Neisseria meningitidis* causes meningococcal MENINGITIS and SEPTICAEMIA. It is divided into three groups: A, B and C; group B accounts for most meningitis cases in the UK, mostly affecting children. *Neisseria gonorrhoeae* causes GONORRHOEA. The bacteria are gram-negative (see GRAM'S STAIN) cocci usually occurring in pairs. A third variety is *Moraxella catarrhalis*: this occurs in the nose and throat and sometimes causes ear infection and low-grade infection of the respiratory tract.

Nematode

A roundworm. (See ASCARIASIS.)

Neomycin

Neomycin is one of the AMINOGLYCOSIDES, derived from *Streptomyces fradiae*. It has a wide antibacterial spectrum, being effective against the majority of gram-negative (see GRAM'S STAIN) bacilli. Its use is limited by the fact that it is liable to cause deafness and kidney damage. Its main use is for application to the skin – either in solution or as an ointment – for the treatment of infection; it is also given by mouth

for the treatment of certain forms of ENTERITIS due to *E. coli*.

Neonatal

Pertaining to the first month of life.

Neonatal Intensive Care

The provision of a dedicated unit with special facilities, including one-to-one nursing and appropriate technology, for caring for premature and seriously ill newborn babies. Paediatricians and neonatologists are involved in the running of such units. Not every maternity unit can provide intensive care: for example, the provision of artificial ventilation, other than as a holding procedure until a baby can be transferred to a better-equipped and better-serviced unit. Such hospitals tend to have special-care baby units, which are capable of looking after the needs of most, but not all, premature or ill babies.

Neonatal Mortality

Neonatal mortality is the mortality of infants under one month of age. In England and Wales this has fallen markedly in recent decades: from more than 28 per 1,000 live births in 1939 to 3.6 in 2002. This improvement can be attributed to various factors: better antenatal supervision of expectant mothers; care to ensure that expectant mothers receive adequate nourishing food; improvements in the management of the complications of pregnancy and of labour; and more skilled resuscitation at birth for those who need it.

Nearly three-quarters of neonatal deaths occur during the first week of life. For this reason, increasing emphasis is being laid on this initial period of life. In Britain, in the last four decades of the 20th century, the number of deaths in the first week of life fell dramatically from 13.2 to just over 2.7 per 1,000 live births. The chief causes of deaths in this period are extreme prematurity (less than 28 weeks' gestation), birth asphyxia with oxygen lack to the brain, and congenital abnormalities. After the first week the commonest cause is infection.

Neonatology

The branch of PAEDIATRICS responsible for the medical care of newborn babies. Problems may be short term – for example, those linked to prematurity – or life-long such as CEREBRAL PALSY. After the first few weeks of life, paediatricians take over the responsibility for any specialist medical care required, with general practitioners looking after the infants' primary-care needs.

Neoplasm

This means literally a 'new formation' and is another word for a benign or non-malignant TUMOUR.

Neostigmine

An ANTICHOLINESTERASE drug which enhances neuromuscular transmission – the passage of chemical messages between nerve and muscle cells – in voluntary and involuntary muscles in patients with the disorder MYASTHENIA GRAVIS. Its effect lasts for about four hours. A disadvantage is that it has a marked cholinergic action – affecting heart rhythm, causing excessive salivation and tear secretion, constricting the BRONCHIOLES and stimulating the gastrointestinal tract.

Nephrectomy

The operation for removal of the kidney. (See KIDNEYS, DISEASES OF.)

Nephritis

Inflammation of the kidneys. (See KIDNEYS, DISEASES OF – Glomerulonephritis.)

Nephroblastoma

Nephroblastoma, or Wilm's tumour, is the commonest kidney tumour in infancy (see also KIDNEYS, DISEASES OF – Tumours of the kidney). It is a malignant tumour, which occurs in around 1 per 10,000 live births. The survival rate with modern treatment (removal of the kidney followed by radiotherapy and chemotherapy) is now around 80 per cent.

Nephrolithiasis

A condition in which CALCULI are present in the kidney.

Nephrology

The branch of medicine concerned with the study and management of kidney disease. A specialist in these diseases is called a nephrologist.

Nephron

Each kidney comprises over a million of these microscopic units which regulate and control the formation of URINE. A tuft of capillaries invaginates the Bowmans capsule, which is the blind-ending tube (GLOMERULUS) of each nephron. Plasma is filtered out of blood and through the Bowmans capsule into the renal tubule. As the filtrate passes along the tubule, most of the water and electrolytes are reabsorbed. The composition is regulated with the retention or addition of certain molecules (e.g. urea, drugs, etc.). The tubules eventually empty the filtrate, which by now is urine, into the renal pelvis from where it flows down the ureters into the bladder. (See KIDNEYS.)

Nephropathy

A description of any damage or disease to the kidneys (see KIDNEYS, DISEASES OF).

Nephropexy

Surgical fixation (to the 12th rib and posterior abdominal wall) of a mobile kidney; this prevents the kidney from descending in the abdomen when the affected person stands up.

Nephroptosis

The condition in which a kidney (see KIDNEYS) is mobile or 'floating' instead of being fixed to the back of the abdominal cavity.

Nephroscope

An endoscopic instrument for examining the inside of the kidney (see KIDNEYS). It is normally passed into the renal pelvis of the organ via a route from the surface of the skin. Instruments can be passed through the nephroscope under direct vision to remove CALCULI (stones) or break them up using ULTRASOUND.

Nephrostomy

Nephrostomy is the operation of making an opening into the kidney (see KIDNEYS) to drain it.

Nephrotic Syndrome

Nephrotic syndrome is one of PROTEINURIA, hypo-albuminaemia and gross OEDEMA. The primary cause is the leak of albumin (see ALBUMINS) through the GLOMERULUS. When this exceeds the liver's ability to synthesise albumin, the plasma level falls and oedema results. The nephrotic syndrome is commonly the result of primary renal glomerular disease (see KIDNEYS, DISEASES OF – Glomerulonephritis). It may also be a result of metabolic diseases such as diabetic glomerular sclerosis and AMYLOIDOSIS. It may be the result of systemic autoimmune diseases such as SYSTEMIC LUPUS ERYTHEMATOSUS (SLE) and POLYARTERITIS NODOSA. It may complicate malignant diseases such as MYELOMATOSIS and Hodgkin's disease (see LYMPHOMA). It is sometimes caused by nephrotoxins such as gold or mercury and certain drugs, and it may be the result of certain infections such as MALARIA and CROHN'S DISEASE.

Nephrotomy

Nephrotomy means the operation of cutting

into the kidney (see KIDNEYS), in search of CALCULI or for other reasons.

Nerve

A nerve is a bundle of conductory fibres called axons (see AXON) that emanate from neurones (see NEURON(E)) – the basic anatomical and functional units of the NERVOUS SYSTEM. Nerves make up the central nervous system (BRAIN and SPINAL CORD) and connect that system to all parts of the body, transmitting information from sensory organs via the peripheral nerves to the centre and returning instructions for action to the relevant muscles and glands.

Nerves vary in size from the large pencil-sized sciatic nerve in the back of the thigh muscles to the single, hair-sized fibres distributed to the skin. A nerve, such as the sciatic, possesses a strong, outer fibrous sheath, called the epineurium, within which lie bundles of nerve-fibres, divided from one another by partitions of fibrous tissue, in which run blood vessels that nourish the nerve. Each of these bundles is surrounded by its own sheath, known as the perineurium, and within the bundle fine partitions of fibrous tissue, known as endoneurium, divide up the bundle into groups of fibres. The finest subdivisions of the nerves are the fibres, and these are of two kinds: medullated and non-medullated fibres. (See NEURON(E) and NERVOUS SYSTEM for more details on structure and functions of neurons and nerves.)

Nerve Block

See ANAESTHESIA – Local anaesthetics.

Nerve Cell

See NEURON(E).

Nerves, Injuries to

These have several causes. Continued or repeated severe pressure may damage a nerve seriously, as in the case of a crutch pressing into the armpit and causing drop-wrist. Bruising due to a blow which drives a superficially placed nerve against a bone may damage, say, the radial nerve behind the upper arm. A wound may sever nerves, along with other structures; this accident is specially liable to occur to the ulnar nerve in front of the wrist when a person accidentally puts a hand and arm through a pane of glass.

Symptoms When a sensory nerve is injured or diseased, sensation is immediately more or less impaired in the part supplied by the nerve. Ulceration or death of the tissue supplied by the

defective nerve may occur. When the nerve in question is a motor one, the muscles governed through it are instantly paralysed. In the latter case, the portion of nerve beyond the injury degenerates and the muscles gradually waste, losing their power of contraction in response to electrical applications. Finally, deformities result and the joints become fixed. This is particularly noticeable when the ulnar nerve is injured, the hand and fingers taking up a claw-like position. The skin may also be affected.

Treatment Damaged or severed (peripheral) nerve fibres should be sewn together, using microsurgery. Careful realignment of the nerve endings gives the fibres an excellent chance of regenerating along the right channels. Full recovery is rare but, with regular physiotherapy to keep paralysed muscles in good shape and to prevent their shortening, the patient can expect to obtain a reasonable return of function after a few weeks, with improvement continuing over several months.

Nervous Breakdown

A non-medical description of a variety of emotional crises ranging from an outburst of hysterical behaviour to a major neurotic illness that may have a lasting effect on an individual's life. Sometimes the term is used to describe an overt psychotic illness – for example, SCHIZOPHRENIA (see also MENTAL ILLNESS; NEUROSIS).

Nervous Impulse

This is transmitted chemically, by the formation at nerve-endings of chemical substances. When, for example, a NERVE to a muscle is stimulated, there appears at the NEURO-MUSCULAR JUNCTION the chemical substance, ACETYLCHOLINE. Acetylcholine also appears at endings of the parasympathetic nerves (see NERVOUS SYSTEM) and transmits the effect of the parasympathetic impulse. When an impulse passes down a sympathetic nerve, the effect of it is transmitted at the nerve-ending by the chemical liberated there: ADRENALINE or an adrenaline-like substance.

Nervous System

This extensive, complex and finely tuned network of billions of specialised cells called neurones (see NEURON(E)) is responsible for maintaining the body's contacts with and responses to the outside world. The network also provides internal communication links – in concert with HORMONES, the body's chemical messengers – between the body's diverse organs and tissues, and, importantly, the BRAIN stores relevant information as memory. Each neurone has a filamentous process of varying length called an AXON along which passes messages in the form of electrochemically generated impulses. Axons are bundled together to form nerves (see NERVE).

The nervous system can be likened to a computer. The central processing unit – which receives, processes and stores information and initiates instructions for bodily activities – is called the central nervous system: this is made up of the brain and SPINAL CORD. The peripheral nervous system – synonymous with the cables that transmit information to and from a computer's processing unit – has two parts: sensory and motor. The former collects information from the body's many sense organs. These respond to touch, temperature, pain, position, smells, sounds and visual images and the information is signalled to the brain via the sensory nerves. When information has been processed centrally, the brain and spinal cord send instructions for action via motor nerves to the 'voluntary' muscles controlling movements and speech, to the 'involuntary' muscles that operate the internal organs such as the heart and intestines, and to the various glands, including the sweat glands in the skin. (Details of the 12 pairs of cranial nerves and the 31 pairs of nerves emanating from the spinal cord are given in respective texts on brain and spinal cord.)

Functional divisions of nervous system
As well as the nervous system's anatomical divisions, the system is divided functionally, into autonomic and somatic parts. The autonomic nervous system, which is split into sympathetic and parasympathetic divisions, deals with the automatic or unconscious control of internal bodily activities such as heartbeat, muscular status of blood vessels, digestion and glandular functions. The somatic system is responsible for the skeletal (voluntary) muscles (see MUSCLE) which carry out intended movements initiated by the brain – for example, the activation of limbs, tongue, vocal cords (speech), anal muscles (defaecation), urethral sphincters (urination) or vaginal muscles (childbirth). In addition, many survival responses – the most powerfully instinctive animal drives, which range from avoiding danger and pain to shivering when cold or sweating when hot – are initiated unconsciously and automatically by the nervous system using the appropriate neural pathways to achieve the particular survival reaction required.

The complex functions of the nervous system include the ability to experience emotions, such as excitement and pleasure, anxiety and frustration, and to undertake intellectual activities. For these experiences an individual can utilise many built-in neurological programmes and he or she can enhance performance through learning – a vital human function that depends on MEMORY, a three stage-process in the brain of registration, storage and recall. The various anatomical and functional divisions of the nervous system that have been unravelled as science has strived to explain how it works may seem confusing. In practical terms, the nervous system works mainly by using automatic or relex reactions (see REFLEX ACTION) to various stimuli (described above), supplemented by voluntary actions triggered by the activity of the conscious (higher) areas of the brain. Some higher functions crucial to human activity – for example, visual perception, thought, memory and speech – are complex and subtle, and the mechanisms are not yet fully understood. But all these complex activities rest on the foundation of relatively simple electrochemical transmissions of impulses through the massive network of billions of specialised cells, the neurones.

Nervous System, Disorders of
The following conditions are discussed under their individual headings: APHASIA; BRAIN, DISEASES OF; CATALEPSY; CHOREA; CRAMP; EPILEPSY; HYSTERIA; LEARNING DISABILITY; MEMORY; MENTAL ILLNESS; MULTIPLE SCLEROSIS (MS); NERVES, INJURIES TO; NEURALGIA; NEURITIS; PARALYSIS; PSYCHOSOMATIC DISEASES; SPINE AND SPINAL CORD, DISEASES AND INJURIES OF; STROKE; TABES.

Nettle-Rash
See URTICARIA.

Neuralgia
Pain which is the result of damage to or irritation of a NERVE. The pain tends to be intermittent, occurring in short bursts. It may be very severe and be located along an identifiable nerve. A particular disorder may give rise to neuralgia, MIGRAINE being an example, and HERPES ZOSTER (shingles) another. Neuralgia may also be caused by disturbance to a particular nerve – for instance, trigeminal neuralgia which affects the sensory nerve supplying most of the face.

Treatment Any obvious underlying cause should be dealt with. Neuralgia may be symptomatically relieved with ANALGESICS. Severe pain may be helped by the analgesic carbamazepine or by destroying (freezing, local alcohol injection or surgery) the affected nerve.

Neural Tube
The structure in the EMBRYO from which the BRAIN and SPINAL CORD develop.

Neural Tube Defects
Congenital abnormalities resulting from the failure of the NEURAL TUBE to form normally. The resulting conditions include SPINA BIFIDA, MENINGOCELE and defects in the bones of the SKULL.

Neurasthenia
An out-of-date term that was used to describe an ill-defined state of nervous exhaustion in which, although the patient suffers from no definite disease, he or she becomes incapable of sustained exertion. The condition which it represented is now believed to be a form of NEUROSIS or psychosomatic disease. It was also used in the past to describe what is now called CHRONIC FATIGUE SYNDROME (CFS).

Neurectomy
An operation in which part of a NERVE is excised: for example, for the relief of NEURALGIA.

Neurilemma
The thin membranous covering which surrounds every nerve-fibre. (See NERVE.)

Neuritis
Inflammation affecting a nerve or nerves which may be localised to one part of the body – as, for instance, in SCIATICA – or which may be general, being then known as multiple neuritis, or POLYNEURITIS. Owing to the fact that the most peripheral parts of the nerves are usually affected in the latter condition (i.e. the fine subdivisions in the substance of the muscles), it is also known as peripheral neuritis.

Causes In cases of localised neuritis, the fibrous sheath of the nerve is usually at fault, the actual nerve-fibres being only secondarily affected. This condition may be due to inflammation spreading into the nerve from surrounding tissues; to cold; or to long-continued irritation by pressure on the nerve. The symptoms produced vary according to the function of the nerve, in the case of sensory nerves being usually neuralgic pain (see NEURALGIA), and in the case of motor nerves some degree of paralysis in the muscles to which the nerves pass.

In polyneuritis, usually due to some general or constitutional cause, the nerve-fibres themselves in the small nerves degenerate and break down. The condition is protracted because, for recovery to occur, the growth of new nerve-fibres from the healthy part of the nerve has to take place. The cause of polyneuritis may be infection by a virus – for example, HERPES ZOSTER – or a bacterium, as in LEPROSY. Neuritis may also be the result of agents such as alcohol, lead or products from industrial or agricultural activities. ORGANOPHOSPHORUS insecticides are believed by some to be a factor in neuritis and other neurological conditions.

Neuroblastoma
A malignant growth comprising embryonic nerve cells. It may start in any part of the AUTONOMIC NERVOUS SYSTEM. The medulla of the adrenal gland (see under ENDOCRINE GLANDS) is a common site; secondary growths develop in other tissues. Neuroblastomas are the most common extracranial solid tumour of childhood. The incidence is around eight cases per one million children. Treatment is by surgery followed by radiotherapy and CYTOTOXIC drugs. About 30 per cent of sufferers survive for at least five years after treatment.

Neurodermatoses
See under SKIN, DISEASES OF.

Neurofibrils
A microscopic strand of CYTOPLASM that occurs in the cell body of a NEURON(E) as well as in the semifluid content of the AXON of a nerve cell.

Neurofibromatosis
See VON RECKLINGHAUSEN'S DISEASE.

Neuroglia
The fine web of tissue and branching cells which supports the nerve-fibres and cells of the nervous system. (See NERVE.)

Neuroleptics
Drugs used to quieten disturbed patients, whether this is the result of brain damage, MANIA, DELIRIUM, agitated DEPRESSION or an acute behavioural disturbance. They relieve the florid PSYCHOTIC symptoms such as hallucinations and thought-disorder in SCHIZOPHRENIA and prevent relapse of this disorder when it is in remission.

Most of these drugs act by blocking DOPAMINE receptors. As a result they can give rise to the extrapyramidal effects of PARKINSONISM and may also cause HYPERPROLACTINAEMIA.

Troublesome side-effects may require control by ANTICHOLINERGIC drugs. The main antipsychotic drugs are: (i) chlorpromazine, methotrimeprazine and promazine, characterised by pronounced sedative effects and a moderate anticholinergic and extrapyramidal effect; (ii) pericyazine, pipothiazine and thioridazine, which have moderate sedative effects and marked anticholinergic effects, but less extrapyramidal effects than the other groups; (iii) fluphenazine, perphenazine, prochlorperazine, sulpiride and trifluoperazine, which have fewer sedative effects and fewer anticholinergic effects, but more pronounced extrapyramidal effects.

Neurology

The branch of medical practice and science which is concerned with the study of the NERVOUS SYSTEM and its disorders. Specialists in neurology – neurologists – examine a patient's nerves, sensory and motor functions and reflexes. They use modern imaging techniques – for example, CT scanning (see COMPUTED TOMOGRAPHY) and MRI – to aid diagnosis. Until relatively recently, many neurological conditions could be treated only with palliative methods. Now there is much improved understanding of the nervous system and its disorders, with closer liaison between psychiatrists (see PSYCHIATRY) and neurologists.

Neuroma

Neuroma means a TUMOUR connected with a NERVE – such tumours being generally composed of fibrous tissue, and of a painful nature.

Neuromuscular Blockade

In clinical practice, the transmission of impulses at the NEUROMUSCULAR JUNCTION may be blocked to paralyse temporarily a patient for a surgical procedure, or to assist treatment on the intensive care unit. There are two main types of drug, both of which competitively block the ACETYLCHOLINE receptors on the motor end plates. (1) Depolarising neuromuscular blocking agents: these act by first producing stimulation at the receptor, and then by blocking it. There are characteristic muscle fasciculations before the rapid onset of paralysis which is of short duration (less than five minutes with the commonly used drug, suxamethonium). The drug is removed from the receptor by the enzyme, CHOLINESTERASE. (2) Non-depolarising neuromuscular blocking agents: these drugs occupy the receptor and prevent acetylcholine from becoming attached to it. However, in sufficiently high concentra-

tions, acetylcholine will compete with the drug and dislodge it from the receptor; the effect of these drugs is reversed by giving an anticholinesterase, which allows the amount of acetylcholine at the neuromuscular junction to build up. These drugs have varying durations of action, but all are slower in onset and of longer duration than the depolarisers.

Neuromuscular Junction

The area where a motor NERVE ends close to the MUSCLE membrane so can initiate muscle contraction. The motor-nerve ending is separated from the motor end plate by the synaptic cleft which is only 50–70 nm wide. When a nerve impulse arrives at the motor-nerve ending, molecules of ACETYLCHOLINE are released which cross the synaptic cleft and attach to receptors on the motor end plate. This initiates depolarisation of the muscle which in turn initiates the process of contraction. Acetylcholinesterase (an ENZYME) rapidly breaks down the molecules of acetylcholine, thus ending their action and freeing the receptor in preparation for the next impulse.

Neuron(e)

Also known as a nerve cell, this is the basic cellular building-block of the NERVOUS SYSTEM, which contains billions of neurones linked in a complex network and acting in different combinations to keep the body informed about the outside world, and then to organise and activate appropriate responses. There are three main types of neurone:

Sensory These carry signals to the central nervous system (CNS) – the BRAIN and SPINAL CORD – from sensory receptors. These receptors respond to different stimuli such as touch, pain, temperature, smells, sounds and light.

Motor These carry signals from the CNS to activate muscles or glands.

Interneurons These provide the interconnecting 'electrical network' within the CNS.

Structure Each neurone comprises a cell body, several branches called dendrites, and a single filamentous fibre called an AXON. Axons may be anything from a few millimetres to a metre long; at their end are several branches acting as terminals through which electrochemical signals are sent to target cells, such as those of muscles, glands or the dendrites of another axon.

Axons of several neurones are grouped

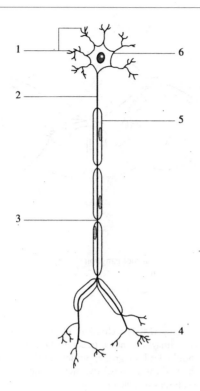

1 dendrites	4 bare axons
2 axon	5 myelin sheath
3 node of Ranvier	6 cell body

Diagram of neurone.

together to form nerve tracts within the brain or spinal cord or nerve-fibres outside the CNS. Each nerve is surrounded by a sheath and contains bundles of fibres. Some fibres are medullated, having a sheath of MYELIN which acts as insulation, preventing nerve impulses from spreading beyond the fibre conveying them.

The cellular part of the neurones makes up the grey matter of the brain and spinal cord – the former containing 600 million neurones. The dendrites meet with similar outgrowths from other neurones to form synapses. White matter is the term used for that part of the system composed of nerve fibres.

Functions of nerves The greater part of the bodily activity originates in the nerve cells (see NERVE). Impulses are sent down the nerves which act simply as transmitters. The impulse causes sudden chemical changes in the muscles as the latter contract (see MUSCLE). The impulses from a sensory ending in the skin pass along a nerve-fibre to affect nerve cells in the spinal cord and brain, where they are perceived as a sensation. An impulse travels at a rate of about 30 metres (100 feet) per second. (See NERVOUS IMPULSE.)

The anterior roots of spinal nerves consist of motor fibres leading to muscles, the posterior roots of sensory fibres coming from the skin. The terms, EFFERENT and AFFERENT, are applied to these roots, because, in addition to motor fibres, fibres controlling blood vessels and secretory glands leave the cord in the anterior roots. The posterior roots contain, in addition to sensory fibres, the nerve-fibres that transmit impulses from muscles, joints and other organs, which among other neurological functions provide the individual with his or her

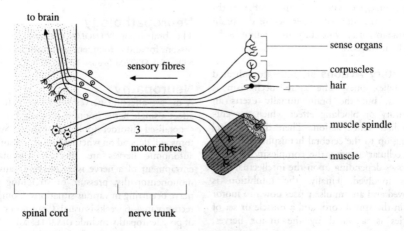

Diagram showing nervous connections between the central nervous system and muscle and skin.

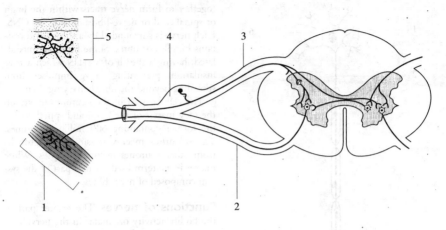

1 muscle	4 dorsal root ganglion
2 ventral root	5 skin
3 dorsal root	

Diagram of a reflex arc.

proprioceptive faculties – the ability to know how various parts of the body are positioned.

The connection between the sensory and motor systems of nerves is important. The simplest form of nerve action is that known as automatic action. In this, a part of the nervous system, controlling, for example, the lungs, makes rhythmic discharges to maintain the regular action of the respiratory muscles. This controlling mechanism may be modified by occasional sensory impressions and chemical changes from various sources.

Reflex action This is an automatic or involuntary activity, prompted by fairly simple neurological circuits, without the subject's consciousness necessarily being involved. Thus a painful pinprick will result in a reflex withdrawal of the affected finger before the brain has time to send a 'voluntary' instruction to the muscles involved.

Voluntary Actions are more complicated than reflex ones. The same mechanism is involved, but the brain initially exerts an inhibitory or blocking effect which prevents immediate reflex action. Then the impulse, passing up to the cerebral hemispheres, stimulates cellular activity, the complexity of these processes depending upon the intellectual processes involved. Finally, the inhibition is removed and an impulse passes down to motor cells in the spinal cord, and a muscle or set of muscles is activated by the motor nerves. (Recent advances in magnetic resonance imaging (MRI) techniques have provided very clear images of nerve tracts in the brain which should lead to greater understanding of how the brain functions.) (See BRAIN; NERVOUS SYSTEM; SPINAL CORD.)

Neuropathic Bladder
A URINARY BLADDER with complete or partial loss of sensation. As there is no sensation of fullness, the individual either develops complete retention of URINE, or the bladder empties automatically – usually every few hours. The condition predisposes affected individuals to urinary-tract infections and back pressure on the KIDNEYS, leading to renal failure. It may be caused by spinal injury, SPINA BIFIDA or any disorder which produces NEUROPATHY.

Neuropathology
The branch of PATHOLOGY that covers the reasons for and consequences of disorders of the NERVOUS SYSTEM (see also NEUROLOGY).

Neuropathy
A disease affecting nerves (see NERVE). It may affect a single nerve (mononeuropathy) or be a generalised disorder (polyneuropathy). Symptoms will depend on whether motor, sensory, or autonomic nerves are affected. Trauma or entrapment of a nerve is a common cause of mononeuropathy, pressure or stretching of a nerve occurring in various situations. Complete recovery in 4–6 weeks is usual. Common causes of polyneuropathy include DIABETES MELLITUS, vitamin B deficiency (often alcohol-associated)

and some viral infections. Genetic and toxic neuropathies are also seen.

Neurosis

A general term applied to mental or emotional disturbance in which, as opposed to PSYCHOSIS, there is no serious disturbance in the perception or understanding of external reality. However, the boundaries between neurosis and psychosis are not always clearly defined. Neuroses are usually classified into anxiety neuroses, depressive neuroses, phobias (see PHOBIA), HYPOCHONDRIASIS, HYSTERIA and obsessional neuroses.

Anxiety neurosis, or anxiety state, constitutes the most common form of neurosis; fortunately it is also among the most responsive to treatment. Once the neurosis develops, sufferers are in a state of persistent anxiety and worry, 'tensed up', always fatigued and unable to sleep at night. In addition, there are often physical complaints – for example, palpitations, sweating, apparent discomfort on swallowing ('globus'), and headache.

Obsessional neuroses are much less common and constitute only about 5 per cent of all neuroses. Like other neuroses, they usually develop in early adult life. (See MENTAL ILLNESS.)

Neurosurgery

Surgery performed on some part of the NERVOUS SYSTEM, whether brain, spinal cord or nerves. Disorders treated by neurosurgeons include damage to the brain, spinal cord and nerves as a result of injury; tumours in the CENTRAL NERVOUS SYSTEM; abnormalities of blood vessels in or supplying blood to the brain – for example, ANEURYSM; brain abscess; bleeding inside the skull; and certain birth defects such as HYDROCEPHALUS and SPINA BIFIDA.

Neurotic

A vague term applied to a person of nervous temperament, whose actions are largely determined by emotions or instincts rather than by reason.

Neurotoxin

A chemical substance that harms nervous tissue, causing symptoms of numbness or weakness of the body part supplied by the damaged NERVE. The venom of some snakes contains neurotoxic substances, and bacteria may produce neurotoxins: examples are those that cause DIPHTHERIA and TETANUS. Arsenic and lead are examples of inorganic neurotoxins.

Neurotransmitter

A chemical substance which transmits the action of a NERVE to a cell (see CELLS). It is released from nerve-endings and transmits the impulse across synapses (see SYNAPSE) to other nerves. In the central nervous system the substances acting as neurotransmitters include ACETYLCHOLINE, NORADRENALINE, DOPAMINE and SEROTONIN. The main transmitter in the peripheral system is acetylcholine, while for the sympathetic system it is noradrenaline. In recent years a new group of neurotransmitters called neuropeptides has been identified, comprising large protein molecules. One of the best-known is that of endorphins, which the brain uses to control pain. (See also NEURON(E); NERVOUS SYSTEM; PAIN.)

Neutron

A neutron is one of the particles that enter into the structure of the atomic nucleus. (See ISOTOPE.)

Neutropenia

A reduction in the number of neutrophil LEUCOCYTES per cubic millimetre of circulating blood to a figure below that found in health. There is still some disagreement over the precise limits of normality, but a count of fewer than 1,500 per mm^3 would be generally accepted as constituting neutropenia. Several infective diseases are characterised by neutropenia, including typhoid fever (see ENTERIC FEVER), INFLUENZA and MEASLES. It may also be induced by certain drugs, including chloramphenicol, the sulphonamides and chlorpromazine.

Neutrophil

A type of leucocyte or white blood cell (see LEUCOCYTES; BLOOD).

NHS

See NATIONAL HEALTH SERVICE (NHS).

NHS Direct

A government-initiated, countrywide, telephone-based helpline which enables members of the public with a potential emergency or inquiry about health to receive counselling over the telephone. They can then be advised on the most appropriate course of action: perhaps an urgent visit to the nearest Accident & Emergency department, a non-urgent visit to the general practitioner, or even self-medication. The intention is to reduce the high workloads of GPs and A&E departments without

endangering patients. NHS Direct is expected to be enhanced to provide:
- links to community pharmacies and social services.
- access to NHS Direct information via the Internet and information points in public sites.
- publication of a guide on health care for dispatch to callers.

NHS Executive
The top management body in the health service. It is part of the Department of Health.

NHS Litigation Authority
See MEDICAL LITIGATION.

NHS Modernisation Board
A group of senior health- and social-care professionals, frontline staff, managers and patients' representatives set up in 2000 to advise the Secretary of State for Health on the implementation of the NHS plan – a ten-year programme for improving the service.

Niclosamide
A widely used anthelmintic drug (see ANTHELMINTICS) for treating TAENIASIS or tapeworm infection.

Nicotinamide
Nicotinamide, the amide of NICOTINIC ACID, is usually used instead of the latter in the treatment of vitamin B deficiency.

Nicotine
An alkaloid which is the principal addictive agent in TOBACCO. The small amount of nicotine in a single cigarette is sufficient to stimulate mental and bodily activities. In larger quantities it acts as a depressant or narcotic – habitual smokers may find its effect sedating. Nicotine works by stimulating the production of a chemical called DOPAMINE, a neurotransmitter or chemical messenger between nerve cells. Nicotine mimics the action of a neurotransmitter called ACETYLCHOLINE. Nerve cells that produce dopamine have acetylcholine-receptor molecules on their surfaces; when these 'nicotine-like' receptors are occupied by acetylcholine molecules, a cell is prompted to produce dopamine. So nicotine itself can artificially stimulate dopamine production. Dopamine is part of the neuronal circuitry that plays a part in the body's perception of pleasure, which is why smoking is enjoyed by many people.

Nicotinic Acid
Nicotinic acid is a member of the vitamin B complex. It is essential for human nutrition, the normal daily requirement for an adult being about 15–20 mg. A deficiency of nicotinic acid is one of the factors in the etiology of PELLAGRA, and either nicotine acid or NICOTINAMIDE is used in the treatment of this condition. Nicotinic acid also reduces the concentration of blood lipids (see HYPERLIPIDAEMIA).

Nidus
A site of infection within the body from which it can spread to other tissues.

Nifedipine
A member of the CALCIUM-CHANNEL BLOCKERS group of cardiovascular drugs. It relaxes vascular smooth muscle and dilates coronary and peripheral arteries. Nifedipine has been used to prevent and treat ANGINA PECTORIS and certain types of HYPERTENSION.

Night Blindness
See under BLINDNESS.

Night Sweats
Copious PERSPIRATION occurring in bed at night and found in conditions such as TUBERCULOSIS, BRUCELLOSIS and lymphomas (see LYMPHOMA), as well as thyrotoxicosis (see under THYROID GLAND, DISEASES OF), anxiety states and menopausal flushes (see MENOPAUSE).

Nipple
The small, sensitive prominence at the tip of each breast (see BREASTS) containing (in women) the small openings through which milk can pass from the milk glands in the breast tissue. The nipple and its surrounding area (the areola) are darker than the adjacent skin. The area becomes darker during pregnancy.

Nipples, Diseases of
See BREASTS, DISEASES OF.

Nitrates
Chemical compounds that have a valuable role in the treatment of ANGINA PECTORIS. They are very effective in dilating the ARTERIES supplying the HEART; their prime benefit, however, is to reduce the return of venous blood to the heart (via the superior and inferior venae cavae), thus reducing the demands on the left ventricle, which pumps deoxygenated blood to the lungs. Undesirable side-effects such as flushing, headache and postural HYPOTENSION may restrict the use of nitrates. Among the nitrate drugs

used is GLYCERYL TRINITRATE which, taken under the tongue (sublingually), provides quick, symptomatic relief of angina, lasting for up to half an hour. Alternative administration can be via a spray product. Isorbide dinitrate taken sublingually is a more stable preparation, suitable for patients who need nitrates infrequently. The drug's effect may last for 12 hours in modified-release form. Patients taking long-acting nitrates or preparations absorbed through the skin (transdermal) may develop TOLERANCE.

Nitrazepam

A tranquilliser introduced as a hypnotic. It is long-acting and may produce drowsiness next day. Addiction can occur. (See TRANQUILLISERS; HYPNOTICS; BENZODIAZEPINES.)

Nitric Oxide (NO)

A naturally occurring chemical that performs a wide range of biological roles. It is involved in the laying down of memories in the BRAIN; in killing viruses, bacteria and cancer cells; and in helping to control blood pressure. NO, comprising a nitrogen atom attached to an oxygen one, is one of the smallest of biologically active compounds as well as having such diverse functions. The chemical is a muscle relaxant and is important in maintaining the heart and circulation in good condition. NO is also the toxic agent released by macrophages (see MACROPHAGE) to kill invading germs and spreading cancer cells. It acts as an essential NEUROTRANSMITTER and protects nerve cells against stress. Researchers are studying how it might be used to treat diseases, for example by using it as an inhaled gas in certain respiratory conditions.

Nitrofurantoin

A synthetic nitrofuran derivative which has a wide range of antibacterial activity and is effective against many gram-positive and gram-negative (see GRAM'S STAIN) micro-organisms. It is used mainly in the treatment of infections of the lower URINARY TRACT.

Nitrogen Mustards

The nitrogen analogues of mustard gas are among the most important ALKYLATING AGENTS used in the treatment of various forms of malignant disease. They include chlormethine, busulphan, chlorambucil and melphalan.

Nitrous Oxide Gas

Also known as laughing gas, this is (at ordinary pressures) a colourless, sweetish-smelling gas. It is used with oxygen to provide relief of pain (see ANALGESICS; PAIN) and mild ANAESTHESIA during childbirth, during painful dental procedures, and at the site of major accidents. It has a rapid action and the effects do not last for long.

Nociceptors

NERVE endings which detect and respond to painful or unpleasant stimuli.

Nocturia

Excess passing of URINE during the night. Among its many causes are glomerulonephritis (see under KIDNEY, DISEASES OF) and enlargement of the PROSTATE GLAND.

Nocturnal Enuresis

The involuntary passing of URINE during sleep. It is a condition predominantly of childhood, and usually genetically determined. Sometimes, however, it is a symptom of anxiety in a child, especially if there has been over-rigorous attempts at toilet-training or hostile or unloving behaviour by a parent. It can also be provoked by apparently unimportant changes in a child's life – for example, moving house. In a small minority of cases it is due to some organic cause such as infection of the genito-urinary tract.

The age at which a child achieves full control of bladder function varies considerably. Such control is sometimes achieved in the second year, but much more commonly not until 2–3 years old. Some children do not normally achieve such control until the fourth, or even fifth, year, so that paediatricians are reluctant to make this diagnosis before a child is aged six.

The approach consists essentially of reassurance and firm but kindly and understanding training. In most cases the use of a 'star chart' and a buzzer alarm which wakens the child should he or she start passing urine is helpful. Where there are relationship or social problems, these need to be considered in treating the child. The few who have urinary infection or irritable bladders may respond to drug treatment.

Those who do not respond may be helped by DDAVP, an analogue of a pituitary hormone, which reduces the amount of urine produced overnight. It is licensed for use for three months at a time. Some children prefer to reserve it for occasions such as sleeping away from home. The antidepressant imipramine can help some children but has to be used cautiously because of side-effects.

For help, contact www.eric.org.uk

Node
The term node is widely used in medicine. For instance, the smaller lymphatic glands are often termed LYMPH NODES. It is also applied to a collection of nerve cells forming a subsidiary nerve centre found in various places in the sympathetic nervous system (see NERVOUS SYSTEM), such as the sinuatrial node and the atrioventricular node which control the beating of the HEART.

Noise
See DEAFNESS; OCCUPATIONAL DISEASES.

Noma
Another name for CANCRUM ORIS.

Nomifensine
See ANTIDEPRESSANT DRUGS.

Non-Accidental Injury (NAI)
(See also CHILD ABUSE). Though NAI has traditionally been seen as abuse against children – and they are still the main victims – such injuries can also be inflicted on vulnerable adults. Adults with learning difficulties, dementias or physical disabilities sufficiently serious as to require institutional care (or who make heavy demands on relatives) are sometimes the victims of NAI. Health professionals, social workers and relatives should bear this possibility in mind when discovering unusual, severe or repeated bruising or fractures in vulnerable adults, even in circumstances where NAI may seem unlikely. (See also MUNCHAUSEN'S SYNDROME; PAEDOPHILIA.)

Non-Conventional Medicine
An umbrella term to describe alternative, complementary, folk and other types of healing practices that are outside the definition of conventional western-type medical practice. (See COMPLEMENTARY AND ALTERNATIVE MEDICINE (CAM).)

Non-Hodgkin's Lymphoma
See LYMPHOMA.

Non-Proprietary Name
See GENERIC DRUG; APPROVED NAMES FOR MEDICINES.

Non-Specific Urethritis (NSU)
An inflammatory condition of the URETHRA due to a cause or causes other than GONORRHOEA. The most common is CHLAMYDIA trachomatis – there has been a rise of over 75 per cent in the incidence in the UK over the past five years to around 70,000 a year. It produces pelvic inflammatory disease in women, which often results in sterility, the risk of ECTOPIC PREGNANCY, and recurrent pelvic pain. Most cases respond well to TETRACYCLINES. Abstinence from sexual intercourse should be observed during treatment and until cure is complete. Children born to infected mothers may have their eyes infected during birth, producing the condition known as ophthalmia neonatorum. This is treated by the application to the eye of chlortetracycline eye ointment. The lungs of such a child may also be infected, resulting in pneumonia.

Non-Steroidal Anti-Inflammatory Drugs (NSAIDs)
These act by inhibiting the formation of PROSTAGLANDINS which are mediators of INFLAMMATION. They act both as ANALGESICS to relieve pain, and as inhibitors of inflammation. Aspirin is a classic example of such a compound. Newer compounds have been synthesised with the aim of producing fewer and less severe side-effects. They are sometimes preferred to aspirin for the treatment of conditions such as RHEUMATOID ARTHRITIS, OSTEOARTHRITIS, sprains, strains and sports injuries. Their main side-effects are gastrointestinal: gastric ulcers and gastric haemorrhage may result (see STOMACH, DISEASES OF). This is because prostaglandins are necessary for the production of the mucous protective coat in the stomach and, when the production of prostaglandin is inhibited, the protection of the stomach is compromised. NSAIDs should therefore be used with caution in patients with DYSPEPSIA and gastric ulceration. The various non-steroidal anti-inflammatory drugs differ little from each other in efficacy, although there is considerable variation in patient response. Ibuprofen is one of the first choices in this group of drugs as it combines good efficacy with a low incidence of side-effects and administration is only required twice daily. Other drugs in this series include diclofenac, fenbufen, fenclofenac, fenoprofen, feprazone, flurbiprofen, indomethacin, indoprofen, ketoprofen, ketorolac, naproxen, piroxicam, sulindac, tiaprofenic acid and tolmetin.

Noradrenaline
A precursor of ADRENALINE in the medulla of the suprarenal glands (see ADRENAL GLANDS). It is also present in the BRAIN. Its main function is to mediate the transmission of impulses in the SYMPATHETIC NERVOUS SYSTEM; it also has a transmitter function in the brain.

Norepinephrine
See NORADRENALINE.

Norethisterone
A synthetic preparation that has the action of PROGESTERONE, but is active when given by mouth.

Norm
The expected value for something measurable. Most people have measurements lying to either side of the norm. Traditionally in medicine, only those lying beyond two standard deviations from the norm are considered likely to be abnormal (approximately 3 per cent of those measured). (See STANDARD DEVIATION.)

Normal
A term used in several different senses. Generally speaking, it is applied to anything which agrees with the regular and established type. In chemistry, the term is applied to solutions of acids or bases of such strength that each litre contains the number of grams corresponding to the molecular weight of the substance in question. In physiology the term 'normal' is applied to solutions of such strength that, when mixed with a body fluid, they are ISOTONIC and cause no disturbance: for example, normal saline solution.

Normoblast
The precursor of an erythrocyte (see ERYTHROCYTES; BLOOD) which still contains the remnant of a NUCLEUS.

Normotensive
Having a BLOOD PRESSURE within the NORMAL range for an individual's age and sex.

Nortriptyline
One of the ANTIDEPRESSANT DRUGS; also a sedative.

Nose
In the course of RESPIRATION, incoming air enters via the nose and is here warmed, moistened, and filtered before entering the lungs. The nose has a protective function, irritant air being expelled by SNEEZING. It is also the organ of SMELL.

Several sinuses (see SINUS) lie concealed in the bones of the SKULL, into which air enters freely by apertures connecting them with the nose. These cavities occupy spaces in the frontal bone over the eyebrow (frontal sinus); in the upper jaw-bone, filling in the angle between the EYE and the nose (maxillary sinus); in the sphenoid bone (sphenoidal sinus); and in the lateral part of the ethmoid bone (ethmoidal sinus). The sinuses drain into the interior of the nose, as does the Eustachian or auditory tube from the middle ear (see EAR).

Nose, Disorders of
Certain skin diseases – particularly CHILBLAIN, ACNE, LUPUS and ERYSIPELAS – tend to affect the NOSE, and may be very annoying. Redness of the skin may be caused by poor circulation in cold weather.

Acute inflammation is generally the result of a viral infection (see COLD, COMMON) affecting the mucous membrane and paranasal sinuses (see SINUSITIS); less commonly it results from the inhalation of irritant gases. Boils may develop just inside the entrance to the nose, causing pain; these are potentially troublesome as infection can spread to the sinuses. HAY FEVER is one distressing form of acute rhinitis.

Malformations are of various kinds. Racial and familial variations in the external nose occur and may be a reason for RHINOPLASTY. Differences in the size and shape of the nose occur, often forming the starting point for chronic inflammation of the nose, perennial rhinitis (all the year round), hay fever, or ASTHMA. More commonly, obstruction results from nasal polyps or adenoids, leading to inhalation through the mouth. Adenoids are an overgrowth of glandular tissue at the back of the throat, into which the nose opens. Polyps are growths of soft jelly-like character: they arise from chronic inflammation associated with allergic rhinitis, chronic sinusitis, asthma, and aspirin abuse. Large polyps can cause erosion of the nasal bones and should be surgically removed.

Bleeding (see HAEMORRHAGE).

Foreign bodies At first these may not cause any symptoms, but in time they can cause obstruction of the affected nostril with a foulsmelling bloody discharge. The problem is common with small children who tend to push small objects into their noses. Foreign bodies require removal, sometimes in hospital. Anyone attempting to remove a foreign body should take care not to push it further into the nose.

Loss of sense of smell, or anosmia, may be temporary or permanent. Temporary anosmia is caused by conditions of the nose which are reversible, whereas permanent

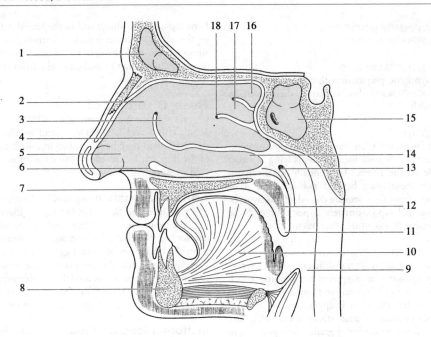

The lateral wall of the right half of the nasal cavity.

1 frontal sinus	10 tongue
2 atrium of middle meatus	11 uvula
3 middle nasal concha	12 soft palate
4 middle meatus	13 auditory tube
5 vestibule	14 inferior nasal concha
6 inferior meatus	15 sphenoidal sinus
7 maxilla	16 sphenoethmoidal recess
8 mandible	and higher nasal concha
9 pharynx	17 superior nasal concha
	18 superior meatus

anosmia is caused by conditions which destroy the OLFACTORY NERVES. Temporary conditions are those such as the common cold, or other inflammatory conditions of the nasal mucosa or the presence of nasal polyps (see above). Permanent anosmia may follow influenzal NEURITIS or it may also follow injuries to the brain and fractures of the skull involving the olfactory nerves.

Injury to nose The commonest injury is a fracture of the nasal bones or displacement of the cartilage that forms the bridge of the nose. The nasal SEPTUM may also be displaced sideways by a lateral blow. Sporting activities, especially boxing and rugby football, are commonly a cause of nasal injury. If a fracture is suspected, or if there is substantial tissue swelling, an X-ray examination is necessary. Resetting a damaged bone should be done either immediately, before swelling makes surgery difficult, or ten days or so later when the swelling has subsided. Results

are usually good, ensuring a clear airway as well as a restored profile. It is not unusual for the cheek-bone to sustain a depressed fracture at the same time as the nose is broken. Careful assessment and prompt surgery are called for. (For more information on fractures, see under BONE, DISORDERS OF).

Rhinitis Inflammation of the MUCOUS MEMBRANE lining the nose. Symptoms include nasal discharge and obstruction, sneezing and sometimes pain in the sinuses. There are several types of rhinitis:

● Allergic – due to allergy to dust, pollen or other airborne particles. Also called hay fever, allergic rhinitis causes a runny nose, sneezing and local congestion. It affects up to 10 per cent of the population and is more common in people suffering from other allergic disorders such as asthma or eczema (see DERMATITIS). Skin tests help to identify the causative ALLERGEN which the sufferer can then try to avoid, although in the case of pollen this is difficult. Decongestant drugs, ANTIHISTAMINE DRUGS, and CORTICO-STEROIDS may help, as can SODIUM CROMO-GLYCATE inhaled regularly during the pollen season. A desensitisation course to a particular allergen sometimes provides long-term relief.

- Atrophic rhinitis is caused by a deterioration in the nasal mucous membrane as a result of chronic bacterial infection, nasal surgery or AGEING. Symptoms include persistent nasal infection and discharge and loss of sense of smell. ANTIBIOTICS and, in some cases, OES-TROGENS alleviate the symptoms.
- Hypertrophic rhinitis results from repeated nasal infection, and is characterised by thickened nasal membranes and congestion of the nasal veins. Removal of thickened mucosa may help severe cases.
- Vasomotor rhinitis occurs when the mucosa becomes oversensitive to stimuli such as pollutants, temperature changes or certain foods or medicines. It may occur as a result of emotional disturbances and is common in pregnancy.
- Viral rhinitis occurs as a result of infection by the common cold virus; treatment is symptomatic. Sinusitis is sometimes a complication.

Nosology
The term applied to scientific classification of diseases.

Nostrils
See NOSE.

Notifiable Diseases
Diseases, usually of an infectious nature, which are required by law to be made known to a health officer or local authority. (See INFEC-TION.) Certain occupational diseases are also notifiable.

Notifiable diseases in the UK (For more information on a specific disease, refer to the separate dictionary entry.)
Acute encephalitis
Acute poliomyelitis
Anthrax
Cholera
Diphtheria
Dysentery (amoebic or bacillary)
Ebola virus disease
Food poisoning
Lassa fever
Leprosy (reported to Chief Medical Officer at the Department of Health)
Leptospirosis
Malaria
Marburg disease
Measles
Meningitis
Meningococcal septicaemia (without meningitis)
Mumps
Ophthalmia neonatorum
Paratyphoid fever
Plague
Rabies
Relapsing fever
Rubella
Scarlet fever.
Smallpox
Tetanus
Tuberculosis
Typhoid fever
Typhus
Viral haemorrhagic fever (including Lassa fever)
Viral hepatitis
Whooping cough
Yellow fever
    Reporting AIDS is voluntary (and in confidence) to the Director, Communicable Diseases Surveillance Centre (PHLS).

NSAIDs
See   NON-STEROIDAL   ANTI-INFLAMMATORY DRUGS (NSAIDS).

NSU
See NON-SPECIFIC URETHRITIS (NSU).

Nucha
The Latin name for the back of the neck. (Adjective – nuchal.)

Nuclear Magnetic Resonance (NMR)
See MAGNETIC RESONANCE IMAGING (MRI).

Nuclear Medicine
The branch of medicine concerned with the use of radioactive material in the diagnosis, investigation and treatment of disease.

Nucleic Acid
A substance constructed out of units known as nucleotides which consist of a purine or pyrimidine base linked to a pentose sugar, which in turn is esterified with phosphoric acid. Two types of nucleic acid occur in nature: deoxyribonucleic acid (DNA) and ribonucleic acid (RNA).

Nucleoside Reverse Transcriptase Inhibitor

See REVERSE TRANSCRIPTASE INHIBITOR.

Nucleus

The central body in a cell, which controls the activities of the latter. (See CELLS.)

Nucleus Pulposus

The inner core of an intervertebral disc. (See SPINAL COLUMN.)

Nullipara

The term applied to a woman who has never borne a child.

Numbness

See TOUCH.

Nursing

Nurses are the largest single group of staff working in the health service. There are more than 330,000 qualified nursing posts in NHS trusts and primary care across the UK. Would-be registered nurses (RNs) do either a three-year diploma programme or a four-year degree. An increasing number of nurses are now acquiring degrees, either as their initial qualification or by studying part-time later in their career. This has led to an often heated debate over the nature of nursing and whether there is now too much emphasis on academic theory at the expense of hands-on care.

Nursing is changing rapidly, and today's nurses are expected to take on an extended role – often performing tasks which were once the sole preserve of doctors, such as diagnosing, prescribing drugs and admitting and discharging patients.

There are four main branches of nursing: adult, child, mental health and learning disability. Student nurses qualify in one of these areas and then apply to go on the nursing register. This is held by nursing's regulatory body, the Council for Nursing and Midwifery. Nurses are expected to abide by the Council's Code of Professional Conduct. The organisation's main role is protecting the public and it is responsible for monitoring standards and dealing with allegations of misconduct. There are more than 637,000 qualified nurses on the Council's register, and this is the main pool from which the NHS and other employers recruit.

The criticisms about nurses' education being too academic, and persisting problems of recruitment of nurses into the NHS, were among factors prompting a strategic government review of the status, training, pay and career opportunities for nurses and other health professionals. The new model emphasises the practical aspects of the education programme with a better response to the needs of patients and the NHS. It also offers nurses a more flexible career path and education linked more closely with practice development and research, so as to provide greater scope for continuing professional education and development.

About 60 per cent of RNs work in NHS hospitals and community trusts. But an increasing number are choosing to work elsewhere, either in the private sector or in jobs such as school nursing, occupational health or for NHS Direct, the nurse-led telephone helpline. Others have dropped out of nursing altogether. The health service is facing a shortage of qualified nurses and many trust employers have resorted to overseas recruitment drives. The government has launched a major nurse recruitment and retention campaign and is promoting family-friendly employment practices to lure those with a nursing qualification currently working outside the NHS back into the workforce. Nursing is a mainly female profession and a third of nurses work part-time.

Nurses' pay has for long compared unfavourably with other professional employment opportunities, despite being determined by an independent Pay Review Body. With the recruitment of nurses a perennial problem, the government's strategy, Making a Difference, is to set up a new pay system offering greater flexibility and opportunities for nurses and other health-service staff. In 2005, a newly qualified staff nurse earned around £16,000 a year, while one of the new grade of consultant nurses could command an annual salary of between £27,000 and £42,000. Nurse consultants were introduced in spring 2000 as a means of allowing nurses to progress up the career ladder while maintaining a clinical role.

The nurse of today is increasingly likely to be part of a multidisciplinary team, working alongside a range of other professionals from doctors and physiotherapists to social workers and teachers. A further sign of the times is that many registered nurses are being asked to act in a supervisory role, delegating tasks to non-registered nurses working as health-care assistants and auxiliaries. In recognition of the latter's increasing role, the Royal College of Nursing, the main professional association and trade union for nurses, has now agreed to extend membership to health-care assistants with a Scottish/National Vocational Qualification at level three.

Midwifery Midwives (see MIDWIFE) are practitioners who offer advice and support to women before, during and after pregnancy. They are regulated by the Council for Nursing and Midwifery (formerly the UK Central Council for Nursing, Midwifery and Health Visiting). Registered nurses can take an 18-month course to become a midwife, and there is also a three-year programme for those who wish to enter the profession directly. Midwifery courses lead to a diploma or degree-level qualification. Most midwives work for the NHS and, as with nursing, there are problems recruiting and retaining staff.

Health visiting Health visitors are registered nurses who work in the community with a range of groups including families, the homeless and older people. They focus on preventing ill-health and offer advice on a range of topics from diet to child behavioural problems. They are employed by health trusts, primary-care groups and primary-care trusts.

Nutrition

The process by which the living organism physiologically absorbs and uses food to ensure growth, energy production and repair of tissues. The science of nutrition includes the study of diets and deficiency diseases (see DIET).

Nystagmus

See under EYE, DISORDERS OF.

Nystatin

An antibiotic, isolated from *Streptomyces noursei*, active against *Candida albicans* (see CANDIDA). It is not absorbed from the gut but is useful in gastrointestinal and skin candidosis.

Oat Cell

A type of cell found in one highly malignant form of lung cancer. The cell is small and either oval or round. The nucleus stains darkly and the cytoplasm is sparse and difficult to identify. Oat-cell, or small-cell, carcinoma of the bronchus is usually caused by smoking, and comprises around 30 per cent of all bronchial cancers. It responds to radiotherapy and chemotherapy but, because the growth has usually spread widely by the time it is diagnosed, the prognosis is poor. Results of surgery are unsatisfactory.

Obesity

A condition in which the energy stores of the body (mainly fat) are too large. It is a prevalent nutritional disorder in prosperous countries – increasingly so among children and young people. The Quetelet Index or BODY MASS INDEX, which relates weight in kilograms (W) to height^2 in metres (H^2), is a widely accepted way of classifying obesity in adults according to severity. For example:

Grade of obesity

	BMI (W/H^2)
III	>40
II	30–40
I	25–29·9
not obese	<25

Causes Whatever the causes of obesity, the fact remains that energy intake (in the form of food and drink) must exceed energy output (in the form of activity and exercise) over a sufficiently long period of time.

Obesity tends to aggregate in families. This has led to the suggestion that some people inherit a 'thrifty' gene which predisposes them to obesity in later life by lowering their energy output. Indeed, patients often attribute their obesity to such a metabolic defect. Total energy output is made up of the resting metabolic rate (RMR), which represents about 70 per cent of the total; the energy cost of physical activity; and thermogenesis, i.e. the increase in energy output in response to food intake, cold exposure, some drugs and psychological influences. In general, obese people are consistently found to have a higher RMR and total energy output, per person – and also when expressed against fat-free mass – than do their lean counterparts. Most obese people do not appear to have a reduced capacity for thermogenesis. Although a genetic component to obesity remains a possibility, it is unlikely to be great or to prevent weight loss from being possible in most patients by reducing energy intake. Environmental influences are believed to be more important in explaining the familial association in obesity.

An inactive lifestyle plays a minor role in the development of obesity, but it is unclear whether people are obese because they are inactive or are inactive because they are obese. For the majority of obese people, the explanation must lie in an excessive energy intake. Unfortunately, it is difficult to demonstrate this directly since the methods used to assess how much people eat are unreliable. For most obese people it seems likely that the defect lies in their failure to regulate energy intake in response to a variety of cognitive factors (e.g. ease of fitting of clothes) in the long term.

Unfortunately, it can be possible to identify by the time of their first birthday, many of the children destined to be obese.

Rarely, obesity has an endocrine basis and is caused by hypothyroidism (see under THYROID GLAND, DISEASES OF), HYPOPITUITARISM, HYPOGONADISM or CUSHING'S SYNDROME.

Symptoms Obesity has adverse effects on MORBIDITY and mortality (see DEATH RATE) which are greatest in young adults and increase with the severity of obesity. It is associated with an increased mortality and/or morbidity from cardiovascular disease, non-insulin-dependent diabetes mellitus, diseases of the gall-bladder, osteoarthritis, hernia, gout and possibly certain cancers (i.e. colon, rectum and prostate in men, and breast, ovary, endometrium and cervix in women). Menstrual irregularities and ovulatory failure are often experienced by obese women. Obese people are also at greater risk when they undergo surgery. With the exception of gallstone formation, weight loss will reduce these health risks.

Treatment Creation of an energy deficit is essential for weight loss to occur, so the initial line of treatment is a slimming diet. An average deficit of 1,000 kcal/day (see CALORIE) will produce a loss of 1 kg of fat/week and should be aimed for. Theoretically, this can be achieved by increasing energy expenditure or reducing energy intake. In practice, a low-energy diet is the usual form of treatment since attempts to increase energy expenditure, either by physical exercise or a thermogenic drug, are relatively ineffective.

Anorectic drugs, gastric stapling and jaw-wiring are sometimes used to treat severe obesity. They are said to aid compliance with a low-energy diet by either reducing hunger (anorectic drugs) or limiting the amount of food the patient can eat. Unfortunately, the long-term effectiveness of gastric stapling is not known, and it is debatable whether the modest reduction in weight achieved by use of anorectic drugs is worthwhile – although a new drug, ORLISTAT, is becoming available that reduces the amount of fat absorbed from food in the gastrointestinal tract. For some grossly obese patients, jaw-wiring can be helpful, but a regain of weight once the wires are removed must be prevented. These procedures carry a risk, so should be done only if an individual's health is in danger.

Obsessive Compulsive Disorder

A mental-health problem which will be experienced at some time by up to 3 per cent of adults. The main feature is the occurrence of spontaneous intrusive thoughts that cause intense anxiety. Many of these thoughts prompt urges, or compulsions, to carry out particular actions in order to reduce the anxiety. One of the commonest obsessions is a fear of dirt and contamination that prompts compulsive cleaning or repeated and unnecessary handwashing. (See MENTAL ILLNESS.)

Obstetrics

The branch of medicine dealing with pregnancy and giving birth. Derived from the Latin word for midwifery (see MIDWIFE), it is closely allied to GYNAECOLOGY. It is concerned with the health of the woman and fetus, from early in pregnancy through to a successful labour and delivery. Pregnancy and childbirth are, however, normal physiological events and for most women they take place without complications. Nevertheless, if something does go wrong, skilled medical care should be immediately available to help the mother and baby achieve a successful outcome. Routine monitoring of pregnancies by midwives and, where necessary, general practitioners or obstetricians is well recognised as a significant contribution to a successful pregnancy and delivery. Such monitoring has been greatly facilitated by advances in ULTRASOUND, AMNIOSCOPY, and amnio- and cordocentesis (see PRENATAL SCREENING OR DIAGNOSIS). Numerous problems may occur at all stages, and early detection, followed rapidly by sensitive and appropriate treatment, is vital. Doctors and nurses can specialise in obstetrics after suitable training. (See also PREGNANCY AND LABOUR.)

Obstipation

Severe CONSTIPATION.

Obstruction of the Bowels

See under INTESTINE, DISEASES OF.

Occiput

The lower and hinder part of the head, where it merges into the neck.

Occlusion

The way that the TEETH fit together when the jaws close. Also the closing or obstruction of a duct, hollow organ, or blood vessel.

Occult

Describing something that is not easily seen. Occult blood in the faeces is present in very small amounts and can be identified only by a chemical test or under the microscope.

Occupational Health, Medicine and Diseases

Occupational health The effect of work on human health, and the impact of workers' health on their work. Although the term encompasses the identification and treatment of specific occupational diseases, occupational health is also an applied and multidisciplinary subject concerned with the prevention of occupational ill-health caused by chemical, biological, physical and psychosocial factors, and the promotion of a healthy and productive workforce.

Occupational health includes both mental and physical health. It is about compliance with health-and-safety-at-work legislation (and common law duties) and about best practice in providing work environments that reduce risks to health and safety to lowest practicable levels. It includes workers' fitness to work, as well as the management of the work environment to accommodate people with disabilities, and procedures to facilitate the return to work of those absent with long-term illness. Occupational health incorporates several professional groups, including occupational physicians, occupational health nurses, occupational hygienists, ergonomists, disability managers, workplace counsellors, health-and-safety practitioners, and workplace physiotherapists.

In the UK, two key statutes provide a

framework for occupational health: the Health and Safety at Work, etc. Act 1974 (HSW Act); and the Disability Discrimination Act 1995 (DDA). The HSW Act states that employers have a duty to protect the health, safety and welfare of their employees and to conduct their business in a way that does not expose others to risks to their health and safety. Employees and self-employed people also have duties under the Act. Modern health-and-safety legislation focuses on assessing and controlling risk rather than prescribing specific actions in different industrial settings. Various regulations made under the HSW Act, such as the Control of Substances Hazardous to Health Regulations, the Manual Handling Operations Regulations and the Noise at Work Regulations, set out duties with regard to different risks, but apply to all employers and follow the general principles of risk assessment and control. Risks should be controlled principally by removing or reducing the hazard at source (for example, by substituting chemicals with safer alternatives, replacing noisy machinery, or automating tasks to avoid heavy lifting). Personal protective equipment, such as gloves and ear defenders, should be seen as a last line of defence after other control measures have been put in place.

The employment provisions of the DDA require employers to avoid discriminatory practice towards disabled people and to make reasonable adjustments to working arrangements where a disabled person is placed at a substantial disadvantage to a non-disabled person. Although the DDA does not require employers to provide access to rehabilitation services – even for those injured or made ill at work – occupational-health practitioners may become involved in programmes to help people get back to work after injury or long-term illness, and many businesses see the retention of valuable staff as an attractive alternative to medical retirement or dismissal on health grounds.

Although a major part of occupational-health practice is concerned with statutory compliance, the workplace is also an important venue for health promotion. Many working people rarely see their general practitioner and, even when they do, there is little time to discuss wider health issues. Occupational-health advisers can fill in this gap by providing, for example, workplace initiatives on stopping smoking, cardiovascular health, diet and self-examination for breast and testicular cancers. Such initiatives are encouraged because of the perceived benefits to staff, to the employing organisation and to the wider public-health agenda. Occupational psychologists recognise

the need for the working population to achieve a 'work-life balance' and the promotion of this is an increasing part of occupational health strategies.

The law requires employers to consult with their staff on health-and-safety matters. However, there is also a growing understanding that successful occupational-health management involves workers directly in the identification of risks and in developing solutions in the workplace. Trade unions play an active role in promoting occupational health through local and national campaigns and by training and advising elected workplace safety representatives.

Occupational medicine The branch of medicine that deals with the control, prevention, diagnosis, treatment and management of ill-health and injuries caused or made worse by work, and with ensuring that workers are fit for the work they do.

Occupational medicine includes: statutory surveillance of workers' exposure to hazardous agents; advice to employers and employees on eliminating or reducing risks to health and safety at work; diagnosis and treatment/management of occupational illness; advice on adapting the working environment to suit the worker, particularly those with disabilities or long-term health problems; and advice on the return to work and, if necessary, rehabilitation of workers absent through illness. Occupational physicians may play a wider role in monitoring the health of workplace populations and in advising employers on controlling health hazards where ill-health trends are observed. They may also conduct epidemiological research (see EPIDEMIOLOGY) on workplace diseases.

Because of the occupational physician's dual role as adviser to both employer and employee, he or she is required to be particularly diligent with regards to the individual worker's medical CONFIDENTIALITY. Occupational physicians need to recognise in any given situation the context they are working in, and to make sure that all parties are aware of this.

Occupational medicine is a medical discipline and thus is only part of the broader field of occupational health. Although there are some specific clinical duties associated with occupational medicine, such as diagnosis of occupational disease and medical screening, occupational physicians are frequently part of a multidisciplinary team that might include, for example, occupational-health nurses, health-and-safety advisers, ergonomists, counsellors and hygienists. Occupational physicians are medical practitioners with a post-registration qualification in occupational medicine. They will have completed a period of supervised in-post training. In the UK, the Faculty of Occupational Medicine of the Royal College of Physicians has three categories of membership, depending on qualifications and experience: associateship (AFOM); membership (MFOM); and fellowship (FFOM).

Occupational diseases Occupational diseases are illnesses that are caused or made worse by work. In their widest sense, they include physical and mental ill-health conditions.

In diagnosing an occupational disease, the clinician will need to examine not just the signs and symptoms of ill-health, but also the occupational history of the patient. This is important not only in discovering the cause, or causes, of the disease (work may be one of a number of factors), but also in making recommendations on how the work should be modified to prevent a recurrence – or, if necessary, in deciding whether or not the worker is able to return to that type of work. The occupational history will help in deciding whether or not other workers are also at risk of developing the condition. It will include information on:
● the nature of the work.
● how the tasks are performed in practice.
● the likelihood of exposure to hazardous agents (physical, chemical, biological and psychosocial).
● what control measures are in place and the extent to which these are adhered to.
● previous occupational and non-occupational exposures.
● whether or not others have reported similar symptoms in relation to the work.

Some conditions – certain skin conditions, for example – may show a close relationship to work, with symptoms appearing directly only after exposure to particular agents or possibly disappearing at weekends or with time away from work. Others, however, may be chronic and can have serious long-term implications for a person's future health and employment.

Statistical information on the prevalence of occupational disease in the UK comes from a variety of sources, including official figures from the Industrial Injuries Scheme (see below) and statutory reporting of occupational disease (also below). Neither of these official schemes provides a representative picture, because the former is restricted to certain prescribed conditions and occupations, and the latter suffers from gross under-reporting. More useful are data from the various schemes that make up the Occupational Diseases Intelligence Network

(ODIN) and from the Labour Force Survey (LFS). ODIN data is generated by the systematic reporting of work-related conditions by clinicians and includes several schemes. Under one scheme, more than 80 per cent of all reported diseases by occupational-health physicians fall into just six of the 42 clinical disease categories: upper-limb disorders; anxiety, depression and stress disorders; contact DERMATITIS; lower-back problems; hearing loss (see DEAFNESS); and ASTHMA. Information from the LFS yields a similar pattern in terms of disease frequency. Its most recent survey found that over 2 million people believed that, in the previous 12 months, they had suffered from an illness caused or made worse by work and that 19.5 million working days were lost as a result. The ten most frequently reported disease categories were:
● stress and mental ill-health (see MENTAL ILLNESS): 515,000 cases.
● back injuries: 508,000.
● upper-limb and neck disorders: 375,000.
● lower respiratory disease: 202,000.
● deafness, TINNITUS or other ear conditions: 170,000.
● lower-limb musculoskeletal conditions: 100,000.
● skin disease: 66,000.
● headache or 'eyestrain': 50,000.
● traumatic injury (includes wounds and fractures from violent attacks at work): 34,000.
● vibration white finger (hand-arm vibration syndrome): 36,000.

A person who develops a chronic occupational disease may be able to sue his or her employer for damages if it can be shown that the employer was negligent in failing to take reasonable care of its employees, or had failed to provide a system of work that would have prevented harmful exposure to a known health hazard. There have been numerous successful claims (either awarded in court, or settled out of court) for damages for back and other musculoskeletal injuries, hand-arm vibration syndrome, noise-induced deafness, asthma, dermatitis, MESOTHELIOMA and ASBESTOSIS. Employers' liability (workers' compensation) insurers are predicting that the biggest future rise in damages claims will be for stress-related illness. In a recent study, funded by the Health and Safety Executive, about 20 per cent of all workers – more than 5 million people in the UK – claimed to be 'very' or 'extremely' stressed at work – a statistic that is likely to have a major impact on the long-term health of the working population.

While victims of occupational disease have

the right to sue their employers for damages, many countries also operate a system of no-fault compensation for the victims of prescribed occupational diseases. In the UK, more than 60 diseases are prescribed under the Industrial Injuries Scheme and a person will automatically be entitled to state compensation for disability connected to one of these conditions, provided that he or she works in one of the occupations for which they are prescribed. The following short list gives an indication of the types of diseases and occupations prescribed under the scheme:

● CARPAL TUNNEL SYNDROME connected to the use of hand-held vibrating tools.
● hearing loss from (amongst others) use of pneumatic percussive tools and chainsaws, working in the vicinity of textile manufacturing or woodworking machines, and work in ships' engine rooms.
● LEPTOSPIROSIS – infection with *Leptospira* (various listed occupations).
● viral HEPATITIS from contact with human blood, blood products or other sources of viral hepatitis.
● LEAD POISONING, from any occupation causing exposure to fumes, dust and vapour from lead or lead products.
● asthma caused by exposure to, among other listed substances, isocyanates, curing agents, solder flux fumes and insects reared for research.
● mesothelioma from exposure to asbestos.

In the UK, employers and the self-employed have a duty to report all occupational injuries (if the employee is off work for three days or more as a result), diseases or dangerous incidents to the relevant enforcing authority (the Health and Safety Executive or local-authority environmental-health department) under the Reporting of Injuries, Diseases and Dangerous Occurrences Regulations 1995 (RIDDOR). Despite this statutory duty, comparatively few diseases are reported so that figures generated from RIDDOR reports do not give a useful indication of the scale of occupational diseases in the UK. The statutory reporting of injuries is much better, presumably because of the clear and acute relationship between a workplace accident and the resultant injury. More than 160,000 injuries are reported under RIDDOR every year compared with just 2,500 or so occupational diseases, a gross underestimate of the true figure.

There are no precise figures for the number of people who die prematurely because of work-related ill-health, and it would be impossible to gauge the exact contribution that work has on, for example, cardiovascular disease and cancers where the causes are multifactorial. The toll would, however, dwarf the number of deaths caused by accidents at work. Around 250 people are killed by accidents at work in the UK each year – mesothelioma, from exposure to asbestos at work, alone kills more than 1,300 people annually.

The following is a sample list of occupational diseases, with brief descriptions of their aetiologies.

Inhaled materials

PNEUMOCONIOSIS covers a group of diseases which cause fibrotic lung disease following the inhalation of dust. Around 250–300 new cases receive benefit each year – mostly due to coal dust with or without silica contamination. SILICOSIS is the more severe disease. The contraction in the size of the coal-mining industry as well as improved dust suppression in the mines have diminished the importance of this disease, whereas asbestos-related diseases now exceed 1,000 per year. Asbestos fibres cause a restrictive lung disease but also are responsible for certain malignant conditions such as pleural and peritoneal mesothelioma and lung cancer. The lung-cancer risk is exacerbated by cigarette-smoking.

Even though the use of asbestos is virtually banned in the UK, many workers remain at risk of exposure because of the vast quantities present in buildings (much of which is not listed in building plans). Carpenters, electricians, plumbers, builders and demolition workers are all liable to exposure from work that disturbs existing asbestos.

OCCUPATIONAL ASTHMA is of increasing importance – not only because of the recognition of new allergic agents (see ALLERGY), but also in the number of reported cases. The following eight substances are most frequently linked to occupational asthma (key occupations in brackets): isocyanates (spray painters, electrical processors); flour and grain (bakers and farmers); wood dust (wood workers); glutaraldehyde (nurses, darkroom technicians); solder/colophony (welders, electronic assembly workers); laboratory animals (technicians, scientists); resins and glues (metal and electrical workers, construction, chemical processors); and latex (nurses, auxiliaries, laboratory technicians).

The disease develops after a short, symptomless period of exposure; symptoms are temporally related to work exposures and relieved by absences from work. Removal of the worker from exposure does not necessarily lead to complete cessation of symptoms. For many agents, there is no relationship with a previous history of ATOPY. Occupational asthma accounts for about 10 per cent of all asthma cases.

DERMATITIS The risk of dermatitis caused by an allergic or irritant reaction to substances used or handled at work is present in a wide variety of jobs. About three-quarters of cases are irritant contact dermatitis due to such agents as acids, alkalis and solvents. Allergic contact dermatitis is a more specific response by susceptible individuals to a range of allergens (see ALLERGEN). The main occupational contact allergens include chromates, nickel, epoxy resins, rubber additives, germicidal agents, dyes, topical anaesthetics and antibiotics as well as certain plants and woods. Latex gloves are a particular cause of occupational dermatitis among health-care and laboratory staff and have resulted in many workers being forced to leave their profession through ill-health. (See also SKIN, DISEASES OF.)

Musculoskeletal disorders Musculoskeletal injuries are by far the most common conditions related to work (see LFS figures, above) and the biggest cause of disability. Although not all work-related, musculoskeletal disorders account for 36.5 per cent of all disabilities among working-age people (compared with less than 4 per cent for sight and hearing impairment). Back pain (all causes – see BACKACHE) has been estimated to cause more than 50 million days lost every year in sickness absence and costs the UK economy up to £5 billion annually as a result of incapacity or disability. Back pain is a particular problem in the health-care sector because of the risk of injury from lifting and moving patients. While the emphasis should be on preventing injuries from occurring, it is now well established that the best way to manage most lower-back injuries is to encourage the patient to continue as normally as possible and to remain at work, or to return as soon as possible even if the patient has some residual back pain. Those who remain off work on long-term sick leave are far less likely ever to return to work.

Aside from back injuries, there are a whole range of conditions affecting the upper limbs, neck and lower limbs. Some have clear aetiologies and clinical signs, while others are less well defined and have multiple causation. Some conditions, such as carpal tunnel syndrome, are prescribed diseases in certain occupations; however, they are not always caused by work (pregnant and older women are more likely to report

carpal tunnel syndrome irrespective of work) and clinicians need to be careful when assigning work as the cause without first considering the evidence. Other conditions may be revealed or made worse by work – such as OSTEOARTHRITIS in the hand. Much attention has focused on injuries caused by repeated movement, excessive force, and awkward postures and these include tenosynovitis (inflammation of a tendon) and epicondylitis. The greatest controversy surrounds upper-limb disorders that do not present obvious tissue or nerve damage but nevertheless give significant pain and discomfort to the individual. These are sometimes referred to as 'repetitive strain injury' or 'diffuse RSI'. The diagnosis of such conditions is controversial, making it difficult for sufferers to pursue claims for compensation through the courts. Psychosocial factors, such as high demands of the job, lack of control and poor social support at work, have been implicated in the development of many upper-limb disorders, and in prevention and management it is important to deal with the psychological as well as the physical risk factors. Occupations known to be at particular risk of work-related upper-limb disorders include poultry processors, packers, electronic assembly workers, data processors, supermarket check-out operators and telephonists. These jobs often contain a number of the relevant exposures of dynamic load, static load, a full or excessive range of movements and awkward postures. (See UPPER LIMB DISORDERS.)

Physical agents A number of physical agents cause occupational ill-health of which the most important is occupational deafness. Workplace noise exposures in excess of 85 decibels for a working day are likely to cause damage to hearing which is initially restricted to the vital frequencies associated with speech – around 3–4 kHz. Protection from such noise is imperative as hearing aids do nothing to ameliorate the neural damage once it has occurred.

Hand-arm vibration syndrome is a disorder of the vascular and/or neural endings in the hands leading to episodic blanching ('white finger') and numbness which is exacerbated by low temperature. The condition, which is caused by vibrating tools such as chain saws and pneumatic hammers, is akin to RAYNAUD'S DISEASE and can be disabling.

Decompression sickness is caused by a rapid change in ambient pressure and is a disease associated with deep-sea divers, tunnel workers and high-flying aviators. Apart from the direct effects of pressure change such as ruptured tympanic membrane or sinus pain, the more serious damage is indirectly due to nitrogen bubbles appearing in the blood and blocking small vessels. Central and peripheral nervous-system damage and bone necrosis are the most dangerous sequelae.

Radiation Non-ionising radiation from lasers or microwaves can cause severe localised heating leading to tissue damage of which cataracts (see under EYE, DISORDERS OF) are a particular variety. Ionising radiation from radioactive sources can cause similar acute tissue damage to the eyes as well as cell damage to rapidly dividing cells in the gut and bone marrow. Longer-term effects include genetic damage and various malignant disorders of which LEUKAEMIA and aplastic ANAEMIA are notable. Particular radioactive isotopes may destroy or induce malignant change in target organs, for example, ^{131}I (thyroid), ^{90}Sr (bone). Outdoor workers may also be at risk of sunburn and skin cancers.

OTHER OCCUPATIONAL CANCERS Occupation is directly responsible for about 5 per cent of all cancers and contributes to a further 5 per cent. Apart from the cancers caused by asbestos and ionising radiation, a number of other occupational exposures can cause human cancer. The International Agency for Research on Cancer regularly reviews the evidence for carcinogenicity of compounds and industrial processes, and its published list of carcinogens is widely accepted as the current state of knowledge. More than 50 agents and processes are listed as class 1 carcinogens. Important occupational carcinogens include asbestos (mesothelioma, lung cancer); polynuclear aromatic hydrocarbons such as mineral oils, soots, tars (skin and lung cancer); the aromatic amines in dyestuffs (bladder cancer); certain hexavalent chromates, arsenic and nickel refining (lung cancer); wood and leather dust (nasal sinus cancer); benzene (leukaemia); and vinyl chloride monomer (angiosarcoma of the liver). It has been estimated that elimination of all known occupational carcinogens, if possible, would lead to an annual saving of 5,000 premature deaths in Britain.

Infections Two broad categories of job carry an occupational risk. These are workers in contact with animals (farmers, veterinary surgeons and slaughtermen) and those in contact with human sources of infection (health-care staff and sewage workers).

Occupational infections include various zoonoses (pathogens transmissible from animals to humans), such as ANTHRAX, *Borrelia burgdorferi* (LYME DISEASE), bovine TUBERCULOSIS, BRUCELLOSIS, *Chlamydia psittaci*, leptospirosis, ORF virus, Q fever, RINGWORM and *Streptococcus suis*. Human pathogens that may be transmissible at work include tuberculosis, and blood-borne pathogens such as viral hepatitis (B and C) and HIV (see AIDS/HIV). Health-care workers at risk of exposure to infected blood and body fluids should be immunised against hapatitis B.

Poisoning The incidence of occupational poisonings has diminished with the substitution of noxious chemicals with safer alternatives, and with the advent of improved containment. However, poisonings owing to accidents at work are still reported, sometimes with fatal consequences. Workers involved in the application of pesticides are particularly at risk if safe procedures are not followed or if equipment is faulty. Exposure to organophosphate pesticides, for example, can lead to breathing difficulties, vomiting, diarrhoea and abdominal cramps, and to other neurological effects including confusion and dizziness. Severe poisonings can lead to death. Exposure can be through ingestion, inhalation and dermal (skin) contact.

Stress and mental health Stress is an adverse reaction to excessive pressures or demands and, in occupational-health terms, is different from the motivational impact often associated with challenging work (some refer to this as 'positive stress'). Stress at work is often linked to increasing demands on workers, although coping can often prevent the development of stress. The causes of occupational stress are multivariate and encompass job characteristics (e.g. long or unsocial working hours, high work demands, imbalance between effort and reward, poorly managed organisational change, lack of control over work, poor social support at work, fear of redundancy and bullying), as well as individual factors (such as personality type, personal circumstances, coping strategies, and availability of psychosocial support outside work). Stress may influence behaviours such as smoking, alcohol consumption, sleep and diet, which may in turn affect people's health. Stress may also have direct effects on the immune system (see IMMUNITY) and lead to a decline in health. Stress may also alter the course and response to treatment of conditions such as cardiovascular disease. As well as these general effects of stress, specific types of disorder may be observed.

Exposure to extremely traumatic incidents at work – such as dealing with a major accident involving multiple loss of life and serious injury (e.g. paramedics at the scene of an explosion or rail crash) – may result in a chronic condition known as post-traumatic stress disorder (PTSD). PTSD is an abnormal psychological reaction to a traumatic event and is characterised by extreme psychological discomfort, such as anxiety or panic when reminded of the causative event; sufferers may be plagued with uncontrollable memories and can feel as if they are going through the trauma again. PTSD is a clinically defined condition in terms of its symptoms and causes and should not be used to include normal short-term reactions to trauma.

Occupational Therapy
The treatment of physical and psychiatric conditions through specific selected activities in order to help people reach their maximum level of function and independence in all aspects of daily life.

Occupational therapists work from hospital and community bases. They do much more than keep patients occupied with diverting hobbies. The arts and crafts still have a place in modern therapy techniques, but these now also include household chores, industrial work, communication techniques, social activities, sports and educational programmes. An occupational therapy department may have facilities for woodwork, metalwork, printing, gardening, cooking, art and drama. Occupational therapists will use any combination of activities to strengthen muscles, increase movement and restore coordination and balance. With mentally ill people, similar activies are used. They help provide order, comfort and support and aim to build up self-confidence. Occupational therapists plan courses of treatment which are individually tailored to the needs of the patient. The aim is to help the patient practise all the activites involved in daily life. (See REHABILITATION.)

The therapists are part of a team including doctors, nurses, social workers, home helps, housing officers, physiotherapists, speech therapists and psychologists. Occupational therapists are mainly employed by the National Health Service and by local-authority social services, and they work in hospitals, special centres and in the handicapped person's own home. State registration is essential for employment as an occupational therapist. There are 15 occupational therapy schools in the United Kingdom where the course leading to the diploma of the College of Occupational Therapists can be followed. The course lasts three academic years. (See also APPENDIX 8: PROFESSIONAL ORGANISATIONS.)

Ochronosis
A rare condition in which the ligaments and cartilages of the body, and sometimes the conjunctiva (see EYE), become stained by dark brown or black pigment. This may occur in chronic carbolic poisoning, or in a congenital disorder of metabolism in which the individual is unable to break down completely the tyrosine of the protein molecule – the intermediate product, homogentisic acid, appearing in the urine, this being known as alkaptonuria.

Oedema
An abnormal accumulation of fluid beneath the skin, or in one or more of the cavities of the body.

Causes Oedema is not a disease, it is a sign – usually of underlying local or systemic disease. It may sometimes be visible as a swelling. Oedema occurs when the normal mechanisms for maintaining a balance between fluid in the tissues and in the blood are upset. That balance depends mainly on the blood pressure that keeps the blood flowing through the circulatory system – thus forcing fluid out of the capillaries – and the osmotic drawing force of the blood proteins which pulls water into the bloodstream. The KIDNEYS also have an essential role in maintaining this balance.

Among the disorders that may disturb this balance are heart failure, NEPHROTIC SYNDROME, kidney failure, CIRRHOSIS of the liver and a diet deficient in protein. Injury may also cause oedema and ascites (fluid in the abdominal cavity) can occur as a result of cirrhosis of the liver or cancer in the abdominal organs.

Treatment The underlying cause of oedema should be treated and, if this is not feasible or effective, the excess fluid should be excreted by boosting the output of the kidney. Restriction of sodium in the diet and the administration of DIURETICS are effective methods of achieving this.

Oedema of the Lungs
This occurs as a result of left ventricular failure (see HEART, DISEASES OF). There is an abrupt increase in the venous and capillary pressure in the pulmonary vessels, followed by flooding of fluid into the interstitial spaces and alveoli. The commonest cause of acute pulmonary oedema is myocardial infarction (see HEART, DISEASES

OF) which reduces the ability of the left ventricular myocardial muscle to handle the blood delivered to it. Pulmonary oedema may result from other causes of left ventricular failure such as HYPERTENSION or valvular disease of the mitral and aortic valves. The initial symptoms are cough with breathlessness and occasionally with wheezing (once called 'cardiac asthma'). The patient becomes extremely short of breath and in a severe attack the patient is pale, sweating and cyanosed and obviously gasping for breath. Frequently, frothy sputum is produced which may be blood-stained. Treatment is with DIURETICS and measures to deal with the myocardial infarction or other underlying cause.

Oedipus Complex

A description used by psychoanalysts of the subconscious attraction of a child for its parent of the opposite sex. This is accompanied by a wish to get rid of the parent of the same sex. The origin of the phrase lies in the Greek story in which Oedipus kills his father without realising who he is, then marries his mother. It has been suggested that the arrest of psychological development at the Oedipal stage may cause NEUROSIS and sexual dysfunction.

Oesophagoscope

An endoscopic instrument for observing the lining of the OESOPHAGUS. (See ENDOSCOPE.)

Oesophagostomy

A surgical operation in which the OESOPHAGUS is opened on to the surface of the neck. The procedure is usually carried out as a temporary measure to facilitate feeding and drinking after an operation on the throat.

Oesophagus

The oesophagus, or gullet, is the muscular tube linking the throat to the stomach, down which passes swallowed food and drink. It consists of three coats: a strong outer coat of muscle-fibres in two layers, the outer running lengthwise, the inner being circular; inside this a loose connective tissue coat containing blood vessels, glands, and nerves; and finally a strong mucous membrane lined by epithelium, which closely resembles that of the mouth and skin. Peristaltic waves (see PERISTALSIS) and mucus secretion from the lining cells help the passage of food.

Oesophagus, Diseases of

Oesophagitis is inflammation of the OESOPHAGUS and may be due to swallowing a corrosive chemical (corrosive oesophagitis) or because the muscles of the lower part of the oesophagus do not work properly (ACHALASIA), allowing the stomach's acidic contents to regurgitate (reflux oesophagitis). HIATUS HERNIA is sometimes associated with the latter condition. Diagnosis can be made by ENDOSCOPY of the oesophagus and/or an X-ray examination using a barium swallow. Treatment of reflux oesophagitis is by an appropriate diet and weight loss. Stricture of the oesophagus can result from swallowing a corrosive fluid and may produce severe narrowing. Such strictures may sometimes be dilated by the use of suitable instruments; otherwise, surgery may be necessary.

A still more serious and frequent cause of oesophageal stricture is that due to cancer, which may occur at any part, but is most common at the lower end, near the entrance into the stomach. The chief symptoms of this condition are increasing difficulty in swallowing, increasing debility, together with enlargement of the glands in the neck. The condition usually occurs in middle age or beyond and around 5,000 people are diagnosed with such cancer every year in the United Kingdom. In many cases treatment can only be palliative, but recent advances in surgery are producing promising results. In some cases treatment with irradiation or anti-cancer drugs produces relief, if not cure. In those in whom neither operation nor radiation can be performed, life may be prolonged and freedom from pain obtained by fluid food which is either swallowed or passed down a tube. In cases of achalasia (see above), the passage of a special bougie down the oesophagus to dilate the sphincter may be effective.

Strictures of the oesophagus may also be produced by the pressure of tumours or aneurysms within the cavity of the chest but external to the gullet.

Finally, difficulty in swallowing sometimes occurs in certain serious nervous diseases from paralysis affecting the nerves supplying the muscular coats of the PHARYNX, which thus loses its propulsive power (bulbar paralysis).

Foreign bodies which lodge in the respiratory part of the throat – i.e. at the entrance to, or in the cavity of, the larynx – set up immediate symptoms of CHOKING. Those which lodge in the gullet, on the contrary, do not usually set up any immediately serious symptoms, although their presence causes considerable discomfort. Medical attention is usually required.

Oestradiol

The name given to the oestrogenic hormone (see OESTROGENS) secreted by the ovarian follicle.

Oestradiol is responsible for the development of the female sexual characteristics, of the BREASTS, and of part of the changes that take place in the UTERUS before MENSTRUATION.

Oestradiol Valerate
See OESTROGENS.

Oestriol
See OESTROGENS.

Oestrogen Receptor
A site on the membrane surrounding a cell (see CELLS) that binds to the hormone OESTRO-GENS. This activates the cell's reaction to the hormone. Anti-oestrogen drugs such as TAM-OXIFEN used to treat breast cancer (see BREASTS, DISEASES OF) prevent the oestrogen from binding to these receptors.

Oestrogens
Natural or synthetic substances that induce the changes in the UTERUS that precede OVU-LATION. They are also responsible for the development of the secondary sex character-istics in women: that is, the physical changes that take place in a girl at puberty, such as enlargement of the BREASTS, appearance of pubic and axillary hair, and the deposition of fat on the thighs and hips. They are used in the management of disturbances of the MENOPAUSE, and also in the treatment of can-cer of the prostate (see PROSTATE GLAND, DIS-EASES OF) and certain cases of cancer of the breast.

The oestrogenic hormones of the ovary are OESTRADIOL and oestrone. The rapid deg-radation of natural oestrogens limits their use as therapeutic agents. Chemical substitution of the steroid molecule, as in ethinyl oestradiol, or the use of a non-steroidal synthetic oestrogen such as STILBOESTROL, greatly reduces the rate of degradation and enhances the therapeutic action. A further development has been the use of compounds which are not actually oestro-genic themselves, but which are slowly metab-olised to oestrogenic substances, or substances such as chlorotrianisene, which are taken up in the body fat and then slowly released into the circulation. There is in fact little to choose between the various synthetic oestrogens. Ethinyl oestradiol is the most potent oral oes-trogen, being 20 times more active than stilboestrol.

Other commonly used oestrogen drugs are dienoestrol and oestrol. The use of oestrogens in hormone replacement therapy (HRT) is dealt with in the entry on the MENOPAUSE.

Oestrone
See OESTROGENS.

Office for National Statistics (ONS)
This is an executive agency of the UK govern-ment formed by an amalgamation in 1990 of the Central Statistical Office and the Office of Population Censuses and Surveys (OPCS). The ONS compiles and publishes statistics on national and local populations, including their social and economic situation and contribu-tions to the country's economy. It also records the demographic patterns of births, marriages and deaths, including the medical cause of death. The former OPCS organised a national ten-yearly census and ONS is carrying on this activity. The census is based on the actual pres-ence of individuals in a house or institutions on a given night. The figures provide government departments and local authorities with infor-mation for planning services.

Ofloxacin
A quinolone drug (see QUINOLONES) used to treat infections in the urinary, respiratory and reproductive tracts.

Ointments
Semi-solid, greasy substances used as EMOL-LIENTS, protectants and as vehicles for topical drug delivery, ointments may be hydrophilic or hydrophobic. The former dissolve in water and usually contain polyethylene glycols. Hydro-phobic ointments do not combine with water and are paraffin-based. Mixing hard and soft paraffins allows stiffness and greasiness to be modified. Pastes are ointments containing a high proportion of inert powder such as starch or zinc oxide which confers stiffness. Pastes are protective and allow precise aplication of drugs to the skin.

Old Age
See AGEING.

Olecranon Process
The large process on the ulnar bone that pro-jects behind the joint of the elbow.

Oleic Acid
The most common of naturally occurring fatty acids, being present in most fats and oils in the form of triglyceride. It is used in the prepar-ation of OINTMENTS, but not eye ointments.

Olfactory Nerves
The nerves of SMELL. Each nerve detects smell

by means of hair-like receptors positioned in the mucous membrane lining the roof of the nasal cavity (see NOSE).

Oligaemia

A diminution of the quantity of blood in the circulation.

Olig(o)-

A prefix which means little or scanty: for example, oliguria, excretion of smaller than normal quantities of urine.

Oligomenorrhoea

Infrequent MENSTRUATION.

Oligospermia

A less-than-normal number of sperm (see SPERMATOZOON) present in each unit volume of seminal fluid (each ml of semen usually contains 20 million sperm). The condition may be permanent or temporary and is a major cause of INFERTILITY in men. It may be caused by ORCHITIS, an undescended testis, or VARICOCELE, and should be investigated.

Oliguria

An abnormally low excretion of URINE, such as occurs in acute NEPHRITIS.

Omentum

A long fold of peritoneal membrane (see PERITONEUM), generally loaded with more or less fat, which hangs down within the cavity of the ABDOMEN in front of the bowels. It is formed by the layers of peritoneum that cover the front and back surfaces of the stomach in their passage from the lower margin of this organ to cover the back and front surfaces of the large intestine. Instead of passing straight from one organ to the other, these layers dip down and form a sort of fourfold apron. This omentum is known as the greater omentum, to distinguish it from two smaller peritoneal folds, one of which passes between the liver and stomach (the hepatogastric omentum), and the other between the liver and duodenum (the hepato-duodenal omentum). Together they are known as the lesser omentum.

Omeprazole

This is a proton-pump inhibitor drug (see PROTON-PUMP INHIBITORS) which inhibits gastric-acid secretion by blocking a key enzyme system in the parietal cells of the STOMACH. The drug is used to treat (short-term) gastric ulcer (see under STOMACH, DISEASES OF) and DUODENAL ULCER, as well as strictures and inflammatory erosion of the oesophagus (see OESOPHAGUS, DISEASES OF).

Omphalocele

Another name for exomphalos – a HERNIA of abdominal organs through the UMBILICUS.

Onchocerciasis

Infestation with the filarial worm, *Onchocerca volvulus*, found in many parts of tropical Africa, in Central and South America, and in the Yemen and Saudi Arabia. After a period of 9–18 months, the young filarial worms, injected into the body by the bite of an infected simulium gnat, mature, mate and start producing young microfilariae. The females live for up to 15 years and during this period each may produce several thousand microfilariae a day. It is these microfilariae, which have a life-span of up to two years, that produce the characteristic features of the disease: an itching rash of the skin and the appearance of nodules in different parts of the body. The worm may invade the optic nerve of the EYE and so cause blindness; hence the name of African river-blindness. Treatment consists of diethylcarbamazine and suramin. An international campaign is now underway in an attempt to destroy simulium in the affected zones.

Oncogenes

GENES found in mammalian cells and viruses that can cause cancer. They are believed to manufacture the proteins that control the division of cells. In certain circumstances this control malfunctions and a normal cell may be changed into one with MALIGNANT properties. Extensive research is being done with oncogenes with the aim of finding ways to prevent or control cancers.

Oncologist

A doctor who specialises in the treatment of cancers (see CANCER; ONCOLOGY). Increasingly, cancer is being treated by multidisciplinary teams which include surgeons, physicians, radiotherapists and oncologists. The latter are non-surgical cancer specialists and are divided into clinical and medical branches: clinical oncologists concentrate mainly on RADIOTHERAPY treatments; medical oncologists are trained in the medical management of cancer patients – diagnosing and classifying cancers and arranging drug, psychosocial and palliative care. The latter claim a pivotal role in liaising with primary-care services, clinical oncologists and those providing palliative care, as well as other medical and surgical colleagues involved in the treatment and care of patients with cancer. With the constant evolution of cancer care and the introduction of new treatments such as GENE THERAPY, the role of oncologists and their relation with other specialists dealing with cancer will also evolve; but the strategic aim will remain to provide patients with up-to-date, comprehensive, coordinated care in hospitals and the community.

Oncology

The management of MALIGNANT disease – a major health problem since successful management requires close liaison between the patient, surgeons, physicians, oncologists, haematologists, paediatricians and other specialists. Diagnosis may involve various investigations and often requires a BIOPSY. Once a diagnosis has been established, treatment may involve surgery, radiotherapy or chemotherapy (or various combinations as required) – see below, and main dictionary entries.

Surgery may be most common, and is often the only treatment, for some gastrointestinal tumours, soft-tissue tumours, gynaecological tumours and advanced cancers of the head and neck.

Radiotherapy uses ionising radiation to kill tumour cells. Radiation is by naturally occurring isotopes (see ISOTOPE) or artificially produced X-RAYS. Germ-cell tumours (see SEMINOMA; TERATOMA) and malignant lymphomas (see LYMPHOMA) appear to be particularly sensitive to irradiation, and many head and neck tumours, gynaecological cancers, and localised cancers of the PROSTATE GLAND and URINARY BLADDER are curable with radiotherapy. It is also a valuable means of reducing pain from bone metastases (see METASTASIS). Unpleasant side-effects are common: chiefly lethargy, loss of appetite and dry, itchy skin symptoms.

Chemotherapy is also an important treatment in germ-cell tumours (see above); in some forms of LEUKAEMIA and lymphoma; in ovarian cancer (following surgery – see OVARIES, DISEASES OF); and in small-cell lung cancer (although most patients die within 18 months – see LUNGS, DISEASES OF). It is also used in some breast cancers (see BREASTS, DISEASES OF); advanced myeloma (see MYELOMATOSIS); sarcomas (see under CANCER); and some childhood cancers (such as WILMS' TUMOUR).

More than 20 substances are in common use, the major classes being ALKYLATING AGENTS (e.g. cyclophosphamide, chlorambucil, busul-

fan); ANTIMETABOLITES (e.g. methotrexate); VINCA ALKALOIDS (e.g. vincristine, vinblastine); and antitumour ANTIBIOTICS (e.g. actinomycin D). Choice of agent and the appropriate regimen requires expert guidance. Common side-effects include nausea and vomiting, bone-marrow suppression and ALOPECIA, with each substance having its own spectrum of unwanted effects.

Good doctor-patient communication, with the sharing of information and bringing the patient into the decision-making process, is vital even if time-consuming and exhausting.

Equally imortant treatment is PALLIATIVE, for example to ensure effective pain or nausea control. Common sources of pain in cancer may involve bone, nerve compression, soft tissue, visceral, myofascial, constipation, muscle spasm, low-back pain, joint pain (e.g. capsulitis) and chronic post-operative pain. Patients may be suffering from more than one pain, all of which should be identified. The aim should be to eliminate pain.

There are three rungs of the analgesic ladder; if one rung fails, the next one should be tried: (1) non-opioid drugs – for example, aspirin, PARACETAMOL, NON-STEROIDAL ANTI-INFLAMMATORY DRUGS (NSAIDS); (2) weak opioids – for example, CODEINE, DIHYDROCODEINE, dextropropoxyphene; (3) strong opioids – for example, MORPHINE, DIAMORPHINE, buprenorphine. Oral treatment is always preferable, unless prevented by severe vomiting. (See also CANCER; ONCOLOGIST; PAIN; PALLIATIVE CARE.)

Onychia

Disease of the nails (see SKIN – Nail; NAILS, DISEASES OF).

Onychogryphosis

A distortion of the nail (see under SKIN) in which it is much thickened, overgrown and twisted on itself. This usually affects a toe-nail and is the result of chronic irritation and inflammation.

Onycholysis

Separation of the nail (see under SKIN) from the nail-bed.

Onychomycosis

A fungus infection of the nail (see under SKIN), caused by CANDIDA or DERMATOPHYTES (see also RINGWORM).

Oöcyte

An immature OVUM. When the cell undergoes MEIOSIS in the ovary it becomes an ovum and is ready for fertilisation by the spermatozoa. Only a small number of the many oöcytes produced survive until PUBERTY, and not all of them will become ova and be ejected into the FALLOPIAN TUBES.

Oögenesis

The production of mature egg cells (ova – see OVUM) by the OVARIES. Germ cells in the ovary multiply to produce oogonia which divide by MEIOSIS to form oöcytes in the FETUS.

Oöphorectomy

Removal, by operation, of an ovary (see OVARIES). When the ovary is removed for the presence of a cyst, the term ovariotomy is usually employed (see OVARIES, DISEASES OF).

Oöphoritis

Another name for ovaritis or inflammation of an ovary (see OVARIES; OVARIES, DISEASES OF).

Oöphoron

Another name for the ovary (see OVARIES).

Operating Microscope

A binocular MICROSCOPE used for MICRO-SURGERY on, for example, the EYE and middle EAR; this microscope is also used for suturing nerves and blood vessels damaged or severed by trauma and for rejoining obstructed FALLOPIAN TUBES in the treatment of INFERTILITY in women.

Operation

A surgical procedure using instruments – or sometimes just the hands; for example, when manipulating a joint or setting a simple fracture. Operations range from simple removal of a small skin lesion under local anaesthetic to a major event such as transplanting a heart which takes several hours and involves many doctors, nurses and technical staff. Increasingly, operations are done on an outpatient or day-bed basis, thus enabling many more patients to be treated than was the case 25 years ago, and permitting them to resume a normal life – often within 24 hours. (See also SURGERY; MINIMALLY INVASIVE SURGERY (MIS).)

Ophthalmia

See under EYE, DISORDERS OF.

Ophthalmologist

A doctor with specialist training in OPHTHALMOLOGY.

Ophthalmology

The study of the structure and function of the EYE and the diagnosis and treatment of the diseases that affect it.

Ophthalmoplegia

Paralysis of the muscles of the EYE. Internal ophthalmoplegia refers to paralysis of the iris and ciliary body; external ophthalmoplegia refers to paralysis of one or all of the muscles that move the eyes.

Ophthalmoscope

An instrument for examining the interior of the EYE. There are different types of ophthalmoscope; all have a light source to illuminate the inside of the eye and a magnifying lens to make examination easier.

Opiate

A preparation of OPIUM.

Opioid

A substance with a pharmacological action that is like that of OPIUM or its derivatives.

Opioid Poisoning

MORPHINE and CODEINE are natural opium ALKALOIDS found in the opium poppy (*Papaver somniferum*). The other opioids are either synthetic or semi-synthetic analogues of these. Their main use is in the treatment of moderate to severe PAIN, but they are also used as antidiarrhoeal and antitussive agents. As a result of induced tolerance (see DEPENDENCE) and great individual variability, the amount of opioid substances required to cause serious consequences varies enormously.

The most common effects of opioid overdose are vomiting, drowsiness, pinpoint pupils, BRADYCARDIA, CONVULSIONS and COMA. Respiratory depression is common and may lead to CYANOSIS and respiratory arrest. HYPOTENSION occurs occasionally and in severe cases non-cardiogenic pulmonary oedema and cardiovascular collapse may occur. Cardiac ARRHYTHMIA may occur with some opioids. Some opioids have a HISTAMINE-releasing effect which may result in an urticarial rash (see URTICARIA), PRURITUS, flushing and hypotension. Activated CHARCOAL should be given following overdose and NALOXONE administered to reverse respiratory depression and deep coma.

Opisthotonos

The name for a position assumed by the body during one of the convulsive seizures of TETANUS. The muscles of the back, by their spasmodic contraction, arch the body in such a way that the person for a time may rest upon the bed only by their heels and head.

Opium

The dried juice of the unripe seed-capsules of the white Indian poppy, *Papaver somniferum.*The action of opium depends upon the 20–25 ALKALOIDS it contains. Of these, the chief is MORPHINE, the amount of which varies from around 9–17 per cent. Other alkaloids include codeine, narcotine, thebaine, papaverine, and naceine.

The importation into Britain of opium is strictly regulated under the Dangerous Drugs Acts. Similar regulations govern the sale and distribution of any preparation of morphine or diamorphine (heroin) stronger than 1 part in 500. (See DEPENDENCE.)

Action The action of opium varies considerably, according to the source of the drug and the preparation used.

In small doses, opium produces a state of gentle excitement, the person finding their imagination more vivid, their thoughts more brilliant, and their power of expression greater than usual. This stage lasts for some hours, and is succeeded by languor. In medicinal doses this stage of excitement is short and is followed by deep sleep. When potentially poisonous doses are taken, sleep comes on quickly, and passes into coma and death (see OPIOID POISONING). The habitual use of opium produces great TOLERANCE, so that opium users require to take large quantities daily before experiencing its pleasurable effects. The need for opium also confers tolerance, so that people suffering great pain may take, with apparently little effect beyond dulling the pain, quantities which at another time would be dangerous.

Opportunistic

A description usually applied to infection resulting from an organism that does not normally cause disease in a healthy individual. It is also used to describe widespread infection by an organism that usually causes local infection. The body's defence mechanism can usually combat these organisms, but if it is impaired – as happens in AIDS/HIV or other immune deficiencies– opportunistic infection, such as PNEUMONIA, may develop. Some viral and fungal infections behave in this way. Antimicrobial treatment is often effective, even though the weakness in the body's defence mechanism cannot be rectified.

Opsonins

Substances present in the SERUM of the blood which act upon bacteria, so as to prepare them for destruction by the white cells of the blood.

Optic

Concerned with the EYE or vision.

Optic Atrophy

A deterioration in the fibres of the optic nerve (see EYE) resulting in partial or complete loss of vision. It may be caused by damage to the nerve from inflammation or injury, or the atrophy may be secondary to disease in the eye.

Optic Chiasma

This is formed by a crossing-over of the two optic nerves (see EYE) which run from the back of the eyeballs to meet in the mid line beneath the brain. Nerve fibres from the nasal part of the retina cross to link up with fibres from the outer part of the retina of the opposite eye. The linked nerves form two separate optic tracts which travel back to the occipital lobes of the brain.

Optic Disc

Otherwise known as the blind spot of the EYE, the disc is the beginning of the optic nerve – the point where nerve fibres from the retina's rods and cones (the light- and colour-sensitive cells) leave the eyeball.

Optician

Someone who fits and sells glasses or contact lenses. An ophthalmic optician (optometrist) is trained to perform eye examinations to test for long- and short-sightedness and to prescribe corrective lenses, but they do not treat disorders of the eye, referring patients with a disorder to a family doctor or ophthalmologist.

Optic Nerve

See EYE.

Optic Neuritis

Inflammation of the optic nerve (see EYE) which may result in sudden loss of part of a person's vision. It is usually accompanied by pain and tenderness on touch. The cause is uncertain, although in some cases it may be a prcursor of MULTIPLE SCLEROSIS (MS): CORTICOSTEROIDS may help by improving the loss of visual acuity, but seems not to check the long-term inflammatory activity.

Oral

An adjective referring to the mouth, or to substances taken by mouth.

Oral Contraceptive

A contraceptive taken by mouth (see CONTRA-CEPTION). It comprises one or more synthetic female hormones, usually an oestrogen (see OESTROGENS), which blocks normal OVULA-TION, and a progestogen which influences the PITUITARY GLAND and thus blocks normal control of the woman's menstrual cycle (see MEN-STRUATION). Progestogens also make the uterus less congenial for the fertilisation of an ovum by the sperm.

Oral Rehydration Therapy (ORT)

This is the essential initial treatment for DIAR-RHOEA, and is particularly valuable for dehydrated children in developing countries ill with diseases such as CHOLERA. A litre of water containing one teaspoonful of salt and eight of sugar, taken by mouth, is readily absorbed. It replaces salts and water lost because of the diarrhoea and usually no other treatment is required.

In developed countries ORT is useful in treating gastroenteritis. There are a number of proprietary preparations, often dispensed as flavoured sachets, including Dioralyte® and Rehydrate®.

Oral Surgery

A branch of surgery that treats deformities, injuries or diseases of the TEETH and JAW, as well as other areas of the face and mouth. Surgeons doing this work are usually qualified dentists who have done further training in oral and maxillofacial surgery.

Orbit

See EYE.

Orchidectomy

Operation for the removal of the testicles (one or both – see TESTICLE) – for example, because of cancer.

Orchidopexy

When testes do not descend into the scrotum, normally in young children (CRYP-TORCHIDISM), an operation is performed to correct this. This is called surgical orchidopexy. The main reason is probably cosmetic; however, a testis which has descended is less likely to become cancerous than one which has not. It is less likely that treatment improves future fertility.

Orchitis

Inflammation of the testicle. (See TESTICLE, DIS-EASES OF.)

Orf

A virus infection of sheep and goats commonly transmitted to farm workers. Red papules on the hands or wrists become vesicular or pustular and resolve spontaneously in a few weeks.

Organ

A collection of different tissues that form a distinct structure in the body with a particular function or functions. The LIVER, for example, comprises a collection of different metabolic cells bound together with connective tissue and liberally supplied with blood vessels; it performs vital functions in the breakdown of substances absorbed from the gastrointestinal tract. Other examples of organs are the KIDNEYS, BRAIN and HEART. (See also TRANSPLANTATION.)

Organic Disease

A term used in contradistinction to the word functional, to indicate that some structural change is responsible for the faulty action of an ORGAN or other part of the body.

Organic Substances

Those which are obtained from animal or vegetable bodies, or which resemble in chemical composition those derived from this source. Organic chemistry has come to mean the chemistry of the carbon compounds.

Organophosphorus

Organophosphorus insecticides act by inhibiting the action of cholinesterase (see ACETYL-CHOLINE). For this reason they are also toxic to humans and must therefore be handled with great care. The most widely used are PARA-THION and MALATHION. Organophosphorus has also been used to make nerve gases (see BIO-LOGICAL WARFARE).

Treatment After contamination with insecticides, decontaminate (remove clothes, wash skin). Those treating should wear gloves, mask, apron and goggles. For symptoms give 2 mg of ATROPINE IV every 30 minutes until full atropinisation (dry mouth, pulse >70). Up to three days' treatment may be needed. Severe poisoning may require pralidoxine mysalate: available from designated centres, this drug should be given intravenously within 24 hours of exposure.

Organ Transplantation

See TRANSPLANTATION.

Orgasm

The climax of sexual intercourse. In men this coincides with ejaculation of the semen when the muscles of the pelvis force the seminal fluid from the prostate into the urethra and out through the urethral orifice. In women, orgasm is typified by irregular contractions of the muscular walls of the vagina followed by relaxation. The sensation is more diffuse in women than in men and tends to last longer with successive orgasms sometimes occurring.

Oriental Sore

This term is a synonym for cutaneous LEISHMANIASIS; others include: Cochin, Delhi, Kandahar, Lahore, Madagascar, Natal, Old World tropical, tropical sore, etc. As with many of the local names for this infection, it is now rarely used.

Orlistat

An inhibitor of the pancreatic enzyme LIPASE, which breaks down fats in food to their constituent parts. By inhibiting lipase, the drug reduces absorption of dietary fat from the INTESTINE. It is used as an ADJUVANT to a modest low-calorie diet in people with a BODY MASS INDEX of 30 kg/m² or more. The drug should be prescribed only if diet alone has, over a period of four consecutive weeks, resulted in a person losing 2.5 kg or more. Orlistat may cause oily liquid faeces, urgency to defecate, excessive wind and, sometimes, headaches, tiredness and anxiety. (See OBESITY.)

Ornithosis

Ornithosis is an infection of birds with the micro-organism known as *Chlamydia psittaci*, which is transmissible to humans.

Oropharynx

The part of the PHARYNX that lies between the soft PALATE and the HYOID bone.

Orphenadrine

A drug used in the treatment of PARKINSONISM.

Orthodontics

Orthodontics is the branch of dentistry concerned with the prevention and treatment of dental irregularities and malocclusion.

Orthopaedics

Originally the general measures, both surgical and mechanical, for the correction or prevention of deformities in children. Now, that branch of medical science dealing with skeletal deformity (congenital or acquired), fractures and infections of bones, replacement of arthritic joints (hips, knees and fingers – see ARTHROPLASTY) and the treatment of bone tumours. (See BONE, DISORDERS OF; JOINTS, DISEASES OF.)

Orthopnoea

A form of difficulty in breathing so severe that the patient cannot bear to lie down, but must sit or stand up. As a rule, it occurs only in serious affections of the heart or lungs.

Orthoptic Treatment

The examination and treatment by exercises of squints and their sequelae (see EYE, DISORDERS OF).

Osgood-Schlatter's Disease

The form of OSTEOCHONDROSIS involving the tibial tubercle – the growing point of the TIBIA. It occurs around PUBERTY, mainly in boys, and first manifests itself by a painful swelling over the tibial tubercle at the upper end of the tibia. The pain is worst during and after exercise. A limp with increasing limitation of movement of the knee-joint develops. The disease usually clears up without treatment. If pain is troublesome, physiotherapy or immobilisation of the knee-joint in a plaster cast for up to eight weeks may be necessary.

Osmosis

The passage of fluids through a semipermeable membrane which separates them, so as to become mixed with one another. Osmotic pressure is a term applied to the strength of the tendency which a fluid shows to do this, and depends largely upon the amount of solid which it holds in solution.

Ossicle

A small bone. The term is usually applied to the three small bones of the middle EAR – malleus, incus, and stapes – that conduct sound from the eardrum to the inner ear.

Ossification

The formation of BONE. In early life, centres appear in the bones previously represented by cartilage or fibrous tissue; and these cells, called osteoblasts, initiate the formation of true bone, which includes the deposition of calcium salts. When a fracture occurs, the bone mends by ossification of the clot which forms between the fragments (see under BONE, DISORDERS OF). In old age, an unnatural process of ossification often takes place in parts which should remain cartilaginous – for example, in the cartilages of the larynx and of the ribs, making these parts unusually brittle.

Osteitis

Osteitis means inflammation in the substance of a BONE. Traumatic osteitis is a condition particularly common in footballers, in which the victim complains of pain in the groin following exercise, particularly if this has involved much hip rotation. Examination reveals difficulty in spreading the legs and marked tenderness over the symphysis pubis. It responds well to rest and the administration of non-steroidal anti-inflammatory drugs (NSAIDS) such as ibuprofen or indomethacin.

Osteitis Deformans

See PAGET'S DISEASE OF BONE.

Osteitis Fibrosa Cystica

A pathological rather than a clinical entity. The term refers to the replacement of BONE by a highly cellular and vascular connective tissue. It is the result of osteoclastic and osteoblastic activity and is due to excessive PARATHYROID activity. It is thus seen in a proportion of patients with primary hyperparathyroidism and in patients with uraemic osteodystrophy; that is, the secondary hyperparathyroidism that occurs in patients with chronic renal disease.

Osteoarthritis

Despite major efforts, it has proved impossible to produce a single clear definition of osteoarthritis and this probably reflects the muddled nature of a concept which will need replacing. Unfortunately, there is confusion because the term is also used to cover joint pain that appears to have a mechanical basis in the absence of clinical or radiographic evidence of CARTILAGE loss.

The primary problem is seen as a change in structure of cartilage and BONE, rather than an inflammatory SYNOVITIS. Osteoarthritis usually implies a loss of the central load-bearing area of articular hyaline cartilage, with outgrowth of cartilage at the articular margin and subsequent ossification to form bony outgrowths known as OSTEOPHYTES. Osteophytes form with increasing age, whether or not there is significant cartilage loss, and in the elderly may lead to local frictional symptoms, and in the spine, to nerve compression.

The condition has a wide range of causes, of which some, like dysplasia and trauma, are known and others have yet to be identified. The main clinical problems occur in the hip and knee. The cartilage loss in the hip usually occurs in the sixth or seventh decade. It may affect both hips in fairly rapid succession, or only one hip; such patients often have no problems in other joints. Cartilage loss in the knee occurs from the fifth decade onwards and is often associated with cartilage loss in small joints in the hand and elsewhere. Cartilage loss in the distal interphalangeal joints of the hand is associated with the formation of bony swellings known as Heberden's nodes.

Treatment Management is largely directed at maintaining activity, with physical and social support as necessary. ANALGESICS may be of some value, particularly in the management of night pain. NON-STEROIDAL ANTI-INFLAMMATORY DRUGS (NSAIDS) may help patients with early-morning stiffness and may also reduce pain on movement and night pain. Their benefit, however, tends to be less marked than in RHEUMATOID ARTHRITIS and their

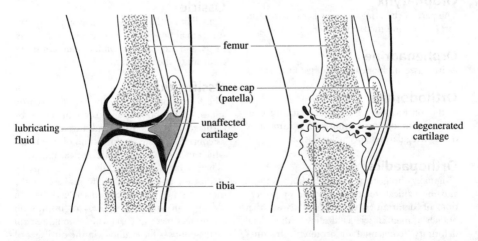

Right lateral view of vertical section through knee-joint: normal joint (left); degenerated joint cartilage and eroded bone surfaces of arthritic knee (right).

long-term usage has considerable toxicity problems. Advanced cartilage loss is best treated by joint replacement. Hip- and knee-joint replacements – with a wide variety of artificial joints – are now common surgical procedures which greatly improve the mobility of affected individuals. (See ARTHROPLASTY.)

People with arthritis and their relatives can obtain help and advice from Arthritis Care.

Osteoblast
A cell responsible for the production of BONE (see OSSIFICATION).

Osteochondritis
Inflammation of both BONE and CARTILAGE. It is a not uncommon cause of BACKACHE in young people, particularly gymnasts.

Osteochondrosis
This includes a group of diseases involving degeneration of the centre of OSSIFICATION (see also BONE) in the growing bones of children and adolescents. They include Kohler's disease, OSGOOD-SCHLATTER'S DISEASE, and PERTHES' DISEASE.

Osteoclast
A cell that resorbs calcified BONE.

Osteocyte
A BONE cell formed from an OSTEOBLAST or bone-forming cell that has stopped its activity. The cell is embedded in the matrix of the bone.

Osteogenesis
See OSSIFICATION.

Osteogenesis Imperfecta
A hereditary disease due to an inherited abnormality of COLLAGEN. It is characterised by extreme fragility of the skeleton, resulting in fractures and deformities. It may be accompanied by blue sclera (the outermost, normally white coat of the eyeball), transparent teeth, hypermobility (excessive range of movement) of the joints, deafness, and dwarfism (shortness of stature). The exact cause is not known, although there is some evidence that it may be associated with collagen formation. Parents of affected children can obtain help and advice from the Brittle Bone Society.

Osteogenic Sarcoma
See OSTEOSARCOMA.

Osteomalacia
Osteomalacia is the adult form of RICKETS. It is due to inadequate mineralisation of osteoid tissue caused by a deficiency of vitamin D. This deficiency may arise because of inadequate intake, or it may be due to impaired absorption such as occurs in intestinal malabsorption. It may also be due to renal disease, as the kidney is responsible for the hydroxylation of cholecalciferol, which has virtually no metabolic action, to dihydroxy-cholecalciferol – the metabolically active form of the vitamin. (See APPENDIX 5: VITAMINS.)

Osteomyelitis
Inflammation of the BONE as a result of infection (see BONE, DISEASES OF).

Osteopathy
A system of treatment by manipulating bones (see BONE) and other parts with the idea of thereby restoring functions in the bodily mechanism that have become deranged. Properly qualified osteopaths are included on the General Council and Register of Osteopaths.

Osteophytes
Bony spurs or projections. They occur most commonly at the margins of areas of bone affected by OSTEOARTHRITIS.

Osteoporosis
See under BONE, DISORDERS OF.

Osteosarcoma
Osteosarcoma, or osteogenic sarcoma, is the most common, and most malignant, tumour of bone (see BONE, DISORDERS OF). It occurs predominantly in older children and young adults; the most common site is at the ends of the long bones of the body – i.e. the femur, tibia and humerus. Treatment is by CHEMOTHERAPY and surgical reconstruction or amputation of the affected limb. The five-year survival rate is over 70 per cent.

Osteotomy
The operation of cutting of a BONE.

Os Trigonum
A small accessory BONE behind the ankle-joint which is present in about 7 per cent of the population. It may be damaged by energetic springing from the toes in ballet, jumping or fast bowling.

OTC
See OVER-THE-COUNTER (OTC).

Otic Barotrauma
Also called aerotitis, this is blockage of the

Eustachian tubes between the middle EAR and the PHARYNX as a result of rapidly changing external air pressure, such as occurs during descent of an aircraft. VALSALVA'S MANOEUVRE – pinching the nose with finger and thumb and attempting to blow hard through the nose – will usually relieve the blockage. People prone to this phenomenon may find nasal decongestants helpful.

Otitis

Inflammation of the EAR. (See EAR, DISEASES OF.)

Otolaryngology

The study, diagnosis and treatment of disorders of the ears, throat and larynx.

Otology

Otology is that branch of medical science which is concerned with disorders and diseases of the organ of hearing – one practising this branch being called an otologist.

Otorhinolaryngology

The study of diseases of the ear, nose, and throat – colloquially referred to as ear, nose and throat (ENT) specialty. The relevant specialist is called an otorhinolaryngologist (US) or ENT surgeon (UK).

Otorrhoea

Discharge from the EAR. (See EAR, DISEASES OF.)

Otosclerosis

See under EAR, DISEASES OF.

Otoscope

See AURISCOPE.

Outpatient

A patient attending a hospital clinic who is not admitted to a bed. Most patients attend an outpatients' department after referral for a specialist opinion by their general practitioner. An increasing number of investigations and treatments, including surgery, are being done on an outpatient basis.

Ovaries

The main female reproductive organs which produce the ova (egg cells – see OVUM) and steroid HORMONES in a regular cycle (see MENSTRUATION) in response to hormones (see GONADOTROPHINS) from the anterior PITUITARY GLAND. Situated one on each side of the uterus in the lower abdomen, each ovary contains numerous follicles within which the ova

develop. Only a small proportion of these reach maturity, when the ovum is described as a Graafian follicle. OVULATION occurs and, if the ovum is fertilised, a pregnancy may develop. (See also ENDOCRINE GLANDS; OESTRADIOL; OESTROGENS; PROGESTERONE.)

Ovaries, Diseases of

Oöphoritis (infection of the ovaries) rarely occurs alone, except in viral infections such as mumps. Usually it is associated with infection of the FALLOPIAN TUBES (SALPINGITIS). It may occur as a complication of a miscarriage, a therapeutic abortion, or the birth of a baby. Cases not associated with pregnancy typically result from sexual activity: the most common organisms involved are Chlamydia, E. coli, and Neisseria gonorrhoea. Cervical swabs should be sent for culture and analgesics given, together with the appropriate antibiotics.

Failure of OVULATION is the cause of INFERTILITY in around a third of couples seeking help with conception. It may also lead to menstrual problems (see MENSTRUATION), such as an irregular menstrual cycle or MENORRHAGIA. An uncommon cause of failure of ovulation is POLYCYSTIC OVARY SYNDROME, often associated with acne, hirsutism, and obesity. Treatment depends on the symptoms. Early ovarian failure is the cause of premature MENOPAUSE. Treatment consists of hormone replacement therapy using a combination of oestrogen and progestogen.

Ovarian cysts (for example, follicular cysts) result from ovulation. They may be symptomless but sometimes cause abdominal pain, pain during intercourse or disturbances in menstruation. Twisting or rupture can cause severe pain, pyrexia (fever) and nausea, and explorative surgery – endoscopic laparotomy – may be needed to establish a diagnosis (symptoms of ECTOPIC PREGNANCY are similar). The ovary may have to be removed. Simple cysts often disappear of their own accord but a large cyst can cause pressure on surrounding structures and therefore should be surgically removed.

In young women the most common benign tumour is a dermoid cyst, while in older women, fibroma (see under UTERUS, DISEASES OF) is more common. All benign tumours should be removed surgically in order to be sure they are not malignant.

Malignant tumours may be primary (arising in the ovary) or secondary (metastases from a cancer developing in another organ). Treatment depends upon the site and type of the primary tumour.

Around 5,000 women a year are diagnosed as

having ovarian cancer in England and Wales. Unfortunately it is not readily detected in its early stages; around 85 per cent of women do not see a doctor until after the tumour has spread. Early tumours present with symptoms similar to benign tumours, while late ones present with abdominal distension, pain and vague gastrointestinal symptoms. The disease is most common in menopausal women. Earlier diagnosis and treatment can be achieved by ULTRA-SOUND screening. Treatment is surgical, aimed at totally removing the tumour mass. Nowadays RADIOTHERAPY is only used for palliation. CHEMOTHERAPY is often given to patients with ovarian metastases, or who have residual disease after surgery. The most active cytotoxic agent is the taxane, PACLITAXEL – especially when it is combined with cisplatin.

Ovariotomy

Also called oöphorectomy. The operation of removal of an ovary (see OVARIES) or an ovarian tumour (see under OVARIES, DISEASES OF).

Overbite

A dental term describing the condition where a person's upper INCISOR teeth vertically overlap the lower incisors. If serious, the person may need orthodontic correction and this is usually done in childhood after the permanent teeth have developed.

Over-The-Counter (OTC)

A description applied in the UK to MEDICINES and drugs that can be obtained from a pharmacist without a doctor's or dentist's prescription. Some medications may be bought from retail outlets other than pharmacists.

Ovulation

The development and release of an OVUM (egg) from the ovary (see OVARIES) into the FALLOPIAN TUBES. Ovulation is initiated by the secretion of luteinising hormone by the anterior PITUITARY GLAND and occurs half way through the menstrual cycle. If the ovum is not fertilised, it is lost during MENSTRUATION.

Ovum

The single cell derived from the female, out of which a future individual arises, after its union with the SPERMATOZOON derived from the male. It is about 35 micrometres in diameter. (See FETUS; OVARIES.)

Oxalic Acid

This is an irritant poison that is used domestically for cleaning purposes. It is also found in many plants including rhubarb and sorrel. Oxalic acid, when swallowed, produces burning of the mouth and throat, vomiting of blood, breathlessness and circulatory collapse. Calcium salts, lime water or milk should be given by mouth. An injection of calcium gluconate is an antidote.

Oxaliplatin

A platinum-based anticancer drug given intravenously for the treatment of colorectal cancer with metastases. It is usually combined with FLUOROURACIL and folinic acid. Side-effects include toxic damage to the nervous system.

Oxalosis

An inherited defect in the body's METABOLISM in which oxalates – a product of metabolism – are deposited in the KIDNEYS and other tissues, ultimately causing failure of the kidneys.

Oxaluria

The presence in the URINE of OXALIC ACID or oxalates, in particular calcium oxalate (see OXALOSIS).

Oxazepam

A benzodiazpine anxiolytic drug (see BENZO-DIAZEPINES; ANXIOLYTICS). Like all benzo-diazepines, oxazepam should be prescribed with caution at the lowest possible dosage for the shortest possible time, as patients can become dependent on it (see DEPENDENCE). The indication for use is short-term relief of severe anxiety, including panic attacks. Oxazepam has an advantage over many diazepams in being shorter acting, and it can be used for patients with impairment of LIVER function. The drug is inappropriate for treatment of DEPRESSION, obsessional states or PSYCHOSIS (see MENTAL ILLNESS).

Oxidant

A molecule that causes biological oxidation in which OXYGEN is added to or electrons removed from a substance. Oxygen-free radicals are highly toxic atoms and chemical groups produced by intracellular activity in various disease processes and by poisons, radiation, smoking and other pollutants. Anti-oxidants such as beta-carotene can neutralise these radicals.

Oximeter

An non-invasive device which can be attached to a patient's skin by an adhesive and records the degree of OXYGEN saturation in their blood, displaying the level on a screen. It also records pulse rate. Oximeters have become essential to safe managament of severe respiratory illness as they provide one measure of the lungs' ability to exchange oxygen and carbon dioxide.

Oximetry

The measurement by an OXIMETER of the proportion of oxygenated HAEMOGLOBIN in the blood.

Oxprenolol

See ADRENERGIC RECEPTORS.

Oxycephaly

A deformity of the skull in which the forehead is high and the top of the head pointed. There is also poor vision and the eyes bulge.

Oxygen

A colourless and odourless gas of molecular weight 32. It constitutes just less than 21 per cent of the earth's atmosphere. As a medical gas, it is supplied in the UK compressed at high pressure (13,600 kilopascals (KPa)) in cylinders which are black with white shoulders. In hospitals, oxygen is often stored as a liquid in insulated tanks and controlled evaporation allows the gas to be supplied via a pipeline at a much lower pressure.

Oxygen is essential for life. It is absorbed via the lungs (see RESPIRATION) and is transported by HAEMOGLOBIN within the ERYTHROCYTES to the tissues. Within the individual cell it is involved in the production of adenosine triphosphate (ATP), a compound that stores chemical energy for muscle cells, by the oxidative metabolism of fats and carbohydrates. HYPOXIA causes anaerobic metabolism with a resulting build-up in LACTIC ACID, the result of muscle cell activity. If severe enough, the lack of ATP causes a breakdown in cellular function and the death of the individual.

When hypoxia occurs, it may be corrected by giving supplemental oxygen. This is usually given via a face mask or nasal prongs or, in severe cases, during ARTIFICIAL VENTILATION OF THE LUNGS. Some indications for oxygen therapy are high altitude, ventilatory failure, heart failure, ANAEMIA, PULMONARY HYPERTENSION, CARBON MONOXIDE (CO) poisoning, anaesthesia and post-operative recovery. In some conditions – e.g. severe infections with anaerobic bacteria and CO poisoning – hyperbaric oxygen therapy has been used.

Oxygen Deficit

In a resting individual the potential OXYGEN supply to the tissues is greater than its consumption. During heavy exercise, the energy required by the tissues is greater than can be supplied by aerobic cellular metabolism and the additional energy is supplied by a biochemical reaction called anaerobic metabolism. There is a build-up of lactate – a product of LACTIC ACID – from anaerobic metabolism which is ultimately oxidised after conversion to citrate and metabolism via the citric acid cycle. The increased amount of oxygen above resting concentrations which needs to be consumed to perform this metabolism is known as the oxygen debt or deficit.

Oxygen Tent

A sheet of plastic put over a hospital bed with OXYGEN fed into it so that a patient can receive oxygen. Such treatment may be for a heart or lung condition in which the normal atmospheric concentration of oxygen is insufficient to enable the person to oxygenate the blood flowing through the lungs to a normal level, so extra oxygen is provided in the patient's immediate surroundings.

Oxygen Toxicity

OXYGEN toxicity in human lungs causes an acute OEDEMA followed by fibrosis and PULMONARY HYPERTENSION. In the neonate, retrolental fibroplasia occurs and central-nervous-system damage may result in the infant having fits. Several factors are involved in toxicity and there is no absolute relationship to time or concentration, although inspired concentrations of under 50 per cent are probably safe for long periods.

Oxyhaemoglobin

The compound formed when the pigment HAEMOGLOBIN in the ERYTHROCYTES (red blood cells) combines with OXYGEN (a reversible reaction). The oxygen is carried in this way from the lungs to the body's tissues where it is released to take part in metabolic activities.

Oxytetracycline

Oxytetracycline is an antibiotic derived from a soil organism, *Streptomyces rimosus*. Its range of antibacterial activity is comparable to that of tetracycline (see TETRACYCLINES).

Oxytocin

Oxytocin is the extract isolated from the pituitary posterior lobe which stimulates the uterine muscle to contract. Oxytocin produced by the PITUITARY GLAND stimulates the flow of milk in breast-feeding mothers. It can also be synthesised. The synthetic form is used to induce or assist labour in pregnancy and childbirth and also to encourage the expelling of the PLACENTA (afterbirth). Sometimes it is given to a woman who has had an incomplete miscarriage (see ABORTION). There have been criticisms that oxytocin is used too often to induce labour for social reasons or for the convenience of obstetric departments. (See also PITUITARY BODY.)

Oxyuriasis

Another name for the threadworm (see ENTEROBIASIS).

Ozaena

A chronic disease of the NOSE of an inflammatory nature, combined with atrophy of the mucous membrane and the formation of extremely foul-smelling crusts in the interior of the nose. (See also NOSE, DISORDERS OF.)

Ozone

A specially active and poisonous form of OXYGEN in which three volumes of the gas are condensed into the space ordinarily occupied by two. It has a characteristic smell and is a strong oxidising agent. Formed when an electrical charge is passed through oxygen or air, it is found at high altitudes in the atmosphere where it screens out much of the sun's ultraviolet radiation. The ozone layer, as it is called, is being damaged by pollutant gases from earth. Unless this damage is reversed, lethal quantities of ultraviolet radiation could penetrate to the earth's surface, further warming the world's climates, with long-term damage to the environment.

O

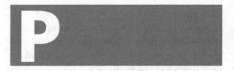

P

Pacemaker
A cardiac or artificial pacemaker is a device that helps a faulty HEART to maintain normal rhythm. It consists of a battery that stimulates the heart by an electric current passed through an insulated wire which is attached either to the surface of the ventricle (epicardial pacemaker) or to the heart lining (endocardial pacemaker). In a normal heart, the regular electrical impulses are initiated by a special area of tissue (sinoatrial node). A cardiac pacemaker is used when a person's sinoatrial node is malfunctioning or when there is interference with the passage of normal impulses. Some devices send out signals at a fixed rate; others monitor the rate and, when it falters in any way, stimulate regular contractions. Implantation is carried out under a local anaesthetic, and the lithium batteries can last for several years. People with pacemakers should avoid any source of powerful electromagnetic radiation – radio or radar transmitters or airport security screens. (See also CARDIAC PACEMAKER.)

Pacinian Corpuscles
Pacinian corpuscles, or lamellated corpuscles, are minute bulbs at the ends of the nerves scattered through the SKIN and subcutaneous tissue, and forming one of the end-organs for sensation.

Packed Cell Volume
That fraction of the blood's total volume made up of red cells. The packed cell volume is found by centrifuging blood in a tube and measuring the depth of the column of red cells as a fraction of the whole column of blood. (See also HAEMATOCRIT.)

Paclitaxel
A CYTOTOXIC drug of the taxane group (see TAXANES). Given by intravenous transfusion, it is used under specialist supervision for the treatment of ovarian cancer (usually following surgery – see OVARIES, DISEASES OF) with or without CISPLATIN. NATIONAL INSTITUTE FOR CLINICAL EXCELLENCE (NICE) guidance in 2001 also recommended that the drug could be used to treat advanced breast cancer (see BREASTS, DISEASES OF) where initial cytotoxic therapy had failed or could not be used. Its use

as first-line treatment is limited to clinical trials.

Side-effects of paclitaxel include hypersensitivity, MYELOSUPPRESSION, cardiac ARRHYTHMIA and peripheral NEUROPATHY. Only a minority of patients respond to the drug, but when it works the results are often long-lasting.

PACS
See PICTURE ARCHIVING AND COMMUNICATIONS SYSTEM (PACS).

Paederasty
A homosexual act between an adult man and a boy or young man (see HOMOSEXUALITY).

Paediatrician
A medical specialist skilled in the care of children's health and diseases.

Paediatrics
Paediatrics means the branch of medicine dealing with diseases of children (see also NEONATOLOGY).

Paedophilia
A perverse sexual attraction to children of either sex. Paedophiles are nearly always male and may have heterosexual, homosexual or bisexual orientation.

In England and Wales, the age of consent for heterosexual and homosexual sex is 16 years; in Northern Ireland, 17 years; and in Scotland the age of consent for heterosexual sex is 12 for a girl and 14 for a boy. However, girls are protected by Section 5 of the Criminal Law (Consolidation) Act 1995 which makes it an offence to have sexual intercourse with a girl aged under 16. For girls under 13, the maximum sentence is life-imprisonment, and between 13 and 16, two years' imprisonment. Homosexual consent in Scotland is 16.

Paedophiles suffer from personality problems rather than overt psychoses (see PSYCHOSIS) and the origins of their behaviour may lie in their own early sexual experiences. Their behaviour often has features of an addiction.

It is of note that most underaged sex is between family members such as stepfather and daughter rather than with a stranger or predatory paedophile.

(See CHILD ABUSE.)

Paget's Disease of Bone
Also called osteitis deformans, this is a chronic disease in which the bones (see BONE) – especially those of the skull, limbs, and spine –

gradually become thick and also soft, causing them to bend. It is said to be the most common form of bone disease in the world, and it is estimated that some 600,000 people in England may suffer from it. It seldom occurs under the age of 40. Pain is its most unpleasant manifestation. The cause is not known, and there is no known cure, but satisfactory results are being obtained from the use of CALCITONIN and a group of drugs known as BISPHOSPHONATES (e.g. etidronate). Those with the disease can obtain help and advice from the National Association for the Relief of Paget's Disease.

Pain

Pain is an unpleasant sensory and emotional experience associated with actual or potential tissue damage, or described in terms of such damage (International Association for the Study of Pain, 1979). Pain is perceived in the cerebral cortex (see BRAIN) and is always subjective. Sometimes sensations that would usually be benign can be perceived as painful – for example, allodynia (extreme tenderness of the skin) or dysaesthesia (unpleasant skin sensations resulting from partial damage to sensory nerve fibres, as in herpes zoster, or shingles).

Acute pain is caused by internal or external injury or disease. It warns the individual that harm or damage is occurring and stimulates them to take avoiding or protective action. With effective treatment of disease or injury and/or the natural healing process, the pain resolves – although some acute pain syndromes may develop into chronic pain (see below). Stimuli which are sufficiently intense potentially to damage tissue will cause the stimulation of specific receptors known as NOCICEPTORS. Damage to tissues releases substances which stimulate the nociceptors. On the surface of the body there is a high density of nociceptors, and each area of the body is supplied by nerves from a particular spinal segment or level: this allows the brain to localise the source of the pain accurately. Pain from internal structures and organs is more difficult to localise and is often felt in some more superficial structure. For example, irritation of the DIAPHRAGM is often felt as pain in the shoulder, as the nerves from both structures enter the SPINAL CORD at the same level (often the structures have developed from the same parts of the embryo). This is known as referred pain.

The impulses from nociceptors travel along nerves to the spinal cord. Within this there is modulation of the pain 'messages' by other incoming sensory modalities, as well as descending input from the brain (Melzack and Walls' gate-control theory). This involves morphine-like molecules (the ENDORPHINS and ENKEPHALINS) amongst many other pain-transmitting and pain-modulating substances. The modified input then passes up the spinal cord through the thalamus to the cerebral cortex. Thus the amount of pain 'felt' may be altered by the emotional state of the individual and by other incoming sensations. Once pain is perceived, then 'action' is taken; this involves withdrawal of the area being damaged, vocalisation, AUTONOMIC NERVOUS SYSTEM response and examination of the painful area. Analysis of the event using memory will occur and appropriate action be taken to reduce pain and treat the damage.

Chronic pain may be defined in several ways: for example, pain resistant to one month's treatment, or pain persisting one month beyond the usual course of an acute illness or injury. Some doctors may also arbitrarily choose the figure of six months. Chronic pain differs from acute pain: the physiological response is different and pain may either be caused by stimuli which do not usually cause the perception of pain, or may arise within nerves or the central nervous system with no apparent external stimulation. It seldom has a physiological protective function in the way acute pain has. Also, chronic pain may be self-perpetuating: if individuals gain a psychological advantage from having pain, they may continue to do so (e.g. gaining attention from family or health professionals, etc.). The nervous system itself alters when pain is long-standing in such a way that it becomes more sensitive to painful inputs and tends to perpetuate the pain.

Treatment The treatment of pain depends upon its nature and cause. Acute pain is generally treated by curing the underlying complaint and prescribing ANALGESICS or using local anaesthetic techniques (see ANAESTHESIA – Local anaesthetics). Many hospitals now have acute pain teams for the management of postoperative and other types of acute pain; chronic pain is often treated in pain clinics. Those involved may include doctors (in Britain, usually anaesthetists), nurses, psychologists and psychiatrists, physiotherapists and complementary therapists. Patients are usually referred from other hospital specialists (although some may be referred by GPs). They will usually have been given a diagnosis and exhausted the medical and surgical treatment of their underlying condition.

All the usual analgesics may be employed, and opioids are often used in the terminal treatment of cancer pain.

ANTICONVULSANTS and ANTIDEPRESSANT DRUGS are also used because they alter the transmission of pain within the central nervous system and may actually treat the chronic pain syndrome.

Many local anaesthetic techniques are used. Myofascial pain – pain affecting muscles and connective tissues – is treated by the injection of local anaesthetic into tender spots, and nerves may be blocked either as a diagnostic procedure or by way of treatment. Epidural anaesthetic injections are also used in the same way, and all these treatments may be repeated at intervals over many months in an attempt to cure or at least reduce the pain. For intractable pain, nerves are sometimes destroyed using injections of alcohol or PHENOL or by applying CRYOTHERAPY or radiofrequency waves. Intractable or terminal pain may be treated by destroying nerves surgically, and, rarely, the pain pathways within the spinal cord are severed by cordotomy (though this is generally only used in terminal care).

ACUPUNCTURE and TRANSCUTANEOUS ELECTRICAL NERVE STIMULATION (TENS) are used for a variety of pain syndromes, particularly myofascial or musculoskeletal pain. It is thought that they work by increasing the release of endorphins and enkephalins (see above). It is possible to implant electrodes within the epidural space to stimulate directly the nerves as they traverse this space before passing into the spinal cord.

Physiotherapy is often used, particularly in the treatment of chronic backache, where pain may be reduced by improving posture and strengthening muscles with careful exercises. Relaxation techniques and psychotherapy are also used both to treat chronic pain and to help patients cope better with their disability.

Some types of chronic pain are caused by injury to sympathetic nerves or may be relieved by interrupting conduction in sympathetic nerves. This may be done in several ways. The nerves may be blocked using local anaesthetic or permanently destroyed using alcohol, phenol or by surgery.

Many of these techniques may be used in the management of cancer pain. Opioid drugs are often used by a variety of routes and methods, and management of these patients concentrates on the control of symptoms and on providing a good quality of life.

Palate

The partition between the cavity of the mouth, below, and that of the nose, above. It consists of the hard palate towards the front, which is composed of a bony plate covered below by the mucous membrane of the mouth, above by that of the nose; and of the soft palate further back, in which a muscular layer, composed of nine small muscles, is similarly covered. The hard palate extends a little further back than the wisdom teeth, and is formed by the maxillary and palate bones. The soft palate is concave towards the mouth and convex towards the nose, and it ends behind in a free border, at the centre of which is the prolongation known as the uvula. When food or air is passing through the mouth, as in the acts of swallowing, coughing, or vomiting, the soft palate is drawn upwards so as to touch the back wall of the throat and shut off the cavity of the nose. Movements of the soft palate, by changing the shape of the mouth and nose cavities, are important in the production of speech.

Palate, Malformations of

The commonest deformity of the PALATE is cleft palate, which is a result of faulty embryonic development in which the two sides of the palate fail to fuse or only fuse in part. If the cleft extends the full length with bilateral clefts at the front of the MAXILLA, it may be accompanied by a cleft lip (also called hare-lip) and disruption in the development of the front teeth. About 1 in 500 babies is born with a cleft lip and 1 in 1,000 has a cleft palate. If the parents are affected, the risk is three times that of the normal population; if one child has a deformity, the risk for a subsequent child is higher. Associated abnormalities include tongue tie, malpositioning of the MANDIBLE and fluid in the middle EAR.

Cleft palate and hare-lip should be rectified by operation, because both are a serious drawback to feeding in early life – while later, hare-lip is a great disfigurement, and the voice may be affected. The lip may be dealt with at any time from the neonatal period to a few weeks, depending on the individual surgeon's view of when the best result is likely to be achieved. Prior to operation, special techniques may be necessary to ensure adequate feeding such as the use of special teats in formula-fed babies. The closure of a large cleft in the palate is a more formidable operation and is better performed when the face has grown somewhat, perhaps at 6–12 months. The operations performed vary greatly in details, but all consist in paring the edges of the gap and drawing the soft parts together across it.

Further operations may be required over the years to improve the appearance of the nose and lip, to make sure that teeth are even, and to improve speech.

Parents of such children can obtain help and advice from the Cleft Lip and Palate Association (CLAPA).

Palilalia

Also called paliphrasia, this means the involuntary repetition of words or sentences. It is a symptom of GILLES DE LA TOURETTE'S SYNDROME.

Palindromic

An adjective describing symptoms or diseases that recur. For example, palindromic rheumatoid arthritis is a condition in which symptoms wax and wane with periods of complete remission.

Palliative

A term applied to treatment that eases the symptoms of a disorder rather than curing the condition. (See also HOSPICE; PALLIATIVE CARE.)

Palliative Care

This is defined as comprehensive care of patients and families facing terminal illness. The care focuses primarily on comfort and support. Such care includes:

- careful control of symptoms, especially PAIN.
- psychosocial and spiritual care.
- a personalised management plan centred on the patient's needs and wishes.
- care that takes into account the family's needs and that is carried into the bereavement period.
- provision of coordinated services in the home, hospital, day-care centre and other facilities used by the patient.

Palliative care should include: managing chronic cancer pain with planned use of common ANALGESICS including opioids (see SYRINGE DRIVERS); planning ahead to preserve as far as possible the patient's autonomy and choice as death approaches and the ability to make decisions may decline; and an understanding and use of artificial feeding and hydration. Palliative care seeks to improve the satisfaction of both patient and family, to identify their needs and, if possible, to reduce the overall cost because the patient can often be looked after at home or in a HOSPICE instead of in hospital.

A well-publicised question that may arise in the context of palliative care is physician-assisted suicide. This subject is referred to in the entry on ETHICS. A request by a patient for accelerated death may suggest that he or she is depressed – a treatable condition – or that the palliative care is inadequate and needs reviewing and, if possible, improving.

Pallidotomy

Also known as pallidectomy, this is a neurosurgical procedure in which the activities of the globus pallidus area of the BRAIN are destroyed or modified. The operation is sometimes used to relieve the symptoms of PARKINSONISM and other neurological conditions in which involuntary movements are a significant and disabling symptom.

Pallor

Unusual paleness of the SKIN caused by a reduced flow of blood or a deficiency in normal pigments. Pallor may be a sign of fright, SHOCK, ANAEMIA, or other diseases.

Palpation

Examination of the surface of the body and the size, shape, and movements of the internal organs, by laying the flat of the hand upon the skin.

Palpebral

Relating to the eyelid (see EYE).

Palpitation

Forcible and/or irregular beating of the HEART such that the person becomes conscious of its action.

Causes As a rule, a person is not conscious of the beating of the heart except when the nervous system is unduly excited. A disorder of the rhythm of the heart (ARRHYTHMIA) may cause palpitations. Sudden emotions, such as fright, or overuse of tobacco, tea, coffee or alcohol may bring it on. Sometimes it may appear in people with organic heart disease.

Symptoms There may simply be a fluttering of the heart and a feeling of faintness, or the heart may be felt pounding and the arteries throbbing, causing great distress. The subject may be conscious of the heart missing beats.

Treatment Although these symptoms can be unpleasant, they do not necessarily signify serious disease. Moderate exercise is a good thing. If the person is a smoker, he or she should stop. Tea, coffee, alcohol or other stimulants should be taken sparingly. If symptoms persist or are severe, the individual should see a doctor and any underlying disorder should be investigated

– including by exercise ECG – and treated. The BETA-ADRENOCEPTOR-BLOCKING DRUGS are the most useful drugs in controlling the palpitations of anxiety and those due to some cardiac arrhythmias.

Palsy

Another name for PARALYSIS. CEREBRAL PALSY involves total or partial paralysis of a limb or limbs due to a perinatal or early infancy brain lesion.

Pan-

A prefix meaning all or completely.

Panacea

Panacea is a term applied to a remedy for all diseases, or more usually to a remedy which benefits many different diseases.

Pancarditis

Inflammation of the pericardium, myocardium, and endocardium at the same time (see HEART – Structure).

Pancreas

A gland situated in the back of the abdomen, at the level of the first and second lumbar vertebrae. It lies behind the lower part of the stomach, an expanded portion – called the head of the pancreas – occupying the bend formed by the duodenum or first part of the small intestine, whilst a long portion – known as the body – extends to the left, ending in the tail which rests against the spleen. A duct runs through the whole gland from left to right, joined by many small branches in its course, and, leaving the head of the gland, unites with the bile duct from the liver to open into the side of the small intestine about 7·5–10 cm (3–4 inches) below the outlet of the stomach.

Scattered through the pancreas are collections of cells known as the ISLETS OF LANGERHANS, of which there are around a million in a normal individual. These do not communicate with the duct of the gland, and the internal secretion of the pancreas – INSULIN – is formed by these cells and absorbed directly into the blood.

Functions The most obvious function of the pancreas is the formation of the pancreatic juice, which is poured into the small intestine after the partially digested food has left the stomach. This is the most important of the digestive juices, is alkaline in reaction, and contains (in addition to various salts) four enzymes (see ENZYME) – TRYPSIN and CHYMOTRYPSIN, which digest proteins; AMYLASE, which converts starchy foods into the disaccharide maltose; and LIPASE, which breaks up fats. (See also DIGESTION.)

Inadequate production of insulin by the islets of Langerhans leads to the condition known as DIABETES MELLITUS. In addition to insulin, another hormone is produced by the pancreas: this is glucagon which has the opposite effect to insulin and raises the blood sugar by promoting the breakdown of liver glycogen.

Pancreas, Disorders of

Diabetes See DIABETES MELLITUS.

Pancreatic cancer The incidence of pancreatic cancer is rising: around 7,000 cases are now diagnosed annually in the UK, accounting for 1–2 per cent of all malignancies. There is an established association with heavy cigarette-smoking, and the cancer is twice as common in patients with diabetes mellitus as compared with the general population. Cancer of the pancreas is hard to diagnose; by the time symptoms occur the tumour may be difficult to treat surgically – with PALLIATIVE bypass surgery the only procedure.

Chronic pancreatitis may be painless; it leads to pancreatic failure causing MALABSORPTION SYNDROME and diabetes mellitus, and the pancreas becomes calcified with shadowing on X-RAYS. The malabsorption is treated by a low-fat diet with pancreatic enzyme supplements; the diabetes with insulin; and pain is treated appropriately. Surgery may be required.

Acute pancreatitis An uncommon disease of the pancreas which may start gradually or suddenly, usually accompanied by severe abdominal pain which often radiates through to the back. Biliary tract disease and alcohol account for 80 per cent of patients admitted with acute pancreatitis, while other causes include drugs (see AZATHIOPRINE and DIURETICS) and infections such as MUMPS. Patients are acutely ill with TACHYCARDIA, fever and low blood pressure; many go into SHOCK. The condition may be mistaken for a perforated PEPTIC ULCER, except that in acute pancreatitis the blood concentration of AMYLASE is raised. The main complication is the formation of a PSEUDOCYST. Treatment includes intravenous feeding, ANTICHOLINERGIC drugs and ANALGESICS. Regular measurements of blood GLUCOSE, CALCIUM, amylase and blood gases are required. Abdominal ULTRASOUND may identify gall-stones (see under GALL-BLADDER, DISEASES OF). If the patient deteriorates, he or she should be admitted for intensive care as haemorrhagic pancreatic necrosis may be developing. LAPAROTOMY and DEBRIDEMENT may be called for. Mortality is 5–10%.

Pancreatin

Pancreatin preparations (often in the form of a powder) contain the four powerful enzymes (see ENZYME), trypsin, chymotrypsin, lipase, and amylase, which continue the digestion of foods started in the stomach (see PANCREAS – Functions; DIGESTION). They are given by mouth for the relief of pancreatic deficiency in conditions such as pancreatitis (see PANCREAS, DISORDERS OF) and CYSTIC FIBROSIS. Pancreatin is also used for the preparation of pre-digested, or so-called peptonised, foods, such as milk and some starchy foods.

Pancreatitis

See PANCREAS, DISORDERS OF.

Pancytopenia

A fall in the number of red ERYTHROCYTES and white LEUCOCYTES, as well as of platelets (see BLOOD – Composition). The condition is found in aplastic ANAEMIA, tumours of the BONE MARROW, enlarged SPLEEN, and other disorders.

Pandemic

An EPIDEMIC that has spread so widely that very many people in different countries are affected. Examples include the Black Death – the epidemic PLAGUE, caused by the bacterium *Yersinia pestis*, that devastated European populations in the Middle Ages, killing more than a third of the people; and the INFLUENZA pandemic of 1919–20 that killed more people than did World War I. AIDS/HIV is currently pandemic.

Panic Attacks

Panic attacks, or panic disorders, are recurrent short episodes of acute distress. Some sufferers may be mentally confused and fear impending death. Initially these attacks tend to occur unexpectedly but, if recurrent, they often become associated with certain places such as a confined space (lift) or among crowds. Symptoms include a feeling of breathing difficulties, including overbreathing, PALPITATION, dizziness, sweating, faintness and pains in the chest. Attacks are usually short (a few minutes) but not often associated with physical illness, although victims may have an anxiety disorder

or PHOBIA. If troublesome or disabling, attacks can be treated symptomatically with short-term ANXIOLYTICS or on a long-term basis with BEHAVIOUR THERAPY.

Panniculitis

Inflammation of the subcutaneous fat (see FAT – Body fat). It may occur anywhere on the body surface.

Pannus

1) Blood vessels growing into the cornea (see EYE) beneath its epithelium. Seen in TRACHOMA and to a lesser extent in patients who are long-term soft-contact-lens wearers.
2) Inflammatory tissue which replaces CARTILAGE in RHEUMATOID ARTHRITIS.

Pantothenic Acid

This plays an important part in the transfer of acetyl groups in the body's METABOLISM and is one of the essential constituents of the diet. The daily requirement is probably around 10 milligrams. It is widely distributed in food stuffs, both animal and vegetable; yeast, liver and egg-yolk are particularly rich sources. (See APPENDIX 5: VITAMINS.)

Papanicolaou Test

See CERVICAL SMEAR.

Papaveretum

The hydrochlorides of ALKALOIDS of OPIUM. Papaveretum relaxes smooth MUSCLE and has the pain-relieving and narcotic effects of MORPHINE, but fewer side-effects. It is largely used to prepare patients for ANAESTHESIA.

Papaverine

A smooth-muscle (see MUSCLE) relaxant once used to treat IMPOTENCE (erectile dysfunction). The drug is injected directly into the corpora caverosa (spongy, blood-filled erectile tissue) of the PENIS. Men with psychogenic or neurological impotence may respond to this treatment. Its use is less common since SILDENAFIL (Viagra®) was introduced for the treatment of erectile dysfunction.

Papilla

A small projection, such as those with which the corium of the skin is covered, and which project into the epidermis and make its union with the corium more intimate; or those covering the tongue and projecting from its surface.

Papillitis

Inflammation of any PAPILLA, but especially of

the prominence formed by the end of the optic nerve in the retina (see EYE) – also known as OPTIC NEURITIS.

Papilloedema

Swelling of the OPTIC DISC of the EYE, specifically due to raised intracranial pressure. It can be seen by examining the back of the eye using an OPHTHALMOSCOPE and is an important sign in managing the care of patients with intracerebral disease such as tumours or MENINGITIS.

Papilloma

Proliferation of epidermis or epithelium (see SKIN) to form a tumour. Benign papillomas are common in the skin and are sometimes viral in origin. Papilloma of the urinary bladder may cause HAEMATURIA.

Papova Viruses

These include the human papilloma viruses (HPV), of which nearly a hundred strains have been identified. HPV cause verrucae (see WARTS) on skin and, less often, on the mucous membranes of mouth, larynx, genitalia and the cervix. Some strains may predispose to eventual cancer.

Papule

Small (less than 5 mm) solid elevation of the skin or mucous membranes. A larger lesion is called a nodule.

Para-

A prefix meaning near, aside from, or beyond.

Para-Amino Salicylic Acid

One of the early antituberculous (see TUBERCU-LOSIS) antibiotics. It tended to cause DYSPEPSIA and has been replaced by newer antituberculous drugs with fewer side-effects. The first-line drugs for tuberculosis are now rifampicin, isoniazid, and ethambutol.

Paracentesis

The puncture by hollow needle or TROCAR and CANNULA of any body cavity (e.g. abdominal, pleural, pericardial), for tapping or aspirating fluid. (See ASPIRATION.)

Paracetamol

(US, acetaminophen.) A non-opioid analgesic (see ANALGESICS) similar in efficacy to aspirin, but without any demonstrable anti-inflammatory activity. It also has the advantage over aspirin of causing less gastric irritation. It is indicated for mild to moderate pain and pyrexia in a dose of 0.5–1g by mouth (maximum 4 doses every 24 hours).

Paracetamol Poisoning

Paracetamol is one of the safest drugs when taken in the correct dosage, but overdose may occur inadvertently or deliberately. Initially there may be no symptoms or there may be nausea, vomiting, abdominal pain and pallor. Then, 16–24 hours after ingestion, liver damage becomes evident and by 72–120 hours the patient may have JAUNDICE, COAGULATION abnormalities, hepatic failure (see LIVER, DIS-EASES OF), renal failure (see KIDNEYS, DISEASES OF), ENCEPHALOPATHY and COMA. Treatment involves the administration of antidotes such as METHIONINE (within 8 hours) orally or intravenous ACETYLCYSTEINE.

An overdose of paracetamol is a common choice of those attempting to commit suicide. Since the government restricted the number of paracetamol tablets an individual may purchase over the counter, the incidence of people taking the drug in overdose with the intention of taking their lives has fallen sharply.

Paradoxical Breathing

The reverse of the normal movements of breathing (see RESPIRATION). The chest wall moves in instead of out when breathing in (inspiration), and out instead of in when breathing out (expiration). The spaces between the ribs are indrawn on inspiration – a symptom seen in children with respiratory distress, say, as a result of ASTHMA or lung infections. Patients with CHRONIC OBSTRUCTIVE PUL-MONARY DISEASE (COPD) often suffer from paradoxical breathing; and trauma to the rib cage, with fractured sternum and ribs, also cause the condition. Treatment is of the underlying cause.

Paraesthesia

A term applied to unusual feelings, apart from mere increase, or loss, of sensation, experienced by a patient without any external cause: for example, hot flushes, numbness, tingling, itching. Various paraesthesiae form a common symptom in some nervous diseases.

Paraffin

The general name used to designate a series of saturated hydrocarbon compounds derived from petroleum. Liquid paraffin is used in the treatment of CONSTIPATION. Externally, the hard and soft paraffins are used in various consistencies, being very useful as OINTMENTS and lubricants.

Paraganglion

One of the small ovoid collections of cells occurring in the walls of the ganglia of the SYMPATHETIC NERVOUS SYSTEM adjacent to the SPINAL CORD. They are CHROMAFFIN cells and sometimes secrete ADRENALINE.

Paragonimiasis

A tropical disease found mainly in the Far East. It is caused by infections of the lungs by a parasitic fluke called *Paragonimus westermani*. The infection is acquired by eating insufficiently cooked shellfish. The affected person has symptoms similar to those of chronic BRONCHITIS; treatment is with the drugs CHLOROQUINE and bithionol.

Paragraphia

Misplacement of words, or of letters in words, or wrong spelling, or use of wrong words in writing as a result of a lesion in the speech region of the BRAIN.

Parainfluenza Viruses

These are included in the paramyxoviruses (see MYXOVIRUSES) and divided into four types, all of which cause infection of the respiratory system (see RESPIRATION). Infection with type 3 begins in May, reaches a maximum in July or August and returns to base-line level in October. Types 1 and 2 are predominantly winter viruses. Children are commonly affected and the manifestations include CROUP, fever, and a rash.

Paraldehyde

A clear, colourless liquid with a penetrating ethereal (see ETHER) odour, paraldehyde may be given by mouth, rectally, or occasionally in intramuscular injection. The drug's prime use is as a hypnotic (see HYPNOTICS) in mentally unstable patients. It is also indicated as an anticonvulsant in STATUS EPILEPTICUS (after initial intravenous DIAZEPAM) and in TETANUS. Its unpleasant taste restricts its use, but this has the advantage that it usually prevents the patient from becoming an addict.

Caution is needed when treating patients with bronchopulmonary disease or liver impairment; and intramuscular injection near the sciatic nerve should be avoided, as it may cause severe CAUSALGIA. Adverse effects include rashes; pain and sterile ABSCESS after intramuscular injection; rectal irritation after ENEMA.

Paralysis

Paralysis, or PALSY, is loss of muscular power due to some disorder of the NERVOUS SYSTEM. Weakness – rather than total movement loss – is sometimes described as paresis. Paralysis may be temporary or permanent and may be accompanied by loss of feeling.

Paralysis due to brain disease The most common form is unilateral palsy, or HEMIPLEGIA, generally arising from cerebral HAEMORRHAGE, THROMBOSIS or EMBOLISM affecting the opposite side of the BRAIN. If all four limbs and trunk are affected, the paralysis is called quadraplegia; if both legs and part of the trunk are affected, it is called paraplegia. Paralysis may also be divided into flaccid (floppy limbs) or spastic (rigid).

In hemiplegia the cause may be an abscess, haemorrhage, thrombosis or TUMOUR in the brain. CEREBRAL PALSY or ENCEPHALITIS are other possible causes. Sometimes damage occurs in the parts of the nervous system responsible for the fine control of muscle movements: the cerebellum and basal ganglion are such areas, and lack of DOPAMINE in the latter causes PARKINSONISM.

Damage or injury Damage to or pressure on the SPINAL CORD may paralyse muscles supplied by nerves below the site of damage. A fractured spine or pressure from a tumour may have this effect. Disorders affecting the cord which can cause paralysis include osteoarthritis of the cervical vertebrae (see BONE, DISORDERS OF), MULTIPLE SCLEROSIS (MS), MYELITIS, POLIOMYELITIS and MENINGITIS. Vitamin B_{12} deficiency (see APPENDIX 5: VITAMINS) may also cause deterioration in the spinal cord (see also SPINE AND SPINAL CORD, DISEASES AND INJURIES OF).

Neuropathies are a group of disorders, some inherited, that damage the peripheral nerves, thus affecting their ability to conduct electrical impulses. This, in turn, causes muscle weakness or paralysis. Among the causes of neuropathies are cancers, DIABETES MELLITUS, liver disease, and the toxic consequences of some drugs or metals – lead being one example.

Disorders of the muscles themselves – for example, muscular dystrophy (see MUSCLES, DISORDERS OF – Myopathy) – can disturb their normal working and so cause partial or complete paralysis of the part(s) affected.

Treatment The aim of treatment should be to remedy the underlying cause – for example, surgical removal of a displaced intervertebral

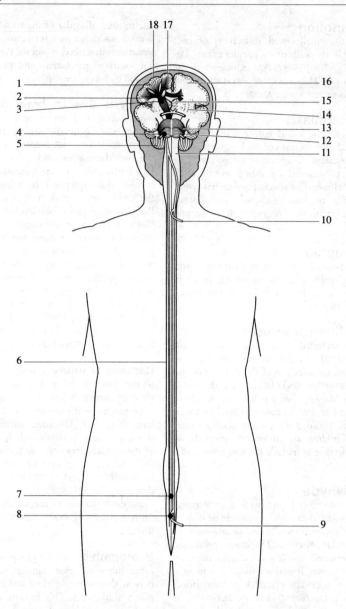

1 position of haemorrhage causing paralysis of left arm
2 position of haemorrhage causing paralysis of face
3 position of haemorrhage causing complete paralysis of left side
4 position of haemorrhage followed by paralysis of left arm and leg with right side of face (crossed paralysis)
5 cerebellum
6 spinal cord
7 position of lesion causing paralysis of both lower limbs (paraplegia)
8 position of lesion, say, from poliomyelitis infection, causing neuromuscular malfunction in the left leg
9 to leg
10 to arm
11 medulla oblongata
12 seventh nerve (facial)
13 pons
14 lentiform nucleus
15 thalamus
16 cerebral hemisphere
17 leg
18 arm

Brain and spinal cord, showing motor paths and positions of injuries causing various forms of paralysis.

disc or treating diabetes mellitus. Sometimes the cause cannot be rectified but, whether treatable or not, physiotherapy is essential to prevent joints from seizing up and to try to maintain some tone in muscles that may be only partly affected. With temporary paralysis, such as can occur after a STROKE, physiotherapy can retrain the sufferers to use their muscles and joints to ensure mobility during and after recovery. Patients with permanent hemiplegia, paraplegia or quadraplegia need highly skilled nursing care, rehabilitative support and resources, and expert help to allow them, if possible, to live at home.

Paralysis agitans
See PARKINSONISM.

Paramedical
A generic title for the professions which work closely with or are reponsible to the medical profession in caring for patients. A paramedical worker, colloquially called a 'paramedic', has skills, experience and qualifications in certain spheres of health care. Examples are ambulance crew – primarily those trained to deal with emergencies; physiotherapists (see PHYSIO-THERAPY); radiographers (see RADIOGRAPHER); and dieticians (see DIETETICS).

Parameter
A measurement of a certain factor – for example, pulse rate, blood pressure, or haemoglobin concentration – that is relevant to a disorder under investigation. Often wrongly used to describe the range of test results.

Paramnesia
A derangement of the MEMORY in which words are used without a comprehension of their meaning; it is also applied to illusions of memory in which a person in good faith imagines and describes experiences which never occurred to him or her.

Paranasal Sinus
Sited within some of the bones of the SKULL, these are spaces filled with air and lined by MUCOUS MEMBRANE. The sinuses comprise frontal and maxillary (a pair of each), ethmoidal (a group of small spaces), and two sphenoid sinuses. They drain into the nasal cavities (see NOSE). When a person has an upper respiratory infection, the sinuses sometimes become infected: this causes pain, purulent discharge from the nose and obstruction of the nasal passages (see SINUSITIS). Generally all that is required is a decongestant and antibiotic but,

occasionally, infection may spread to produce a cerebral abscess or cerebral venous sinus thrombosis (see BRAIN, DISEASES OF).

Paranoia
A condition whose main characteristic is the delusion (see DELUSIONS) that other people are (in an unclear way) connected to the affected individual. A sufferer from paranoia constructs a complex of beliefs based on his or her interpretation of chance remarks or events. Persecution, love, jealousy and self-grandeur are among the emotions evoked. Acute paranoia – a history of less than six months – may be the result of drastic changes in a person's environment, such as war, imprisonment, famine or even leaving home for the first time. Chronic paranoia may be caused by brain damage, substance abuse (including alcohol and cannbis), SCHIZOPHRENIA or severe DEPRESSION. Those affected may become constantly suspicious and angry and tend to live an isolated existence, exhibiting difficult and odd behaviour. Often believing themselves to be normal, they do not seek treatment. If treated early with antipsychotic drugs, they often recover; if not, the delusions and accompanying erratic behaviour become entrenched. (See MENTAL ILLNESS.)

Paraparesis
A disorder or injury of the NERVOUS SYSTEM in which the affected individual suffers from weakness in both legs and sometimes of the muscles in the lower trunk.

Paraphasia
Misplacement of words, or use of wrong words, in speech as a result of a lesion in the speech region of the BRAIN.

Paraphimosis
The constriction of the PENIS behind the glans by an abnormally tight foreskin that has been retracted. The condition causes swelling and severe pain. Sometimes the foreskin can be returned by manual manipulation after an ice pack has been applied to the glans or a topical local anaesthetic applied. Sometimes an operation to cut the foreskin is required.

Paraphrenia
A form of PARANOIA. (See also MENTAL ILLNESS.)

Paraplegia
PARALYSIS of the lower limbs, accompanied generally by paralysis of bladder and rectum.

Parapsychology

The branch of PSYCHOLOGY that studies extra-sensory perception. This includes precognition (seeing into the future); psychokinesis (a supposed ability of some people to move or change the state of objects by thinking); telepathy (communicating thoughts from one person to another); and clairvoyance (the ability to visualise events at a distance). These phenomena have no scientific explanation and some of these 'abilities' may be manifestations of mental illness such as SCHIZOPHRENIA.

Paraquat

A contact herbicide widely used in agriculture and horticulture. People using paraquat should be careful to protect their eyes and skin so as not to come into contact with it: a mouthful is enough to kill, and the substance is involved in around 40 suicides annually in the UK. Its major misuse has resulted from its being decanted from the professional pack into soft-drink bottles and kept in the kitchen. Medical assistance should be obtained as soon as possible, as some victims of poisoning may require hospital inpatient care, including renal DIALYSIS. Several medical centres have been set up throughout the country to provide treatment in cases of paraquat poisoning. Details of these can be obtained from the National Poisons Information Service.

Parasite

An organism which lives in or on another organism, known as the host. A parasite derives all its nourishment from the host but provides no benefits in return. It may damage the host's bodily functions and in extreme cases cause the death of the host. Human parasites include WORMS, fungi (see FUNGUS), BACTERIA and viruses (see VIRUS).

Parasiticide

A general term applied to agents or substances destructive to parasites (see PARASITE).

Parasuicide

Non-fatal self-poisoning or self-injury, or attempted suicide. It is most common in the 12–15 age group. As a rule, the intention is not to commit suicide but to sound a cry for help to resolve an acute domestic, social or personal upset.

Parasympathetic Nervous System

That part of the AUTONOMIC NERVOUS SYSTEM which is connected with the BRAIN and SPINAL CORD through certain nerve centres in the midbrain, medulla, and lower end of the cord. The nerves from these centres are carried in the third, seventh, ninth and tenth cranial nerves and the second, third and fourth sacral nerves. The action of the parasympathetic system is usually antagonistic to that of the sympathetic system. Thus it inhibits the action of the HEART and augments the action of the INTESTINE; whereas the sympathetic augments the action of the heart and inhibits that of the intestine. (See diagram of sympathetic and parasympathetic nervous systems under NERVOUS SYSTEM.)

Parasympathomimetic

A drug that stimulates the PARASYMPATHETIC NERVOUS SYSTEM. The actions of such drugs resemble those of ACETYLCHOLINE. Those cholinergic actions include stimulation of musculoskeletal muscle, reduction in the heart rate, greater tension in involuntary (or smooth) muscle, increasing glandular secretions such as saliva, and constriction of the pupil of the EYE. MYASTHENIA GRAVIS, GLAUCOMA, certain disorders of the cardiovascular system, and intestinal or bladder malfunction are among the conditions for which cholinergic drugs are prescribed.

Parathion

One of the ORGANOPHOSPHORUS insecticides. It is highly toxic to humans and must therefore be handled with the utmost care.

Parathyroid

The grouping of four small glands, about 5 mm in diameter, which lie to the side of and behind the THYROID GLAND. These glands regulate the metabolism of calcium and of phosphorus. If for any reason there is a deficiency of the secretion of the parathyroid glands, the amount of calcium in the blood falls too low and the amount of phosphorus increases. The result is the condition known as TETANY characterised by restlessness and muscle spasms – sometimes severe. The condition is checked by the injection of calcium gluconate, which causes an increase in the amount of calcium in the blood.

The most common cause of this condition (hypoparathyroidism) is accidental injury to or removal of the glands during the operation of thyroidectomy for the treatment of Graves' disease (see THYROID GLAND, DISEASES OF – Thyrotoxicosis). If there is over-production of the parathyroids, there will be an increase of calcium in the blood: this extra calcium is drawn from the bones, causing cysts to form with resulting bone fragility. This cystic disease of bone is known as OSTEITIS FIBROSA CYSTICA. Tumours of the parathyroid glands result in this overactivity of the parathyroid hormone, and the resulting increase in the amount of calcium in the blood leads to the formation of stones in the kidneys. The only available treatment is surgical removal of the tumour. Increased activity of the parathyroid glands, or hyperparathyroidism, may cause stones in the kidneys. (See KIDNEYS, DISEASES OF.)

Paratyphoid Fever
See ENTERIC FEVER.

Parenchyma
A term meaning originally all the soft tissues of internal organs except their supporting structures, although now reserved for the secreting cells of the glandular organs.

Parenteral
Administration of drugs by any route other than by the mouth or by the bowel – for example, by intramuscular or intravenous injection or infusion.

Parenteral Nutrition
In severely ill patients – especially those who have had major surgery or those with SEPSIS, burns, acute pancreatitis (see PANCREAS, DISORDERS OF) and renal failure – the body's reserves of protein become exhausted. This results in weight loss; reduction in muscle mass; a fall in the serum albumin (see ALBUMINS) and LYMPHOCYTE count; and an impairment of cellular IMMUNITY. Severely ill patients are unable to take adequate food by mouth to repair the body protein loss so that enteral or parenteral nutrition is required. Enteral feeding is through the gastrointestinal tract with the aid of a nasogastric tube; parenteral nutrition involves the provision of carbohydrate, fat and proteins by intravenous administration.

The preferred route for the infusion of hyperosmolar solutions is via a central venous catheter (see CATHETERS). If parenteral nutrition is required for more than two weeks, it is advisable to use a long-term type of catheter such as the Broviac, Hickman or extra-corporeal type, which is made of silastic material and is inserted via a long subcutaneous tunnel; this not only helps to fix the catheter but also minimises the risk of ascending infection.

Dextrose is considered the best source of carbohydrate and may be used as a 20 per cent or 50 per cent solution. AMINO ACIDS should be in the laevo form and should contain the cor-

rect proportion of essential (indispensable) and non-essential amino acids. Preparations are available with or without electrolytes and with or without fat emulsions.

The main hazards of intravenous feeding are blood-borne infections made possible by continued direct access to the circulation, and biochemical abnormalities related to the composition of the solutions infused. The continuous use of hypertonic solutions of glucose can cause HYPERGLYCAEMIA and glycosuria and the resultant POLYURIA may lead to dehydration. Treatment with INSULIN is needed when hyperosmolality occurs, and in addition the water and sodium deficits will require to be corrected.

Paresis
A state of partial PARALYSIS.

Parietal
The term applied to anything pertaining to the wall of a cavity: for example, parietal pleura, the part of the pleural membrane which lines the wall of the chest.

Parietal Bone
Either one of a pair of bones that form the top and sides of the cranium of the SKULL.

Parietal Lobe
A major section of each cerebral hemisphere (see BRAIN). The two lobes lie under the parietal bones and contain the sensory cortex.

Parkinsonism
Parkinsonism, or paralysis agitans, is a progressive disease of insidious onset usually occurring in the second half of life; it is much more common in men than in women. Degenerative changes in the basal ganglia (see BASAL GANGLION) lead to a deficiency in the NEUROTRANSMITTER, DOPAMINE – or occasionally in other neurotransmitters – and it is this deficiency that is responsible for most cases.

The clinical picture is characterised by TREMOR, rigidity and poverty of spontaneous movements. The loss of natural play of expression in the face produces a mask-like expression. Rigidity of the larynx, tongue and lips produces a flat, expressionless voice. The most common symptom is tremor, often affecting one hand, spreading to the leg on the same side, then to the other limbs. It is more pronounced in resting limbs and is exaggerated by excitement, stopping during sleep. It may interfere with eating and dressing. Limb rigidity leads to an increasing tendency to stoop. The patient has a shuffling walk with a peculiar running gait.

Treatment Several drugs are used to keep the condition under control. None is curative, all have side-effects, and finding the most suitable one for any individual depends largely on understanding cooperation between family doctor and patient. Dopaminergic and antimuscarinic (see ANTIMUSCARINE) drugs are used in treatment. Levodopa, a precursor of dopamine, is a long-used example of the former; it produces spectacular improvement in one-fifth and moderate improvement in two-fifths of patients. Benzhexol hydrochloride is one of several antimuscarinic drugs used in Parkinson's disease; selegiline is a monoamine-oxidase inhibitor used in severe parkinsonism in conjunction with levodopa to reduce 'end-of-dose' deterioration. Adverse effects include HYPOTENSION, nausea and vomiting, confusion, and agitation. Some drugs used to treat other disorders produce Parkinsonian side-effects. Patients seeking further advice and help, together with their relatives, are advised to contact the Parkinson's Disease Society of the UK.

Paronychia

The term applied to inflammation near the nail (see under SKIN). The infection, usually caused by *Staphyloccous aureus* (see STAPHYLOCOCCUS), may affect the tissues around the nail, including its root, and sometimes spreads to the pulp of the affected finger or toe. The tendons that run along the back of the infected digit may occasionally become infected. Acute paronychia is the most common type, with local pain and tenderness and swelling of the nail fold. Treatment is with ANTIBIOTICS or, if an ABSCESS forms, local surgery to release any pus. Sometimes infection may be caused by a virus, against which antibiotics are ineffective. If viral infection persists then antiviral drugs may eradicate it.

Chronic paronychia occurs with reinfection of the nail bed. This is usually because the person's hands are regularly immersed in water, making the skin vulnerable to infection. The finger should be kept dry and a dry dressing applied accompanied by a course of antibiotics – FLUCLOXACILLIN or a cephalosporin.

Parosmia

A perverted sense of SMELL; everything may smell unpleasant to the affected individual. The most common cause is some septic condition of the nasal passages (see NOSE), but the condition may occasionally be due to a lesion in the BRAIN involving the centre responsible for the sense of smell.

Parotid Gland

One of the SALIVARY GLANDS. It is situated just in front of the ear, and its duct runs forwards across the cheek to open into the interior of the mouth on a little projection opposite the second last tooth of the upper row. The parotid gland is generally the first of the salivary glands to become enlarged in MUMPS.

Parotitis

Inflammation of the PAROTID GLAND caused by infection or by many AUTOIMMUNE DISORDERS. Epidemic parotitis is another name for MUMPS.

Paroxetine

One of the ANTIDEPRESSANT DRUGS in the SELECTIVE SEROTONIN-REUPTAKE INHIBITORS (SSRIS) group. (See also MENTAL ILLNESS.)

Paroxysm

A sudden temporary attack that may take the form of a convulsion or spasm. It may also occur when a patient with a disease suddenly deteriorates.

Parrot Disease

See PSITTACOSIS.

Parthenogenesis

Non-sexual reproduction. In other words, development of the OVUM into an individual without fertilisation by a SPERMATOZOON. It is common in plants and has been produced in animals experimentally.

Partogram

A method of recording the degree of dilatation, or opening, of the cervix (or neck) of the UTERUS in labour (see PREGNANCY AND LABOUR) to assess how labour is progressing.

Parturition

Labour – see PREGNANCY AND LABOUR.

Parvoviruses

(from *parvus*, Latin for small) is a group of viruses responsible for outbreaks of WINTER VOMITING DISEASE. One strain is the cause of ERYTHEMA infectiosum (slapped-cheek syndrome).

PAS

A commonly used abbreviation for PARA-AMINO SALICYLIC ACID.

Passive Movement

A movement induced by someone other than

the patient. Physiotherapists (see PHYSIO-THERAPY) manipulate joints by passive movement in order to retain and encourage function of a nerve or muscle that is not working normally because of injury or disease.

Pastes
See OINTMENTS.

Pasteurella
A group of bacilli. They are essentially animal parasites (see PARASITE) that under certain conditions are transmitted to humans, and include the micro-organism responsible for PLAGUE and TULARAEMIA.

Pasteurisation
A method of sterilising milk (see also MILK – Preparation of milk). In many parts of the world, pasteurisation has done away with milk-borne infections, of which the most serious is bovine TUBERCULOSIS, affecting the glands, bones and joints of children. Other infections conveyed by milk are SCARLET FEVER, DIPHTHERIA, ENTERIC FEVER (typhoid and paratyphoid), undulant fever (BRUCELLOSIS), and food poisoning (e.g. from CAMPYLOBACTER, or the toxins of the STAPHYLOCOCCUS).

High-temperature short-time (HTST) pasteurisation consists of heating the milk at a temperature not less than 71·7 °C (161 °F) for at least 15 seconds, followed by immediate cooling to a temperature of not more than 10 °C (50 °F).

Low-temperature pasteurisation, or 'holder' process, consists in maintaining the milk for at least half an hour at a temperature between 63 and 65 °C (145–150 °F), followed by immediate cooling to a temperature of not more that 10 °C (50 °F). This has the effect of considerably reducing the number of bacteria contained in the milk, and of preventing the diseases conveyed by milk as referred to above.

Patch Test
This is used to identify possible substances that may be causing a patient's ALLERGY. Small amounts of different substances are placed on the skin – usually of the back or arm. If the patient is allergic then a red flare and swelling will appear, usually within about 15 minutes. Sometimes the reaction may take longer – up to three days – to develop.

Patella
Also known as the knee-cap, this is a flat bone

shaped somewhat like an oyster-shell, lying in the tendon of the extensor muscle of the thigh, and protecting the knee-joint in front. (See also KNEE.)

Patellar Reflex
See REFLEX ACTION.

Patellar Tendinitis
Also known as jumper's knee. Inflammation of the tendon of the extensor muscle of the thigh, in which the PATELLA or knee-cap is secured. Usually the result of injury or excessive use or stress – for example, in athletic training – symptoms include pain, tenderness and sometimes restricted movement of the parent muscle. Treatment may include NON-STEROIDAL ANTI-INFLAMMATORY DRUGS (NSAIDS), ULTRASOUND treatment and PHYSIOTHERAPY, and, if persistent, injection of a corticosteroid drug (see CORTICOSTEROIDS) around the tendon.

Patent
In the medical context, a term meaning open – for example, patent DUCTUS ARTERIOSUS. The term is also used for proprietary MEDICINES which, because of the research and cost involved in producing many of them, are protected by a patent. This means that without an agreement, no company or organisation other than the patent-holder can produce the substance.

Patent Ductus Arteriosus
See DUCTUS ARTERIOSUS.

Patho-
A prefix indicating relationship to a disease – for example, PATHOLOGY, a study of disease.

Pathogenesis
The ways in which a disease or disorder starts and develops. The term applies in particular to the physiological and cellular activities that are involved in the mode of origin and development of the condition.

Pathogenic
This term means disease-producing, and is a term applied, for example, to bacteria capable of causing disease.

Pathogens
Micro-organisms that cause diseases, parasitising plants, animals and humans (see PARASITE). Some organisms are frequently PATHOGENIC, whereas others rarely cause disease. Opportunistic pathogens are those which rarely cause

serious infection in healthy people but can do so in patients with weakened immune systems (immunocompromised – see IMMUNITY). Pathogens include BACTERIA, viruses (see VIRUS), prions (see PRION), fungi (see FUNGUS), PROTOZOA and metazoa (multicellular microorganisms called HELMINTHS or worms). The pathogenicity of an organism is called its virulence, which is measured by the number of organisms required to cause disease. The 50 per cent of lethal dose (LD$_{50}$) is the quantity of a particular pathogen needed to cause infection in half of the hosts invaded.

Pathognomonic

A term applied to signs or symptoms which are especially characteristic of certain diseases, and on the presence or absence of which the diagnosis depends. Thus the discovery of the *Mycobacterium tuberculosis* in the sputum is said to be pathognomonic of pulmonary tuberculosis.

Pathology

The science which deals with the causes of, and changes produced in the body by, disease.

Patient

A person with injury, physical or mental disorder or disease, or abnormality who comes into the care of a health professional or of an institution responsible for providing care to such persons. Professions more politically correct than medicine have adopted the term 'client' – perhaps due to a misunderstanding of the meaning of the word, patient (*I wait upon, i.e. I consult*).

Patient Choice

See ETHICS.

Patient Consent

See ETHICS.

Patient-Controlled Analgesia

A technique whereby a patient can deliver an analgesic substance (see ANALGESICS) in amounts related to the extent of the PAIN that he or she is suffering. For example, to combat post-operative pain, some hospitals use devices which allow patients to give themselves small intravenous amounts of opiates when they are needed. Pain is more effectively controlled if it is not allowed to reach a high level, a situation which tends to happen when patients receive analgesics only on ward drug rounds or when they ask the nursing staff for them.

Patient Empowerment

At a personal level, the engagement of individuals in decisions about their health and about the diagnosis, treatment and after-care of their illness, injuries and other disorders. At a public level, the engagement of all members of the public in the planning, provision and performance of their health-care services. Traditionally, at both personal and public levels, the patient has generally been regarded as naturally subordinate to the politicians and managers who plan and run the health-care system(s), and to health professionals and medical institutions who provide personal health care. The public and patients are increasingly unwilling to accept this traditional model and are asserting themselves, for example through patient help groups, complaints, litigation and local political action with the aim of securing changes in how health care is organised and a much greater say in their own care.

Paul-Bunnell Test

A test for MONONUCLEOSIS which is based upon the fact that patients with this disease develop ANTIBODIES which agglutinate sheep red blood cells.

Peak Flow Meter

A device that measures the rate at which an individual can expel air from the LUNGS. This is an indication of the reserve in the capacity of the lungs. Narrowed airways (bronchospasm) slow the rate at which air can be expelled; the peak flow meter can assess the severity of the condition. ASTHMA causes bronchospasm and the device can measure the effectiveness of treatment with BRONCHODILATOR drugs; this should be done regularly to monitor the progress of the disease.

Pectin

A polysaccharide substance allied to STARCH, contained in fruits and plants, and forming the basis of vegetable jelly. It has been used as a TRANSFUSION fluid in place of blood in cases of haemorrhage and shock.

Pectoral

Anything pertaining to the chest, or a remedy used in treating chest troubles.

Pectoriloquy

The resonance of the voice, when spoken or whispered words can be clearly heard through the stethoscope placed on the chest wall. It is a sign of consolidation, or of a cavity, in the lung.

Pedicle

A narrow tube of tissue formed by folded skin which links a piece of tissue used for surgical grafting to its site of origin. A pedicle graft is used by the surgeon – usually a reconstructive/ plastic surgeon – when the site under repair is unsuitable for an independent graft, usually because the blood supply at the recipient site is inadequate. (See RECONSTRUCTIVE (PLASTIC) SURGERY.)

A pedicle is also found occurring between a tumour and its tissue of origin, and the term is used in anatomy to refer to any slim tubular process.

Pediculocide

A substance that kills *Pediculosis capitis* – head louse (see under PEDICULOSIS).

Pediculosis

Infestation with lice, of which three species infect humans:

Pediculus humanus var. capitis (head louse) affects the scalp in children or adults, particularly in females. The adult louse may visit many heads in one day, especially in schoolgirls. It lays its eggs on the scalp hair and the resulting 'nit' grows out with the hair. Secondary infection owing to scratching is common in severe infestations, causing enlarged lymph glands in the posterior neck and some general debility. The lice and nits can be killed by applications of MALATHION 0.5 per cent lotion or PERMETHRIN 1 per cent lotion. After the hair is washed, application of a conditioner allows nits to be removed with a fine nit comb.

Pediculus pubis (crab louse) is broader and shorter than the head louse and less mobile. Usually transmitted sexually, it is found in the pubic area but may infect eyelashes and other body hair. It is easily seen, as are the large nits attached to the public hair: permethrin and malathion lotions are effective.

Pediculus humanus var. corporis (body louse) differs from the head and crab louse in that it lives in clothing and only goes on to the body to feed. Infestation is found in vagabonds, armies in the field, or prisoners in conditions where even minimal hygiene is impossible. The lice are found in the seams of clothing together with multiple eggs. Typically excoriation and pigmentation are seen on the back of the infested person. Replacement of clothing or autoclaving or hot ironing of the clothes is curative.

Peduncle

A stalk-like structure that usually acts as a support.

Peer Review

The procedures used by doctors and scientists to review the work, decisions and writings of their professional colleagues – peer groups. Reviewers of scientific papers are commonly called referees, and papers submitted to medical and scientific journals for publication are customarily reviewed by one or more experts in the subject(s) dealt with in the paper. The aim is to improve the quality of the study by pointing out potential pitfalls or errors to the author(s), or to assist medical-journal editors in deciding which papers to prioritise for publication. Evidence that peer review is effective is mixed. Applications for research grants are also usually subjected to peer review. (See also RESEARCH FRAUD AND MISCONDUCT.)

Pellagra

A potentially fatal nutritional disorder caused by a deficiency of vitamin B complex (niacin). The symptoms are DERMATITIS, diarrhoea and DEMENTIA. The deficiency occurs mainly in poor people in developing countries where maize is a prime constituent of the diet. Nicotinic acid in maize is in a bound form that the consumer cannot utilise. Further, maize is deficient in the amino acid, tryptophan, from which the human body can make nicotinic acid (see AMINO ACIDS).

Treatment The disease is prevented or cured by adding to the diet, foods such as fresh meat, eggs, milk, liver, and yeast extracts, as well as nicotinic acid – in addition to improving the general conditions of life.

Pelvic Inflammatory Disease (PID)

An infection of the endometrium (membraneous lining) of the UTERUS, FALLOPIAN TUBES and adjacent structures caused by the ascent of micro-organisms from the vulva and vagina. Around 100,000 women develop PID each year in the UK; most of those affected are under 25 years of age. Infection is commonly associated with sexual intercourse; *Chlamydia trachomatis* (see CHLAMYDIA) and *Neisseria gonorrhoeae* (see NEISSERIACEAE) are the most common pathogens. Although these bacteria initiate PID, opportunistic bacteria such as STREPTOCOCCUS and bacteroides often replace them.

The infection may be silent – with no obvious symptoms – or symptoms may be troublesome, for example, vaginal discharge and sometimes a palpable mass in the lower abdomen. If a LAPAROSCOPY is done – usually by endoscopic examination – overt evidence of PID is found in around 65 per cent of suspected cases.

PID may be confused with APPENDICITIS, ECTOPIC PREGNANCY – and PID is a common cause of such pregnancies – ovarian cyst (see OVARIES, DISEASES OF) and inflammatory disorders of the intestines. Treatment is with a combination of ANTIBIOTICS that are active against the likely pathogens, accompanied by ANALGESICS. Patients may become seriously ill and require hospital care, where surgery is sometimes required if conservative management is unsuccessful. All women who have PID should be screened for sexually transmitted disease and, if this is present, should be referred with their partner(s) to a genito-urinary medicine clinic. Up to 20 per cent of women who have PID become infertile, and there is a seven- to ten-fold greater risk of an ectopic pregnancy occurring.

Pelvimetry

Measurement of the internal dimensions of the PELVIS. The four diameters measured are: transverse, anterioposterior, and left and right oblique. These measurements help to establish whether a fetus can be delivered normally. If the outlet is abnormally small, the mother will have to be delivered by CAESAREAN SECTION.

Pelvis

The bony pelvis consists of the two hip bones, one on each side, with the sacrum and coccyx behind. It connects the lower limbs with the spine. In the female it is shallower than in the male and the ilia are more widely separated, giving great breadth to the hips of the woman; the inlet is more circular and the outlet larger; whilst the angle beneath the pubic bones (sub-pubic angle), which is an acute angle in the male, is obtuse in the female. All these points are of importance in connection with child-bearing.

The contents of the pelvis are the urinary bladder and rectum in both sexes; in addition the male has the seminal vesicles and the prostate gland surrounding the neck of the bladder, whilst the female has the womb, ovaries, and their appendages.

A second meaning is as in renal pelvis – that part of the collecting system proximal to the URETER which collects urine from the renal pyramids (see KIDNEYS).

Pemphigoid

See PEMPHIGUS.

Pemphigus

Autoimmune disease of the SKIN in which the cells of the epidermis lose their adhesion to each other, resulting in blister formation.

Pemphigus vulgaris is a serious form affecting skin and MUCOUS MEMBRANE. It affects young and middle-aged people with widespread blistering, erosion and crusting of the skin. Extensive involvement of the lips, mouth and throat interfere with nutrition. Untreated, it is eventually fatal, but the disease can now be controlled by large doses of oral CORTICOSTEROIDS and other immunosuppressive drugs. MORBIDITY from the adverse effects of steroids is a serious problem, but some patients are eventually cured.

Pemphigus foliaceus is seen in the elderly; the blistering is more superficial in the epidermis. It may be very widespread, but is not life-threatening because mucous membranes are not affected. Topical corticosteroids will sometimes control the eruption, but in severe cases treatment is as for pemphigus vulgaris.

Pemphigoid is a variant where the blistering occurs because of separation of the epidermis and dermis. Mucosae are rarely affected and the disease affects mainly the arms and legs in the elderly. Treatment is as for pemphigus but smaller doses of corticosteroids usually suffice.

Penicillamine

A metabolite of PENICILLIN which is one of the CHELATING AGENTS. It is sometimes used in RHEUMATOID ARTHRITIS that has not responded to the first-line remedies and it is particularly useful when the disease is complicated by VASCULITIS. Penicillamine is also used as an antidote to poisoning by heavy metals, particularly copper and lead, as it is able to bind these metals and so remove their toxic effects. Because of its ability to bind copper it is also used in WILSON'S DISEASE where there is a deficiency in the copper-binding protein so that copper is able to become deposited in the brain and liver, damaging these tissues.

Penicillin

The name given by Sir Alexander Fleming, in 1929, to an antibacterial substance produced by the mould *Penicillium notatum*. The story of penicillin is one of the most dramatic in the history of medicine, and its introduction into medicine initiated a new era in therapeutics comparable only to the introduction of ANAES-THESIA by Morton and Simpson and of ANTI-SEPTICS by Pasteur and Lister. The two great advantages of penicillin are that it is active against a large range of bacteria and that, even in large doses, it is non-toxic. Penicillin diffuses well into body tissues and fluids and is excreted in the urine, but it penetrates poorly into the cerebrospinal fluid.

Penicillin is a beta-lactam antibiotic, one of a group of drugs that also includes CEPHA-LOSPORINS. Drugs of this group have a four-part beta-lactam ring in their molecular structure and they act by interfering with the cell-wall growth of mutliplying bacteria.

Among the organisms to which it has been, and often still is, active are: streptococcus, pneumococcus, meningococcus, gonococcus, and the organisms responsible for syphilis and for gas gangrene (for more information on these organisms and the diseases they cause, refer to the separate dictionary entries). Most bacteria of the genus staphylococcus are now resistant because they produce an enzyme called PENI-CILLINASE that destroys the antibiotic. A particular problem has been the evolution of strains resistant to methicillin – a derivative originally designed to conquer the resistance problem. These bacteria, known as METHICILLIN-RESISTANT STAPHYLOCOCCUS AUREUS (MRSA), are an increasing problem, especially after major surgery. Some are also resistant to other antibiotics such as vancomycin.

An important side-effect of penicillins is hypersensitivity which causes rashes and sometimes ANAPHYLAXIS, which can be fatal.

Forms of penicillin These include the following broad groups: benzylpenicillin and phenoxymethyl-penicillin; penicillinase-resistant penicillins; broad-spectrum penicillins; antipseudomonal penicillins; and mecillinams.

BENZYLPENICILLIN is given intramuscularly, and is the form that is used when a rapid action is required.

PHENOXYMETHYLPENICILLIN (also called penicillin V) is given by mouth and used in treating such disorders as TONSILLITIS.

AMPICILLIN, a broad-spectrum antibiotic, is another of the penicillins derived by semi-synthesis from the penicillin nucleus. It, too, is active when taken by mouth, but its special feature is that it is active against gram-negative (see GRAM'S STAIN) micro-organisms such as E. coli and the salmonellae. It has been superceded by amoxicillin to the extent that prescriptions for ampicillin written by GPs in the UK to be dis-

pensed to children have fallen by 95 per cent in the last ten years.

CARBENICILLIN, a semi-synthetic penicillin, this must be given by injection, which may be painful. Its main use is in dealing with infections due to *Pseudomonas pyocanea*. It is the only penicillin active against this micro-organism which can be better dealt with by certain non-penicillin antibiotics.

PIPERACILLIN AND TICARCILLIN are carboxy-penicillins used to treat infections caused by *Pseudomonas aeruginosa* and Proteus spp.

FLUCLOXACILLIN, also a semi-synthetic penicillin, is active against penicillin-resistant staphylococci and has the practical advantage of being active when taken by mouth.

TEMOCILLIN is another penicillinase-resistant penicillin, effective against most gram-negative bacteria.

AMOXICILLIN is an oral semi-synthetic penicillin with the same range of action as ampicillin but less likely to cause side-effects.

MECILLINAM is of value in the treatment of infections with salmonellae (see FOOD POISON-ING), including typhoid fever, and with E. coli (see ESCHERICHIA). It is given by injection. There is a derivative, pivmecillinam, which can be taken by mouth.

TICARCILLIN is a carboxypenicillin used mainly for serious infections caused by *Pseudomonas aeruginosa*, though it is also active against some gram-negative bacilli. Ticarcillin is available only in combination with clarulanic acid.

Penicillinase

A bacterial ENZYME capable of neutralising the antibacterial properties of PENICILLIN and other beta-lactam antibiotics such as the CEPHA-LOSPORINS. Most staphylococci are now resistant to benzylpenicillin because they produce this enzyme; cloxacillin, flucloxacillin and temocillin are not inactivated.

Penis

The male organ through which the tubular URETHRA runs from the neck of the URINARY BLADDER to the exterior at the meatus or opening. URINE and SEMEN are discharged along the urethra, which is surrounded by three cylindrical bodies of erectile tissue, two of which (corpora cavernosa) lie adjacent to each other along the upper length of the penis and one (corpus spongiosum) lies beneath them. Normally the penis hangs down in a flaccid state in front of the SCROTUM. When a man is sexually aroused the erectile tissue, which is of spongy constituency and well supplied with small blood vessels, becomes engorged with blood.

This makes the penis erect and ready for insertion into the woman's vagina in sexual intercourse. The end of the penis, the glans, is covered by a loose fold of skin – the foreskin or PREPUCE – which retracts when the organ is erect. The foreskin is sometimes removed for cultural or medical reasons.

A common congenital disorder of the penis is HYPOSPADIAS, in which the urethra opens somewhere along the under side; it can be repaired surgically. BALANITIS is inflammation of the glans and foreskin. (See also REPRODUCTIVE SYSTEM; EJACULATION; IMPOTENCE; PRIAPISM.)

Pentamidine
A drug that is used in the prevention and treatment of African trypanosomiasis (see SLEEPING SICKNESS), and in the treatment of LEISHMANIASIS.

Pepsin
An ENZYME found in the gastric juice which digests proteins, converting them into peptides (see PEPTIDE) and AMINO ACIDS. It is used in the preparation of predigested foods (PEPTONISED FOODS), or, more frequently, taken orally after meals. Available as a white powder or liquid, it is prepared from the mucous membrane of cow, sheep, or pig stomachs.

Peptic Ulcer
The term commonly applied to ulcers in the stomach and duodenum. (See DUODENAL ULCER; STOMACH, DISEASES OF.)

Peptide
A compound formed by the union of two or more AMINO ACIDS.

Peptonised Foods
Foods which have been predigested by PANCREATIN and thereby rendered more digestible.

Percussion
An aid to diagnosis practised by striking the patient's body with the fingers, in such a way as to make it give out a note. It was introduced in 1761 by Leopold Auenbrugger (1722–1809) of Vienna, the son of an innkeeper, who derived the idea from the habit of his father tapping casks of wine to ascertain how much wine they contained. According to the degree of dullness or resonance of the note, an opinion can be formed as to the state of CONSOLIDATION of air-containing organs, the presence of abnormal cavities in organs, and the dimensions of solid and air-containing organs, which happen to lie next to one another. Still more valuable evidence is given by AUSCULTATION.

Percutaneous
Any method of administering remedies by passing them through the SKIN, as by rubbing in an ointment or applying a patch containing a drug.

Percutaneous Transhepatic Cholangiopancreatography (PTC)
A technique for displaying the bile ducts (see BILE DUCT) and pancreatic ducts (see PANCREAS) with radio-opaque dyes. These are introduced via a catheter (see CATHETERS) inserted into the ducts through an incision in the skin. An X-ray is then taken of the area.

Percutaneous Transluminal Coronary Angioplasty
A treatment for a stenosed (restricted) coronary artery (see ARTERIES). A balloon-tipped catheter (see CATHETERS) is passed through an incision in the skin of the chest into the artery of the HEART that has developed stenosis (narrowing). The balloon is aligned with the stenosed section and then inflated to dilate the coronary artery and allow the blood to flow more freely.

Perforation
The perforation of one of the hollow organs of the abdomen or major blood vessels may occur spontaneously in the case of an ulcer or an advanced tumour, or may be secondary to trauma such as a knife wound or penetrating injury from a traffic or industrial accident. Whatever the cause, perforation is a surgical emergency. The intestinal contents, which contain large numbers of bacteria, pass freely out into the abdominal cavity and cause a severe chemical or bacterial PERITONITIS. This is usually accompanied by severe abdominal pain, collapse or even death. There may also be evidence of free fluid or gas within the abdominal cavity. Surgical intervention, to repair the leak and wash out the contamination, is often necessary. Perforation or rupture of major blood vessels, whether from disease or injury, is an acute emergency for which urgent surgical repair is usually necessary. Perforation of hollow structures elsewhere than in the abdomen – for example, the heart or oesophagus – may be caused by congenital weaknesses, disease or injury. Treatment is usually surgical but depends on the cause.

Perfusion

The transfer of fluid through a tissue. For example, when blood passes through the lung tissue, dissolved oxygen perfuses from the moist air in the alveoli to the blood. Fluid may also be deliberately introduced into a tissue by injecting it into the blood vessels supplying the tissue. It is used as a sign of how adequate the circulation is at the time of illness. Poor peripheral perfusion, a sign of circulatory collapse or shock, is recognised by pressing on the skin to force blood from capillaries. The time it takes for them to refill and the skin to become pink is noted: more than 5 seconds, and the circulation is likely to be compromised.

Peri-

A prefix meaning around.

Periarteritis Nodosa

See POLYARTERITIS NODOSA.

Pericarditis

Acute or chronic inflammation of the PERI-CARDIUM, the membranous sac that surrounds the HEART. It may occur on its own or as part of PANCARDITIS, when inflammation also affects the MYOCARDIUM and ENDOCARDIUM (membranous lining of the inside of the heart). Various causes include virus infection, cancer and URAEMIA. (See also HEART, DISEASES OF.)

Pericardium

The smooth membrane that surrounds the HEART.

Perichondritis

Inflammation of CARTILAGE and the tissue surrounding it, usually as a result of chronic infection.

Perimetritis

A localised inflammation of the PERITONEUM surrounding the UTERUS.

Perimetry

A test of the visual fields of the EYE that assesses the extent of peripheral vision. The procedure does not normally form part of a routine test of vision but can be of value in assessing neurological diseases such as tumour of the brain.

Perinatal

A term applied to the period starting a few weeks before birth, the birth itself and the week or two following it.

Perinatal Mortality

Perinatal mortality consists of deaths of the FETUS after the 28th week of pregnancy and deaths of the newborn child during the first week of life. Today, more individuals die within a few hours of birth than during the following 40 years. It is therefore not surprising that the perinatal mortality rate, which is the number of such deaths per 1,000 total births, is a valuable indicator of the quality of care provided for the mother and her newborn baby. In 2002, the perinatal mortality rate was 7.87 in the United Kingdom compared with 11.4 in 1982 – and over 30 in the early 1960s.

The causes of perinatal mortality include extreme prematurity, intrapartum anoxia (that is, difficulty in the birth of the baby, resulting in lack of oxygen), congenital abnormalities of the baby, and antepartum anoxia (that is, conditions in the terminal stages of pregnancy preventing the fetus from getting sufficient oxygen). The most common cause of perinatal death is some complication of placenta, cord or membranes. The next most common is congenital abnormality. Intrauterine hypoxia and birth asphyxia comprise the third most common cause.

Perineum

Popularly called the crotch, or crutch, this is the region situated between the opening of the bowel behind and of the genital organs in front. In women it becomes stretched in childbirth, and the vaginal opening may tear or need to be cut (see EPISIOTOMY) to facilitate delivery of the baby.

Period

See MENSTRUATION.

Periodontal

An adjective that relates to the tissues around the TEETH.

Periodontal Membrane

See TEETH.

Perioperative Cell Salvage

A method of autologous blood TRANSFUSION – using a patient's own blood, salvaged during a surgical operation – instead of conventional blood-bank transfusion.

Periosteum

The membrane surrounding a BONE. The periosteum carries blood vessels and nerves for the nutrition and development of the bone. When it is irritated, an increased deposit of bone takes place beneath it; if it is destroyed, the bone may cease to grow and a portion may die and separate as a sequestrum.

Periostitis

Periostitis means inflammation on the surface of a BONE, affecting the PERIOSTEUM. (See BONE, DISORDERS OF.)

Peripheral-Blood Stem-Cell Transplants

These have almost completely replaced BONE MARROW TRANSPLANT, used to treat malignancies such as LEUKAEMIA and LYMPHOMA for the past 20 years. The high doses of CHEMOTHERAPY or RADIOTHERAPY used to treat these diseases destroy the bone marrow which contains stem cells from which all the blood cells derive. In 1989 stem cells were found in the blood during recovery from chemotherapy. By giving growth factors (cytokines), the number of stem cells in the blood increased for about three to four days. In a peripheral-blood stem-cell transplant, these cells can be separated from the peripheral blood, without a general anaesthetic. The cells taken by either method are then frozen and returned intravenously after the chemotherapy or radiotherapy is completed. Once transplanted, the stem cells usually take less than three weeks to repopulate the blood, compared to a month or more for a bone marrow transplant. This means that there is less risk of infection or bleeding during the recovery from the transplant. The whole procedure has a mortality risk of less than 5 per cent – half the risk of a bone marrow transplant.

Peripheral Nervous System

See NERVOUS SYSTEM.

Peripheral Neuritis

Inflammation of the nerves (see NERVE) in the outlying parts of the body. (See NEURITIS.)

Peripheral Vascular Disease

The narrowing of the blood vessels in the legs and, less commonly, in the arms. Blood flow is restricted, with pain occurring in the affected area. If the blood supply is seriously reduced, GANGRENE of the tissues supplied by the affected vessel(s) may occur and the limb may need to be amputated. The common cause is ATHEROSCLEROSIS which may be brought on by HYPERTENSION, excessively fatty diet, poorly controlled DIABETES MELLITUS or smoking – the latter being the biggest risk factor, with 90 per cent of affected patients having been moderate to heavy smokers. Stopping smoking is essential; adequate exercise and a low-fat diet

are important measures. Surgery may be required.

Peristalsis

The worm-like movement by which the stomach and bowels propel their contents. It consists of alternate waves of relaxation and contraction in successive parts of the intestinal tube. Any obstruction to the movement of the contents causes these contractions to become more forcible and are often accompanied by the severe form of pain known as COLIC.

Peritoneoscopy

See LAPAROTOMY.

Peritoneum

The serous membrane of the abdominal cavity. The parietal peritoneum lines the walls of the abdomen and the visceral peritoneum covers the abdominal organs. The two are continuous with one another at the back of the abdomen and form a complicated closed sac (see MESENTERY; OMENTUM). A small amount of fluid is always present to lubricate the membrane, while a large amount collects in conditions associated with OEDEMA or in PERITONITIS.

Peritonitis

Inflammation of the PERITONEUM. It may be acute or chronic, localised or generally diffused, and its severity and danger may vary according to the cause.

Acute peritonitis generally arises because bacteria enter the peritoneal cavity, from penetrating wounds, e.g. stabs, from the exterior or from the abdominal organs. Hence conditions leading to perforation of the STOMACH, INTESTINE, BILE DUCT, URINARY BLADDER, and other hollow organs such as gastric ulcer (see STOMACH, DISEASES OF), typhoid fever (see ENTERIC FEVER), gall-stones (see under GALL-BLADDER, DISEASES OF), rupture of the bladder, strangulated HERNIA, and obstructions of the bowels, may lead to peritonitis. Numerous bacteria may cause the inflammation, most common being *E. coli*, streptococci and the gonococcus.

The symptoms usually begin with a RIGOR together with fever, vomiting, severe abdominal pain and tenderness. Shock develops and the abdominal wall becomes rigid. If untreated the patient usually dies. Urgent hospital admission is required. X-ray examination may show gas in the peritoneal cavity. Treatment consists of intravenous fluids, antibiotics and surgical repair of the causative condition. Such treatment, together with strong analgesics is usually successful if started soon enough.

Peritonsillar Abscess

The term applied to a collection of pus or an ABSCESS which occurs complicating an attack of TONSILLITIS. The collection of pus forms between the tonsil and the superior constrictor muscle of the pharynx. This condition is also known as quinsy; treatment drainage of the abscess and the administration of appropriate antibiotics.

Permethrin

Along with phenothrin, this is a largely non-toxic pyrethroid insecticide, effective in SCABIES and lice infestations. Resistance may develop to these insecticides and also to MALATHION and CARBARYL, in which case topical treatment should be alternated among the different varieties.

Pernicious Anaemia

An autoimmune disease in which sensitised lymphocytes (see LYMPHOCYTE) destroy the parietal cells of the STOMACH. These cells normally produce intrinsic factor, which is the carrier protein for vitamin B_{12} that permits its absorption in the terminal ileum. Without intrinsic factor, vitamin B_{12} cannot be absorbed and this gives rise to a macrocytic ANAEMIA. The skin and mucosa become pale and the tongue smooth and atrophic. A peripheral NEUROPATHY is often present, causing paraesthesiae (see under TOUCH), numbness and even ATAXIA. The more severe neurological complication of sub-acute combined degeneration of the cord is fortunately more rare. The anaemia gets its name from the fact that before the discovery of vitamin B_{12} it was uniformly fatal. Now a monthly injection of vitamin B_{12} is all that is required to keep the patient healthy.

Peroneal

The name given to structures, such as the muscles, and nerves, on the outer or fibular side of the leg.

Perphenazine

See PHENOTHIAZINES.

Perseveration

Perseveration is the senseless repetition of words or deeds by a person with a disordered mind.

Persistent Vegetative State (PVS)

PVS may occur in patients with severe brain damage from HYPOXIA or injury. Patients do not display any awareness of their surroundings, and are unable to communicate. Sleep alternates with apparent wakefulness, when some reflexes (see REFLEX ACTION) may be present: for example, patients' eyes may reflexly follow or respond to sound, their limbs can reflexly withdraw from pain, and their hands can reflexly grope or grasp. Patients can breathe spontaneously, and retain normal heart and kidney function, although they are doubly incontinent (see INCONTINENCE).

For a diagnosis of PVS to be made, the state should have continued for more than a predefined period, usually one month. Half of patients die within 2–6 months, but some can survive for longer with artificial feeding. To assess a person's level of consciousness, a numerical marking system rated according to various functions – eye opening, motor and verbal responses – has been established called the GLASGOW COMA SCALE.

The ETHICS of keeping patients alive with artificial support are controversial. In the UK, a legal ruling is usually needed for artificial support to be withdrawn after a diagnosis of PVS has been made. The chances of regaining consciousness after one year are slim and, even if patients do recover, they are usually left with severe neurological disability.

PVS must be distinguished from conditions which appear similar. These include the 'LOCKED-IN SYNDROME' which is the result of damage to the brain stem (see BRAIN). Patients with this syndrome are conscious but unable to speak or move except for certain eye movements and blinking. The psychiatric state of CATATONIA is another condition in which the patient retains consciousness and will usually recover.

Personality Disorder

Condition in which the individual fails to learn from experience or to adapt to changes. The outcome is impaired social functioning and personal distress. There are three broad overlapping groups. One group is characterised by eccentric behaviour with paranoid or schizoid overtones. The second group shows dramatic and emotional behaviour with self-centredness and antisocial behaviour as typical components of the disorder. In the third group, anxiety and fear are the main characteristics, which are accompanied by dependency and compulsive behaviour. These disorders are not classed as illnesses but psychotherapy and behavioural therapy may help. The individuals affected are notoriously resistant to any help that is offered, tending to blame other people, circumstances or bad luck for their persistent difficulties. (See MENTAL ILLNESS; MULTIPLE PERSONALITY DISORDER; MUNCHAUSEN'S SYNDROME.)

Perspiration

Commonly called sweat, it is an excretion from the SKIN, produced by microscopic sweat-glands, of which there are around 2·5 million, scattered over the surface. There are two different types of sweat-glands, known as eccrine and apocrine. Insensible (that is unnoticed) perspiration takes place constantly by evaporation from the openings of the sweat-glands, well over a litre a day being produced. Sensible perspiration (that is, obvious) – to which the term 'sweat' is usually confined – occurs with physical exertion and raised body temperature: up to 3 litres an hour may be produced for short periods. Normal sweating maintains the body within its customary temperature range and ensures that the skin is kept adequately hydrated – for example, properly hydrated skin of the palm helps the effectiveness of a person's normal grip.

The chief object of perspiration is to maintain an even body temperature by regulating the heat lost from the body surface. Sweating is therefore increased by internally produced heat, such as muscular activity, or external heat. It is controlled by two types of nerves: vasomotor, which regulate the local blood flow, and secretory (part of the sympathetic nervous system) which directly influence secretion.

Eccrine sweat is a faintly acid, watery fluid containing less than 2 per cent of solids. The eccrine sweat-glands in humans are situated in greatest numbers on the soles of the feet and palms of the hands, and with a magnifying glass their minute openings or pores can be seen in rows occupying the summit of each ridge in the skin. Perspiration is most abundant in these regions, although it also occurs all over the body.

Apocrine sweat-glands These start functioning at puberty and are found in the armpits, the eyelids, around the anus in association with the external genitalia, and in the areola and nipple of the breast. (The glands that produce wax in the ear are modified apocrine glands.) The flow of apocrine sweat is evoked by emotional stimuli such as fear, anger, or sexual excitement.

Abnormalities of perspiration Decreased sweating may occur in the early stages

of fever, in diabetes, and in some forms of glomerulonephritis (see KIDNEYS, DISEASES OF). Some people are unable to sweat copiously, and are prone to HEAT STROKE.

EXCESSIVE SWEATING, OR HYPERIDROSIS, may be caused by fever, hyperthyroidism (see THYROID GLAND, DISEASES OF), obesity, diabetes mellitus, or an anxiety state. Offensive perspiration, or bromidrosis, commonly occurs on the hands and feet or in the armpits, and is due to bacterial decomposition of skin secretions. A few people, however, sweat over their whole body surface. For most of those affected, it is the palmar and/or axillary hyperhidrosis that is the major problem.

Conventional treatment is with an ANTICHOLINERGIC drug. This blocks the action of ACETYLCHOLINE (a neurotransmitter secreted by nerve-cell endings) which relaxes some involuntary muscles and tightens others, controlling the action of sweat-glands. But patients often stop treatment because they get an uncomfortably dry mouth. Aluminium chloride hexahydrate is a topical treatment, but this can cause skin irritation and soreness. Such antiperspirants may help patients with moderate hyperhidrosis, but those severely affected may need either surgery or injections of BOTULINUM TOXIN to destroy the relevant sympathetic nerves to the zones of excessive sweating.

Perthes' Disease

A condition of the hip in children, due to death and fragmentation of the epiphysis (or spongy extremity) of the head of the femur. The cause is not known. The disease occurs in the 4–10 year age-group, with a peak between the ages of six and eight; it is ten times more common in boys than girls, and is bilateral in 10 per cent of cases. The initial sign is a lurching gait with a limp, accompanied by pain. Treatment consists of limiting aggressive sporting activity which may cause intact overlying CARTILAGE to loosen. Where there are no mechanical symptoms and MRI scanning shows that the cartilage is intact, only minor activity modification may be necesssary – but for several months or even years. Any breach in the cartilage is dealt with at ARTHROSCOPY by fixing or trimming any loose flaps. Eventually the disease burns itself out.

Pertussis

Another name for WHOOPING-COUGH.

Pes Cavus

Known popularly as claw-foot, this is a deformity in which the foot has an abnormally high arch and the tips of the toes are turned under.

Pes cavus may be present at birth or it can be caused by disruption of or damage to the blood and nerve supplies to the foot muscles. The use of a specially made insole in the shoe may help, but surgery is sometimes needed.

Pes Planus
The technical name for FLAT-FOOT.

Pessaries
(1) A plastic device placed in the VAGINA designed to support a displaced UTERUS.
(2) A suppository suitably shaped for insertion into the vagina. Made of oil of theobromine or a glycerin basis, they are used for applying local treatment to the vagina.

Pesticides
Any substance or mixture of substances intended for preventing or controlling unwanted species of plants and animals. This includes any substances intended for use as plant-growth regulators, defoliants or desiccants. The main groups of pesticides are: herbicides to control weeds; insecticides to control insects; and fungicides to control or prevent fungal disease.

Petechiae
Small red MACULES due to haemorrhage in the skin. They may be caused by trauma – such as by tight pressure, as in strangulation – or even by the effect of violent coughing. Bleeding and clotting disorders may provoke petechiae, and they are a feature of many childhood viral infections. Most importantly they may be a sign of SEPTICAEMIA due to a meningococcus (see NEISSERIACEAE).

Pethidine Hydrochloride
A synthetic analgesic and antispasmodic drug, which is used in the treatment of painful and spasmodic conditions in place of morphine and atropine. A prompt but short-lasting analgesic, it has less of a constipating effect than morphine but is less potent. Useful for analgesia during childbirth because it produces less respiratory depression in the baby than other opioids. Pethidine is one of the CONTROLLED DRUGS.

Petit Mal
An out-of-date term for less severe type of epileptic seizure (see EPILEPSY) that occurs usually in children or adolescents but less often in adults. The type of seizure is now referred to as an absence attack.

Petri Dishes
Shallow, circular glass dishes, usually 10 cm in diameter, which are used in bacteriology laboratories for the growth of micro-organisms.

PET Scanning
Positron-emission tomography is a NUCLEAR MEDICINE diagnostic technique that works by identifying positrons – positively charged electrons – given off by substances labelled with radioactive varieties of elements. The result is three-dimensional images that identify metabolic and chemical activities of tissues, especially brain tissues. The images provide information about tissue and organ functions, and can be collated with structural images using COMPUTED TOMOGRAPHY or magnetic resonance imaging (MRI). The equipment is very expensive and available only in selected hospitals in the United Kingdom. The technique is especially valuable in the assessment of neurological disorders.

Peyer's Patches
Peyer's patches are conglomerations of lymphoid nodules in the ileum, or lower part of the small INTESTINE. They play an important part in the defence of the body against bacterial invasion, as in typhoid fever (see ENTERIC FEVER).

Peyronie's Disease
Painful and deformed erection of the PENIS caused by the formation of fibrous tissue. The cause is unknown but it may be associated with DUPUYTREN'S CONTRACTURE. The condition may be improved by surgery.

pH
A measurement of the concentration of hydrogen ions in a solution that is calculated as a negative logarithm. A neutral solution has a pH of 7·0 and this figure falls for a solution with increasing acidity and rises if the alkalinity increases. Measuring the pH of arterial blood has a major role in managing serious respiratory or cardiac disease including SHOCK and SEPTICAEMIA.

Phaeochromocytoma
A disorder in which a vascular tumour of the adrenal medulla (see ADRENAL GLANDS) develops. The tumour may also affect the structurally similar tissues associated with the chain of sympathetic nerves. There is uncontrolled and irregular secretion of ADRENALINE and NORADRENALINE with the result that the patient suffers from episodes of high blood

pressure (HYPERTENSION), raised heart rate, and headache. Surgery to remove the tumour may be possible; if not, drug treatment may help.

Phagocyte

Cells – including monocytes (a variety of LEUCOCYTES) in the blood and macrophages (see MACROPHAGE) in the tissues – that envelop and digest BACTERIA cells, cell debris and other small particles. Phagocytes are an essential part of the body's defence mechanisms.

Phagocytosis

A process by which BACTERIA and other foreign particles in the body are ingested by monocytes in the blood and macrophages in the tissues (see under PHAGOCYTE) that envelop and digest bacteria, cells, cell debris and other small particles. Phagocytes are an essential part of the body's defence mechanisms.

Phalanx

(Plural: phalanges.) The name given to any one of the small bones of the fingers and toes. The phalanges are 14 in number in each hand and foot – the thumb and great toe possessing only two each, whilst each of the other fingers and toes has three.

Phallus

An alternative name for the PENIS, this word may also be used to describe a penis-like object. In embryology the phallus is the rudimentary penis before the urethral duct has completely developed.

Phantasy

The term applied to an imaginary appearance or daydream.

Phantom Limb

Following the AMPUTATION of a limb, it is usual for the patient to experience sensations as if the limb were still present. This condition is referred to as a phantom limb. In most patients the sensation passes off in time.

Pharmacists

Health professionals trained in the preparation and dispensing of medicines; in England, Scotland and Wales they are registered (after acquiring the relevant professional qualifications) by the Royal Pharmaceutical Society. Northern Ireland has its own registration body. Registered pharmacists are a vital branch of health care. They dispense P (pharmacy-only) and POM (prescription-only medicines) products; those working in community (retail) pharmacies also sell over-the-counter (OTC) drugs, providing, where appropriate, advice on their use. (See also MEDICINES.)

Pharmacists work in hospitals (NHS and private) and in community pharmacies, as well as in the pharmaceutical industry where they conduct research and prepare and test pharmaceutical products. They have particular expertise on the use of drugs: for instance, the way in which one medicinal compound can affect another and their possible adverse effects; and they advise doctors and patients on these aspects. The NHS is also encouraging community pharmacists to offer the public advice on the treatment of simple illnesses such as coughs, colds, headaches and stomach upsets. Hospital pharmacists are salaried employees of the NHS but community pharmacists enter into contract with the service, the terms of which are negotiated centrally between pharmacists' representatives and the health departments. Hospital pharmacists are now invited by the COMMITTEE ON SAFETY OF MEDICINES (CSM) to report suspected adverse drug reactions under the 'Yellow Card' scheme in the same way as doctors.

Pharmacogenetics

See PHARMACOGENOMICS.

Pharmacogenomics

Also called pharmacogenetics – the use of human genetic variations to optimise the discovery and development of drugs and the treatment of patients. The human race varies much more in its genetic make-up than has previously been realised; these variations in GENES and their PROTEIN products could be utilised to provide safer and more effective drugs. Genes affect drug absorption, distribution, METABOLISM and excretion. Drugs are designed and prescribed on the basis of a population's needs, but patients comprise a diverse range of individuals. For example, nearly one-third of patients fail to respond to the cholesterol-reducing group of drugs, the STATINS. Around half do not respond to the tricyclic ANTIDEPRESSANT DRUGS. Over 80 per cent of patients' responses to drugs depends on their genetics: this genetic variation needs to be identified so as to make the prescription of drugs more effective, and technology for analysing genetic variants is progressing. Assessing drug effectiveness, however, is not simple because the health and diets of individuals are different and this can affect the response to a drug. Even so, the genetic identification of people who would or would not respond to a particular drug should benefit patients by ensuring a more accurately targeted drug and by reducing the risks to a person of side-effects from taking a drug that would not work. There would also be substantial economic savings.

Pharmacokinetics

The way in which the body deals with a drug. This includes the drug's absorption, distribution in the tissues, METABOLISM, and excretion.

Pharmacology

The branch of science that deals with the discovery and development of drugs. Those working in it (pharmacologists, doctors, scientists and laboratory technicians) determine the chemical structure and composition of drugs and how these act in the body. They assess the use of drugs in the prevention and treatment of diseases, their side-effects and likely toxicity. This work takes place in universities, hospitals and, in particular, the pharmaceutical industry. The latter has expanded tremendously during the 20th century and in Britain it is now one of the largest business sectors, not only providing the NHS with most of its pharmaceutical requirements but also exporting many medicines to other countries.

Pharmacologists not only research for new drugs, but also look for ways of synthesising them on a large scale. Most importantly, they organise with clinicians the thorough testing of drugs to ensure that these are safe to use, additionally helping to monitor the effects of drugs in regular use so as to identify unforeseen side-effects. Doctors and hospital pharmacists have a special reporting system ('Yellow Cards') under which they notify the government's MEDICINES CONTROL AGENCY of any untoward consequences of drug treatments on their patients (see also MEDICINES).

Pharmacopoeia

An official publication dealing with the recognised drugs and giving their doses, preparations, sources, and tests. Most countries have a pharmacopoeia of their own. That for Great Britain and Ireland is prepared by the British Pharmacopoeia Commission under the direction of the Medicines Commission. Many hospitals and medical schools have a small pharmacopoeia of their own, giving the prescriptions most commonly dispensed in that particular hospital or school. The *British National Formulary* is a compact authoritative volume for those concerned with the prescribing or dispensing of medicines.

Pharmacy

The term applied to the practice of preparing and compounding medicines, or to a place where this is carried out.

Pharyngitis

An inflammatory condition affecting the wall of the PHARYNX or the throat proper. It is most commonly due to a viral upper respiratory tract infection, and may be confined to the pharynx or may also involve the rest of the upper respiratory tract – i.e. the nose and the larynx. The mucous membrane is red and glazed with enlarged lymph-follicles scattered over it. The patient's throat feels sore and swallowing may be uncomfortable. Only symptomatic treatment, such as the use of analgesic drugs or lozenges and gargles, is necessary for viral pharyngitis, which usually is a stage in the development of a cold, or (less often, but more seriously) INFLUENZA. MONONUCLEOSIS may also start with pharyngitis. Streptococcal bacteria – linked to SCARLET FEVER – also cause the condition.

Pharynx

Another name for the throat. The term throat is popularly applied to the region about the front of the neck generally, but in its strict sense it means the irregular cavity into which the nose and mouth open above, from which the larynx and gullet open below, and in which the channel for the air and that for the food cross one another. In its upper part, the EUSTACHIAN TUBES open one on either side, and between them on the back wall grows a mass of glandular tissue – adenoids (see NOSE, DISORDERS OF).

Phenazocine Hydrobromide

A powerful analgesic which can be given under the tongue if nausea and vomiting are a problem.

Phenelzine

An example of the widely used ANTIDEPRESSANT DRUGS which are classified as MONOAMINE OXIDASE INHIBITORS (MAOIS). The drug is particularly useful because its stimulant effect is less than that of most other MAOIs.

Phenindione

A synthetic anticoagulant (see ANTICOAGULANTS). Given by mouth, it is used to prevent the formation of clots in the blood in rheumatic heart disease and atrial fibrillation (see HEART, DISEASES OF); as prophylaxis after insertion of a prosthetic heart valve; and as prophylaxis and treatment of venous thrombosis and pulmonary embolism. It is slower in action than WARFARIN, not achieving its full anticoagulant effect until up to 48 hours after the initial dose. The drug should be avoided in patients with renal or hepatic impairment, and whenever severe hypersensitivity reactions have previously occurred. Adverse effects include rashes, fever, LEUCOPENIA, AGRANULOCYTOSIS, diarrhoea and pink urine; breast feeding should be avoided.

Phenobarbitone
The *British Pharmacopoeia* name for one of the most widely used of all the group of drugs called BARBITURATES. It was mainly used in combination with PHENYTOIN SODIUM as an anticonvulsant drug in the control of EPILEPSY, but has been superceded largely by newer and safer anti-epileptic drugs.

Phenol
Another name for CARBOLIC ACID.

Phenothiazines
A group of major antipsychotic drugs, colloquially called 'TRANQUILLISERS', widely used to treat psychoses (see PSYCHOSIS). They can be divided into three main groups. Chlorpromazine, methotrimeprazine and promazine are examples of group 1, usually characterised by their sedative effects and moderate antimuscarinic and extrapyramidal side-effects. Group 2 includes pericyazine, pipothiazine and thioridazine, which have moderate sedative effects but significant antimuscarinic action and modest extrapyramidal side-effects. Fluphenazine, perphenazine, prochlorperazine and trifluoperazine comprise group 3. Their sedative effects are less than for the other groups and they have little antimuscarinic action; they have marked extrapyramidal side-effects.

Uses Phenothiazines should be prescribed and used with care. The drugs differ in predominant actions and side-effects; selection depends on the extent of sedation required and the susceptibility of the patient to extrapyramidal side-effects. The differences between the drugs, however, are less important than the variabilities in patients' responses. Patients should not be prescribed more than one antipsychotic drug at a time. In the short term these therapeutically powerful drugs can be used to calm disturbed patients, whatever the underlying condition (which might have a physical or psychiatric basis). They also alleviate acute anxiety and some have antidepressant properties, while others worsen DEPRESSION (see also MENTAL ILLNESS).

Phenothrin
See PERMETHRIN.

Phenotype
An individual's characteristics as determined by the interaction between his or her genotype – quota of GENES – and the environment.

Phenoxybenzamine
An alpha-adrenoceptor blocking drug (see ADRENERGIC RECEPTORS) used in the treatment of HYPERTENSION caused by PHAEOCHROMOCYTOMA.

Phenoxymethylpenicillin
See under PENICILLIN.

Phenylalanine
A natural amino acid (see AMINO ACIDS) essential for growth in infants, and for nitrogen metabolism in adults.

Phenylketonuria
Commonly referred to as PKU, this is one of the less common, but very severe, forms of mental deficiency. The incidence in populations of European origin is around 1 in 15,000 births. The condition is due to the inability of the baby to metabolise the amino acid, phenylalanine (see AMINO ACIDS). In the UK, every newborn baby is screened for PKU by testing a spot of their blood collected by the midwife. A positive diagnosis leads to lifelong treatment with a diet low in phenylalanine, with a good chance that the infant will grow up mentally normal. Parents of children with phenylketonuria can obtain help and information from the National Society for Phenylketonuria (UK) Ltd. (See also METABOLIC DISORDERS; GENETIC DISORDERS – Recessive genes.)

Phenytoin Sodium
An older drug for the treatment of EPILEPSY. It is not now widely used, as it is difficult to determine the precise dose to avoid ill-effects and long-term use leads to changes to the facial appearance. However, the drug is still used for the quick control of an apparently uncontrollable epileptic fit, and after head injury or neurosurgery.

Pheromones
Chemicals produced and emitted by an individual which produce changes in the social or sexual behaviour when perceived by other individuals of the same species. The precise role of these odours – for it is by their smell that they are recognised – in humans is still not clear, but

there is growing evidence of the part they play in the animal kingdom. Thus, if a strange male rat is put into a group of female rats, this may cause death of the fetus in any pregnant rats, and this is attributed to the pheromones emitted by the male rat.

Phimosis

Tightness of the foreskin (PREPUCE) which prevents it from being pulled back over the underlying head (glans) of the PENIS. Some phimosis is normal in uncircumcised males until they are six months old. The condition may, however, persist, eventually causing problems with urination. BALANITIS may occur because the inside of the foreskin cannot be properly washed. There may be an increased risk of cancer of the penis. In adolescents and adults with phimosis, erection of the penis is painful. CIRCUMCISION is the treatment.

Phlebitis

Inflammation of a vein. (See VEINS; VEINS, DISEASES OF.)

Phlebography

The study of the VEINS, particularly by means of X-rays after the veins have been injected with a radio-opaque substance.

Phlebolith

The term applied to a small stone formed in a vein (see VEINS) as a result of calcification of a THROMBUS.

Phlebotomy

A traditional name for the operation of bloodletting by opening a vein. (See VEINS; VENESECTION.)

Phlegm

A popular name for MUCUS, particularly that secreted in the air passages. (See BRONCHITIS; EXPECTORANTS.)

Phlyctenule

A HYPERSENSITIVITY reaction of the conjunctiva (see EYE). At the turn of the century the most common cause was TUBERCULOSIS; nowadays it is most commonly due to hypersensitivity to staphylococci (see STAPHYLOCOCCUS).

Phobia

An irrational fear of particular objects or situations. A well-known American medical dictionary lists more than 200 'examples' of phobias, ranging, alphabetically, from fear of air to fear of writing. Included in the list are phobophobia (fear of phobias) and triskaidekaphobia (fear of having 13 sitting at table).

Phobia is a form of obsession, and not uncommonly one of the features of anxiety. Treatment is behavioural therapy complemented in some patients with ANTIDEPRESSANT DRUGS. Care is needed, as some sufferers can become psychologically dependent on the drugs used to treat them (see DEPENDENCE). Those who suffer from what can be a most distressing condition can obtain help and advice from the Phobics Society. (See also MENTAL ILLNESS.)

Phocomelia

This is a great reduction in the size of the proximal parts of the limbs. In extreme cases the hands and feet may spring directly from the trunk. A rare condition, it occurred most commonly in children whose mothers took THALIDOMIDE in early pregnancy.

Pholcodine

An OPIOID cough suppressant similar to CODEINE; it is not, however, potent enough to suppress severe coughs and is also constipating.

Phonation

The production of vocal sounds – in particular, speech.

Phonocardiograph

An instrument for the graphic recording of heart sounds and murmurs.

Phosphates

Salts of phosphoric acid. As this substance is contained in many articles of food as well as in bone, the nuclei of cells, and the nervous system, phosphates are constantly excreted in the URINE. The continued use of an excess of food containing alkalis, such as green vegetables, and still more the presence in the urine of bacteria which lead to its decomposition, produce the necessary change from the natural mild acidity to alkalinity, and lead to the deposit of phosphates and to their collection into stones.

Phosphaturia

The presence in the URINE of a large amount of PHOSPHATES.

Phospholipid

A LIPID, the molecule of which contains a chemical derivative of PHOSPHORUS called phosphate. This type of lipid, which includes cephalins, lecithins and plasmalogens, is found in all tissues and organs, especially the BRAIN. Phospholipids are produced in the LIVER and

and take part in many of the body's metabolic activities (see METABOLISM).

Phosphorus

A non-metallic element whose compounds are widely found in plant and animal tissues. In humans, this element is largely concentrated in BONE. Some phosphorus-containing compounds such as ADENOSINE TRIPHOSPHATE (ATP) and creatine phosphate are essential participants in the conversion and storage of energy that are part of the body's METABOLISM. Pure phosphorus is toxic.

Phosphorus Burns

Phosphorus compounds are used in chemical laboratories, some industrial processes, matches, fireworks and in certain types of aerial bombs and artillery shells. If particles of phosphorus settle on or become embedded in the skin, the resulting burn should be treated with a 2 per cent solution of sodium bicarbonate, followed by application of a 1 per cent solution of copper sulphate.

Photochemotherapy

A form of treatment in which deliberate exposure to a photosensitising drug and ultraviolet light benefits certain skin diseases, particularly PSORIASIS and T-cell LYMPHOMA. A psoralen is the photoactive agent which reacts with long-wave ultraviolet light (UVA), giving the acronym, PUVA therapy.

Photocoagulation

Coagulation of the tissues of the retina (see EYE) by laser, for treatment of diseases of the retina such as diabetic retinopathy (see under EYE, DISORDERS OF – Retina, disorders of).

Photodermatoses

Diseases of the SKIN for which sunlight is partially or wholly responsible. In sufficient dosage, short-wave ultraviolet light (UVB – see ULTRAVIOLET RAYS (UVR)) always causes ERYTHEMA. Higher doses progressively cause OEDEMA and blistering; this is acute sunburn. Graduated exposure to UVB causes pigmentation (tanning). Prolonged chronic exposure to sunlight eventually accelerates ageing of the exposed skin with LENTIGO formation and loss of COLLAGEN and elastic tissue. After decades of such exposure, epidermal DYSPLASIA and CANCER may supervene.

Drugs given orally or topically may induce phototoxic reactions of various types. Thus, TETRACYCLINES exaggerate sunburn reactions. and the diuretic FRUSEMIDE may cause blistering reactions. Psoralens induce erythema and pigmentation. AMIODARONE also induces pigmentation. (See also PHOTOCHEMOTHERAPY.)

Phytophotodermatitis is a streaky, blistering photodermatosis typically seen on the limbs of children playing in grassy meadows in summer. The phototoxic reaction is caused by psoralens in weeds.

Berlocque dermatitis is a pattern of streaky pigmentation usually seen on women's necks, caused by a reaction to psoralens in perfumes.

Certain rare metabolic diseases may lead to photosensitisation. They include the PORPHYRIAS and PELLAGRA. Other skin diseases such as lupus erythematosus (see under LUPUS) and ROSACEA may be aggravated by light exposure. Sometimes, in the absence of any of these factors, some people spontaneously develop a sensitivity to light causing various patterns of DERMATITIS or URTICARIA. The most common pattern is 'polymorphic light eruption' which typically appears within a day or two of arrival at a sunny holiday destination and persists until departure. Continuously exposed areas, such as the hands and face, may be 'hardened' and unaffected.

Treatment Appropriate clothing and headgear, sunscreen creams and lotions are the main preventative measures.

Photodynamic Therapy

This comprises a photosensitising agent (one activated by light), which accumulates in malignant tissue, and a source of light that activates the photosensitiser, triggering it to generate highly reactive oxygen compounds that destroy malignant cells. One such photosensitiser is temoporfin. Photodynamic therapy is used to treat various types of malignancy; a recognised complication is photosensitivity, when a patient may suffer burns after transient exposure to sunlight. Photodynamic therapy is increasingly used and photosensitivity reactions may also become more common.

Photophobia

Sensitivity to light. It can occur in MIGRAINE, disorders of the eye, or in MENINGITIS.

Photopsia

This is a description of the flashing lights which are a not uncommon AURA preceding an attack of MIGRAINE.

Photosensitivity

Abnormal reaction to sunlight. The condition usually occurs as a skin rash appearing in response to light falling on the skin, and it may be caused by substances that have been eaten or applied to the skin. These are called photosensitisers and may be dyes, chemicals in soaps, or drugs. Sometimes plants act as photosensitisers – for example, buttercups and mustard. The condition may occur in some illnesses such as lupus erythematosus (see under LUPUS).

Photosynthesis

The method by which green plants and some bacteria produce CARBOHYDRATE from water and carbon dioxide. They use energy absorbed from the sun's rays by a green pigment in the organism called chlorophyll. Photosynthesis is one of the earth's fundamental biological processes. As well as converting the carbon dioxide into the essential biological compound carbohydrate, the process removes the gas from the atmosphere where, if it builds to excess, the atmospheric temperature rises, thus contributing to global warming.

Phrenic Nerve

The NERVE which chiefly supplies the DIA-PHRAGM. A phrenic nerve arises on each side of the SPINAL CORD from the third, fourth and fifth cervical spinal nerves; both follow a long course down the neck, and through the chest to the diaphragm. They play a key part in RESPIR-ATION through control of the diaphragm. Injury to one nerve paralyses one half of the diaphragm. Occasionally the phrenic nerve may be surgically crushed as part of the treatment to repair a HIATUS HERNIA or, rarely, to stop intractable hiccups.

Phrenology

A quack method, common in the Victorian era, allegedly to study the mind and character of individuals from the shape of the head. As the shape of the head has been shown to depend chiefly upon accidental characteristics, such as the size of the air spaces in the bones, and not upon development of special areas in the contained brain, there is no scientific basis for the practice.

Phthisis

A historical term means wasting, and was applied to that progressive enfeeblement and loss of weight that arose from tuberculous disease of all kinds, but especially from the disease as it affected the lungs (see TUBERCULOSIS).

Physical Examination

That part of a patient's consultation with a doctor in which the doctor looks, feels (palpates) and listens to (auscultates) various parts of the patient's body. Along with the history of the patient's symptoms, this enables the doctor to assess the patient's condition and decide whether an immediate diagnosis is possible or whether laboratory or imaging investigations are needed to reach a diagnosis. A full physical examination may take 30 minutes or more. Physical examination, along with certain standard investigations, is done when a person attends for a 'preventive' check-up of his or her state of health.

Physical Medicine

A medical specialty founded in 1931 and recognised by the Royal College of Physicians of London in 1972. Physical-medicine specialists started by treating rheumatic diseases; subsequently their work developed to include the diagnosis and rehabilitation of people with physical handicaps. The specialty has now been combined with that of RHEUMATOLOGY. (See also PHYSIOTHERAPY.)

Physician-Assisted Suicide

See SUICIDE.

Physiology

Physiology is the branch of medical science that deals with the healthy functions of different organs, and the changes that the whole body undergoes in the course of its activities. The teaching of physiology is a basic part of the medical student's initial education.

Physiotherapy

An important treatment involving the use of physical measures, such as exercise, heat, manipulation and remedial exercises in the treatment of disease. An alternative name is PHYSICAL MEDICINE. It is an essential part of the rehabilitation of convalescent or disabled patients. Those who practise physiotherapy – physiotherapists – have a recognised training and, on successful completion of this, are placed on the profession's official register (see APPENDIX 8: PROFESSIONAL ORGANISATIONS.)

Physostigmine

Also known as eserine. An alkaloid (see ALKAL-OIDS) obtained from Calabar bean, the seed of *Physostigma venenosum*, a climbing plant of West Africa. Its action depends on the presence of two alkaloids, the one known as physostigmine or eserine, the other as calabarine, the former of these being much the more important.

Action Physostigmine produces the same effect as stimulation of the PARASYMPATHETIC NERVOUS SYSTEM: i.e. it constricts the pupil of the eye, stimulates the gut, increases the secretion of saliva, stimulates the bladder, and increases the irritability of voluntary muscle. In poisonous doses it brings on a general paralysis.

Uses It is used in medicine in the form of eye drops or ointment to treat GLAUCOMA.

Phytomenadione
The *British Pharmacopoeia* name for vitamin K. (See APPENDIX 5: VITAMINS.)

Pia Mater
The membrane closely investing the BRAIN and SPINAL CORD, in which run blood vessels for the nourishment of these organs.

Pica
This is the Latin for magpie and is used to describe an abnormal craving for unusual foods. It is not uncommon in pregnancy. Among the unusual substances for which pregnant women have developed a craving are soap, clay pipes, bed linen, charcoal, ashes – and almost every imaginable food stuff taken in excess. In primitive races, the presence of pica is taken as an indication that the growing fetus requires such food. It is also not uncommon in children in whom, previously, it was an important cause of LEAD POISONING due to ingestion of paint flakes. (See also APPETITE.)

Picorna Viruses
These infectious agents derive their name from pico (small) and from RNA (because they contain ribonuleic acid). They are a group of viruses which includes the ENTEROVIRUSES and the RHINOVIRUSES.

Picric Acid
A yellow crystalline solid substance which is used as a fixative for tissues being prepared for examination under a microscope; it is also used as a dye.

Picture Archiving and Communications System (PACS)
The use of digital imaging systems to replace conventional X-ray pictures and other imaging techniques. Though expensive to operate, digital imaging and storage systems offer promising possibilities for transmission of clinical images within and between hospitals and community health-care units, providing fast access and remote working that will benefit patients and health-care staff alike. When security and confidentiality are assured, images could be transferred via the Internet and teleradiology. In future, hospitals might be able to eliminate the costly physical transfer and storage of X-ray films. The integration of PACS with hospital information systems in the NHS will (hopefully) facilitate the introduction of electronic radiology.

Pigeon Breast
See CHEST, DEFORMITIES OF.

Pigment
The term applied to the colouring matter of various secretions, blood, etc.; also to any medicinal preparation of thick consistency intended for painting on the skin or mucous membranes.

Piles
See HAEMORRHOIDS.

Pills
Small round masses containing active drugs held together by syrup, gum, glycerin, or adhesive vegetable extracts. They are sometimes without coating, being merely rolled in French chalk, but often they are covered with sugar or gelatin. Many people use the term interchangeably with tablets, and 'the pill' has come to represent oral contraceptives.

Pilocarpine
An alkaloid (see ALKALOIDS) derived from the leaves of *Pilocarpus microphyllus* (jaborandi). It produces the same effects as stimulation of the PARASYMPATHETIC NERVOUS SYSTEM: i.e. it has exactly the opposite effect to ATROPINE, but cannot be used in the treatment of atropine poisoning as it does not antagonise the action of poisonous doses of atropine on the brain. Its main use today is in the form of eye drops to decrease the pressure inside the eyeball in GLAUCOMA.

Pilonoidal Sinus
A SINUS that contains hairs, usually occurring in the cleft between the buttocks. It may get infected and cause considerable pain. Treatment is by antibiotics and, if necessary, surgical removal.

Pimples
Technically known as papules, these are small, raised and inflamed areas on the SKIN. On the

face, the most common cause is ACNE. BOILS (FURUNCULOSIS) start as hard pimples. The eruption of SMALLPOX and that of CHICKENPOX begin also with pimples. (See also SKIN, DISEASES OF.)

Pineal Gland

A small reddish structure, 10 mm in length and shaped somewhat like a pine cone (hence its name), situated on the upper part of the midbrain (see BRAIN). Many theories have been expounded as to its function, but there is increasing evidence that, in some animals at least, it is affected by light and plays a part in hibernation and in controlling sexual activity and the colour of the skin. This it seems to do by means of a substance it produces known as MELATONIN. There is also growing evidence that it may play a part in controlling the circadian rhythms of the body – the natural variations in physiological activities throughout the 24-hour day.

Pinna

The part of the EAR, formed of cartilage and skin, that is external to the head. In animals it is an important element in detecting the direction of sound.

Pins and Needles

A form of PARAESTHESIA, or disturbed sensation, such as may occur, for example, in NEURITIS or POLYNEURITIS.

Pint

A measure of quantity containing 16 fluid ounces (wine measure) or 20 fluid ounces (Imperial measure). The metric equivalent is 568 millilitres. (See APPENDIX 6: MEASUREMENTS IN MEDICINE.)

Pinworm

See ENTEROBIASIS.

Piperacillin

A ureidopenicillin with a broad spectrum of antibacterial activity. The drug is active against the serious infective agent *Pseudomonas aeruginosa*. (See PENICILLIN.)

Piperazine

A drug used for the treatment of threadworms (see ENTEROBIASIS) and ASCARIASIS.

Pipothiazine

An antipsychotic drug for maintenance treatment of SCHIZOPHRENIA. It is given as a depot injection that lasts four weeks. (See NEUROLEPTICS; MENTAL ILLNESS.)

Piroxicam

An intermediate risk, oral non-steroidal anti-inflammatory drug (see NON-STEROIDAL ANTI-INFLAMMATORY DRUGS (NSAIDS)) with prolonged action. Used to treat pain and inflammation in RHEUMATOID ARTHRITIS, other musculoskeletal disorders, and acute GOUT.

Pituitary Gland

Also known as the pituitary body and the hypophysis, this is an ovoid structure, weighing around 0·5 gram in the adult. It is attached to the base of the BRAIN, and lies in the depression in the base of the skull known as the sella turcica. The anterior part is called the adenohypophysis and the posterior part the neurohypophysis. The gland is connected to the HYPOTHALAMUS of the brain by a stalk known as the hypophyseal or pituitary stalk.

The pituitary gland is the most important ductless, or endocrine, gland in the body. (See

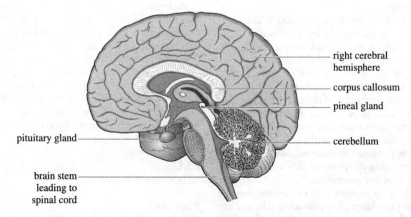

Vertical cross-section of brain seen from the left showing positions of pineal and pituitary glands.

ENDOCRINE GLANDS.) It exerts overall control of the endocrine system through the media of a series of hormones which it produces. The adenohypophysis produces trophic hormones (that is, they work by stimulating or inhibiting other endocrine glands) and have therefore been given names ending with 'trophic' or 'trophin'. The thyrotrophic hormone, or thyroid-stimulating hormone (TSH), exerts a powerful influence over the activity of the THYROID GLAND. The ADRENOCORTICOTROPHIC HORMONE (ACTH) stimulates the cortex of the adrenal glands. GROWTH HORMONE, also known as somatotrophin (SMH), controls the growth of the body. There are also two gonadotrophic hormones which play a vital part in the control of the gonads: these are the follicle-stimulating hormone (FSH), and the luteinising hormone (LH) which is also known as the interstitial-cell-stimulating hormone (ICSH) – see GONADOTROPHINS. The lactogenic hormone, also known as prolactin, mammotrophin and luteotrophin, induces lactation.

The neurohypophysis produces two hormones. One is oxytocin, which is widely used because of its stimulating effect on contraction of the UTERUS. The other is VASOPRESSIN, or the antidiuretic hormone (ADH), which acts on the renal tubules and the collecting tubules (see KIDNEYS) to increase the amount of water that they normally absorb.

Pituitary-Linked Disorders

ACROMEGALY or gigantism is the result of the overactivity of, or tumour formation of cells in, the adenohypophysis which produces GROWTH HORMONE (see also PITUITARY GLAND). If this overactivity occurs after growth has ceased, acromegaly arises, in which there is gross overgrowth of the ears, nose, jaws, and hands and feet. DWARFISM may be due to lack of growth hormone.

DIABETES INSIPIDUS, a condition characterised by the passing of a large volume of URINE every day, is due to lack of the antidiuretic hormone (see VASOPRESSIN). Enhanced production of the ADRENOCORTICOTROPHIC HORMONE (ACTH) leads to CUSHING'S SYNDROME. Excessive production of PROLACTIN by micro or macro adenomas (benign tumours) leads to hyperprolactinaemia and consequent AMENORRHOEA and GALACTORRHOEA. Some adenomas do not produce any hormone but cause effects by damaging the pituitary cells and inhibiting their hormone production.

The most sensitive cells to extrinsic pressure are the gonadotrophin-producing cells and the growth-hormone producing cells, so that if the tumour occurs in childhood, growth hormone will be suppressed and growth will slow. Gonadotrophin hormone suppression will prevent the development of puberty and, if the tumour occurs after puberty, will result in amenorrhoea in the female and lack of LIBIDO in both sexes. The thyroid-stimulating hormone cells are the next to suffer and the pressure effects on these cells will result in hypothyroidism (see under THYROID GLAND, DISEASES OF).

Fortunately the ACTH-producing cells are the most resistant to extrinsic pressure and this is teleologically sound as ACTH is the one pituitary hormone that is essential to life. However, these cells can suffer damage from intracellular tumours, and adrenocortical insufficiency is not uncommon.

Information about these disorders may be obtained from the Pituitary Foundation.

Pityriasis

A skin disorder typified by a bran-like desquamation (flaking). There are several varieties including P. alba, rosea, versicolor (fungal caused) and rubra (exfoliative dermatitis).

Pityriasis alba is a mild form of chronic eczema (see DERMATITIS) occurring mainly in children on the face and in young adults on the upper arms. It is characterised by round or oval flaky patches which are paler than the surrounding skin due to partial loss of MELANIN pigment. The appearance is more dramatic in dark-skinned or suntanned subjects. Moisturising cream often suffices, but 1 per cent HYDROCORTISONE cream is more effective.

Pityriasis rosea is a common self-limiting eruption seen mainly in young adults. It usually begins as a solitary red flaky patch (often misdiagnosed as ringworm). Within a week this 'herald patch' is followed by a profuse symmetrical eruption of smaller rose-pink, flaky, oval lesions on the trunk and neck but largely sparing the limbs and face. Itching is variable. The eruption usually peaks within 3 weeks and fades away leaving collarettes of scale, disappearing within 6–7 weeks. It rarely recurs and a viral cause is suspected but not proved. It is not contagious and there is no specific treatment, but crotamiton cream (Eurax) may relieve discomfort.

PKU

See PHENYLKETONURIA.

Placebo

Placebo is the Latin for 'I will please' and

implies giving an inactive treatment. Traditionally, placebos were used to pacify without actually benefiting the patient. They were inactive, often highly coloured, substances formerly given to please or gratify the patient but without pharmacological benefit. Nowadays they are used in controlled studies, approved by ETHICS COMMITTEES and with patient consent, to determine the efficacy of drugs.

However, pharmacologically inert compounds can relieve symptoms, and this is called the placebo effect. The reassurance that is associated with placebo administration is accompanied by measurable changes in body function which are affected through autonomic pathways and humoral mechanisms. Alterations in blood pressure and pulse frequency are especially common. Placebos have the ability to relieve a variety of symptoms in a consistent proportion of the population – in some studies in as many as 30 per cent. Some patients with symptoms such as pain or cough will respond to placebo medications, and an even higher proportion of patients with psychological symptoms such as anxiety or insomnia may benefit. In judging the effectiveness of a drug, the comparison must be with a placebo rather than with no treatment at all.

Placenta

The thick, spongy, disc-like mass of tissue which connects the EMBRYO with the inner surface of the UTERUS, the embryo otherwise lying free in the amniotic fluid (see AMNION). The placenta is mainly a new structure growing with the embryo, but, when it separates, a portion of the inner surface of the womb – called the maternal placenta – comes away with it. It is mainly composed of loops of veins belonging to the embryo, lying in blood-sinuses, in which circulates maternal blood. Thus, although no mixing of the blood of embryo and mother takes place, there is ample opportunity for the exchange of fluids, gases, and the nutrients brought by the mother's blood. The width of the full-sized placenta is about 20 cm (8 inches), its thickness 2·5 cm (1 inch). One surface is rough and studded with villi, which consist of the loops of fetal veins; the other is smooth, and has implanted in its centre the umbilical cord, or navel string, which is about as thick as a finger and 50 cm (20 inches) long. It contains two arteries and a vein, enters the fetus at the navel, and forms the sole connection between the bodies of mother and fetus. The name 'afterbirth' is given to the structure because it is expelled from the womb in the

third stage of labour (see PREGNANCY AND LABOUR).

Placenta Praevia

Implantation of the PLACENTA in the bottom part of the UTERUS adjacent to or over the CERVIX. The condition may cause few problems during pregnancy or labour; it may, however, cause vaginal bleeding late in pregnancy or hinder vaginal delivery of the baby and this may necessitate obstetric intervention.

Placentography

The procedure of rendering the PLACENTA visible by means of X-rays. This can be done either by using what is known as soft-tissue radiography, or by injecting a radio-opaque substance into the bloodstream or into the amniotic cavity (see AMNION). The procedure has some risk to both mother and fetus, and is carried out under expert supervision. It can help to assess the cause of antepartum haemorrhage. The placenta and fetus can now be visualised by the non-invasive and safe method of ULTRASOUND.

Plague

This infection – also known as bubonic plague – is caused by the bacterium *Yersinis pestis*. Plague remains a major infection in many tropical countries.

The reservoir for the bacillus in urban infection lies in the black rat (*Rattus rattus*), and less importantly the brown (sewer) rat (*Rattus norvegicus*). It is conveyed to humans by the rat flea, usually *Xenopsylla cheopis*. *Y. pestis* multiplies in the gastrointestinal tract of the flea, which may remain infectious for up to six weeks. In the pneumonic form (see below), human-to-human transmission can occur by droplet infection. Many lower mammals (apart from the rat) can also act as a reservoir in sylvatic transmission which remains a major problem in the US (mostly in the south-western States); ground-squirrels, rock-squirrels, prairie dogs, bobcats, chipmunks, etc. can be affected.

Clinically, symptoms usually begin 2–8 days after infection; disease begins with fever, headache, lassitude, and aching limbs. In over two-thirds of patients, enlarged glands (buboes) appear – usually in the groin, but also in the axillae and cervical neck; this constitutes bubonic plague. Haemorrhages may be present beneath the skin causing gangrenous patches and occasionally ulcers; these lesions led to the epithet 'Black Death'. In a favourable case, fever abates after about a week, and the buboes discharge foul-smelling pus. In a rapidly fatal form

P

(septicaemic plague), haematogenous transmission produces mortality in a high percentage of cases. Pneumonic plague is associated with pneumonic consolidation (person-to-person transmission) and death often ensues on the fourth or fifth day. (The nursery rhyme 'Ring-o-ring o' roses, a pocketful o' posies, atishoo! atishoo!, we all fall down' is considered to have originated in the 17th century and refers to this form of the disease.) In addition, meningitic and pharyngeal forms of the disease can occur; these are unusual. Diagnosis consists of demonstration of the causative organism.

Treatment is with tetracycline or doxycycline; a range of other antibiotics is also effective. Plague remains (together with CHOLERA and YELLOW FEVER) a quarantinable disease. Contacts should be disinfected with insecticide powder; clothes, skins, soft merchandise, etc. which have been in contact with the infection can remain infectious for several months; suspect items should be destroyed or disinfected with an insecticide. Ships must be carefully checked for presence of rats; the rationale of anchoring a distance from the quay prevents access of vermin. (See also EPIDEMIC; PANDEMIC; NOTIFIABLE DISEASES.)

Plantar
Describing anything related to the sole of the foot.

Plantar Dermatosis
A common form of eczema (see DERMATITIS) of the soles of the feet typically seen in boys with an atopic (see ATOPY) background who constantly wear trainers.

Plantar Fasciitis
See FASCIITIS.

Plaque
(1) A coating of the TEETH which forms as a result of poor mouth and dental hygiene. It consists of food debris and bacteria; later, calcium salts will be deposited in it to form calculus. It is therefore associated with both caries and periodontal disease (see TEETH, DISORDERS OF – Caries of the teeth).
(2) Raised patch on the skin resulting from the merging or enlargement of papules (see PAPULE; PIMPLES).

Plasma
The name applied to the straw-coloured fluid portion of the BLOOD composed of a solution of various inorganic salts of sodium, potassium, calcium, etc., as well as SERUM and fibrinogen,

the material which produces clotting (see COAGULATION). When the plasma is clotted, the thinner fluid separating from the clot is the serum.

Plasma Cells
These are cells that produce ANTIBODIES and occur in bone-forming tissue as well as the lining of the gastrointestinal tract and the lungs. The cells develop in LYMPH NODES, SPLEEN and BONE MARROW when T-lymphocytes (see IMMUNITY) are stimulated by antigens (see ANTIGEN) to produce the precursor cells from which plasma cells originate.

Plasma Exchange
Also known as plasmapheresis. The removal of the circulating PLASMA from the patient. It is done by removing blood from a patient and returning the red cells with a plasma expander. The plasma exchange is carried out through an in-dwelling CANNULA in the femoral vein, and the red cells and plasma are separated by a hemonetics separator. Usually a sequence of three or four sessions is undertaken, at each of which 2–3 litres of plasma are removed. The lost plasma can either be replaced by human serum albumin (see ALBUMINS) or a plasma expander.

In autoimmune disorders, disease is due to damage wrought by circulating ANTIBODIES or sensitised lymphocytes (see LYMPHOCYTE). If the disease is due to circulating humoral antibodies, removal of these antibodies from the body should theoretically relieve the disorder. This is the principle on which plasma exchange was used in the management of autoimmune diseases due to circulating antibodies. Such disorders include Goodpasture's syndrome, SYSTEMIC LUPUS ERYTHEMATOSUS (SLE) and MYASTHENIA GRAVIS. One of the problems in the use of plasma exchange in the treatment of such diseases is that the body responds to the removal of an antibody from the circulation by enhanced production of that antibody by the immune system. It is therefore necessary to suppress this homeostatic response with cytotoxic drugs such as AZATHIOPRINE. Nevertheless, remissions can be achieved in autoimmune diseases due to circulating antibodies by the process of plasma exchange.

Plasmapheresis
See PLASMA EXCHANGE.

Plasma Transfusion
This procedure is sometimes used instead of blood TRANSFUSION. PLASMA – the fluid part of

blood from which the cells have been separated – may be dried and in powder form kept almost indefinitely; when wanted it is reconstituted by adding sterile distilled water. In powder form it can be transported easily and over long distances. Transfusion of plasma is especially useful in the treatment of SHOCK. One advantage of plasma transfusion is that it is not necessary to carry out testing of blood groups before using it.

Plasmids
A generic description of any discrete agents in cells that have genetic functions. They include plasmagenes (self-reproducing copies of a nuclear gene existing outside the cell nucleus) and viruses.

Plasmin
Also called fibrinolysin, this is an ENZYME that digests the protein FIBRIN. It dissolves blood clots (see COAGULATION) and so is present in the blood in the form of PLASMINOGEN, an inactive precursor.

Plasminogen
A precursor of PLASMIN, an ENZYME that digests the protein FIBRIN – the main constituent of blood clots (see COAGULATION). When tissue is damaged, activators are released which provoke the conversion of plasminogen into plasmin.

Plasmodium
The general term applied to minute protoplasmic cells, and particularly to those which cause MALARIA and allied diseases.

Plaster of Paris
A form of calcium sulphate, which, after soaking in water, sets firmly. For this reason it is widely used as a form of splinting in the treatment of fractures, for producing casts to immobilise parts of the body, and for dental models. Splints are made with bandages impregnated with plaster and a suitable adhesive. Its great advantage, compared with an ordinary splint, is that it can be moulded to the shape of the limb.

Plastic Surgery
See RECONSTRUCTIVE (PLASTIC) SURGERY.

Platelets
Blood platelets, or thrombocytes, are small spherical bodies in the BLOOD, which play an important part in the process of its COAGULATION. Normally, there are around 300,000 per cubic millimetre of blood.

Plethora
A condition of fullness of the blood vessels in a particular part or in the whole body. This results in a florid, red appearance of the affected area, particularly the face. The volume of blood may be increased (POLYCYTHAEMIA) or the blood vessels beneath the skin may be dilated. Plethoric lung fields are seen on X-rays of patients with left-to-right shunts through the heart wall (see SEPTAL DEFECT).

Plethysmograph
An apparatus for estimating changes in the size of any part placed in the apparatus; in this way changes in the volume of blood in a part can be measured.

Pleura
The name of the membrane which, on either side of the chest, forms a covering for one lung. The two pleurae are distinct, though they touch one another for a short distance behind the breast-bone. (See LUNGS.)

Pleural Cavity
The normally restricted space between the parietal and the visceral PLEURA, which slide over one another as the individual breathes in and out. If gas or fluid are introduced as a result of injury or infection, the pleural surfaces are separated and the pleural space increases in volume. This usually causes breathing difficulties.

Pleurisy
Inflammation of the PLEURA or serous membrane investing the lung and lining the inner surface of the ribs. It is a common condition, and may be either acute or chronic, the latter being usually tuberculous in origin (see TUBERCULOSIS).

Many cases of pleurisy are associated with only a little effusion, the inflammation consisting chiefly in exudation of FIBRIN: to this form the term 'dry pleurisy' is applied. Further, pleurisy may be limited to a very small area – or, on the contrary, may affect, throughout a greater or less extent, the pleural surfaces of both lungs.

Causes Pleurisy is often associated with other forms of inflammatory disease within the chest, more particularly PNEUMONIA, BRONCHIECTASIS, and tuberculosis; it occasionally accompanies PERICARDITIS. It may also be due to carcinoma of the lung, or be secondary to abdominal infections such as subphrenic abscess. Further, wounds or injuries of the thoracic walls are apt to set up pleurisy.

Symptoms The symptoms of pleurisy vary, being generally well marked, but sometimes obscure.

DRY PLEURISY In the case of dry pleurisy, which is, on the whole, the milder form, the chief symptom is a sharp pain in the side, felt especially on breathing. Fever may or may not be present. There is a slight, dry cough, and breathing is quicker than normal and shallow.

PLEURISY WITH EFFUSION is usually more severe than dry pleurisy, and, although it may in some cases develop insidiously, it is in general ushered in sharply by shivering and fever, like other acute inflammatory diseases. Pain is felt in the side or breast, of a severe cutting or stabbing character. A dry cough usually occurs and breathing is painful and difficult.

Treatment The treatment varies greatly with the form and severity of the attack. Bed rest, antibiotics, analgesics and antipyretics are advisable. A large pleural effusion may need to be drained via an aspiration needle.

Pleurodynia

Also known as BORNHOLM DISEASE. A painful condition of the chest wall, it is usually the result of an infection of coxsackie virus B (see COXSACKIE VIRUSES) and may occur in epidemics (see EPIDEMIC). Fever, sore throat, headache and malaise are typical but the condition is self-limiting, subsiding within a few days.

Plexus

A network of nerves or vessels: for example, the brachial and sacral plexuses of nerves and the choroid plexus of veins within the brain.

Plumbism

Another name for LEAD POISONING.

Plummer-Vinson Syndrome

Hypochromic ANAEMIA and difficulty in swallowing due to an oesophageal web.

Pneumo-

A prefix relating to the LUNGS or to air. Examples are PNEUMONIA, PNEUMONECTOMY and PNEUMOPERITONEUM.

Pneumococcus

A type of streptococcal bacterium (see STREPTOCOCCUS) which can cause otitis media (see EAR, DISEASES OF – Diseases of the middle ear), TONSILLITIS, PNEUMONIA, MENINGITIS and SEPTICAEMIA. It is usually sensitive to PENICILLIN.

Pneumoconiosis

The general name applied to a chronic form of inflammation of the LUNGS which is liable to affect people who constantly inhale irritating particles at work. It has been defined by the Industrial Injuries Advisory Council as: 'Permanent alteration of lung structure due to the inhalation of mineral dust and the tissue reactions of the lung to its presence, but does not include bronchitis and emphysema.' Some of the tradespeople liable to suffer are stonemasons, potters, steel-grinders, coal-miners, millers, and workers in cotton, flax, or wool mills. (See also OCCUPATIONAL HEALTH, MEDICINE AND DISEASES; TUBERCULOSIS.)

Pneumocystis Pneumonia

PNEUMONIA caused by a species of the genus of PROTOZOA, a parasitic micro-organism. *Pneumocystis carinii* causes an opportunistic infection in the lung which is dangerous to people whose immune system is impaired (see IMMUNITY), thus reducing their resistance to infections. People with AIDS/HIV or LEUKAEMIA have impaired immune systems and *P. carinii* is a major cause of death in the former. Fever, dry cough and breathlessness are among the symptoms; treatment is with high doses of antibiotic drugs such as CO-TRIMOXAZOLE or PENTAMIDINE.

Pneumonectomy

The operation of removing an entire lung (see LUNGS) in such diseases as BRONCHIECTASIS, TUBERCULOSIS, and cancer of the lung.

Pneumonia

Pneumonia is an inflammation of the lung tissue (see LUNGS) caused by infection. It can occur without underlying lung or general disease, or in patients with an underlying condition that makes them susceptible.

Pneumonia with no predisposing cause – community-acquired pneumonia – is caused most often by *Streptococcus pneumoniae* (PNEUMOCOCCUS). The other most common causes are viruses, *Mycoplasma pneumoniae* and *Legionella* species (Legionnaire's disease). Another cause, *Chlamydia psittaci*, may be associated with exposure to perching birds.

In patients with underlying lung disease, such as CHRONIC OBSTRUCTIVE PULMONARY DISEASE (COPD) or BRONCHIECTASIS as in CYSTIC FIBROSIS, other organisms such as *Haemophilus influenzae*, *Klebsiella*, *Escherichia coli* and *Pseudomonas aeruginosa* are more prominent. In patients in hospital with severe underlying disease, pneumonia, often caused by gram-negative bacteria (see GRAM'S STAIN), is commonly the terminal event.

In patients with an immune system suppressed by pregnancy and labour, infection with HIV, CHEMOTHERAPY or immunosuppressive drugs after organ transplantation, a wider range of opportunistic organisms needs to be considered. Some of these organisms such as CYTOMEGALOVIRUS (CMV) or the fungus *Pneumocystis carinii* rarely cause disease in immunocompetent individuals – those whose body's immune (defence) system is effective.

TUBERCULOSIS is another cause of pneumonia, although the pattern of lung involvement and the more chronic course usually differentiate it from other causes of pneumonia.

Symptoms The common symptoms of pneumonia are cough, fever (sometimes with RIGOR), pleuritic chest pain (see PLEURISY) and shortness of breath. SPUTUM may not be present at first but later may be purulent or reddish (rusty).

Examination of the chest may show the typical signs of consolidation of an area of lung. The solid lung in which the alveoli are filled with inflammatory exudate is dull to percussion but transmits sounds better than air-containing lung, giving rise to the signs of bronchial breathing and increased conduction of voice sounds to the stethoscope or palpating hand.

The chest X-ray in pneumonia shows opacities corresponding to the consolidated lung. This may have a lobar distribution fitting with limitation to one area of the lung, or have a less confluent scattered distribution in bronchopneumonia. Blood tests usually show a raised white cell (LEUCOCYTES) count. The organism responsible for the pneumonia can often be identified from culture of the sputum or the blood, or from blood tests for the specific ANTIBODIES produced in response to the infection.

Treatment The treatment of pneumonia involves appropriate antibiotics together with oxygen, pain relief and management of any complications that may arise. When treatment is started, the causative organism has often not been identified so that the antibiotic choice is made on the basis of the clinical features, prevalent organisms and their sensitivities. In severe cases of community-acquired pneumonia (see above), this will often be a PENICILLIN or one of the CEPHALOSPORINS to cover *Strep. pneumoniae* together with a macrolide such as ERYTHROMYCIN. Pleuritic pain will need analgesia to allow deep breathing and coughing; oxygen may be needed as judged by the oxygen saturation or blood gas measurement.

Possible complications of pneumonia are local changes such as lung abscess, pleural effusion or EMPYEMA and general problems such as cardiovascular collapse and abnormalities of kidney or liver function. Appropriate treatment should result in complete resolution of the lung changes but some FIBROSIS in the lung may remain. Pneumonia can be a severe illness in previously fit people and it may take some months to return to full fitness.

Pneumonitis
An inflammation of the lung (see LUNGS) due to chemical or physical agents.

Pneumoperitoneum
A collection of air in the peritoneal cavity (see PERITONEUM). Air introduced into the peritoneal cavity collects under the diaphragm which is thus raised and collapses the lungs. This procedure was sometimes carried out in the treatment of pulmonary tuberculosis in the pre-antibiotic days as an alternative to artificial PNEUMOTHORAX.

Pneumothorax
A collection of air in the pleural cavity, into which it has gained entrance by a defect in the lung or a wound in the chest wall. When air enters the chest, the lung immediately collapses towards the centre of the chest; but, air being absorbed from the pleural cavity, the lung expands again within a short time. (See LUNGS, DISEASES OF.)

Tension pneumothorax is a life-threatening condition in which the air in the hemithorax is under such pressure that it forces the heart to the other side and compresses the still-inflated lung on the other side. It must be promptly relieved by inserting a hollow tube into the pleural cavity – a chest drain.

Artificial pneumothorax was an operation often performed in the pre-antibiotic days to treat pulmonary tuberculosis. Air was run into the pleural cavity to cause collapse of one lung, which rested it and allowed cavities in it to heal.

Podagra
Another name for GOUT affecting the foot.

Podophyllin
A resin derived from podophyllum plants, its active agent, podophyllotoxin, in alcoholic solution is used to treat genital WARTS. Paints, creams and impregnated plasters are used for calluses and warts elsewhere.

Poikilocytosis

This is a term used to describe the variation seen in the shape of red blood cells in some disorders of the BONE MARROW.

Poisons

A poison is any substance which, if absorbed by, introduced into or applied to a living organism, may cause illness or death. The term 'toxin' is often used to refer to a poison of biological origin. Toxins are therefore a subgroup of poisons, but often little distinction is made between the terms. The study of the effects of poisons is toxicology and the effects of toxins, toxinology.

The concept of the dose-response is important for understanding the risk of exposure to a particular substance. This is embodied in a statement by Paracelsus (c.1493–1541): 'All substances are poisons; there is none which is not a poison. The right dose differentiates a poison and a remedy.'

Poisoning may occur in a variety of ways: deliberate – SUICIDE, substance abuse or murder; accidental – including accidental overdose of medicines; occupational; and environmental – including exposure during fire.

Ingestion is the most common route of exposure, but poisoning may also occur through inhalation, absorption through the skin, by injection and through bites and stings of venomous animals. Poisoning may be described as acute, where a single exposure produces clinical effects with a relatively rapid onset; or chronic, where prolonged or repeated exposures may produce clinical effects which may be insidious in onset, cumulative and in some cases permanent.

Diagnosis of poisoning is usually by circumstantial evidence or elimination of other causes of the clinical condition of the patient. Some substances (e.g. opioids) produce a characteristic clinical picture in overdose that can help with diagnosis. In some patients laboratory analysis of body fluids or the substance taken may be useful to determine or confirm the offending agent. Routine assays are not necessary. For a very small number of poisons, such as paracetamol, aspirin, iron and lead, the management of the patient may depend on measuring the amount of poison in the bloodstream.

Accurate statistics on the incidence of poisoning in the UK are lacking. Mortality figures are more reliable than morbidity statistics; annually, well over 100,000 cases of poisoning are admitted to hospital. The annual number of deaths from poisoning is relatively small – about 300 – and in most cases patients die before reaching hospital. Currently, CAR-BON MONOXIDE (CO) is by far the most common cause of death due to poisoning. The most common agents involved in intentional or accidental poisoning are drugs, particularly ANALGESICS, ANTIDEPRESSANT DRUGS and SEDATIVES. Alcohol is also commonly taken by adults, usually in combination with drugs. Children frequently swallow household cleaners, white spirit, plant material – such as belladonna (deadly nightshade) and certain mushrooms; for example, death cap and fly agaric – aftershave and perfume as well as drugs. If possible, the suspect container, drug or plant should be taken with the victim to the hospital or doctor. The use of child-resistant containers has reduced the number of admissions of children to hospital for treatment. Bixtrex® is an intensely bitter-tasting agent which is often added to products to discourage ingestion; however, not everybody is able to taste it, nor has any beneficial effect been proven.

Treatment of poisoning usually begins with decontamination procedures. For ingested substances this may involve making the patient sick or washing the stomach out (GASTRIC LAVAGE): this is usually only worthwhile if performed soon after ingestion. It should be emphasised that salt (sodium chloride) water must never be given to induce vomiting, since this procedure is dangerous and has caused death. For substances spilt on the skin, the affected area should immediately be thoroughly washed and all contaminated clothing removed. Following eye exposure, the affected eye/s should be thoroughly irrigated with saline or water.

Treatment thereafter is generally symptomatic and supportive, with maintenance of the victim's respiratory, neurological and cardiovascular systems and, where appropriate, monitoring of their fluid and electrolyte balance and hepatic and renal function. There are specific antidotes for a few substances: the most important of these are PARACETAMOL, iron, cyanide (see CYANIDE POISONING), opioids (see OPIOID), DIGOXIN, insecticides and some heavy metals. Heavy-metal poisoning is treated with CHELATING AGENTS – chemical compounds that form complexes by binding metal ions: desferrioxamine and pencillinamine are two such agents. The number of people presenting with paracetamol overdose – a common drug used for attempted suicide – has fallen sharply since restrictions were placed on its over-the-counter sales.

When a patient presents with an illness thought to be caused by exposure to substances at work, further exposure should be limited or prevented and investigations undertaken to determine the source and extent of the problem. Acutely poisoned workers will usually go to hospital, but those suffering from chronic exposure may attend their GP with non-specific symptoms (see OCCUPATIONAL HEALTH, MEDICINE AND DISEASES).

In recent years, legislation has been enacted in the UK to improve safety in the workplace and to ensure that data on the hazardous constituents and effects of chemicals are more readily available. These official controls include the Control of Substances Hazardous to Health (COSHH) and the Chemicals (Hazard Information and Packaging) Regulations (CHIP) and are UK legislation in response to European Union directives.

The National Poisons Information Service is a 24-hour emergency telephone service available to the medical profession and provides information on the likely effects of numerous agents and advice on the management of the poisoned patient. The telephone numbers are available in the medical literature. In the UK this is not a public-access service. People who believe they, or their relatives, have been poisoned should seek medical advice from their GPs or attend their local hospital.

Toxbase The National Poisons Information Service provides a primary clinical toxicology database on the Internet: www.spib.axl.co.uk. This website provides information about routine diagnosis, treatment and management of people exposed to drugs, household products and industrial and agricultural products. (See also APPENDIX 1: BASIC FIRST AID.)

Poliomyelitis

Once known as infantile paralysis, this disease is caused by a viral infection involving the BRAIN and SPINAL CORD. Since the development of effective vaccines in the 1950s (see IMMUNISATION), polio has been practically eliminated in most developed countries. People who have not been fully vaccinated, however, may get the disease: it remains a serious risk for unvaccinated travellers to Africa, Asia or southern Europe. Most reported cases are now from sub-Saharan Africa.

Pathology There are three types of virus, infection spreading by the stools-contaminated hands-mouth route. Children are most susceptible.

One attack usually produces permanent immunity, and second attacks are rare. The virus typically affects the anterior horn cells of the spinal cord, especially those in the lumbar region; the grey matter of the brain stem and cortex may also be damaged.

Vaccination is given to infants at two, three and four months: a booster dose is given at around the age of five. The vaccine contains all three types of polio virus. Two types of vaccine are available: inactivated polio virus (IPV) contains dead virus and is administered by injections; oral polio vaccine (OPV) contains live, harmless strains. The latter is used in the United Kingdom.

Symptoms The incubation period is around 7–14 days, the onset being marked by a mild fever and headache which improves after a few days. In around 85 per cent of infected children there is no further progression, but in some – after approximately one week – the symptoms recur, together with neck stiffness and signs of meningeal irritation (see MENINGES). Weakness of individual muscle groups is common, and may progress – to a variable extent, depending on the distribution of the virus – to widespread PARALYSIS. Involvement of the diaphragm and intercostal muscles may lead to respiratory failure and rapid death unless artificial respiration is provided. Involvement of the cranial nerves and brain may lead to nystagmus (see under EYE, DISORDERS OF), hoarseness and difficulty in swallowing, and CONVULSIONS may occur in young children. The CEREBROSPINAL FLUID shows an early increase in lymphocytes, followed by a rise in protein concentration.

Treatment There is no effective drug treatment for the infection. Treatment involves early bed rest, followed by PHYSIOTHERAPY and orthopaedic measures as required. At the onset of respiratory difficulties a TRACHEOSTOMY and artificial ventilation should be started. (In the 1950s, when polio epidemics were occurring, respiratory difficulties were treated by placing patients in an 'iron lung' – a large, airtight, cylindrical container in which the air pressure was raised and lowered to simulate normal breathing.) In cases of severe paralysis with persistent wasting of the limbs, surgery may be necessary to minimise the resulting disability.

Pollex

A Latin term for thumb.

Polyarteritis Nodosa

Also known as periarteritis nodosa. A rare but potentially serious disease, probably caused by a disturbance of the immune system (see IMMUNITY). Prolonged fever and obscure symptoms referable to any system of the body are associated with local areas of inflammation along the arteries, giving rise to nodules in their walls. Large doses of CORTICOSTEROIDS, coupled with IMMUNOSUPPRESSANT treatment, usually curtail the disorder. Recovery occurs in about 50 per cent of cases.

Polyarthritis

A rheumatic disorder – usually caused by RHEUMATOID ARTHRITIS – that affects several joints in the body. The joints are stiff, painful and swollen. Different joints may be affected at the same time or in various sequences.

Polychromasia

Also polychromatophilia; terms applied to an abnormal reaction of the red blood cells in severe ANAEMIA. They have a bluish tinge instead of the normal red colour in a blood film stained by the usual method. It is a sign that the cell is not fully developed.

Polychromatophilia

See POLYCHROMASIA.

Polycystic Disease of the Kidney

An inherited disease in which the KIDNEYS contain many cysts. These grow in size until normal kidney tissue is largely destroyed. Cysts may also occur in other organs such as the liver. In adults, the disease will cause HYPERTENSION and kidney failure. There is also a juvenile form. There is no effective treatment, although symptoms can be alleviated by DIALYSIS and sometimes kidney transplant (see TRANSPLANTATION).

Polycystic Ovary Syndrome

Characterised by scanty (or absent) MENSTRUATION, INFERTILITY, hirsutism (excessive hairiness) and OBESITY and the sufferers often have multiple cysts in their OVARIES.

The condition is caused by an imbalance between LUTEINISING HORMONE (LH) and FOLLICLE-STIMULATING HORMONE (FSH); this imbalance stops OVULATION and varies the TESTOSTERONE output of the ovaries. The treatment may be with CLOMIPHENE; with a PROGESTOGEN drug; with LUTEINISING HORMONE-RELEASING HORMONE (LHRH); or with oral contraceptives (see under CONTRACEPTION – Non-barrier methods). The treatment chosen depends on the severity of the disease and whether the woman wants to conceive. Rarely a section of ovarian tissue is surgically removed.

Polycythaemia

A rise in the amount of HAEMOGLOBIN in the blood. This may be caused by an excess in the number of ERYTHROCYTES produced in the BONE MARROW or to a fall in the total volume of PLASMA in the circulatory system. It may also be a response to reduced oxygen levels – for example, among people living at high altitudes – or to liver or kidney disease: this type is called secondary polycythaemia.

The disorder may, however, occur for no obvious reason and is then called polycythaemia vera. This type develops mainly in people over 40 and about 400 people develop the disorder every year in the United Kingdom. The blood thickens, the sufferer may develop high blood pressure, flushing, headaches, itching and an enlarged spleen. A stroke may occur later in the disease process. Treatment of polycythaemia vera is by regular removal of blood by VENESECTION, sometimes in combination with an anticancer drug. Secondary polycythaemia is treated by remedying the underlying cause.

Polycythaemia rubra vera A disorder in which the red blood cells increase in number along with an increase in the number of white blood cells and platelets. The cause is unknown. Severe cases may require treatment with CYTOTOXIC drugs or RADIOTHERAPY.

Polydactyly

The presence of extra, or supernumerary, fingers or toes.

Polydipsia

Excessive thirst, which is a symptom of DIABETES MELLITUS and some other diseases.

Polyenes

Antifungal agents that include AMPHOTERICIN (given by intravenous injection in the treatment of systemic ASPERGILLOSIS) and NYSTATIN, applied topically for fungus infection of the skin, mouth and other mucous membranes.

Polygene

One of several GENES that between them control a single characteristic in an individual. With each polygene exerting a slight effect, the genetic outcome is the consequence of 'group action'. The hereditary characteristics produced in this way are usually those of a quantitative type – for instance, an individual's height.

Polymorph

(Diminutive of polymorphonuclear leucocyte.) A name applied to certain white corpuscles of the blood which have a nucleus of irregular and varied shape. These form between 70 and 75 per cent of all the white corpuscles. (See BLOOD.)

Polymyalgia Rheumatica

A form of rheumatism characterised by gross early-morning stiffness, which tends to ease off during the day, and pain in the shoulders and sometimes around the hips. It affects women more than men, and is rare under the age of 60. The cause is still obscure. It responds well to PREDNISOLONE, but treatment may need to be long continued. On the other hand the condition is not progressive and does not lead to disability.

Polymyositis

A connective-tissue disease affecting the muscles throughout the body. This rare disorder, which is associated with DERMATOMYOSITIS, may be acute or chronic but it usually affects the muscles of the shoulders or hip areas. The muscles weaken and are tender to the touch. Diffuse inflammatory changes occur and symptomatic relief may be obtained with CORTICOSTEROIDS.

Polymyxin

A group of antibiotics derived from various species of *Bacillus polymyxa*. One variety, colistin, is used to sterilise the bowels before surgery as it is not absorbed when given by mouth. The drugs are sometimes used in topical applications for infections of the skin, eye and ear.

Polyneuritis

An inflammatory condition of nerves in various parts of the body. (See NEURITIS.)

Polyp

See POLYPUS.

Polypeptide

A molecule in which several AMINO ACIDS are joined together by peptide bonds. PROTEIN molecules are polypeptides.

Polypharmacy

A term applied to the administration of too many drugs to one person. Sometimes combinations of drugs are an effective means of treatment, reducing the risk of drug resistance. Polypharmacy, however, worsens the risk of drug interactions and of adverse effects, especially in the elderly.

Polypill

A suggestion by two epidemiologists, made in the *British Medical Journal* in 2003, that many lives could be saved if all persons aged over 55 took a daily combination pill they termed the polypill. Its components would be ASPIRIN, a CHOLESTEROL-lowering agent, FOLIC ACID and two blood-pressure-lowering agents. The suggestion caused a massive correspondence as it implied treating a whole population rather than individuals considered to be at special risk.

Polyposis

The presence of a crop, or large number, of polypi (see POLYPUS). The most important form of polyposis is that known as familial polyposis coli. This is a hereditary disease characterised by the presence of large numbers of polypoid tumours in the large bowel. Every child born to an affected parent stands a fifty-fifty chance of developing the disease. Its importance is that sooner or later one or more of these tumours undergoes cancerous change. If the affected gut is removed surgically before this occurs, and preferably before the age of 20, the results are excellent.

Polypus

or polyp (plural: polypi). A general name applied to tumours which are attached by a stalk to the surface from which they spring. The term refers only to the shape of the growth and has nothing to do with its structure or nature. Most polypi are of a simple nature, although malignant polypi are also found. The usual structure of a polypus is that of a fine fibrous core covered with epithelium resembling that of the surrounding surface. The sites in which polypi are most usually found are the interior of the nose, the outer meatus of the ear, and the interior of the womb, bladder, or bowels (see POLYPOSIS).

Their removal is generally easy, as they are simply twisted off, or cut off, by some form of snare or ligature. (The tissue removed should be checked for malignant cells.) Those which are situated in the interior of the bladder or bowels, and whose presence is usually recognised because blood appears in the urine or stools, require a more serious operation – usually an endoscopic examination (see ENDOSCOPE).

Polysaccharide

A CARBOHYDRATE comprising several monosaccharides linked in long chains. Polysaccharides store energy – as starch in plants and glycogen in animals – and they also for structural parts of plants (as cellulose) and animals (as mucopolysaccharides).

Polyuria

The production of excessive amounts of URINE (1,500 ml or thereabout is the usual daily quantity). It is a symptom of DIABETES MELLITUS, DIABETES INSIPIDUS and chronic renal failure.

Pompholyx

See DERMATITIS.

Popliteal Space

The name given to the region behind the knee. The muscles attached to the bones immediately above and below the knee bound a diamond-shaped space through which pass the main artery and vein of the limb (known in this part of their course as the popliteal artery and vein); the tibial and common peroneal nerves (which continue the sciatic nerve from the thigh down to the leg); the external saphenous vein; and several small nerves and lymphatic vessels. The muscles – which bound the upper angle of the space and which are attached to the leg bones by strong prominent tendons – are known as the hamstrings. The lower angle of the space lies between the two heads of the gastrocnemius muscle, which makes up the main bulk of the calf of the leg.

Poppy

Two species are used in medicine: *Papaver somniferum*, the white opium-poppy (see OPIUM), and *Papaver rhoeas*, the red corn-poppy. The corn-poppy is chiefly used as a colouring agent, its syrup being a brilliant crimson colour.

Pore

A small opening. The word is usually used to describe an opening in the skin that releases sweat or sebum, a waxy material secreted by the sebaceous glands in the SKIN.

Porphyrias

A group of rare inherited ENZYME diseases in which disorders of the metabolic pathways leading to the synthesis of HAEM cause excessive production of haem precursors called PORPHYRINS by the bone marrow or liver. The excess porphyrins in the blood mainly affect the skin, causing PHOTOSENSITIVITY, or the central nervous system, causing various neuro-psychiatric disorders. Excess porphyrins can be detected in blood, urine and faeces. Usually porphyrias are genetically determined, but one form is due to alcoholic liver disease. The commonest form, porphyria cutanea tarda, affects up to 1 in

5,000 people in some countries. The British king, George III, suffered from porphyria, a disorder unrecognised in the 18th century.

Porphyrins

Complex organic compounds which are sensitive to light and form the basis of respiratory pigments – for example, haemoglobin and myoglobin. Porphyrins are crucial to many metabolic oxidation/reduction reactions in animals, plants, and micro-organisms.

Portal Hypertension

Raised blood pressure in the PORTAL VEIN entering the LIVER. This results in increased pressure in the veins of the oesophagus and upper stomach and these grow in size to form varices – dilated tortuous veins. Sometimes these varices rupture, causing bleeding into the oesophagus. The raised pressure also causes fluid to collect in the abdomen and form ASCITES. The commonest reason for portal hypertension is cirrhosis (fibrosis) of the liver (see LIVER, DISEASES OF). THROMBOSIS in the portal vein may also be a cause. Treatment requires the cause to be tackled, but bleeding from ruptured vessels may be stopped by injecting a sclerosant or hardening solution into and around the veins. Sometimes a surgical shunt may be done to divert blood from the portal vein to another blood vessel.

Portal System

A vein or collection of veins which finish at both ends in a bed of capillary blood vessels. An important example is the hepatic portal system, comprising the portal vein and its tributaries. Blood from the stomach, pancreas, spleen and intestines drains into the veins that join up to comprise the portal vein into the liver, where it branches into sinusoids.

Portal Vein

The vein which carries to the LIVER, blood that has been circulating in many of the abdominal organs. It is peculiar among the veins of the body in that it ends by breaking up into a capillary network instead of carrying the blood directly to the heart – a peculiarity which it shares only with certain small vessels in the kidneys. The PORTAL SYSTEM begins below in the haemorrhoidal plexus of veins around the lower end of the rectum; from this point, along the whole length of the intestines, the blood is collected into an inferior mesenteric vein upon the left, and a superior mesenteric vein upon the right side. The inferior mesenteric vein empties into the splenic vein, and the latter, uniting with the superior mesenteric vein immediately above the pancreas, forms the portal vein. The portal vein is joined by veins from the stomach and gall-bladder, and finally divides into two branches which sink into the right and left lobes of the liver. (For their further course, see LIVER).

The organs from which the portal vein collects the blood are the large and small intestines, the stomach, spleen, pancreas, and gall-bladder.

Port Wine Stain

See NAEVUS.

Positron-Emission Tomography (PET)

See PET SCANNING.

Possetting

The technical term used to describe the quite common habit of healthy babies to regurgitate, or bring up, small amounts of the meal they have just taken. Its name derives from possett, an 18th century drink made from porridge and sherry.

Post-

A prefix signifying after or behind.

Post-Coital Contraception

Action taken to prevent CONCEPTION after sexual intercourse. The type of contraception may be hormonal, or it may be an intrauterine device (see below, and under CONTRACEPTION). Pregnancy after intercourse without contraception – or where contraception has failed as a result, for example, of a leaking condom – may be avoided with a course of 'morning-after' contraceptive pills. Such preparations usually contain an oestrogen (see OESTROGENS) and a PROGESTOGEN. Two doses should be taken within 72 hours of 'unprotected' intercourse. An alternative for the woman is to take a high dose of oestrogen on its own. The aim is to postpone OVULATION and to affect the lining of the UTERUS so that the egg is unable to implant itself.

Intrauterine contraceptive device (IUCD)

This, in effect, is a form of post-coital contraception. The IUCD is a plastic shape up to 3 cm long around which copper wire is wound, carrying plastic thread from its tail. Colloquially known as a coil, it acts by inhibiting implantation and may also impair migration of sperm. Devices need changing every 3–5 years. Coils have generally replaced the larger, non-copper-bearing 'inert' types of IUCD, which caused more complications but did not

need changing (so are sometimes still found *in situ*). They tend to be chosen as a method of contraception (6 per cent) by older, parous women in stable relationships, with a generally low problem rate.

Nevertheless, certain problems do occur with IUCDs, the following being the most common:

- They tend to be expelled by the uterus in women who have never conceived, or by a uterus distorted by, say, fibroids.
- ECTOPIC PREGNANCY is more likely.
- They are associated with pelvic infection and INFERTILITY, following SEXUALLY TRANSMITTED DISEASES (STDS) – or possibly introduced during insertion.
- They often produce heavy, painful periods (see MENSTRUATION), and women at high risk of these problems (e.g. women who are HIV positive [see AIDS/HIV], or with WILSON'S DISEASE or cardiac lesions) should generally be excluded – unless the IUCD is inserted under antibiotic cover.

Post-Coital Test

A test for INFERTILITY. A specimen of cervical mucus, taken up to 24 hours after coitus (during the post-ovulatory phase of the menstrual cycle), is examined microscopically to assess the motility of the sperms. If motility is above a certain level, then sperms and mucus are not interacting abnormally – thus eliminating one cause of sterility.

Post-Mortem Examination

Also called an autopsy (and less commonly, necropsy), this is an examination of a body to discover the causes of death. Such an examination is sometimes required by law. An unnatural death; a death occurring in suspicious circumstances; or a death when a doctor feels unable to complete a certificate about the cause – all must be reported to the CORONER (in Scotland, to the procurator fiscal). He or she may order an autopsy to be carried out as part of the inquiry into cause of death. Sometimes doctors may request the permission of relatives to perform a post-mortem so that they may discover something of value for the improvement of medical care. Relatives may refuse consent. (See also DEATH, CAUSES OF.)

Post-Operative

The period after an operation, the patient's condition after operation, or any investigations or treatment during this time.

Post-Partum

The term applied to anything happening

immediately after childbirth: for example, post-partum haemorrhage. (See also PREGNANCY AND LABOUR.)

Post-Traumatic Stress Disorder (PTSD)

A term introduced to PSYCHIATRY in 1980 after the Vietnam War. It is one of several psychiatric disorders that can develop in people exposed to severe trauma, such as a major physical injury, participation in warfare, assault or rape, or any event in which there is major loss of life or a threat of loss of life. Most people exposed to trauma do not develop psychiatric disorder; however, some develop immediate distress and, occasionally, the reaction can be delayed for many months. Someone with PTSD has regular recurrences of memories or images of the stressful event ('flashbacks'), especially when reminded of it. Insomnia, feelings of guilt and isolation, an inability to concentrate and irritability may result. DEPRESSION is very common. Support from friends and family is probably the best management, but those who do not recover quickly can be helped by antidepressants and psychological treatments such as COGNITIVE BEHAVIOUR THERAPY. Over the past few years, PTSD has featured increasingly in compensation litigation.

Postural Drainage

Facilitation of the drainage of secretions from dilated bronchi of the LUNGS. The patient lies on an inclined plane, head downwards, and is encouraged to cough up as much secretion from the lungs as possible. The precise position depends on which part of the lungs is affected. It may need to be carried out for up to three hours daily in divided periods. It is of particular value in BRONCHIECTASIS and lung abscess (see LUNGS, DISEASES OF).

Post-Viral Fatigue Syndrome

See MYALGIC ENCEPHALOMYELITIS (ME).

Potassium

A metal which, on account of its great affinity for other substances, is not found in a pure state in nature. Its salts are widely used in medicine but, as their action depends in general not on their metallic radical but upon the acid with which it is combined, their uses vary greatly and are described elsewhere. All salts of potassium depress the heart's action as a result of action by the potassium ion.

Potassium-Channel Activators

Drugs that have the ability to dilate ARTERIES and VEINS and are used to relieve pain in ANGINA of the HEART. Nicorandil is the main example.

Potassium Permanganate

A salt of the metallic element POTASSIUM. It is used as a skin antiseptic (see ANTISEPTICS) and for cleaning wounds; its astringent effect is useful in the treatment of DERMATITIS. It should not be taken internally because the compound is poisonous.

Pott's Disease

A traditional name often applied to the angular curvature of the spine which results from tuberculous disease. (See SPINE AND SPINAL CORD, DISEASES AND INJURIES OF.) The disease is named after Percivall Pott, an English surgeon (1714–88), who first described the condition.

Pott's Fracture

A variety of fractures around the ankle, accompanied by a varying degree of dislocation of the ankle. In all cases the fibula is fractured. Named after Percivall Pott, who suffered from this fracture and was the first to describe it (see BONE, DISORDERS OF), it is often mistaken for a simple sprain of the ankle.

Pouchitis

A rare chronic inflammatory disease in the ileal pouch, which remains after a patient has had intestinal resection because of INFLAMMATORY BOWEL DISEASE (IBD). Metronidazole and oral PROBIOTICS are effective treatments.

Poultices

(See also FOMENTATION.) Soft, moist applications to the surface of the body, generally used hot to soothe pain due to inflammation and to promote resolution.

Poupart's Ligament

Also known as the inguinal ligament, it is the strong ligament lying in the boundary between the anterior abdominal wall and the front of the thigh.

Praziquantel

An effective drug against all human schistosomes which has a broad spectrum of activity and low toxicity (see SCHISTOSOMIASIS).

Pre-

A prefix meaning before.

Precipitin

An antibody (see ANTIBODIES) that combines

with an ANTIGEN and forms the immune complex as a precipitate. The reaction is used in some diagnostic serological tests to identify antigens in the serum.

Precordial Region
The area on the centre and towards the left side of the chest, lying in front of the heart.

Prednisolone
A derivative of CORTISONE, which is five or six times as active as cortisone and has less of the salt- and water-retaining properties of cortisone. It is given by mouth.

Prednisone
This corticosteroid drug has a similar level of glucocorticoid activity as PREDNISOLONE and is converted to prednisolone in the liver. Though prednisone is still in use, prednisolone is the most commonly used oral corticosteroid for long-term anti-inflammatory treatment. (See CORTICOSTEROIDS; GLUCOCORTICOIDS.)

Pre-Eclampsia
A complication of pregnancy (see PREGNANCY AND LABOUR), of unknown cause, which in severe cases may proceed to ECLAMPSIA. It is characterised by HYPERTENSION, renal impairment, OEDEMA, often with PROTEINURIA and disseminated intravascular coagulation. It usually occurs in the second half of pregnancy – mild cases (without proteinuria) occurring in about 10 per cent of pregnancies, severe cases in about 2 per cent. Predisposing factors include a first pregnancy, or pregnancy by a new partner; a family history of pre-eclampsia, hypertension, or other cardiovascular disorders; and pre-existing hypertension or DIABETES MELLITUS. Increased incidence with lower socio-economic class may be linked to diet or to failure to attend for antenatal care. Although less common in smokers, fetal outlook is worse. Multiple pregnancy and HYDATIDIFORM MOLE, together with hydrops fetalis (see HAEMOLYTIC DISEASE OF THE NEWBORN), predispose to early and severe pre-eclampsia.

Treatment Severe pre-eclampsia is an emergency, and urgent admission to hospital should be arranged. Treatment should be given to control the hypertension; the fetal heart rate carefully monitored; and in very severe cases urgent CAESAREAN SECTION may be necessary.

Pregnancy and Labour

Pregnancy The time when a woman carries a developing baby in her UTERUS. For the first 12 weeks (the first trimester) the baby is known as an EMBRYO, after which it is referred to as the FETUS.

Pregnancy lasts about 280 days and is calculated from the first day of the last menstrual period – see MENSTRUATION. Pregnancy-testing kits rely on the presence of the hormone beta HUMAN CHORIONIC GONADOTROPHIN (b HCG) which is excreted in the woman's urine as early as 30 days from the last menstrual period. The estimated date of delivery can be accurately estimated from the size of the developing fetus measured by ULTRASOUND (see also below) between seven and 24 weeks. 'Term' refers to the time that the baby is due; this can range from 38 weeks to 41 completed weeks.

Physical changes occur in early pregnancy – periods stop and the abdomen enlarges. The breasts swell, with the veins becoming prominent and the nipples darkening. About two in three women will have nausea with a few experiencing such severe vomiting as to require hospital admission for rehydration.

Antenatal care The aim of antenatal care is to ensure a safe outcome for both mother and child; it is provided by midwives (see MIDWIFE) and doctors. Formal antenatal care began in Edinburgh in the 1930s with the recognition that all aspects of pregnancy – normal and abnormal – warranted surveillance. Cooperation between general practitioners, midwives and obstetricians is now established, with pregnancies that are likely to progress normally being cared for in the community and only those needing special intervention being cared for in a hospital setting.

The initial visit (or booking) in the first half of pregnancy will record the history of past events and the results of tests, with the aim of categorising the patients into normal or not. Screening tests including blood checks and ultrasound scans are a routine part of antenatal care. The first ultrasound scan is done at about 11 weeks to date the pregnancy, with a further one done at 20 weeks – the anomaly scan – to assess the baby's structure. Some obstetric units will check the growth of the baby with one further scan later in the pregnancy or, in the case of twin pregnancies (see below), many scans throughout. The routine blood tests include checks for ANAEMIA, DIABETES MELLITUS, sickle-cell disease and THALASSAEMIA, as well as for the blood group. Evidence of past infections is also looked for; tests for RUBELLA (German measles) and SYPHILIS are routine, whereas tests for human immunodeficiency virus (see AIDS/

P

HIV below) and HEPATITIS are being offered as optional, although there is compelling evidence that knowledge of the mother's infection status is beneficial to the baby.

Traditional antenatal care consists of regular appointments, initially every four weeks until 34 weeks, then fortnightly or weekly. At each visit the mother's weight, urine and blood pressure are checked, and assessment of fetal growth and position is done by palpating the uterus. Around two-thirds of pregnancies and labours are normal: in the remainder, doctors and midwives need to increase the frequency of surveillance so as to prevent or deal with maternal and fetal problems.

Common complications of pregnancy

Some of the more common complications of pregnancy are listed below.

As well as early detection of medical complications, antenatal visits aim to be supportive and include emotional and educational care. Women with uncomplicated pregnancies are increasingly being managed by midwives and general practitioners in the community and only coming to the hospital doctors should they develop a problem. A small number will opt for a home delivery, but facilities for providing such a service are not always available in the UK.

Women requiring more intensive surveillance have their management targeted to the specific problems encountered. Cardiologists will see mothers-to-be with heart conditions, and those at risk of diabetes are cared for in designated clinics with specialist staff. Those women needing more frequent surveillance than standard antenatal care can be looked after in maternity day centres. These typically include women with mildly raised blood pressure or those with small babies. Fetal medicine units have specialists who are highly skilled in ultrasound scanning and specialise in the diagnosis and management of abnormal babies still in the uterus.

ECTOPIC PREGNANCY Chronic abdominal discomfort early in pregnancy may be caused by unruptured ectopic pregnancy, when, rarely, the fertilised OVUM starts developing in the Fallopian tube (see FALLOPIAN TUBES) instead of the uterus. The patient needs hospital treatment and LAPAROSCOPY. A ruptured ectopic pregnancy causes acute abdominal symptoms and collapse, and the woman will require urgent abdominal surgery.

URINARY TRACT INFECTIONS These affect around 2 per cent of pregnant women and are detected by a laboratory test of a mid-stream specimen of urine. In pregnancy, symptoms of these infections do not necessarily resemble those experienced by non-pregnant women. As they can cause uterine irritability and possible premature labour (see below), it is important to find and treat them appropriately.

ANAEMIA is more prevalent in patients who are vegetarian or on a poor diet. Iron supplements are usually given to women who have low concentrations of HAEMOGLOBIN in their blood (less than 10.5 g/dl) or who are at risk of becoming low in iron, from bleeding, twin pregnancies and those with placenta previa (see below).

ANTEPARTUM HAEMORRHAGE Early in pregnancy, vaginal bleedings may be due to a spontaneous or an incomplete therapeutic ABORTION. Bleeding from the genital tract between 24 completed weeks of pregnancy and the start of labour is called antepartum haemorrhage. The most common site is where the PLACENTA is attached to the wall of the uterus. If the placenta separates before delivery, bleeding occurs in the exposed 'bed'. When the placenta is positioned in the upper part of the uterus it is called an abruption.

PLACENTA PRAEVIA is sited in the lower part and blocks or partly blocks the cervix (neck of the womb); it can be identified at about the 34th week. Ten per cent of episodes of antepartum bleeding are caused by placenta previa, and it may be associated with bleeding at delivery. This potentially serious complication is diagnosed by ultrasound scanning and may require a caesarean section (see below) at delivery.

INCREASED BLOOD PRESSURE, associated with protein in the urine and swelling of the limbs, is part of a condition known as PRE-ECLAMPSIA. This occurs in the second half of pregnancy in about 1 in 10 women expecting their first baby, and is mostly very mild and of no consequence to the pregnancy. However, some women can develop extremely high blood pressures which can adversely affect the fetus and cause epileptic-type seizures and bleeding disorders in the mother. This serious condition is called ECLAMPSIA. For this reason a pregnant woman with raised blood pressure or PROTEIN in her urine is carefully evaluated with blood tests, often in the maternity day assessment unit. The condition can be stopped by delivery of the baby, and this will be done if the mother's or the fetus's life is in danger. If the condition is milder, and the baby not mature enough for a safe delivery, then drugs can be used to control the blood pressure.

MISCARRIAGE Also called spontaneous abortion, miscarriage is the loss of the fetus. There are several types:

- threatened miscarriage is one in which some vaginal bleeding occurs, the uterus is enlarged, but the cervix remains closed and pregnancy usually proceeds.
- inevitable miscarriage usually occurs before the 16th week and is typified by extensive blood loss through an opened cervix and cramp-like abdominal pain; some products of conception are lost but the developing placental area (decidua) is retained and an operation may be necessary to clear the womb.
- missed miscarriages, in which the embryo dies and is absorbed, but the decidua (placental area of uterine wall) remains and may cause abdominal discomfort and discharge of old blood.

THERAPEUTIC ABORTION is performed on more than 170,000 women annually in England and Wales. Sometimes the woman may not have arranged the procedure through the usual health-care channels, so that a doctor may see a patient with vaginal bleeding, abdominal discomfort or pain, and open cervix – symptoms which suggest that the decidua and a blood clot have been retained; these retained products will need to be removed by curettage.

Septic abortions are now much less common in Britain than before the Abortion Act (1967) permitted abortion in specified circumstances. The cause is the passage of infective organisms from the vagina into the uterus, with *Escherichia coli* and *Streptococcus faecalis* the most common pathogenic agents. The woman has abdominal pain, heavy bleeding, usually fever and sometimes she is in shock. The cause is usually an incomplete abortion or one induced in unsterile circumstances. Antibiotics and curettage are the treatment.

INTRAUTERINE GROWTH RETARDATION describes a slowing of the baby's growth. This can be diagnosed by ultrasound scanning, although there is a considerable margin of error in estimates of fetal weight. Trends in growth are favoured over one-off scan results alone.

GESTATIONAL DIABETES is a condition that is more common in women who are overweight or have a family member with diabetes. If high concentrations of blood sugar are found, efforts are made to correct it as the babies can become very fat (macrosomia), making delivery more difficult. A low-sugar diet is usually enough to control the blood concentration of sugars; however some women need small doses of INSULIN to achieve control.

FETAL ABNORMALITIES can be detected before birth using ultrasound. Some of these defects are obvious, such as the absence of kidneys, a condition incompatible with life outside the womb. These women can be offered a termination of their pregnancy. However, more commonly, the pattern of problems can only hint at an abnormality and closer examination is needed, particularly in the diagnosis of chromosomal deformities such as DOWN'S (DOWN) SYNDROME (trisomy 21 or presence of three 21 chromosomes instead of two).

Chromosomal abnormalities can be definitively diagnosed only by cell sampling such as amniocentesis (obtaining amniotic fluid – see AMNION – from around the baby) done at 15 weeks onwards, and chorionic villus sampling (sampling a small part of the placenta) – another technique which can be done from 12 weeks onwards. Both have a small risk of miscarriage associated with them; consequently, they are confined to women at higher risk of having an abnormal fetus.

Biochemical markers present in the pregnant woman's blood at different stages of pregnancy may have undergone changes in those carrying an abnormal fetus. The first such marker to be routinely used was a high concentration of alpha-fetol protein in babies with SPINA BIFIDA (defects in the covering of the spinal cord). Fuller research has identified a range of diagnostic markers which are useful, and, in conjunction with other factors such as age, ethnic group and ultrasound findings, can provide a predictive guide to the obstetrician – in consultation with the woman – as to whether or not to proceed to an invasive test. These tests include pregnancy-associated plasma protein assessed from a blood sample taken at 12 weeks and four blood tests at 15–22 weeks – alpha-fetol protein, beta human chorionic gonadotrophin, unconjugated oestriol and inhibin A. Ultrasound itself can reveal physical findings in the fetus, which can be more common in certain abnormalities. Swelling in the neck region of an embryo in early pregnancy (increased nuchal thickness) has good predictive value on its own, although its accuracy is improved in combination with the biochemical markers. The effectiveness of prenatal diagnosis is rapidly evolving, the aim being to make the diagnosis as early in the pregnancy as possible to help the parents make more informed choices.

MULTIPLE PREGNANCIES In the UK, one in 95 deliveries is of twins, while the prevalence of triplets is one in 10,000 and quadruplets around one in 500,000. Racial variations occur, with African women having a prevalence rate of one in 30 deliveries for twins and Japanese women a much lower rate than the UK figure. Multiple pregnancies occur more often in older women, and in the UK the prevalence of fertility treatments, many of these being given to older women, has raised the incidence. There is now an official limit of three eggs being transferred to a woman undergoing ASSISTED CONCEPTION (gamete intrafallopian transfer, or GIFT).

Multiple pregnancies are now usually diagnosed as a result of routine ultrasound scans between 16 and 20 weeks of pregnancy. The increased size of the uterus results in the mother having more or worse pregnancy-related conditions such as nausea, abdominal discomfort, backache and varicose veins. Some congenital abnormalities in the fetus occur more frequently in twins: NEURAL TUBE defects, abnormalities of the heart and the incidence of TURNER'S SYNDROME and KLINEFELTER'S SYNDROME are examples. Such abnormalities may be detected by ultrasound scans or amniocentesis. High maternal blood pressure and anaemia are commoner in women with multiple pregnancies (see above).

The growth rates of multiple fetuses vary, but the difference between them and single fetuses are not that great until the later stages of pregnancy. Preterm labour is commoner in multiple pregnancies: the median length of pregnancy is 40 weeks for singletons, 37 for twins and 33 for triplets. Low birth-weights are usually the result of early delivery rather than abnormalities in growth rates. Women with multiple pregnancies require more frequent and vigilant antenatal assessments, with their carers being alert to the signs of preterm labour occurring.

CEPHALOPELVIC DISPROPORTION Disparity between the size of the fetus and the mother's pelvis is not common in the UK but is a significant problem in the developing world. Disparity is classified as absolute, when there is no possibility of delivery, and relative, when the baby is large but delivery (usually after a difficult labour) is possible. Causes of absolute disparity include: a large baby – heavier than 5 kg at birth; fetal HYDROCEPHALUS; and an abnormal maternal pelvis. The latter may be congenital, the result of trauma or a contraction in pelvic size because of OSTEOMALACIA early in life. Disproportion should be suspected if in late pregnancy the fetal head has not 'engaged' in the pelvis. Sometimes a closely supervised 'trial of labour' may result in a successful, if prolonged, delivery. Otherwise a caesarean section (see below) is necessary.

UNUSUAL POSITIONS AND PRESENTATIONS OF THE BABY In most pregnant women the baby fits into the maternal pelvis head-first in what is called the occipito-anterior position, with the baby's face pointing towards the back of the pelvis. Sometimes, however, the head may face the other way, or enter the pelvis transversely – or, rarely, the baby's neck is flexed backwards with the brow or face presenting to the neck of the womb. Some malpositions will correct naturally; others can be manipulated abdominally during pregnancy to a better position. If, however, the mother starts labour with the baby's head badly positioned or with the buttocks instead of the head presenting (breech position), the labour will usually be longer and more difficult and may require intervention using special obstetric forceps to assist in extracting the baby. If progress is poor and the fetus distressed, caesarean section may be necessary.

HIV INFECTION Pregnant women who are HIV positive (see HIV; AIDS/HIV) should be taking antiviral drugs in the final four to five months of pregnancy, so as to reduce the risk of infecting the baby *in utero* and during birth by around 50 per cent. Additional antiviral treatment is given before delivery; the infection risk to the baby can be further reduced – by about 40 per cent – if delivery is by caesarean section. The mother may prefer to have the baby normally, in which case great care should be taken not to damage the baby's skin during delivery. The infection risk to the baby is even further reduced if it is not breast fed. If all preventive precautions are taken, the overall risk of the infant becoming infected is cut to under 5 per cent.

Premature birth This is a birth that takes place before the end of the normal period of gestation, usually before 37 weeks. In practice, however, it is defined as a birth that takes place when the baby weighs less than 2·5 kilograms (5½ pounds). Between 5 and 10 per cent of babies are born prematurely, and in around 40 per cent of premature births the cause is unknown. Pre-eclampsia is the most common known cause; others include hypertension, chronic kidney disease, heart disease and diabetes mellitus. Multiple pregnancy is another cause. In the vast majority of cases the aim of management is to prolong the pregnancy and so improve the outlook for the unborn child. This consists essentially of rest in bed and sedation, but there are now several drugs, such as RITODRINE, that may be used to suppress the activity of the uterus and so help to delay premature labour. Prematurity was once a prime cause of infant mortality but modern medical care has greatly improved survival rates in developing countries.

Labour Also known by the traditional terms parturition, childbirth or delivery, this is the process by which the baby and subsequently the placenta are expelled from the mother's body. The onset of labour is often preceded by a 'show' – the loss of the mucus and blood plug from the cervix, or neck of the womb; this passes down the vagina to the exterior. The time before the beginning of labour is called the 'latent phase' and characteristically lasts 24 hours or more in a first pregnancy. Labour itself is defined by regular, painful contractions which cause dilation of the neck of the womb and descent of the fetal head. 'Breaking of the waters' is the loss of amniotic fluid vaginally and can occur any time in the delivery process.

Labour itself is divided into three stages: the first is from the onset of labour to full (10 cm) dilation of the neck of the womb. This stage varies in length, ideally taking no more than one hour per centimetre of dilation. Progress is monitored by regular vaginal examinations, usually every four hours. Fetal well-being is observed by intermittent or continuous monitoring of the fetal heart rate in relation to the timing and frequency of the contractions. The print-out is called a cardiotocograph. Abnormalities of the fetal heart rate may suggest fetal distress and may warrant intervention. In women having their first baby (primigravidae), the common cause of a slow labour is uncoordinated contractions which can be overcome by giving either of the drugs PROSTAGLANDIN or OXYTOCIN, which provoke contractions of the uterine muscle, by an intravenous drip. Labours which progress slowly or not at all may be due to abnormal positioning of the fetus or too large a fetus, when prostaglandin or oxytocin is used much more cautiously.

The second stage of labour is from full cervical dilation to the delivery of the baby. At this stage the mother often experiences an irresistible urge to push the baby out, and a combination of strong coordinated uterine contractions and maternal effort gradually moves the baby down the birth canal. This stage usually lasts under an hour but can take longer. Delay, exhaustion of the mother or distress of the fetus may necessitate intervention by the midwife or doctor. This may mean enlarging the vaginal opening with an EPISIOTOMY (cutting of the perineal outlet – see below) or assisting the delivery with specially designed obstetric forceps or a vacuum extractor (ven-

touse). If the cervix is not completely dilated or open and the head not descended, then an emergency caesarean section may need to be done to deliver the baby. This procedure involves delivering the baby and placenta through an incision in the mother's abdomen. It is sometimes necessary to deliver by planned or elective caesarean section: for example, if the placenta is low in the uterus – called placenta praevia – making a vaginal delivery dangerous.

The third stage occurs when the placenta (or afterbirth) is delivered, which is usually about 10–20 minutes after the baby. An injection of ergometrine and oxytocin is often given to women to prevent bleeding.

Pain relief in labour varies according to the mother's needs. For uncomplicated labours, massage, reassurance by a birth attendant, and a warm bath and mobilisation may be enough for some women. However, some labours are painful, particularly if the woman is tired or anxious or is having her first baby. In these cases other forms of analgesia are available, ranging from inhalation of NITROUS OXIDE GAS, injection of PETHIDINE HYDROCHLORIDE or similar narcotic, and regional local anaesthetic (see ANAESTHESIA).

Once a woman has delivered, care continues to ensure her and the baby's safety. The midwives are involved in checking that the uterus returns to its normal size and that there is no infection or heavy bleeding, as well as caring for stitches if needed. The normal blood loss after birth is called lochia and generally is light, lasting up to six weeks. Midwives offer support with breast feeding and care of the infant and will visit the parents at home routinely for up to two weeks.

Some complications of labour

All operative deliveries in the UK are now done in hospitals, and are performed if a spontaneous birth is expected to pose a bigger risk to the mother or her child than a specialist-assisted one. Operative deliveries include caesarean section, forceps-assisted deliveries and those in which vacuum extraction (ventouse) is used. CAESAREAN SECTION Absolute indications for this procedure, which is used to deliver over 15 per cent of babies in Britain, are cephalopelvic disproportion and extensive placenta praevia, both discussed above. Otherwise the decision to undertake caesarean section depends on the clinical judgement of the specialist and the views of the mother. The rise in the proportion of this type of intervention (from 5 per cent in the 1930s to its present level of over 23 per cent

P

of the 600,000 or so annual deliveries in England) has been put down to defensive medicine – namely, the doctor's fear of litigation (initiated often because the parents believe that the baby's health has suffered because the mother had an avoidably difficult 'natural' labour). In Britain, over 60 per cent of women who have had a caesarean section try a vaginal delivery in a succeeding pregnancy, with about two-thirds of these being successful. Indications for the operation include:

- absolute and relative cephalopelvic disproportion.
- placenta previa.
- fetal distress.
- prolapsed umbilical cord – this endangers the viability of the fetus because the vital supply of oxygen and nutrients is interrupted.
- malpresentation of the fetus such as breech or transverse lie in the womb.
- unsatisfactory previous pregnancies or deliveries.
- a request from the mother.

Caesarean sections are usually performed using regional block anaesthesia induced by a spinal or epidural injection. This results in loss of feeling in the lower part of the body; the mother is conscious and the baby not exposed to potential risks from volatile anaesthetic gases inhaled by the mother during general anaesthesia. Post-operative complications are higher with general anaesthesia, but maternal anxiety and the likelihood that the operation might be complicated and difficult are indications for using it. A general anaesthetic may also be required for an acute obstetric emergency. At operation the mother's lower abdomen is opened and then her uterus opened slowly with a transverse incision and the baby carefully extracted. A transverse incision is used in preference to the traditional vertical one as it enables the woman to have a vaginal delivery in any future pregnancy with a much smaller risk of uterine rupture. Women are usually allowed to get up within 24 hours and are discharged after four or five days.

FORCEPS AND VENTOUSE DELIVERIES Obstetric forceps are made in several forms, but all are basically a pair of curved blades shaped so that they can obtain a purchase on the baby's head, thus enabling the operator to apply traction and (usually) speed up delivery. (Sometimes they are used to slow down progress of the head.) A ventouse or vacuum extractor comprises an egg-cup-shaped metal or plastic head, ranging from 40 to 60 mm in diameter with a hollow tube attached through which air is extracted by a foot-operated vacuum pump. The instrument is placed on the descending head, creating a negative pressure on the skin of the scalp and enabling the operator to pull the head down. In mainland Europe, vacuum extraction is generally preferred to forceps for assisting natural deliveries, being used in around 5 per cent of all deliveries. Forceps have a greater risk of causing damage to the baby's scalp and brain than vacuum extraction, although properly used, both types should not cause any serious damage to the baby.

Episiotomy Normal and assisted deliveries put the tissues of the genital tract under strain. The PERINEUM is less elastic than the vagina and, if it seems to be splitting as the baby's head

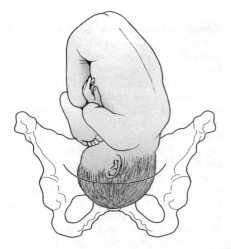 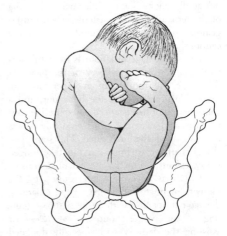

Cephalic (left) and breech (right) presentation of fetus in maternal pelvis at term.

moves down the birth canal, it may be necessary to cut the perineal tissue – a procedure called an episiotomy – to limit damage. This is a simple operation done under local anaesthetic. It should be done only if there is a specific indication; these include:

● to hasten the second stage of labour if the fetus is distressed.

● to facilitate the use of forceps or vacuum extractor.

● to enlarge a perineum that is restricted because of unyielding tissue, perhaps because of a scar from a previous labour.

Midwives as well as obstetricians are trained to undertake and repair (with sutures) episiotomies.

(For organisations which offer advice and information on various aspects of childbirth, including eclampsia, breast feeding and multiple births, see APPENDIX 2: ADDRESSES: SOURCES OF INFORMATION, ADVICE, SUPPORT AND SELF-HELP.)

Psychological and social problems

Any previously existing mental-health problems may worsen under the stress of pregnancy and childbirth, and a woman's socio-economic circumstances may be an influential factor. Mood swings are common in pregnant women and mothers of new babies; sympathetic support from staff and relations will usually remedy the situation. If postnatal depression lasts for more than a week or two the use of mild ANTI-DEPRESSANT DRUGS may be justified. If depression persists, referral to a psychiatrist may be advisable. Rarely, severe psychiatric problems – puerperal psychosis – may develop during or after pregnancy and referral to an appropriate psychiatric unit is then essential. If the mother's social circumstances are unsatisfactory, advice should be sought from social services departments. Mothers may also need advice on benefits to which they are entitled and how to claim them. Benefits Agency offices or Citizens' Advice Bureaux as well as antenatal clinics are useful sources of information.

Pregnancy Tests

There are several tests for pregnancy (see PREGNANCY AND LABOUR) in its early stages, and these can be done on blood or urine; some of the urine tests may be carried out at home. Most tests are based on the detection of HUMAN CHORIONIC GONADOTROPHIN (HCG) in the woman's urine. They are nearly 100 per cent accurate and may show positive as early as 30 days after the first day of the last normal period.

The haemagglutination inhibition test This, and the subsequent tests to be mentioned, are known as immunological tests. They are based upon the effect of the urine from a pregnant woman upon the interaction of red blood cells, which have been sensitised to human gonadotrophin, and anti-gonadotrophin serum. They have the great practical advantage of being performed in a test-tube or even on a slide. Because of their ease and speed of performance, a result can be obtained in two hours.

Enzyme-linked immunosorbent assay (ELISA) This is the basis of many of the pregnancy-testing kits obtainable from pharmacies. It is a highly sensitive antibody test and can detect very low concentrations of human chorionic gonadotrophin. Positive results show up as early as ten days after fertilisation – namely, four days before the first missed period.

Ultrasound The fetal sac can be detected by ULTRASOUND from five weeks, and a fetal echo at around six or seven weeks (see also PRENATAL SCREENING OR DIAGNOSIS).

Pregnandiol

The excretion product of the hormone, PROGESTERONE, manufactured by the corpus luteum of the ovary (see OVARIES). Pregnandiol is excreted in the urine during the second half of the menstrual period, and its excretion rises steadily throughout pregnancy.

Premature Beat

See ECTOPIC BEAT.

Premature Birth

See ABORTION; FETUS; PREGNANCY AND LABOUR.

Premature Ejaculation

A disorder in which EJACULATION of semen occurs before or immediately after the penis penetrates the vagina during sexual intercourse. The most common sexual problem in men, persistent premature ejaculation may have psychological causes, although many adolescents and some adults experience it occasionally. Sexual counselling may help to alleviate the condition.

Premedication

A drug or drugs given to a patient to produce sedation before an operation, whether this is done under a local or general anaesthetic. A narcotic analgesic drug (see NARCOTICS;

ANALGESICS) is usually used, as this relieves pain as well as anxiety. An antisecretory drug is often added to reduce the secretions in the airways and thus lessen the risk associated with general anaesthesia. Premedication reduces the amount of anaesthetic needed to make the patient unconscious.

Premenstrual Syndrome

This has been defined as 'any combination of emotional or physical features which occur cyclically in a woman before MENSTRUATION, and which regress or disappear during menstruation'. It is characterised by mood-changes, discomfort, swelling and tenderness in the breasts, swelling of the legs, a bloated feeling in the abdomen, headache, fatigue and constipation. The mood-changes range from irritability and mild depression to outbursts of violence. It may last for 3–14 days. How common it is is not known, as only the more severe cases are seen by doctors, but it has been estimated that one in ten of all menstruating women suffer from it severely enough to require treatment. The cause is not known, but it is probably due to some upset of the hormonal balance of the body. In view of the multiplicity of causes that have been put forward, it is not surprising that there is an equal multiplicity of treatments. Among these, one of the most widely used is PROGESTERONE. Others include pyridoxine, danazol, and gamma linolenic acid available in the form of oil of evening primrose. Whatever drug may be prescribed, counselling is equally essential and, in many cases, is all that is required.

Premolar

The two TEETH on each side of the jaw positioned between the canines and the molars in the adult. The teeth are used with the molars for holding and grinding food.

Prenatal Screening or Diagnosis

Prenatal screening of fetal abnormalities may be the result of screening tests carried out on most or all pregnant women, or as the result of specific diagnostic tests performed to detect specific conditions. Prenatal diagnosis is important as it will identify babies who might need medical or surgical treatment before or soon after birth. In addition, it may also detect severe abnormalities for which parents might decide to have a therapeutic ABORTION.

ULTRASOUND scanning is probably the most widely used diagnostic tool in obstetric practice. It can detect structural abnormalities such as SPINA BIFIDA and CLEFT PALATE and even cardiac and renal problems. A series of scans can assess whether the baby is growing at a normal rate; ultrasound may also be used to assist with other diagnostic tests (e.g. AMNIOCENTESIS – see below).

Tests on the mother's blood can also diagnose fetal abnormalities. Alphafetoprotein (AFP) is produced by babies and 'leaks' into the AMNIOTIC FLUID and is absorbed by the mother. In spina bifida and other neural-tube defects there is increased leakage of AFP, and a blood test at 16 weeks' gestation can detect a raised level which suggests the presence of these abnormalities.

The triple test, also performed at 16 weeks, measures AFP and two hormones – HUMAN CHORIONIC GONADOTROPHIN and unconjugated OESTRADIOL – and is used in diagnosing DOWN'S (DOWN) SYNDROME.

Amniocentesis involves inserting a needle through the mother's abdominal wall into the uterus to remove a sample of amniotic fluid at 16–18 weeks. Examination of the fluid and the cells it contains is used in the diagnosis of Down's syndrome and other inherited disorders. The test carries a small risk of miscarriage.

Chorionic villus sampling may be used to diagnose various inherited conditions. A small amount of tissue from the developing PLACENTA is removed for analysis: this test has the advantages of having a lower incidence of miscarriage than amniocentesis and is carried out at an earlier stage (9–13 weeks).

Analysis of a blood sample removed from the umbilical cord (cordocentesis) may diagnose infections in the uterus, blood disorders or inherited conditions.

Direct observation of the fetus via a viewing instrument called a fetoscope is also used diagnostically and will detect structural abnormalities.

Most tests have a recognised incidence of false positive and negative results and are therefore usually cross-checked with another test. Counselling of the parents about prenatal tests is important. This allows them to make an informed choice which may not necessarily involve terminating the pregnancy if an abnormality is found. (See PREGNANCY AND LABOUR.)

Prepuce

Also known as the foreskin, this is the free fold of skin that overlaps the glans PENIS and retracts when the penis becomes erect. It is the part that is removed at CIRCUMCISION.

Presbyacusis

DEAFNESS that comes on with increasing years. It is caused by increasing loss of elasticity in the hearing mechanism, combined with the slowing-down of the mental processes that accompanies old age. It is characterised by particular difficulty in hearing high notes such as the telephone and the voices of women and children. Hearing in a background of noise is also affected. Modern, miniaturised, transistor 'within-the-ear' hearing aids are now available that are proving helpful in making life more bearable for the elderly in this respect. (See also AGEING; HEARING AIDS.)

Presbyopia

See ACCOMMODATION; EYE, DISORDERS OF.

Prescribed Diseases

A collection of industrial diseases which provide those with a disease legal entitlement to welfare benefits. Examples are DEAFNESS from excessive noise in the workplace; ANTHRAX from farming; PNEUMOCONIOSIS from industrially generated dust (coal mining); and LEAD POISONING from the handling of chemicals. (See also OCCUPATIONAL HEALTH, MEDICINE AND DISEASES.)

Prescription

The written direction for drugs for medicinal use, given by the doctor, dentist and (for some drugs) nurse to the patient, for dispensation by the pharmacist. Drugs should only be prescribed when essential for treatment, and when any possible risks involved to the patient (and fetus in cases of pregnancy) are outweighed by the potential benefits of giving the drug. When possible, non-proprietary, or generic, titles should be prescribed; by allowing the pharmacist to dispense any equivalent drug this avoids delay for the patient, as well as reducing the cost to the Health Service. Dosage is generally stated in metric units, and both the amount and frequency should be carefully explained to the patient by the doctor, and clearly written when the drug is dispensed (see also DOSAGE; DRUGS). Strict adherence to the Misuse of Drugs Act 1973 is necessary to restrict the inappropriate prescription and abuse of drugs, particularly CONTROLLED DRUGS. Full details of drugs available on NHS prescription are given in the *British National Formulary*, which is published by the British Medical Association and the Royal Pharmaceutical Society of Great Britain twice a year and distributed to all NHS doctors by the government. Careful monitoring of prescribing in the UK is carried out by a government-appointed agency.

Computer-generated prescriptions

The Royal College of General Practitioners has issued guidelines on the use of computer-generated prescriptions for drugs other than controlled drugs. The guidelines include rules on giving the patient's name, address and date of birth with the responsible prescribing doctor's name at the bottom, along with his or her surgery address and telephone number. The prescription has to be signed by the doctor. Several other requirements are included to minimise the risk of prescription-tampering, fraud or the inclusion of identifiable confidential information. Full details of the guidelines appear in the *British National Formulary*, published every six months.

Presenile

Describing the condition of premature AGEING. The mental and physical faculties are adversely affected in presenility to an extent that does not usually occur until old age. (See also DEMENTIA.)

Presentation

The appearance in labour of some particular part of the child's body at the mouth of the uterus (see PREGNANCY AND LABOUR). This is a head presentation in 96 per cent of cases, but in a certain number the breech (or buttocks) may present, or the face, or foot, or even a part of the trunk in cases of cross-birth.

The term is also used for the symptoms or signs with which a patient first brings to a doctor.

Pressor

An agent that raises the BLOOD PRESSURE.

Pressure Sores

See ULCER – Decubitus ulcer.

Prevalence

An epidemiological term describing the proportion of a defined group in the population having a condition at one point in time. It is an appropriate measure only in relatively stable conditions – for example, chronic bronchitis – and is not suitable for measuring acute illnesses.

Preventive Medicine

The term 'preventive medicine' may be used both in a general 'lay' sense and to cover a specific range of activities carried out by health professionals. The definition and scope vary from country to country. Some people use the term widely and almost synonymously with 'public health'; others limit its use to specific measures directed at individuals, such as an immunisation against an infectious disease, preferring other terms such as 'health promotion' for educational activities and 'health protection' to cover consumer-protection regulations such as food inspection. The preventive approach is an essential component of a broader public-health strategy, and, for example, in relation to diet and physical activity a normal part of the lifestyle of many in the population.

In Britain, for instance, preventive medicine is usually taken to encompass a range of activities whose purpose is:
● to reduce the chance of a person contracting a disease or becoming disabled.
● to identify either an increased susceptibility to develop a disease, or an early manifestation of a disease at a stage which will still allow treatment to be effective.

The American College of Preventive Medicine (1983) defined it as 'a specialised field of medical practice composed of distinct disciplines which utilise skills focusing on the health of defined populations in order to promote and maintain health and well-being and to prevent disease, disability and premature death'.

However defined, the spectrum of activities encompassed by preventive medicine is wide and includes actions, such as counselling about lifestyle, where there may not be a clear cut-off between a preventive and a curative act. For example, advice about smoking and exercise to a recent victim of a myocardial infarction (see under HEART, DISEASES OF) is both essential to treatment and preventive against a future attack. Action aimed at a whole population – such as the addition of fluoride to drinking-water to protect against dental caries (see under TEETH, DISORDERS OF) – is part of a population-based public-health strategy but would also be widely regarded as preventive medicine.

A common and widely accepted classification of preventive medicine is as follows:

Primary prevention which aims at the complete avoidance of a disease (for example, by immunising a child against an infectious disease – see IMMUNISATION).

Secondary prevention which aims at detecting and curing a disease at an early stage before it has caused any symptoms. This requires 'screening' procedures to detect either the early pre-symptomatic condition, or a risk factor which may lead to it. (An example of the former is cervical cytology, where a sample of cells is scraped from the cervix of the UTERUS and examined microscopically for abnormality.

An example of the latter is CHOLESTEROL measurement as part of assessing an individual's risk of developing ischaemic heart disease (see under HEART, DISEASES OF). If it is significantly raised, dietary or drug treatment can be advised.)

Tertiary prevention aims at minimising the consequences for a patient who already has the disease (e.g. advising people to take more exercise and stop smoking after a heart attack).

Many prefer to limit the term 'preventive medicine' to primary and secondary prevention, emphasising the focus on risk-reducing interventions targeted at 'well' individuals. Others prefer the wider emphasis because of the importance of a preventive approach in reducing further disability by recognising and treating symptoms early. This can be particularly important in older people, where, for example, vigorous treatment of an orthopaedic problem can enable the patient to maintain physical mobility with all the benefits to health that brings. Whether primary, secondary or tertiary prevention, some form of screening question or test is normally necessary to identify a problem.

The range and extent of opportunities for prevention are expanding as research identifies the causes of diseases and more effective treatment becomes feasible. Inevitably there is economic and political debate about the cost-effectiveness of prevention versus cure, as well as about the ETHICS. The situation varies in relation to the natural history of the specific disease. Some conditions can easily be prevented but once contracted cannot be cured (e.g. RABIES); others are easily cured but are not yet preventable.

Screening Screening involves carrying out tests either to identify a treatable disease at a very early stage, before it has caused symptoms or damage; or to identify a risk factor which can lead to a disease. The tests might be by simple questioning (e.g. 'Do you smoke cigarettes?' – this predicts a considerable increase in the risk of chronic bronchitis, heart disease, bronchial cancer and many other diseases, and enables targeted advice and help to stop smoking to be given). Other screening tests involve carrying out complex special investigations such as blood tests or the microscopic investigations of cells – for example, for precancerous changes.

Many conditions can be identified at an early stage before they cause symptoms or signs of disease and in time for effective treatment to be carried out. Inevitably, some of the screening tests proposed can be expensive (particularly if used in large populations), painful or inaccurate and may not improve the results of treatment. Screening can also provoke considerable anxiety in those waiting for tests or results. Therefore, over the years considerable research has been carried out into the appropriateness and ethics of screening, and the World Health Organisation in 1968 identified a set of rules for evaluating screening tests:

- The condition sought should be an important health problem, for which there should be an accepted treatment for patients with recognised disease.
- Facilities for diagnosis and treatment should be available if a case is found.
- The screening test or examination must be suitable and valid. A false positive test will cause massive anxiety and also considerable expense in proving that there is no disease. Similarly, false negatives can lead people to be reassured and to ignore serious symptoms until too late. If large numbers of positive tests or false positives occur during a screening programme, health services can be swamped.
- The test, and any treatment as a possible result, should be acceptable. For example, there is little point in screening for a fetal abnormality which, if found, would lead to a recommendation for termination if the mother will refuse it on religious or moral grounds.
- Screening tests also need to be considered from an economic perspective and the cost of case-finding (including diagnosis and treatment of patients diagnosed) balanced in relation to possible expenditure on medical care as a whole.
- Finally the programme should reflect the natural history of the disease, and case-finding should normally be a continuing process and not a 'once for all' project.

If these rules are followed, considerable benefits can result from well-planned and well-managed screening programmes, and they form an important part of any health-care system. The extent to which manipulation of genetic material will be added to more traditional approaches such as counselling, immunisation and drug treatment cannot yet be predicted but, as time goes by, it is often likely to be ethical and social controls which limit developments rather than technical and scientific limits.

Priapism

A persisting painful ERECTION of the PENIS occurring without sexual stimulation. It is a rare but acute condition that requires immediate treatment. The cause is the failure of blood to drain from the spongy corpus caversonum tissues of the penis, thus maintaining an erection. This may happen because of infection, damage to the nerves controlling the blood vessels, or a clotting defect in the blood.

Prickly Heat

See MILIARIA.

Primary Care Trust

See GENERAL PRACTITIONER (GP)

Primary Health Care

Sometimes called primary medical care, this is the care provided by a GENERAL PRACTITIONER (GP) – traditionally entitled the family doctor – or other health professionals who have first contact with a patient needing or wanting medical attention. In the NHS, the primary health-care services include those provided by the general, dental, ophthalmic and pharmaceutical services as well as the family doctor service. Community health services provided outside the hospitals also offer some primary health care.

Primidone

A barbiturate-related drug (see BARBITURATES) used to treat all forms of EPILEPSY, except in sufferers who do not have seizures.

Primigravida

A woman who is undergoing her first pregnancy (see PREGNANCY AND LABOUR).

Primipara

The term applied to a woman who has given birth, or is giving birth, to her first child (see PREGNANCY AND LABOUR).

Prion

An aberrant variety of one of the proteins, called PrP, in a brain cell. The result of a gene mutation (see GENES), prions are stable, resistant to radiation and impervious to the normal cellular processes of degradation. They seem to react with normal PrP, turning it into an abnormal type that then accumulates in brain tissue. Prions are believed to be the infectious agents that cause a group of serious neurological disorders called spongiform encephalopathies. CREUTZFELDT-JAKOB DISEASE (CJD), the new variant of CJD linked with BOVINE SPONGIFORM ENCEPHALOPATHY (BSE), and KURU – a neurological disorder found in a cannibal tribe in New Guinea – are all diseases in this group that occur in humans. The prion disorders have a long latent period between infection and manifestation of symptoms; they are hard to diagnose until autopsy and there is no cure as yet.

Private Health Care

The provision of medical and dental care to patients who pay for the care either directly, through private medical insurance, or through employer-funded private insurance. In the UK, most patients are treated and cared for by the community- or hospital-based NHS. Although not forbidden to do so, few NHS general practitioners see private patients. NHS consultants are – within certain prescribed circumstances – allowed to treat private patients and many, especially surgeons, do so; but consultations and treatment are usually done on private-health premises. Some NHS hospitals have private facilities attached, but most private care is carried out in separate, privately run clinics and hospitals.

Certain specialties – for example, orthopaedic and reconstructive/cosmetic surgery and mental health – attract more private patients than others, such as paediatrics or medicine for the elderly. The standards of clinical care are generally the same in the two systems, but private patients can see the specialist of their choice at a time convenient to them. Waiting times for consultations and treatment are short and, when in hospital, private patients usually have their own room, telephone, TV, open visiting hours, etc.

A substantial proportion of private medical-care services are those provided for elderly people requiring regular nursing care and some medical supervision. The distinction between residential care and nursing care for the elderly is often blurred, but the government policy of providing means-tested state funding only for people genuinely needing regular nursing care – a system operated by local-authority social-service departments in England and Wales – has necessitated clearer definitions of the facilities provided for the elderly by private organisations. The strict criteria for state support (especially in England), the budget-conscious approach of local authorities when negotiating fees with private nursing homes, and the fact that NHS hospital trusts also have to pay for some patients discharged to such homes (to free-up hospital beds for new admissions) have led to intense financial pressures on private facilities for the elderly. This has caused the closure of many homes, which, in turn, is worsening the level of BED-BLOCKING by elderly patients who do not require hospital-intensity nursing but who lack family support in the community and cannot afford private care.

Pro-
A prefix meaning forwards.

Probe
A slender, flexible instrument, usually made of metal, designed for introduction into a wound or cavity – to explore its depth and direction, to discover the presence of foreign bodies, or to introduce medicinal substances.

Probenecid
A benzoic-acid derivative which interferes with the excretion by the KIDNEYS of certain compounds, including PENICILLIN and PARA-AMINO SALICYLIC ACID. Probenecid and was originally introduced into medicine for this reason, as a means of increasing and maintaining the concentration of penicillin in the body; it is also used to treat chronic GOUT.

Probiotics
Viable BACTERIA that colonise the intestine and alter the microflora and their metabolic activities, with a presumed beneficial effect for the host. Many probiotics are LACTIC ACID bacteria – for example, LACTOBACILLUS or bifidobacterium. Not all probiotics have the same properties or effectiveness. To be effective, a probiotic must survive passage through the stomach – an acid environment – and successfully colonise in the intestines, even when antibiotics are present. Research suggests that probiotics ameliorate the symptoms of childhood and travellers' DIARRHOEA, reducing the period of acute symptoms – particularly if the infection is caused by one of the ROTAVIRUSES.

Procainamide Hydrochloride
A derivative of PROCAINE, used to treat certain cardiac arrythmias (irregularities in the heartbeat).

Procaine
Once used widely as a local anaesthetic, but rarely so now.

Procarbazine
An antineoplastic drug used mainly to treat Hodgkin's disease (see under LYMPHOMA). It acts by interfering with the process of MITOSIS, the method by which the cells of the body, including tumours, reproduce themselves.

Prochlorperazine

Prochlorperazine is an antipsychotic phenothiazine drug (see NEUROLEPTICS). It is also an effective drug for the prevention or treatment of vomiting, and has therefore been used in the treatment of MENIÈRE'S DISEASE.

Procidentia

Another term for PROLAPSE.

Proctalgia

'Nerve pain' in the ANUS or RECTUM, without any local disease to account for it. Proctalgia fugax is a condition more common in men, characterised by cramp-like pains in the rectum and occasionally accompanied by a feeling of faintness. Occurring at night and lasting up to 15 minutes, the cause is unknown, but is probably due to muscle spasm. Rapid relief may be achieved by taking food or drink, exerting perineal pressure (including inserting a finger into the rectum), or sucking a 1 mg tablet of GLYCERYL TRINITRATE.

Proctitis

Inflammation situated about the RECTUM or ANUS.

Prodromata

A term applied to the earliest symptoms of a disease, or those which give warning of its presence.

Progeria

Premature old age (see also AGEING).

Progesterone

The hormone of the CORPUS LUTEUM of the ovary (see OVARIES). After the escape of the OVUM from the ruptured follicle, the corpus luteum secretes progesterone, which stimulates the growth and secretion of the endometrial glands of the UTERUS during the 14 days before MENSTRUATION. In the event of pregnancy, the secretion of progesterone continues until the baby's birth. (See also NORETHISTERONE; PREGNANDIOL; CONTRACEPTION.)

Progestogen

One of a naturally occurring or synthetically produced group of steroid HORMONES, including PROGESTERONE, that help to maintain normal pregnancy. Progestogens are used in contraceptives (see CONTRACEPTION) and are useful in treating AMENORRHOEA, premenstrual tension, and abnormal uterine bleeding.

Prognathism

Abnormal protusion of the lower JAW, or sometimes of both jaws. The condition may make biting and chewing difficult, in which case corrective surgery is necessary.

Prognosis

The term applied to a forecast as to the probable result of an illness or disease, particularly with regard to the prospect of recovery.

Proguanil Hydrochloride

A synthetic antimalarial drug usually used with CHLOROQUINE to prevent infection with MALARIA. Occasionally the drug is used to treat uncomplicated falciparum malaria in combination with atovaquone.

Prolactin

Prolactin is the pituitary hormone (see PITUITARY GLAND) which initiates lactation. The development of the breasts during pregnancy is ascribed to the action of OESTROGENS; prolactin starts them secreting. If lactation does not occur or fails, it may be started by injection of prolactin.

The secretion of prolactin is normally kept under tonic inhibition by the secretion of DOPAMINE which inhibits prolactin. This is formed in the HYPOTHALAMUS and secreted into the portal capillaries of the pituitary stalk to reach the anterior pituitary cells. Drugs that deplete the brain stores of dopamine or antagonise dopamine at receptor level will cause HYPERPROLACTINAEMIA and hence the secretion of milk from the breast and AMENORRHOEA. METHYLDOPA and RESERPINE deplete brain stores of dopamine and the PHENOTHIAZINES act as dopamine antagonists at receptor level. Other causes of excess secretion of prolactin are pituitary tumours, which may be minute and are then called microadenomas, or may actually enlarge the pituitary fossa and are then called macroadenomas. The most common cause of hyperprolactinaemia is a pituitary tumour. The patient may present with infertility – because patients with hyperprolactinaemia do not ovulate – or with amenorrhea and even GALACTORRHOEA.

BROMOCRIPTINE is a dopamine agonist. Treatment with bromocriptine will therefore control hyperprolactinaemia, restoring normal menstruation and ovulation and suppressing galactorrhoea. If the cause of hyperprolactinaemia is an adenomatous growth in the pituitary gland, surgical treatment should be considered.

Prolapse

Displacement of an organ or structure from its normal position. The term is applied chiefly to downward displacements of the RECTUM and UTERUS.

Prolapsed Intervertebral Disc

The SPINAL COLUMN is built up of a series of bones, known as vertebrae, placed one upon the other. Between these vertebrae lies a series of thick discs of fibro-cartilage known as intervertebral discs. Each disc consists of an outer portion known as the anulus fibrosus, and an inner core known as the nucleus pulposus. The function of these discs is to give flexibility and resiliency to the spinal column and to act as buffers against undue jarring. In other words, they are most efficient shock-absorbers. They may, however, PROLAPSE, or protrude, between the two adjacent vertebrae. If this should happen they press on the neighbouring spinal nerve and cause pain. As the most common sites of protrusion are between the last two lumbar vertebrae and between the last lumbar vertebra and the sacrum, this means that the pain occurs in the back, causing LUMBAGO, or down the course of the sciatic nerve causing SCIATICA. The prolapse is most likely to occur in middle age, which suggests that it may be associated with degeneration of the disc involved, but it can occur in early adult life as well. It usually occurs when the individual is performing some form of exercise which involves bending or twisting, as in gardening. The onset of pain may be acute and sudden, or gradual and more chronic in intensity. (See also INTERVERTEBRAL DISC.)

Treatment varies, depending (amongst other things) on the severity of the condition. In the acute phase, rest in bed is advisable, along with ANALGESICS. Later, exercise and physiotherapy are helpful, and in some cases manipulation of the spine brings relief by allowing the herniated, or prolapsed, disc to slip back into position. The injection of a local anaesthetic into the spine (epidural ANAESTHESIA) is yet another measure that often helps the more chronic cases. If those measures fail, surgery to remove the prolapsed disc may be necessary, but the patient's condition should be carefully reviewed before surgery is considered since success is not certain. An alternative form of treatment is the injection into the disc of chymopapain, an ENZYME obtained from the paw-paw, which dissolves the disc.

Promazine

A phenothiazine drug used to tranquillise disturbed patients (see NEUROLEPTICS).

Promethazine Hydrochloride

A widely used antihistamine drug with a prolonged action and a pronounced sedative effect. (See ANTIHISTAMINE DRUGS.)

Promethazine Theoclate

A drug that is widely used in the alleviation or prevention of sea-sickness (see MOTION (TRAVEL) SICKNESS).

Pronation

The movement whereby the bones of the forearm are crossed and the palm of the hand faces downwards.

Prone

Lying with the face down, or positioning the arm and hand so that the palm faces downwards.

Prophylaxis

Treatment or action adopted with the view of warding off disease.

Propofol

A drug used intravenously to induce general ANAESTHESIA. Propofol may be used by intravenous infusion to maintain anaesthesia; it is also useful for sedating patients in intensive care.

Propranolol Hydrochloride

One of the BETA-ADRENOCEPTOR-BLOCKING DRUGS, propranolol hydrochloride is used in the treatment of ANGINA PECTORIS, myocardial infarction (see under HEART, DISEASES OF), certain abnormal rhythms of the heart, and high blood pressure (HYPERTENSION). It also prevents attacks of MIGRAINE, and is used for certain anxiety states – particularly those associated with unpleasant bodily sensations, such as palpitations. (See also ADRENERGIC RECEPTORS.)

Proprietary Name

The trade name of a drug registered by the pharmaceutical company which has developed and patented it. This protects the name, ingredients and manufacturing technique for a set period of time, and helps the company to recoup the often costly research and development needed to produce and test the drug. Doctors may prescribe a drug by its trade name or by its official, approved name, although the

NHS encourages the latter. (See GENERIC DRUG; PATENT.)

Proprioceptors

Sensory nerve endings in the muscles, tendons and joints which signal to the brain their position relative to the outside world and the state of contraction of the muscle. During movement, a regular flow of information to the brain from the proprioceptors, the eyes and ears ensures that actions are coordinated and the body's balance maintained.

Proptometer

See EXOPHTHALMOMETER.

Proptosis

A condition in which the EYE protrudes from the orbit. Some causes include thyroid disorders (see THYROID GLAND, DISEASES OF), tumours within the orbit, inflammation or infection of the orbit. Proptosis due to endocrine abnormality (e.g. thyroid problems) is known as EXOPHTHALMOS.

Propylthiouracil

An oral antithyroid drug given daily to a person with HYPERTHYROIDISM. It interferes with the body's production of thyroid hormones.

Prospective Study

Research in which patients are studied from the first contact with a doctor or hospital regarding their illness – as opposed to a retrospective study, in which notes are obtained of a group of patients already treated or under treatment. The advantage is that before the study is undertaken, decisions can be made on what criteria determine who should enter the study, what information to collect and how many patients are needed to provide a meaningful result. The results of prospective studies are regarded as likely to be far more accurate than those from retrospective studies, where missing data and both reearcher and patient bias can colour the results.

Prostacyclin

A prostaglandin (see PROSTAGLANDINS) produced by the endothelial lining of the blood vessels. It inhibits the aggregation of PLATELETS, and thereby reduces the likelihood of the blood clotting. It is also a strong vasodilator (see VASODILATORS).

Prostaglandins

Those natural substances, so-called because they were first discovered in the SEMEN and thought to arise in the PROSTATE GLAND, are a group of fatty-acid substances with a wide range of activity. The richest known source is semen, but they are also present in many other parts of the body. Their precise mode of action is not yet clear, but they are potent stimulators of muscle contraction and they are also potent VASODILATORS. They cause contraction of the UTERUS and have been used to induce labour (see PREGNANCY AND LABOUR); they are also being used as a means of inducing therapeutic abortions (see ABORTION).

Prostaglandins play an important part in the production of PAIN, and it is now known that ASPIRIN relieves pain by virtue of the fact that it prevents, or antagonises, the formation of certain prostaglandins. In addition, they play some, although as yet incompletely defined, part in producing inflammatory changes. (See INFLAMMATION; NON-STEROIDAL ANTI-INFLAMMATORY DRUGS (NSAIDS).)

Thus prostaglandins have potent biological effects, but their instability and rapid metabolism make them short-acting. They are produced but not stored by most living cells and act locally. The two most important prostaglandins are prostacycline and thromboxane: prostacycline is a vasodilator and an inhibitor of platelet aggregation; thromboxanes have the opposite effects and cause vasoconstriction and platelet aggregation. The NSAIDs act by blocking an ENZYME called cyclo-oxygenase which converts arachidonic acid to the precursors of the various prostaglandins. Despite their potent pharmacological properties, the role of prostaglandins in current therapeutics is limited and controversial. They have been used most successfully as an inhibitor of platelet aggregation in extra-corporeal haemoperfusion systems. The problems with the prostacyclines is that they have to be given intravenously as they are inactive by mouth, and continuous infusion is required because the drug is rapidly eliminated with a half-life of minutes. Side-effects tend to be severe because the drug is usually given at the highest dose the patient can tolerate. The hope for the future lies in the exploitation of the compound to generate, synthetically, stable orally active prostacycline analogues which will inhibit platelet aggregation and hence thrombotic events, and yet have minimal effects on the heart and blood vessels.

Prostate Gland

This is an accessory sex gland in males which is wrapped round the URETHRA as this tube leaves the URINARY BLADDER. Opening into the urethra, the gland secretes an alkaline fluid during ejaculation and is a constituent of SEMEN. The gland grows during adolescence and is sensitive to the concentrations of sex hormones.

Prostate Gland, Diseases of

Disease of the PROSTATE GLAND can affect the flow of URINE so that patients present with urological symptoms.

Prostatitis This can be either acute or chronic. Acute prostatitis is caused by a bacterial infection, while chronic prostatitis may follow on from an acute attack, arise insidiously, or be non-bacterial in origin.

Symptoms Typically the patient has pain in the PERINEUM, groins, or supra pubic region, and pain on EJACULATION. He may also have urinary frequency, and urgency.

Treatment Acute and chronic prostatitis are treated with a prolonged course of antibiotics. Patients with chronic prostatitis may also require anti-inflammatory drugs, and antidepressants.

Prostatic enlargement This is the result of benign prostatic hyperplasia (BPH), causing enlargement of the prostate. The exact cause of this enlargement is unknown, but it affects 50 per cent of men between 40 and 59 years and 95 per cent of men over 70 years.

Symptoms These are urinary hesitancy, poor urinary stream, terminal dribbling, frequency and urgency of urination and the need to pass urine at night (nocturia). The diagnosis is made from the patient's history; a digital examination of the prostate gland via the rectum to assess enlargement; and analysis of the urinary flow rate.

Treatment This can be with tablets, which either shrink the prostate – an anti-androgen drug such as finasteride – or relax the urinary sphincter muscle during urination. For more severe symptoms the prostate can be removed surgically, by transurethral resection of prostate (TURP), using either electrocautery or laser energy. A new treatment is the use of microwaves to heat up and shrink the enlarged gland.

Cancer Cancer of the prostate is the fourth most common cause of death from cancer in northern European males: more than 10,000 cases are diagnosed every year in the UK and the incidence is rising by 3 per cent annually.

Little is known about the cause, but the majority of prostate cancers require the male hormones, androgens, to grow.

Symptoms These are similar to those resulting from benign prostatic hypertrophy (see above). Spread of the cancer to bones can cause pain. The use of a blood test measuring the amount of an ANTIGEN, PROSTATE SPECIFIC ANTIGEN (PSA), can be helpful in making the diagnosis – as can an ULTRASOUND scan of the prostate.

Treatment This could be surgical, with removal of the prostate (either via an abdominal incision, total prostatectomy, or transurethrally), or could be by radiotherapy. In more advanced cancers, treatment with anti-androgen drugs, such as cyprotexone acetate or certain oestrogens, is used to inhibit the growth of the cancer.

Prostate Specific Antigen (PSA)

An ENZYME produced by glandular tissue in the PROSTATE GLAND. When the gland enlarges (see PROSTATE, DISEASES OF), greater amounts of PSA are secreted, raising the concentration of the enzyme in the blood. This is especially so in cancer of the prostate, and testing the level of PSA is an indicator that the disease may be present. There is much controversy about the use of PSA as a screening test. Its proponents claim that its use reduces deaths from prostate cancer; its opponents suggest that it does this only by bringing to light many cases that needed no treatment and would not have caused death in any case. Further, if the level of PSA is very high, the disease is already advanced; where the result is equivocal it is uncertain whether the benefits of treatment outweigh the risks.

Prostatectomy

An operation to remove part or all of the PROSTATE GLAND. The most common method is transurethral prostatectomy (TURP) carried out during cytoscopy. A very enlarged prostate may need to be removed by a retropubic prostatectomy. After several weeks, most patients are able to resume normal activity including sexual intercourse.

Prostatis

See under PROSTATE GLAND, DISEASES OF.

Prostatism

The condition induced by benign enlargement of the PROSTATE GLAND.

Prosthesis

An artificial replacement of a missing or mal-functioning body part. Examples include false legs or arms fitted after AMPUTATION (see below); artificial heart valves; artificial heart devices; COCHLEAR IMPLANTS to improve hearing; a bio-artificial PANCREAS (containing live pancreatic cells from pigs) now under development to treat DIABETES MELLITUS; artificial bone; and (under development) artifical lungs. Cosmetic prostheses such as artifical eyes, teeth, noses and breasts are in widespread use.

Development of such mechanical and bio-mechanical devices points the way to a much wider use of effective prostheses, enabling people who would previously have died or been severely handicapped to lead normal or near normal lives. The technical hazards that have already been overcome provide a sound foundation for future successes. Progress so far in producing prostheses should also ensure that organ replacement is free from the serious ethical problems that surround the use of genetic manipulation to cure or prevent serious diseases (see ETHICS).

Limbs These are best made to meet the individual's requirements but can be obtained 'off the shelf'. Artificial joints normally comprise complex mechanisms to stimulate flexion and rotation movements. Leg prostheses are generally more useful than those for arms, because leg movements are easier to duplicate than those of the arm. Modern electronic circuitry that enables nerve impulses to be picked up and converted into appropriate movements is greatly improving the effectiveness of limb prostheses.

Eyes Artificial eyes are worn both for appearance and for psychological reasons. They are made of glass or plastic, and are thin shells of a boat-shape, representing the front half of the eye which has been removed. The stump which is left has still the eye-muscles in it, and so the artificial eye still has the power of moving with the other. A glass eye has to be replaced by a new one every year. Plastic eyes have the advantage of being more comfortable to wear, being more durable, and being unbreakable. Research is taking place aimed at creating a silicon chip that stimulates the visual cortex and thus helps to restore sight to the blind.

Dental prostheses is any artificial replacement of a tooth. There are three main types: a crown, a bridge and a denture. A crown is the replacement of the part of a tooth which sticks through the gum. It is fixed to the remaining part of the tooth and may be made of metal, porcelain, plastic or a combination of these. A bridge is the replacement of two or three missing teeth and is usually fixed in place. The replacement teeth are held in position by being joined to one or more crowns on the adjacent teeth. A denture is a removable prosthesis used to replace some or all the teeth. The teeth are made of plastic or porcelain and the base may be of plastic or metal. Removable teeth may be held more firmly by means of implants.

Heart The surgical replacement of stenosed or malfunctioning heart-valves with metal or plastic, human or pig valves has been routinely carried out for many years. So too has been the insertion into patients with abnormal heart rhythms of battery-driven artificial pacemakers (see CARDIAC PACEMAKER) to restore normal function. The replacement of a faulty heart with an artificial one is altogether more challenging. The first working attempt to create an artificial heart took place in the early 1980s. Called the Jarvik-7, it had serious drawbacks: patients had to be permanently connected to apparatus the size of an anaesthetic trolley; and it caused deaths from infection and clotting of the blood. As a result, artificial hearts have been used primarily as bridging devices to keep patients alive until a suitable donor heart for transplantation can be found. Recent work in North America, however, is developing artificial hearts made of titanium and dacron. One type is planted into the chest cavity next to the patient's own heart to assist it in its vital function of pumping blood around the body. Another replaces the heart completely. Eventually, it is probable that artificial hearts will replace heart transplants as the treatment of choice in patients with serious heart disorders.

Liver Artificial livers work in a similar way to kidney dialysis machines (see DIALYSIS). Blood is removed from the body and passed through a machine where it is cleaned and treated and then returned to the patient. The core of the device comprises several thousand flexible membrane tubules on which live liver cells (from pigs or people) have been cultured. There is an exchange of biological molecules and water with the 'circulating' blood, and the membrane also screens the 'foreign' cells from the patient's immune system, thus preventing any antagonistic immune reaction in the recipient.

P

Nose The making of a new nose is the oldest known operation in plastic surgery, Hindu records of such operations dating back to 1,000 BC. Loss of a nose may be due to eroding disease, war wounds, gun-shot wounds or dog bites. In essence the operation is the same as that practised a thousand years before Christ: namely the use of a skin graft, brought down from the forehead. Alternative sources of the skin graft today are skin from the arm, chest or abdomen. As a means of support, the new nose is built round a graft of bone or of cartilage from the ear.

Protease

A digestive ENZYME – also known as a proteolytic enzyme – that breaks down PROTEIN in food as part of the digestive process. The complex protein molecules are reduced to their constituent AMINO ACIDS.

Protease Inhibitors

A new group of drugs which, in combination with antiviral agents, are used to treat AIDS (see AIDS/HIV). They inhibit the activity of PROTEASE, an enzyme produced by HIV, and which breaks down proteins. The drugs have recently been introduced: those in use are indinavir, nelfinavir, ritonavir and saquinavir.

Protein

The term applies to members of a group of non-crystallisable nitrogenous substances widely distributed in the animal and vegetable kingdoms, and forming the characteristic materials of their tissues and fluids. They are essentially combinations of AMINO ACIDS. They mostly dissolve in water and are coagulated by heat and various chemical substances. Typical examples of protein substances are white of egg and gelatin.

Proteins constitute an essential part of the diet as a source of energy, and for the replacement of protein lost in the wear and tear of daily life. Their essential constituent from this point of view is the nitrogen which they contain. To be absorbed, or digested, proteins have to be broken down into their constituent amino acids. The adult human body can maintain nitrogenous equilibrium on a mixture of eight amino acids, which are therefore known as the essential (or indispensable) amino acids. They are isoleucine, leucine, lysine, methionine, phenylalanine, threonine, tryptophan and valine. In addition, infants require histidine.

Proteinuria

A condition in which proteins, principally ALBUMINS, are present in the URINE. It is often a symptom of serious heart or kidney disease, although some normal people have mild and transient proteinuria after exercise.

Causes

KIDNEY DISEASE is the most important cause of proteinuria, and in some cases the discovery of proteinuria may be the first evidence of such disease. This is why an examination of the urine for the presence of albumin constitutes an essential part of every medical examination. Almost any form of kidney disease will cause proteinuria, but the most frequent form to do this is glomerulonephritis (see under KIDNEYS, DISEASES OF). In the subacute (or nephrotic) stage of glomerulonephritis, the most marked proteinuria of all may be found. Proteinuria is also found in infections of the kidney (pyelitis) as well as in infections of the bladder (cystitis) and of the urethra (urethritis).

PREGNANCY The development of proteinuria in pregnancy requires investigation, as it may be the first sign of one of the most dangerous complications of pregnancy: toxaemia of pregnancy (PRE-ECLAMPSIA and ECLAMPSIA) and glomerulonephritis. Proteinuria may also result from the contamination of urine with vaginal secretions. (See also PREGNANCY AND LABOUR.)

CARDIOVASCULAR DISORDERS are commonly accompanied by proteinuria, particularly when the right side of the heart is failing. In severe cases of failure, accompanied by OEDEMA, the proteinuria may be marked. (See also HEART, DISEASES OF.)

FEVER often causes proteinuria, even though there is no actual kidney disease. The proteinuria disappears soon after the temperature becomes normal. (See also PYREXIA.)

DRUGS AND POISONS These include arsenic, lead, mercury, gold, copaiba, salicylic acid and quinine.

ANAEMIA A trace of albumin may be found in the urine in severe anaemia.

POSTURAL OR ORTHOSTATIC ALBUMINURIA This type is important because, if its true cause is unrecognised, it may be taken as a sign of kidney disease. The significance of postural proteinuria is unclear: it is more common among young people and is absent when the person is recumbent – hence the importance of testing a urine sample that is taken before rising in the morning.

Treatment The treatment is that of the underlying disease. (See KIDNEYS, DISEASES OF.)

Proteolysis

The mechanism by which complex PROTEIN molecules are broken down by digestive enzymes (see PROTEASE) in the stomach and small intestine. The constituent AMINO ACIDS are then absorbed into the bloodstream.

Prothrombin

An inactive substance in the blood PLASMA that is the precursor of the ENZYME, thrombin, which clots the blood. The conversion occurs when a blood vessel is damaged and the process of blood COAGULATION occurs.

Proton Pump

A key enzyme system in the parietal cells of the mucosal lining of the stomach: hydrogen ions are produced which acidify the stomach's secretions and convert pepsinogen to PEPSIN, an active participant in the digestion of food.

Proton-Pump Inhibitors

These are drugs that inhibit the production of acid in the stomach by blocking a key enzyme system, known as the PROTON PUMP, of the parietal cells of the stomach. The drugs include omeprazole, lansoprazole and pantoprazole, and they are the treatment of choice for oesophagitis (erosion and stricture – see under OESOPHAGUS, DISEASES OF); for the short-term treatment for gastric ulcer (see under STOMACH, DISEASES OF) and DUODENAL ULCER; and, in combination with ANTIBIOTICS, for the eradication of *Helicobacter pylori*.

Protoplasm

The viscid, translucent, glue-like material containing fine granules and composed mainly of proteins, which makes up the essential material of plant and animal cells and has the properties of life.

Protozoa

A simple, primitive animal comprising a single cell. Protozoa are microscopic in size but are much larger than BACTERIA. Most protozoa live freely, but around 30 are parasitic in humans causing disease such as amoebiasis (see DYSENTERY) and GIARDIASIS (intestinal infections), MALARIA, kala-azar (see LEISHMANIASIS) and SLEEPING SICKNESS. Some protozoa are able to excrete, respire, and absorb food particles and they may move around like a mobile jelly or by means of flagellae.

Protriptyline

One of the tricyclic ANTIDEPRESSANT DRUGS. (See MENTAL ILLNESS.)

Proximal

A term of comparison applied to structures which are nearer the centre of the body or the median line as opposed to more distal, or distant, structures.

Prozac

See FLUOXETINE.

Prurigo

An intensely itching form of eczema (see DERMATITIS) in which LICHEN takes a nodular form.

Pruritus

Another name for itching, it is a common symptom with many causes. It may accompany obvious skin disease such as URTICARIA, eczema (see DERMATITIS) or SCABIES. Pruritus may be systemic in origin and can be caused by advanced hepatic (liver) or renal (kidney) failure, uncontrolled DIABETES MELLITUS, or HYPERTHYROIDISM. It may be due to drugs and certain forms of malignancy – for example, Hodgkin's disease (see LYMPHOMA). Anxiety or depression may also cause pruritus. Pruritus ani, itching round the ANUS, is a common troublesome condition: it may be caused by obsessive efforts to keep this area clean; soft toilet paper and gentle cleansing once daily should be sufficient. A weak anal sphincter, skin tags, and HAEMORRHOIDS may also cause itching, and these conditions should be treated.

Treatment The first aim is to identify and treat the cause, whether local or systemic. Once the cause has been dealt with, symptomatic treatment may be required to break the cycle of itching, scratching and itching; topical steroid ointments and occlusive dressings help to prevent scratching. For dry skin, emollients (see OINTMENTS) are useful. Local anaesthetics (see under ANAESTHESIA) provide relief but may cause allergic reactions, and systemic ANTIHISTAMINE DRUGS at night can help.

Prussic Acid Poisoning

See CYANIDE POISONING.

Pseudocyesis

Pseudocyesis means spurious or false pregnancy, a condition characterised by enlargement of the abdomen, and even enlargement of the breasts and early-morning sickness – the woman being quite convinced that she is pregnant.

Pseudocyst

A space within an organ without a defined

lining and which contains fluid. Patients with chronic pancreatitis (see PANCREAS, DISORDERS OF) sometimes develop these pseudocysts which fill with pancreatic juice containing enzymes produced by the gland. Abdominal pain usually results; treatment is by surgical draining.

Pseudohermaphrodite

A person in whom the gonads (testes or ovaries – see GONAD) of only one sex are present in the body but in whom the external GENITALIA may not be obviously male or female. The condition is a result of a hormonal imbalance and can normally be treated by appropriate surgery and hormone drugs. (See also HERMAPHRODITE.)

Pseudohypertrophic Muscular Dystrophy

A condition in which certain muscles enlarge owing to a fatty and fibrous degeneration, giving a false appearance of increased strength.

Pseudomonas Aeruginosa

A pathogenic bacterium of the genus pseudomonas – rod-like, motile gram-negative bacteria (see GRAM'S STAIN) – that occurs in pus from wounds and is associated with urinary tract infections. The bacteria mostly live in soil and decomposing organic matter and help to recycle nitrogen in nature. Most of the bacteria in this genus are harmless to humans.

Pseudoxanthoma Elasticum

This is a hereditary disorder of elastic tissue. Degenerating elastic tissue in the skin produces lesions which look like soft yellow papules. Elastic tissue in the eye and blood vessels is also involved, giving rise to visual impairment, raised blood pressure and haemorrhages.

Psittacosis

Also called parrot disease. An infectious disease of parrots and other exotic birds which may be transmitted to humans and is caused by the micro-organism *Chlamydia psittaci*. It presents as PNEUMONIA or a systemic illness in which the patient has an enlarged spleen and liver and PNEUMONITIS. Tetracycline is an effective treatment, but relapses may occur.

Psoas

A powerful muscle which arises from the front of the vertebral column in the lumbar region, and passes down, round the pelvis and through the groin, to be attached to the inner side of the thigh-bone not far from its upper end. The act of sitting up from a recumbent posture, or that of bending the thigh on the abdomen, is mainly accomplished by the contraction of this muscle. Disease of the spine in the lumbar region may produce an ABSCESS which lies within the sheath of this muscle and makes its way down to the front of the thigh. Such an abscess is known as a psoas abscess.

Psoralens

See PHOTOCHEMOTHERAPY; PHOTODERMATOSES.

Psoriasis

This chronic, relapsing inflammatory skin disease is extremely common, affecting about 2 per cent of the UK population. Frequently it is mild and trivial, affecting only the points of the elbows or knees and the scalp, but in a substantial minority of sufferers the disease is much more widespread and causes considerable discomfort and social embarrassment. Rarely, it can be universal and even life-threatening.

The predisposition to psoriasis is genetic, multiple genes being involved, but postnatal factors such as acute infection, hormonal disturbance, pregnancy and drugs can influence or provoke it. The sexes are equally affected and onset is most common in the second or third decade of life.

The psoriatic lesion is dull red, scaly and well defined. Scale is shed constantly, either in tiny pieces or as large plaques. The scalp is usually affected but the disease does not cause significant hair loss. The fingernails may be pitted or ridged and the toenails grossly thickened. Several clinical patterns occur: in guttate psoriasis, a sudden explosion of multiple tiny lesions may follow a streptococcal throat infection, especially in children. Larger lesions are characteristic of discoid (plaque) psoriasis, the usual adult form. In the elderly the plaques may be mainly in the large body folds – flexural psoriasis. Rarely, psoriasis may be universal (psoriatic erythroderma), or a sterile pustular eruption may supervene (pustular psoriasis).

Mucous membranes in the mouth and elsewhere are not affected. Psoriasis does not affect internal organs, but in about 1 per cent of subjects an inflammatory joint disease (psoriatic arthritis) may be associated with the condition.

Treatment There is no absolute cure, but several agents used topically are of value including coal-tar extracts, DITHRANOL, CORTICOSTEROIDS and synthetic derivatives of vitamins A and D. Ultraviolet B phototherapy (and natural sunlight) benefits most but not all psoriatics. Systemic therapy, including PHOTOCHEMOTHERAPY, is reserved for severe forms of psoriasis. METHOTREXATE, CICLOSPORIN A and oral RETINOIDS are the most effective drugs, but they are potentially dangerous and require expert monitoring.

Patient information may be obtained through the Psoriasis Association.

Psyche

The mind or soul of an individual and his or her mental – in contrast to the physical – functioning.

Psychedelic Drugs

Drugs, such as CANNABIS and LYSERGIC ACID DIETHYLAMIDE (LSD), that expand consciousness and perception. (See DEPENDENCE.)

Psychiatry

That branch of medical science which treats mental disorder and disease and also helps with the management of people with learning disabilities (see LEARNING DISABILITY; MENTAL ILLNESS).

Psychoanalysis

The term applied to the theories and practice of the school of psychology originating with Freud and developed by Jung and other psychotherapists (see PSYCHOLOGY). It depends upon the theory that states of disordered mental health have been produced by a repression in the subconscious of painful memories or of conflicting instincts, thus absorbing the individual's mental energy and diverting attention from normal mental activities.

Psychoanalysis aims at discovering these repressed memories, which are responsible for the diversion of mental power and of which the affected person usually is only dimly aware or quite unaware. The fundamental method of psychoanalytical treatment is the free expression of thoughts, ideas and fantasies on the part of the patient. To facilitate this, the analyst uses techniques to relax the patient and maintains a neutral attitude to his or her problems. In the course of analysis the patient will re-explore his or her early emotional attitudes and tensions.

The fundamental conception of psychoanalysis, although hard to prove by orthodox scientific methods and therefore challenged by some psychiatrists, has been widely adopted and developed by other schools of psychology. Freud's work changed the attitudes of the scientific community and the public to the problems of the neurotic, the morbidly anxious, the fearful and to the mental and emotional develoment of the child.

Psychogeriatrics

The branch of PSYCHIATRY that investigates, diagnoses and treats the mental-health problems of old people. Psychogeriatricians work in close co-operation with physicians for the care of the elderly, and with other health professionals and social workers in this branch of medicine.

Psychologist

Psychologists have a graduate degree in PSYCHOLOGY, followed by an accredited postgraduate training leading to chartered status. There are a number of different branches related to the various applications psychology has to different fields of work.

Types of psychologist

EDUCATIONAL PSYCHOLOGISTS Working in schools and in local education authorities, they are concerned with children's learning and development. They carry out tasks aimed at improving children's learning and helping teachers to become more aware of social factors that affect teaching and learning. Chartered educational psychlogists have a graduate degree in psychology and also a teaching qualification, with experience; in addition they have completed a one-year postgraduate course in educational psychology with supervised experience.

COUNSELLING PSYCHOLOGISTS apply psychology to working in collaboration with people across a range of human problems. For example, helping people to manage difficult life events, relationship issues, BEREAVEMENT and issues raised by mental-health problems. Their usual route to qualify is completing a three-year postgraduate training in counselling psychotherapy.

CLINICAL PSYCHOLOGISTS have completed a three-year doctorate training course as well as having their first degree in psychology. They work in health and care settings. Their aim is to reduce psychological distress and to promote psychological well-being. They work with individuals, families, groups and organisations: the individuals are people who have problems such as anxiety, DEPRESSION, serious and enduring MENTAL ILLNESS, brain injuries, addiction, child and family problems, LEARNING DISABILITY and the after-effects of trauma. They provide various types of treatment, for example COGNITIVE BEHAVIOUR THERAPY and family therapy, based on psychological theories and research. They also carry out research, training, consultation with other professionals involved with clients, and supervision of colleagues.

(See also NEUROSIS; PSYCHOTHERAPY.)

FORENSIC PSYCHOLOGISTS work in the

P

criminal and justice fields, applying psycho-logical theory to aspects of legal processes in courts, criminal investigation, and understand-ing and treating psychological problems associ-ated with criminal behaviour. They will have completed an accredited training course in forensic psychology.

HEALTH PSYCHOLOGISTS apply psychological methods to studying behaviour relevant to health, illness and care including health promo-tion and education.

OCCUPATIONAL PSYCHOLOGISTS are concerned with how people perform at work and how organisations function. They work in manage-ment, personnel, selection and careers advice. They have a postgraduate degee in occupational psychology and will have had to undertake three years' supervised practice.

Psychology

The scientific study of people: how they think, and how and why they act, react and interact as they do. It covers such matters as memory, rational and irrational thought, intelligence, learning, personality, perceptions and emo-tions. There are different schools of psychology, varying both in attitude and in methods of working. The main groups consist of the intro-spectionist Freudian, Jungian and Adlerian schools, and the gestaltist, behaviourist and cognitive schools. Although many practical psychologists deny belonging to any specific school, contemporary psychology in general favours the cognitive schools, although many are sub-specialities based on practical consider-ations. (See also FREUDIAN THEORY; JUNGIAN ANALYSIS; ADLER; GESTALTISM; PSYCHOLOGIST.)

Psychometrics

The use of standardised psychological tests to measure differences in functions – for example, intelligence and personality – in individuals.

Psychoneurosis

A general term applied to various functional disorders of the nervous system. (See NEUROSIS.)

Psychopathic

Psychopathic disorder is defined by the Mental Health Act 1983 as a persistent disorder or dis-ability of mind (whether or not including sig-nificant impairment of intelligence) which results in abnormally aggressive or seriously irresponsible conduct. The cardinal features are as follows: (1) Absence of normal feelings for other people such as love, affection, sympathy and condolence. (2) A tendency to antisocial impulsive acts with no forethought of the con-sequences. (3) A failure to learn by experience and to be deterred from crime by punishment. (4) Absence of any other form of mental disorder that would explain the unusual behaviour. The corresponding American ter-minology is 'antisocial personality disorder'. (See MENTAL ILLNESS.)

Psychosexual

Relating to the relationships between the behavioural, emotional, mental and physiological characteristics of sex or sexual development.

Psychosis

One of a group of mental disorders in which the affected person loses contact with reality. Thought processes are so disturbed that the per-son does not always realise that he or she is ill. Symptoms include DELUSIONS, HALLUCIN-ATIONS, loss of emotion, MANIA, DEPRESSION, poverty of thought and seriously abnormal behaviour. Psychoses include SCHIZOPHRENIA, MANIC DEPRESSION and organically based mental disorders. (See also MENTAL ILLNESS.)

Psychosomatic Diseases

Taken at face value, the term 'psychosomatic' simply means the interaction of psyche (mind) and soma (body). As such it is a non-controversial concept that points out the many ways in which psychological factors affect the expression of physical disorder and vice-versa. Few doubt that stress makes many physical ill-nesses worse, at least as far as symptoms are concerned. There are also few physical illnesses in which the outcome is not made worse by psychological factors: depression after a heart attack, for example, has a worse effect on prog-nosis than even smoking. A little more prob-lematic is the very popular belief that stress causes relapses of physical disorders, such as cancer; some studies have found this to be the case, others not.

However, calling a condition psychosomatic implies something more – the primacy of the psyche over the soma. Going back to the influential theories and practice of PSYCHO-ANALYSIS as expounded from the 1930s, many diseases have been proposed as the result of psy-chological factors.These have included PEPTIC ULCER, ULCERATIVE COLITIS, ASTHMA, PSOR-IASIS and others. In this view, much physical disorder is due to repressed or excessive emo-tions. Likewise it is also argued that whereas some people express psychological distress via psychological symptoms (such as anxiety, depression and so on), others develop physical symptoms instead – and that they are also at greater risk of physical disease.

The trouble with this view is that medical advances repeatedly show that it goes too far. Stress certainly causes physical symptoms – for example, DYSPEPSIA – but the belief that it caused peptic ulcers vanished with the discovery of the true cause: colonisation of the stomach by the bacterium, *Helicobacter pylori*. Of course, stress and social adversity affect the risk of many diseases. For example, the incidence of heart disease among UK government employees (civil servants) has been shown to be influenced by their social class and their degree of job satisfaction. But we do not know how this works. Some argue that social adversity and stress influence how the heart functions ('He died of a broken heart'). Stress can also affect IMMUNITY but it cannot cause AIDS/HIV and we do not know if there is a link running from stress to abnormal immune function to actual illness.

We can say that psychological factors provoke physical symptoms, and often even explain how this can happen. For example, when you are anxious you produce more epinephrine (adrenaline), which gives rise to chest pain, 'butterflies in the stomach' and PALPITATION. These symptoms are not 'all in the mind', even if the trigger is a psychological one. People who are depressed are more likely to experience nearly every physical symptom there is, but especially pain and fatigue. Taken as a whole, psychologically induced symptoms are an enormous burden on the NHS and probably responsible for more doctor visits and sickness absence than any other single cause. Also we can be confident that social adversity and stress powerfully influence the outcome of many illnesses; likewise, a vast range of unhealthy activities and behaviours such as smoking, excessive alcohol intake, excessive eating, and so on. But we must be careful not to assume that our emotions directly cause our illnesses.

Psychosurgery

This was introduced in 1936 by Egas Moniz, Professor of Medicine in Lisbon University, for the surgical treatment of certain psychoses (see PSYCHOSIS). For his work in this field he shared the Nobel prize in 1949. The original operation, known as leucotomy, consisted of cutting white fibres in the frontal lobe of the BRAIN. It was accompanied by certain hazards such as persistent EPILEPSY and undesirable changes in personality; pre-frontal leucotomy is now regarded as obsolete. Modern stereotactic surgery may be indicated in certain intractable psychiatric illnesses in which the patient is chronically incapacitated, especially where there is a high suicide risk. Patients are only considered for psychosurgery when they have failed to respond to routine therapies. One contraindication is marked histrionic or antisocial personality. The conditions in which a favourable response has been obtained are intractable and chronic obsessional neuroses (see NEUROSIS), anxiety states and severe chronic DEPRESSION.

Psychosurgery is now rare in Britain. The Mental Health Act 1983 requires not only consent by the patient – confirmed by an independent doctor, and two other representatives of the Mental Health Act Commission – but also that the Commission's appointed medical representative also advise on the likelihood of the treatment alleviating or preventing a deterioration in the patient's condition.

Psychotherapy

A psychological rather than physical method for the treatment of psychological and psychiatric disorders (see PSYCHOLOGY; PSYCHIATRY). Almost every type of disease or injury has a mental aspect, even if this relates only to the pain or discomfort that it causes. In some diseases, and with some temperaments, the mental factor is much more pronounced than in others; for such cases psychotherapy is particularly important. The chief methods employed all depend on the client-therapist relationship being of prime importance.

Suggestion is a commonly employed method, used in almost every department of medicine. It may consist, in its simplest form, merely of emphasising that the patient's health is better, so that this idea becomes fixed in the patient's mind. A suggestion of efficacy may be conveyed by the physical properties of a medicine or by the appearance of some apparatus used in treatment. Again, suggestion may be conveyed emotionally, as in religious healing. Sometimes a therapeutic suggestion may be made to the patient in a hypnotic state (see HYPNOTISM).

Analysis consists in the elucidation of the half-conscious or subconscious repressed memories or instincts that are responsible for some cases of mental disorder or personal conflicts.

Group therapy is a method whereby patients are treated in small groups and encouraged to participate actively in the discussion which ensues amongst themselves and the participating therapists. A modification of group therapy is drama therapy. Large group therapy also exists.

Education and employment may be important factors in rehabilitative psychotherapy.

Supportive therapy consists of sympathetically reviewing the patient's situation with him or her, and encouraging the patient to identify and solve problems.

Short-term supportive psychotherapy is aimed at stabilising and strengthening the psychological defence mechanisms of those patients who are confronted by a crisis which threatens to overwhelm their ability to cope, or who are struggling with the aftermath of major life events.

Long-term supportive psychotherapy is needed for patients with personality disorders or recurrent psychotic states, where the aim of treatment is to prevent deterioration and help the patient to achieve an optimal adaptation, making the most of his or her psychological assets. Such patients may find more profound and unstructured forms of therapy distressing.

Behavioural therapy and cognitive therapy, often carried out by psychologists, attempt to clarify with the patient specific features of behaviour or mental outlook respectively, and to identify step-by-step methods that the patient can use for controlling the disorder. Behaviour therapy is commonly used for AGORAPHOBIA and other phobias, and cognitive therapy has been used for depression and anxiety. (See MENTAL ILLNESS.)

Psychotic
Adjective describing PSYCHOSIS or noun referring to someone with a psychosis.

Psychotropic
Affecting the mind. Psychotropic drugs include HALLUCINOGENS, HYPNOTICS or sleeping drugs, sedatives, TRANQUILLISERS and NEUROLEPTICS (antipsychotic drugs).

PTC
See PERCUTANEOUS TRANSHEPATIC CHOLANGIOPANCREATOGRAPHY (PTC).

Pterygium
A degenerative disorder of the conjunctiva (see EYE) which grows over the cornea medially and laterally. The overgrowths look like wings. They are commonly seen in people who live in areas of bright sunlight, particularly when reflected from deserts or snowfields. Treatment involves excision of the overgrowth. (See also EYE, DISORDERS OF.)

Ptosis
See EYE, DISORDERS OF.

Ptyalin
The name of the ENZYME contained in the SALIVA, by which starchy materials are changed into sugar, and so prepared for absorption. It is identical to the AMYLASE of pancreatic juice. (See DIGESTION; PANCREAS.)

Puberty
The change that takes place when childhood passes into manhood or womanhood. This change is generally a very definite one, occurring at about the age of 14 years, although it is modified by race, climate, and bodily health so that it may appear a year or two earlier or several years later. At this time, the sexual functions attain their full development; the contour of the body changes from a childish to a more rounded womanly, or sturdy manly, form; and great changes take place in the mode of thought and feeling.

In girls, puberty is marked by the onset of MENSTRUATION and development of the BREASTS. The latter is usually the first sign of puberty to appear, and may occur from nine years onwards; most girls show signs of breast development by the age of 13. The time from the beginning of breast development to the onset of menstruation is usually around two years but may range from six months to five years. The first sign of puberty in boys is an increase in testicular and penile size (see TESTICLE; PENIS) between the age of ten and 14. The LARYNX enlarges in boys, so that the voice – after going through a period of 'breaking' – finally assumes the deep manly pitch. Hair appears on the pubis and later in the armpits in both boys and girls, whilst in the former it also begins to grow on the upper lip, and skin eruptions are not uncommon on the face (see ACNE).

The period is one of transition from a physical and mental point of view. Puberty is not to be regarded as a physiological 'coming of age', for full development is usually achieved in the early 20s.

Pubis
Pubis is the bone that forms the front part of the pelvis. The pubic bones of opposite sides

meet in the symphysis and protect the bladder from the front.

Public Health

Individuals with health problems go to their doctor, are diagnosed and prescribed treatment. Public-health doctors use epidemiological studies (see EPIDEMIOLOGY, and below) to diagnose the causes of health problems in populations and to plan services to treat the health and disease problems identified. Their concern is often focused particularly on those who are disadvantaged or marginalised, and on the delivery of safe, effective and accessible health care: however, to achieve their goal of better health and well-being for everybody, they must also influence decision-makers across the whole community.

Central to an understanding of public health is recognition that public-health practitioners are concerned not just with individuals, but also with whole populations – and that improving health care plays only a part of public-health improvement. The health of populations (public health) is also dependent on many factors such as the social, economic and physical environment in which the people live and the nutrition and health care available to them.

For thousands of years, a fundamental feature of civilisations has been to seek to improve the health of the population and protect it from disease. This has led to the development of legal frameworks which differ widely from country to country, depending on their social and political development. All are concerned to stop the spread of infectious diseases, and to maintain the safety of urban food and water supplies and waste disposal. Most are also associated with housing standards, some form of poverty relief, and basic health care. Some trading standards are often covered, at least in relation to the sale and distribution of poisons and drugs, and to controls on industrial and transport safety – for example, in relation to drinking and driving and car design. Although these varied functions protect the public health and were often originally developed to improve it, most are managerially and professionally separated from today's public-health departments. So public-health professionals in the NHS, armed with evidence of the cause of a disease problem, must frequently act as advocates for health across many agencies where they play no formal management part. They must also seek to build alliances and add a health perspective to the policies of other services wherever possible.

Epidemiology is the principal diagnostic method of public health. It is defined as the study of the distribution and determinants of health-related states in specified populations, and the application of this study to the control of health problems. Public-health practitioners also draw on many other skills, such as those of statisticians, sociologists, anthropologists, economists and policy analysts in identifying and trying to resolve the health problems of the societies they serve. Treatments proposed are likely to extend well beyond the clinic or hospital and may include recommendations for measures to resolve poverty, improve sanitation or housing, control pollution, change lifestyles such as smoking, improve nutrition, or change health services. At times of acute EPIDEMIC, public-health doctors have considerable legal powers granted to enable them to prevent infection from spreading. At other times their work may be more concerned with monitoring, reporting, planning and managing services, and advocating policy changes to politicians so that health is promoted.

The term 'the public health' can relate to the state of health of the population, and be represented by measures such as MORTALITY indices (e.g. perinatal or infant mortality and standardised mortality rates), life expectancy, or measures of MORBIDITY (illness). These can be compared across areas and even countries. Sometimes people refer to a pubic health-care system; this is a publicly funded service, the primary aim of which is to improve health by the use of population-based measures. They may include or be separate from private health-care services for which individuals pay. The structure of these systems varies from country to country, reflecting different social composition and political priorities. There are, however, some general elements that can be identified:

Surveillance The collection, collation and analysis of data to provide useful information about the distribution and causes of health and disease and related factors in populations. These activities form the basis of epidemiology, which is the diagnostic backbone of public-health practice.

Intervention The design, advocacy and implementation of policies to improve health. This may be through the provison of PREVENTIVE MEDICINE, environmental measures, influencing the behaviour of individuals, or the provision of appropriate services to limit disability and handicap. It will lead to advocacy for health, promoting change in many areas of policy including, for example, taxation and improved housing and employment opportunities.

Evaluation Assessment of the first two steps to assess their impact in terms of effectiveness, efficiency, acceptability, accessibility, value for money or other indicators of quality. This enables the programme to be reviewed and changed as necessary.

The practice of public health The situation in the United Kingdom will be described as, even though systems vary, it will give a general impression of the type of work covered.

HISTORY   Initially,   public-health   practice related to food, the urban environment and the control of infectious diseases. Early examples include rules in the Bible about avoiding certain foods. These were probably based on practical experience, had gradually been adopted as sensible behaviour, become part of culture and finally been incorporated into religious laws. Other examples are the regulations about quarantine for PLAGUE and LEPROSY in the Middle Ages, vaccination against SMALLPOX introduced by William Jenner, and Lind's use of citrus fruits to prevent SCURVY at sea in the 18th century.

It was during the 19th century, in response to the health problems arising from the rapid growth of urban life, that the foundations of a public-health system were created. The 'sanitary' concept was fundamental to these developments. This suggested that overcrowding in insanitary conditions was the cause of most disease epidemics and that improved sanitation measures such as sewerage and clean water supplies would prevent them. Action to introduce such measures were often initiated only after epidemics spread out of the slums and into wealthier and more powerful families. Other problems such as the stench of the River Thames outside the Houses of Parliament also led to a demand for effective sanitary control measures. Successive public-health laws were passed by Parliament, initially about sanitation and housing, and then, as scientific knowledge grew, about bacterial infections.

In the middle of the 19th century the first medical officers of health were appointed with responsibility to report regularly and advise local government about the measures needed to control disease and improve health. Their scope and responsibility widened as society changed and took on a wider welfare role. After more than a century they changed as part of the reforms of the NHS and local government in

the 1960s and became more narrowly focused within the health-care system and its management. Increased recognition of the multifactorial causes, costs and limitations of treatment of conditions such as cancer and heart disease, and the emergence of new problems such as AIDS/HIV and BOVINE SPONGIFORM ENCEPHALOPATHY (BSE) have again showed the importance of prevention and a broader approach to health. With it has come recognition that, while disease may be the justification for action, a narrow disease-treatment-based approach is not always the most effective or economic solution. The role of the director of public health (the successor to the medical officer of health) is again being expanded, and in 1997 – for the first time in the UK – a government Minister for Public Health was appointed. This reflects not only a greater priority for public health, but also a concern that the health effects of policy should be considered across all parts of government.

(See also ENVIRONMENT AND HEALTH.)

Public Health Laboratory Service (PHLS)

A statutory organisation that is part of the NHS. It comprises ten laboratory groups and two centres in the UK, with central coordination from PHLS headquarters. The service provides diagnostic-testing facilities for cases of suspected infectious disease. The remit of the PHLS (which was set up during World War II and then absorbed into the NHS) is now based on legislation approved in 1977 and 1979. Its overall purpose was to protect the population from infection by maintaining a national capability of high quality for the detection, diagnosis, surveillance, protection and control of infections and communicable diseases. It provided microbiology services to hospitals, family doctors and local authorities as well as providing national reference facilities. In 2001 it was incorporated into the newly established NATIONAL INFECTION CONTROL AND HEALTH PROTECTION AGENCY.

Pudendal Nerve

The nerve that operates the lowest muscles of the floor of the PELVIS and also the anal SPHINCTER muscle. It may be damaged in childbirth, resulting in INCONTINENCE.

Pudendum

The external genital organs. The term is usually used to describe those of the female (see VULVA).

Puerperal Depression

Also called postnatal DEPRESSION, this is the state of depression that may affect women soon after they have given birth. The condition often occurs suddenly a day or so after the birth. Many women suffer from it and usually they can be managed with sympathetic support. If, however, the depression – sometimes called 'maternal blues' – persists for ten days or more, mild ANTIDEPRESSANT DRUGS are usually effective. If not, psychiatric advice is recommended. (See PREGNANCY AND LABOUR.)

Puerperal Sepsis

An infection, once called puerperal fever, that starts in the genital tract within ten days after childbirth, miscarriage or abortion (see PREGNANCY AND LABOUR). Once a scourge of childbirth, with many women dying from the infection, the past 50 years have seen a dramatic decline in its incidence in developed countries, with only 1–3 per cent of women having babies now being affected. This decline is due to much better maternity care and the advent of ANTIBIOTICS. Infection usually starts in the VAGINA and is caused by the bacteria that normally live in it: they can cause harm because of the mother's lowered resistance, or when part of the PLACENTA has been retained in the genital tract. The infection usually spreads to the UTERUS and sometimes to the FALLOPIAN TUBES. Sometimes bacteria may enter the vagina from other parts of the body.

Fever, an offensive-smelling post-partum vaginal discharge (lochia) and pain in the lower abdomen are the main features. Untreated, the women may develop SALPINGITIS, PERITONITIS and septicaemia. Antibiotics are used to treat the infection and any retained placental tissue must be removed.

Puerperium

The period which elapses after the birth of a child until the mother is again restored to her ordinary health. It is generally regarded as lasting for a month. One of the main changes to occur is the enormous decrease in size that takes place in the muscular wall of the womb. There are often AFTERPAINS during the first day in women who have borne several children, less often after a first child. The discharge is blood-stained for the first two or three days, then clearer till the end of the first week, before stopping within two or three weeks. The breasts, which have already enlarged before the birth of the child, secrete milk more copiously, and there should be a plentiful supply on the third day of the puerperium. (See also PREGNANCY AND LABOUR.)

Management The mother should start practising exercises to help ensure that the stretched abdominal muscles regain their normal tone. There is no need for any restriction of diet, but care must be taken to ensure an adequate intake of fluid, including at least 580 ml (a pint) of milk a day.

Milk, as already stated, appears copiously on the third day, but this is preceded by a secretion from the breast, known as colostrum, which is of value to the newborn child. The child should therefore be put to the breasts within 6–8 hours of being born. This also stimulates both the breasts and the natural changes taking place during this period. Suckling is beneficial for both child and mother and encourages bonding between the two.

Pulmonary

Relating to the LUNGS.

Pulmonary Diseases

See LUNGS, DISEASES OF.

Pulmonary Embolism

The condition in which an embolus (see EMBOLISM), or clot, is lodged in the LUNGS. The source of the clot is usually the veins of the lower abdomen or legs, in which clot formation has occurred as a result of the occurrence of DEEP VEIN THROMBOSIS (DVT) – THROMBOPHLEBITIS (see VEINS, DISEASES OF). Thrombophlebitis, with or without pulmonary embolism, is a not uncommon complication of surgical operations, especially in older patients. This is one reason why nowadays such patients are got up out of bed as quickly as possible, or, alternatively, are encouraged to move and exercise their legs regularly in bed. Long periods of sitting, particularly when travelling, can cause DVT with the risk of pulmonary embolism. The severity of a pulmonary embolism, which is characterised by the sudden onset of pain in the chest, with or without the coughing up of blood, and a varying degree of SHOCK, depends upon the size of the clot. If large enough, it may prove immediately fatal; in other cases, immediate operation may be needed to remove the clot; whilst in less severe cases anticoagulant treatment, in the form of HEPARIN, is given to prevent extension of the clot. For some operations, such as hip-joint replacements, with a high risk of deep-vein thrombosis in the leg, heparin is given for several days post-operatively.

P

Pulmonary Fibrosis

A condition which may develop in both LUNGS (interstitial pulmonary fibrosis) or part of one lung. Scarring and thickening of lung tissues occur as a consequence of previous lung inflammation, which may have been caused by PNEUMONIA or TUBERCULOSIS. Symptoms include cough and breathlessness and diagnosis is confirmed with a chest X-ray. The patient's underlying condition should be treated, but the damage already done to lung tissue is usually irreversible. (See also ALVEOLITIS.)

Pulmonary Function Tests

Tests to assess how the LUNGS are functioning. They range from simple spirometry (measuring breathing capacity) to sophisticated physiological assessments.

Static lung volumes and capacities can be measured: these include vital capacity – the maximum volume of air that can be exhaled slowly and completely after a maximum deep breath; forced vital capacity is a similar manoeuvre using maximal forceful exhalation and can be measured along with expiratory flow rates using simple spirometry; total lung capacity is the total volume of air in the chest after a deep breath in; functional residual capacity is the volume of air in the lungs at the end of a normal expiration, with all respiratory muscles relaxed.

Dynamic lung volumes and flow rates reflect the state of the airways. The forced expiratory volume (FEV) is the amount of air forcefully exhaled during the first second after a full breath – it normally accounts for over 75 per cent of the vital capacity. Maximal voluntary ventilation is calculated by asking the patient to breathe as deeply and quickly as possible for 12 seconds; this test can be used to check the internal consistency of other tests and the extent of co-operation by the patient, important when assessing possible neuromuscular weakness affecting respiration. There are several other more sophisticated tests which may not be necessary when assessing most patients. Measurement of arterial blood gases is also an important part of any assessment of lung function.

Pulmonary Hypertension

In this condition, increased resistance to the blood flow through the LUNGS occurs. This is usually the result of lung disease, and the consequence is an increase in pulmonary artery pressure and in the pressure in the right side of the heart and in the veins bringing blood to the heart. Chronic BRONCHITIS or EMPHYSEMA commonly constrict the small arteries in the lungs, thus causing pulmonary HYPERTENSION. (See also EISENMENGER SYNDROME.)

Pulmonary Oedema

Collection of water in the lungs caused by left ventricular failure or MITRAL STENOSIS which produces back pressure in the LUNGS, thus forcing fluid into the tissues. (See HEART, DISEASES OF.)

Pulmonary Stenosis

A disorder of the HEART in which obstruction of the outflow of blood from the right ventricle occurs. Narrowing of the pulmonary valve at the exit of the right ventricle and narrowing of the pulmonary artery may cause obstruction. The condition is usually congenital, although it may be caused by RHEUMATIC FEVER. In the congenital condition, pulmonary stenosis may occur with other heart defects and is then known as Fallot's tetralogy. Breathlessness and enlargement of the heart and eventual heart failure may be the consequence of pulmonary stenosis. Surgery is usually necessary to remove the obstruction.

Pulmonary Surfactant

Naturally produced in the LUNGS by cells called pneumocytes, this substance is a mixture of phospholipids (see PHOSPHOLIPID) and LIPO-PROTEINS. Present in fluid lining the alveoli (see ALVEOLUS) in the lungs, their action helps maintain their patency. Premature babies may have a deficiency of surfactant, a disorder which causes severe breathing difficulties – RESPIRATORY DISTRESS SYNDROME or hyaline membrane disease – and HYPOXIA. They will need urgent respiratory support, which includes oxygen and the administration (via an endotracheal tube) of a specially prepared surfactant such as beractant (bovine lung extract) or edfosceril palmitate.

Pulp

See under TEETH.

Pulsation

Also known as throbbing. An appearance seen or felt naturally below the fourth and fifth ribs on the left side, where the heart lies, and also at every point where an artery lies close beneath the surface. In other situations, it may be a sign of ANEURYSM. In thin people, pulsation can often be seen and felt in the upper part of the abdomen, due to the throbbing of the normal abdominal AORTA.

Pulse

If the tip of one finger is laid on the front of the forearm, about 2·5 cm (one inch) above the wrist, and about 1 cm (half an inch) from the outer edge, the pulsations of the radial artery can be felt. This is known as the pulse, but a pulse can be felt wherever an artery of large or medium size lies near the surface.

The cause of the pulsation lies in the fact that, at each heartbeat, 80–90 millilitres of blood are driven into the AORTA, and a fluid wave, distending the vessels as it passes, is transmitted along the ARTERIES all over the body. This pulsation falls away as the arteries grow smaller, and is finally lost in the minute capillaries, where a steady pressure is maintained. For this reason, the blood in the veins flows steadily on without any pulsation. Immediately after the wave has passed, the artery, by virtue of its great elasticity, regains its former size. The nature of this wave helps the doctor to assess the state of the artery and the action of the heart.

The pulse rate is usually about 70 per minute, but it may vary in health from 50 to 100, and is quicker in childhood and slower in old age than in middle life; it is low (at rest) in physically fit athletes or other sports people. Fever causes the rate to rise, sometimes to 120 beats a minute or more.

In childhood and youth the vessel wall is so thin that, when sufficient pressure is made to expel the blood from it, the artery can no longer be felt. In old age, however, and in some degenerative diseases, the vessel wall becomes so thick that it may be felt like a piece of whipcord rolling beneath the finger.

Different types of heart disease have special features of the pulse associated with them. In atrial FIBRILLATION the great character is irregularity. In patients with an incompetent AORTIC VALVE the pulse is characterised by a sharp rise and sudden collapse. (See HEART, DISEASES OF.)

An instrument known as the SPHYGMO-GRAPH registers the arterial waves and a polygraph (an instrument that obtains simultaneous tracings from several different sources such as radial and jugular pulse, apex beat of the heart and ELECTROCARDIOGRAM (ECG)) enables tracings to be taken from the pulse at the wrist and from the veins in the neck and simultaneous events in the two compared.

The pressure of the blood in various arteries is estimated by a SPHYGMOMANOMETER. (See BLOOD PRESSURE.)

Pulse Oximetry

Measurement of OXYGEN saturation of HAEMOGLOBIN in a blood sample using a non-invasive device called a spectrophotometer.

Pulsus Paradoxus

A big fall in a person's systolic BLOOD PRESSURE when he or she breathes in. It may occur in conditions such as constrictive PERICARDITIS and pericardial effusion, when the normal pumping action of the heart is hindered. ASTHMA may also cause pulsus paradoxus, as can CHRONIC OBSTRUCTIVE PULMONARY DISEASE (COPD).

Punctate Basophilia

See BASOPHILIA.

Punctum

See EYE – Eyelids.

Puncture

Description of a wound made by a sharp object, such as a knife, or by a surgical instrument. Puncture wounds, whether accidental (e.g. from a car accident) or deliberate (e.g. from a fight), are potentially dangerous. Despite an often small entry hole, serious damage may have been done to underlying tissues – for example, HEART, LUNGS, LIVER, or large blood vessel – and surgical exploration may be required to assess the extent of the injury. Punctures through the skin are also done deliberately in medicine to extract fluid or tissue through a hollow needle so that it can be examined in the laboratory. LUMBAR PUNCTURE, where cerebrospinal fluid is withdrawn, is one example.

Pupil

See EYE.

Purgatives

See LAXATIVES.

Purkinje Cells

Large specialised nerve cells occurring in great numbers in the cortex (superficial layer of grey matter) of the cerebellum of the BRAIN. They have a flask-shaped body, an AXON and branching tree-like extensions called dendrites, which extend towards the surface of the brain (see NEURON(E)).

Purpura

A skin rash caused by bleeding into the skin from capillary blood vessels. The discrete purple spots of the rash are called purpuric spots or, if very small, petechiae. The disorder may be caused by capillary defects (non-thrombocytopenic purpura) or be due to a deficiency of PLATELETS in the blood (thrombocytopenic purpura). Most worryingly, the rash may be due to a fulminant form of meningococcal SEPTICAEMIA called purpura fulminans. (See also HENOCH-SCHÖNLEIN PURPURA; IDIOPATHIC THROMBOCYTOPENIC PURPURA (ITP); THROMBOCYTOPENIA.).

Purulent
Containing, comprising or forming PUS.

Pus
Pus is a thick, white, yellow or greenish fluid, found in abscesses (see ABSCESS), ulcers, and on inflamed and discharging surfaces generally. Its colour and consistency are due to the presence of white blood corpuscles, and superficial cells of granulation tissue or of a mucous membrane which die and are shed off in consequence of the inflammatory process (see PHAGOCYTOSIS). Bacteria that normally produce pus are STREPTOCOCCUS, PNEUMOCOCCUS and ESCHERICHIA coli.

Pustule
A small collection of PUS. Malignant pustule is one of the forms of ANTHRAX.

Putrefaction
The change that takes place in the bodies of plants and animals after death, whereby they are ultimately reduced to carbonic acid gas, ammonia, and other simple substances. The change is almost entirely due to the action of bacteria, and, in the course of the process, various offensive and poisonous intermediate substances are formed. In the case of the human body, putrescine, cadaverine, and other alkaloids are among these intermediate products.

Putrid Fever
An old name for typhus fever (see ENTERIC FEVER).

PUVA
See PHOTOCHEMOTHERAPY; PSORIASIS.

PVS
See PERSISTENT VEGETATIVE STATE (PVS).

Pyaemia
A form of blood-poisoning in which abscesses (see ABSCESS) appear in various parts of the body. (See also SEPTICAEMIA.)

Pyelitis
A term describing inflammation of the pelvis of the kidney. In fact, the inflammation usually affects the whole kidney tissue and the description should be PYELONEPHRITIS.

Pyelogram
See INTRAVENOUS PYELOGRAM (UROGRAM).

Pyelography
The process whereby the KIDNEYS are rendered radio-opaque, and therefore visible on an X-ray film. It constitutes a most important part of the examination of a patient with kidney disease. (See SODIUM DIATRIZOATE.)

Pyelolithotomy
Surgery to remove a stone from the kidney (see KIDNEYS, DISEASES OF) via an incision in the pelvis of the kidney.

Pyelonephritis
Inflammation of the kidney (see KIDNEYS), usually the result of bacterial infection. The inflammation may be acute or chronic. Acute pyelonephritis comes on suddenly, is commoner in women, and tends to occur when they are pregnant. Infection usually spreads up the URETER from the URINARY BLADDER which has become infected (CYSTITIS). Fevers, chills and backache are the usual presenting symptoms. ANTIBIOTICS should be given, and in severe cases the intravenous route may be necessary. SEPTICAEMIA is an occasional complication.

Chronic pyelonephritis may start in childhood, and the usual cause is back flow of urine from the bladder into one of the ureters – perhaps because of a congenital deformity of the valve where the ureter drains into the bladder. Constant urine reflux results in recurrent infection of the kidney and damage to its tissue. Full investigation of the urinary tract is essential and, if an abnormality is detected, surgery may well be required to remedy it. HYPERTENSION and renal failure may be serious complications of pyelonephritis (see also KIDNEYS, DISEASES OF).

Pylephlebitis
Inflammation of the PORTAL VEIN. A rare but serious disorder, it usually results from the spread of infection within the abdomen – for example, appendicitis. The patient may develop liver abscesses and ASCITES. Treatment is by ANTIBIOTICS and surgery.

Pyloric Stenosis
Narrowing of the PYLORUS, the muscular exit

from the STOMACH. It is usually the result of a
pyloric ulcer or cancer near the exit of the
stomach. Food is delayed when passing from
the stomach to the duodenum and vomiting
occurs. The stomach may become distended
and peristalsis (muscular movement) may be
seen through the abdominal wall. Unless surgically treated the patient will steadily deteriorate,
losing weight, becoming dehydrated and developing ALKALOSIS.

A related condition, congenital hypertrophic
pyloric stenosis, occurs in babies (commonly
boys) about 3–5 weeks old, and surgery produces a complete cure.

Pyloromyotomy
Also called Ramstedt's operation, this is a surgical procedure to divide the muscle around the
outlet of the stomach (PYLORUS). It is done –
usually on babies – to relieve the obstruction
caused at the outlet by congenital PYLORIC
STENOSIS.

Pylorospasm
Spasm of the pyloric portion of the STOMACH.
This interferes with the passage of food in a
normal, gentle fashion into the intestine, causing the pain that comes on from half an hour
to three hours after meals; it is associated with
severe disorders of digestion. It is often produced by an ulcer of the stomach or
duodenum.

Pylorus
The lower opening of the STOMACH, through
which the softened and partially digested food
passes into the small INTESTINE.

Pyo-
A prefix attached to the name of various diseases to indicate cases in which PUS is formed,
such as pyonephrosis.

Pyoderma Gangrenosum
This is a disorder in which large ulcerating
lesions appear suddenly and dramatically in the
skin. It is the result of underlying VASCULITIS. It
is usually the result of inflammatory bowel disease such as ULCERATIVE COLITIS or CROHN'S
DISEASE but can be associated with RHEUMA-
TOID ARTHRITIS.

Pyogenic
Pyogenic is a term applied to those bacteria
which cause the formation of PUS and so lead to
the formation of abscesses (see ABSCESS).
Although many bacteria have this property, the
most common cause of abscess is one of

the rounded forms of bacterium (e.g.
streptococcus).

Pyorrhoea
Any copious discharge of PUS. For pyorrhoea
alveolaris, see under TEETH, DISORDERS OF.

Pyrazinamide
An antituberculous drug used in combination,
usually with RIFAMPICIN and ISONIAZID, as the
treatment regime for TUBERCULOSIS. It penetrates the MENINGES so is valuable in treating
tuberculous MENINGITIS. The drug is sometimes associated with liver damage and liver
function tests should be done before using it.

Pyrexia
See FEVER.

Pyridoxine
Pyridoxine, or vitamin B, plays an important
part in the metabolism of a number of AMINO
ACIDS. Deficiency leads to ATROPHY of the EPI-
DERMIS, the hair follicles, and the SEBACEOUS
glands, and peripheral NEURITIS may also occur.
Young infants are more susceptible to pyridoxine deficiency than adults: they begin to lose
weight and develop a hypochromic ANAEMIA;
irritability and CONVULSIONS may also occur.
Liver, yeast and cereals are relatively rich sources
of the vitamin; fish is a moderately rich source,
but vegetables and milk contain little. The minimal daily requirement in the diet is probably
about 2 mg. (See APPENDIX 5: VITAMINS.)

Pyrimethamine
An antimalarial drug used with either sulfadoxine or DAPSONE to treat *Plasmodium falciparum
malariae* (see MALARIA). It should not be used
for PROPHYLAXIS because of potentially severe
side-effects when used in the long term.

Pyromania
A powerful urge in a person to set things on fire.
Affected individuals, more commonly males,
are called pyromaniacs. They usually have a history of fascination with fire since childhood and
obtain pleasure or relief of tension from causing
fires. Treatment is difficult and pyromaniacs
commonly end up in the courts.

Pyrosis
See WATERBRASH.

Pyuria
The presence of PUS in the URINE, in consequence of inflammation situated in the KID-
NEYS, URINARY BLADDER or other part of the
urinary tract.

Q

QALY
This is an outcome measure of health care devised by health economists in the 1980s, and stands for Quality Adjusted Life Year. It takes a year of healthy life expectancy to be worth a grade of 1, and a year of unhealthy life expectancy to be worth less than 1. The worse the forecast of an unhealthy person's quality of life, the lower will be his or her rating. If someone is expected to live five years in a healthy state, the grading will be 5; ten years of life estimated to be only 25 per cent healthy will rate as 2·5 QALYs. The measure has proved controversial but nevertheless is an indication of the likely cost-effectiveness of a particular treatment, and can contribute to assessing whether or not a proposed or actual treatment or procedure is worthwhile – both for patients and for the economy.

Q Fever
A disease of worldwide distribution due to the organism *Coxiella burneti*. It is characterised by fever, severe headache and often PNEUMONIA. It was first described in 1937 amongst abattoir workers in Brisbane. The disease was given the name 'Q' fever, the Q (as in question mark) referring to the unknown cause of the disease when first described.

The principal reservoir of human infection in Britain is probably cattle and sheep in which the infection is usually sub-clinical. The diagnosis is confirmed by the detection of serum antibodies to *Coxiella burneti*. The organism is sensitive to tetracycline.

QRS Complex
The section of an ELECTROCARDIOGRAM (ECG) that precedes the S-T segment and registers contraction of the VENTRICLE of the HEART.

Q-T Interval
The interval in an ELECTROCARDIOGRAM (ECG) that registers the electrical activity generated during ventricular contraction of the HEART.

Quack
Colloquial description of an unqualified person claiming to be a medical doctor.

Quadrantanopia
Inability to see in one quarter of the visual field.

Homonymous quadrantanopia is loss of vision in the same quarter of the field in each EYE.

Quadriceps
(More accurately quadriceps femoris) – the large, four-headed muscle occupying the front and sides of the thigh, which straightens the leg at the knee-joint and maintains the body in an upright position. It comprises the rectus femoris, vastus lateralis, vastus intermedius and vastus medialis.

Quadriplegia
PARALYSIS of the four limbs of the body.

Quadruplets
See MULTIPLE BIRTHS.

Quantitative Digital Radiography
A radiological technique for detecting osteoporosis (see BONE, DISORDERS OF) in which a beam of X-rays is directed at the bone-area under investigation – normally the spine and hip – and the CALCIUM density measured. If the calcium content is low, preventive treatment can be started to reduce the likelihood of fractures occurring.

Quarantine
The principle of preventing the spread of infectious disease by which people, baggage, merchandise, and so forth likely to be infected or coming from an infected locality are isolated at frontiers or ports until their harmlessness has been proven to the satisfaction of the authorities. (See INFECTION.)

Originally quarantine, as its name implies, involved detention for 40 days; but the period now covers the incubation period of the disease, the presence of which is suspected.

Numerous international conferences upon the subject have been held with the view of arriving at a uniform practice as regards quarantine in different countries. The diseases to which quarantine applies are CHOLERA, YELLOW FEVER, PLAGUE, SMALLPOX, TYPHUS FEVER and RELAPSING FEVER.

The general practice with regard to quarantine is that when a serious disease breaks out in any country, the government of that country notifies surrounding governments as to the ports and other places that have become centres of infection. Any people travelling from these centres and attempting to enter another country, are subject to measures prescribed in the appropriate regulations. These measures vary with the disease involved.

Quartan Fever
Description of intermittent fever with paroxysms developing every fourth day. Usually applied to MALARIA.

Quickening
The first movements of a FETUS in the womb as experienced by the mother, usually around the 16th week of pregnancy (see PREGNANCY AND LABOUR).

Quiescent
The description applied to a disease in an individual which is in an inactive phase and so likely to be undiagnosed.

Quinghaosu
A herbal drug used for two millennia in China to treat MALARIA. Its action derives from sesquiterpene lactone, a substance that cuts the number of blood-borne malarial parasites.

Quinidine
An alkaloid (see ALKALOIDS) obtained from cinchona bark and closely related in chemical composition and in action to QUININE. It is commonly used in the form of quinidine sulphate to treat cardiac irregularities such as supraventricular tachycardia and ventricular arrhythmias (see HEART, DISEASES OF).

Quinine
An alkaloid (see ALKALOIDS) obtained from the bark of various species of cinchona trees. This bark is mainly derived from Peru and neighbouring parts of South America and the East Indies. Other alkaloids and acid substances are also derived from cinchona bark, such as QUINIDINE and cinchonine.

Quinine is generally used in the form of one of its salts, such as the sulphate of quinine, or dihydrochloride of quinine. All are sparingly soluble in water, much more so when taken along with an acid.

Action Quinine is a powerful antiseptic (see ANTISEPTICS). Its best-known action is in checking the recurrence of attacks of MALARIA, as it destroys malarial parasites in the blood. In fevers it acts as an antipyretic (see ANTIPYRETICS).

Among its side-effects are ringing in the ears, temporary impairment of vision, and sometimes disturbance of kidney function leading to renal failure.

Uses The most important use of quinine is its original one in malaria, attacks of which it quickly cuts short or prevents altogether. It has been largely replaced by more effective and less toxic antimalarial drugs; however, development of malarial parasites resistant to newer drugs has revived the use of quinine. For intravenous injection, when this is necessary in cases of malaria, a soluble form of quinine, the dihydrochloride, is used. Quinine can also be given in combination with other antimalarial drugs on medical advice. The drug is sometimes used in the treatment of cramps.

Quinolones
A group of chemically related synthetic ANTIBIOTICS. Examples include nalidixic acid, cinoxacin and norfloxocin which are effective in treating uncomplicated urinary-tract, respiratory-tract and gastrointestinal infections. They are usually effective against gram-negative and gram-positive bacteria (see GRAM'S STAIN). Many staphylococci – including METHICILLIN-RESISTANT STAPHYLOCOCCUS AUREUS (MRSA) – are resistant to quinolones. This group of drugs has a range of potentially troublesome side-effects including nausea, vomiting, DYSPEPSIA, abdominal pain, diarrhoea, dizziness, sleep disorders and PRURITUS.

Quinsy
A corruption of 'cynanche', this is an old name for a PERITONSILLAR ABSCESS.

Quintuplets
See MULTIPLE BIRTHS.

R

Rabies

An acute and potentially fatal disease, caused by a rhabdovirus called *Lyssavirus*, which affects the nervous system of animals, particularly carnivora, and may be communicated from them to humans. Infection from person to person is very rare, but those in attendance on a case should take precautions to avoid being bitten or allowing themselves to be contaminated by the patient's saliva, as this contains the causative virus.

The disease is ENDEMIC in dogs and wolves in some countries; an EPIDEMIC may occasionally occur. It also occurs in foxes, coyotes and skunks, as well as in vampire bats. Thanks to QUARANTINE measures, since 1897 rabies has been rare in Great Britain, which still retains strict measures (the Rabies Act) to prevent the entry of infected animals into the country, including a six-month quarantine period and vaccination (see IMMUNISATION). This policy was relaxed somewhat in 2001 with the launch of the Pet Travel Scheme; this allows cats and dogs to enter the UK from specified countries without the need for quarantine, as long as stringent conditions as to microchipping and vaccinations are met. Full details can be obtained from the Department for the Environment, Food and Rural Affairs (DEFRA) or from a veterinary surgeon engaged in operating the scheme. Six months has to elapse between vaccination against rabies and a positive blood test before the 'pet passport' can be issued.

Rabies is highly infectious from the bite of an animal already affected, but the chance of infection from different animals varies. Thus only about one person in every four bitten by rabid dogs contracts rabies, whilst the bites of rabid wolves and cats almost invariably produce disease.

Symptoms In animals there are two types of the disease: mad rabies and dumb rabies. In the former, the dog (or other animal) runs about, snapping at objects and other animals, unable to rest; in the latter, which is also the final stage of the mad type, the limbs become paralysed and the dog crawls about or lies still.

In humans the incubation period is usually 6–8 weeks, but may be as short as ten days or as long as two years. The disease begins with mental symptoms, the person becoming irritable, restless and depressed. Fever and DYSPHAGIA follow. The irritability passes into a form of MANIA and the victim has great difficulty in swallowing either food or drink.

Treatment The best treatment is, of course, preventive. Local treatment consists of immediate, thorough and careful cleansing of the wound-surfaces and surrounding skin. This is followed by a course of rabies vaccine therapy.

Only people bitten (or in certain circumstances, licked) by a rabid animal or by one thought to be infected with rabies need treatment; this is with rabies vaccine and antiserum and one of the IMMUNOGLOBULINS. A person previously vaccinated against rabies who is subsequently bitten by a rabid animal should be given three or four doses of the vaccine. The vaccine is also used to give protection to those liable to infection, such as kennel-workers and veterinary surgeons. Those who develop the disease require intensive care with ventilatory support, despite which the death rate is very high.

RAD

A unit of ionising RADIATION absorbed by an individual. The acronym stands for radiation absorbed dose.

Radial Artery

This artery arises from the brachial artery at the level of the neck of the radius. It passes down the forearm to the wrist, where it is easily palpated laterally. It then winds around the wrist to the palm of the hand to supply the fingers. (See ARTERIES.)

Radial Nerve

This NERVE arises from the BRACHIAL plexus in the axilla. At first descending posteriorly and then anteriorly, it ends just above the elbow by dividing into the superficial radial and interosseous nerves. It supplies motor function to the muscles which extend the arm, wrist, and some fingers, and supplies sensation to parts of the posterior and lateral aspects of the arm, forearm and hand.

Radiation

Energy in the form of waves or particles. Radiation is mainly electromagnetic and is broadly classified as ionising and non-ionising. The former can propel ions from an atom; these have an electrical charge and can combine chemically with each other. Ionisation occurring in molecules that have a key function in living tissue can cause biological damage which may affect existing tissue or cause mutations in the GENES of germ-cell nuclei (see GAMETE; CELLS). Non-ionising radiation agitates the constituent atoms of nuclei but is insufficiently powerful to produce ions.

Ionising radiation comprises X-RAYS, GAMMA RAYS and particle radiation. X-rays are part of the continuous electromagnetic-wave spectrum: this also includes gamma rays, infra-red radiation, ultraviolet light and visible light. They have a very short wavelength and very high frequency, and their ability to penetrate matter depends upon the electrical energy generating them. X-rays that are generated by 100,000 volts can pass through body tissue and are used to produce images – popularly known as X-rays. X-rays, generated at several million volts can destroy tissue and are used in RADIOTHERAPY for killing cancer cells. Gamma rays are similar to X-rays but are produced by the decay of radioactive materials. Particle radiation, which can be produced electrically or by radioactive decay, comprises parts of atoms which have mass as well as (usually) an electrical charge.

Non-ionising radiation includes ultraviolet light, radio waves, magnetic fields and ULTRASOUND. Magnetic fields are used in magnetic resonance imaging (MRI) and ultrasound, which is inaudible high-frequency sound waves, and is used for both diagnoses and treatment in medicine.

Radiation Sickness

The term applied to the nausea, vomiting and loss of appetite which may follow exposure to RADIATION – for example, at work – or the use of RADIOTHERAPY in the treatment of cancer and other diseases. People exposed to radiation at work should have that exposure carefully monitored so it does not exceed safety limits. Doses of radiation given during radiotherapy treatment are carefully measured: even so, patients may suffer side-effects. The phenothiazine group of tranquillisers, such as CHLORPROMAZINE, as well as the ANTIHISTAMINE DRUGS, are of value in the prevention and treatment of radiation sickness.

Radiculopathy

Radiculopathy is damage to the roots of nerves where they enter or leave the SPINAL CORD. Causes include ARTHRITIS of the spine, thickening of the MENINGES, and DIABETES MELLITUS. Symptoms include pain, PARAESTHESIA, numbness and wasting of muscles supplied by the nerves. Treatment is of the underlying cause.

Radioactive Isotopes

See ISOTOPE.

Radioactivity

Breakdown of the nuclei of some elements resulting in the emission of energy in the form of alpha, beta and gamma rays. Because of this particle emission, the elements decay into other elements. Radium and uranium are naturally occurring radioactive elements. RADIOTHERAPY treatment utilises artificially produced isotopes (alternative forms of an element) such as iodine-131 and cobalt-60.

Radiographer

An individual trained in the techniques of taking X-ray pictures (see X-RAYS) of areas of the body is known as a diagnostic radiographer. One who is trained to treat patients with RADIOTHERAPY is a therapeutic radiographer.

Radiography

Diagnostic radiography is the technique of examining parts of the body by passing X-RAYS through them to produce images on fluorescent screens or photographic plates.

Radioimmunoassay

A technique introduced in 1960 which enables the minute quantities of natural substances in the blood such as HORMONES to be measured. A radioimmunoassay depends upon the ability of an unlabelled hormone to inhibit, by simple competition, the binding of isotopically labelled hormone by specific ANTIBODIES. The requirements for a radioimmunoassay include adequate amounts of the hormone; a method for labelling the hormone with a radioactive isotope; the production of satisfactory antibodies; and a technique for separating antibody-bound from free hormone. Radioimmunoassay is more sensitive than the best bioassay for a given hormone, and the most sensitive radioimmunoassays permit the detection of picogram (pg = 10^{-12}g) and femtogram (fg = 10^{-15}g) amounts of material.

Radiology

See X-RAYS.

Radionuclide

Radionuclide is another word for a radioactive ISOTOPE. These isotopes are used in a scanning technique of body tissues. Different types of tissue – and normal or abnormal tissues – absorb varying amounts of the isotopes; these differences are detected, recorded and displayed on a screen.

Radio-Opaque

Substances which absorb X-RAYS, rather than transmitting them, appear white on X-ray film and are described as radio-opaque. This is true of bones, teeth, certain types of gall-stones, renal stones and contrast media used to enhance the accuracy of radiographic imaging.

Radiotherapy

The treatment of disease (mainly CANCER) with penetrating RADIATION. For many years RADIUM and X-RAYS were the only sources available, but developments in knowledge led to the use of powerful X-rays, beta rays or gamma rays, either produced by linear accelerator machines or given off by radioactive isotopes (see ISOTOPE). The latter is rarely used now.

Beams of radiation may be directed at the tumour from a distance, or radioactive material – in the form of needles, wires or pellets – may be implanted in the body. Sometimes germ-cell tumours (see SEMINOMA; TERATOMA) and lymphomas (see LYMPHOMA) are particularly sensitive to irradiation which therefore forms a major part of management, particularly for localised disease. Many head and neck tumours, gynaecological cancers, and localised prostate and bladder cancers are curable with radiotherapy. Radiotherapy is also valuable in PALLIATIVE CARE, chiefly the reduction of pain from bone metastases (see METASTASIS). Side-effects are potentially hazardous and these have to be balanced against the substantial potential benefits. Depending upon the type of therapy and doses used, generalised effects include lethargy and loss of appetite, while localised effects – depending on the area treated – include dry, itchy skin; oral infection (e.g. thrush – see CANDIDA); bowel problems; and DYSURIA.

Radium

The radiations of radium consist of: (1) alpha rays, which are positively charged helium nuclei; (2) beta rays – negatively charged electrons; (3) gamma rays, similar to X-RAYS but of shorter wavelength. These days the use of radium is largely restricted to the treatment of carcinoma of the neck of the womb, the tongue, and the lips. Neither X-rays nor radium supersede active surgical measures when these are available for the complete removal of a tumour.

Radius

The outer of the two bones in the forearm.

Râle

See CREPITATIONS.

Raloxifene

A drug used to prevent and treat postmenopausal osteoporosis (see under BONE, DISORDERS OF). Its action differs from hormone-replacement drugs in that it does not modify the symptoms of the MENOPAUSE.

Randomised Controlled Trial

A method of comparing the results between two or more groups of patients intentionally subjected to different methods of treatment – or sometimes of prevention. Those subjects entering the trial have to give their informed permission. They are allocated to their respective groups using random numbers, with one group (controls) receiving no active treatment, instead receiving either PLACEBO or a traditional treatment. Preferably, neither the subject nor the assessor should know which 'regimen' is allocated to which subject: this is known as a double-blind trial.

Ranitidine

An H$_2$-receptor antagonist drug used in the treatment of DUODENAL ULCER by reducing the hyperacidity of the gastric juice. The drug blocks the production of histamine produced by mast cells in the stomach lining. Histamine stimulates the acid-secreting cells in the stomach. Ranitidine, like other H$_2$-blocking drugs, should be used in combination with an antibiotic drug to treat ulcers caused by *Helicobacter pylori* infection in the stomach. The drug should be given for up to eight weeks with repeat courses if ulcers recur.

Ranula

A swelling which occasionally appears beneath the tongue, caused by a collection of saliva in the distended duct of a salivary gland. (See also MOUTH, DISEASES OF.)

Rape

A criminal offence in which sexual intercourse takes place with an unwilling partner, female or male, under threat of force or violence. Reported rape cases have increased in number in recent years, but it is hard to know whether this is because the incidence of rape has increased or because the victims – women and men – are more willing to report the crime. A more sympathetic and understanding approach by the police, courts and society generally has resulted in the provision of greater support for victims who are usually severely traumatised psychologically as well as physically. It is argued that rape is motivated by a desire to dominate rather than simply an attempt to achieve sexual gratification. The majority of rapes are probably unreported because of the victims' shame, anxiety about publicity and fear that the rapist will take reprisals. It is legally recognised that rape can happen within marriage. There are moves to make court proceedings less traumatic for victims, whose attackers are often known to them.

Anxiety, DEPRESSION and POST-TRAUMATIC STRESS DISORDER (PTSD) are common after rape: many victims are now given help by rape crisis counselling. A recent report suggests that in at least 50 per cent of reported rapes, the attacker was known to, or had been a friend of, the victim. The deliberate misuse of alcohol or drugs to reduce a potential victim's resistance seems to be increasing (see DRUG ASSISTED RAPE; FLUNITRAZEPAM.)

Raphe
A ridge or furrow between the halves of an organ.

Rarefaction
Diminution in the density of a BONE as a result of withdrawal of calcium salts from it. (See BONE, DISORDERS OF – Osteoporosis.)

Rash
See ERUPTION.

Rat-Bite Fever
An infectious disease following the bite of a rat. There are two causative organisms – *Spirillum minus* and *Actinobacillus muris* – and the incubation period depends upon which is involved. In the case of the former it is 5–30 days; in the case of the latter it is 2–10 days. The disease is characterised by fever, a characteristic skin rash and often muscular or joint pains. It responds well to PENICILLIN.

Raynaud's Disease
So called after Maurice Raynaud (1834–81), the Paris physician who published a thesis on the subject in 1862. This is a condition in which the circulation (see CIRCULATORY SYSTEM OF THE BLOOD) becomes suddenly obstructed in outlying parts of the body. It is supposed to be due to spasm of the smaller arteries in the affected part, as the result of them responding abnormally to impulses from the SYMPATHETIC NERVOUS SYSTEM. Its effects are increased both by cold and by various diseases involving the blood vessels.

Symptoms The condition is most commonly confined to the occurrence of 'dead fingers' – the fingers (or the toes, ears, or nose) becoming white, numb, and waxy-looking. This condition may last for some minutes, or may not pass off for several hours, or even for a day or two.

Treatment People who are subject to these attacks should be careful in winter to protect the feet and hands from cold, and should always use warm water when washing the hands. In addition, the whole body should be kept warm, as spasm of the arterioles in the feet and hands may be induced by chilling of the body. Sufferers should not smoke. VASODILATORS are helpful, especially the calcium antagonists. In all patients who do not respond to such medical treatment, surgery should be considered in the form of sympathectomy: i.e. cutting of the sympathetic nerves to the affected part. This results in dilatation of the arterioles and hence an improved blood supply. This operation is more successful in the case of the feet than in the case of the hands.

RCN
Stands for Royal College of Nursing.

Reactive Arthritis
An aseptic (that is, not involving infection) ARTHRITIS secondary to an episode of infection elsewhere in the body. It often occurs in association with ENTERITIS caused by salmonella (see FOOD POISONING) and certain SHIGELLA strains, and in both YERSINEA and CAMPYLOBACTER enteritis. Non-gonococcal urethritis, usually due to CHLAMYDIA, is another cause of reactive arthritis; Reiter's syndrome is a particularly florid form, characterised by mucocutaneous and ocular lesions.

The SYNOVITIS usually starts acutely and is frequently asymmetrical, with the knees and ankles most commonly affected. Often there are inflammatory lesions of tendon sheaths and entheses (bone and muscle functions) such as plantar fasciitis (see FASCIITIS). The severity and duration of the acute episode are extremely variable. Individuals with the histocompatibility antigen HLA B27 are particularly prone to severe attacks.

Read Codes
These form an agreed UK thesaurus of healthcare terminology named after the general practitioner who devised them initially in the 1970s. The coding system provides a basis for computerised clinical records that can be shared across professional and administrative boundaries. Such records have essential safeguards for

security and confidentiality. The codes accommodate the different views of specialists, but use simple terms without any loss of the fine detail necessary in specialist terminology. The Read Codes are being merged with the world's other leading coding and classification system: the College of American Pathologists' Systemised Nomenclature of Medicine (SNOMED-RT).

Receptor
(1) Organs, which may consist of one cell or a small group of cells, that respond to different forms of external or internal stimuli by conveying impulses down nerves to the CENTRAL NERVOUS SYSTEM, alerting it to changes in the internal or external environment.
(2) A small, discrete area on the cell membrane or within the cell with which molecules or molecular complexes (e.g. hormones, drugs, and other chemical messengers) interact. When this interaction takes place it initiates a change in the working of the cell.

Recessive
Tending to recede. In genetic terms, a recessive gene is one whose expression remains dormant if paired with an unlike allele. The trait will only be manifest in an individual homozygous for the recessive gene. (See GENES.)

Recombinant DNA
DNA or deoxyribonucleic acid containing GENES from various sources that have been combined by GENETIC ENGINEERING.

Recombinant DNA Technology
See GENETIC ENGINEERING.

Reconstructive (Plastic) Surgery
Reconstructive surgery on the skin and underlying tissues that have been damaged or lost as a result of disease or injury. Congenital malformations are also remedied using reconstructive surgery. Surgeons graft healthy skin from another part of the body to repair skin damaged or destroyed by burns or injuries. New techniques are under development for growing new skin in the laboratory to be used in reconstructive surgery. Surgeons also repair damage using skin flaps prepared in another part of the body – for example, a skin flap from the arm may be used to repair a badly injured nose or face. Reconstructive surgery is also used to repair the consequences of an operation for cancer of, say, the neck or the jaw. Plastic surgeons undertake cosmetic surgery to improve the appearance of noses, breasts, abdomens and faces.

Recovered Memory Syndrome
See REPRESSED MEMORY THERAPY.

Recovery Position
If an individual is unconscious – whether as a result of accident or illness or when in the postoperative recovery unit – but is breathing and has a pulse, he or she should be placed in the recovery position. The individual is turned on his or her side to allow the tongue to fall forwards and so reduce the likelihood of pharyngeal obstruction (see PHARYNX). Fluid in the mouth can also drain outwards instead of into the TRACHEA and LUNGS. The person can lie on either side with upper or lower leg flexed. Sometimes the semi-prone position is used; this gives better drainage from the mouth and greater stability during transport, but makes it more difficult to observe the face, colour or breathing. (See APPENDIX 1: BASIC FIRST AID.)

Recrudescence
The reappearance of a disease after a period without signs or symptoms of its presence.

Rectum
The last part of the large INTESTINE. It pursues a more or less straight course downwards through the cavity of the pelvis, lying against the sacrum at the back of this cavity. This section of the intestine is about 23 cm (9 inches) long: its first part is freely movable and corresponds to the upper three pieces of the sacrum; the second part corresponds to the lower two pieces of the sacrum and the coccyx; whilst the third part, known also as the anal canal, is about 25 mm (1 inch) long, runs downwards and backwards, and is kept tightly closed by the internal and external SPHINCTER muscles which surround it. The opening to the exterior is known as the ANUS. The structure of the rectum is similar to that of the rest of the intestine.

Rectum, Diseases of
The following are described under their separate dictionary entries: FAECES; HAEMORRHOIDS; FISTULA; DIARRHOEA; CONSTIPATION.

Imperforate anus, or absence of the anus, may occur in newly born children, and the condition is relieved by operation.

Itching at the anal opening is common and can be troublesome. It may be due to slight abrasions, to piles, to the presence of threadworms (see ENTEROBIASIS), and/or to anal sex. The anal area should be bathed once or twice a day; clothing should be loose and smooth. Local application of soothing preparations containing mild astringents (bismuth subgallate, zinc oxide and hamamelis) and CORTICOSTEROIDS may provide symptomatic relief. Proprietary preparations contain lubricants, VASOCONSTRICTORS and mild ANTISEPTICS.

Pain on defaecation is commonly caused by a small ulcer or fissure, or by an engorged haemorrhoid (pile). Haemorrhoids may also cause an aching pain in the rectum. (See also PROCTALGIA.)

Abscess in the cellular tissue at the side of the rectum – known from its position as an ischio-rectal abscess – is fairly common and may produce a fistula. Treatment is by ANTIBIOTICS and, if necessary, surgery to drain the abscess.

Prolapse or protrusion of the rectum is sometimes found in children, usually between the ages of six months and two years. This is generally a temporary disorder. Straining at defaecation by adults can cause the lining of the rectum to protrude outside the anus, resulting in discomfort, discharge and bleeding. Treatment of the underlying constipation is essential as well as local symptomatic measures (see above). Haemorrhoids sometimes prolapse. If a return to normal bowel habits with the production of soft faeces fails to restore the rectum to normal, surgery to remove the haemorrhoids may be necessary. If prolapse of the rectum recurs, despite a return to normal bowel habits, surgery may be required to rectify it.

Tumours of small size situated on the skin near the opening of the bowel, and consisting of nodules, tags of skin, or cauliflower-like excrescences, are common, and may give rise to pain, itching and watery discharges. These are easily removed if necessary. Polypi (see POLYPUS) occasionally develop within the rectum, and may give rise to no pain, although they may cause frequent discharges of blood. Like polypi elsewhere, they may often be removed by a minor operation. (See also POLYPOSIS.)

Cancer of the rectum and colon is the commonest malignancy in the gastrointestinal tract: around 17,000 people a year die from these conditions in the United Kingdom. Rectal cancer is more common in men than in women; colonic cancer is more common in women. Rectal cancer is a disease of later life, seldom affecting young people, and its appearance is

generally insidious. The tumour begins commonly in the mucous membrane, its structure resembling that of the glands with which the membrane is furnished, and it quickly infiltrates the other coats of the intestine and then invades neighbouring organs. Secondary growths in most cases occur soon in the lymphatic glands within the abdomen and in the liver. The symptoms appear gradually and consist of diarrhoea, alternating with attacks of constipation, and, later on, discharges of blood or blood-stained fluid from the bowels, together with weight loss and weakness. A growth can be well advanced before it causes much disturbance. Treatment is surgical and usually this consists of removal of the whole of the rectum and the distal two-thirds of the sigmoid colon, and the establishment of a COLOSTOMY. Depending upon the extent of the tumour, approximately 50 per cent of the patients who have this operation are alive and well after five years. In some cases in which the growth occurs in the upper part of the rectum, it is now possible to remove the growth and preserve the anus so that the patient is saved the discomfort of having a colostomy. RADIOTHERAPY and CHEMOTHERAPY may also be necessary.

Recurrent Laryngeal Nerve
A branch of the vagus NERVE which leaves the latter low down in its course, and – hooking around the right subclavian artery on the right side and round the arch of the aorta on the left – runs up again into the neck, where it enters the larynx and supplies branches to the muscles which control the vocal cords.

Red Blood Cell
See ERYTHROCYTES; BLOOD.

Red Cross
See FIRST AID.

Reduction
The manipulation of part of the body from an abnormal position to the correct one (e.g. fractures, dislocations or hernias).

Reduction Division
See MEIOSIS.

Referred Pain
Pain felt in one part of the body which is actually arising from a distant site (e.g. pain from the diaphragm is felt at the shoulder tip). This occurs because both sites develop from similar embryological tissue and therefore have

common pain pathways in the CENTRAL NER-
VOUS SYSTEM. (See also PAIN.)

Reflex Action

One of the simplest forms of activity of the
nervous system. (For the mechanism upon
which it depends, see NERVOUS SYSTEM; NEUR-
ON(E).) Reflex acts are divided usually into three
classes.

Superficial reflexes comprise the sudden
movements which result when the skin is
brushed or pricked, such as the movement of
the toes that results from stroking the sole of
the foot.

Deep reflexes depend upon the state of
mild contraction in which muscles are constantly maintained when at rest, and are
obtained, as in the case of the knee-jerk (see
below), by sharply tapping the tendon of the
muscle in question.

Visceral reflexes are those connected with
various organs, such as the narrowing of the
pupil when a bright light is directed upon the
EYE, and the contraction of the URINARY BLAD-
DER when distended by urine.

Faults in these reflexes give valuable evidence
as to the presence and site of neurological disorders. Thus, absence of the knee-jerk, when
the patellar tendon is tapped, means some
interference with the sensory nerve, nerve-cells,
or motor nerve upon which the act depends –
as, for example, in POLIOMYELITIS, or peripheral NEURITIS; whilst an exaggerated jerk
implies that the controlling influence exerted by
the BRAIN upon this reflex mechanism has been
cut off – as, for example, by a tumour high up
in the SPINAL CORD, or in the disease known as
MULTIPLE SCLEROSIS (MS).

Reflux

Fluid flowing in the opposite direction to normal (i.e. back flow). Often refers to regurgitation of stomach contents into the OESOPHAGUS
(see also OESOPHAGUS, DISEASES OF), or of urine
from the URINARY BLADDER back into the
ureters (see URETER).

Refraction

The deviation of rays of light on passing from
one transparent medium into another of different density. The refractive surfaces of the EYE
are the anterior surface of the cornea (which
accounts for approximately two-thirds of the
focusing or refractive power of the eye), and
the lens (one-third of the focusing power of the

eye). The refractive power of the lens can
change, whereas that of the cornea is fixed. (For
errors of refraction, see under EYE, DISORDERS
OF.)

Refractory

Unresponsive or resistant to treatment.

Regimen

A course of treatment – possibly combining
drugs, exercise, diet, etc. – designed to bring
about an improvement in health.

Regional Anaesthesia

See ANAESTHESIA – Local anaesthetics.

Regional Ileitis

See ILEITIS.

Registrar

(1) Divided into specialist registrar and GP
registrar, this is a training grade for NHS doctors. After a period in this grade – usually 3–6
years – they may be appointed as GP principals or gain a certificate of specialist training
and be able to apply for NHS consultant
posts (provided they have passed the appropriate higher examinations). In 2004 there were
almost 15,000 specialist registrars in the UK
and more than 1,800 GP registrars. Registrar
numbers are also regulated by the government
to achieve a balance between the numbers in
training and the likely number of vacancies
for career-grade doctors or dentists in the
future.
(2) A public official responsible for registering
births, deaths, and marriages.

Regulation of Health Professions

Professional staff working in health care are
registered with and regulated by several statutory bodies: doctors by the GENERAL MEDICAL
COUNCIL (GMC); dentists by the GENERAL DEN-
TAL COUNCIL; nurses and midwives by the
Council for Nursing and Midwifery, formerly
the UK Central Council for Nursing, Midwifery and Health Visiting (see NURSING);
PHARMACISTS by the Royal Pharmaceutical
Society; and the professions supplementary to
medicine (chiropody, dietetics, medical laboratory sciences, occupational therapy, orthoptics, physiotherapy and radiography) by the
Council for Professions Supplementary to
Medicine. In 2002, the Council for the Regulation of Health Care Professions was set up
as a statutory body that will promote co-
operation between and give advice to existing

R

regulatory bodies, provide a quality-control mechanism, and play a part in promoting the interests of patients. The new Council is accountable to a Select Committee of Parliament and is a non-ministerial government department similar in status to the FOOD STANDARDS AGENCY. It has the right to scrutinise the decisions of its constituent bodies and can apply for judicial review if it feels that a judgement by a disciplinary committee has been too lenient.

Regurgitation

Regurgitation is a term used in various connections in medicine. For instance, in diseases of the HEART it is used to indicate a condition in which, as the result of valvular disease, the blood does not entirely pass on from the atria of the heart to the ventricles, or from the ventricles into the arteries. The defective valve is said to be incompetent, and a certain amount of blood leaks past it, or regurgitates back, into the cavity from which it has been driven. (See HEART, DISEASES OF.)

The term is also applied to the return to the mouth of food already swallowed and present in the gullet or stomach (see also REFLUX).

Rehabilitation

The restoration to health and working capacity of a person incapacitated by disease – mental or physical – or by injury. Treatment usually includes OCCUPATIONAL THERAPY, PHYSIOTHERAPY and PSYCHOTHERAPY depending upon the type of disease or injury. Rehabilitation is commonly carried out at special centres, either on a daily or a residential basis. This allows different types of specialists to co-operate in the patient's rehabilitation. (See also DISABLED PERSONS.)

Reiter's Syndrome

A condition probably caused by an immunological response to a virus (see IMMUNITY), in which the patient has URETHRITIS, ARTHRITIS and conjunctivitis (see under EYE, DISORDERS OF). The skin may also be affected by horny areas which develop in it. The disorder was first described by a German physician, H. Reiter (1881–1969); it is more common in men than in women, and is the most common cause of arthritis in young men. It usually develops in people who have a genetic predisposition for it: around 80 per cent of sufferers have the HLA B27 tissue type. Treatment is symptomatic with ANALGESICS and NON-STEROIDAL ANTI-INFLAMMATORY DRUGS (NSAIDS). (See also REACTIVE ARTHRITIS.)

Rejection

A term used in transplant medicine (see TRANSPLANTATION) to describe the body's immunological response to foreign tissue (see IMMUNITY). Various drugs, such as CICLOSPORIN A, can be used to dampen the host's response to a graft or organ transplant and reduce the risk of rejection.

Relapse

The return of a disease that a patient has had and apparently recovered from. It may also be a worsening of a disease from which a person is still recovering.

Relapsing Fever

So-called because of the characteristic temperature chart showing recurring bouts of fever, this is an infectious disease caused by SPIROCHAETE. There are two main forms of the disease.

Louse-borne relapsing fever is an EPIDEMIC disease, usually associated with wars and famines, which has occurred in practically every country in the world. For long confused with TYPHUS FEVER and typhoid fever (see ENTERIC FEVER), it was not until the 1870s that the causal organism was described by Obermeier. It is now known as the *Borrelia recurrentis*, a motile spiral organism 10–20 micrometres in length. The organism is transmitted from person to person by the louse, *Pediculus humanus*.

Symptoms The incubation period is up to 12 days (but usually seven). The onset is sudden, with high temperature, generalised aches and pains, and nose-bleeding. In about half of cases, a rash appears at an early stage, beginning in the neck and spreading down over the trunk and arms. JAUNDICE may occur; and both the LIVER and the SPLEEN are enlarged. The temperature subsides after five or six days, to rise again in about a week. There may be up to four such relapses (see the introductory paragraph above).

Treatment Preventive measures are the same as those for typhus. Rest in bed is essential, as are good nursing and a light, nourishing diet. There is usually a quick response to PENICILLIN; the TETRACYCLINES and CHLORAMPHENICOL are also effective. Following such treatment the incidence of relapse is about 15 per cent. The mortality rate is low, except in a starved population.

Tick-borne relapsing fever is an ENDEMIC disease which occurs in most tropical and sub-tropical countries. The causative organism is *Borrelia duttoni*, which is transmitted by a tick, *Ornithodorus moubata*. David Livingstone suggested that it was a tick-borne disease, but it was not until 1905 that Dutton and Todd produced the definitive evidence.

Symptoms The main differences from the louse-borne disease are: (*a*) the incubation period is usually shorter, 3–6 days (but may be as short as two days or as long as 12); (*b*) the febrile period is usually shorter, and the afebrile periods are more variable in duration, sometimes only lasting for a day or two; (*c*) relapses are much more numerous.

Treatment Preventive measures are more difficult to carry out than in the case of the louse-borne infection. Protective clothing should always be worn in 'tick country', and old, heavily infected houses should be destroyed. Curative treatment is the same as for the louse-borne infection.

Relate Marriage Guidance
The idea of a marriage-guidance council came from a group of doctors, clergy and social workers who were concerned for the welfare of marriage. It is based upon two major concepts: that marriage provides the best possible way for a man and woman to live together and rear their children; and that the counsellors share a basic respect for the unique personality of the individual and his (or her) right to make his (or her) own decisions. The organisation consists of between 120 and 130 Marriage Guidance Councils throughout the country, comprising about 1,250 counsellors. These Councils are affiliated to Relate National Marriage Guidance, which is responsible for the selection, training and continued supervision of all counsellors. Anyone seeking help can telephone or write for an appointment. No fees are charged, but those receiving help are encouraged to donate what they can.

Relaxation Therapy
This is a treatment in which patients are helped to reduce their levels of anxiety by reducing their muscle tone. It can be used on its own or in conjunction with a broader PSYCHOTHERAPY regime. The technique guides people on how to cope with stressful situations and deal with phobias – see PHOBIA.

Relenza
See ZANAMOVIR.

Remission
A period when a disease has responded to treatment and there are no signs or symptoms present.

Remittent Fever
The term applied to the form of fever in which, during remissions (see REMISSION), the temperature falls, but not to normal.

REM Sleep
Rapid-eye-movement is a stage during SLEEP in which the eyes are seen to move rapidly beneath the lids and during which dreaming occurs. It occurs for several minutes at a time approximately every 100 minutes.

Renal
Related to the KIDNEYS.

Renal Cell Carcinoma
See HYPERNEPHROMA.

Renal Diseases
See KIDNEYS, DISEASES OF.

Renal Tubule
See KIDNEYS.

Renin
An ENZYME produced by the kidney (see KIDNEYS) and released into the blood in response to STRESS. Renin reacts with a compound produced by the liver to produce ANGIOTENSIN. This causes blood vessels to constrict and raises the blood pressure. If too much renin is produced, this results in renal HYPERTENSION.

Rennin
A milk-coagulating ENZYME produced by the lining of the stomach. Rennin converts milk protein (caseinogen) into insoluble casein, thus ensuring that milk stays in the stomach for some time, during which it can be digested by various enzymes before passing into the small intestine.

Renography
The radiological examination of the KIDNEYS using a gamma camera. This is a device that can follow the course of an injected radioactive (see RADIOACTIVITY) compound which is concentrated and excreted by the kidneys. This provides information on kidney function.

Repetitive Strain Injury (RSI)
See UPPER LIMB DISORDERS.

Repressed Memory Therapy
Also called recovered memory syndrome, this

treatment was developed in the wake of the widespread exposure in the 1980s and 90s of the frequency of child sexual abuse. A controversial concept emerged in the USA, picked up later by some experts in the UK, that abused children sometimes suppress their unpleasant memories, and that subsequent PSYCHO-THERAPY could help some victims to recover these memories – thus possibly aiding rehabilitation. This recall of 'repressed' memories, however, was believed by some psychiatrists to be, in effect, a false memory implanted into the victim's subconscious by the psychotherapy itself – or perhaps invented by the individual for personal motives.

In 1997 the Royal College of Psychiatrists in the UK produced a comprehensive report which was sceptical about the notion that the awareness of recurrent severe sexual abuse in children could be pushed entirely out of consciousness. The authors did not believe that events could remain inaccessible to conscious memory for decades, allegedly provoking vague non-specific symptoms to be recovered during psychotherapy with resolution of the symptoms. Supporting evidence pointed to the lack of any empirical proof that unconscious dissociation of unpleasant memories from conscious awareness occurred to protect the individual. Furthermore, experimental and natural events had shown that false memories, created through suggestion or influence, could be implanted. Many individuals who had claimed to have recovered memories of abuse subsequently withdrew and, often, non-specific symptoms allegedly linked to suppression worsened rather than improved as therapy to unlock memories proceeded. The conclusion is that recovered memory therapy should be viewed with great caution.

Reproductive System

A collective term for all the organs involved in sexual reproduction. In the female these are the OVARIES, FALLOPIAN TUBES, UTERUS, VAGINA and VULVA. In the male these are the testes (see TESTICLE), VAS DEFERENS, SEMINAL VESICLES, URETHRA and PENIS.

Research

In medicine, the collation and assessment of existing facts and knowledge, and the critical systematic investigation of the normal and abnormal functioning of the body, along with the EPIDEMIOLOGY of diseases and disorders affecting it – the aim being to increase the sum of knowledge in respect of the prevention, diagnosis and treatment of disease.

Ethics of research Although Britain has had legislation governing aspects of research on animals since the 19th century, there is no overarching statute regulating research on humans and human material. Such activity is covered in law by the vaguely defined common-law concept of consent, and by piecemeal legislation such as the DATA PROTECTION ACT 1998 and the HUMAN FERTILISATION & EMBRYOLOGY ACT 1990. Nevertheless, extensive and very detailed ethical guidance on aspects of research has been published by a wide range of national and international organisations (see ETHICS COMMITTEES). Several basic principles feature in all statements about research ethics: these include the importance of ensuring that research is independently and rigorously scrutinised by appropriately constituted ethics committees; verifying that any risk to the research subject is reasonable in relation to the anticipated benefit; and ensuring that all efforts are made to minimise possible harm. The research subject's willingness to tolerate some risk does not relieve researchers of the responsibility of making sure that all risks are kept to a minimum. Above all, a key feature of ethical research has involved seeking informed consent from research participants. This rule, initially applied to actual involvement by human subjects in research, has gradually been extended to include seeking informed consent from patients or from their relatives to the use of data and to the use of human organs and tissue in research, including after POST-MORTEM EXAMINATION. (See also EVIDENCE-BASED MEDICINE.)

Research Fraud and Misconduct

Research misconduct is defined as behaviour by a researcher that falls short of good ethical and scientific standards – whether or not this be intentional. For example, the same data may be sent for publication to more than one medical journal, which might have the effect of their being counted twice in any META-ANALYSIS or systematic review; or the data may be 'salami sliced' to try to make the maximum number of publications, even though the data may overlap. Fraud in the context of research is defined as the generation of false data with the intent to deceive. It is much less frequent than carelessness, but its incidence is estimated as between 0.1 and 1 per cent. A figure of 1 per cent means that, in the United Kingdom at any one time, maybe 30 studies are being conducted, or their results published, which could contain false information. Examples include forged ethics-committee approval, patient signatures and diary cards; fabricated figures and results;

invention of non-existent patient subjects; or sharing one electrocardiogram or blood sample amongst many subjects.

Research fraud should be first suspected by a clinical-trial monitor who recognises that data are not genuine, or by a quality-assurance auditor who cannot reconcile data in clinical-trial report forms with original patient records. Unfortunately, it often comes to light by chance. There may be suspicious similarities between data ostensibly coming from more than one source, or visits may have been recorded when it was known that the clinic was shut. Statistical analysis of a likely irregularity will frequently confirm such suspicion. The motivation for fraud is usually greed, but a desire to publish at all costs, to be the original author of a medical breakthrough, to bolster applications for research grants, or to strengthen a bid for more departmental resources are other recognised reasons for committing fraud.

In the USA, those proved to have committed fraud are debarred from receiving federal funds for research purposes or from undertaking government-funded therapeutic research. The four Nordic countries (Denmark, Finland, Norway and Sweden) have committees on research dishonesty that investigate all cases of suspected research misconduct. In the United Kingdom, an informal system operated by the pharmaceutical industry, using the disciplinary mechanism of the General Medical Council (GMC), has led to more than 16 doctors in the past ten years being disciplined for having committed research fraud. Editors of many of the world's leading medical journals have united to form the Committee on Publishing Ethics, which advises doctors on proper practice and assists them in retracting or refusing to publish articles found or known to be false. (See ETHICS; ETHICS COMMITTEES.) Where an author does not offer a satisfactory explanation, the matter is passed to his or her institution to investigate; where an editor or the committee is not satisfied with the result they may pass the complaint to the appropriate regulatory body, such as the GMC in Britain.

Resection
The name of an operation in which a part of some organ is removed, as, for example, the resection of a fragment of dead bone or of a diseased section of intestine.

Reserpine
An alkaloid (see ALKALOIDS) obtained from the root of rauwolfia that has been and continues to

be used as an anti-hypertensive (see HYPERTEN-SION) and a tranquillising agent.

Reserve Volume
The additional amount of air that a person could breathe in or out if he or she were not using the full capacity of their LUNGS. (See also LUNG VOLUMES.)

Residual Volume
The amount of air left in the LUNGS after an individual has breathed out as much as possible. It is a measure of lung function: for example, in a person with EMPHYSEMA the residual volume is increased. (See RESPIRATION; LUNG VOLUMES.)

Resistance
In a medical context, resistance has several meanings. The walls of blood vessels exert resistance to the flow of blood and this rises as the diameters of the vessels diminish. This in turn leads to a rise in blood pressure: the phenomenon may be physiological or pathological.

Resistance may also mean the extent of the body's IMMUNITY – an indication of its ability to withstand disease. Another meaning relates to the development of resistance in a bacterium (see BACTERIA) to the effects on it of ANTIBIOTICS.

In PSYCHOANALYSIS, resistance refers to the blocking-off from a person's consciousness of repressed emotions and memories. A psychoanalyst helps the patient to break this resistance and bring the repressed material out into the open. (See also REPRESSED MEMORY THERAPY.)

Resistin
A new hormone (see HORMONES) recently identified by researchers in the United States. It links OBESITY to type 2 diabetes (see DIABETES MELLITUS – Non-insulin dependent diabetes mellitus (NIDDM)) and its name is based on its action – namely, resistance to INSULIN. This resistance is a hallmark of this type of diabetes and is manifested throughout the body. THIAZOLIDINEDIONE DRUGS, a new class of antidiabetic drugs that lower insulin resistance, are mediated by receptors which are abundant in fat cells, and the researchers claim to have identified a fat-cell PROTEIN that may be responsible for this and which they believe to be a hormone; it was also found in high concentrations in diabetic mice.

Resolution
A term applied to infective processes, to indicate a natural subsidence of the INFLAMMATION

without the formation of PUS. Thus a pneumonic lung is said to 'resolve' when the material exuded into it is absorbed into the blood and lymph, so that recovery takes place naturally; an inflamed area is said to resolve when the inflammation diminishes and no abscess forms; a glandular enlargement is said to resolve when it decreases in size without suppuration. Resolution is also used to describe the extent to which individual details – for example, cell structures – can be identified by the eye when using a light microscope.

Resonance

The lengthening and intensification of sound produced by striking the body over an air-containing structure such as the lung. Decrease of resonance is called dullness and increase of resonance is called hyper-resonance. The process of striking the chest or other part of the body to discover its degree of resonance is called PERCUSSION, and according to the note obtained, an opinion can be formed as to the state of consolidation of air-containing organs, the presence of abnormal cavities, and the dimensions and relations of solid and air-containing organs lying together. (See also AUSCULTATION.)

Resorcinol

A white, crystalline, antiseptic substance soluble in water, alcohol and oils. It can be used in combination with sulphur to treat ACNE.

Respiration

The process in which air passes into and out of the lungs so that the blood can absorb oxygen and give off carbon dioxide and water. This occurs 18 times a minute in a healthy adult at rest and is called the respiratory rate. An individual breathes more than 25,000 times a day and during this time inhales around 16 kg of air.

Mechanism of respiration For the structure of the respiratory apparatus, see AIR PASSAGES; CHEST; LUNGS. The air passes rhythmically into and out of the air passages, and mixes with the air already in the lungs, these two movements being known as inspiration and expiration.

INSPIRATION is due to a muscular effort which enlarges the chest, so that the lungs have to expand in order to fill up the vacuum that would otherwise be left, the air entering these organs by the air passages. The increase of the chest in size from above downwards is mainly due to the diaphragm, the muscular fibres of

which contract and reduce its domed shape and cause it to descend, pushing down the abdominal organs beneath it.

EXPIRATION is an elastic recoil, the diaphragm rising and the ribs sinking into the position that they naturally occupy, when muscular contraction is finished. Occasionally, forced expiration may occur, involving powerful muscles of the abdomen and thorax; this is typically seen in forcible coughing.

Nervous control Respiration is usually either an automatic or a REFLEX ACTION, each expiration sending up sensory impulses to the CENTRAL NERVOUS SYSTEM, from which impulses are sent down various other nerves to the muscles that produce inspiration. Several centres govern the rate and force of the breathing, although all are presided over by a chief respiratory centre in the medulla oblongata (see under BRAIN – Divisions). This in turn is controlled by the higher centres in the cerebral hemispheres, so that breathing can be voluntarily stopped or quickened.

Quantity of air The lungs do not completely empty themselves at each expiration and refill at each inspiration. With each breath, less than one-tenth of the total air in the lungs passes out and is replaced by the same quantity of fresh air, which mixes with the stale air in the lungs. This renewal, which in quiet breathing amounts to about 500 millilitres, is known as the tidal air. By a special inspiratory effort, an individual can draw in about 3,000 millilitres, this amount being known as complemental air. By a special expiratory effort, too, after an ordinary breath one can expel much more than the tidal air from the lungs – this extra amount being known as the supplemental or reserve air, and amounting to about 1,300 millilitres. If an individual takes as deep an inspiration as possible and then makes a forced expiration, the amount expired is known as the vital capacity, and amounts to around 4,000 millilitres in a healthy adult male of average size. Figures for women are about 25 per cent lower. The vital capacity varies with size, sex, age and ethnic origin.

Over and above the vital capacity, the lungs contain air which cannot be expelled; this is known as residual air, and amounts to another 1,500 millilitres.

Tests of respiratory efficiency are used to assess lung function in health and disease. Pulmonary-function tests, as they are known, include spirometry (see SPIROMETER), PEAK FLOW METER (which measures the rate at which a

R

person can expel air from the lungs, thus testing vital capacity and the extent of BRONCHOS-PASM), and measurements of the concentration of oxygen and carbon dioxide in the blood. (See also LUNG VOLUMES.)

Abnormal forms of respiration Apart from mere changes in rate and force, respiration is modified in several ways, either involuntarily or voluntarily. SNORING, or stertorous breathing, is due to a flaccid state of the soft palate causing it to vibrate as the air passes into the throat, or simply to sleeping with the mouth open, which has a similar effect. COUGH is a series of violent expirations, at each of which the larynx is suddenly opened after the pressure of air in the lungs has risen considerably; its object is to expel some irritating substance from the air passages. SNEEZING is a single sudden expiration, which differs from coughing in that the sudden rush of air is directed by the soft palate up into the nose in order to expel some source of irritation from this narrow passage. CHEYNE-STOKES BREATHING is a type of breathing found in persons suffering from stroke, heart disease, and some other conditions, in which death is impending; it consists in an alternate dying away and gradual strengthening of the inspirations. Other disorders of breathing are found in CROUP and in ASTHMA.

Respiratory Arrest

Sudden stoppage of breathing which results from any process that strongly suppresses the function of the brain's respiratory centre. It leads to lack of oxygen in the tissues and, if not remedied, to cardiac arrest, brain damage, COMA and death. Treatment is artificial respiration (see APPENDIX 1: BASIC FIRST AID) and, if necessary, artificial ventilation. Causes of respiratory arrest include cardiac arrest, electrical injury, overdose of narcotic drugs, prolonged seizures (EPILEPSY), serious head injury, STROKE or inhalation of noxious material that causes respiratory failure.

Respiratory Distress Syndrome

This may occur in adults as ACUTE RESPIRATORY DISTRESS SYNDROME (ARDS), or in newborn children, when it is also known as HYALINE MEMBRANE DISEASE. The adult syndrome consists of PULMONARY OEDEMA of non-cardiac origin. The process begins when tissue damage stimulates the autonomic nervous system, releases vasoactive substances, precipitates complement activation, and produces abnormalities of the clotting cascade – the serial process that leads to clotting of the blood (see COAGULATION). The activation of complement causes white cells to lodge in the pulmonary capillaries where they release substances which damage the pulmonary endothelium.

Respiratory distress syndrome is a complication of SHOCK, systemic SEPSIS and viral respiratory infections. It was first described in 1967, and – despite advances with assisted ventilation – remains a serious disease with a mortality of more than 50 per cent. The maintenance of adequate circulating blood volume, peripheral PERFUSION, acid-base balance and arterial oxygenation is important, and assisted ventilation should be instituted early.

In newborns the mechanism is diferent, being provoked by an inability of the lungs to manufacture SURFACTANT.

Respiratory Syncytial Virus (RSV)

Usually known as RSV, this is one of the MYXOVIRUSES. It is among the major causes of BRONCHIOLITIS and PNEUMONIA among infants aged under 6 months; its incidence has been increasing, possibly due to atmospheric pollution.

Respiratory System

All the organs and tissues associated with the act of RESPIRATION or breathing. The term includes the nasal cavity (see NOSE) and PHARYNX, along with the LARYNX, TRACHEA, bronchi (see BRONCHUS), BRONCHIOLES and LUNGS. The DIAPHRAGM and other muscles, such as those between the RIBS, are also part of the respiratory system which is responsible for oxygenating the blood and removing carbon dioxide from it.

Restless Legs Syndrome

A condition in which the patient experiences unpleasant sensations, and occasionally involuntary movements, in the legs when at rest, especially at night. No pathological changes have been identified. It is sometimes indicative of iron-deficiency ANAEMIA, but in many cases the cause remains a mystery and the variety of cures offered are a testimony to this. Some anti-epileptic drugs are said to help (see EPILEPSY).

Restriction Enzyme

An endonuclease ENZYME, extracted from BACTERIA, that is used to cut DNA into short segments – a process essential in GENETIC ENGINEERING.

Resuscitation

See APPENDIX 1: BASIC FIRST AID. See also DNR.

Retardation

Slowing down; developmental delay. Psycho-motor retardation is a significant slowing down of speech and activity which eventually leads to a person being unable to cope with daily activities or to maintain personal hygiene. It is a symptom of severe DEPRESSION.

Retching

Retching is an ineffectual form of VOMITING.

Retention of Urine

See URINE RETENTION.

Reticulocytes

These are newly formed red blood corpuscles, in which a fine network can be demonstrated by special staining methods. Where a large number are present, one can infer that the patient is recovering from ANAEMIA – for example, after a previous bleed (HAEMOR-RHAGE) or as a result of treatment of iron deficiency.

Reticulo-Endothelial System

This consists of highly specialised cells scattered throughout the body, but found mainly in the SPLEEN, BONE MARROW, LIVER, and LYMPH nodes or glands. Their main function is the ingestion of red blood cells and the conversion of HAEMOGLOBIN to BILIRUBIN. They are also able to ingest bacteria and foreign colloidal particles.

Retina

See EYE.

Retina, Disorders of

See EYE, DISORDERS OF.

Retinoblastoma

A rare malignant growth of the retina (see EYE) which occurs in infants. It can sometimes be discovered at birth because shining a light in the baby's pupil produces a white reflection rather than a red one. Alternatively, the infant may present with a SQUINT or a mass in the abdomen. In 25 per cent of cases there is a family history of the condition and abnormality of chromosome 13 is common (see CHROMO-SOMES). It is treated by removing the eye or, if affecting both eyes, by laser PHOTOCOAGULA-TION with or without RADIOTHERAPY.

Retinoic Acid

A synthetic vitamin A derivative. (See APPENDIX 5: VITAMINS.)

Retinoids

Any one of a collection of drugs that are derived from vitamin A (see APPENDIX 5: VITAMINS). They can be taken orally or applied topically, and affect the skin by causing drying and peeling, with a reduction in the production of SEBUM. These properties are useful in the treatment of ACNE and PSORIASIS.

Retinol

Retinol is the official chemical name of vitamin A. (See APPENDIX 5: VITAMINS.)

Retinopathy

See EYE, DISORDERS OF – Retina, disorders of.

Retractor

An instrument for pulling apart the edges of an incision to allow better surgical access to the organs and tissues being operated on.

Retro-

A prefix signifying behind or turned backwards.

Retrobulbar Neuritis

Inflammation of the optic nerve behind (rather than within) the EYE. It usually occurs in young adults and presents with a rapid deterioration in vision over a few hours. Colour vision is also impaired. Usually vision recovers over a few weeks, but colour vision may be permanently lost. It can be associated with certain viral illnesses and with MULTIPLE SCLEROSIS (MS). (See also EYE, DISORDERS OF.)

Retrograde

Movement in a contrary or backward direction from normal (e.g. a retrograde pyelogram introduces dye into the pelvis of the kidney by passing it up the ureters).

Retropharyngeal Abscess

An ABSCESS occurring in the cellular tissue behind the throat (PHARYNX). It is the result in general of disease in the upper part of the SPINAL COLUMN.

Retrospective Study

The opposite of a PROSPECTIVE STUDY, involving a historical review of the characteristics of a collection of people to assess MORBIDITY, often by obtaining and analysing their casenotes. The procedure is commonly used in studying the EPIDEMIOLOGY of disease.

Retrospectoscope

A mock-humorous term used by doctors to imply that one can always see things more clearly after the event than at the time. One danger of making a judgement on the competence of a doctor treating a patient is that it is easier to know what was the right thing to have done once you know the end of the story.

Retroversion
An abnormal position of the UTERUS, occurring in about 20 per cent of women, in which its long axis is pivoted backwards in relation to the CERVIX UTERI and VAGINA instead of forwards.

Retrovirus
A VIRUS containing ribonucleic acid (RNA) which is able to change its genetic material into deoxyribonucleic acid (DNA) using an ENZYME called reverse transcriptase. This conversion enables the retrovirus to become integrated into the host cell's DNA. Retroviruses are believed to be involved in the development of some cancers; they are also associated with disorders linked with an impaired immune system (see IMMUNITY). HIV is a retrovirus.

Retroviruses are also used in the development of gene therapy (see GENETIC ENGINEERING).

Revalidation
The periodic assessment of a doctor's professional competence. Revalidation began in the UK in 2004, to ensure that those doctors on the Medical Register of the GENERAL MEDICAL COUNCIL (GMC) as active practitioners are capable of providing appropriate standards of medical care. The process depends, amongst other things, upon the doctor being able to demonstrate that he or she has maintained a continuing programme of professional development: 'lifelong learning'.

Reverse Transcriptase
An ENZYME, usually found in retroviruses (see RETROVIRUS), that catalyses the manufacture of DNA from RNA, enabling the viral RNA to amalgamate with the DNA of the infected host.

Reverse Transcriptase Inhibitor
An agent that prevents the action of the viral ENZYME, REVERSE TRANSCRIPTASE, so disrupting the virus's colonisation of its target host. The reverse transcriptase inhibitor ZIDOVUDINE is used (in combination with other agents) to treat HIV infection.

Reye's Syndrome
A condition, now rare, which occurs predominantly in young children following a viral infection of the upper respiratory tract or a viral infection such as CHICKENPOX or INFLUENZA.

The cause is not known, but there is evidence that ASPIRIN may also play a part in its causation. Doctors recommend that children should be given PARACETAMOL in place of aspirin. The initial feature is severe, persistent vomiting and fever. This is followed by outbursts of wild behaviour, DELIRIUM and CONVULSIONS terminating in COMA and death, often from liver failure. The MORTALITY rate is around 23 per cent, and 50 per cent of the survivors may have persistent mental or neurological disturbances. The younger the patient, the higher the death rate and the more common the permanent residual effects. Since aspirin has no longer been licensed for use in children and young people the incidence of the condition has fallen dramatcally. Some cases, previously thought to be Reye's syndrome, have subsequently turned out to have been due to certain inherited metabolic diseases and to be unconnected with aspirin.

Rhabdoviruses
A group of viruses which includes the RABIES virus.

Rhesus Factor
See BLOOD GROUPS.

Rheumatic Fever
An acute febrile illness, usually seen in children, which may include ARTHRALGIA, ARTHRITIS, CHOREA, carditis (see below) and rash (see ERUPTION). The illness has been shown to follow a beta-haemolytic streptococcal infection (see STREPTOCOCCUS).

Rheumatic fever is now extremely uncommon in developed countries, but remains common in developing areas. Diagnosis is based on the presence of two or more major manifestations – endocarditis (see under HEART, DISEASES OF), POLYARTHRITIS, chorea, ERYTHEMA marginatum, subcutaneous nodules – or one major and two or more minor ones – fever, arthralgia, previous attacks, raised ESR, raised white blood cell count, and ELECTROCARDIOGRAM (ECG) changes. Evidence of previous infection with streptococcus is also a criterion.

Clinical features Fever is high, with attacks of shivering or rigor. Joint pain and swelling (arthralgia) may affect the knee, ankle, wrist or shoulder and may migrate from one joint to another. TACHYCARDIA may indicate cardiac involvement. Subcutaneous nodules may occur, particularly over the back of the wrist or over the elbow or knee. Erythema marginatum is a red rash, looking like the outline of a map, characteristic of the condition.

Cardiac involvement includes PERICARDITIS, ENDOCARDITIS, and MYOCARDITIS. The main long-term complication is damage to the mitral and aortic valves (see HEART).

The chief neurological problem is chorea (St Vitus's dance) which may develop after the acute symptoms have subsided.

Chronic rheumatic heart disease occurs subsequently in at least half of those who have had rheumatic fever with carditis. The heart valve usually involved is the mitral; less commonly the aortic, tricuspid and pulmonary. The lesions may take 10–20 years to develop in developed countries but sooner elsewhere. The heart valves progressively fibrose and fibrosis may also develop in the myocardium and pericardium. The outcome is either mitral stenosis or mitral regurgitation and the subsequent malfunction of this or other heart valves affected is chronic failure in the functioning of the heart. (see HEART, DISEASES OF).

Treatment Eradication of streptococcal infection is essential. Other features are treated symptomatically. PARACETAMOL may be preferred to ASPIRIN as an antipyretic in young children. One of the NON-STEROIDAL ANTI-INFLAMMATORY DRUGS (NSAIDS) may benefit the joint symptoms. CORTICOSTEROIDS may be indicated for more serious complications.

Patients who have developed cardiac-valve abnormalities require antibiotic prophylaxis during dental treatment and other procedures where bacteria may enter the bloodstream. Secondary cardiac problems may occur several decades later and require replacement of affected heart valves.

Rheumatism

An obsolete medical term which no longer has a defined meaning. It remains a lay term covering any painful condition of the muscles and/or joints of the arms, legs or spine.

Rheumatoid Arthritis

A chronic inflammation of the synovial lining (see SYNOVIAL MEMBRANE) of several joints, tendon sheaths or bursae which is not due to SEPSIS or a reaction to URIC ACID crystals. It is distinguished from other patterns of inflammatory arthritis by the symmetrical involvement of a large number of peripheral joints; by the common blood-finding of rheumatoid factor antibody; by the presence of bony erosions around joints; and, in a few, by the presence of subcutaneous nodules with necrobiotic (decaying) centres.

Causes There is a major immunogenetic predisposition to rheumatoid arthritis in people carrying the HLA-DR4 antigen (see HLA SYSTEM). Other minor immunogenetic factors have also been implicated. In addition, there is a degree of familial clustering which suggests other unidentified genetic factors. Genetic factors cannot alone explain aetiology, and environmental and chance factors must be important, but these have yet to be identified.

Epidemiology Rheumatoid arthritis more commonly occurs in women from the age of 30 onwards, the sex ratio being approximately 4:1. Typical rheumatoid arthritis may occur in adolescence, but in childhood chronic SYNOVITIS usually takes one of a number of different patterns, classified under juvenile chronic arthritis.

Pathology The primary lesion is an inflammation of the synovial membrane of joints. The synovial fluid becomes diluted with inflammatory exudate: if this persists for months it leads to progressive destruction of articular CARTILAGE and BONE. Cartilage is replaced by inflammatory tissue known as pannus; a similar tissue invades bone to form erosions. Synovitis also affects tendon sheaths, and may lead to adhesion fibrosis or attrition and rupture of tendons. Subcutaneous and other bursae may be involved. Necrobiotic nodules also occur at sites outside synovium, including the subcutaneous tissues, the lungs, the pericardium and the pleura.

Clinical features Rheumatoid arthritis varies from the very mild to the severely disabling. Many mild cases probably go undiagnosed. At least 50 per cent of patients continue to lead a reasonably normal life; around 25 per cent are significantly disabled in terms of work and leisure activities; and a minority become markedly disabled and are limited in their independence. There is often an early acute phase, followed by substantial remission, but in other patients gradual step-wise deterioration may occur, with progressive involvement of an increasing number of joints.

The diagnosis of rheumatoid arthritis is largely based on clinical symptoms and signs. Approximately 70 per cent of patients have rheumatoid factor ANTIBODIES in the SERUM but, because of the large number of false positives and false negatives, this test has very little value in clinical practice. It may be a useful pointer to a worse prognosis in early cases if the level is high. X-RAYS may help in diagnosing early cases and are particularly helpful when considering surgery or possible complications such as pathological fracture. Patients commonly develop ANAEMIA, which may be partly due to gastrointestinal blood loss from anti-inflammatory drug treatment (see below).

Treatment involves physical, pharmacological, and surgical measures, together with psychological and social support tailored to the individual patient's needs. Regular activity should be maintained. Resting of certain joints such as the wrist with splints may be helpful at night or to assist prolonged manual activities. Sound footwear is important. Early use of anti-rheumatic drugs reduces long-term disability. Drug treatment includes simple ANALGESICS, NON-STEROIDAL ANTI-INFLAMMATORY DRUGS (NSAIDS), and slow-acting drugs including GOLD SALTS (in the form of SODIUM AUROTHIOMALATE), PENICILLAMINE, SULFASALAZINE, METHOTREXATE and AZATHIOPRINE.

The non-steroidal agents are largely effective in reducing pain and early-morning stiffness, and have no effect on the chronic inflammatory process. It is important, especially in the elderly, to explain to patients the adverse effects of NSAIDs, the dosage of which can be cut by prescribing paracetamol at the same time. Combinations of anti-rheumatic drugs seem better than single agents. The slow-acting drugs take approximately three months to act but have a more global effect on chronic inflammation, with a greater reduction in swelling and an associated fall in erythrocyte sedimentation rate (ESR) and rise in the level of HAEMOGLOBIN. Local CORTICOSTEROIDS are useful, given into individual joints. Systemic corticosteroids carry serious problems if continued long term, but may be useful under special circumstances. Much research is currently going on into the use of tumour necrosis factor antagonists such as INFLIXIMAB and etanercept, but their precise role remains uncertain.

Rheumatology
The medical speciality concerned with the study and management of diseases of the JOINTS and CONNECTIVE TISSUE.

Rh Factor
See BLOOD GROUPS.

Rhinitis
Inflammation of the mucous membrane of the NOSE. (See also NOSE, DISORDERS OF.)

Rhinophyma
The condition characterised by swelling of the NOSE due to enormous enlargement of the sebaceous glands which may develop in the later stages of ROSACEA.

Rhinoplasty
Repair of the NOSE or modification of its shape by operation. This operation is performed by reconstructive and ENT (ear, nose and throat) surgeons alike. It may involve alteration of the bony skeleton of the nose and/or alteration of the SEPTUM (septorhinoplasty). It is mostly performed for cosmetic reasons; however, any disease process or injury which has caused a defect in the nose may be repaired as well. The latter problem would usually involve the utilisation of some form of skin flap, whereas this would not be required for cosmetic surgical purposes.

Rhinorrhoea
The persistent discharge of watery mucus from the NOSE. This is a usual symptom as a result of COMMON COLD or consequent upon ALLERGY (perennial rhinitis and HAY FEVER).

Rhinoviruses
A large group of viruses; to date around 80 distinct rhinoviruses have been identified. Their practical importance is that some of them are responsible for around one-quarter of the cases of the COMMON COLD.

Rhizotomy
The surgical operation of cutting a nerve root, as, for example, to relieve the pain of TRIGEMINAL NEURALGIA.

Rhonchi
A description of the harsh cooing, hissing, or whistling sounds (wheezing) heard by AUSCULTATION over the bronchial tubes when they are the seat of infection. (See BRONCHITIS.)

Rhythm Method
A method of CONTRACEPTION which attempts to prevent conception by avoiding intercourse during the fertile part of the menstrual cycle. (See MENSTRUATION; SAFE PERIOD.)

Ribavirin
Also known as tribavirin, this drug inhibits a wide variety of DNA and RNA viruses. It is administered by inhalation to treat severe BRONCHIOLITIS caused by RESPIRATORY SYNCYTIAL VIRUS (RSV), particularly in infants who also have congenital heart disease. It is not used in uncomplicated bronchiolitis as its benefits

are arguable in that circumstance: the babies are likely to recover without treatment.

Ribavarin, along with INTERFERON alpha-2b, is given orally to treat patients with chronic HEPATITIS C infection. It is also used to treat LASSA FEVER.

Riboflavin

The *British Pharmacopoeia* name for what used to be known as vitamin B$_2$. The minimal daily requirement for an adult is 1·5–3 mg, but is greater during pregnancy and lactation. Deficiency in the diet is thought to cause inflammation of the substance of the cornea (see EYE), sores on the lips, especially at the angles of the mouth (CHEILOSIS), and DERMATITIS. (See APPENDIX 5: VITAMINS.)

Ribonucleic Acid

See RNA.

Ribosome

Granules either found free within the cell, or attached to a reticular network within the cell's endoplasm (the inner part of a cell's cytoplasm – see CELLS). Consisting of approximately 65 per cent RNA and 35 per cent PROTEIN, they are the sites where protein is made.

Ribozyme

Sections of deoxyribonucleic acid (DNA) – the principal molecule in a cell carrying genetic information – that act as enzymes (see ENZYME). The function of a ribozyme is to transform the messages encoded in DNA into proteins (see PROTEIN), using its property of catalysing chemical reactions in a cell. Most ribozymes act only on other pieces of ribonucleic acid (RNA), editing the messenger type that carries instructions to the parts of the cell that makes proteins. This editing ability is being used by scientists researching ways of correcting faulty GENES which can cause inherited disorders. The aim is to persuade the ribozyme to inhibit the messenger RNA to prevent production of the faulty gene. Ribozymes might also be used to disrupt infectious agents, such as viruses, which rely on RNA to invade body cells.

Ribs

The bones, 12 on each side, which enclose the cavity of the chest. The upper seven are joined to the breast-bone by their costal cartilages and are therefore known as true ribs. The lower five do not reach the breast-bone, and are therefore known as false ribs. Of the latter, the eighth, ninth and tenth are joined by their costal cartilages, each one to the rib immediately above it,

while the 11th and 12th are free from any such connection and are therefore known as floating ribs. Each rib has a head, by which it is joined to the upper part of the body of the vertebra with which it corresponds, as well as to the vertebra immediately above. The greater part of the bone is made up of the shaft, which runs at first outwards and at the angle turns sharply forwards. On the lower margin of the shaft is a groove, which lodges the corresponding intercostal artery and nerve.

Rice-Water

A useful diluent drink for invalids, similar to barley-water.

Rickets

A disease of childhood characterised chiefly by a softened condition of the bones (see BONE), and by other evidence of poor nutrition.

Causes This disease is the result of deficiency of vitamin D in the diet. Healthy bones cannot be built up without calcium (or lime) salts, and the body cannot use these salts in the absence of vitamin D. Want of sunlight and fresh air in the dwellings where children are reared is also of importance. Once a common condition in industrial areas, it had almost disappeared in Great Britain but has recurred in recent years, largely amongst children of Asian and African origin.

The periosteum – the membrane enveloping the bones – becomes inflamed, and the bone formed beneath it is defective in lime salts and very soft. Changes also occur at the growing part of the bone, the epiphyseal plate.

Symptoms The symptoms of rickets most usually appear towards the end of the first year, and rarely after the age of five. The children are often 'snuffly' and miserable.

Gradually, changes in the shape of the bones becomes visible, first chiefly noticed at the ends of the long bones. The softened bones also tend to become distorted, the legs bending outwards and forwards so the child becomes bow-legged or knock-kneed. Changes occur in the ribs ('rickets rosary') and cranial bones, while teeth appear late and decay or fall out.

The disease usually ends in recovery with more or less of deformity and dwarfing – the bones, although altered in shape, becoming ultimately ossified.

Treatment The specific remedy is vitamin D in the form of calciferol (vitamin D$_2$). A full diet is of course essential, with emphasis upon a sufficient supply of milk. Rickets is very rare in breast-fed children but it is a wise precaution to give breast-fed babies supplementary vitamin D. After the child is weaned, the provision of suitable food is vital, supplemented with some source of vitamin D. Regular exposure to sunlight is desirable. Controversy exists as to whether vitamin D should be added in the manufacture of flour, particularly of types used by the Asian community.

Deficiency of vitamin D in adults results in osteomalacia (see under BONE, DISORDERS OF). (See also APPENDIX 5: VITAMINS.)

Rickettsia

The general term given to a group of micro-organisms which are intermediate between BACTERIA and viruses (see VIRUS). They are the causal agents of TYPHUS FEVER and a number of typhus-like diseases, such as ROCKY MOUNTAIN SPOTTED FEVER, Japanese River fever, and scrub typhus. These micro-organisms are usually conveyed to man by lice, fleas, ticks, and mites.

Visceral rickettsia is a disease transmitted by mites from an infected house mouse, which occurs in the USA, South Africa, Korea and the former Soviet Union. The causal organism is *Rickettsia akari*. The incubation period is 7–14 days and the characteristic features are fever, headache, and a non-irritating rash on the face, trunk and extremities. The disease is non-fatal and responds rapidly to TETRACYCLINES.

Rifampicin

An antibiotic derived from *Streptomyces mediterranei*, rifampicin is a key component of the treatment of TUBERCULOSIS. Like ISONIAZID, it should always be included unless there is a specific contraindication. It is also valuable in the treatment of BRUCELLOSIS, LEGIONNAIRE'S DISEASE, serious staphylococcal (see STAPHYLOCOCCUS) infections and LEPROSY. It is also given to contacts of certain forms of childhood MENINGITIS.

Rifampicin is given by mouth; during the first two months it often causes transient disturbance of LIVER function, with raised concentrations of serum transaminases, but usually treatment need not be interrupted. In patients with pre-existing liver disease more severe toxicity may occur, and liver function should be carefully monitored both before starting and during rifampicin treatment. It induces hepatic enzymes which accelerate the metabolism of various drugs including ANTICOAGULANTS, SULPHONYLUREAS, PHENYTOIN SODIUM, CORTICOSTEROIDS and OESTROGENS. The

effectiveness of oral contraceptives is reduced and alternative family-planning advice should be offered.

Rifampicin should be avoided during pregnancy and breast feeding, and extra caution should be applied if there is renal impairment, JAUNDICE or PORPHYRIAS. Adverse effects include gastrointestinal symptoms, influenza-like symptoms, collapse and SHOCK, haemolytic ANAEMIA, acute flushing and URTICARIA; body secretions may be coloured red.

Rift Valley Fever

A virus disease, caused by a phlebovirus and transmitted by mosquitoes, at one time confined to sub-Saharan Africa and predominantly found in domestic animals such as cattle, sheep and goats. The only humans affected were veterinary surgeons, butchers and others exposed to heavy infection by direct contact with infected animals; these usually recovered. In the 1970s the disease flared up in Egypt, probably owing to a more virulent virus. The illness in humans is characterised by fever, haemorrhages, ENCEPHALITIS and involvement of the EYE. An effective vaccine protects both animals and human beings against the disease (see IMMUNISATION).

Rigidity

Stiffness, resistance to movement. The term is often used in NEUROLOGY – for example, limb rigidity is a sign of PARKINSONISM. Smooth rigidity is described as being 'plastic' and jerky rigidity as 'cogwheel'.

Rigor

Shivering. If prolonged, it is generally accompanied by fever, and may be a sign of the onset of some acute disease such as INFLUENZA, PNEUMONIA, or some internal inflammation. Rigor mortis is the name given to the stiffness that ensues soon after death. (See DEATH, SIGNS OF; MUSCLE.)

Ring Block

A local anaesthetic agent (see ANAESTHESIA) injected into the circumference of the base of a digit. It numbs the nerves of the finger or toe and so permits minor surgery to be performed. Care must be taken to avoid damage to local blood vessels which can lead to GANGRENE.

Ringworm

Ringworm, or tinea, is the name given to inflammatory rashes caused by DERMATOPHYTES of the genera microsporum, epidermophyton and trichophyton. These fungi can infect skin, hair and nails. The important clinical patterns are:

Tinea capitis Usually seen in children in Britain and caused by microsporum species of human or animal (frequently a kitten) origin. Typically, patches of ALOPECIA are seen with broken-off hair stumps which fluoresce bright green under an ultraviolet (Wood's) lamp. In Asia a chronic, scarring alopecia may be caused by a specific trichophyton (favus).

Tinea corporis is usually due to trichophyton species and forms ringed (hence 'ringworm') patches of redness and scaling on the trunk or limbs.

Tinea pedis (athlete's foot) is caused by epidermophyton or trichophyton species. Its minor form manifests as itching, scaling or blistering in the lateral toe clefts. More severe forms can be extensive on the sole. *Trichophyton rubrum* can cause a chronic, dry, scaling inflammation of the foot, eventually extending into the nails and on to the soles and top of the foot which may persist for years if untreated.

Tinea cruris typically causes a 'butterfly' rash on the upper inner thighs in young adult males. It is usually caused by spread from the feet.

Tinea unguium (onychomycosis) Affecting the nails, especially of the toes, *T. rubrum* is the usual cause and may persist for decades.

Tinea barbae This rash of the face and beard is rare. It may be very inflammatory and is usually contracted from cattle by farm workers.

Treatment Tinea of the toe clefts and groin will usually respond to an antifungal cream containing terbinafine or an azole. Tinea capitis, barbae, extensive tinea corporis and all nail infections require oral treatment with terbinafine or itraconazole (a triazole antifungal agent taken orally and used for candidiasis of the mouth, throat and vulgovaginal area as well as for ringworm) which have largely superseded the earlier treatment with the antiobiotic griseofulvin. (See FUNGAL AND YEAST INFECTIONS.)

Rinnes Test

A hearing test in which a vibrating tuning fork is placed on the mastoid process (see EAR). When the subject can no longer hear the ring-

ing, it is placed beside the ear. Normal subjects can then hear the noise once more, but in people with conductive DEAFNESS, air conduction does not persist after bone conduction has ceased. It can help to distinguish between nerve (sensorineural) and conduction deafness.

Ripple Beds

A development of the conventional air-beds. Their essential feature is a mattress which is alternately pressurised by a compressor to create a gentle rippling effect along the entire length of the mattress. This provides a continuous massaging motion which stimulates the circulation and helps to maintain the nutrition of the skin, thereby reducing the risk of bed sores (see ULCER – Decubitus ulcer).

Risk Factor

An environmental or genetic factor which makes the occurrence of a disease in an individual more likely. For example, male sex, OBESITY, smoking and high blood pressure (HYPERTENSION) are all risk factors for ischaemic heart disease (see under HEART, DISEASES OF).

Risk Management

A predictive technique for identifying potential untoward occurrences. It has been in use in certain industries (such as nuclear power generation) for many years and was introduced to the NHS in 1991 when self-governing trusts were first set up. The reasons were, firstly, that Crown immunity had been removed from the health service in 1988, so that ceased to be immune from prosecution for non-compliance with health and safety legislation; secondly, because trusts were responsible for their own liabilities and any consequential costs. Risk management starts with three simple questions:
- what can go wrong?
- how likely is it to happen?
- how bad would it be if it happened?

The combined answers allow an estimate to be made of the risk. Given the scope for clinical mishaps in the NHS – let alone staff and corporate risks – the need for a credible, operational risk strategy is substantial.

Risk Register

The term is used in two ways. Firstly, it may comprise a list of infants whose obstetric and/or perinatal history suggests they might be at risk of illness or serious abnormality such as LEARNING DISABILITY.

Secondly – and more commonly termed the 'At-risk register' – this is a list held by social-service departments, and accessible to doctors in A&E departments, of children whom a local-authority social-services case conference has deemed to have been harmed or to be at risk of harm from mental, physical or sexual abuse (see also CHILD ABUSE).

Risus Sardonicus
The term used for describing the facial appearance when the muscles of the forehead and the face go into spasm in TETANUS, giving the effect of a sardonic grin.

Ritalin
See METHYLPHENIDATE.

Ritodrine
A beta$_2$-adrenoceptor-stimulating drug that relaxes uterine muscle (see UTERUS). It is used in selected women close to term to inhibit the onset of labour for at least 48 hours. This allows for the implementation of measures to improve the perinatal health of the infant, including making arrangements for transfer to a neonatal intensive-care facility. (See PREGNANCY AND LABOUR – Premature birth.)

Rivastigmine
An acetylcholinesterase inhibitor used in the treatment of ALZHEIMER'S DISEASE. Treatment should be under the supervision of a specialist and the drug should be started at a low dose because of potential side-effects.

RNA
RNA is the abbreviation for ribonucleic acid, one of the two types of NUCLEIC ACID that exist in nature. It is present in both the cytoplasm and nucleus of the CELLS of the body, but principally in the former. With DNA it is an essential component of the genetic code. It exists in three categories known, respectively, as ribosomal (r), transfer (t), and messenger (m) RNA. Genetic information resides in the linear sequence of nucleotides (see NUCLEIC ACID) in DNA and is transcribed into messenger RNA before protein is synthesised. In the language of the computer, the genetic code consists of 64 three-letter code-words, or codons. The code in DNA is comparable to a tape which contains information written linearly in the form of these codons, each of which is the code for one of the 20 AMINO ACIDS from which proteins are made. The genetic information encoded in DNA is used to programme the manufacture of proteins (see PROTEIN) in two stages.

In the first, the information is transcribed from DNA on to a molecule of mRNA. In the second, the messenger RNA-intermediary transports the information to the protein-manufacturing centres of the cell where the information is translated from the linear sequence of codons in the RNA into a linear sequence of amino acids which are concurrently converted into protein. (See also GENES.)

Rocky Mountain Spotted Fever
A fever of the typhus group (see TYPHUS FEVER). It received its name from the fact that it was first reported in the Rocky Mountain States of the United States; these are still the most heavily infected areas, but the fever is now found in all parts of the US. The causative organism is *Rickettsia rickettsi*, which is transmitted to humans by tics.

Rodent Ulcer
A chronic form of BASAL CELL CARCINOMA, the most common form of skin cancer.

Rohypnol
See FLUNITRAZEPAM.

Rombergism
A term applied to marked unsteadiness when a person stands with the eyes shut. It is found as a symptom in some nervous diseases, such as peripheral NEUROPATHY and tabes dorsalis (neurosyphilis).

Root Filling
Also called root-canal therapy, this is the treatment given when the nerve of a tooth (see TEETH) has been exposed while the tooth is being prepared for a filling, or if it has died or become infected. The nerve debris is removed and, when the chamber is clear of infection, an inert material is inserted to seal off the root.

Rorschach Test
A psychological test (see PSYCHOLOGY) for investigating personality and disorders of personality. Also called the 'ink blot test', it is now rarely used. It was devised by a Swiss psychiatrist, Hermann Rorschach (1884–1922), who determined individuals' reactions to a series of symmetrical ink-blots, ten in number and standardised by him.

Rosacea
Common chronic inflammation of the facial skin, this condition is seen in middle and late life. Redness, obvious dilatation of venules and crops of ACNE-like papules and pustules affect mainly the central forehead, cheeks, nose and chin. A keratoconjunctivitis (combined

inflammation of the cornea and conjunctiva of the EYE) may be associated. Subjects flush easily, especially after alcohol or hot drinks. Eventually the affected areas may become thickened and oedematous, and in men, proliferation of fibrous and sebaceous tissue may lead to gross thickening and enlargement of the nose (RHINOPHYMA).

Treatment Long-term, low-dose, oral tetracycline (see ANTIBIOTICS; TETRACYCLINES) is the treatment of choice. In mild cases, METRONIDAZOLE gel can be helpful. Potent topical CORTICOSTEROIDS are contraindicated and make rosacea worse.

Roseola Infantum
A transient EXANTHEM of toddlers. Mild malaise is followed by a RUBELLA-like rash. It is caused by herpes virus 6 (see HERPES VIRUSES).

Rotator Cuff
A musculo-tendinous structure that helps to stabilise the shoulder-joint. The cuff may be damaged as a result of a fall; complete rupture requires surgical treatment and intensive PHYSIOTHERAPY.

Rotaviruses
A group of viruses (so-called because of their wheel-like structure: *rota* is Latin for wheel) which are a common cause of GASTROENTERITIS in infants (see also DIARRHOEA). They cause from 25 to 80 per cent of childhood diarrhoea in different parts of the world, and in the United Kingdom they are responsible for 60–65 per cent of cases. They infect only the cells lining the small intestine. In the UK, death from rotavirus is rare.

Roughage
Dietary fibre is that part of food which cannot be digested in the gastrointestinal tract, although it can be metabolised in the colon by the micro-organisms there. Roughage falls into four groups: cellulose, hemicelluloses, lignins and pectins, found in unrefined foods such as wholemeal cereals and flour, root vegetables, nuts and fruit. It has long been known to affect bowel function, probably because of its capacity to hold water in a gel-like form. It plays an important role in the prevention of CONSTIPATION, DIVERTICULOSIS, IRRITABLE BOWEL SYNDROME (IBS), APPENDICITIS, DIABETES MELLITUS and cancer of the colon (see INTESTINE). At present, many western diets do not contain enough roughage.

Rouleaux
The term applied to the heaps into which red blood corpuscles (ERYTHROCYTES) collect as seen under the microscope.

Roundworms
See ASCARIASIS.

Rous Sarcoma
A malignant tumour of fowls which is caused by a virus. This tumour has been the subject of much experimental work on the nature of CANCER.

Royal College of Nursing (RCN)
See APPENDIX 8: PROFESSIONAL ORGANISATIONS.

RSI
Repetitive strain injury – see UPPER LIMB DISORDERS.

RSV
See RESPIRATORY SYNCYTIAL VIRUS (RSV).

Rubella
Rubella, or German measles, is an acute infectious disease of a mild type, which may sometimes be difficult to differentiate from mild forms of MEASLES and SCARLET FEVER.

Cause A virus spread by close contact with infected individuals. Rubella is infectious for a week before the rash appears and at least four days afterwards. It occurs in epidemics (see EPIDEMIC) every three years or so, predominantly in the winter and spring. Children are more likely to be affected than infants. One attack gives permanent IMMUNITY. The incubation period is usually 14–21 days.

Symptoms are very mild, and the disease is not at all serious. On the day of onset there may be shivering, headache, slight CATARRH with sneezing, coughing and sore throat, with very slight fever – not above 37·8 °C (100 °F). At the same time the glands of the neck become enlarged. Within 24 hours of the onset a pink, slightly raised eruption appears, first on the face or neck, then on the chest, and the second day spreads all over the body. The clinical signs and symptoms of many other viral infections are indistinguishable from rubella so a precise diagnosis cannot be made without taking samples (such as saliva) for antibody testing, but this is rarely done in practice.

An attack of German measles during the early months of pregnancy may be responsible for CONGENITAL defects in the FETUS (for information on fetal abnormalities, see under PREGNANCY AND LABOUR). The incidence of such defects is not precisely known, but probably around 20 per cent of children whose mothers have had German measles in the first three months of the pregnancy are born with congenital defects. These defects take a variety of forms, but the most important ones are: low birth weight with retarded physical development; malformations of the HEART; cataract (see under EYE, DISORDERS OF); and DEAFNESS.

Treatment There is no specific treatment. Children who develop the disease should not return to school until they have recovered, and in any case not before four days have passed from the onset of the rash.

In view of the possible dangerous effect of the disease upon the fetus, particular care should be taken to isolate pregnant mothers from contact with infected subjects. As the risk is particularly high during the first 16 weeks of pregnancy, any pregnant mother exposed to infection during this period should be given an intramuscular injection of GAMMA-GLOBULIN. A vaccine is available to protect an individual against rubella (see IMMUNISATION).

In the United Kingdom it is NHS policy for all children to have the combined measles, mumps and rubella vaccine (see MMR VACCINE), subject to parental consent. All women of childbearing age, who have been shown by a simple laboratory test not to have had the disease, should be vaccinated, provided that the woman is not pregnant at the time and has not been exposed to the risk of pregnancy during the previous eight weeks.

Rupture
A popular name for HERNIA.

Ryle's Tube
See NASOGASTRIC TUBE.

R

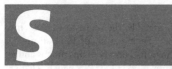

S

Sabin Vaccine

Introduced in 1962, the attenuated live oral vaccine (Sabin) against POLIOMYELITIS replaced the previous inactivated vaccine introduced in 1956 (see SALK VACCINE).

Saccharine

A sweetening agent that is 400 times as sweet as cane sugar, but with no energy content. Apart from its rather bitter aftertaste, it has practically no effect on the tissues, and escapes from the body unchanged. Destroyed by heat, saccharine is not used in cooking, but is an important component of all diabetic and low-calorie diets.

Saccharomyces

Another name for YEAST.

Sacral Nerves

The five pairs of spinal nerves that leave the SPINAL COLUMN in the sacral area. They carry motor and sensory fibres from the anal and genital regions and from both legs.

Sacral Vertebrae

The five fused vertebrae that link the thoracic spine and the coccyx and form the sacrum (see SPINAL COLUMN).

Sacroileitis

(See SACROILIAC JOINT.) Inflammation of one or both sacroiliac joints, which lie between the sacrum and the iliac bones. The condition may be the result of RHEUMATOID ARTHRITIS, ankylosing spondylitis (see under SPINE AND SPINAL CORD, DISEASES AND INJURIES OF), REITER'S SYNDROME, or the arthritis that occurs with PSORIASIS or infection. Sacroileitis causes pain in the lower back, buttocks, thighs, and groin. Stiffness may occur with ankylosing spondylitis. NON-STEROIDAL ANTI-INFLAMMATORY DRUGS (NSAIDS) relieve the symptoms. If the cause is infection, antibiotics should be used.

Sacroiliac Joint

One of a pair of joints between each side of the SACRUM and each ILIUM. Strong ligaments between the ilium and the sacrum stabilise the joint, permitting little movement. Childbirth or strenuous sporting activities may strain the joint, causing pain in the lower part of the back and buttocks. Such strains may take a long time to mend; PHYSIOTHERAPY is the treatment. The joint(s) may become inflamed (see SACROILEITIS).

Sacrum

The portion of the SPINAL COLUMN near its lower end. The sacrum consists of five vertebrae fused together to form a broad triangular bone which lies between the two haunch-bones and forms the back wall of the pelvis.

Sadism

The term applied to a form of sexual perversion, in which satisfaction is derived from the infliction of cruelty upon another person. The condition is commoner in men than in women and is sometimes linked with MASOCHISM (a wish to be hurt or abused).

Safe Period

That period during the menstrual cycle (see MENSTRUATION) when fertilisation of the OVUM is unlikely to occur. OVULATION usually occurs about 15 days before the onset of the menstrual period. A woman is commonly believed to be fertile for about 11 days in each menstrual cycle – in other words, on the day of ovulation and for five days before and five days after this; this would be the eighth to the 18th day of the usual 28-day menstrual cycle. Outside this fertile period is the SAFE PERIOD: the first week and the last ten days of the menstrual cycle. On the other hand, there is increasing evidence that the safest period is the last few days before menstruation. In the case of irregular menstruation it is not possible to calculate the safe period. In any event, the safety is not absolute. (See also CONTRACEPTION.)

Safety of Drugs

The COMMITTEE ON SAFETY OF MEDICINES (CSM) has the function of scrutinising the efficacy, quality and safety of new DRUGS before clinical trials and before marketing, as well as the surveillance of each drug after marketing so that adverse reactions are monitored and documented, and warnings issued as required. Early clinical trials of a drug can only be carried out after a clinical-trial certificate has been issued by the licensing authority.

The major defect in this system is the difficulty in obtaining reports of adverse reactions. Evidence suggests that at most, about 10 per cent of such reactions are reported. One method of trying to obtain this information is the 'yellow card' system. It is so called because it is based on the distribution of yellow cards to all doctors, pharmacists and dentists, on which they are asked to report any adverse reaction happening to someone taking a drug, whether or not they think it is the cause. Alternatively the CSM has a Freephone line and on-line computer facilities (ADROIT) for practitioners to use. Even though the annual number of adverse reactions reported in this way has risen from around 5,000 in 1975 to more than 18,000, this is probably fewer than the number actually occurring.

Two further committees in this safety screen are the Joint Committee on Vaccination and Immunisation and the Adverse Reactions to Vaccines and Immunological Substances Committee.

Sagittal
The term applied to a structure or section running from front to back in the body.

Salaam Attacks
See INFANTILE SPASMS.

Salbutamol
A short-acting selective beta$_2$-adrenoceptor stimulant delivered via a metered-dose aerosol inhaler, a powder inhaler or through a nebuliser to control symptoms of ASTHMA. If stimulant inhalation is needed more than twice a day to control asthma attacks, prophylactic treatment should be considered including, in severe cases, oral CORTICOSTEROIDS. Salbutamol relaxes the muscles which cause bronchial spasms in the lungs – the prime symptom of asthma. There are other similar preparations such as terbutaline.

Salicylic Acid
A crystalline substance sparingly soluble in water that is used externally in ointments and pastes. It has antifungal properties and helps to loosen and remove scales. In high concentrations it is useful in treatment of verrucae (WARTS) and corns (see CORNS AND BUNIONS).

Saline
Normal saline is a solution containing 0·9 per cent of sodium chloride (common salt). Saline is used clinically to dilute drugs given by injection; it is also given as an intravenous infusion to restore blood volume if blood loss from accident or operation is not too serious, or to tide a patient over until PLASMA or blood for TRANSFUSION becomes available.

Saline is also given orally to severely dehydrated children or adults suffering from diarrhoea and, in particular, CHOLERA.

Saliva
The fluid secreted by the SALIVARY GLANDS into the mouth. The ingestion of food stimulates saliva production. Saliva contains mucus and an ENZYME known as PTYALIN, which changes starch into dextrose and maltose (see DIGESTION); also many cells of different types. About 750 millilitres are produced daily.

The principal function of saliva is to aid in the initial processes of digestion, and it is essential for the process of mastication (chewing), whereby food is reduced to an homogeneous mass before being swallowed. In addition, the ptyalin in the saliva initiates the digestion of starch in the food.

An excessive flow of saliva known as salivation occurs as the result of taking certain drugs. Salivation also occurs as the result of irritation in the mouth – as for instance, in the teething child – and from DYSPEPSIA. Deficiency of saliva is known as XEROSTOMIA.

Salivary Glands
The glands (see GLAND) situated near, and opening into, the cavity of the mouth, by which the SALIVA is manufactured. They include the parotid gland, placed in the deep space that lies between the ear and the angle of the jaw; the submandibular gland, lying beneath the horizontal part of the jaw-bone; and the sublingual gland, which lies beneath the tongue.

Each gland is made up of branching tubes closely packed together, and supported by strong connective tissue. These tubes are lined by large cells that secrete the saliva, and ducts transfer the saliva to openings in the mouth. The parotid gland secretes a clear fluid containing the ENZYME, PTYALIN; in the sublingual gland they mainly produce mucus, whilst the submandibular gland contains cells of both types.

Salk Vaccine
A vaccine obtained by treating the POLIOMYELITIS virus with formalin. This prevents the virus from causing the disease but allows it to stimulate the production of ANTIBODIES. Salk vaccine is given by injection and protects the recipient against the disease. (See also IMMUNISATION.)

Salmonella Infections
See FOOD POISONING; ENTERIC FEVER; DYSENTERY.

Salmon Patches
See NAEVUS – Naevus simplex.

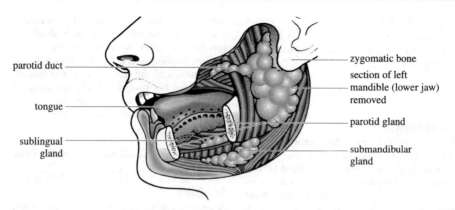

parotid duct

tongue

sublingual
gland

zygomatic bone

section of left
mandible (lower jaw)
removed

parotid gland

submandibular
gland

Cutaway diagram of left side of face showing position of salivary glands in relation to tongue and lower jaw.

Salpingitis

Inflammation situated in the FALLOPIAN TUBES; these run from the OVARIES to the UTERUS and carry the ova or eggs. The disorder is commonly caused by infection spreading upwards from the VAGINA, cervix or uterus. It is one feature of PELVIC INFLAMMATORY DISEASE (PID). Salpingitis is potentially serious and requires treatment with antibiotics and sometimes surgery to drain any PUS or, in persistent infections, to remove the Fallopian tubes.

Salpingo-

A prefix indicating a connection with either the FALLOPIAN TUBES or the EUSTACHIAN TUBES.

Salpingography

Radiography (see X-RAYS) of one or both FALLOPIAN TUBES after radio-opaque material has been injected into them via the UTERUS.

Salpingo-Oöphorectomy

Surgical removal of a Fallopian tube (see FALLOPIAN TUBES) and its accompanying ovary (see OVARIES).

Salt

The substance produced by the replacement of the acidic hydrogen of an acid by a metal or basic radical. It is also a synonym for common salt or sodium chloride. Sodium chloride is a vital constituent of cells, and a proper balance between it and other salts in the cells and body tissues is important for their viability.

Sandfly Fever

This is a short, sharp fever occurring in many parts of the tropics and subtropics, including most of the Mediterranean littoral. It is due to a virus, called phlebovirus, conveyed by the bite of a small hairy midge or sandfly (*Phlebotomus papatasi*). The incubation period is 3–7 days.

Symptoms There are headache, feverishness, general sensations like those of INFLUENZA, flushed face and bloodshot eyes, but no signs of CATARRH. The fever passes off in three days, but the patient may take some time to convalesce.

Treatment As there is no specific remedy, PROPHYLAXIS is important. This consists of the spraying of rooms with an insecticide such as GAMMEXANE; the application of insect repellents such as dimethyl phthalate to the exposed parts of the body (e.g. ankles, wrists and face), particularly at sunset; and the use of sandfly nets at night. Once the infection is acquired, treatment consists of rest in bed, light diet and aspirin and codeine.

Sanguineous

This term means containing blood.

Sanitary Protection

Disposable sanitary towels or tampons (see TAMPON) used to protect clothing from bloodstains during MENSTRUATION. They are available in different absorbencies to meet women's individual needs.

Saphenous

The name given to the two large superficial veins of the leg. The small saphenous vein, which runs up the outside and back of the leg, joins the deep veins at the bend of the knee; the great saphenous vein – the longest vein in the body, which has a course from the inner ankle to the groin – is especially subject, with its branches, to become the site of VARICOSE VEINS.

Saprophyte

An organism which lives usually upon decaying and dead matter and produces its decomposition.

Sarco-

A prefix signifying flesh or fleshy.

Sarcoidosis

An uncommon chronic inflammatory disease of unknown origin which can affect many organs, particularly the SKIN, eyes (see EYE) and LUNGS. Commonly, it presents as ERYTHEMA nodosum in association with lymph-gland enlargement within the chest. In the eyes it causes UVEITIS. BIOPSY of affected tissue allows diagnosis, which is confirmed by a KVEIM TEST. Often sarcoidosis is self-limiting, but in severe cases oral CORTICOSTEROIDS may be needed.

Sarcoma

See CANCER.

Sarcoptes

Mites which infest humans and animals. *Sarcoptes scabei hominis* causes human SCABIES. Other species infest dogs (sarcoptic mange), cats and birds.

SARS

In 2003, an outbreak occurred of a previously unrecognised illness – termed SARS, or severe acute respiratory syndrome. It was caused by infection with a newly identified coronavirus, *SARS-COV*. Infection produced an illness with PNEUMONIA as a prominent feature, but some patients developed other events such as loss of appetite, diarrhoea and bleeding from the stomach. Many of those who developed the disease were health-care workers and the contagion rate was vey high.

Exceptional isolation procedures became necessary as the EPIDEMIC threatened to spread worldwide from its origin in Hong Kong. For example, patients were concentrated in individual hospitals which were turned into isolation units with a 'no visiting' policy. Staff and other patients exposed to those with the disease were quarantined (see QUARANTINE) in the special units. All non-urgent hospital inpatient care was cancelled, and potential contacts were closely screened. Travel restrictions were put in place. These measures, coordinated by the World Health Organisation, brought the epidemic under control.

Scab

The crust which forms on superficial injured areas. It is composed of FIBRIN, which is exuded from the raw surface, together with blood corpuscles and epithelial cells entangled in its meshes. Healing takes place naturally under this protection, and the scab dries up and falls off when healing is complete. Scabs appearing on the face without any previous abrasion are usually caused by an infection (see IMPETIGO).

Scabicide

A drug that eliminates the mites which cause SCABIES.

Scabies

A common contagious itching disease caused by *Sarcoptes scabei hominis* (see SARCOPTES) which can live only on human skin. The fertilised female burrows into the skin surface, creating a tunnel within the stratum corneum in which she deposits 2–3 eggs per day, as well as faecal pellets which contain the ALLERGEN which initiates the immune reaction responsible for symptoms. The adult female is just visible. Eggs hatch within 3–4 days, producing larvae. After successive moults these become adult mites and the 15-day lifecycle re-starts. A rapid build-up of mite numbers is not noticed by the host until an immune response induces itching after about six weeks. Subsequently, scratching reduces the adult mites to a dozen or fewer. Scabies is spread by skin-to-skin contact, usually via the hands: it thus spreads in a family or sexual setting. Though most common in young adults, scabies can affect any age-group.

Typically the patient complains of widespread severe itching, worse when the body is warm after a bath or in bed. Burrows are visible as wavy black lines 3–5 mm long in the skin of the hands, wrists or sides of the feet. The intensity of the rash depends on the immune response. Papules, pustules, crusts and excoriations are seen on the hands and there may be a widespread eczematous (see DERMATITIS) or urticarial (see URTICARIA) rash elsewhere. Papules or even nodules on the PENIS and SCROTUM are characteristic. In infants, burrows occur on the palms and soles. Diminished immune response in old age, DOWN'S (DOWN) SYNDROME, etc. lead to a type of scabies which is less itching and more scaly. Rarely, absence of immune response causes a mite-saturated, generalised scaly dermatitis (Norwegian scabies). Admission of such a patient to hospital may result in an outbreak of scabies in other patients, staff and visitors caused by mite-infested airborne scale.

Treatment MALATHION 0·5 per cent aqueous

lotion, or PERMETHRIN 5 per cent cream, applied to the whole body, except the head, for 24 hours and then washed off cures the infection. In infants the head and neck should be included. The secondary eruption may take 2–3 weeks to settle completely and 10 per cent crotamiton cream is used during this period. It is essential that all intimate contacts be treated simultaneously. FOMITES need not be treated.

Scalded-Skin Syndrome
In infants, certain staphylococcal bacteria (see STAPHYLOCOCCUS) can cause an acute toxic illness in which the subject develops sheets of bright ERYTHEMA, accompanied by shedding of layers of outer epidermis. The result is similar to a hot-water scald. The condition responds promptly to appropriate antibiotic therapy. Drug reactions, especially from sulphonamides, may cause a similar syndrome in adults. In drug-induced forms, mucosae are also affected and the disease is often fatal.

Scalds
See BURNS AND SCALDS.

Scalp
The soft covering of the SKULL on the top of the head. It consists of five layers, which from the surface inwards are as follows: the skin, from which grows hair; next a subcutaneous layer of fat; thirdly, a tough fibrous membrane known as the epicranium; fourthly, a loose layer of connective tissue attaching the epicranium to the deepest layer, and permitting the free movement of the scalp; and, finally, another fibrous layer clinging closely to the skull, and known as the pericranium.

Scalpel
A small, straight, surgical knife.

Scanning Speech
A speech disorder in which articulated syllables are wrongly spaced and each is given the same vocal emphasis. The condition occurs as a result of disease in the cerebellum (see BRAIN) or its connecting nerves. (See also VOICE AND SPEECH.)

Scanning Techniques
Ways of producing images of body organs that record, process and analyse sound waves, radio waves or X-RAYS passing through or generated by the body's tissues. ULTRASOUND scanning using high-frequency, inaudible sound waves directed at the area of the body being studied is the most generally used scanning procedure. Sound waves are reflected more powerfully by some structures than others, and a pattern of those reflections is detected and shown on a screen. Other screening methods include COMPUTED TOMOGRAPHY, magnetic resonance imaging (MRI), positron emission tomography (PET SCANNING) and RADIONUCLIDE scanning, which measures the differential uptake of radioactive materials in the body's tissues.

Scaphoid Bone
The outside bone on the thumb side of the HAND in the row of carpal (wrist) bones nearest to the forearm. Fracture of the scaphoid is a common wrist injury that usually occurs when someone falls on to their outstretched hand. The fracture may not be diagnosed at first (even an X-ray may not be abnormal). Pain in and permanent damage to the wrist can occur.

Scapula
The scientific name for the shoulder-blade. (See SHOULDER.)

Scar
The name applied to a healed wound, ulcer or breach of tissue. A scar consists essentially of fibrous tissue, covered by an imperfect formation of epidermis in the case of scars on the surface of the skin. The fibrous tissue is produced by the connective tissue that migrates to the wound in the course of its repair (see WOUNDS). Gradually this fibrous tissue contracts, becomes more dense, and loses its blood vessels, leaving a hard white scar. (See also KELOID.)

Scarlet Fever
This disorder is caused by the erythrogenic toxin of the STREPTOCOCCUS. The symptoms of PYREXIA, headache, vomiting and a punctate erythematous rash (see ERYTHEMA) follow a streptococcal infection of the throat or even a wound. The rash is symmetrical and does not itch. The skin subsequently peels.

Symptoms The period of incubation (i.e. the time elapsing between the reception of infection and the development of symptoms) varies somewhat. In most cases it lasts only two to three days, but in occasional cases the patient may take a week to develop his or her first symptoms. The occurrence of fever is usually short and sharp, with rapid rise of temperature to 40 °C (104 °F), shivering, vomiting, headache, sore throat and marked increase in the rate of the pulse. In young children, CONVULSIONS or DELIRIUM may precede the fever. The rash usually appears within 24 hours of the onset of fever and lasts about a week.

Complications The most common and serious of these is glomerulonephritis (see under KIDNEYS, DISEASES OF), which may arise during any period in the course of the fever, but particularly when DESQUAMATION occurs. Occasionally the patient develops chronic glomerulonephritis. Another complication is infection of the middle ear (otitis media – see under EAR, DISEASES OF). Other disorders affecting the heart and lungs occasionally arise in connection with scarlet fever, the chief of these being ENDOCARDITIS, which may lay the foundation of valvular disease of the heart later in life. ARTHRITIS may produce swelling and pain in the smaller rather than in the larger joints; this complication usually occurs in the second week of illness. Scarlet fever, which is now a mild disease in most patients, should be treated with PENICILLIN.

Schistomicide
A drug used to treat SCHISTOSOMIASIS. Praziquantel is the drug of choice, with a combination of effectiveness, broad-activity spectrum and few side-effects.

Schistosomiasis
Also known as BILHARZIASIS. This infection results from one of the human *Schistosoma* species. It is common in Africa, South America, the Far East, Middle East, and, to a limited extent, the Caribbean. The life-cycle is dependent on fresh-water snails which act as the intermediate host for the fluke; the cercarial stage of the fluke enters via intact human skin and matures in the portal circulation. Clinically, 'swimmers' itch' may occur at the site of cercarial skin penetration. Acute schistosomiasis (Katayama fever) can result in fever, an urticarial rash (see URTICARIA), and enlargement of LIVER and SPLEEN. The adult male is about 12 mm and the female 24 mm in length.

S. haematobium causes CYSTITIS and haematuria – passage of blood in the urine; bladder cancer and ureteric obstruction, giving rise to hydronephrosis and kidney failure, are long-term sequelae in a severe case. *S. mansoni* can cause colonic symptoms and in a severe case, POLYPOSIS of the COLON; diarrhoea, which may be bloody, can be a presenting feature. In a heavy infection, eggs surrounded by granulomas are deposited in the liver, giving rise to extensive damage (pipe-stem fibrosis) associated with PORTAL HYPERTENSION, oesophageal varices, etc. However, unlike in CIRRHOSIS, hepato-

cellular function is preserved until late in the disease. *S. japonicum* (which is confined to the Far East, especially Indonesia) behaves similarly to *S. mansoni* infection; liver involvement is often more severe.

Diagnosis can be made by microscopic examination of URINE or FAECES. The characteristic eggs are usually detectable. Alternatively, rectal or liver BIOPSY are of value. Serological tests, including an ELISA (see ENZYME-LINKED IMMUNOSORBENT ASSAY (ELISA)), have now largely replaced invasive procedures used in making a parasitological diagnosis.

Treatment CHEMOTHERAPY has been revolutionised by the introduction of praziquantel (administered orally); this compound has no serious side-effects, although its cost may limit its use in developing countries. Oxamniquine is cheaper and effective in *S. mansoni* infection, although evidence of resistance has been recorded in several countries. Metriphonate is also relatively cheap and is of value in *S. haematobium* infection. Prevention is by complete avoidance of exposure to contaminated water; all travellers to infected areas should know about this disease. It is increasing in frequency as new expanses of fresh water appear as a result of irrigation schemes and dam projects. Molluscicides can be employed for snail-control.

Schizo-
A prefix signifying splitting.

Schizogony
An asexual phase in the life-cycle of a sporozoan (see SPOROZOA) that occurs in red blood cells or liver cells.

Schizophrenia
An overall title for a group of psychiatric disorders typfied by disturbances in thinking, behaviour and emotional response. Despite its inaccurate colloquial description as 'split personality', schizophrenia should not be confused with MULTIPLE PERSONALITY DISORDER. The illness is disabling, running a protracted course that usually results in ill-health and, often, personality change. Schizophrenia is really a collection of symptoms and signs, but there is no specific diagnostic test for it. Similarity in the early stages to other mental disorders, such as MANIC DEPRESSION, means that the diagnosis may not be confirmed until its response to treatment and its outcome can be assessed and other diseases excluded.

Causes There is an inherited element: parents, children or siblings of schizophrenic sufferers have a one in ten chance of developing the disorder; a twin has a 50 per cent chance if the other twin has schizophrenia. Some BRAIN disorders such as temporal lobe EPILEPSY, tumours and ENCEPHALITIS seem to be linked with schizophrenia. Certain drugs – for example, AMPHETAMINES – can precipitate schizophrenia and DOPAMINE-blocking drugs often relieve schizophrenic symptoms. Stress may worsen schizophrenia and recreational drugs may trigger an attack.

Symptoms These usually develop gradually until the individual's behaviour becomes so distrubing or debilitating that work, relationships and basic activities such as eating and sleeping are interrupted. The patient may have disturbed perception with auditory HALLUCINATIONS, illogical thought-processes and DELUSIONS; low-key emotions ('flat affect'); a sense of being invaded or controlled by outside forces; a lack of INSIGHT and inability to acknowledge reality; lethargy and/or agitation; a disrespect for personal appearance and hygiene; and a tendency to act strangely. Violence is rare although some sufferers commit violent acts which they believe their 'inner voices' have commanded.

Relatives and friends may try to cope with the affected person at home, but as severe episodes may last several months and require regular administration of powerful drugs – patients are not always good at taking their medication – hospital admission may be necessary.

Treatment So far there is no cure for schizophrenia. Since the 1950s, however, a group of drugs called antipsychotics – also described as NEUROLEPTICS or major tranquillisers – have relieved florid symptoms such as thought disorder, hallucinations and delusions as well as preventing relapses, thus allowing many people to leave psychiatric hospitals and live more independently outside. Only some of these drugs have a tranquillising effect, but their sedative properties can calm patients with an acute attack. CHLORPROMAZINE is one such drug and is commonly used when treatment starts or to deal with an emergency. Halperidol, trifluoperazine and pimozide are other drugs in the group; these have less sedative effects so are useful in treating those whose prominent symptoms are apathy and lethargy.

The antipsychotics' mode of action is by blocking the activity of DOPAMINE, the chemical messenger in the brain that is faulty in schizophrenia. The drugs quicken the onset and prolong the remission of the disorder, and it is

very important that patients take them indefinitely. This is easier to ensure when a patient is in hospital or in a stable domestic environment.

CLOZAPINE – a newer, atypical antipsychotic drug – is used for treating schizophrenic patients unresponsive to, or intolerant of, conventional antipsychotics. It may cause AGRANULOCYTOSIS and use is confined to patients registered with the Clorazil (the drug's registered name) Patient Monitoring Service. Amisulpride, olanzapine, quetiapine, risperidone, sertindole and zotepine are other antipsychotic drugs described as 'atypical' by the *British National Formulary*; they may be better tolerated than other antipsychotics, and their varying properties mean that they can be targeted at patients with a particular grouping of symptoms. They should, however, be used with caution.

The welcome long-term shift of mentally ill patients from large hospitals to community care (often in small units) has, because of a lack of resources, led to some schizophrenic patients not being properly supervised with the result that they fail to take their medication regularly. This leads to a recurrence of symptoms and there have been occasional episodes of such patients in community care becoming a danger to themselves and to the public.

The antipsychotic drugs are powerful agents and have a range of potentially troubling side-effects. These include blurred vision, constipation, dizziness, dry mouth, limb restlessness, shaking, stiffness, weight gain, and in the long term, TARDIVE DYSKINESIA (abnormal movements and walking) which affects about 20 per cent of those under treatment. Some drugs can be given by long-term depot injection: these include compounds of flupenthixol, zuclopenthixol and haloperidol.

Prognosis About 25 per cent of sufferers recover fully from their first attack. Another 25 per cent are disabled by chronic schizophrenia, never recover and are unable to live independently. The remainder are between these extremes. There is a high risk of suicide.

Schwann Cell

The cells that produce the MYELIN sheath of the AXON of a medullated NERVE. They are wrapped around a segment of the axon, forming concentric layers.

Sciatica

Pain in the distribution of the sciatic nerve. It is often accompanied by pain in the back, or LUMBAGO. In the majority of cases, however, it is due to a PROLAPSED INTERVERTEBRAL DISC in the lower part of the SPINAL CORD. What probably happens is that degenerative changes take place in the annulus fibrosus (see SPINAL COLUMN) as a result of some special strain – caused, for example, by heavy lifting – or spontaneously. The cushioning disc between the two neighbouring vertebral bodies slips through the rent in the annulus fibrosus, and presses on the neighbouring roots, thus causing the pain. The precise distribution of the pain will thus depend on which of the nerve roots are affected. As a rule, the pain is felt in the buttock, the back of the thigh and the outside and front of the leg, sometimes extending on to the top of the foot, the back of the thigh and the calf, and then along the outer border of the foot towards the little toe.

Rare causes include a tumour in the spine or spinal column, tuberculosis of the spine, ankylosing spondylitis (see SPINE AND SPINAL CORD, DISEASES AND INJURIES OF) or a tumour in one of the organs in the pelvis such as the UTERUS.

Treatment consists essentially of rest in bed in the early stages until the acute phase is over. ANALGESICS, such as aspirin and codeine, are given to relieve the pain. Expert opinion varies as to the desirability of wearing a PLASTER OF PARIS jacket or a specially made corset; also, as to the desirability of manipulation of the spine and operation. Surgeons are selective about which patients might benefit from a LAMINECTOMY (removal of the protruding disc).

Scirrhus
A hard form of cancer containing fibrous tissue.

Sclera
See EYE.

Scleritis
See under EYE, DISORDERS OF.

Scleroderma
A rare autoimmune disease. Scleroderma circumscriptum (morphoea) affects the skin, usually of the trunk, producing indurated plaques which resolve over many years. The more serious systemic form of scleroderma usually begins with RAYNAUD'S DISEASE, eventually producing a deforming hardening and clawing of the hands. Later the face and sometimes the internal organs, particularly the gastrointestinal tract and kidneys, may be affected.

Sclerosis
This term means literally hardening, and is applied to conditions in which portions of organs harden and lose their function as the result of an excessive production of CONNECTIVE TISSUE. The term is especially applied to a change of this type taking place in the nervous system. (See MULTIPLE SCLEROSIS (MS)).

Sclerotherapy
A treatment that involves injecting varicose veins (see VEINS, DISEASES OF) with a sclerosing fluid. This causes fibrosis of the lining of the vein and its eventual obliteration. Sclerotherapy is also used to treat varicose veins in the legs, anus (HAEMORRHOIDS) and at the junction of the OESOPHAGUS with the stomach.

Scoliosis
The name applied to curvature of the spine. (See SPINE AND SPINAL CORD, DISEASES AND INJURIES OF.)

Scorbutic
This is an adjective characterising SCURVY; typically swollen, spongy gums that bleed easily, and spontaneous haemorrhages and bruising anywhere in the body.

Scotoma
An area of blindness in the field of vision.

Screening Test
The screening of apparently healthy people to identify those who may have treatable diseases. Cervical smears are done when screening women to detect if they have cancer or precancer of the neck of the womb (cervix). Newborn babies are screened for hip dislocation. Screening tests are not designed to diagnose individual persons, but rather to divide a population into a large number at low risk and a small number at high risk of a condition. This allows clinicians to concentrate on a sub-section of the population. All screening tests produce false negative and false positive results, a problem often misunderstood by those at the receiving end. Factors to be assessed when planning screening procedures include the severity, frequency and distribution of the disease, and the availability and effectiveness of treatment. Convenience, safety, sensitivity and cost should also be assessed. In the United Kingdom the government has supported the extension of screening procedures for breast cancer, cervical cancer, hypertension and diabetes. (See PREVENTIVE MEDICINE.)

Scrivener's Palsy
Another name for writer's cramp (see MUSCLES, DISORDERS OF).

Scrofula

This is a traditional term for TUBERCULOSIS of the lymph glands in the neck. It was formerly known in England as 'king's evil', from the belief that the touch of the sovereign could effect a cure. This superstition can be traced back to the time of Edward the Confessor in England, and to a much earlier period in France. The disease, which is treated with antituberculous drugs, is now rare in developed societies and usually affects young children.

Scrombotoxin Poisoning

This occurs from eating poorly preserved scromboid fish such as tuna, mackerel and other members of the mackerel family. In such fish, a toxic histamine-like substance is produced by the action of bacteria or histidine, a normal component of fish flesh. This toxin produces nausea, vomiting, headache, upper abdominal pain, difficulty in swallowing, thirst, itching and sometimes URTICARIA. The condition settles as a rule in 12 hours. ANTI-HISTAMINE DRUGS sometimes ameliorate the condition.

Scrotum

The pouch of skin and fibrous tissue, positioned outside the abdomen behind the root of the PENIS, within which the testicles (see TES-TICLE) are suspended. It consists of a purse-like fold of skin, within which each testicle has a separate investment of muscle fibres, several layers of fibrous tissue, and a serous membrane known as the tunica vaginalis. The extra-abdominal site means that the production and storage of sperm (see SPERMATOZOON) in the testicles is at a lower temperature than internal body heat. Temperature control is facilitated by contraction and relaxation of the scrotal muscles.

Scrum-Pox

A popular name for a contagious condition of the face affecting rugby football players. It is most likely to occur in forwards as a result of face-to-face contact with individuals with the infection in the opposing side of the scrum. Other possible sources of infection are changing rooms and communal baths. The condition may take the form of IMPETIGO or HERPES SIMPLEX.

Scurf

See DANDRUFF.

Scurvy

Scurvy, or scorbitus, is caused by deficiency of vitamin C (ascorbic acid – see APPENDIX 5: VIT-AMINS) and is now rarely seen in developed countries except in people on poor diets, such as homeless down-and-outs. Ascorbic acid is a water-soluble vitamin derived from citrus fruits, potatoes and green vegetables. Nowadays woody haemorrhagic OEDEMA of the legs is the usual way in which the disease presents. The former classic disease of sailors living on salt beef and biscuits was characterised by bleeding of the gums, loss of teeth, haemorrhage into joints, ANAEMIA, lethargy and DEPRESSION. The introduction of fresh lime juice into the sea-man's diet in 1795 eliminated scurvy in the Royal Navy. Vitamin C is curative.

Sea-Sickness

See MOTION (TRAVEL) SICKNESS.

Seasonal Affective Disorder Syndrome

Known colloquially as SADS, this is a disorder in which an affected individual's mood changes with the seasons. He or she is commonly depressed in winter, picking up again in the spring. The diagnosis is controversial and its prevalence is not known. The mood-change is probably related to light, with MELATONIN playing a key role. (See also MEN-TAL ILLNESS.)

Sebaceous Cyst

A misnomer applied to epidermoid cysts of the skin whose contents are kerateous not sebaceous. The common 'wen' of the scalp arises from follicular epithelium and is similar.

Sebaceous Glands

The minute glands situated alongside hairs and opening into the follicles of the latter a short distance below the point at which the hairs emerge on the surface. These glands secrete an oily material, and are especially large upon the nose, where their openings form pits that are easily visible. In the mouth the glands open directly on the mucosal surface. (See also SKIN.)

Seborrhoea

Excessive production of SEBUM; it occurs in ACNE vulgaris.

Sebum

The secretion of the SEBACEOUS GLANDS. It acts as a natural lubricant of the hair and skin and protects the skin from the effects of moisture or excessive dryness. It may also have antibacterial action.

Secondary Prevention

The early detection of disease that reduces or prevents its serious outcome. Routine regular examination of particular age-groups – for example, children or the elderly – and screening tests are examples of secondary prevention.

Secondary Sexual Characteristics

The physical characteristics that develop during PUBERTY as the body matures sexually. Girls' breasts and genitals increase in size, and, like boys, they grow pubic hair. Boys also grow facial hair, their voice breaks and their genitals grow to adult size.

Secretin

A hormone (see HORMONES) secreted by the mucous membrane of the duodenum, the first part of the small INTESTINE, when food comes in contact with it. On being carried by the blood to the PANCREAS, it stimulates the secretion of pancreatic juice.

Secretion

The term applied to the material formed by a GLAND as the result of its activity. For example, saliva is the secretion of the salivary glands; gastric juice that of the glands in the stomach wall; bile that of the liver. Some secretions consist apparently of waste material which is of no further use in the chemistry of the body. These secretions are often spoken of as excretions: for example, the URINE and the sweat – see PERSPIRATION. (For further details, see ENDOCRINE GLANDS, and also under the headings of the various organs.)

Section

(1) A thin slice of a tissue specimen taken for examination under a microscope.
(2) The act of cutting in surgery; for example, an abdominal section is done to explore the abdomen.
(3) The issuing of an order under the United Kingdom's Mental Health Act to admit someone compulsorily to a psychiatric hospital.

Secundines

Another name for the afterbirth, consisting of the PLACENTA and membranes expelled in the final stage of labour (see PREGNANCY AND LABOUR).

Sedation

The production of a calm and peaceful state of mind, especially by the use of SEDATIVES. The aim is to reduce abnormal anxiety and bring aggressive behaviour under control. Sedation is also a part of the preparation of a patient for surgery or for any procedure that may be frightening or uncomfortable.

Sedatives

Drugs and other measures which have a calming effect, reducing tension and anxiety. They include ANXIOLYTICS and HYPNOTICS (usually given in smaller doses than is needed to induce sleep).

Sedimentation Rate

See ESR.

Seizure

Also called a FIT, this is a sudden burst of uncontrolled electrical activity in the BRAIN. A seizure may be generalised or partial: in the former, abnormal electrical activity may affect the whole brain, resulting in unconsciousness and characteristic of EPILEPSY; in partial seizures, abnormal electrical activity occurs in one part of the brain. HALLUCINATIONS may occur and localised symptoms include muscular twitching or a tingling sensation in a small area of the face, arm, leg or trunk. Different neurological or medical disorders may cause seizures: for example, STROKE, brain tumour, head injury, infection or metabolic disturbance (see METABOLISM; METABOLIC DISORDERS). People dependent on alcohol may suffer seizures if they stop drinking. Treatment is of the underlying condition coupled with antiepileptic drgus such as CARBAMAZEPINE, lamotrigine, SODIUM VALPROATE or PHENYTOIN SODIUM.

Selective Serotonin-Reuptake Inhibitors (SSRIs)

These ANTIDEPRESSANT DRUGS have few antimuscarinic effects (see ANTIMUSCARINE), but do have adverse effects of their own – predominantly gastrointestinal. They are, however, much safer in overdose than the tricyclic antidepressants, which is a major advantage in patients who are potentially suicidal. Examples are citalopram, used to treat panic disorders, as well as depressive illness; FLUOXETINE; and PAROXETINE. (See also MENTAL ILLNESS.)

Selegiline

A monoamine-oxidase-B-inhibiting drug used in conjunction with LEVODOPA to treat severe PARKINSONISM. Early treatment with selegiline may delay the need to give the patient levodopa, but at present there is no firm evidence that it slows down the progression of the disease.

Selenium Sulphide

This is used as a shampoo in the treatment of dandruff and seborrhoeic DERMATITIS of the scalp. In view of its potential toxicity it should only be used under medical supervision. It must never be applied to inflamed areas of the scalp, and it must not be allowed to get into the eyes as it may cause conjunctivitis or keratitis. It is also used in the treatment of tinea versicolor (see RINGWORM).

Self-Poisoning

See POISONS.

Sella Turcica

The deep hollow on the upper surface of the sphenoid bone in which the PITUITARY GLAND is enclosed.

Semen

Fluid produced by the male on ejaculation from the penis at sexual orgasm. Each ejaculate contains up to 500 million spermatozoa (male germ cells) suspended in a fluid that is secreted by the PROSTATE GLAND, seminal vesicles (see TESTICLE), and Cowper's glands – a pair of small glands (also called the bulbo-urethral glands) that open into the URETHRA at the base of the penis. Semen, or seminal fluid, contains a form of sugar (fructose) essential for the motility of sperm. The hormone TESTOSTERONE is a key element in the production of sperm and of seminal fluid.

Semilunar Cartilages

Two crescentic layers of fibro-cartilage on the outer and inner edges of the knee-joint, which form hollows on the upper surface of the tibia in which the condyles at the lower end of the femur rest. The inner cartilage is especially liable to be displaced by a sudden and violent movement at the KNEE.

Seminal Vesicle

One of the small paired sacs lying on either side of the male URETHRA, which collect and store spermatozoa. (See TESTICLE.)

Seminiferous Tubules

The long tortuous tubules that form much of the testis (see TESTICLE) and carry the SEMEN to the URETHRA.

Seminoma

A malignant tumour of the testis (see TESTICLE) that appears as an often painless swelling. This tumour usually occurs in an older age-group of men than does TERATOMA. The treatment is surgical removal. (See also TESTICLE, DISEASES OF.)

Senile Dementia

DEMENTIA was traditionally divided into presenile and senile types; this is increasingly recognised as an arbitrary division of a condition in which there is a general and often slow decline in mental capabilities. Around 10 per cent of people over 65 years of age and 20 per cent over 75 are affected by dementing illness, but people under 65 may also be affected. Treatable causes such as brain tumour, head injury, ENCEPHALITIS and alcoholism are commoner in younger people. Other causes such as cerebrovascular disease – which is a major factor, especially among older people – or ALZHEIMER'S DISEASE are not readily treatable, although ANTIHYPERTENSIVE DRUGS for the former disorder may help, and symptomatic treatment for both is possible.

Individuals with dementia suffer a gradual deterioration of memory and of the ability to grasp what is happening around them. They often cover up their early failings and the condition may first become apparent as a result of emotional outbursts or uncharacteristic behaviour in public. Eventually personal habits and speech deteriorate and they become thoroughly confused and difficult to look after. Treatment is primarily a matter of ameliorating the symptoms, coupled with a sympathetic handling of the sufferer and the relatives. Admission to hospital or nursing home may be necessary if relatives are unable to look after the patient at home. (See also MEDICINE OF THE AGEING.)

Senility

See AGEING.

Senna

The leaves of various species of *Cassia senna*. It is one of the most active of the simple laxative drugs (see LAXATIVES). Senna is excreted in the urine, giving it a dark red or yellow colour. In the case of nursing mothers, some of the drug is excreted in the milk and may affect the infant. A standardised preparation of senna, Senokot®, is widely used for the management of constipation in children and old people. A side-effect of senna is HYPOKALAEMIA; like other laxatives, it should not be used too often.

Sensation

See PAIN; TOUCH.

Sensitisation
See ALLERGY; ANAPHYLAXIS.

Sensitivity
The extent to which a SCREENING TEST detects the proportion of true cases of the disease being screened.

Sensory
Description applied to the part of the nervous system dedicated to bringing information on sensations affecting the body to the brain. The opposite of sensory nerves is motor nerves; these carry instructions for action to the voluntary muscles in the body.

Sensory Cortex
See BRAIN.

Sensory Deprivation
A substantial reduction in the volume of SENSORY information impinging on the body – for instance, sitting in a dark, silent room. Prolonged deprivation is potentially harmful as the body needs constant stimulation in order to function normally. The main input organs are the eyes, ears, skin and nose. The absence of sensations disorients a person and results in neurological dysfunction. Some interrogation techniques involve sensory deprivation to 'soften up' the individual being questioned.

Sepsis
Poisoning by the products of the growth of micro-organisms in the body, the general symptoms which accompany it are those of INFLAMMATION. Sepsis is prevented by the various procedures mentioned under ASEPSIS, and is treated locally with ANTISEPTICS and systemically with ANTIBIOTICS.

Septal Defect
A congenital abnormality of the HEART affecting about 260 babies in every 100,000, in which there is a hole in the septum – the dividing wall – between the left and right sides of the heart. The effects of the defect depend upon its size and position. A defect in the wall between the atria (upper chambers of the heart) is called an atrial septal defect, and that between the ventricles, a ventricular septal defect – the most common form (25 per cent of all defects). Both defects allow blood to circulate from the left side of the heart, where pressures are highest, to the right. This abnormal flow of blood is described as a 'shunt' and the result is that too much blood flows into the lungs. PULMONARY HYPERTENSION occurs and, if the shunt is large,

heart failure may develop. A small septal defect may not need treatment but a large one will need to be repaired surgically.

Septicaemia
A serious condition caused by the presence of micro-organisms in the bloodstream. A very high temperature may be the only sign, but there is often associated shivering (rigor), profuse sweating and pains in the joints and muscles. If the condition is not brought to a halt by the early use of high-dose antibiotics, preferably given intravenously, SEPTIC SHOCK may supervene and the patient's life be put at risk. Any infected area of the body may progress to septicaemia if untreated.

Septic Arthritis
Infection in a joint which becomes warm, swollen and sore, with restricted movement. The infectious agent may enter the joint as a result of a penetrating wound or via the bloodstream. The condition is treated by ARTHROTOMY or ARTHROSCOPY, joint irrigation and ANTIBIOTICS. Unless treated, the articular CARTILAGE of the joint is destroyed, resulting in a painful, deformed and sometimes immobile joint. (See ARTHRITIS.)

Septic Shock
A dangerous disorder characterised by a severe fall in blood pressure and damage to the body tissues as a result of SEPTICAEMIA. The toxins from the septicaemia cause widespread damage to tissue, provoke clotting in small blood vessels, and seriously disturb the circulation. The kidneys, lungs and heart are particularly affected. The condition occurs most commonly in people who already have a chronic disease such as cancer, CIRRHOSIS of the liver or DIABETES MELLITUS. Septic shock may also develop in patients with immunodeficiency illnesses such as AIDS (see AIDS/HIV). The symptoms are those of septicaemia, coupled with those of SHOCK: cold, cyanotic limbs; fast, thready pulse; and a lowered blood pressure. Septic shock requires urgent treatment with ANTIBIOTICS, intravenous fluids and oxygen, and may require the use of drugs to maintain blood pressure and cardiac function, artificial ventilation and/or renal DIALYSIS.

Septum
A dividing wall within a structure in the body. Examples are the divisions between the chambers of the heart, and the layer of bone and cartilage that separates the two nostrils of the nose.

Sequelae

The term applied to symptoms or effects which are liable to follow certain diseases. For example, BRONCHITIS and other chest complaints may be sequelae of MEASLES; heart disease is often a sequelae of RHEUMATIC FEVER; PARALYSIS may follow DIPHTHERIA.

Sequestrum

A fragment of dead bone cast off from the living bone in the process of NECROSIS. (See also BONE, DISORDERS OF.) A sequestrum often remains in contact with, and partly enveloped by, newly formed bone, so that a SINUS is produced; a constant discharge goes on until the dead bone is removed.

Seroconversion

The production of specific ANTIBODIES to antigens (see ANTIGEN) present in the body. This may happen as a result of infection by a virus, or IMMUNISATION with a VACCINE. Thus, if blood has been tested before the event there may be little or no evidence of antibody to the condition in question; but when a sample is taken 1–2 weeks later there may be a high level of antibody confirming that recent infection has taken place. Sometimes this is the only way to prove that a particular infection has occurred or that a vaccination has 'taken'.

Serotonin

Also known as 5-hydroxytryptamine, this is a substance widely distributed in the body tissue, but especially in the PLATELETS in the blood, the lining of the gastrointestinal tract, and the BRAIN. Serotonin is believed to have a similar function to that of HISTAMINE in INFLAMMATION. In the gut it inhibits gastric secretion and stimulates smooth (involuntary) muscle in the walls of the INTESTINE. Serotonin participates in the transmission of nerve impulses and may have a function in controlling mood and states of consciousness. (See also SELECTIVE SEROTONIN-REUPTAKE INHIBITORS (SSRIS).)

Serotype

A classification of a substance according to its serological activity. This is done in the context of the antigens (see ANTIGEN) that it contains, or the ANTIBODIES it may provoke. Micro-organisms of the same species may be classified according to the different antigens that they produce.

Serous

Relating to, containing or resembling SERUM.

Serous Membranes

These are smooth, transparent membranes that line certain large cavities of the body. The chief serous membranes are the PERITONEUM, lining the cavity of the abdomen; the pleurae (see PLEURA), one of which lines each side of the chest, surrounding the corresponding lung; the PERICARDIUM, in which the heart lies; and the tunica vaginalis on each side, enclosing a testicle. The name of these membranes is derived from the fact that the surface is moistened by thin fluid derived from the serum of blood or LYMPH. Every serous membrane consists of a visceral portion, which closely envelops the organs concerned, and a parietal portion, which adheres to the wall of the cavity. These two portions are continuous with one another so as to form a closed sac, and the opposing surfaces are close together, separated only by a little fluid. This arrangement enables the organs in question to move freely within the cavities containing them. For further details, see under PERITONEUM.

Serpiginous

A term describing a creeping or extending skin lesion such as an ULCER.

Serum

The fluid which separates from blood, LYMPH, and other body fluids when clotting occurs (see COAGULATION; HAEMORRHAGE). PLASMA is the fluid of the blood, including FIBRIN, which carries the circulating blood cells and PLATELETS.

Serum is a clear, yellowish fluid containing around 7 per cent proteins and globulins, small quantities of salts, fat, sugar, urea, and uric acid, and even smaller quantities of immunoglobulins, essential in the prevention of disease (see IMMUNITY; IMMUNOLOGY). The serum given in the commonly used vaccines is generally derived from horses' blood, after they have been subjected to a long course of treatment.

Serum Sickness

A hypersensitivity reaction due to circulating antigen-antibody complexes (see ANTIGEN; ANTIBODIES), so-called because it was a not uncommon reaction to the administration of foreign SERUM which used to be given as a form of passive IMMUNITY before the days of antibiotics. By definition, it is a manifestation of sensitivity to serum – but the same clinical and pathological picture can occur 1–3 weeks after the administration of drugs such as PENICILLIN and STREPTOMYCIN. It is characterised by fever, ARTHRALGIA and LYMPHADENOPATHY and is usually self-limiting as it resolves when the supply of antigen is used up.

Serum Therapy
See IMMUNOLOGY.

Sesamoid Bones
Rounded nodules of bone usually embedded in tendon. They are usually a few millimetres in diameter, but some are larger, such as the PATELLA, or knee-cap.

Sessile
A growth or tumour that has no stalk.

Severe Acute Respiratory Syndrome (SARS)
See SARS.

Sevoflurane
A quick-acting volatile liquid anaesthetic (see ANAESTHESIA). Emergence and recovery from anaesthetic are rapid, and early post-operative measures to control pain are advised.

Sex Change
A major surgical operation, usually coupled with the appropriate hormone treatment (see HORMONES), to change a person's anatomical sex. The operation is done on transsexual individuals or in those whose sexual organs are neither totally female nor male. Male-to-female sex change is the more common. Such operations should not be performed without rigorous physical and mental assessment of the individual, and should be accompanied by extensive counselling. Some subjects make a satisfactory adjustment to the change of anatomical sex, while others may suffer serious psychological problems. Hormone therapy may need to be continued for life.

Sex Chromosomes
In humans there are 23 pairs of CHROMOSOMES. Male and female differ in respect of one pair. In the nucleus of female cells, the two members of the pair are identical and are called X chromosomes. In the male nucleus there is one X chromosome paired with a dissimilar, differently sized chromosome called the Y chromosome. In the sex cells, after MEIOSIS, all cells in the female contain a single X chromosome. In the male, half will contain an X chromosome and half a Y chromosome. If a sperm with an X chromosome fertilises an ovum (which, as stated, must have an X chromosome) the offspring will be female; if a sperm with a Y chromosome fertilises the ovum

the offspring will be male. It is the sex chromosomes which determine the sex of an individual.

Sometimes during cell division chromosomes may be lost or duplicated, or abnormalities in the structure of individual chromosomes may occur. The surprising fact is the infrequency of such errors. About one in 200 live-born babies has an abnormality of development caused by a chromosome, and two-thirds of these involve the sex chromosomes. There is little doubt that the frequency of these abnormalities in the early embryo is much higher, but because of the serious nature of the defect, early spontaneous ABORTION occurs.

Chromosome studies on such early abortions show that half have chromosome abnormalities, with errors of autosomes being three times as common as sex chromosome anomalies. Two of the most common abnormalities in such fetuses are triploidy with 69 chromosomes and trisomy of chromosome 16. These two anomalies almost always cause spontaneous abortion. Abnormalities of chromosome structure may arise because of:

Deletion   Where a segment of a chromosome is lost.

Inversion   Where a segment of a chromosome becomes detached and re-attached the other way around. GENES will then appear in the wrong order and thus will not correspond with their opposite numbers on homologous chromosomes.

Duplication   Where a segment of a chromosome is included twice over. One chromosome will have too little nuclear material and one too much. The individual inheriting too little may be non-viable and the one with too much may be abnormal.

Translocation   Where chromosomes of different pairs exchange segments.

Errors in division of centromere   Sometimes the centromere divides transversely instead of longitudinally. If the centromere is not central, one of the daughter chromosomes will arise from the two short arms of the parent chromosome and the other from the two long arms. These abnormal daughter chromosomes are called isochromosomes.

These changes have important bearings on heredity, as the effect of a gene depends not only upon its nature but also upon its position on the chromosome with reference to other genes. Genes do not act in isolation but against the background of other genes. Each gene normally has its own position on the chromosome, and this corresponds precisely with the positon of its allele on the homologous chromosome of the pair. Each member of a pair of chromosomes will normally carry precisely the same number of genes in exactly the same order. Characteristic clinical syndromes, due to abnormalities of chromosome structure, are less constant than those due to loss or gain of a complete chromosome. This is because the degree of deletion, inversion and duplication is inconstant. However, translocation between chromosomes 15 and 21 of the parent is associated with a familial form of mongolism (see DOWN'S (DOWN) SYNDROME) in the offspring, and deletion of part of an X chromosome may result in TURNER'S SYNDROME.

Non-disjunction Whilst alterations in the structure of chromosomes arise as a result of deletion or translocation, alterations in the number of chromosomes usually arise as a result of non-disjunction occurring during maturation of the parental gametes (germ cells). The two chromosomes of each pair (homologous chromosomes) may fail to come together at the beginning of meiosis and continue to lie free. If one chromosome then passes to each pole of the spindle, normal gametes may result; but if both chromosomes pass to one pole and neither to the other, two kinds of abnormal gametes will be produced. One kind of gamete will contain both chromosomes of the pair, and the other gamete will contain neither. Whilst this results in serious disease when the autosomes are involved, the loss or gain of sex chromosomes seems to be well tolerated. The loss of an autosome is incompatible with life and the malformation produced by a gain of an autosome is proportional to the size of the extra chromosome carried.

Only a few instances of a gain of an autosome are known. An additional chromosome 21 (one of the smallest autosomes) results in mongolism, and trisomy of chromosome 13 and 18 is associated with severe mental, skeletal and congenital cardiac defects. Diseases resulting from a gain of a sex chromosome are not as severe. A normal ovum contains 22 autosomes and an X sex chromosome. A normal sperm contains 22 autosomes and either an X or a Y sex chromosome. Thus, as a result of non-disjunction of the X chromosome at the first meiotic division during the formation of female gametes, the ovum may contain two X chromosomes or none at all, whilst in the male the sperm may contain both X and Y chromosomes

(XY) or none at all. (See also CHROMOSOMES; GENES.)

Sex Education

Information given to children and young adults about sexual relationships. Evidence suggests that young people want more information about the emotional aspects of sexual relationships, and about homosexuality and AIDS/HIV. There is growing concern about sexual risk-taking behaviour among adolescents, many of whom feel that sex education was provided too late for them. Although most parents or guardians provide some guidance by the age of 16, friends, magazines, television and films are a more significant source of information. Schools have been targeted as a place to address and possibly limit risky behaviour because they are geared towards increasing knowledge and improving skills, and have a captive audience of young adults. There are concerns that the conditions in schools may not be ideal: class time is limited; teachers are often not trained in handling sensitive subjects; and considerable controversy surrounds teaching about subjects such as homosexuality.

Sex education in schools is regarded as an effective way of reducing teenaged pregnancy, especially when linked with contraceptive services. Several studies have shown that it does not cause an increase in sexual activity and may even delay the onset of sexual relationships and lessen the number of partners. Programmes taught by youth agencies may be even more effective than those taught in the classroom – possibly because teaching takes place in small groups of volunteer participants, and the programmes are tailored to their target populations. Despite improvements in sex education, the United Kingdom has the highest incidence of teenaged pregnancies in the European Community.

Sex education, including information about AIDS/HIV and other sexually transmitted infections (STIs), is compulsory in all state-maintained secondary schools in England and Wales. The National Curriculum includes only biological aspects of AIDS/HIV, STIs and human sexual behaviour.

All maintained schools must have a written statement of their policy, which is available to parents. The local education authority, governing body and headteacher should ensure that sex education encourages pupils to have due regard to moral considerations and the value of family life. Sex-education policies and practices are monitored by the Office for Standards in Education (OFSTED) and the Office of HM

Chief Inspector of Schools (OHMCI) as part of school inspections.

Sex Hormones

These HORMONES control the development of primary and secondary sexual characteristics. They also regulate sex-related functions – for example, menstruation and the production of sperm and eggs. The three main types of sex hormone are androgens, or male sex hormones (see ANDROGEN); OESTROGENS, or female sex hormones; and progesterones, which are involved in pregnancy (see PROGESTERONE).

Sex-Linked Inheritance

The way in which a characteristic or an illness determined by the SEX CHROMOSOMES in an individual's cells is passed on to the succeeding generation. Men have one X and one Y sex chromosome and women have two X chromosomes. Disorders that result from an abnormal number of sex chromosomes include KLINEFELTER'S SYNDROME, which affects only men, and TURNER'S SYNDROME, which affects mainly women. Recessive GENES on the X chromosome cause most other sex-linked characteristics; in women these may well be masked because one of their two X chromosomes carries a normal (dominant) gene. In men, who have just one X chromosome, no such masking occurs – so more men than women are affected by X-linked characteristics or diseases. (See also HEREDITY.)

Sex Therapy

The counselling and treatment of individuals with psychosexual dysfunction (see SEXUAL DYSFUNCTION). Around half of couples experience some type of sexual problem during their relationships, and for most of them the difficulties are psychological. Sexual therapy is usually given to both partners, but sometimes individual counselling is necessary. Couples may sometimes find that group therapy is helpful. Therapy has proved effective especially for women with VAGINISMUS (spasm of vaginal muscles), men with PREMATURE EJACULATION or IMPOTENCE, and men and women who fail to achieve ORGASM.

Sexual Abuse

See CHILD ABUSE.

Sexual Deviation

Any type of pleasurable sexual practice which society regards as abnormal. Deviation may be related to the activity, such as EXHIBITIONISM or sadomasochistic sex (see SADISM; MASOCHISM); or to the sexual object, for example, shoes or clothes (fetishism). Different cultures have different values, and treatment is probably not required unless the deviation is antisocial or harmful to the participant(s). Aversion therapy, or the conditioning of a person's behaviour, may help if treatment is considered necessary.

Sexual Dysfunction

Inadequate sexual response may be due to a lack of sexual desire (LIBIDO) or to an inadequate performance; or it may be that there is a lack of satisfaction or ORGASM. Lack of sexual desire may be due to any generalised illness or endocrine disorder, or to the taking of drugs that antagonise endocrine function (see ENDOCRINE GLANDS). Disorders of performance in men can occur during arousal, penetration and EJACULATION. In the female, DYSPAREUNIA and VAGINISMUS are the main disorders of performance. DIABETES MELLITUS can cause a neuropathy which results in loss of erection. IMPOTENCE can follow nerve damage from operations on the PROSTATE GLAND and lower bowel, and can be the result of neurological diseases affecting the autonomic system (see NERVOUS SYSTEM). Disorders of satisfaction include, in men, impotence, emission without forceful ejaculation and pleasureless ejaculation. In women such disorders range from the absence of the congestive genital response to absence of orgasm. Erectile dysfunction in men can sometimes be treated with SILDENAFIL CITRATE (Viagra®), a drug that recent research suggests may also be helpful to women with reduced libido and/or inability to achieve orgasm.

Sexual dysfunction may be due to physical or psychiatric disease, or it may be the result of the administration of drugs. The main group of drugs likely to cause sexual problems are the ANTICONVULSANTS, the ANTIHYPERTENSIVE DRUGS, and drugs such as metoclopramide that induce HYPERPROLACTINAEMIA. The benzodiazepine TRANQUILLISERS can reduce libido and cause failure of erection. Tricyclic ANTIDEPRESSANT DRUGS may cause failure of erection and clomipramine may delay or abolish ejaculation by blockade of alpha-adrenergic receptors. The MONOAMINE OXIDASE INHIBITORS (MAOIS) often inhibit ejaculation. The PHENOTHIAZINES reduce sexual desire and arousal and may cause difficulty in maintaining an erection. The antihypertensive drug, methyldopa, causes impotence in over 20 per cent of patients on large doses. The beta-adrenoceptor-blockers and the DIURETICS can also cause impotence. The main psychiatric causes of sexual dysfunction include stress, depression and guilt.

Sexually Transmitted Diseases (STDs)

Sexually transmitted diseases – traditionally called venereal diseases – are infections transmitted by sexual intercourse (heterosexual and homosexual). In the United Kingdom they are treated in genito-urinary medicine (GUM) clinics. The incidences of these diseases are more common among people who have several sexual partners, as STDs are very infectious; some of the major STDs, particularly AIDS/HIV, are also transmitted by blood and so can result from needle-sharing by drug addicts, or by TRANSFUSION. The 'traditional' STDs – SYPHILIS, GONORRHOEA and CHANCROID – now comprise only 10 per cent of all such diseases treated in STD clinics: these clinics also treat patients with CHLAMYDIA, TRICHOMONIASIS, HERPES GENITALIS, MOLLUSCUM CONTAGIOSUM and genital WARTS. SCABIES and pubic lice (see PEDICULOSIS – *Pediculus pubis*) can also be transmitted by sexual intercourse, and HEPATITIS B is also recognised as an STD.

The incidence of STDs rose sharply during World War II but the advent of PENICILLIN and subsequent antibiotics meant that syphilis and gonorrhoea could be treated effectively. The arrival of oral contraception and more tolerant public attitudes to sexual activities resulted in an increase in the incidence of sexually transmitted infections. The diagnosis of NON-SPECIFIC URETHRITIS (NSU), once given to many patients whose symptoms were not due to the traditional recognised infections, was in the 1970s realised to be wrong, as the condition was proved to be the result of infection by chlamydia.

Most STDs are treatable, but herpes is an infection that could become chronic, while hepatitis B and, of course, AIDS/HIV are potentially fatal – although treatment of HIV is now proving more effective. As well as the treatment and subsequent monitoring of patients with STDs, one of the important functions of clinics has been the tracing, treatment and follow-up of sexual contacts of infected individuals, a procedure that is conducted confidentially.

Apart from AIDS/HIV, the incidence of STDs fell during the 1980s; however in some countries the agents causing syphilis and gonorrhoea began to develop resistance to antibiotics, which showed the continued importance of practising safe sex – in particular by restricting the number of sexual partners and ensuring the regular use of condoms. In the United Kingdom the rates per million of the male population infected by syphilis rose from 8.8 in 1991 to 9.7 in 1999; in females the figures were 4.0 to 4.5, respectively. For gonorrhoea, the figures for men were 399.4 in 1991 and 385 in 1999, with women also showing a reduction, from 216.5 to 171.3. In 1991, 552.6 per million of men had chlamydia, a figure which rose to 829.5 in 1999; for women in the same period the incidence also rose, from 622.5 to 1,077.1 per million. For genital herpes simplex virus, the infection rate for men fell from 236.6 per million to 227.7, whereas the figures for women showed a rise, 258.5 to 357. The incidence of AIDS/HIV is given under the relevant entry. (These figures are based on information in *United Kingdom Health Statistics*, 2001 edition, UKHSI, published by the Office of National Statistics.)

Shaken Impact Syndrome

A type of non-accidental head-injury to infants. A study published in 2000 (*Lancet*, 4 November) suggests that almost 25 out of 100,000 children under a year old sustain brain damage from shaken impact syndrome, even if they do not strike any hard surface. So, of around 685,000 babies in this age-group in Britain, as many as 170 a year may suffer injury from violent shaking. The median age for admission to hospital for the condition in Scotland was 2.2 months in the 18 months from July 1998. A Swedish report has concluded that children at risk from CHILD ABUSE can be identified and the incidence reduced by legislation banning corporal punishment. (See also NON-ACCIDENTAL INJURY (NAI).)

Shellfish Poisoning

In the United Kingdom this occurs in two main forms. Shellfish may be the cause of typhoid fever (see ENTERIC FEVER) as a result of their contamination by sewage containing the causative organism. They may also be responsible for what is known as paralytic shellfish poisoning. This is caused by a toxin, or poison, known as saxotoxin, which is present in certain planktons which, under unusual conditions, multiply rapidly, giving rise to what are known as 'red tides'. In these circumstances the toxin accumulates in mussels, cockles and scallops which feed by filtering plankton. The manifestations of such poisoning are loss of feeling in the hands, tingling of the tongue, weakness of the arms and legs, and difficulty in breathing. There is also growing evidence that some shellfish poisoning may be due to a virus infection. (See also FOOD POISONING.)

Sheltered Housing

Accommodation that has been adapted to cater for the special requirements of those elderly people who can largely look after themselves but benefit from some discreet supervision. The accommodation is usually a small flat, and a warden will supervise a group of flats. Meals and other services may be provided, and the payment system varies depending on whether the accommodation is privately owned or run by a local social-services department.

Shigella

The name given to a group of rod-shaped, gram-negative bacteria (see GRAM'S STAIN) that are the cause of bacillary DYSENTERY.

Shingles

See HERPES ZOSTER.

Shin Splints

See MEDIAL TIBIAL SYNDROME.

Shock

A state of acute circulatory failure in which the heart's output of blood is inadequate to provide normal PERFUSION of the major organs. It is accompanied by a fall in arterial blood pressure and is characterised by systemic arterial hypotension (arterial blood pressure less than 80 mm of mercury), sweating and signs of VASOCONSTRICTION (for example, pallor, CYANOSIS, a cold clammy skin and a low-volume pulse). These signs may be associated with clinical evidence of poor tissue perfusion, for example to the brain and kidneys, leading to mental apathy, confusion or restlessness and OLIGURIA.

Shock may result from loss of blood or plasma volume. This may occur as a result of haemorrhage or severe diarrhoea and vomiting. It may also result from peripheral pooling of blood due to such causes as TOXAEMIA or ANAPHYLAXIS. The toxaemia is commonly the result of a SEPTICAEMIA in which leakage through capillaries reduces circulating blood volume. Another form is called cardogenic shock, and is due to failure of the heart as a pump. It is most commonly seen as a result of myocardial infarction (see under HEART, DISEASES OF).

If failure of adequate blood flow to vital organs is prolonged, the effects can be disastrous. The ischaemic intestine permits the transfer of toxic bacterial products and proteins across its wall into the blood; renal ISCHAEMIA

prevents the maintenance of a normal electrolyte and acid-base balance.

Treatment If the shock is a result of haemorrhage or diarrhoea or vomiting, replacement of blood, lost fluid and electrolytes is of prime importance. If it is due to septicaemia, treatment of the infection is of paramount importance, and in addition, intravenous fluids and vasopressor drugs will be required. Cardiogenic shock is treated by attention to the underlying cause. Full intensive care is likely to be required, and artificial ventilation and DIALYSIS may both be needed.

Shock Lung

See ACUTE RESPIRATORY DISTRESS SYNDROME (ARDS).

Shock Therapy

See ELECTROCONVULSIVE THERAPY (ECT).

Short-Sight

A condition in which objects near at hand are seen clearly, while objects at a distance are blurred. The condition is technically known as myopia. (See EYE, DISORDERS OF – Errors of refraction; VISION.)

Short Stature

See DWARFISM.

Shoulder

The joint formed by the upper end of the HUMERUS and the shoulder-blade or SCAPULA. The acromion process of the scapula and the outer end of the collar-bone (see CLAVICLE) form a protective bony arch above the joint, and from this arch the wide and thick deltoid muscle passes downwards, protecting the outer surface of the joint and giving to the shoulder its rounded character. The joint itself is of the ball-and-socket variety, the rounded head of the humerus being received into the hollow glenoid cavity of the scapula, which is further deepened by a rim of cartilage. One tendon of the biceps muscle passes through the joint, grooving the humerus deeply, and being attached to the upper edge of the glenoid cavity. The joint is surrounded by a loose fibrous capsule, strengthened at certain places by ligamentous bands. The main strength of the joint comes from the powerful muscles that unite the upper arm with the scapula, clavicle and ribs.

Shoulder-blade or scapula. A flat bone, about as large as the flat hand and fingers, placed on the upper and back part of the

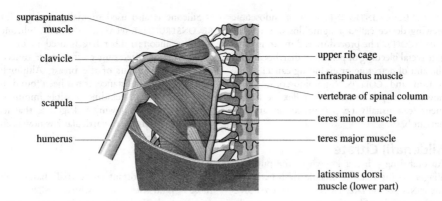

supraspinatus muscle

clavicle

scapula

humerus

upper rib cage

infraspinatus muscle

vertebrae of spinal column

teres minor muscle

teres major muscle

latissimus dorsi muscle (lower part)

Posterior view of musculoskeletal structure of left shoulder.

thorax. Many of the large muscles that move the arm are attached to it. It is not in contact with the ribs, and its only attachment to the trunk of the body is through a joint between its acromion process and the clavicle on the tip of the shoulder and by the powerful muscles which suspend it from the backbone and ribs. With the arm hanging by the side, the scapula extends from the second to the seventh rib, but, as the arm is raised and lowered, it slides freely over the back of the chest. On the rear surface of the bone is a strong process, the spine of the scapula. This arches upwards and forwards into the acromion process. The latter forms the bony prominence on the top of the shoulder, where it unites in a joint with the outer end of the clavicle.

Shunt

Passage of blood through a channel that is not its normal one. This may occur as a result of a congenital deformity (see SEPTAL DEFECT) or of surgery – for example, a porto-caval shunt in which the main portal vein is joined up to the inferior vena cava.

Sialagogues

Substances which produce a copious flow of SALIVA.

Sialorrhoea

Also called ptyalism, this is the excessive production of SALIVA. It occurs in various nervous disorders, such as PARKINSONISM; poisoning by MERCURY or mushrooms; or RABIES infection.

Siamese Twins

See CONJOINED TWINS; MULTIPLE BIRTHS.

Sibling

A brother or sister. Sibling rivalry is the term

applied to the intense competition that sometimes occurs between brothers and/or sisters. The birth of a new baby in the family may prompt jealousy and rivalry that can persist throughout life.

Sickle-Cell Anaemia

See under ANAEMIA.

Sickness

See VOMITING; MOTION (TRAVEL) SICKNESS.

Side-Effects

This refers to an effect of a drug which is not that which doctor and patient require. Some side-effects are almost inevitable: for example, drowsiness with older ANTIHISTAMINE DRUGS; others are very rare, such as REYE'S SYNDROME with ASPIRIN. Some can be predicted to occur if the dose is raised, while others may occur at the lowest of doses due to the individual patient's susceptibility. In deciding whether to prescribe or take a drug, a balance must always be struck between its benefits and risks. (See also MEDICINES – Safe use of medicines.)

Siderosis

Chronic FIBROSIS of the LUNGS occurring in iron-workers and due to the inhalation of fine iron particles. The term is also applied to the condition in which there is an excessive deposit of iron in the tissues of the body.

SIDS

See SUDDEN INFANT DEATH SYNDROME (SIDS).

Sight

See VISION.

Sigmoidoscopy

Examination of the RECTUM and sigmoid

COLON (see also INTESTINE) with an endoscopic viewing device called a sigmoidoscope (see also ENDOSCOPE). The procedure is done to investigate rectal bleeding or persistent diarrhoea, with the aim of detecting or excluding cancer of the rectum and COLITIS. Sigmoidoscopy, which nowadays is performed with a flexible instrument, can usually be performed on an outpatient basis.

Sildenafil Citrate

An oral drug – better known to the public as Viagra® – for treating erectile dysfunction of the PENIS (see also ERECTION; SEXUAL DYSFUNCTION). Sildenafil citrate was originally developed to treat ANGINA PECTORIS; during clinical trials, patients reported that they were having more erections than before taking the drug. Clinical trials were then conducted on 4,000 men, and 70 per cent of them found sildenafil effective. The men, of an average age of 55 years, had experienced erectile problems for around five years before taking part in the trials. The medical conditions associated with their problems included high blood pressure, high concentrations of CHOLESTEROL, DIABETES MELLITUS, surgery and psychological disorders. Among side-effects, headache was the most common; others included facial flushing, indigestion and a stuffy nose. The drug is a vasodilator so that blood flow to the penis is enhanced. It works in response to sexual stimulation and has no properties as an aphrodisiac; nor does it provoke sexual fantasies. Sildenafil must not be taken with drugs containing nitrates such as GLYCERYL TRINITRATE or isosorbide trinitrate as the subject may suffer a sudden fall in blood pressure. Nitrates inhaled for recreational use (poppers) have a similar effect. Recent research suggests that the drug may help women with low LIBIDO or who have difficulty in achieving ORGASM.

Silica

A major constituent of the earth's crust. Its main danger to health arises from free silica, present mainly as quartz and flint and as an important constituent of granite, sandstone and slate. (See SILICOSIS.)

Silicones

Organic compounds of silicone, with a structure of alternate atoms of silicone and oxygen, and organic groups – such as methyl and phenyl – attached to the silicone atoms. As they produce a flexible and stable water-repellent film on the skin, they are used as BARRIER CREAMS.

Silicone is also used to make implants for RECONSTRUCTIVE (PLASTIC) SURGERY. Silicone oil in a silicone rubber bag is used in breast reconstruction after surgery for breast cancer, and for enlargement of the breast. Although usually an inert substance, it has been found to cause side-effects, including possible immunological reactions following leakages, so that its use in breast surgery in particular has now been restricted.

Silicosis

The most important industrial hazard in those industries in which SILICA is encountered: in other words, the pottery industry, the sandstone industry, sandblasting, metal-grinding, the tin-mining industry, and anthracite coal-mines. It is a specific form of PNEUMOCONIOSIS caused by the inhalation of free silica. Among pottery workers the condition has for long been known as potter's asthma, whilst in the cutlery industry it was known as grinder's rot. For the production of silicosis, the particles of silica must measure 0·5–5 micrometres in diameter, and they must be inhaled into the alveoli (air sacs) of the lungs, where they produce FIBROSIS. This diminishes the efficiency of the lungs, resulting in slowly progressive shortness of breath. The main danger of silicosis, however, is that it is liable to be complicated by TUBERCULOSIS.

The incidence of silicosis is steadily being reduced by various measures which diminish the risk of inhaling silica dust. These include adequate ventilation to draw off the dust; the suppression of dust by the use of water; the wearing of respirators where the risk is particularly great and it is not possible to reduce the amount of dust – for example, in sand-blasting; and periodic medical examination of workpeople exposed to risk. Fewer than 100 new cases a year are diagnosed now in the United Kingdom. (See also OCCUPATIONAL HEALTH, MEDICINE AND DISEASES.)

Simmonds' Disease

A rare condition in which wasting of the skin and the bones, IMPOTENCE, and loss of hair (ALOPECIA) occur as a result of destruction of the PITUITARY GLAND.

Simvastatin

One of the STATINS – a group of LIPID-lowering drugs which are effective – in combination with a low CHOLESTEROL diet – in reducing the incidence of heart attacks (see HEART, DISEASES OF – Coronary thrombosis).

Singer's Nodule

A small excrescence on the vocal cords (see LARYNX) which causes hoarseness. This tends to develop in people who abuse their voices – for example, singers, or people who shout excessively.

Sinoatrial Node

This is the natural pacemaker of the HEART, and comprises a collection of specialised muscle cells in the wall of the upper chamber (atrium) of the heart. The cells initiate electrical impulses at a rate of up to 100 a minute. These impulses stimulate the muscles of the heart to contract. The rate is altered by the effects of certain hormones and various impulses from the nervous system. Damage or disease of the node affects the regular beating of the heart. (See also CARDIAC PACEMAKER.)

Sinus

A term applied to narrow cavities of various kinds, occurring naturally in the body, or resulting from disease. Thus it is applied to the air-containing cavities which are found in the frontal, ethmoidal, sphenoidal and maxillary bones of the SKULL, and which communicate with the NOSE. The function of these paranasal sinuses, as they are known, is doubtful, but they do lighten the skull and add resonance to the voice. They enlarge considerably around puberty and in this way are a factor in the alteration of the size and shape of the face. The term is also used in connection with the wide spaces through which the blood circulates in the membranes (MENINGES) of the BRAIN. Cavities which are produced when an ABSCESS has burst, but remain unhealed, are also known as sinuses (see also FISTULA).

Sinusitis

Sinusitis is inflammation of the mucosal lining of a SINUS. The term is usually applied to inflammation of the sinuses in the face. Most cases occur as a result of infection spreading to the sinuses from the NOSE along the passages that drain mucus secreted by the linings of the sinuses to the nose. The bacterial infection usually follows a viral infection of the upper respiratory tract. Treatment with ANTIBIOTICS is usually effective but the condition tends to recur. If the episodes are severe, they can be disabling, with bad headaches. Surgery is sometimes necessary to drain the sinuses. Rarely, sinusitis may lead to cerebral abscess or venous sinus thrombosis.

Sinusoid

A small blood vessel like an enlarged capillary (see CAPILLARIES) occurring, for example, in the LIVER, which contains a large number of them. The sinusoids in the liver are drained by the hepatic veins.

Sinus Tachycardia

A regular heart rate of 100 or more beats a minute, caused by increased electrical activity in the SINOATRIAL NODE (see also HEART). This level of tachycardia is normal during and just after exercise, and may also be caused by stress or anxiety. If tachycardia persists when the person is resting, it may be due to underlying disease such as thyrotoxicosis (see under THYROID GLAND, DISEASES OF) and investigation is advisable.

SI Units

The international system of measurement-units used throughout the sciences. SI units, which derive from metres, kilograms, and seconds, comprise seven basic units and two supplementary ones. Among the other base units are ampere (electric current) and mole (amount of a substance at molecular level). Derived SI units include joule (energy), pascal (pressure), becquerel (activity), and newton (force). (See APPENDIX 6: MEASUREMENTS IN MEDICINE.)

Sjogren's Syndrome

A disorder of CONNECTIVE TISSUE, with dryness of the mouth (xerostomia) and dryness of the eye (kerato conjunctivitis sicca) occurring in association with RHEUMATOID ARTHRITIS. It occurs in approximately 10 per cent of patients with the latter condition, but it can occur – and frequently does so – independently of rheumatoid disease. The lack of tears gives rise to symptoms of dryness and grittiness of the eyes; the dry mouth can occasionally be so severe as to cause a DYSPHAGIA. The disease is due to the autoimmune destruction of the SALIVARY GLANDS and the lacrimal glands (see EYE – Lacrimal apparatus). The disorder is usually associated with specific HLA antigen (see HLA SYSTEM). Treatment is unsatisfactory and is limited to oral and ocular hygiene as well as the provision of artificial tears in the form of cellulose eye drops.

Skeletal Muscle

Muscle under a person's voluntary control (see MUSCLE; VOLUNTARY MUSCLE).

Skeleton

The comprehensive term applied to the hard structures that support or protect the softer tissues of the body. Many animals are possessed of an exoskeleton, consisting of superficial plates of bone, horn, or the like; but in humans the skeleton is entirely an endoskeleton, covered everywhere by soft parts and consisting mainly of bones, but in places also of cartilage. The chief positions in which cartilage is found in place of bone are the larynx and the front of the chest. (For details of the skeleton, see BONE.)

Skin

The membrane which envelops the outer surface of the body, meeting at the body's various orifices, with the mucous membrane lining the internal cavities.

Structure

CORIUM The foundation layer. It overlies the subcutaneous fat and varies in thickness from 0·5–3.0 mm. Many nerves run through the corium: these have key roles in the sensations of touch, pain and temperature (see NEURON(E)). Blood vessels nourish the skin and are primarily responsible for regulating the body temperature. Hairs are bedded in the corium, piercing the epidermis (see below) to cover the skin in varying amounts in different parts of the body. The sweat glands are also in the corium and their ducts lead to the surface. The fibrous tissue of the corium comprises interlocking white fibrous elastic bundles. The corium contains many folds, especially over joints and on the palms of hands and soles of feet with the epidermis following the contours. These are permanent throughout life and provide unique fingerprinting identification.

HAIR Each one has a root and shaft, and its varying tone originates from pigment scattered throughout it. Bundles of smooth muscle (arrectores pilorum) are attached to the root and on contraction cause the hair to stand vertical.

GLANDS These occur in great numbers in the skin. SEBACEOUS GLANDS secrete a fatty substance and sweat glands a clear watery fluid (see PERSPIRATION). The former are made up of a bunch of small sacs producing fatty material that reaches the surface via the hair follicle. Around three million sweat or sudoriparous glands occur all over the body surface; sited below the sebaceous glands they are unconnected to the hairs.

EPIDERMIS This forms the outer layer of skin and is the cellular layer covering the body surface: it has no blood vessels and its thickness varies from 1 mm on the palms and soles to 0·1 mm on the face. Its outer, impervious, horny layer comprises several thicknesses of flat cells

(pierced only by hairs and sweat-gland openings) that are constantly rubbed off as small white scales; they are replaced by growing cells from below. The next, clear layer forms a type of membrane below which the granular stratum cells are changing from their origins as keratinocytes in the germinative zone, where fine sensory nerves also terminate. The basal layer of the germinative zone contains melanocytes which produce the pigment MELANIN, the cause of skin tanning.

Nail A modification of skin, being analogous to the horny layer, but its cells are harder and more adherent. Under the horny nail is the nail bed, comprising the well-vascularised corium (see above) and the germinative zone. Growth occurs at the nail root at a rate of around 0·5 mm a week – a rate that increases in later years of life.

Skin functions By its ability to control sweating and open or close dermal blood vessels, the skin plays a crucial role in maintaining a constant body temperature. Its toughness protects the body from mechanical injury. The epidermis is a two-way barrier: it prevents the entry of noxious chemicals and microbes, and prevents the loss of body contents, especially water, electrolytes and proteins. It restricts electrical conductivity and to a limited extent protects against ultraviolet radiation.

The Langerhans' cells in the epidermis are the outposts of the immune system (see IMMUNITY), just as the sensory nerves in the skin are the outposts of the nervous system. Skin has a social function in its ability to signal emotions such as fear or anger. Lastly it has a role in the synthesis of vitamin D.

Skin, Diseases of

They may be local to the SKIN, or a manifestation of systemic disorders – inherited or acquired. Some major types are described below.

Others appear under their appropriate alphabetical headings: ACNE; ALBINISM; ALOPECIA; ALOPECIA AREATA; APHTHOUS ULCER; BASAL CELL CARCINOMA; BOILS (FURUNCULOSIS); BOWEN'S DISEASE; CALLOSITIES; CANDIDA; CHEILOSIS; CHEIRAPOMPHOLYX; DANDRUFF; DERMATOFIBROMA; DERMATOMYOSITIS; DERMATOPHYTES; DERMOGRAPHISM; ECTHYMA; ERYSIPELAS; ERYTHEMA; ERYTHRASMA; ERYTHRODERMA; ESCHAR; EXANTHEM; FUNGAL AND YEAST INFECTIONS; HAND, FOOT AND MOUTH DISEASE; HERPES GENITALIS; HERPES SIMPLEX; HERPES ZOSTER; IMPETIGO; INTERTRIGO; KELOID; KERATOSIS;

LARVA MIGRANS; LICHEN; LUPUS; MADURA FOOT; MELANOMA; MILIARIA; MOLLUSCUM CONTAGIOSUM; MOLE; MYCOSIS FUNGOIDES; NAEVUS; ORF; PEDICULOSIS; PEMPHIGUS; PHOTOCHEMOTHERAPY; PHOTODERMATOSES; PITYRIASIS; PORPHYRIAS; PRURITUS; PSORIASIS; RINGWORM; ROSACEA; SARCOIDOSIS; SCABIES; SCLERODERMA; URTICARIA; VITILIGO; WARTS; XANTHOMATA.

Skin cancer Primary cancer is common and chronic exposure to ultraviolet light is the most important cause. BASAL CELL CARCINOMA is the most common form; squamous cell carcinoma is less common and presents as a growing, usually painless nodule which may ulcerate. Squamous cancer may spread to regional lymph glands and metastasise, unlike basal cell cancer. Occupational exposure to chemical carcinogens may cause squamous carcinoma – for example, cancer from pitch warts or the scrotal carcinoma of chimney sweeps exposed to coal dust in earlier centuries. Squamous carcinoma of the lip is associated with clay-pipe smoking.

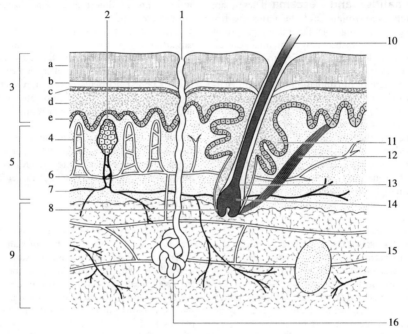

1 sweat gland duct
2 tactile corpuscle in corium
3 epidermis
   (a) stratum corneum
   (b) stratum lucidum
   (c) stratum granulosum
   (d) stratum spinosum
   (e) stratum basale
4 fascicular papilla in corium
5 corium
6 blood vessel
7 nerve
8 bulb of hair
9 subcutaneous fat
10 hair
11 sebaceous gland
12 arrectores pilorum muscle
13 medulla of hair
14 papilla of hair
15 pacinian corpuscle
16 body of sweat gland

Vertical section through the skin including hair and sweat glands.

Cancer may arise from the population of melanocytes of the skin (see MELANOCYTE; MELANOMA).

Apart from these three most frequent forms of skin cancer, various forms of cancer can arise from cells of the dermis, of which LYMPHOMA is the most important (see also MYCOSIS FUNGOIDES).

Lastly, secondary deposits from internal cancer, particularly from the breast, may metastasise to the skin.

Dermatitis and eczema These are broadly synonymous, and the terms are frequently interchangeable. Eczema is a pattern of inflammation with many potential causes. Dermatitis is commonly used to suggest an eczema caused by external factors; it is a common pattern of inflammation of the skin characterised by redness and swelling, vesiculation (see VESICLE), and scaling with intense itching and often exudation (weeping). Fissuring, thickening (lichenification – see LICHEN) and secondary bacterial infection may follow. Dermatitis can affect any part of the body. It may be genetically detemined or due to other 'internal' factors, such as venous HYPERTENSION in a leg, or stress. Often it is 'external' in origin – due to strong irritants or chemical allergens. (See also ALLERGY; ALLERGEN.)

ATOPIC DERMATITIS is genetic in origin and usually begins in infancy. It may persist for years, and ASTHMA, allergic RHINITIS and conjunctivitis (see under EYE, DISORDERS OF) – 'hay fever' – may be associated. Atopic children tend to have multiple allergies, especially to inhaled allergens such as house-dust mite, cat and dog dander and pollens. Allergy to foods is less common but potentially more dangerous, especially if to nuts, when it can cause acute URTICARIA or even ANAPHYLAXIS. Atopic subjects are particularly prone to persistent and multiple verrucae (see WARTS) and mollusca (see MOLLUSCUM CONTAGIOSUM) and to severe HERPES SIMPLEX infections. (See also ATOPY.)

EXFOLIATE DERMATITIS (PITYRIASIS RUBRA) Generalised exfoliation and scaling of the skin, commonly with ERYTHEMA. Drugs may cause it, or the disorder may be linked with other skin diseases such as benign dermatoses and lupus erythematosus (see under LUPUS).

SUMMER POMPHOLYX is an acute vesicular eczema of the palms and soles recurring every summer. Inhaled allergens are a frequent cause.

VENOUS (STASIS) DERMATITIS begins on a lower calf, often in association with PURPURA, swelling and sometimes ulceration. Chronic venous hypertension in the leg, consequent on valvular incompetence in the deep leg veins owing to previous deep vein thrombosis (see VEINS, DISEASES OF), is the usual cause.

NEURODERMATITIS A pattern of well-defined plaques of lichenified eczema particularly seen on the neck, ulnar forearms or sides of the calves in subjects under emotional stress.

IRRITANT CONTACT DERMATITIS Most often seen in an industrial setting (occupational dermatitis), it is due to damage by strong chemicals such as cutting oils, cement, detergents and solvents. In almost all cases the hands are most severely affected.

ALLERGIC CONTACT DERMATITIS, in contrast, can affect any part of the body depending on the cause – for example, the face (cosmetics), hands (plants, occupational allergens) or soles (rubber boots). Particularly common allergens include metals (nickel and chromate), rubber additives, and adhesives (epoxy resins).

Treatment Avoidance of irritants and contact allergens, liberal use of EMOLLIENTS, and topical application of corticosteroid creams and ointments (see CORTICOSTEROIDS) are central.

Skin-Grafting

An operation in which large breaches of SKIN surface due to wounding, burns or ulceration are closed by TRANSPLANTATION of skin from other parts. There are three methods by which this is done. Most frequently the epidermis only is transplanted, using a method introduced by Reverdin and by Thiersch, and known by their names. For this purpose, a broad strip of epidermis is shaved off the thigh or upper arm, after the part has been carefully sterilised, and is transferred bodily to the raw or ulcerated surface, or is cut into smaller strips and laid upon it. A second method is for small pieces of the skin in its whole thickness to be removed from the arm and thigh, or even from other people, and then implanted and bound upon the raw surface. (This method has the disadvantage that the true skin must contract at the spot from which the graft is taken, leaving an unsightly scar.) When very large areas require to be covered, a third method is commonly used. A large flap of skin, amply sufficient to cover the gap, is raised from a neighbouring or distant part of the body, in such a way that it remains attached along one margin, so that blood vessels can still enter and nourish it. It is then turned so as to cover the gap; or, if it be situated on a distant part, the two parts are brought together and fixed in this position until the flap grows firmly to its new bed. The old connection of the flap is then severed, leaving it growing in its new place.

Researchers are having success in growing human skin in the laboratory for grafting on to people who have been badly burned and have insufficient intact skin surface to provide an autologous graft (one provided by the recipient of the graft). Other techniques being researched are the use of specially treated shark skin and the production of artificial skin.

Skull

This is the collection of 22 flat and irregularly shaped bones which protect the brain and form the face (see BONE).

Arrangement of the bones In childhood, the bones are independent, gradually fusing together by sutures, and in old age fusing completely so that the cranium forms a solid bony case. At the time of birth the growth of several bones of the infant's head has not been quite completed, so that six soft spots, or fontanellas, present; here the brain is covered only by skin and membranes, and the pulsations of its blood vessels may be seen. One of these spots, the anterior fontanelle, does not close completely until the child is 18 months to 2½ years old.

Parts of the skull The cranium, enclosing the brain, consists of eight bones, while the face, which forms a bony framework for the eyes, nose and mouth, consists of 14 bones. These two parts can be detached.

Shape of the skull The development of large central hemispheres of the brain in humans has influenced the skull shape. Unlike in other mammals, the cranium extends above as well as behind the face which therefore looks forwards. The skull's proportions change with age: the cranium in children is larger in comparison with the face – one-eighth of the whole head – than is the case in adults, where sizes are about the same. Old age reduces the size of the face because of the loss of teeth and absorption of their bony sockets. Women's skulls tend to be lighter and smoother with less obvious protuberances than those in men.

Slapped Cheek Syndrome

See ERYTHEMA – Erythema infectiosum.

SLE

See SYSTEMIC LUPUS ERYTHEMATOSUS (SLE).

Sleep

Sleep is a state which alternates with wakefulness, and in which awareness and responsiveness to the environment are reduced. It is not, however, uniform and can be divided into two main states differentiated according to electrical recordings of brain activity (EEG), of the muscles (EMG), and of the eye movements (EOG).

Non-rapid-eye-movement (NREM) sleep This is subdivided into four stages, of which stage 1 is the lightest and stage 4 the deepest. The activity of the cerebral cortex (see BRAIN) is diminished and the body's functions are mainly regulated by brain-stem activity. The metabolic rate is reduced; in keeping with this the temperature falls, respiration is reduced, cardiac output, heart rate, and blood pressure fall, and activity of the sympathetic nervous system is reduced. NREM sleep normally occurs at the onset of sleep except in neonates. During adult life, the duration – particularly of stages 3 and 4 – of NREM sleep becomes less, and very little of this deep sleep occurs after the age of 60 years.

NREM sleep has been thought to have several functions, such as energy conservation and growth. Growth hormone is produced in bursts during stages 3 and 4, and more cell division occurs during this type of sleep than during wakefulness. A controversial proposal has been that processing of information acquired during wakefulness occurs during NREM sleep.

Rapid-eye-movement (REM) sleep This is characterised by the presence of rapid eye movements and a reduction in muscle tone. Cerebral cortical activity is prominent and its blood flow increased. This activity is, however, different from wakefulness and may cause irregular movements of the body as well as of the eyes. Most dreams occur in REM sleep: these may represent a process of reorganising mental associations after the period of wakefulness. The analysis of the content of dreams has been subject to a variety of interpretations, but no consensus view has evolved.

Physiological changes, such as a fall in temperature and blood pressure, take place just before sleep and continue during the early stages of NREM sleep. There is an intrinsic rhythm of sleep which in most subjects has a periodicity of around 25 hours. This can be modified by external factors to bring it into line with the 24-hour day. Two peaks of a tendency to sleep have been identified, and these usually occur between around 14.00–18.00 hours, and

02.00–06.00 hours. There are, however, differences according to age, in that, for instance, infants sleep for most of the 24 hours; during adolescence there is also an increase in the duration of sleep. Sleep requirements fall later in life, but there are wide genetic differences in the amount of sleep that people require and also the time at which they fall asleep most readily.

The internal clock can be disturbed by a variety of external factors which include irregular sleeping habits due, for instance, to shift work or jet lag. Sleep is also more likely to occur after physical exertion, reading and social activity. The duration and intensity of exposure to light can also modify sleep profoundly. Light promotes wakefulness and is the main factor that adjusts the 25-hour internal rhythm to the 24-hour daily cycle. Neural connections from the retina of the EYE act on an area in the brain called the supra-chiasmatic nucleus which stimulates the pineal gland which produces MELATONIN. This is thought to trigger the range of neurological and metabolic processes that characterise sleep.

Sleep Apnoeas

A sleep apnoea is conventionally defined as the cessation of breathing for ten seconds or more. Apnoeas, which affect around 5 per cent of adults and are markedly more common in men, may occur as frequently as 400 times per night. They can be due to a failure of the physiological drive to breathe (central sleep apnoeas) but much more often are due to a transient obstruction of the airway between the level of the soft PALATE and the LARYNX (obstructive sleep apnoeas) when the airway dilator muscles over-relax. Any factor such as alcohol or sedative drugs that accentuates this, or that makes the airway narrower (such as obesity or large TON-SILS), will tend to cause sleep apnoeas.

Vigorous respiratory movements are made to overcome the obstruction during each apnoea. These are associated with snoring and snorting noises. The apnoea ends with a mini-arousal from sleep. As a result, sleep becomes fragmented and sleep deprivation, manifested as sleepiness during the day, is common. This may result in accidents – for instance, at work or while driving – and sleep apnoea is also linked with an increased risk of STROKE, heart attacks and HYPERTENSION.

The diagnosis of sleep apnoea has recently been facilitated by linking specially designed software with ELECTROCARDIOGRAPHY performed during sleep, with minimal disturbance of the subject.

Initial treatment is directed at correcting the cause (e.g. obesity), but if the apnoeas persist or are severe a nasal mask and pump which introduces air under slight pressure into the upper airway (continuous positive airway pressure, CPAP) is almost invariably effective.

Sleep, Disorders of

There are three main groups of SLEEP disorders:

Parasomnias   These include medical disorders such as ASTHMA, ANGINA PECTORIS or EPILEPSY which are made worse by sleep, and a range of behavioural alterations which are usually related to a specific sleep stage or to a change from one state of sleep to another. Sleepwalking, night terrors, and nightmares are examples.

Insomnia   Insomnia is defined as a difficulty in initiating or maintaining sleep. It affects around 15 per cent of the population at any one time, and is often due to a poor pre-sleep routine (e.g. taking excessive stimulants such as caffeine); unsatisfactory sleep due to poor environments such as an uncomfortable bed or a cold or noisy bedroom; anxiety and/or depression; or occasionally to a physical problem – for example, pain – or a medical disorder associated with sleep such as obstructive SLEEP APNOEAS or periodic limb movements.

Excessive daytime sleepiness   This is usually due to sleep deprivation caused either by inadequate duration of sleep, or by poor quality of sleep. The individual's lifestyle is often a cause and modification of this may relieve the problem. Other common causes of excessive daytime sleepiness are depression, obstructive sleep apnoeas, periodic limb movements, excessive alcohol or other drug intake, and, less commonly, NARCOLEPSY.

Sleeping Sickness

There are two major forms of the disease: *Trypanosoma brucei gambiense* is confined to west and central Africa, and *T.b. rhodesiense* to central, east, and south-east Africa. The infection is caused by the bite of tsetse fly (*Glossina* spp.). Clinically, a trypanosomal CHANCRE may develop at the site of the tsetse-fly bite. After introduction into the bloodstream, the parasite develops in blood and lymphatic glands. After the blood stage, it enters the central nervous system, causing characteristic neurological sequelae (see below). Infection may be followed by a generalised macular papular reaction. In *T.b. gambiense* infection, enlarged glands in the neck (Winterbottom's sign) may be striking. Onset of disease is accompanied by fever, progressive ANAEMIA, and enlarged glands; these signs and symptoms are followed by increasing lethargy, slowing of mentality, and physical weakness, and give way to headache and an increasing tendency to sleep. These symptoms are caused by proliferation of parasites in the patient's cerebral blood vessels; this is accompanied by inflammatory changes and disorganisation of nervous tissue. Patients become emaciated and develop bed sores. Death finally takes place either as a result of gross emaciation or of an intercurrent infection.

Diagnosis is by detection of trypanosomes in a blood specimen or, alternatively, a sample of cerebrospinal fluid. Serological tests are of great value in diagnosis.

Treatment is with suramine or pentamidine; when cerebral involvement has ensued, melarsoprol – which penetrates the blood-brain barrier – is of value. In *T.b. gambiense* infection, eflornithine has recently given encouraging results; however, this form of CHEMOTHERAPY is not effective in a *T.b. rhodesiense* infection. From the point of view of prevention, control of the tsetse-fly population is crucial; even so, only a very small percentage of these vectors is infected with *Trypanosoma* spp.

Sling
A hanging bandage for the support of injured or diseased parts. Slings are generally applied for support of the upper limb, in which case the limb is suspended from the neck. The lower limb may also be supported in a sling from an iron cage placed upon the bed on which the patient lies, the object usually being to aid the circulation, and so quicken the healing of ulcers on the leg.

Slipped Disc
The popular name for a PROLAPSED INTER-VERTEBRAL DISC. (See also SPINAL COLUMN; SCIATICA.)

Slough
Slough (pronounced 'sluff') is dead tissue separated by natural processes from the living body. The term is applied to hard external parts which the lower animals cast off naturally in the course of growth, like the skin of snakes or the shell of crabs. In humans, however, the process is generally associated with disease, and is then known as GANGRENE. Sloughs may be of very small size, as in the case of the core of a boil, or they may include a whole limb; but in general a slough involves a limited area of skin or of the

underlying tissues. The process of separation of a slough is described under gangrene.

Small-Bowel Transplantantion
Before the advent of small-bowel transplants, long-term intravenous feeding (total parenteral nutrition or TPN) was the last option for patients with chronic intestinal failure. Most recipients are children, and small-bowel transplantation is currently reserved for patients unable to continue on long-term parenteral nutrition. The main constraints to small-bowel transplantation are the intensity of rejection (necessitating high levels of immunosuppression), and the lack of donors who are the same size as the recipient (a particular problem for children).

Small-Cell Carcinoma
See OAT CELL.

Smallpox
So-called to distinguish the disease from syphilis, the great pox (pox being the plural of pock, the Old English term for a PUSTULE), is also known as variola (from *varus*, the Latin for pimple). It is an acute, highly infectious disease due to a virus. Once it was one of the major killing diseases; however, in the 1960s the World Health Organisation undertook an eradication scheme by means of mass VACCINATION. As a result, the last naturally occurring case was recorded in October 1977, and on 8 May 1980 the World Health Assembly confirmed that smallpox has finally been eradicated from the world.

Smegma
A thick, cheesy secretion formed by the SEBACEOUS GLANDS of the glans penis (see PENIS). A bacillus, closely resembling the tubercle bacillus morphologically, develops readily in this secretion.

Smell
The sense of smell is picked up in what is known as the olfactory areas of the NOSE. Each of these is about 3 square centimetres in area and contains 50 million olfactory, or smelling, cells. They lie, one on either side, at the highest part of each nasal cavity. This is why we have to sniff if we want to smell anything carefully, as in ordinary quiet breathing only a few eddies of the air we breathe in reaches an olfactory area. From these olfactory cells the olfactory nerves (one on each side) run up to the olfactory bulbs underneath the frontal lobe of the BRAIN, and here the

impulse is translated into what we describe as smell.

Smoke Inhalation

Smoke is made up of small particles of carbon in hot air and gases. The particles are covered with organic chemicals and smoke may also contain carbon monoxide and acids. When smoke is inhaled, the effects on breathing may be immediate or delayed, depending upon the density of smoke and its composition. Laryngeal stridor (obstruction of the LARYNX), lack of oxygen and PULMONARY OEDEMA are life-threatening symptoms that require urgent treatment. Immediate removal of the victim from the smoke is imperative, as is the administration of oxygen. The victim may require admission to an intensive-care unit.

Smoking

See TOBACCO.

Smooth Muscle

Muscle under the 'involuntary' control of the autonomic nervous system (see MUSCLE; NERVOUS SYSTEM).

Snake-Bite

See BITES AND STINGS.

Snapping Finger

See TRIGGER FINGER.

Sneezing

A sudden expulsion of air through the NOSE, designed to expel irritating materials from the upper air passages. In sneezing, a powerful expiratory effort is made; the vocal cords (see VOICE AND SPEECH; LARYNX) are kept shut until the pressure in the chest has risen high; and air is then suddenly allowed to escape upwards, being directed into the back of the nose by the soft PALATE. One sneeze projects 10,000 to 100,000 droplets a distance of up to 10 metres at a rate of over 60 kilometres an hour. As such droplets may contain micro-organisms, it is clear what an important part sneezing plays in transmitting infections such as the COMMON COLD. Although usually transitory, sneezing may persist for days on end – up to 204 days have been recorded.

Sneezing may be caused by the presence of irritating particles in the nose, such as snuff, or the pollen of grasses and flowers. It is also an early symptom of colds, INFLUENZA, MEASLES, and HAY FEVER, being then accompanied or followed by running at the nose (RHINITIS).

Snellen Chart

The most commonly used chart for testing the acuity of distant VISION. The chart comprises rows of capital letters, with the letters in each row being smaller than those in the one above. The top line of large letters can be seen by a normally sighted person standing 60 metres away. The subject under test sits 6 metres from the screen and, if he or she can read the 6-metre line of letters, his or her visual acuity is normal at 6/6.

Snoring

This is usually attributed to vibrations of the soft PALATE, but there is evidence that the main fault lies in the edge of the posterior pillars of the FAUCES which vibrate noisily. Mouth-breathing is necessary for snoring, but not all mouth-breathers snore. The principal cause is blockage of the nose, such as occurs during the course of the common cold or chronic nasal CATARRH; such blockage also occurs in some cases of deviation of the nasal SEPTUM or nasal polypi (see NOSE, DISORDERS OF). In children, mouth-breathing, with resulting snoring, is often due to enlarged TONSILS and adenoids. A further cause of snoring is loss of tone in the soft palate and surrounding tissues due to smoking, overwork, fatigue, obesity, and general poor health. One in eight people are said to snore regularly. The intensity, or loudness, of snoring is in the range of 40–69 decibels. (Pneumatic drills register between 70 and 90 decibels.) Bouts of snoring sometimes alternate with SLEEP APNOEAS.

Treatment therefore consists of the removal of any of these causes of mouth-breathing that may be present. Should this not succeed in preventing snoring, then measures should be taken to prevent the sufferer from sleeping lying on his or her back, as this is a habit strongly conducive to snoring. Simple measures include sleeping with several pillows, so that the head is raised quite considerably when asleep; alternatively, a small pillow may be put under the nape of the neck. If all these measures fail it may be worth trying the traditional method of sewing a hairbrush, or some other hard object such as a stone, into the back of the snorer's pyjamas. Thus, if they turn on their back, they are quickly awakened. (See also STERTOR.)

Snow Blindness

Damage caused to the cornea of an unprotected EYE by the reflection of the sun's rays from snow. ULTRAVIOLET RAYS (UVR) are the damaging agent and people going out in snow and sunlight should wear protective goggles. The condition is painful but resolves if the eyes are covered with pads for a day or two. Prolonged exposure may seriously damage the cornea and impair vision.

Snuffles

The traditional name applied to noisy breathing in children due to the constant presence of nasal discharge. (For treatment, see under NOSE, DISORDERS OF.)

Social Classes

As factors such as the cause of death and the incidence of diseases vary in different social strata, the Registrar-General evolved the following social classification, which has now been in official use for many years:

Class I Professional occupations, such as lawyers, clergymen, and commissioned officers in the Armed Forces.

Class II Intermediate occupations, such as teachers, managers and nurses.

Class III N: non-manual – for example, clerical workers.

Class III M: skilled manual occupations such as miners and bricklayers.

Class IV Partly skilled occupations, such as agricultural workers.

Class V Unskilled occupations, such as building and dock labourers.

Social Medicine

See PUBLIC HEALTH.

Sodium

A metal, the salts of which are white, crystalline, and very soluble. The fluids of the body contain naturally a considerable quantity of sodium chloride.

Sodium carbonate, commonly known as soda or washing soda, has a powerful softening action upon the tissues.

Sodium bicarbonate, or baking soda, is used as an antacid (see ANTACIDS) in relieving indigestion associated with increased acidity of the gastric secretion.

The citrate and the acetate of sodium are used as DIURETICS.

Sodium Aurothiomalate

A gold compound given by deep intramuscular injection in the treatment of RHEUMATOID ARTHRITIS in children and adults. Known as a second-line or disease-modifying antirheumatoid drug, its therapeutic effect may take up to six months to achieve a full response. If this fails to happen, the drug should be stopped. If the patient responds, treatment may be continued at increasingly long intervals (up to four weeks) for as long as five years. Gold treatment is particularly useful for palindromic arthritis in which the disease comes and goes.

Sodium Chloride

The chemical name for common salt (see SODIUM).

Sodium Cromoglycate

Used in the prophylaxis of ASTHMA, it is administered by inhalation and can reduce the incidence of asthmatic attacks but is of no value in the treatment of an acute attack. It acts by preventing the release of pharmacological mediators of BRONCHOSPASM, particularly HISTAMINE, by stabilising mast-cell membranes. It is of particular use in patients whose asthma has an allergic basis; children over four may respond better than adults. It is less potent than inhaled steroids. The dose frequency is adjusted to the patient's response but is usually administered by inhalation four times daily. Sodium cromoglycate is also used in the prophylaxis of allergic RHINITIS and to treat allergic conjunctivitis (see under EYE, DISORDERS OF).

Sodium Diatrizoate

An organic iodine salt that is radio-opaque and therefore used as a contrast medium to outline various organs in the body in X-ray films (see X-RAYS). It is given intravenously. Its main use is in PYELOGRAPHY – that is, in rendering the kidneys radio-opaque – but it is also used to outline the blood vessels (ANGIOGRAPHY) and the gall-bladder and bile ducts (CHOLANGIOGRAPHY).

Sodium Hypochlorite

A disinfectant by virtue of the fact that it gives off chlorine. For domestic use – as, for example, for sterilising baby feeding bottles – it is available in a variety of proprietary preparations.

Sodium Valproate

A drug of first choice for the treatment of several forms of EPILEPSY, including primary generalised epilepsy, generalised absences and myoclonic seizures; it may also be tried in atypical absence, atonic and tonic seizures. Usually taken orally, the drug has shown promising initial results from controlled trials in partial epilepsy. It probably has similar efficacy to CARBAMAZEPINE and PHENYTOIN SODIUM.

Sodium valproate has widespread metabolic effects and may have dose-related side-effects. There has been concern over severe hepatic and pancreatic toxicity, but such adverse effects are rare. Other adverse effects include digestive upsets, drowsiness, muscle incoordination and skin rashes. Rare reports have been given of behavioural disturbances, with occasional aggression. Initiation and withdrawal of treatment should always be slow. Patients should reduce their alcohol intake; any other drugs they are taking that are metabolised by the liver should be carefully monitored.

Sodomy

Sexual intercourse in which the penis penetrates the anus and the rectum. Sodomy may occur between men, between a man and a woman, or between a man and an animal (bestiality).

Solar Plexus

A large network of sympathetic nerves and ganglia situated in the abdomen behind the stomach, where it surrounds the coeliac artery. Branches of the VAGUS nerve – the most important part of the PARASYMPATHETIC NERVOUS SYSTEM – lead into the solar plexus, which in turn distributes branches to the stomach, intestines and several other abdominal organs. A severe blow in the solar plexus may cause temporary unconsciousness.

Solution

A liquid preparation containing one or more soluble drugs, usually dissolved in water.

Solvent Abuse (Misuse)

Also known as volatile-substance abuse, this is the deliberate inhalation of intoxicating fumes given off by some volatile liquids. Glue-sniffing was the most common type of solvent abuse, but inhalation of fuel gases such as butane, especially in the form of lighter refills, is now a greater problem and has become common among children – particularly teenagers. Solvents or volatile substances are applied to a piece of cloth or put into a plastic bag and inhaled, sometimes until the person loses consciousness. He or she may become acutely intoxicated; chronic abusers may suffer from ulcers and rashes over the face as well as damage to peripheral nerves. Death can occur, probably as a result of an abnormal rhythm of the heart. TOL-

ERANCE to the volatile substances may develop over months, but acute intoxication may lead to aggressive and impulsive behaviour. Treatment of addiction is difficult and requires professional counselling. Victims with acute symptoms require urgent medical attention. In Britain, most solvent misusers are males under 20 years of age. Around 150 deaths occur every year. (See also DEPENDENCE.)

Somatic

(1) A term describing tissues of the body that do not form any part of the reproductive process. A somatic MUTATION cannot be passed on to the next generation.

(2) It is also used to refer to the body rather than the mind (see PSYCHOSOMATIC DISEASES).

Somatoform Diseases

A group of disorders in which the affected individuals suffer from repeated physical symptoms for which no physical cause can be discovered. Somatisation is the process by which a person's psychological needs are expressed in the form of physical symptoms. (See also PSYCHOSOMATIC DISEASES.)

Somatostatin

Also known as the growth-hormone-release-inhibiting factor, this is a hormone secreted by the HYPOTHALAMUS and some non-nervous tissues (including the gastrointestinal tract and pancreas). It stops the pituitary-releasing somatotrophin – GROWTH HORMONE. Somatostatin and growth-hormone-releasing hormone are controlled by complicated neural mechanisms linked to exercise, sleep patterns, stress, NEUROTRANSMITTERS and blood GLUCOSE.

Somatotype

The physical build of a person. Attempts have been made to link body build with personality type, but with no great success. One approach is to classify people as endomorphs (heavy physique and sociable personality); mesomorphs (strong, muscular build with well-developed bones linked with a physically adventurous temperament); and ectomorphs (thin and lightly built with an introspective nature).

Somnambulism

Sleep-walking. (See SLEEP.)

Soporifics

Soporifics are measures which induce SLEEP. (See also HYPNOTICS.)

Sore

Sore is a popular term for ULCER.

Sore Throat

A raw sensation at the back of the throat. A common symptom, the cause is usually PHARYNGITIS, sometimes TONSILLITIS. It is often the presenting symptom of colds, INFLUENZA, LARYNGITIS and infectious MONONUCLEOSIS. Sore throats caused by streptococcal infection (see STREPTOCOCCUS) should be treated with antibiotics, as should other bacteria-initiated sore throats; otherwise, symptomatic treatment with analgesics and antiseptic gargles is sufficient for this usually self-limiting condition.

Sotalol

See BETA-ADRENOCEPTOR-BLOCKING DRUGS.

Sound

A rod with a curve at one end used to explore body cavities such as the bladder, or to dilate strictures in the urethra or other channels in the body. (See URINARY BLADDER, DISEASES OF.)

Soya Bean

The bean of *Glycine soja*, a leguminous plant related to peas and beans. It has a high protein and fat content. Starch is almost completely absent and there is much mineral matter, for example a variable but large amount of iron: 6·7 to 30 mg per 100 grams of soya flour compared with 1 mg in white flour and 3 mg in 100 grams of wholemeal flour. It is a good source of thiamine and riboflavine, and of vitamin A in the form of carotene. It is used in infant formulas, especially for those babies thought to have cows' milk protein intolerance.

Space Medicine

A medical specialty dealing with the physiological, PSYCHOLOGICAL and pathological consequences of space flight in which the body has to cope with unusual variations in gravitational forces, including weightlessness, a constricted environment, prolonged close contact with work colleagues in very demanding technical circumstances, and sustained periods of emotional pressure including fear. Enormous progress has been made in providing astronauts with as normal an environment as possible, and they have to undergo prolonged physical and mental training before embarking on space travel.

Spanish Fly

A popular term for cantharides, which is used as a blistering agent.

Spasm

An involuntary, and, in severe cases, painful contraction of a muscle or of a hollow organ with a muscular wall. Spasm may be due to affections in the muscle where the spasm takes place, or it may originate in some disturbance of that part of the nervous system which controls the spasmodically acting muscles. Spasms of a general nature are usually spoken of as CONVULSIONS; spasms of a painful nature are known as cramp (see under MUSCLES, DISORDERS OF) when they affect the muscles of the limbs, and as COLIC when they are situated in the stomach, intestines, ureters or bile duct, or other organs of the abdomen. Spasm of the heart is called ANGINA PECTORIS, and is both a serious and an agonising condition. When the spasm is a prolonged firm contraction, it is spoken of as tonic spasm; when it consists of a series of twitches or quick alternate contractions and relaxations, it is known as clonic spasm. Spasm is a symptom of many diseases.

Spasmodic Torticollis

A chronic condition in which the neck is rotated or deviated laterally, forwards, or backwards, often with additional jerking or tremor. It is a form of focal DYSTONIA, and should not be confused with the far commoner transient condition of acute painful wry-neck.

Spastic

A term applied to any condition showing increased muscle tone: for example, spastic gait, or spastic colon (see IRRITABLE BOWEL SYNDROME (IBS)). This is especially associated with some disease affecting the upper part of the NERVOUS SYSTEM connected with movement (upper neuron), so that its controlling influence is lost and the muscles become overexcitable.

Spatula

A flat, knife-like instrument used for spreading plasters and ointments, and also for depressing the tongue when the throat is being examined.

Specialist

A doctor or other health professional who has trained to develop a particular skill: for example, surgery, cardiac medicine, accident and emergency care, care of the ageing, or radiology. As new medical techniques and treatments are developed, so new specialties evolve to provide them. Specialists have to pass recognised examinations as well as be certified that they have undergone appropriate education and hands-on training. Once qualified, they are expected to continue their education and training to ensure that their skills are kept up-to-date. For doctors, the GENERAL MEDICAL COUNCIL (GMC), which is responsible for overseeing the training and registration of all medical doctors in the UK, also notes in its annual *Medical Register* those doctors who have completed appropriate specialist training. Doctors who have qualified and trained overseas have to pass appropriate GMC tests before they can practise in the UK.

Specificity

An epidemiological term (see EPIDEMIOLOGY) describing the extent to which a SCREENING TEST for the presence of the precursors of disease – for example, pre-malignant cells in the cervix – throws up false positives. A specific test has few false positives.

Speculum

An instrument designed to aid the examination of the various openings on the surface of the body. Many specula are provided with small electric lamps so placed as to light up the cavity of the mouth, ear, nose, rectum or vagina.

Speech Disorders

These may be of physical or psychological origin – or a combination of both. Difficulties may arise at various stages of development: due to problems during pregnancy; at birth; caused by childhood illnesses; or as a result of delayed development. Congenital defects such as CLEFT PALATE or lip may make speech unintelligible until major surgery is performed, thus discouraging talking and delaying development. Recurrent ear infections may make hearing difficult; the child's experience of speech is thus limited, with similar results. Childhood DYSPHASIA occurs if the language-development area of the BRAIN develops abnormally; specialist education and SPEECH THERAPY may then be required.

Dumbness is the inability to pronounce the sounds that make up words. DEAFNESS is the most important cause, being due to a congenital brain defect, or acquired brain disease, such as tertiary SYPHILIS. When hearing is normal or only mildly impaired, dumbness may be due to a structural defect such as tongue-tie or enlarged tonsils and adenoids, or to inefficient voice control, resulting in lisping or lalling. Increased tension is a common cause of STAMMERING; speech disorders may occasionally be of psychological origin.

Normal speech may be lost in adulthood as a result of a STROKE or head injury. Excessive use of the voice may be an occupational hazard; and throat cancer may require a LARYNGECTOMY,

with subsequent help in communication. Severe psychiatric disturbance may be accompanied by impaired social and communication skills. (See also VOICE AND SPEECH.)

Treatment The underlying cause of the problem should be diagnosed as early as possible; psychological and other specialist investigations should be carried out as required, and any physical defect should be repaired. People who are deaf and unable to speak should start training in lip-reading as soon as possible, and special educational methods aimed at acquiring a modulated voice should similarly be started in early childhood – provided by the local authority, and continued as required. Various types of speech therapy or PSYCHOTHERAPY may be appropriate, alone or in conjunction with other treatments, and often the final result may be highly satisfying, with a good command of language and speech being obtained.

Help and advice may be obtained from AFASIC (Unlocking Speech and Language).

Speech Therapy

Professionally trained speech therapists assist, diagnose and treat the whole spectrum of acquired or developmental communication disorders. They work in medical and education establishments, often in an advisory or consultative capacity. The medical conditions in which speech therapy is employed include: dysgraphia, DYSLEXIA, DYSARTHRIA, DYSPHASIA, DYSPHONIA, DYSPRAXIA, AUTISM, BELL'S PALSY, CEREBRAL PALSY, DEAFNESS, disordered language, delayed speech, disordered speech, DOWN'S (DOWN) SYNDROME, LARYNGECTOMY, LEARNING DISABILITY, MACROGLOSSIA, MOTOR NEURONE DISEASE (MND), malformations of the PALATE, PARKINSONISM, STAMMERING, STROKE and disorders of voice production.

Speech therapists form a small independent profession, most of whom work for the National Health Service in community clinics, general practices and hospitals. They may also work in schools or in units for the handicapped, paediatric assessment centres, language units attached to primary schools, adult training centres and day centres for the elderly.

A speech therapist undergoes a four-year degree course which covers the study of disorders of communication in children and adults, phonetics and linguistics, anatomy and physiology, psychology and many other related subjects. Further information on training can be obtained from the College of Speech Therapists.

If the parents of a child are concerned about

their child's speech, they may approach a speech therapist for assessment and guidance. Their general practitioner will be able to give them local addresses or they should contact the district speech therapist. Adults are usually referred by hospital consultants.

The College of Speech Therapists keeps a register of all those who have passed a recognised degree or equivalent qualification in speech therapy. It will be able to direct you to your nearest NHS or private speech therapist.

Sperm
See SPERMATOZOON.

Spermatic
The name applied to the blood vessels and other structures associated with the TESTICLE.

Spermatic Cord
This comprises the VAS DEFERENS, nerves and blood vessels, and it runs from the cavity of the ABDOMEN to the TESTICLE in the SCROTUM.

Spermatogenesis
The production of mature sperm (see SPERMATOZOON) in the testis (see TESTICLE). The sperm cells originate from the outermost layer of the seminiferous tubules in the testis: these multiply throughout reproductive life and are transformed into mature spermatozoa, a process that takes up to 80 days.

Spermatorrhoea
The passage of SEMEN without erection of the PENIS or ORGASM.

Spermatozoa
See SPERMATOZOON.

Spermatozoon
(Plural: spermatozoa.) This is the male sex or germ cell which unites with the OVUM to form the EMBRYO or fetus. It is a highly mobile cell approximately 4 micrometres in length – much smaller than an ovum, which is about 35 micrometres in diameter. Each millilitre of SEMEN contains on average about 100 million spermatozoa, and the average volume of semen discharged during ejaculation in sexual intercourse is 2–4 ml. (Some recent research suggests that male fertility is falling because of a reduction in the production of viable spermatozoa – possibly due to environmental factors, including the discharge of hormones used for agricultural purposes and for human hormonal contraception.)

Once ejaculated during intercourse the spermatozoon travels at a rate of 1·5–3 millimetres a minute and remains mobile for several days after insemination, but quickly loses its potency for fertilisation. As it takes only about 70 minutes to reach the ovarian end of the uterine tube, it is assumed that there must be factors other than its own mobility, such as contraction of the muscle of the womb and uterine tube, that speed it on its way.

Spermicide
Contraceptive preparations that kill sperm. They may be in the form of gels, pessaries, cream or foam and should be used with a barrier contraceptive such as a diaphragm or a condom. (See CONTRACEPTION.)

Sphenoid
A bone lying in the centre of the base of the SKULL, and supporting the others like a wedge or keystone.

Sphincter
A circular muscle which surrounds the opening from an organ, and, by maintaining a constant state of moderate contraction, prevents the escape of the contents of the organ. Sphincters close the outlet from the URINARY BLADDER and RECTUM, and in certain nervous diseases their action is interfered with, so that the power to relax or to keep moderately contracted is lost, and retention or INCONTINENCE of the evacuation results.

Sphygmograph
An instrument for recording the PULSE.

Sphygmomanometer
The traditional device for measuring blood pressure in clinical practice, devised by Riva-Rocci and Korotkoff about a century ago. Measurement depends on accurate transmission and interpretation of the pulse wave to an artery. The sphygmomanometer is of two types, mercury and aneroid. The former is more accurate. Both have some features in common – an inflation-deflation system, an occluding bladder encased in a cuff, and the use of AUSCULTATION with a STETHOSCOPE. The mercury sphygmomanometer consists of a pneumatic armlet which is connected via a rubber tube with an air-pressure pump and a measuring gauge comprising a glass column containing mercury. The armlet is bound around the upper arm and pumped up sufficiently to obliterate the pulse felt at the wrist or heard by auscultation of the artery at the bend of the elbow. The pressure, measured in millimetres of mercury

S

(mm Hg), registered at this point on the gauge is regarded as the pressure of the blood at each heartbeat (ventricular contraction). This is called the systolic pressure. The cuff is then slowly deflated by releasing the valve on the air pump and the pressure at which the sound heard in the artery suddenly changes its character marks the diastolic pressure. Aneroid sphygmomanometers register pressure through an intricate bellows and lever system which is more susceptible than the mercury type to the bumps and jolts of everyday use which reduce its inaccuracy.

While mercury sphygmomanometers are simple, accurate and easily serviced, there is concern about possible mercury toxicity for users, those servicing the devices and the environment. Use of them has already been banned in some European hospitals. Although it may be a few years before they are widely replaced, automated blood-pressure-measuring devices will increasingly be in routine use. A wide variety of ambulatory blood-pressure-measuring devices are already available and may be fitted in general practice or hospital settings, where the patient is advised on the technique. Blood-pressure readings can be taken half-hourly – or more often, if required – with little disturbance of the patient's daily activities or sleep. (See also BLOOD PRESSURE; HYPERTENSION.)

Spina Bifida

This is one of the most common of the congenital (present at birth) malformations. It is one of the three types of neural-tube anomaly, the other two being ANENCEPHALY and cranium bifidum. It takes two main forms – spina bifida occulta being much the commoner. There is a deficit in the posterior part of the SPINAL COLUMN, usually in the LUMBAR region, and it is generally asymptomatic unless the underlying spinal cord is affected. Occasionally it is associated with a hairy patch or birthmark on the back, and a few children develop a mild spastic gait or bladder problems.

Much more serious is spina bifida cystica, in which the spinal-wall defect is accompanied by a protrusion of the spinal cord. This may take two forms: a meningocele, in which the MENINGES, containing CEREBROSPINAL FLUID, protrude through the defect; and a meningo-myelocele, in which the protrusion contains spinal cord and nerves.

Meningocele is less common and has a good prognosis. HYDROCEPHALUS and neurological problems affecting the legs are rare, although the bladder may be affected. Treatment consists of surgery which may be in the first few days of life or much later depending upon the precise situation; long-term follow-up is necessary to pick up any neurological problems that may develop during subsequent growth of the spine.

Meningomyelocele is much more serious and more common, accounting for 90 per cent of all cases. Usually affecting the lumbo-sacral region, the range of severity may vary considerably and, while early surgery with careful attention in a minor case may achieve good mobility, normal bladder function and intellect, a more extensive protrusion may cause complete ANAESTHESIA of the skin, with increased risk of trauma; extensive paralysis of the trunk and limbs, with severe deformities; and paralysis and insensitivity of the bladder and bowel. Involuntary movements may be present, and hydrocephalus occurs in 80 per cent of cases. The decision to operate can only be made after a full examination of the infant to determine the extent of the defect and any co-existent congenital abnormalities. The child's potential can then be estimated, and appropriate treatment discussed with the parents. Carefully selected patients should receive long-term treatment in a special centre, where full attention can be paid to all their various problems.

There is growing evidence of the value of vitamin supplements before and during pregnancy in reducing the incidence of spina bifida. Parents of affected infants may obtain help, advice, and encouragement from the Association for Spina Bifida and Hydrocephalus which has branches throughout the country, or the Scottish Spina Bifida Association.

Spinal Anaesthesia
See under ANAESTHESIA.

Spinal Column
Also known as the spine, this forms an important part of the skeleton, acting both as the rigid pillar which supports the upper parts of the body and as a protection to the SPINAL CORD and nerves arising from it. The spinal column is built up of a number of bones placed one upon another, which, in consequence of having a slight degree of turning-movement, are known as the vertebrae. The possession of a spinal cord supported by a vertebral column distinguishes the higher animals from the lower types, and is why they are called vertebrates. Of the vertebrates, humans alone stand absolutely erect, and this erect carriage of the body gives to the skull and vertebral column certain distinctive characters.

The human backbone is about 70 cm (28

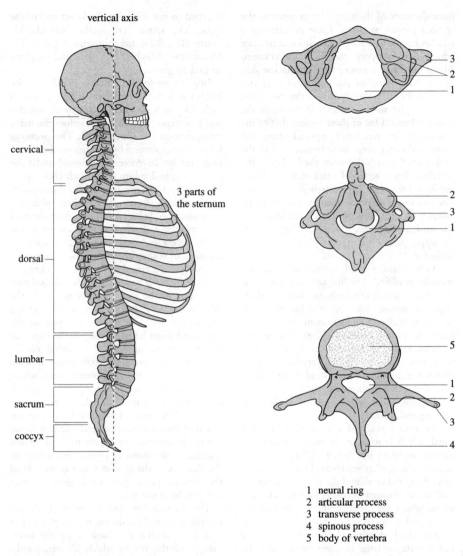

vertical axis

cervical

3 parts of
the sternum

dorsal

lumbar

sacrum

coccyx

1 neural ring
2 articular process
3 transverse process
4 spinous process
5 body of vertebra

The atlas (first cervical vertebra) and axis (second cervical vertebra) vertebrae and a lumbar vertebra seen from above. (Top) the spinal column.

inches) in length, and varies little in full-grown people; differences in height depend mainly upon the length of the lower limbs. The number of vertebrae is 33 in children, although in adult life five of these fuse together to form the sacrum, and the lowest four unite in the coccyx, so that the number of separate bones is reduced to 26. Of these there are seven in the neck, known as cervical vertebrae; 12 with ribs attached, in the region of the thorax known as thoracic or dorsal vertebrae; five in the loins, called lumbar vertebrae; five fused to form the sacrum; and four joined in the coccyx. These

numbers are expressed in a formula thus: C7, D12, L5, S5, Coc4=33.

Although the vertebrae in each of these regions have distinguishing features, all the vertebrae are constructed on the same general plan. Each has a thick, rounded, bony part in front, known as the body, and these bodies form the main thickness of the column. Behind the body of each is a ring of bone, the neural ring, these rings placed one above another forming the bony canal which lodges the spinal cord. From each side of the ring a short process of bone known as the transverse process stands out, and from the back of the ring a larger process, the spinous process, projects. These processes give attachment to the strong ligaments and muscles which unite, support, and bend the column. The spines can be seen or felt beneath the skin of the back lying in the centre of a groove between the muscular masses of the two sides, and they give to the column its name of the spinal column. One of these spines, that of the seventh cervical vertebra, is especially large and forms a distinct bony prominence, where the neck joins the back. Between the bodies of the vertebrae lies a series of thick discs of fibro-cartilage known as intervertebral discs. Each disc consists of an outer portion, known as the annulus fibrosus, and an inner core, known as the nucleus pulposus. These 23 discs provide the upper part of the spine with pliability and resilience.

The first and second cervical vertebrae are specially modified. The first vertebra, known as the atlas, is devoid of a body, but has a specially large and strong ring with two hollows upon which the skull rests, thus allowing forward and backward movements (nodding). The second vertebra, known as the axis, has a pivot on its body which fits into the first vertebra and thus allows free rotation of the head from side to side. The spinal column has four natural curves (see diagram) which help to cushion the shocks of walking and running.

The neural rings of the vertebrae form a canal, which is wide in the neck, smaller and almost round in the dorsal region, and wide again in the lumbar vertebrae. Down the canal runs the spinal cord, and the nerves leaving the cord do so through openings between the vertebrae which are produced by notches on the upper and lower margins of each ring. The intervertebral foramina formed by these notches are so large in comparison with the nerves passing through them that there is no chance of pressure upon the latter, except in very serious injuries which dislocate and fracture the spine.

Spinal Cord

This is the lower portion of the CENTRAL NERVOUS SYSTEM which is situated within the SPINAL COLUMN. Above, it forms the direct continuation of the medulla oblongata, this part of the BRAIN changing its name to spinal cord at the foramen magnum, the large opening in the base of the skull through which it passes into the spinal canal. Below, the spinal cord extends to about the upper border of the second lumbar vertebra, where it tapers off into a fine thread, known as the filum terminale, that is attached to the coccyx at the lower end of the spine. The spinal cord is thus considerably shorter than the spinal column, being only 37–45 cm (15–18 inches) in length, and weighing around 30 grams.

In its course from the base of the skull to the lumbar region, the cord gives off 31 nerves on each side, each of which arises by an anterior and a posterior root that join before the nerve emerges from the spinal canal. The openings for the nerves formed by notches on the ring of each vertebra have been mentioned under the entry for spinal column. To reach these openings, the upper nerves pass almost directly outwards, whilst lower down their obliquity increases, until below the point where the cord ends there is a sheaf of nerves, known as the cauda equina, running downwards to leave the spinal canal at their appropriate openings.

The cord is a cylinder, about the thickness of the little finger. It has two slightly enlarged portions, one in the lower part of the neck, the other at the last dorsal vertebra; and from these thickenings arise the nerves that pass to the upper and lower limbs. The upper four cervical nerves unite to produce the cervical plexus. From this the muscles and skin of the neck are mainly supplied, and the phrenic nerve, which runs down through the lower part of the neck and the chest to innervate the diaphragm, is given off. The brachial plexus is formed by the union of the lower four cervical and first dorsal nerves. In addition to nerves to some of the muscles in the shoulder region, and others to the skin about the shoulder and inner side of the arm, the plexus gives off large nerves that proceed down the arm.

The thoracic or dorsal nerves, with the exception of the first, do not form a plexus, but each runs around the chest along the lower margin of the rib to which it corresponds, whilst the lower six extend on to the abdomen.

The lumbar plexus is formed by the upper four lumbar nerves, and its branches are distributed to the lower part of the abdomen, and front and inner side of the thigh.

The sacral plexus is formed by parts of the fourth and fifth lumbar nerves, and the upper three and part of the fourth sacral nerves. Much of the plexus is collected into the sciatic nerves, the largest in the body, which go to the legs.

The sympathetic system is joined by a pair of small branches given off from each spinal nerve, close to the spine. This system consists of two parts, first, a pair of cords running down on the side and front of the spine, and containing on each side three ganglia in the neck, and beneath this a ganglion opposite each vertebra. From these two ganglionated cords numerous branches are given off, and these unite to form the second part – namely, plexuses connected with various internal organs, and provided with numerous large and irregularly placed ganglia. The chief of these plexuses are the cardiac plexus, the solar or epigastric plexus, the diaphragmatic, suprarenal, renal, spermatic, or ovarian, aortic, hypogastric and pelvic plexuses.

The spinal cord, like the brain, is surrounded by three membranes: the dura mater, arachnoid mater, and pia mater, from without inwards. The arrangement of the dura and arachnoid is much looser in the case of the cord than their application to the brain. The dura especially forms a wide tube which is separated from the cord by fluid and from the vertebral canal by blood vessels and fat, this arrangement protecting the cord from pressure in any ordinary movements of the spine.

In section the spinal cord consists partly of grey, but mainly of white, matter. It differs from the upper parts of the brain in that the white matter (largely) in the cord is arranged on the surface, surrounding a mass of grey matter (largely neurons – see NEURON(E)), while in the brain the grey matter is superficial. The arrangement of grey matter, as seen in a section across the cord, resembles the letter H. Each half of the cord possesses an anterior and a posterior horn, the masses of the two sides being joined by a wide posterior grey commissure. In the middle of this commissure lies the central canal of the cord, a small tube which is the continuation of the ventricles in the brain. The horns of grey matter reach almost to the surface of the cord, and from their ends arise the roots of the nerves that leave the cord. The white matter is divided almost completely into two halves by a posterior septum and anterior fissure and is further split into anterior, lateral and posterior columns.

Functions The cord is, in part, a receiver and originator of nerve impulses, and in part a conductor of such impulses along fibres which pass through it to and from the brain. The cord contains centres able to receive sensory impressions and initiate motor instructions. These control blood-vessel diameters, eye-pupil size, sweating and breathing. The brain exerts an overall controlling influence and, before any incoming sensation can affect consciousness, it is usually 'filtered' through the brain.

Many of these centres act autonomously. Other cells of the cord are capable of originating movements in response to impulses brought

direct to them through sensory nerves, such activity being known as REFLEX ACTION. (For a fuller description of the activities of the spinal cord, see NEURON(E) – Reflex action.)

The posterior column of the cord consists of the fasciculus gracilis and the fasciculus cuneatus, both conveying sensory impressions upwards. The lateral column contains the ventral and the dorsal spino-cerebellar tracts passing to the cerebellum, the crossed pyramidal tract of motor fibres carrying outgoing impulses downwards together with the rubro-spinal, the spino-thalamic, the spino-tectal, and the postero-lateral tracts. And, finally, the anterior column contains the direct pyramidal tract of motor fibres and an anterior mixed zone. The pyramidal tracts have the best-known course. Starting from cells near the central sulcus on the brain, the motor nerve-fibres run down through the internal capsule, pons, and medulla, in the lower part of which many of those coming from the right side of the brain cross to the left side of the spinal cord, and vice versa. Thence the fibres run down in the crossed pyramidal tract to end beside nerve-cells in the anterior horn of the cord. From these nerve-cells other fibres pass outwards to form the nerves that go direct to the muscles. Thus the motor nerve path from brain to muscle is divided into two sections of neurons, of which the upper exerts a controlling influence upon the lower, while the lower is concerned in maintaining the muscle in a state of health and good nutrition, and in directly calling it into action. (See also NERVE; NERVOUS SYSTEM.)

Spine and Spinal Cord, Diseases and Injuries of

Scoliosis A condition where the spine is curved to one side (the spine is normally straight when seen from behind). The deformity may be mobile and reversible, or fixed; if fixed it is accompanied by vertebral rotation and does not disappear with changes in posture. Fixed scoliosis is idiopathic (of unknown cause) in 65–80 per cent of cases. There are three main types: the infantile type occurs in boys under three and in 90 per cent of cases resolves spontaneously; the juvenile type affects 4–9 year olds and tends to be progressive. The most common type is adolescent idiopathic scoliosis; girls are affected in 90 per cent of cases and the incidence is 4 per cent. Treatment may be conservative with a fixed brace, or surgical fusion may be needed if the curve is greater than 45 degrees. Scoliosis can occur as a congenital condition and in neuromuscular diseases where there is muscle imbalance, such as in FRIEDREICH'S ATAXIA.

Kyphosis is a backward curvature of the spine causing a hump back. It may be postural and reversible in obese people and tall adolescent girls who stoop, but it may also be fixed. Scheuermann's disease is the term applied to adolescent kyphosis. It is more common in girls. Senile kyphosis occurs in elderly people who probably have osteoporosis (bone weakening) and vertebral collapse.

Disc degeneration is a normal consequence of AGEING. The disc loses its resiliance and becomes unable to withstand pressure. Rupture (prolapse) of the disc may occur with physical stress. The disc between the fourth and fifth lumbar vertebrae is most commonly involved. The jelly-like central nucleus pulposus is usually pushed out backwards, forcing the annulus fibrosus to put pressure on the nerves as they leave the spinal canal. (See PROLAPSED INTERVERTEBRAL DISC.)

Ankylosing spondylitis is an arthritic disorder of the spine in young adults, mostly men. It is a familial condition which starts with lumbar pain and stiffness which progresses to involve the whole spine. The discs and ligaments are replaced by fibrous tissue, making the spine rigid. Treatment is physiotherapy and anti-inflammatory drugs to try to keep the spine supple for as long as possible.

A National Association for Ankylosing Spondylitis has been formed which is open to those with the disease, their families, friends and doctors.

Spondylosis is a term which covers disc degeneration and joint degeneration in the back. OSTEOARTHRITIS is usually implicated. Pain is commonly felt in the neck and lumbar regions and in these areas the joints may become unstable. This may put pressure on the nerves leaving the spinal canal, and in the lumbar region, pain is generally felt in the distribution of the sciatic nerve – down the back of the leg. In the neck the pain may be felt down the arm. Treatment is physiotherapy; often a neck collar or lumbar support helps. Rarely surgery is needed to remove the pressure from the nerves.

Spondylolisthesis means that the spine is shifted forward. This is nearly always in the lower lumbar region and may be familial, or due to degeneration in the joints. Pressure may be put on the cauda equina. The usual complaint is of pain after exercise. Treatment is bed rest in a bad attack with surgery indicated only if there are worrying signs of cord compression.

Spinal stenosis is due to a narrowing of the spinal canal which means that the nerves become squashed together. This causes numbness with pins and needles (paraesthia) in the legs. COMPUTED TOMOGRAPHY and nuclear magnetic resonance imaging scans can show the amount of cord compression. If improving posture does not help, surgical decompression may be needed.

Whiplash injuries occur to the neck, usually as the result of a car accident when the head and neck are thrown backwards and then forwards rapidly. This causes pain and stiffness in the neck; the arm and shoulder may feel numb. Often a support collar relieves the pain but recovery commonly takes between 18 months to three years.

Transection of the cord occurs usually as a result of trauma when the vertebral column protecting the spinal cord is fractured and becomes unstable. The cord may be concussed or it may have become sheared by the trauma and not recover (transected). Spinal concussion usually recovers after 12 hours. If the cord is transected the patient remains paralysed. (See PARALYSIS.)

Spiramycin
One of the MACROLIDES isolated from *Streptomyces ambofaciens* which is used under strict conditions for the treatment of TOXOPLASMOSIS.

Spirillum
A form of micro-organism of wavy or spiral shape. (See MICROBIOLOGY.)

Spirit
A strong solution of ALCOHOL in water. Proof spirit is one containing 57 per cent of alcohol by volume or 49 per cent by weight, and is so-named because it can stand the proof of just catching fire. Rectified spirit contains 90 per cent of alcohol by volume or over 85 per cent by weight. Methylated spirit (also known as wood naphtha or wood spirit) is distilled from wood; when taken internally it is a dangerous poison producing NEURITIS, especially neuritis of the optic nerves which may result in blindness. Methylated spirit is used to harden the skin for the prevention of bed sores and foot soreness.

Spiritual Pain

Spiritual pain is what may be felt when one of a person's four key spiritual relationships (with other people, with oneself, with the world around, or with 'Life' itself) is traumatised or broken. A bad trauma in one of the first three relationships can lead to damage to the last of them – that of the relationship with Life itself. For example, a wife deserted by her husband for another woman may not only feel devastated by the loss of her partner around the place, but may also feel a pain caused by the shattering of her beliefs about life (about faithfulness, hope, love, security, etc.). It is as if there is a picture at the centre of each person of what life should be about – whether or not held in a frame by a belief in God; this picture can be smashed by a particular trauma, so that nothing makes sense any more. The individual cannot get things together; everything loses its meaning. This shattering of someone's picture of life is the source of the deepest pain in any spiritual trauma. The connection is often made between spiritual pain and meaninglessness. If the shattering of the picture, on the other hand, is done by the individual – for instance, by breaking his or her own moral or religious code – the pain may take the form of guilt and associated feelings. Hence, the therapist will be intent upon helping a client to recognise and come to terms with this 'pain beneath the pain'.

Spirochaete

An order of bacteria which has a spiral form. (See MICROBIOLOGY.)

Spirometer

A device to test how the lung is working (see also PULMONARY FUNCTION TESTS) to assess the effects of lung disease or the progress of treatment – a procedure called spirometry. The spirometer records the total volume of air breathed out – the forced vital capacity. The machine also records the volume of air breathed out in one second – the forced expiratory volume. In diseases such as ASTHMA, in which the airways are obstructed, the ratio of the forced expiratory volume to the forced vital capacity is reduced. (See RESPIRATION.)

Spironolactone

One of the group of substances known as spirolactones. These are steroids similar to ALDOSTERONE in structure which competitively act as inhibitors of it; they can thus antagonise the action of aldosterone in the renal tubules. As there is evidence that there is an increased output of aldosterone in oedematous conditions (see OEDEMA) – such as congestive heart failure, which accentuates the oedema – spironolactone is used, along with other DIURETICS.

Splanchnic

Anything belonging to the internal organs of the body, as distinguished from its framework.

Spleen

An organ deeply placed in the abdomen and a major constituent of the RETICULO-ENDOTHELIAL SYSTEM.

Position and size The spleen lies behind the stomach, high up on the left side of the abdomen, and corresponds to the position of the ninth, tenth and 11th ribs, from which it is separated by the diaphragm. It is a soft, highly vascular, plum-coloured organ, and has a smooth surface. It is usually about 12·5–15 cm (5–6 inches) in length, and weighs about 170 grams or more. In diseased conditions the organ may reach a weight of 8–9 kg.

Structure The spleen is enveloped by peritoneal membrane beneath which is a strong elastic tunic, composed partly of fibrous tissue

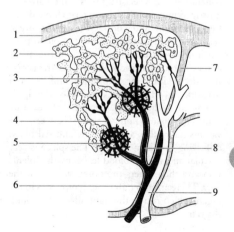

1 capsule
2 venous sinuses
3 arterial capillaries ending in sinuses
4 small arteries
5 Malphigi corpuscles
6 artery
7 trabecula of capsule
8 central artery of Malphigi corpuscle
9 vein

Cross-section of cone of tissue from spleen.

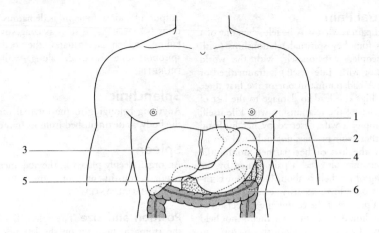

1 oesophagus
2 stomach
3 liver
4 spleen
5 pancreas
6 transverse colon

Position of spleen in relation to other abdominal organs.

containing many elastic fibres, and partly of unstriped muscle. This elastic coat allows of the free expansion and contraction of the organ according to the varying amount of blood present in it. From the inner surface of the membrane, fibrous partitions known as trabeculae run down into the substance and form a network in which the dark spleen pulp is contained. The pulp consists of delicate connective-tissue fibres passing between the various trabeculae, and of white and red blood cells lying in this meshwork. The spleen is very vascular and venous blood leaves by the splenic vein and then enters the portal vein from the liver. There are also numerous lymphatics in the organ, which run in the trabeculae or surround the veins.

Functions The organ produces lymphocytes (see LYMPHOCYTE) and acts as a reservoir of red blood cells for use in emergencies. It is also one of the sites for the manufacture of red blood cells in the fetus, but not after birth. Useless or worn-out red and white blood cells and blood PLATELETS are broken up by this organ. This results in the production of BILIRUBIN, which is conveyed to the liver, and of iron, which is used in the bone marrow for the production of new red blood cells.

Spleen, Diseases of

In certain diseases associated with marked changes in the blood, such as LEUKAEMIA and MALARIA, the SPLEEN becomes chronically enlarged. In some of the acute infectious diseases, it becomes congested and acutely enlarged: for example, in typhoid fever (see ENTERIC FEVER), ANTHRAX and infectious MONONUCLEOSIS. Rupture of the spleen may occur, like rupture of other internal organs, in consequence of extreme violence – but in malarious countries, where many people have the spleen greatly enlarged and softened as the result of malaria, rupture of this organ occasionally occurs following even a light blow to the left side of the abdomen. The spleen, in consequence of its structure, bleeds excessively when torn, so that this accident is generally followed by collapse, signs of internal haemorrhage – and death if not dealt with promptly by operation.

Splenectomy

Removal of the SPLEEN. This operation may be necessary if the spleen has been severely injured, or in the treatment of the severe form of acholuric JAUNDICE or autoimmune thrombocytopenic PURPURA.

Splenomegaly
Enlargement of the SPLEEN beyond its normal size.

Splinter Haemorrhages
Linear bleeding under the fingernails. Although they may result from injury, they are a useful physical sign of infective ENDOCARDITIS.

Splints
Supports for an injured or wounded part. They are most commonly employed in cases in which a bone is fractured, and consist then of some rigid substance designed to take the place of the broken bone in maintaining the shape of the limb, as well as to keep the broken ends at rest and in contact and so ensure their union. Splints are most commonly made of wood, either shaped to the limb or consisting merely of strips of wood about the width of the injured limb, and carefully padded with wool or similar soft material. Splints are also made of metal, poroplastic felt, leather, and cotton stiffened with plaster of Paris, as well as other materials. Splints may be improvised for first-aid out of walking-sticks, rifles, broom-handles, branches, folded-up newspapers, and in fact anything of suitable length and rigidity. (See also BONE, DISORDERS OF – Bone fractures.)

Spondylitis
Another name for ARTHRITIS of the spine (see SPINE AND SPINAL CORD, DISEASES AND INJURIES OF).

Spondylolisthesis
See SPINE AND SPINAL CORD, DISEASES AND INJURIES OF.

Spondylosis
See SPINE AND SPINAL CORD, DISEASES AND INJURIES OF.

Spongiform Encephalopathy
A disease of the neurological system caused by a PRION. Spongy degeneration of the BRAIN occurs with progressive DEMENTIA. Known examples of the disorder in humans are CREUTZFELDT-JAKOB DISEASE (CJD) and KURU. Among animals, scrapie in sheep and BOVINE SPONGIFORM ENCEPHALOPATHY (BSE) are caused by slow viruses. The latter has occurred as an outbreak in cattle over the past decade or so, probably as a result of cattle being fed processed offal from infected animals. Some people have developed a form of CJD from eating infected beef.

Sporadic
The term applied to cases of disease occurring here and there, as opposed to EPIDEMIC outbreaks.

Spore
Part of the lifecycle of certain BACTERIA when the vegetative cell is encapsulated and metabolism falls to a low level. The spore is resistant to changes in the environment and, when these are unfavourable, the spore remains dormant; when they improve, it starts to grow. Certain dangerous bacteria, such as CLOSTRIDIUM, produce resistant ubiquitous spores, so sterilisation procedures need to be very effective.

Sporozoa
The name of a group of parasitic PROTOZOA which includes the parasitic *Plasmodium* that causes MALARIA. The life-cycles of sporozoa are complex, often with sexual and asexual stages.

Sporozoites
Sporozoites is one cell type of the many that are formed during the life-cycle of SPOROZOA. In the case of MALARIA, sporozoites pass into the salivary glands of the mosquito and and are the infecting agent of the human host when the insect next feeds on human blood.

Sports Medicine
The field of medicine concerned with physical fitness and the diagnosis and treatment of both acute and chronic sports injuries sustained during training and competition. Acute injuries are extremely common in contact sports, and their initial treatment is similar to that of those sustained in other ways, such as falls and road traffic incidents. Tears of the muscles (see MUSCLES, DISORDERS OF), CONNECTIVE TISSUE and LIGAMENTS which are partial (sprains) are initially treated with rest, ice, compression, and elevation (RICE) of the affected part. Complete tears (rupture) of ligaments (see diagrams) or muscles, or fractures (see BONE, DISORDERS OF – Bone fractures) require more prolonged immobilisation, often in plaster, or surgical intervention may be considered. The rehabilitation of injured athletes requires special expertise – an early graded return to activity gives the best long-term results, but doing too much too soon runs the risk of exacerbating the original injury.

Chronic (overuse) injuries affecting the bones (see BONE), tendons (see TENDON) or BURSAE of the JOINTS are common in many sports. Examples include chronic INFLAMMATION of the common extensor tendon where it

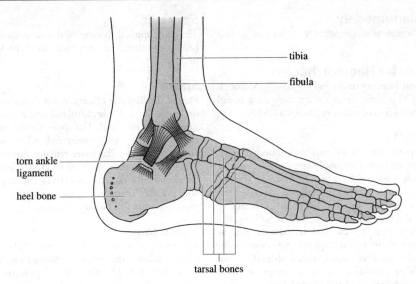

tibia

fibula

torn ankle ligament

heel bone

tarsal bones

Torn ankle ligament.

attaches to the later EPICONDYLE of the humerus – common in throwers and racquet sportspeople – and stress fractures of the TIBIA or METATARSAL BONES of the foot in runners. After an initial period of rest, management often involves coaching that enables the athlete to perform the repetitive movement in a less injury-susceptible manner.

Exercise physiology is the science of measuring athletic performance and physical fitness for exercise. This knowledge is applied to devising and supervising training regimens based on scientific principles. Physical fitness depends upon the rate at which the body can deliver oxygen to the muscles, known as the VO_2max, which is technically difficult to measure. The PULSE rate during and after a bout of exercise serves as a good proxy of this measurement.

Regulation of sport Sports medicine's role is to minimise hazards for participants by, for example, framing rule-changes which forbid collapsing the scrum, which has reduced the risk of neck injury in rugby; and in the detection of the use of drugs taken to enhance athletic performance. Such attempts to gain an edge in competition undermine the sporting ideal and are banned by leading sports regulatory bodies. The Olympic Movement Anti-Doping Code lists prohibited substances and methods that could be used to enhance performance. These include some prohibited in certain circumstances as well as those completely banned. The latter include:

- stimulants such as AMPHETAMINES, bromantan, caffeine, carphedon, COCAINE, EPHEDRINE and certain beta-2 agonists.
- NARCOTICS such as DIAMORPHINE (heroin), MORPHINE, METHADONE HYDROCHLORIDE and PETHIDINE HYDROCHLORIDE.
- ANABOLIC STEROIDS such as methandione, NANDROLONE, stanazol, TESTOSTERONE, clenbuterol, androstenedone and certain beta-2 agonists.
- peptide HORMONES, mimetics and analogues such as GROWTH HORMONE, CORTICOTROPHIN, CHORIONIC GONADOTROPHIC HORMONE, pituitary and synthetic GONADOTROPHINS, ERYTHROPOIETIN and INSULIN.

(The list produced above is not comprehensive: full details are available from the governing bodies of relevant sports.) Among banned methods are blood doping (pre-competition administration of an athlete's own previously provided and stored blood), administration of artificial oxygen carriers or plasma expanders. Also forbidden is any pharmacological, chemical or physical manipulation to affect the results of authorised testing.

Drug use can be detected by analysis of the URINE, but testing only at the time of competition is unlikely to detect drug use designed to enhance early-season training; hence random testing of competitive athletes is also used.

The increasing professionalism and competitiveness (among amateurs and juveniles as well as professionals) in sports sometimes results in pressures on participants to get fit quickly after injury or illness. This can lead to

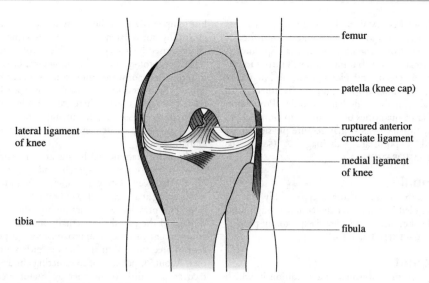

femur

patella (knee cap)

ruptured anterior cruciate ligament

medial ligament of knee

lateral ligament of knee

tibia

fibula

Anterior view of right knee-joint.

players returning to their activity before they are properly fit – sometimes by using physical or pharmaceutical aids. This practice can adversely affect their long-term physical capabilities and perhaps their general health.

Spots Before the Eyes

Also called FLOATERS, these can arise from a variety of causes including inflammation and bleeding in the eye, or preceding a retina detachment. They may also occur for a variety of totally harmless reasons. (See EYE, DISORDERS OF.)

Spotted Fever

See MENINGITIS; EPIDEMIC; TYPHUS FEVER.

Sprains

Injuries in the neighbourhood of joints, consisting usually in tearing of a ligament with effusion of blood. (See JOINTS, DISEASES OF.)

Sprue

A disease occurring most commonly in patients in or from the tropics, and characterised by diarrhoea with large, fatty stools; ANAEMIA; sore tongue; and weight loss. Its manifestations resemble those of non-tropical sprue, or gluten enteropathy, and COELIAC DISEASE.

Causes Tropical sprue is thought to be due to an inborn error of metabolism, characterised primarily by an inability to absorb fats from the intestines. Its epidemiological pattern suggests that an infection such as DYSENTERY may be the precipitating factor. Subsequently there is inter-

ference with the absorption of carbohydrates, vitamins, and minerals, leading to anaemia and HYPOCALCAEMIA.

Symptoms Of gradual or rapid onset, there is initial weakness, soreness of the tongue, difficulty swallowing, indigestion, diarrhoea and poor appetite. Anaemia is typically macrocytic, and mild HYPOGLYCAEMIA may occur. Untreated, the patient steadily loses weight and, unless appropriate treatment is started early, death may be expected because of exhaustion and some intercurrent infection.

Treatment This consists of bed rest, a high-protein diet (initially skimmed milk), and treatment of the anaemia and any other deficiencies present. Minimum fat should be given to sufferers, who should also take folic acid and cyanocobalamin for the anaemia; large vitamin-B-complex supplements (such as Marmite®) are helpful. Vitamins A and D, together with calcium supplements, help to raise the concentration of calcium in the blood. A long convalescence is often required, which may lead to marked depression, and patients should be sent home to a temperate climate.

Non-tropical sprue is the result of GLUTEN hypersensitivty and is treated with a gluten-free diet.

Sputum

The mucous secretions from the mouth, throat or back of the nose. Sputum is also expectorated by coughing from the lower air passages. Its production may be increased by respiratory-tract allergy (ASTHMA) or by breathing-in irritants such as tobacco smoke, smoke from a fire, or fumes from chemical materials. Sputum is normally white, but infection will turn it to yellow or green, and blood from the lungs may produce pink frothy sputum. Treatment is to deal with the underlying disorder. Production of large quantities of sputum – for instance, in BRONCHIECTASIS – may require physiotherapy and postural drainage. (See also EXPECTORATION.)

Squill

A herbal extract (from a type of lily) that is included in some over-the-counter cough remedies because of its believed expectorant properties (see EXPECTORATION).

Squint

Squint, or strabismus, is a condition in which the visual axes of each EYE are not directed simultaneously at the same fixation point (i.e. each eye is not pointing at the same object at the same time). Squints may be: (*a*) Paralytic, where one or more of the muscles, or their nerve supply, is damaged; this type usually results in double vision. (*b*) Non-paralytic, where the muscles and nerves are normal. It is usually found in children. This type of squint can either result in poor vision, or occasionally may result from poor vision.

Squints may be convergent (where one eye 'turns in') or divergent (one eye 'turns out'). Vertical squints can also occur but are less common. All squints should be seen by an eye specialist as soon as possible. Some squints can be corrected by exercises or spectacles; others require surgery.

SSRIs

See SELECTIVE SEROTONIN-REUPTAKE INHIBITORS (SSRIS).

Stabs

See WOUNDS.

Staghorn Calculus

A branched renal stone formed in the image of the collecting system of the kidney (see KIDNEYS). It fills the calyces and pelvis and is commonly associated with an infection of the urine, particularly *Proteus vulgaris*. The calculus may lead to pyonephrosis and an ABSCESS of the kidney.

Stammering

A disruption of the forward flow of speech. The individual knows what he or she wants to say, but temporarily loses the ability to execute linguistically formulated speech. Stammering is characterised by a silent or audible involuntary repetition/prolongation of an utterance, be it a sound, syllable or word. Sometimes it is accompanied by accessory behaviours, or speech-related struggle. Usually there are indications or the report of an accompanying emotional state, involving excitement, tension, fear or embarrassment.

Idiopathic stammering begins at some time between the onset of speech and puberty, mostly between 2–5 years of age. Acquired stammering at a later age due to brain damage is rare. The prevalence of stammering (the percentage of the population actually stammering at any point in time) is approximately 0·9 per cent. Three times as many boys as girls stammer. About 70 per cent of stammering children recover with little or no therapy. Stammerers have not been shown to demonstrate differences in personality from non-stammerers; there are, however, indications that at least some stammerers show minimal differences from fluent speakers in cerebral processing of verbal material.

There is a genetic predisposition towards stammering. The risk of stammering among first-degree relatives of stammerers is more than three times the population risk. In 77 per cent of identical twins, either both stammer or both are fluent. Only 33 per cent of non-identical twins agree in this way. As there are identical twins who differ for stammering, environmental factors must be important for some stammerers. There are relatively large numbers of stammerers in highly competitive societies, where status and prestige are important and high standards of speech competence are valued.

Different treatments have been demonstrated to produce considerable benefit, their basic outline being similar. A long period of time is spent in training stammerers to speak in a different way (fluency-shaping techniques). This may include slowing down the rate of speech, gentle onset of utterance, continuous flow with correct juncturing, etc. When the targets have been achieved within the clinic, a series of planned speech assignments outside the clinic is undertaken. In these assignments, and initially in everyday situations, the fluency-enchancing techniques have to be used conscientiously. Gradually speech is shaped towards normality requiring less and less effort. Therapy may also include some work on attitude change (i.e. helping the client to see him or herself as a fluent speaker) and possibly general communicative skills training.

For information about organisations concerned with stammering, see Appendix 2.

Standard Deviation

A statistical measure of the spread of observations about their arithmetic mean. It is a measure regularly used in working out the results of trials about clinical treatment.

Stannosis

The form of PNEUMOCONIOSIS caused by the inhalation of stannous (tin) oxide, which occurs in tin-ore mining.

Stanozolol

See ANABOLIC STEROIDS.

Stapedectomy

An operation on the middle EAR to remove the STAPES and replace it with an artificial alternative. The procedure is aimed at treating DEAFNESS caused by otosclerosis in which the stapes becomes fixed by an overgrowth of bone, preventing it from transmitting sound. Stapedectomy improves hearing in around 90 per cent of those people who have the operation. (See EAR, DISEASES OF.)

Stapes

The innermost of the small trio of bones in the middle EAR. It is stirrup-shaped, articulates with the incus, and is linked to the oval window of the inner ear.

Staphylococcus

Staphylococcus is a genus of gram-positive bacterium (see GRAM'S STAIN; BACTERIA) which under the microscope appears in small masses like bunches of grapes. It is one of the most common infectious micro-organisms and is found, for example, in the PUS discharged from BOILS (FURUNCULOSIS). (See also MICROBIOLOGY.)

Starch

A substance belonging to that group of carbohydrate known as the amyloses. It is the form in which utilisable CARBOHYDRATE is stored in granules within the seeds and roots of many plants.

Starch is converted into sugar when treated with heat in presence of a dilute acid. It is changed largely into dextrin when exposed to a considerable degree of dry heat, as in toasting bread; and a similar change into dextrin and malt-sugar takes place under the action of vari-ous enzymes (see ENZYME) such as the PTYALIN of the SALIVA. Starch forms a chief constituent of the carbohydrate foods (see DIET); and in the process of digestion, the above-mentioned change takes place to prepare it for absorption. It is also slowly broken down in the process of cooking.

Starch is used as a constituent of dusting powders for application to chafed or irritable areas of the skin.

Starvation

A condition that results from a lack of food for a long time. The person suffers weight loss and changes in the body's METABOLISM, with production of potentially harmful chemicals called ketones (see KETONE) and ACETONE. Sometimes starvation may occur as a result of an eating disorder (see EATING DISORDERS – Anorexia nervosa). In cases of slow starvation, the vitality of the tissues is reduced and they become more liable to tuberculosis and other diseases. (See also FASTING.)

Stasis

A term applied to stoppage of the flow of blood in the vessels or of the food materials down the intestinal canal.

STAT

An abbreviation (for statim) meaning straightaway – usually applying to a request by a doctor for a drug to be given without delay.

Statins

A group of LIPID-lowering drugs used to treat primary hypercholesterolaemia – a condition in which the concentrations of LIPOPROTEINS in the blood plasma are raised, increasing the likelihood of affected individuals developing coronary heart disease. Statins act by competitively inhibiting an ENZYME called 3-hydroxy-3-methylglutaryl coenzyme A (HMG CoA) reductase. This enzyme plays a part in the synthesis of CHOLESTEROL, particularly in the LIVER. Statins are more effective than other classes of drugs in lowering body concentrations of LDL-cholesterol but less effective than fibrates in reducing triglyceride concentration. Their use results in significant reductions in heart attacks (myocardial infarctions) and other adverse cardiovascular events, such as STROKE. Recent research shows that drugs which reduce lipid concentrations may prevent as many as one-third of myocardial infarctions and deaths from coronary disease. Statins are valuable in preventing coronary events in patients at increased risk of those conditions. They should

S

be used in conjunction with other preventive measures such as low-fat diets, reduction in alcohol consumption, taking exercise and stopping smoking. Among statin drugs available are atorvastatin, cerivastatin sodium, fluvastatin, pracastatin sodium and simvasatin. (See HEART, DISEASES OF; HYPERLIPIDAEMIA.)

Status Asthmaticus
Repeated attacks of ASTHMA, with no respite between the spasms, usually lasting for more than 24 hours. The patient is seriously distressed and, untreated, the condition may lead to death from respiratory failure and exhaustion. Continuous or very frequent use of nebulised bronchodilators, intravenous corticosteroid treatment, and other skilled medical care are urgently required.

Status Epilepticus
Repeated epileptic fits (see EPILEPSY) with no return to consciousness between them. Breathing stops between each fit and the body is deprived of oxygen which causes damage to the brain. Urgent medical attention is required to control the condition, or the patient may suffer permanent brain damage.

STD(s)
See SEXUALLY TRANSMITTED DISEASES (STDS).

Steatoma
A fatty, cystic tumour.

Steatorrhoea
Any condition characterised by the passing of stools (FAECES) containing an excess of FAT. (See MALABSORPTION SYNDROME.)

Stem Cell
Stem CELLS develop a few days after an egg (ovum) is fertilised by a spermatozoon and starts developing to form an EMBRYO. These master cells are crucial to the development of a normal embryo. They contain a specialised ENZYME that gives them the facility to divide indefinitely, developing into the many different specialised cells that comprise the various tissues in the body – for example, skin, blood, muscle, glands or nerves.

In a highly significant advance in research, a scientific team in the United States obtained stem cells from newly formed human embryos – donated by women who had become pregnant after successful *in vitro* fertilisation – and successfully cultivated these cells in the laboratory. This achievement opened the way to replicating in the laboratory, the various specialised

cells that develop naturally in the body. UK government legislation constrains the use of human embryos in research (see ETHICS) and the ethical aspects of taking this stem-cell culture technique forwards will have to be resolved. Nevertheless, this discovery points the biological way to the use of genetic engineering in selecting differentiated specialised cells from which replacement tissues could be grown for use as transplants to rectify absent or damaged tissues in the human body.

Research into potential use of stem cells has raised expectations that in the long term they may prove to be an effective regenerative treatment for a wide range of disorders including PARKINSONISM, ALZHEIMER'S DISEASE, type-2 diabetes (see under DIABETES MELLITUS), myocardial infarction (see HEART, DISEASES OF), severe burns, osteoporosis (see under BONE, DISORDERS OF) and the regeneration of blood to replace the need for BONE MARROW TRANSPLANT. Recent research has shown that adult stem cells may also be stimulated to produce new cell lines. If successful, this would eliminate the need to use embryos and thus resolve existing ethical dilemmas over the use of stem cells.

Stenosis
An unnatural narrowing in any passage or orifice of the body. The word is especially used in connection with the four openings of the HEART at which the valves are situated. (See HEART, DISEASES OF.)

Stent
A surgical device used to assist the healing of an operative anastamosis – a joining-up of two structures. A splint is left inside the lumen of a duct and this drains the contents.

Stereognosis
The faculty of recognising the solidity of objects, and thus their nature, by handling them.

Stereotaxis
The procedure using computer-controlled X-ray images whereby precise localisation in space is achieved. It is applied to that branch of surgery known as stereotactic neurosurgery, in which the surgeon is able to localise precisely those areas of the brain on which he or she wishes to operate.

Sterilisation
Sterilisation means either (1) the process of rendering various objects – such as those which

come in contact with wounds, and various foods – free from microbes, or (2) the process of rendering a person incapable of producing children.

The manner of sterilising bedding, furniture, and the like, after contact with a case of infectious disease, is given under DISINFECTION; whilst the sterilisation of instruments, dressings, and skin surfaces, necessary before surgical procedures, is mentioned in the same article and also under ANTISEPTICS, ASEPSIS, and WOUNDS. For general purposes, one of the cheapest and most effective agents is boiling water or steam.

Bacteriological sterilisation may be effected in many ways, and different methods are used in different cases.

Reproductive sterilisation In women, this is performed by ligating (cutting) and then tying the FALLOPIAN TUBES – the tubes that carry the OVUM from the ovary (see OVARIES) to the UTERUS. Alternatively, the tubes may be sealed-off by means of plastic and silicone clips or rings. The technique is usually performed (by LAPAROSCOPY) through a small incision, or cut, in the lower abdominal wall. It has no effect on sexual or menstrual function, and, unlike the comparable operation in men, it is immediately effective. The sterilisation is usually permanent (around 0·05 pregnancies occur for every 100 women years of use), but occasionally the two cut ends of the Fallopian tubes reunite, and pregnancy is then again possible. Removal of the uterus and/or the ovaries also sterilises a woman but such procedures are only used when there is some special reason, such as the presence of a tumour.

The operation for sterilising men is known as VASECTOMY.

Sterility
The state of (1) being free of infectious agents or (2) permanent INFERTILITY.

Sternum
The scientific name for the breastbone. This is a long, flat, bony plate that comprises the central part of the chest. Made up of three parts: an upper triangular piece (manubrium); a middle part (the body); and at the bottom end the small, flexible xiphoid process. The two clavicles articulate to the manubrium. Seven pairs of costal cartilages link the sternum to the ribs. The sternum is very strong and a powerful blow is needed to fracture it: such an injury may damage the underlying heart and lungs.

Steroid
The group name for compounds that resemble CHOLESTEROL chemically. The group includes the sex hormones, the hormones of the adrenal cortex, and bile acids. They have a powerful influence on the normal functioning of the body, and natural and synthetic steroids are used in the treatment of many disorders. (See CORTICOSTEROIDS; ENDOCRINE GLANDS.)

Stertor
Stertor is a form of noisy breathing, similar to SNORING, and usually due to flapping of the soft PALATE. Whereas ordinary snoring results from sleeping with the mouth open, stertor is the result of paralysis of the soft palate: this may be the result of a stroke, suffocation, concussion, drunkenness, or poisoning by OPIUM or chloroform. In severe cases of paralysis, the tongue may loll back against the back of the throat, resulting in a very loud sound. In such cases breathing may be rapidly relieved by pulling the lower jaw forwards, pulling the tongue out of the mouth, or turning the person on to one side.

Stethoscope
An instrument used for listening to the sounds produced by the action of the lungs, heart, and other internal organs. (See AUSCULTATION.)

Stevens-Johnson Syndrome
See ERYTHEMA – Erythema multiforme.

Stiffness
A condition which may be due to a change in the joints, ligaments, tendons, or muscles, or to the influence of the nervous system over the muscles of the part affected. Stiffness is associated with various forms of arthritis or muscular disorders and with the effects of injuries to joints, tendons and muscles. Stiffness of the neck muscles resulting in bending the head backwards, and of the hamstring muscles, causing difficulty in straightening the lower limbs, is a sign of MENINGITIS. Stiffness or spasticity also occurs in certain diseases of the central nervous system.

Treatment is of the underlying disease or injury. Mild stiffness can be treated symptomatically with local warmth and ANALGESICS. PHYSIOTHERAPY is helpful in relieving stiffness as a result of muscle or joint injuries.

Stigma
Any spot or impression upon the SKIN. The term, stigmas of degeneration, is applied to

physical defects that are found in people with learning disabilities (see LEARNING DISABILITY).

Stilboestrol

A synthetic oestrogen (see OESTROGENS). Its physiological actions are closely similar to those of the natural ovarian hormone, and it has the great merit of being active when taken by mouth. The drug may help patients suffering from cancer of the PROSTATE GLAND, inducing in some cases regression of the primary tumour and of secondary deposits in bone.

Stilboestrol Diphosphate

See OESTROGENS.

Stilet

A stilet, or stilette, is the delicate probe or the wire used to clear a catheter (see CATHETERS) or hollow needle.

Stillbirth

A stillborn child is 'any child which has issued forth from its mother after the 24th week of pregnancy and which did not at any time after being completely expelled from its mother, breathe or show any other sign of life'. In the United Kingdom in 2002 the number of still-births and deaths at under one week of age (PERINATAL MORTALITY) was 5.6 per 1,000 live births.

Still's Disease

Or juvenile rheumatoid arthritis – see JUVENILE IDIOPATHIC ARTHRITIS (JIA).

Stimulant

A drug or other agent that prompts the activity of a body system or function. For example, the sight and smell of food stimulates salivation, and the rods and cones in the retina of the eye are stimulated by light. Another example is the use of amphetamines and caffeine to stimulate the central nervous system and make an individual more alert and active – or, if taken in excess, hyperactive. In treatment procedures, electrical stimulation may be used to bring muscles into action. Aromatics, spices and bitters are traditional stimulants of digestive processes.

Stings

See BITES AND STINGS.

Stitch

A popular name for a sharp pain in the side. It is generally due to cramp (see MUSCLES, DIS-

ORDERS OF) following unusually hard exertion, but care must be taken that this trivial condition is not taken for PLEURISY or for a fractured rib. The word is also used to mean the repair of skin following surgery or any other trauma.

St John's Wort

A herbal remedy which has achieved popularity as a treatment for mild depression. It may, however, induce the production of enzymes (see ENZYME) that metabolise drugs, and several important interactions have been identified which may result in unwanted side-effects, even when treatment with St John's Wort is stopped.

Stokes-Adams Syndrome

A term applied to a condition in which slowness of the PULSE is associated with attacks of unconsciousness, and which is due to ARRHYTHMIA of the cardiac muscle or even complete heart block. Usually the heart returns to normal rhythm after a short period, but patients who suffer from the condition are commonly provided with a PACEMAKER to maintain normal cardiac function (see also CARDIAC PACEMAKER).

Stoma

A stoma refers to an opening constructed when the bowel has to be brought to the skin surface to convey gastrointestinal contents to the exterior. It is derived from the Greek word meaning mouth. In the United Kingdom there are about 100,000 patients with a COLOSTOMY, 10,000 with an ILEOSTOMY and some 2,000 with a urostomy, in which the ureters (see URETER) are brought to the skin surface. They may be undertaken because of malignancy of the colon or rectum (see INTESTINE) or as a result of inflammatory bowel diseases such as CROHN'S DISEASE. Urostomies usually take the form of an isolated loop of ilium into which the ureters have been implanted and which in its turn is either brought to the skin's surface or converted into an artificial bladder. This is undertaken because of bladder cancer or because of neurological diseases of the bladder. The stomas drain into appliances such as disposable plastic bags. Most of the modern appliances collect the effluent of the stoma without any leak or odour.

Patients with stomas often find explanatory booklets helpful: *Living with your Colostomy* and *Understanding Colostomy* are examples. They are published by the British Colostomy Association.

Stomach

This is a distensible, sac-like organ with an

average adult capacity of 1·5 litres situated in the upper abdomen. It is positioned between the OESOPHAGUS and DUODENUM, lying just beneath the DIAPHRAGM to the right of the SPLEEN and partly under the LIVER. The stomach is a part of the gastrointestinal tract with its walls formed of layers of longitudinal and circular muscles and lined by glandular cells that secrete gastric juice. It is well supplied with blood vessels as well as nerves from the autonomic system which enter via the phrenic nerve. The exit of the stomach is guarded by a ring of muscle called the pyloric sphincter which controls the passage of food into the duodenum.

Function   As well as the stomach's prime role in physically and physiologically breaking down the food delivered via the oesophagus, it also acts as a storage organ – a function that enables people to eat three or four times a day instead of every 30 minutes or so as their metabolic needs would otherwise demand. Gastric secretion is stimulated by the sight and smell of food and its subsequent arrival in the stomach. The secretions, which contain mucus and hydrochloric acid (the latter produced by parietal cells), ster-

ilise the food; pepsin, a digestive ENZYME in the gastric juices, breaks down the protein in food. The juices also contain intrinsic factor, vital for the absorption of vitamin B_{12} when the chyle – as the stomach contents are called – reaches the intestine. This chyle is of creamy consistency and is the end product of enzymic action and rhythmic contractions of the stomach's muscles every 30 seconds or so. Food remains in the stomach for varying lengths of time depending upon its quantity and nature. At regular intervals a bolus of chyle is forced into the duodenum by contractions of the stomach muscles coordinated with relaxation of the pyloric sphincter.

Stomach, Diseases of

Gastritis is the description for several unrelated diseases of the gastric mucosa.

Acute gastritis is an inflammatory reaction of the gastric mucosa to various precipitating factors, ranging from physical and chemical injury to infections. Acute gastritis (especially of the antral mucosas) may well represent a reaction to infection by a bacterium called *Helicobacter pylori*. The inflammatory changes usually

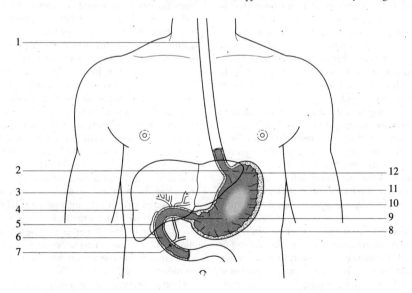

1 oesophagus	7 common bile duct entering
2 cardiac orifice of stomach	duodenum at ampulla of vater
3 lesser curvature of stomach	8 antrum of stomach
4 liver (right lobe)	9 pylorus
5 gall bladder	10 fundus of stomach
6 duodenum	11 cardia of stomach
	12 liver (left lobe)

Interior of stomach.

go after appropriate antibiotic treatment for the *H. pylori* infection.

Acute and chronic inflammation occurs in response to chemical damage of the gastric mucosa. For example, REFLUX of duodenal contents may predispose to inflammatory acute and chronic gastritis. Similarly, multiple small erosions or single or multiple ulcers have resulted from consumption of chemicals, especialy aspirin and antirheumatic NON-STEROIDAL ANTI-INFLAMMATORY DRUGS (NSAIDS).

Acute gastritis may cause anorexia, nausea, upper abdominal pain and, if erosive, haemorrhage. Treatment involves removal of the offending cause.

Chronic gastritis Accumulation of cells called round cells in the gastric mucosal characterises chronic gastritis. Most patients with chronic gastritis have no symptoms, and treatment of *H. pylori* infection usually cures the condition.

Atrophic gastritis A few patients with chronic gastritis may develop atrophic gastritis. With or without inflammatory change, this disorder is common in western countries. The incidence increases with age, and more than 50 per cent of people over 50 may have it. A more complete and uniform type of ATROPHY, called 'gastric atrophy', characterises a familial disease called PERNICIOUS ANAEMIA. The cause of the latter disease is not known but it may be an autoimmune disorder.

Since atrophy of the corpus mucosa results in loss of acid- and pepsin-secreting cells, gastric secretion is reduced or absent. Patients with pernicious anaemia or severe atrophic gastritis of the corpus mucosa may secrete too little intrinsic factor for absorption of vitamin B_{12} and so can develop severe neurological disease (subacute combined degeneration of the spinal cord).

Patients with atrophic gastritis often have bacterial colonisation of the upper alimentary tract, with increased concentration of nitrite and carcinogenic N-nitroso compounds. These, coupled with excess growth of mucosal cells, may be linked to cancer. In chronic corpus gastritis, the risk of gastric cancer is about 3–4 times that of the general population.

Postgastrectomy mucosa The mucosa of the gastric remnant after surgical removal of the distal part of the stomach is usually inflamed and atrophic, and is also premalignant, with the risk of gastric cancer being very much greater than for patients with duodenal ulcer who have not had surgery.

Stress gastritis Acute stress gastritis develops, sometimes within hours, in individuals who have undergone severe physical trauma, BURNS (Curling ulcers), severe SEPSIS or major diseases such as heart attacks, strokes, intracranial trauma or operations (Cushing's ulcers). The disorder presents with multiple superficial erosions or ulcers of the gastric mucosa, with HAEMATEMESIS and MELAENA and sometimes with perforation when the acute ulcers erode through the stomach wall. Treatment involves inhibition of gastric secretion with intravenous infusion of an H_2-receptor-antagonist drug such as RANITIDINE or FAMO-TIDINE, so that the gastric contents remain at a near neutral pH. Despite treatment, a few patients continue to bleed and may then require radical gastric surgery.

Gastric ulcer Gastric ulcers were common in young women during the 19th century, markedly fell in frequency in many western countries during the first half of the 20th century, but remained common in coastal northern Norway, Japan, in young Australian women, and in some Andean populations. During the latter half of this century, gastric ulcers have again become more frequent in the West, with a peak incidence between 55 and 65 years.

The cause is not known. The two factors most strongly associated with the development of duodenal ulcers – gastric-acid production and gastric infection with *H. pylori* bacteria – are not nearly as strongly associated with gastric ulcers. The latter occur with increased frequency in individuals who take aspirin or NSAIDs. In healthy individuals who take NSAIDs, as many as 6 per cent develop a gastric ulcer during the first week of treatment, while in patients with rheumatoid arthritis who are being treated long term with drugs, gastric ulcers occur in 20–40 per cent. The cause is inhibition of the enzyme cyclo-oxygenase, which in turn inhibits the production of repair-promoting PROSTAGLANDINS.

Gastric ulcers occur especially on the lesser curve of the stomach. The ulcers may erode through the whole thickness of the gastric wall, perforating into the peritoneal cavity or penetrating into liver, pancreas or colon.

Gastric ulcers usually present with a history of epigastric pain of less than one year. The pain tends to be associated with anorexia and may be aggravated by food, although patients with 'prepyloric' ulcers may obtain relief from eating or taking antacid preparations. Patients with gastric ulcers also complain of nausea and vomiting, and lose weight.

The principal complications of gastric ulcer are haemorrhage from arterial erosion, or perforation into the peritoneal cavity resulting in PERITONITIS, abscess or fistula.

Aproximately one in two gastric ulcers heal 'spontaneously' in 2–3 months; however, up to 80 per cent of the patients relapse within 12 months. Repeated recurrence and rehealing results in scar tissue around the ulcer; this may cause a circumferential narrowing – a condition called 'hour-glass stomach'.

The diagnosis of gastric ulcer is confirmed by ENDOSCOPY. All patients with gastric ulcers should have multiple biopsies (see BIOPSY) to exclude the presence of malignant cells. Even after healing, gastric ulcers should be endoscopically monitored for a year.

Treatment of gastric ulcers is relatively simple: a course of one of the H₂ RECEPTOR ANTAGONISTS heals gastric ulcers in 3 months. In patients who relapse, long-term indefinite treatment with an H₂ receptor antagonist such as ranitidine may be necessary since the ulcers tend to recur. Recently it has been claimed that gastric ulcers can be healed with a combination of a bismuth salt or a gastric secretory inhibitor – for example, one of the PROTON PUMP INHIBITORS such as omeprazole or lansoprazole – together with two antibiotics such as AMOXYCILLIN and METRONIDAZOLE. The long-term outcome of such treatment is not known. Partial gastrectomy, which used to be a regular treatment for gastric ulcers, is now much more rarely done unless the ulcer(s) contain precancerous cells.

Cancer of the stomach Cancer of the stomach is common and dangerous and, worldwide, accounts for approximately one in six of all deaths from cancer. There are marked geographical differences in frequency, with a very high incidence in Japan and low incidence in the USA. In the United Kingdom around 33 cases per 100,000 population are diagnosed annually. Studies have shown that environmental factors, rather than hereditary ones, are mainly responsible for the development of gastric cancer. Diet, including highly salted, pickled and smoked foods, and high concentrations of nitrate in food and drinking water, may well be responsible for the environmental effects.

Most gastric ulcers arise in abnormal gastric mucosa. The three mucosal disorders which especially predispose to gastric cancer include pernicious anaemia, postgastrectomy mucosa, and atrophic gastritis (see above). Around 90 per cent of gastric cancers have the microscopic appearance of abnormal mucosal cells (and are called 'adenocarcinomas'). Most of the remainder look like endocrine cells of lymphoid tissue, although tumours with mixed microscopic appearance are common.

Early gastric cancer may be symptomless and, in countries like Japan with a high frequency of the disease, is often diagnosed during routine screening of the population. In more advanced cancers, upper abdominal pain, loss of appetite and loss of weight occur. Many present with obstructive symptoms, such as vomiting (when the pylorus is obstructed) or difficulty with swallowing. METASTASIS is obvious in up to two-thirds of patients and its presence contraindicates surgical cure. The diagnosis is made by endoscopic examination of the stomach and biopsy of abnormal-looking areas of mucosa. Treatment is surgical, often with additional chemotherapy and radiotherapy.

Stomach Tube

A soft rubber or plastic tube with rounded end, and usually about 75 cm (30 inches) in length, which is used for washing out the stomach when it contains some poisonous material. (See GASTRIC LAVAGE.) A narrower tube, 90 cm (36 inches) in length, is used to obtain a sample of gastric juice for examination. Such a tube can also be allowed to pass out of the stomach into the duodenum so that the contents of the upper part of the small intestine are similarly obtained for analysis.

Stomach Washout

See GASTRIC LAVAGE.

Stomatitis

Inflammation or ulceration of the mouth. (See MOUTH, DISEASES OF.)

-Stomy

A suffix signifying formation of an opening in an organ by operation: for example, COLOSTOMY.

Stone

See URINARY BLADDER, DISEASES OF; GALL-BLADDER, DISEASES OF.

Stools

See FAECES.

Strabismus

See SQUINT.

Strain

Stretching or tearing of muscle fibres caused by subjecting them to sudden pulling. Bleeding into the muscle causes pain and swelling and sometimes muscle spasm. Application of ice packs and strapping, coupled with a day or two's rest and analgesics, are usually sufficient to remedy most strains. Sometimes anti-inflammatory drugs or physiotherapy may be required.

Strangulation

The constriction of a passage or tube in the body that blocks the blood flow and disturbs the working of the affected organ. It is usually caused by compression or twisting. Strangulation customarily occurs when part of the INTESTINE herniates either inside the abdomen or outside as in an inguinal HERNIA. If a section of the intestine twists, this may strangulate and is known as a VOLVULUS.

Strangulation of a person's neck, either with a ligature or with the hands, obstructs the jugular veins in the neck, preventing the normal outflow of blood from the brain and head. The TRACHEA is also compressed, cutting off the supply of air to the lungs. The combination of these effects leads to HYPOXIA and damage to the brain. If not quickly relieved, unconsciousness and death follow. Strangulation may be deliberate or accidental – the latter being a particular hazard for children, for example, when playing with a rope. Removal of the constriction, artificial respiration, and medical attention are urgently necessary.

Strangury

A condition in which there is constant desire to pass water, accompanied by a straining sensation, though only a few drops can be voided. It is a symptom of inflammation in the urinary tract.

Strapping

The application of strips of adhesive plaster, one overlapping the other, so as to cover and exert pressure on an area of the body. This treatment is used in cases of injury or disease when it is desired to keep a part at rest: for example, strapping may be applied to the chest in cases of pleurisy and fracture of the ribs. Also, it is often used to prevent the movement of joints which are sprained or otherwise injured.

Strep Throat

An infection of the throat with STREPTOCOC-CUS bacteria: it is most common in children and symptoms range from minor discomfort to sore throat, fever, general malaise and enlarged LYMPH nodes in the neck. If symptoms are severe the infection may lead to SCARLET FEVER. PENICILLIN is the treatment of choice.

Streptococcus

Streptococcus is a variety of gram-positive bacterium (see GRAM'S STAIN; BACTERIA) which under the microscope has much the appearance of a string of beads. Most species are saprophytic (see SAPROPHYTE); a few are PATHOGENIC and these include haemolytic types which can destroy red blood cells in a culture of blood agar. This offers a method of classifying the varying streptococcal strains. Alpha-haemolytic streptococci are usually associated with bacterial ENDOCARDITIS. SCARLET FEVER is caused by a β-haemolytic streptococcus called *S. pyogenes*. *S. pneumoniae*, also called PNEUMOCOCCUS, causes respiratory-tract infections, including PNEUMONIA. *S. pyogenes* may on its own, or with other bacteria, cause severe NECROTISING FASCIITIS or CELLULITIS in which oedema and death of subcutaneous tissues occur. The infection can spread very rapidly and, unless urgently treated with ANTIBIOTICS and sometimes surgery, death may quickly result. This spread is related to the ability of *S. pyogenes* to produce toxic substances called exotoxins. Although drug-resistant forms are occurring, streptococcal infections usually respond to treatment with antibiotics.

Streptokinase

An ENZYME produced by certain streptococci (see STREPTOCOCCUS). It acts as a PLASMINO-GEN activator, and hence enhances FIBRINOLY-SIS. The most important use of streptokinase is in the treatment of myocardial infarction (see HEART, DISEASES OF) in the first 12 hours after the initial diagnosis. Subsequently, use of this thrombolytic drug should be under hospital supervision. It is given intravenously, in hospital by infusion. It may be given as an infusion to treat severe THROMBOSIS or EMBOLISM, particularly when they occur in a limb, and in deep venous thrombosis. Being antigenic and very expensive it is rarely used for more than two days, and is followed by anticoagulation therapy. The chief risk is haemorrhage, so an antifibrinolytic such as aminocaproic acid should always be available.

Streptomycin

Streptomycin is an antibacterial substance obtained from the soil mould, *Streptomyces griseus,* first isolated in 1944 and the first antibiotic to be effective against the tubercle bacillus. It was once routinely used to treat TUBERCULOSIS; because of side-effects and the development of other drugs, it is now rarely used except for in cases of resistant tuberculosis.

One of the AMINOGLYCOSIDES, streptomycin has two disadvantages. The most important of these is the tendency of organisms to become resistant to it. This means that the administration of this antibiotic must be carefully supervised to ensure that correct dosage is being used. The other disadvantage is that streptomycin produces toxic effects, especially disturbance of the vestibular and hearing apparatus. This may result in DEAFNESS, VERTIGO, and TINNITUS. Whilst in many cases these toxic manifestations disappear when the antibiotic is withdrawn, they may be permanent. For this reason therefore streptomycin must always be used with special care.

Stress

Any factor or event that threatens a person's health or adversely affects his or her normal functioning. Injury, disease or worry are common examples; others include internal conflicts, emotive life events – such as the death of a close relative or friend, the birth of a baby, separation or divorce – pressures at work or a hostile environment such as war or famine. Some individuals seem to be more prone than others to develop medical problems related to stress.

Stress prompts the body to raise its output of HORMONES such as ADRENALINE and CORTISOL, causing changes in blood pressure, heart rate and metabolism. These are physiological responses intended to improve a person's physical and mental performance – the 'fight or flight' reaction to fear. Stress may, however, disrupt the ability to cope. Constant or recurrent exposure to stress may produce symptoms such as anxiety, depression, headaches, indigestion, diarrhoea, palpitations and general malaise (see POST-TRAUMATIC STRESS DISORDER (PTSD)). Treatment can be difficult and prolonged; counselling can help as can ANXIOLYTICS or ANTIDEPRESSANT DRUGS – but a change in job or lifestyle may be necessary in some circumstances.

Stress Fractures

Stress fractures are comparatively common in sportspeople. They tend to occur when an undue amount of exercise is taken – that is, an amount of exercise which an individual is not capable of coping with in his or her state of training. The main initial feature is pain over the affected bone that has been subjected to abnormal physical stress. This is usually insidious in onset, and worse at night and during and after exercise. It is accompanied by tenderness, and a lump may be felt over the affected site. X-ray evidence only appears after several weeks. Treatment consists of rest, some form of external support, and in the initial stage ANALGESICS to deaden or kill the pain. (See also BONE, DISORDERS OF – Bone fractures.)

Striae

Stretch-marks seen in the skin, common in adolescent boys and girls owing to stretching of the skin by rapid growth (striae distensae). In boys, striae occur around the shoulders and thighs; in girls the breasts and hips are affected. In both sexes horizontal striae on the back may be mistaken for signs of trauma. Striae are common in women in late pregnancy, especially on the lower abdomen (striae gravidarum). Injudicious prolonged use of potent topical CORTICOSTEROIDS can induce striae, particularly about the groins, inner thighs or armpits. Prolonged high-dose oral STEROID therapy may cause widespread striae.

Stricture

A narrowing in any of the natural passages of the body, such as the GULLET, the bowel, or the URETHRA. It may be due to the development of some growth in the wall of the passage affected, or to pressure upon it by such a growth in some neighbouring organ, but in the majority of cases a stricture is the result of previous ulceration on the inner surface of the passage, followed by contraction of the scar. (See INTESTINE, DISEASES OF; URETHRA, DISEASES OF.)

Stridor

A noise associated with inspiration due to narrowing of the upper airway, in particular the LARYNX.

Stroke

Stroke, or cerebrovascular accident (CVA), is sudden damage to BRAIN tissue caused either by a lack of blood supply or rupture of a blood vessel (see ISCHAEMIC STROKE). The affected brain cells die and the parts of the body they control or receive sensory messages from cease to function.

Causes Blood supply to the brain may be interrupted by arteries furring up with ATHEROSCLEROSIS (which is accelerated by HYPERTENSION and DIABETES MELLITUS, both of which are associated with a higher incidence of strokes) or being occluded by blood clots arising from distant organs such as infected heart valves or larger clots in the heart (see BLOOD CLOT; THROMBOSIS). Hearts with an irregular rhythm are especially prone to develop clots. Patients with thick or viscous blood, clotting disorders or those with inflamed arteries – for example, in SYSTEMIC LUPUS ERYTHEMATOSUS (SLE) – are particularly in danger of having strokes. Bleeding into the brain arises from areas of weakened blood vessels, many of which may be congenital.

Symptoms Minor episodes due to temporary lack of blood supply and oxygen (called TRANSIENT ISCHAEMIC ATTACKS OR EPISODES (TIA, TIE)) are manifested by short-lived weakness or numbness in an arm or leg and may precede a major stroke. Strokes cause sudden weakness or complete paralysis of the muscles controlled by the part of the brain affected, as well as sensory changes (e.g. numbness or tingling). In the worst cases these symptoms and signs may be accompanied by loss of consciousness. If the stroke affects the area of the brain controlling the larynx and throat, the patient may suffer slurring or loss of speech with difficulty in initiating swallowing. When the face is involved, the mouth may droop and the patient dribble. Strokes caused by haemorrhage may be preceded by headaches. Rarely, CVAs are complicated by epileptic fits (see EPILEPSY). If, on the other hand, numerous small clots develop in the brain rather than one major event, this may manifest itself as a gradual deterioration in the patient's mental function, leading to DEMENTIA.

Investigations Tests on the heart or COMPUTED TOMOGRAPHY or ultrasonic scans (see ULTRASOUND) on arteries in the neck may indicate the original sites of distantly arising clots. Blood tests may show increased thickness or tendency to clotting, and the diagnosis of general medical conditions can explain the presence of inflamed arteries which are prone to block. Special brain X-rays show the position and size of the damaged brain tissue and can usually distinguish between a clot or infarct and a rupture of and haemorrhage from a blood vessel in the brain.

Management It is better to prevent a stroke than try to cure it. The control of a person's diabetes or high blood pressure will reduce the risk of a stroke. Treatment with ANTICOAGULANTS prevents the formation of clots; regular small doses of aspirin stop platelets clumping together to form plugs in blood vessels. Both treatments reduce the likelihood of minor transient ischaemic episodes proceeding to a major stroke.

Once the latter has occurred, there is no effective treatment to reduce the damage to brain tissue. Function will return to the affected part of the body only if and when the brain recovers and messages are again sent down the appropriate nerves. Simple movements are more likely to recover than delicate ones, and sophisticated functions have the worst outlook. Thus, movement of the thigh may improve more easily than fine movements of fingers, and any speech impairment is more likely to be permanent. A rehabilitation team can help to compensate for any disabilities the subject may have. Physiotherapists maintain muscle tone and joint flexibility, whilst waiting for power to return; occupational therapists advise about functional problems and supply equipment to help patients overcome their disabilities; and speech therapists help with difficulties in swallowing, improve the clarity of remaining speech or offer alternative methods of communication. District nurses or home helps can provide support to those caring for victims of stroke at home. Advice about strokes may be obtained from the Stroke Association.

Stroma
The name applied to the tissue which forms the framework and covering of an organ.

Strongyloidiasis
This infection is caused by nematode worms of the genus *Strongyloides* spp. – the great majority being from *S. stercoralis*. This helminth is present throughout most tropical and subtropical countries; a single case report has been made in England – about an individual who had not been exposed to such an environment. Larvae usually penetrate intact skin, especially the feet (as with hookworm infection). Unlike hookworm infection, eggs mature and hatch in the lower gastrointestinal tract; thus larvae can immediately re-enter the circulation in the colo-rectum or perianal region, setting up an auto-infection cycle. Therefore, infection can continue for the remaining lifespan of the individual. Severe malnutrition may be a predisposing factor to infection, as was the case in prisoners of war in south-east Asia during World War II.

Whilst an infected patient is frequently asymptomatic, heavy infection can cause jejunal mucosal abnormalities, and an absorptive defect, with weight loss. During the migratory phase an itchy linear rash (larva currens) may be present on the lower abdomen, buttocks, and groins; this gives rise to recurrent transient itching. In an immunosuppressed individual, the 'hyperinfection syndrome' may ensue; migratory larvae invade all organs and tissues, including the lungs and brain. Associated with this widespread infection, the patient may develop an *Enterobacteriacae* spp. SEPTICAEMIA; this, together with *S. stercoralis* larvae, produces a MENINGOENCEPHALITIS. There is no evidence that this syndrome is more common in patients with HIV infection.

Diagnosis consists of visualisation of *S. stercoralis* (larvae or adults) in a jejunal biopsy-section or aspirate. Larvae may also be demonstrable in a faecal sample, especially following culture. Eosinophilia may be present in peripheral blood, during the invasive stage of infection. Chemotherapy consists of albendazole. The formerly used benzimidazole compound, thiabendazole, is now rarely prescribed in an uncomplicated infection due to unpleasant side-effects; even so, in the 'hyperinfection syndrome' it probably remains the more effective of the two compounds.

Strychnine

An alkaloid (see ALKALOIDS) derived from *Strychnos nux-vomica*, the seeds of an East Indian tree, as well as from the seeds of several other closely allied trees and shrubs. It is a white crystalline body possessed of an intensely bitter taste, more bitter perhaps than that of any other substance, and it is not very soluble in water. It stimulates all parts of the nervous system, and was at one time widely used for this purpose. Strychnine poisoning is fortunately rare. It shows itself in CONVULSIONS, which come on very speedily after the person has taken the poison. The mental faculties remain unaffected, and the symptoms end in death or recovery within a few hours.

Treatment The patient should be kept quiet. Artificial respiration may be necessary and intravenous BENZODIAZEPINES to prevent convulsions may also be needed. (See POISONS; also APPENDIX 2: ADDRESSES: SOURCES OF INFORMATION, ADVICE, SUPPORT AND SELF-HELP.)

Stupor

See UNCONSCIOUSNESS.

Stuttering

See STAMMERING.

St Vitus's Dance

An obsolete name for CHOREA.

Stye

See under EYE, DISORDERS OF.

Styptics

Applications which check bleeding, either by making the blood vessels contract more firmly or by causing rapid clotting in the blood (see COAGULATION). Some possess both modes of action.

Sub-

Prefix signifying under, near, or moderately.

Subacute

The description applied to a disease the duration of which lies between ACUTE and chronic (see CHRONIC DISORDER). An example is subacute ENDOCARDITIS, a disorder that may not be diagnosed for several weeks or months, during which time it can severely damage valves in the heart.

Subacute Combined Degeneration of the Cord

A degenerative condition of the SPINAL CORD which most commonly occurs as a complication of PERNICIOUS ANAEMIA. The motor and sensory nerves in the cord are damaged, causing spasticity of the limbs and an unsteady gait. Treatment is with vitamin B_{12} (see APPENDIX 5: VITAMINS).

Subacute Sclerosing Panencephalitis

A rare complication of MEASLES due to infection of the brain with the measles virus. It develops 2–18 years after the onset of the measles, and is characterised by mental deterioration leading on to CONVULSIONS, COMA and death. The annual incidence in Britain is about one per million of the childhood population. The risk of its developing is 5–25 times greater after measles than after measles vaccination (see MMR VACCINE; IMMUNISATION).

Subarachnoid Haemorrhage

A haemorrhage into the subarachnoid space in the BRAIN. It is usually the result of rupture of an ANEURYSM on the CIRCLE OF WILLIS. Head injury or intense physical exercise occasionally cause subarachnoid haemorrhage; the diagnosis is confirmed by CT scan or by identifying blood in the CEREBROSPINAL FLUID at LUMBAR PUNCTURE. Cerebral ANGIOGRAPHY will usually pinpoint the site of bleeding. Treatment is bed rest, life-support measures and procedures to reduce blood pressure; sometimes surgery is carried out but not usually until several weeks after the acute episode. About 30 per cent of patients recover fully, whilst some have residual disabilities such as EPILEPSY, mental deterioration or paralysis. About 50 per cent of those affected die.

Subarachnoid Space
The space between the arachnoid and the pia mater – two of the membranes covering the BRAIN. (See also MENINGES.)

Subclavian
The name applied to a large artery and vein which pass to the upper arm between the collarbone and the first rib.

Subclinical
A description of a disease that is suspected but which has not developed sufficiently or is too mild in form to produce clear signs and symptoms in an individual. Even so, damage may be caused to tissues and organs.

Subconscious
A state of being partially conscious, or the condition in which mental processes occur and outside objects and events are perceived with the mind nearly or quite unconscious of them. Such subconscious impressions or events may be forgotten at the time but may nevertheless exert a continued influence over the conscious mind, or may at a subsequent time come fully into consciousness. Much importance is attached to the influence of painful or unpleasant experiences which, although forgotten, continue to influence the mind; these may be a factor in the development of anxiety states. This injurious influence may be reduced when the subconscious impressions come fully into consciousness and are then remembered and clearly seen in their relative importance.

Subcutaneous
Anything pertaining to the loose cellular tissue beneath the SKIN: for example, a subcutaneous injection (see HYPODERMIC).

Subdural
Relating to the space between the strong outer layer of the MENINGES, the membranes which cover the BRAIN, and the arachnoid, which is the middle layer of the meninges. A subdural haemorrhage occurs when bleeding takes place

into this space. The trapped blood forms a large blood clot or haematoma within the skull and this causes pressure on the underlying brain. Bleeding may occur slowly as the result of disease or suddenly as the result of injury. Headaches, confusion and drowsiness result, sometimes with paralysis. Medical attention is required urgently if a serious haematoma occurs soon after injury.

Subinvolution
A term used to indicate that the womb (see UTERUS) has failed to undergo the usual involution, or decrease in size, which naturally takes place within one month after a child is born.

Subjective
A term applied to symptoms, and sensations, perceived only by the affected individual. For example, numbness is a purely subjective sensation, whilst the jerk given by the leg on tapping the tendon of the knee is an objective sign.

Sublimation
The conversion of a solid substance into a vapour and its recondensation. The term is also used in a mental sense for the process of converting instinctive sexual desires to new aims and objects devoid of sexual significance.

Subluxation
A partial dislocation of a joint; the term is sometimes applied to a sprain.

Submucosa
The layer of CONNECTIVE TISSUE that occurs under a MUCOUS MEMBRANE – for example, in the intestinal wall.

Subphrenic Abscess
An ABSCESS that develops under the DIAPHRAGM, usually on the right side of the abdomen between the liver and the diaphragm. The cause may be an organ that has perforated – for instance, a peptic ulcer in the stomach or intestine. An abscess may also occur after an abdominal operation, usually when the bowel or stomach has been operated on. Antibiotics and sometimes surgery are the method of treatment.

Substrate
A compound on which an ENZYME acts: for instance, ribonucleic acid (RNA) is the substrate for ribonuclease (an enzyme that catalyses the breakdown of ribonucleic acid, a cellular compound involved in the synthesis of PROTEIN).

Succussion

See THRILL. A clinical technique in which a patient suspected of having excessive fluid in a body cavity – usually the stomach or pleural cavity – is gently shaken in order to elicit splashing sounds.

Suckling

See INFANT FEEDING.

Sucrose

Cane sugar.

Suction

The use of a reduction in pressure to clear away fluids or other material through a tube. Suction is used to remove blood from the site of a surgical operation; it is commonly necessary to remove secretions from the airways of newly born babies to help them breathe.

Sudden Infant Death Syndrome (SIDS)

Sudden infant death syndrome, or cot death, refers to the unexpected death – usually during sleep – of an apparently healthy baby. Well over 1,500 such cases are thought to have occurred in the United Kingdom each year until 1992, when government advice was issued about laying babies on their backs. The figure was 192 in 2002 and continues to fall. Boys are affected more than girls, and over half of these deaths occur at the age of 2–6 months. More common in lower social classes, the incidence is highest in the winter; most of the infants have been bottle-fed (see also INFANT FEEDING).

Causes These are unknown, with possible multiple aetiology. Prematurity and low birth-weight may play a role. The sleeping position of a baby and an over-warm environment may be major factors, since deaths have fallen sharply since mothers were officially advised to place babies on their backs and not to overheat them. Some deaths are probably the result of respiratory infections, usually viral, which may stop breathing in at-risk infants, while others may result from the infant becoming smothered in a soft pillow. Faults in the baby's central breathing control system (central APNOEA) may be a factor. Other possible factors include poor socioeconomic environment; vitamin E deficiency; or smoking, drug addiction or anaemia in the mother. Help and advice may be obtained from the Foundation for the Study of Infant Deaths and the Cot Death Society.

Sudek's Atrophy

Osteoporosis (see under BONE, DISORDERS OF) in the hand or foot which develops quickly as a result of injury, infection or malignant growth.

Sudorifics

Drugs and other agents which produce copious PERSPIRATION.

Suffocation

See ASPHYXIA; CHOKING.

Suicide

Self-destruction as an intentional act. Attempted suicide is when death does not take place, despite an attempt by the person concerned to kill him or herself; parasuicide is the term describing an attempt at suicide that is really an act to draw attention to the perceived problems of the individual involved.

Societies vary in the degree to which they tolerate individuals acting intentionally to cause their own death. Apart from among some native peoples, particularly the Innuit, suicide is generally viewed pejoratively in modern societies. Major religious movements, including Catholicism, Judaism and Islam, have traditionally regarded suicide as a sin. Nevertheless, it is a growing phenomenon, particularly among the young, and so has become a serious public health problem. It is estimated that suicide among young people has tripled – at least – during the past 45 years. Worldwide, suicide is the second major cause of death (after tuberculosis) for women between the ages of 15 and 44, and the fourth major killer of men in the same age-group (after traffic accidents, tuberculosis and violence). The risk of suicide rises sharply in old age. Globally, there are estimated to be between ten and 25 suicide attempts for each completed suicide.

In the United Kingdom, suicide accounts for 20 per cent of all deaths of young people. Around 6,000 suicides are reported annually in the UK, of which approximately 75 per cent are by men. In the late 1990s the suicide rate in England, Wales and Northern Ireland fell, but increased in Scotland and the Republic of Ireland. Attempted suicide became significantly more common, particularly among people under the age of 25: among adolescents in the UK, for example, it is estimated that there are about 19,000 suicide attempts annually. Follow-up studies of teenagers who attempt suicide by an overdose show that up to 11 per cent will succeed in killing themselves over the following few years. In young people, factors linked to suicide and attempted suicide include alcohol or drug abuse, unemployment, physical or sexual abuse, and the fact of being in custody. (In the mid-1990s, 20 per cent of all prison suicides were by people under 21.)

Apart from the young, those at highest risk of dying by suicide include health professionals, pharmacists, vets and farmers. Self-poisoning (see POISONS) is the common method used by health professionals for whom high stress levels, together with relatively easy access to means, are important factors. The World Health Organisation has outlined six basic steps for the prevention of suicide, focusing particularly on reducing the availability of common methods. Although suicide is not a criminal offence in the UK, assisting suicide is a crime carrying a potential sentence of 14 years' imprisonment. There are several dilemmas faced by health professionals if they believe that a patient is considering suicide: one is that the provision of information to the patient may make them an accessory (see below). A dilemma after suicide is the common demand from insurers for medical information, although, ethically, the duty of confidentiality extends beyond the patient's death (see ETHICS). (Legally, some disclosure is permitted to those with a claim arising from the patient's death.) Life-insurance contracts generally render invalid any claim by the heirs on the policy of an individual who commits suicide, so that disclosure by a doctor often creates tensions with the relatives. Non-disclosure of relevant medical information, however, may result in a fraudulent insurance claim being made.

Physician-assisted suicide Although controversial, a special legal exemption applies to doctors in a few countries who assist terminally ill patients to kill themselves. Oregon in the United States legalised physician-assisted suicide in 1997, where it still occurs; assisted suicide was briefly legal in the Australian Northern Territory in 1996 but the legislation was repealed. (It is also practised, but not legally authorised, in the Netherlands and Switzerland.)

In the UK there have been unsuccessful parliamentary attempts to legalise assisted suicide, such as the 1997 Doctor Assisted Dying Bill. In law, a distinction is made between killing people with their consent (classified as murder) and assisting them to commit suicide (a statutory offence under the Suicide Act 1961). The distinction is between acting as a perpetrator and as an accessory. Doctors may be judged to have aided and abetted a suicide if they knowingly provide the means – or even if they simply provide advice about the toxicity of medication and tell patients the lethal dosage. Some argue that the distinction between EUTHANASIA and physician-assisted suicide has no moral or practical relevance, particularly if patients are too disabled to act themselves. In theory, patients retain ultimate control in cases of assisted suicide, whereas control rests with the doctor in euthanasia. Surveys of health professionals appear to indicate a feeling by some that less responsibility or culpability attaches to assisting suicide than to euthanasia. In a recent UK court case (2002), a judge declared that a mentally alert woman on a permanent life-support regime in hospital had a right to ask for the support system to be switched off. (See also MENTAL ILLNESS.)

Sulcus
The term applied to any groove or furrow, but especially to a fissure of the BRAIN.

Sulfadiazine
A highly active drug which in moderate dosage produces a high and persistent blood concentration. It is relatively non-toxic and is sometimes used to prevent the recurrence of RHEUMATIC FEVER.

Sulfamethoxazole
has been used in combination with TRIMETHOPRIM (as co-trimoxazole) to treat infections of the URINARY TRACT. Increasing bacterial resistance to sulphonamides and the incidence of side-effects means that caution is needed in prescribing co-trimoxazole.

Sulfasalazine
A chemical combination of sulphapyridine and 5-aminosalicylic acid. It is used to treat ULCERATIVE COLITIS (valuable as oral therapy for mild symptomatic disease; also available as suppositories for rectal disease) and RHEUMATOID ARTHRITIS. The salicylate part is now available alone in drugs such as mesalazine and olsalazine. Several reports of blood dyscrasias from patients taking these drugs have prompted the COMMITTEE ON SAFETY OF MEDICINES (CSM) to recommend that patients with unexplained blood disorders should stop treatment and be given an immediate blood count.

Sulfinpyrazone
A derivative of phenylbutazone which is of value in the prophylaxis and treatment of GOUT.

S

Sulphonylureas

Sulphonylureas are sulphonamide derivatives which lower the blood sugar when they are given by mouth by enhancing the production of INSULIN. They are effective in treating DIABETES MELLITUS only when some residual pancreatic beta-cell function is present. All may lead to HYPOGLYCAEMIA if given in overdose and this is particularly common when long-acting sulphonylureas are given to elderly patients. There is no evidence for any difference in the effectiveness of the various sulphonylureas. TOLBUTAMIDE was the first of the sulphonlyurea drugs; it has a short duration of action and is usually given twice daily. CHLOR-PROPAMIDE has a more prolonged action and only needs to be given once daily, but its prolonged action causes more side-effects – including sensitivity reactions. Other oral hypoglycaemic agents of this family include glibenclamide, which has a duration of action intermediate between tolbutamide and chlorpropamide and also produces side-effects (in about 30 per cent of outpatients, according to a recent study). Other sulphonlyureas include acetohexamide, glibornuride, gliclazide, glipizide, gliquidone and tolazamide. Glymidine is a related compound with a similar action to the sulphonylureas. It is particularly useful in patients who are hypersensitive to sulphonylureas.

Sulphonylureas are best avoided in patients who are overweight, as they tend to stimulate the appetite and aggravate obesity. They should be used with caution in patients with hepatic or renal disease. Side-effects are infrequent and usually not severe, the most common being epigastric discomfort with occasional nausea, vomiting and anorexia. In about 10 per cent of patients, chlorpropamide and tolbutamide may cause facial flushing after drinking alcohol. Some patients are hypersensitive to oral hypoglycaemic agents and develop rashes which may progress to ERYTHEMA multiforme and exfoliative DERMATITIS. These reactions usually appear in the first 6–8 weeks of treatment.

Sulphur

Chemical combinations of this substance were once applied topically because of their antimicrobial activity; they are no longer used.

Sumatriptan

A drug used in the treatment of MIGRAINE attacks. Given by subcutaneous injection, it provides quick relief of pain, acting on the same receptors as 5-hydroxytryptamine – a neuro-transmitter and vasoconstrictor agent. It may also be taken orally, but sumatriptan should not be used within 24 hours of treatment with ERGOTAMINE, the standard antimigraine treatment.

Summer Diarrhoea

See DIARRHOEA; INFANT FEEDING.

Sunburn

See PHOTODERMATOSES.

Super-

A prefix signifying above, or implying excess.

Superficial

Positioned near the surface: for example, superficial blood vessels or capillaries lie just beneath the skin, and by contracting and expanding help to regulate body TEMPERATURE.

Supination

Supination means the turning of the forearm and hand so that the palm faces upwards.

Supine

Lying on the back, face upwards; or the position of the forearm where the hand lies face upwards.

Suppository

A drug preparation in solid, bullet-like form, which is inserted into the RECTUM (or the VAGINA, when it is called a pessary). This method of using drugs may be chosen for various reasons. For example, the suppository, as in the case of glycerin suppositories, may be used to produce an aperient action. Other suppositories, such as those of MORPHINE, are used to reduce pain and check the action of the bowels. Suppositories are useful when the patient is unable to take oral medication and when no suitable preparation is available for injection.

Suppression

(1) The stopping of any physiological activity.
(2) A psychological defence mechanism by which an individual intentionally refuses to acknowledge an idea or memory that he or she finds distasteful or unpleasant.
(3) A treatment that stops the visible signs of an illness or holds back its usual progress.

Suppuration

The process of PUS formation. When pus forms on a raw surface the process is called ulceration, whilst a deep-seated collection of pus is known as an ABSCESS. (See also INFLAMMATION; PHAGOCYTOSIS; ULCER; WOUNDS.)

Supra-

A prefix signifying above or upon.

Suprapubic

An operation in which the abdomen is opened in its lower part, immediately above the pubic bones. It was a common approach for removal of the PROSTATE GLAND but is now used less often, as transurethral PROSTATECTOMY has become the standard procedure. (See also LITHOTOMY.)

Suprarenal Glands

See ADRENAL GLANDS.

Supraventricular Tachycardia

An unusually fast but regular beating of the HEART occurring for periods that may last several hours or days. In most people with this abnormality the heart rate is between 140 and 180 beats a minute; rarely, the rate may rise as high as 250–300 beats. The condition occurs when abnormal electrical impulses that arise in the upper chambers (atria) of the heart override the normal control centre – the sinoatrial node – for the heartbeat. Symptoms usually include breathlessness, palpitations, pain in the chest and fainting. An ELECTROCARDIOGRAM (ECG) is taken to help make the diagnosis. An acute episode can sometimes be stopped by VALSAVA'S MANOEUVRE or by drinking cold water. Anti-arrhythmic drugs (see ARRHYTHMIA) such as adenosine and digoxin are used to treat recurrent attacks. Occasionally, a severe attack may need to be treated with an electric shock to the heart: this is known as DEFIBRILLATION.

Suramin

A drug used to treat trypanosomiasis or SLEEPING SICKNESS. Side-effects vary in frequency and intensity and are sometimes serious. They include nausea, vomiting, SHOCK and occasionally loss of consciousness.

Surfactant

A surface-active agent lining the alveoli (see ALVEOLUS) of the LUNGS, which plays an essential part in RESPIRATION by preventing the alveoli from collapsing at the end of expiration. Absence, or lack, of surfactant is one of the factors responsible for HYALINE MEMBRANE DISEASE, and it is now being used in the treatment of this condition by means of instillation into the trachea.

Surgery

That branch of medicine involved in the treatment of injuries, deformities or individual diseases by operation or manipulation. It incorporates: general surgery; specialised techniques such as CRYOSURGERY, MICROSURGERY, MINIMALLY INVASIVE SURGERY (MIS), or minimal access (keyhole) surgery, and stereotactic sugery (see STEREOTAXIS); and surgery associated with the main specialties, especially cardiothoracic surgery, gastroenterology, GYNAECOLOGY, NEUROLOGY, OBSTETRICS, ONCOLOGY, OPHTHALMOLOGY, ORTHOPAEDICS, TRANSPLANTATION surgery, RECONSTRUCTIVE (PLASTIC) SURGERY, and UROLOGY. Remotely controlled surgery using televisual and robotic techniques is also being developed.

It takes up to 15 years to train a surgeon from the time at which he or she enters medical school; after graduating as a doctor a surgeon has to pass a comprehensive two-stage examination to become a fellow of one of the five recognised colleges of surgeons in the UK and Ireland.

Surgery is carried out in specially designed operating theatres. Whereas it used to necessitate days and sometimes weeks of inpatient hospital care, many patients are now treated as day patients, often under local anaesthesia, being admitted in the morning and discharged later in the day.

More complex surgery, such as transplantation and neurosurgery, usually necessitates patients being nursed post-operatively in high-dependency units (see INTENSIVE THERAPY UNIT (ITU)) before being transferred to ordinary recovery wards. Successful surgery requires close co-operation between surgeons, physicians and radiologists as well as anaesthetists (see ANAESTHESIA), whose sophisticated techniques enable surgeons to undertake long and complex operations that were unthinkable 30 or more years ago. Surgical treatment of cancers is usually done in collaboration with oncologists. Successful surgery is also dependent on the skills of supporting staff comprising nurses and operating-theatre technicians and the availability of up-to-date facilities.

Surrogate

A term applied in medicine to a substance used as a substitute for another. The term is also applied to a woman who agrees to become pregnant and give birth to a child on the understanding that she will give up the child to the parents who have contracted with her for the surrogacy arrangement. When *in vitro* fertilisation (IVF – see under ASSISTED CONCEPTION) proved successful, it became possible to transfer a fertilised egg to a 'uterus of choice'. Artificial insemination of the potential surrogate mother using sperm from the putative 'father' is also practised. Surrogacy has thrown up a host of ethical and legal problems which have yet to be satisfactorily resolved.

Susceptibility
A reduced ability to combat an illness, usually an infection. The patient may be in poor general health, or immunisation or disease may have affected his or her defence mechanisms. For example, a person with AIDS is particularly susceptible to infection.

Suture
A word used in both an anatomical and a surgical sense. (1) Anatomically, suture is a type of immovable joint, found particularly in the SKULL, including the coronal suture (between the frontal and parietal bones); the lamboidal suture (between the parietal and occipital bones); and the sagittal suture (between the two parietal bones). (2) Surgically the word refers either to the technique of closing a wound, or to the material used. Stitching methods have been developed for gastrointestinal, neurological, dermatological and other forms of surgery, and include laser surgery and removable clips or staples. The material used is generally divided into monofilament, twisted or braided. Absorbable sutures – used for internal stitching – include catgut, Vicryl® and Dexon®. Non-absorbable sutures include silk, nylon and prolene. The type used and time of suture-removal depend upon the site and general state of the patient. Those patients on steroids who have a malignant or infective disorder heal slowly, and their sutures may need to stay in for 14 days or more instead of the usual 5–8 days.

Swab
A term applied to a small piece of gauze, lint or similar material used for wiping out the mouth of a patient or for drying out a wound. The term is also applied to a tuft of sterilised cotton-wool wrapped round a wire and enclosed in a sterile glass tube used for obtaining a sample – for example, from the throat or from wounds – for bacteriological examination.

Swan-Ganz Catheter
(See also CATHETERS.) A flexible tube with a double lumen and a small balloon at its distal end. It is introduced into a vein in the arm and advanced until the end of the catheter is in the right atrium (see HEART). The balloon is then inflated with air through one lumen and this enables the bloodstream to propel the catheter through the right ventricle to the pulmonary artery. The balloon is deflated and the catheter can then record the pulmonary artery pressure. When the balloon is inflated, the tip is isolated from the pulmonary artery and measures the left atrial pressure. These measurements are important in the management of patients with circulatory failure, as under these circumstances the central venous pressure or the right atrial pressure is an unreliable guide to fluid-replacement.

Sweat
See PERSPIRATION.

Sweat Glands
See SKIN.

Sweetbread
A traditional term applied to several glands used for food, including the THYMUS GLAND of young animals (neck sweetbread), the PANCREAS (stomach sweetbread), and the testis (see TESTICLE).

Sycosis Barbae
(Barber's itch.) A chronic staphylococcal folliculitis (infection of the hair follicles with staphylococci bacteria – see STAPHYLOCOCCUS) of the beard area in males, causing a papulo-pustular inflammation clearly centred on hair follicles. It must be distinguished from RINGWORM infection of the face and hair follicles (tinea barbae) and from pseudo-folliculitis due to ingrowing hairs. Topical and oral anti-staphyloccocal antibiotics are effective.

Sydenham's Chorea
Also called St Vitus's dance, this type of CHOREA is a disease of the central nervous system that occurs after RHEUMATIC FEVER – up to six months later – and is probably an inflammatory complication of a β-haemolytic streptococcal infection (see STREPTOCOCCUS). The patient presents with jerky, purposeless, involuntary movements of a limb and tongue, similar to the symptoms of CEREBRAL PALSY. Chorea is best treated as a transitory reversible form of cerebral palsy. The disorder usually lasts 6–8 months and residual symptoms are rare.

Sympathetic
A term applied to certain diseases or symptoms which arise in one part of the body in consequence of disease in some distant part. Inflammation may arise in one eye, in consequence of injury to the other, by the spread of

organisms along the lymphatic channels connecting the two, and is then known as sympathetic inflammation. PAIN also may be of a sympathetic nature.

Sympathetic Nervous System

Part of the AUTONOMIC NERVOUS SYSTEM. It consists of scattered collections of grey matter known as ganglia, united by an irregular network of nerve-fibres; those portions where the ganglia are placed most closely and where the network of fibres is especially dense being known as plexuses. The chief part of the sympathetic system consists of two ganglionated cords that run through the neck, chest, and abdomen, lying close in front of the spine. In conjunction with the other part of the autonomic nervous system – the parasympathetic – this part controls many of the body's involuntary activities involving glands, organs and other tissues. (For further details, see NERVOUS SYSTEM.)

Sympathomimetic Drugs

These drugs stimulate the activity of the SYMPATHETIC NERVOUS SYSTEM. There are three groups: inotropic and vasoconstrictor sympathomimetics, and those used for cardiopulmonary resuscitation. The properties of these drugs vary according to whether they act on alpha or beta adrenergic receptors.

Inotropics act on beta receptors in heart muscle (see HEART), increasing its contractility and sometimes the heart rate. DOBUTAMINE and DOPAMINE are cardiac stimulants, while dopexamine acts on heart muscle and, via peripheral dopamine receptors, increases the excretion of URINE. ISOPRENALINE is used only as emergency treatment of heart block (interruption of the heart's conduction) or severe slowing of the heart rate (bradycardia).

Vasoconstrictor sympathomimetics These drugs temporarily raise the BLOOD PRESSURE by constricting peripheral blood vessels. Sometimes they are used as a speedy way of raising blood pressure when other treatment has failed. EPHEDRINE and methoxamine hydrochloride are examples of this type of sympathomimetic.

Cardiopulmonary resuscitation ADRENALINE (epinephrine) is given intravenously in cardiac arrest, and other drugs used include ATROPINE and CALCIUM.

Symphysis

An anatomical description of a joint in which two bones are connected by strong fibrous cartilage. One example is the joint between the two pubic bones in the front of the pelvis; another, the joint between the upper and middle parts of the breastbone.

Symptom

A term applied to any evidence of disease. The term, physical sign, is generally applied to evidence of disease of which the patient does not complain but which is elicited upon examination. For the symptoms indicative of the various diseases, see under the headings of each disease.

Syn-

A prefix signifying union.

Synapse

The term applied to the anatomical relation of one NEURON(E) (nerve cell) with another which is effected at various points by contact of their branching processes. The two neurons do not come directly into contact, but the release of a chemical NEUROTRANSMITTER by one neuronal AXON is followed by this chemical travelling across the synapse and firing off the signal along another nerve. A signal can be sent across a synapse in one direction only, from presynaptic or postsynaptic membranes. Synapses are divided into excitatory and inhibitory types. When a neurotransmitter travels across an excitatory synapse it usually provokes the receptor neuron into initiating an electrical impulse. Inhibitory synapses cool down the excitation of the adjacent neurons. Drugs that influence the NERVOUS SYSTEM usually do so by affecting the release or modification of the neurotransmitters passing across the synapse.

Syncope

Another word for fainting – a loss of consciousness due to a fall in BLOOD PRESSURE. This may result because the cardiac output has become reduced, or because the peripheral resistance provided by the arterioles has decreased. The simple faint or vaso-vagal attack is a result of a failure to maintain an adequate venous return of blood to the heart. This is likely to occur after prolonged periods of standing, particularly if one is standing still or if the climatic conditions are hot. It can also result from an unpleasant or painful experience. Pallor, sweating and a slow pulse are characteristic. Recovery is immediate when the venous return is restored by lying flat.

Syncope can also result when the venous return to the heart is impaired as a result of a rise in intrathoracic pressure. This may happen after prolonged vigorous coughing – the so-called COUGH SYNCOPE – or when elderly men with prostatic hypertrophy strain to empty their bladder. This is known as micturition syncope. Syncope is particularly likely to occur when the arterial blood pressure is unusually low. This may result from overtreatment of HYPERTENSION with drugs or it may be the result of diseases, such as ADDISON'S DISEASE, which are associated with low blood pressures. It is important that syncope be distinguished from EPILEPSY.

Syndactyly
A congenital condition in which two or more fingers or toes are fused together to a varying extent. The condition is popularly known as WEBBED FINGERS (or toes).

Syndrome
A term applied to a group of symptoms occurring together regularly, and thus constituting a disease to which some particular name is given: for example, CUSHING'S SYNDROME comprising obesity, hypertension, purple striae and osteoporosis; or KORSAKOFF'S SYNDROME, comprising loss of appreciation of time and place combined with talkativeness, forming signs of alcoholic delirium.

Synechiae
Adhesions between the iris (see EYE) and adjacent structures (e.g. cornea, lens). They usually arise as a result of inflammation of the iris.

Synergist
(1) A muscle that works in concert with an AGONIST muscle to perform a certain movement.
(2) An agent, for example a drug, that acts with another to produce a result that is greater than adding together the separate effects of the two agents. Synergism in drug treatment may be beneficial, as in the case of combined LEVODOPA and SELEGILINE, a selective monoamine oxidase inhibitor (see MONOAMINE OXIDASE INHIBITORS (MAOIS), in the treatment of PARKINSONISM. It may be potentially dangerous, however, as when MAOIs boost the effects of BARBITURATES.

Synostosis
The term applied to a union by bony material of adjacent bones which are normally separate.

Synovectomy
Surgical removal of the synovium (see SYNOVIAL

MEMBRANE) to treat troublesome SYNOVITIS. The operation is not normally done until other treatments have failed.

Synovial Membrane
This forms the lining of the soft parts that enclose the cavity of a joint. (See JOINTS.)

Synovitis
Inflammation of the membrane lining a joint (see JOINTS). It is usually painful and accompanied by effusion of fluid within the synovial sac of the joint. It is found in RHEUMATOID ARTHRITIS, various injuries and inflammations of joints, and in the chronic form in TUBERCULOSIS. Treatment of synovitis is with rest, splinting, ANALGESICS and NON-STEROIDAL ANTI-INFLAMMATORY DRUGS (NSAIDS). Infection should be treated with ANTIBIOTICS. If the joint fails to respond, surgery (SYNOVECTOMY) may be needed. (See also JOINTS, DISEASES OF.)

Synovium
See SYNOVIAL MEMBRANE.

Synthetic
A term applied to substances produced by chemical processes in the laboratory or by artificial building-up.

Syphilis
A sexually transmitted or CONGENITAL disease (the latter variety is now rare). Because in most cases the disease is acquired as a result of sexual intercourse with an infected individual, syphilis is classed as one of the SEXUALLY TRANSMITTED DISEASES (STDS). It normally affects only human beings.

Today, around 40 million new cases are notified annually in the world, and this is probably an underestimate. In the UK the annual incidence of new cases of syphilis diagnosed in NHS genito-urinary medicine clinics has risen from 8.8 to 9.7 per million of male population between 1991 and 1999; among women the figures were 4.0 to 4.5 per million. The infection is most common in homosexual men (see HOMOSEXUALITY).

Causes The causative organism is the *Treponema pallidum*, a long, thread-like wavy organism with pointed tapering ends. It is found in large numbers in the sores in the primary stage of the disease and in the skin lesions in the secondary stage.

Syphilis may be acquired from people already suffering from the disease, or it may be congenital. The acquired form is usually got by sexual intercourse, kissing or other intimate bodily contact. The epithelium covering the general surface of the skin seems to be an efficient protection, but the infective material penetrates mucous membranes. The acquired form of the disease is infectious from contact with sores, both in its primary and secondary stages; infants suffering from the congenital form are also highly infectious. Accordingly, anyone frequently handling such an infant is at risk of infection, although the mother may handle the baby with impunity.

Symptoms The acquired form of the disease is commonly divided into three stages – primary, secondary, and tertiary (although the latter is much less common than it was 50 years ago). The clinical manifestations are varied and are sometimes confused with those of other diseases. There are several laboratory tests for confirming the diagnosis.

The incubation period ranges from ten to 90 days, although most frequently it is around four weeks. Then, a small persistent ULCER appears at the site of infection, which is accompanied by a typical cartilaginous hardness of the tissues immediately around and beneath it. This, which is known as the primary sore (or chancre), may be very much inflamed, or it may be so small as to pass almost or quite unnoticed. A few days later, the lymphatic glands in its neighbourhood, and then those all over the body, become swollen and hard. This condition lasts for several weeks before the sore slowly heals and the glands subside. After a variable period – usually about two months from the date of infection – the secondary symptoms appear and resemble the symptoms of an ordinary FEVER, with pyrexia, loss of appetite, vague pains through the body, and a faint red rash seen best upon the front of the chest. People with syphilis are infectious in the primary and secondary stages but not in the latent or tertiary stages.

In untreated or inadequately treated cases, manifestations of the tertiary stage develop after the lapse of some months or even years: this is known as the latent period. These consist in the growth, at various sites throughout the body, of masses of granulation tissue known as gummas. These gummas may appear as hard nodules in the skin, or form tumour-like masses in the muscles, or produce thickening of bones. They may develop in the brain and spinal cord, where their presence causes very serious symptoms. Gummas yield readily, as a rule, to appropriate treatment, and generally disappear speedily.

Still later, effects are apt to follow, such as disease of the arteries, leading to ANEURYSM (see also ARTERIES, DISEASES OF), to STROKE, and to mental deterioration (see MENTAL ILLNESS); also certain nervous diseases, of which tabes dorsalis and general paralysis are the chief.

The congenital form of syphilis, now rare, may affect the child before birth, leading then as a rule to miscarriage or to a stillbirth if born at full time. Alternatively he (or she) may show the first symptoms a few weeks after birth, the appearances then corresponding to the secondary manifestations of the acquired form.

Laboratory confirmation of a clinical diagnosis is done by identifying active spirochaetes (see SPIROCHAETE) in a smear taken at the site of the initial chancre, and by blood tests such as the treponomal antibody absorption tests. These tests are strongly positive at the secondary stage, and in patients with neurosyphilis the tests may have to be done on CEREBROSPINAL FLUID.

Treatment Any person with syphilis is a source of infection, and should take precautions not to spread it. PENICILLIN is the drug of choice in the disease in all its stages, but resistant strains of the *Treponema pallidum* have emerged and are causing problems, especially in developing countries. Treatment must be instituted as soon as possible after infection is acquired: (1) a full course of treatment is essential in every case, no matter how mild the disease may appear to be; (2) periodic blood examinations must be carried out on every patient for at least two years after he or she has been apparently cured.

Prevention is important and promiscuous hetero- or homosexual intercourse involves a risk of infection. Condoms provide some, but not complete protection. Infection can be avoided by maintaining a monogamous relationship.

Syringe

An instrument for injecting fluid into, or withdrawing fluid from, a body cavity, tissue or blood. Syringes come in different sizes and some are specially designed for use in a particular site – for example, for withdrawing CEREBROSPINAL FLUID. The basic design is the same: a calibrated barrel with a plunger at one end, while the other end has a nozzle to which a hollow needle can be attached. Most syringes are disposable, plastic, presterilised and packed in sealed containers. Injections can be given under the skin, into muscle, into a vein or into the cerebrospinal fluid. The term hypodermic, though literally meaning under the skin, is now used to describe most syringes.

Syringe Drivers

Battery or mains electrically driven portable devices into which a SYRINGE can be loaded to give a continuous INFUSION to patients who need regular treatment to control severe pain, or to newborns where the volume to be given is critical and difficult to control with other devices.

Syringomyelia

A rare disease affecting the SPINAL CORD, in which irregular cavities form, surrounded by an excessive amount of the connective tissue of the central nervous system. These cavities encroach upon the nerve-tracts in the cord, producing especially loss of the sense of pain or of that for heat and cold in parts of the limbs, although the sensation of touch is retained. Another occasional symptom is wasting of certain muscles in the limbs. Changes affecting outlying parts like the fingers are also found. Because of their insensitiveness to pain, these are often burnt or injured; troublesome ulcers, or loss of parts of the fingers, may result. The condition of the spinal cord is probably present at birth, although the symptoms do not usually appear until adulthood. The disease is slowly progressive, although sudden exacerbations may occur after a cough, a sneeze, or sudden straining. Treatment is supportive for this progressive disorder.

Systemic

A description of something – for example, a drug – that affects the whole body and not just part of it.

Systemic Lupus Erythematosus (SLE)

A serious and potentially fatal autoimmune disease occurring predominantly in women (see also LUPUS – Lupus erythematosus). The disorder is found worldwide, although its incidence is higher in some ethnic groups such as Afro-Caribbeans and Chinese. The body's immune system attacks CONNECTIVE TISSUE, causing severe inflammation. As connective tissue is widely distributed, the skin and many organs are affected. Recent research suggests that the autoimmune response is triggered by a failure in the body's mechanism for clearing up the debris of dead cells. The affected person lacks an ENZYME called D Nase 1 which degrades DNA. This discovery should enable people who are at high risk of developing SLE to be detected and treated early with D Nase 1. Sunlight, viral infections and certain drugs can induce some of the symptoms, especially in older people. Symptoms of SLE – and also of discoid lupus erythematosus (DLE) – come and go with varying levels of severity. SLE produces characteristic red, blotchy rash over the cheeks and bridge of the nose. Patients feel ill, are fatigued and feverish with appetite loss, nausea, joint pain and loss of weight. Some develop ARTHRITIS, ANAEMIA, kidney failure, neurological or psychiatric problems, PLEURISY and PERICARDITIS.

Treatment D Nase 1 offers promising possibilities for treating SLE. Recognised treatment has been aimed at reducing inflammation and alleviating symptoms. NON-STEROIDAL ANTI-INFLAMMATORY DRUGS (NSAIDS) help to reduce joint pains; anti-malarial drugs reduce the skin rash; and CORTICOSTEROIDS combat fever, pleurisy and neurological symptoms. If patients develop serious kidney or neurological damage, CYTOTOXIC immunosuppressant drugs should be given, The disease is life-threatening if the kidneys are seriously affected; otherwise the prospect for people with SLE has improved greatly in recent years.

Systole

The contraction of the HEART. It alternates with the resting phase, known as DIASTOLE. The two occupy, respectively, about one-third and two-thirds of the cycle of heart action.

Systolic Pressure

See BLOOD PRESSURE.

Tabes

This means, literally, a wasting disease, and is a traditional name applied to various diseases such as tabes dorsalis (tertiary SYPHILIS) and TUBERCULOSIS accompanied by enlargement of glands (see GLAND).

Tablet

A solid, disc-like preparation made by compression of a powder and containing a drug or drugs mixed usually with sugar and other material. Tablets are widely used because of their convenience and accurate dosage.

TAB Vaccine

A combined VACCINE administered to produce IMMUNITY against typhoid and paratyphoid A and B (see ENTERIC FEVER). (See also IMMUNISATION.)

Tacalcitol

A recently introduced, once-daily topical preparation for the treatment of plaque PSORIASIS.

Tachycardia

A rise in the heart rate above the normal range at rest – 60–100 beats a minute – sometimes accompanied by irregularities in rhythm (ARRHYTHMIA). Sinus tachycardia may occur with exercise or emotional excitement, but it may be the result of a feverish illness. (See also HEART, DISEASES OF.)

Tachyphylaxis

Rapidly developing TOLERANCE to a drug.

Tachypnoea

Unusually rapid breathing.

Tacrolimus

An IMMUNOSUPPRESSANT drug used for primary immunosuppression in recipients of kidney or liver transplants (see TRANSPLANTATION) where the natural rejection process has been resistant to conventional immunosuppression regimens such as CORTICOSTEROIDS, AZATHIO-PRINE and CICLOSPORIN A. It is also used, with caution, in some severe cases of eczema (see DERMATITIS).

Tactile

Perceptible to, pertaining to or related to the sense of TOUCH.

Taenia

A parasitic tapeworm that infects several animals including humans (see TAENIASIS).

Taeniasis

A parasitic disorder caused by taeniae or tapeworms.

In the case of infestation with *Taenia saginata*, the host may not have any symptoms and only become aware that he or she is infested upon sight of the tapeworm – or rather, part of it – in the stools (FAECES). In the case of *Taenia solium* the outlook is more serious because the eggs, when swallowed, are liable to migrate into the tissues of the body (as they do in the pig) and cause hydatid cysts. If these occur in the muscles they may cause little trouble but, if they occur in the brain or liver, they can prove very serious.

Hydatid cysts often grow to a great size, budding off smaller cysts in their interior. The symptoms produced by a hydatid cyst depend mainly upon the effects of its size and consequent pressure.

Treatment of tapeworm infestation is the administration (on a named-patient basis) of niclosamide or praziquantal. Hydatid disease is treated by surgical removal, sometimes in coordination with albendazole.

Talc

Talc is a soft mineral consisting of magnesium silicate. It is much used as an ingredient of dusting powders.

Talipes

Also known colloquially as club-foot, this is a deformity apparent at birth, affecting the ankle and foot: the foot is twisted at the ankle-joint so that the sole does not rest on the ground when standing. The heel may be pulled up so that the individual walks on the toes (talipes equinus); the toes may be bent up and the heel used for walking (talipes calcaneus); the sole may be twisted inwards (varus) or outwards (valgus); or the individual may have a combination of deformities (equinovarus). The condition is probably the result of genetic predisposition with an environmental trigger. In the UK the incidence is one in 1,000 live births and talipes is more common in boys than in girls, with 10 per cent of sufferers having a first-degree relative with the same condition. Clinically, there are two types of congenital talipes equinovarus (CTEV): a milder form – resolving CTEV – in which full correction to the normal position is relatively easily achieved; and a more severe type – resistant CTEV – which is harder to correct; and the infant has reduced calf-muscle bulk and abnormally shaped bones.

Treatment should be started at birth with the foot corrected to an improved position and then maintained in plaster of Paris or strapping – a procedure performed weekly or more often. If the deformity is not corrected by around six weeks of age, a decision has to be made about whether to carry out surgical correction. If a deformity persists to maturity, a triple arthrodosis – fusion of three affected joints – may be required.

Talus
The square-shaped bone which forms the lower part of the ankle-joint and unites the leg bones to the foot.

Tamoxifen
An OESTROGENS receptor antagonist – namely, the drug blocks the action of oestrogen – which is the treatment of choice for breast cancer (see BREASTS, DISEASES OF) in postmenopausal women in conjunction with LUMPECTOMY or partial or complete MASTECTOMY. Around 30 per cent of patients in whom breast cancer has spread to adjacent glands or beyond respond to this hormonal treatment. In patients with tumours that are oestrogen-sensitive, the positive response to tamoxifen is 60 per cent; those tumours that are not oestrogen-sensitive are much less likely to respond to the drug. Tamoxifen increases both survival rates and the period between the diagnosis of the tumour and appearance of metastatic growth (see METASTASIS) in tumours sensitive to it. The drug has fewer adverse effects than most others used for treating breast cancer. Patients in whom the cancer has spread to the bone(s) may suffer pain with tamoxifen treatment.

Tamoxifen is also used to treat INFERTILITY, being taken on certain days of the menstrual cycle (see MENSTRUATION).

Tampon
A plug of compressed gauze or cotton wool inserted into a wound or orifice to arrest bleeding. Also inserted into the VAGINA to absorb the flow of blood during MENSTRUATION. Infected tampons may cause TOXIC SHOCK SYNDROME,

a potentially dangerous but fortunately uncommon reaction.

Tamponade
A potentially life-threatening compression of the HEART by the accumulation of fluid in the pericardial sac (see PERICARDIUM) – for example, blood after a penetrating knife wound. This is characterised by TACHYCARDIA, PULSUS PARADOXUS, low blood pressure, raised pressure in the jugular vein, and abnormally quiet heart sounds.

Treatment consists of draining the fluid (which may be blood or an effusion) and treating the underlying cause.

Tannin
Tannin, or tannic acid, is an uncrystallisable white powder, soluble in water or glycerin. It is extracted from oak galls in large amount, but it is also present in almost all vegetable infusions. Tannic acid acts as an astringent.

Tantulum
A heavy metal that is used in surgery because it is easy to mould and does not corrode. It is particularly suitable for repairing defects in the SKULL bones.

Tapeworm
See TAENIASIS.

Tapotement
A MASSAGE technique in which a part of the body is hit repeatedly and quickly with the hands. The technique is useful in helping patients with BRONCHITIS to loosen the MUCUS in the air passages of their lungs, thus helping them to cough it up.

Tapping
The popular name for the withdrawal of OEDEMA fluid from the cavities or the subcutaneous tissues of the body. (See also ASPIRATION.)

Tardive Dyskinesia
Also known as orofacial DYSKINESIA, this is characterised by involuntary chewing and grimacing, usually the result of years of taking ANTIPSYCHOTIC DRUGS, particularly in the elderly when these drugs are sometimes used to sedate troublesome patients.

Target Cell
Abnormal ERYTHROCYTES which are large and 'floppy' and have a ringed appearance, similar

to that of a target, when stained and viewed under the microscope. This change from normal may occur with iron-deficiency ANAEMIA, liver disease, a small SPLEEN, haemoglobinopathies (disorders of HAEMOGLOBIN), and THALASSAEMIA.

A target cell is also a cell that is the focus of attack by macrophages (killer cells – see MACROPHAGE) or ANTIBODIES; it may also be the site of action of a specific hormone (see HORMONES).

Target Organ

The specific organ (or tissue) at which a hormone (see HORMONES), drug or other agent is aimed to bring about its physiological or pharmacological effect.

Tars

Complex oily mixtures derived from coal or wood (pine). Prolonged exposure to some crude tars occupationally may lead to multiple cutaneous warty lesions (pitch warts). Squamous carcinoma may supervene. More refined extracts of tar are used in dermatological therapy, especially in PSORIASIS.

Tarsal

Of or pertaining to the TARSUS of the foot and ankle – this comprises TALUS, calcaneus navicular, cuboid and three cuneiform bones – or eyelid (see EYE).

Tarsus

The region of the instep with its seven bones, the chief of which are the TALUS supporting the leg-bones and the CALCANEUS or heel-bone, the others being the navicular, cuboid, and three cuneiform bones.

Tartar

A concretion that forms on the TEETH near the margin of the gum, consisting chiefly of phosphate of lime deposited from the saliva. Mixed with this are food particles, and this is an ideal medium for bacteria to flourish in. Regular brushing of the teeth is a preventive measure. Dentists or dental hygienists routinely remove tartar, because it gives rise to wasting of the gums and loosening of the teeth.

Taste

See TONGUE.

Tattooing

This has been a cult, or fashion, since the earliest days of history. Apart from the mixed motives for its use, it has a therapeutic use in

matching the colour of skin grafts (see GRAFT). It is performed by implanting particles of colour pigment into the deeper layer of the skin known as the corium (see SKIN). This is done by means of a needle or needles. The main medical hazard of tattooing is infection, particularly HEPATITIS. The tattooed person may also become allergic to one of the pigments used, particularly cinnabar. Removal, which should be done by a plastic surgeon, always leaves a residual scar, and often needs to be followed by a skin graft. Removal is not allowed under the National Health Service unless there is some medical reason: for example, allergic reactions to it. Other methods of removal are by CRYOSURGERY, DERMABRASION and laser surgery. These, too, must only be carried out under skilled medical supervision.

In order to reduce the health hazards, tattooists – along with acupuncturists, cosmetic skin-piercers and hair electrolysers – are required by UK legislation to register their premises with health and local authorities before starting business. The practitioners have to satisfy the authorities that adequate precautions have been taken to prevent the transmission of infections.

Taxanes

A group of CYTOTOXIC drugs administered intravenously for the treatment of advanced ovarian cancer (see OVARIES, DISEASES OF) and secondary spread of breast cancer (see BREASTS, DISEASES OF). Given under specialist supervision in hospital, taxanes are not effective for all patients but results are encouraging when they do respond. Side-effects include HYPERSENSITIVITY, MYELOSUPPRESSION, cardiac ARRHYTHMIA, and peripheral NEUROPATHY. Examples of the taxanes are PACLITAXEL and DOCETAXEL.

Taxis

The method of pushing back, into the abdominal cavity, a loop of bowel which has passed through the wall in consequence of a rupture.

Tay Sachs Disease

An inherited recessive condition in which there is abnormal accumulation of lipids (see LIPID) in the BRAIN. The result is blindness, mental retardation and death in early childhood. The disease can usually be prevented by genetic counselling in those communities in which the disease is known to occur.

Tazarotene

A RETINOIDS preparation recently introduced for the topical treatment of PSORIASIS. It is applied in the evening and continued for up to six weeks. Tazarotene is not suitable for those aged under 18.

T-Cell Lymphoma
See LYMPHOMA.

Tears
See EYE – Lacrimal apparatus.

Technetium-99
An ISOTOPE of the artificial element technetium. It emits gamma rays and is used as a tracer in building up a scintigraphic radioactive image of organs such as the brain.

Teeth
Hard organs developed from the mucous membranes of the mouth and embedded in the jawbones, used to bite and grind food and to aid clarity of speech.

Structure Each tooth is composed of enamel, dentine, cement, pulp and periodontal membrane.

ENAMEL is the almost translucent material which covers the crown of a tooth. It is the most highly calcified material in the body, 96–97 per cent being composed of calcified salts. It is arranged from millions of long, six-sided prisms set on end on the dentine (see below), and is thickest over the biting surface of the tooth. With increasing age or the ingestion of abrasive foods the teeth may be worn away on the surface, so that the dentine becomes visible. The outer sides of some teeth may be worn away by bad tooth-brushing technique.

DENTINE is a dense yellowish-white material from which the bulk and the basic shape of a tooth are formed. It is like ivory and is harder than bone but softer than enamel. The crown of the tooth is covered by the hard protective enamel and the root is covered by a bone-like substance called cement. Decay can erode dentine faster than enamel (see TEETH, DISORDERS OF – Caries of the teeth).

CEMENT or cementum is a thin bone-like material which covers the roots of teeth and helps hold them in the bone. Fibres of the periodontal membrane (see below) are embedded in the cement and the bone. When the gums recede, part of the cement may be exposed and the cells die. Once this has happened, the periodontal membrane can no longer be attached to the tooth and, if sufficient cement is destroyed, the tooth-support will be so weakened that the tooth will become loose.

PULP This is the inner core of the tooth and is

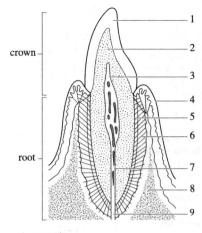

1 enamel
2 dentine
3 pulp (contains blood vessels and nerves)
4 gingiva (gum)
5 cementum
6 periodontal membrane
7 pulp canal
8 bone
9 apical foramen

Vertical section through incisor tooth.

composed of a highly vascular, delicate fibrous tissue with many fine nerve-fibres. The pulp is very sensitive to temperature variation and to touch. If the pulp becomes exposed it will become infected and usually cannot overcome this. Root-canal treatment or extraction of the tooth may be necessary.

PERIODONTAL MEMBRANE This is a layer of fibrous tissue arranged in groups of fibres which surround and support the root of a tooth in a bone socket. The fibres are interspersed with blood vessels and nerves. Loss of the membrane leads to loss of the tooth. The membrane can release and re-attach the fibres to allow the tooth to move when it erupts, or (to correct dental deformities) is being moved by orthodontic springs.

Arrangement and form Teeth are present in most mammals and nearly all have two sets: a temporary or milk set, followed by a permanent or adult set. In some animals, like the toothed whale, all the teeth are similar; but in humans there are four different shapes: incisors, canines (eye-teeth), premolars (bicuspids), and molars. The incisors are chisel-shaped and the canine is pointed. Premolars have two cusps on the crown (one medial to the other) and molars have at least four cusps. They are arranged together in an arch in each jaw and the

maxilla

mandible

8   7   6   5   4   3   2   1

1 central incisor
2 lateral incisor
3 canine
4 1st premolar
5 2nd premolar
6 1st molar
7 2nd molar
8 3rd molar

The permanent teeth of the left side of upper and lower jaws.

cusps of opposing teeth interdigitate. Some herbivores have no upper anterior teeth but use a pad of gum instead. As each arch is symmetrical, the teeth in an upper and lower quadrant can be used to identify the animal. In humans, the quadrants are the same: in other words, in the child there are two incisors, one canine and two molars (total teeth 20); in the adult there are two incisors, one canine, two premolars and three molars (total 32). This mixture of tooth-form suggests that humans are omnivorous. Anatomically the crown of the tooth has mesial and distal surfaces which touch the tooth next to it. The mesial surface is the one nearer to the centre line and the distal is the further away. The biting surface is called the incisal edge for the anterior teeth and the occlusal surface for the posteriors.

Development The first stage in the formation of the teeth is the appearance of a downgrowth of EPITHELIUM into the underlying

mesoderm. This is the dental lamina, and from it ten smaller swellings in each jaw appear. These become bell-shaped and enclose a part of the mesoderm, the cells of which become specialised and are called the dental papillae. The epithelial cells produce enamel and the dental papilla forms the dentine, cement and pulp. At a fixed time the teeth start to erupt and a root is formed. Before the deciduous teeth erupt, the permanent teeth form, medial to them. In due course the deciduous roots resorb and the permanent teeth are then able to push the crowns out and erupt themselves. If this process is disturbed, the permanent teeth may be displaced and appear in an abnormal position or be impacted.

Eruption of teeth is in a definite order and at a fixed time, although there may be a few months' leeway in either direction which is of no significance. Excessive delay is found in some congenital disorders such as CRETINISM. It may also be associated with local abnormalities of the jaws such as cysts, malformed teeth and supernumerary teeth.

The usual order of eruption of deciduous teeth is:

Middle incisors	6–8 months
Lateral incisors	8–10 months
First molars	12–16 months
Canines (eye-teeth)	16–20 months
Second molars	20–30 months

The usual order of eruption of permanent teeth is:

First molars	6–7 years
Middle incisors	6–8 years
Lateral incisors	7–9 years
Canines	9–12 years
First and second premolars	10–12 years
Second molars	11–13 years
Third molars (wisdom teeth)	17–21 years

T

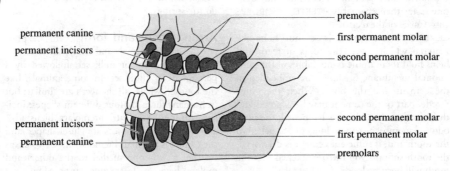

permanent canine
permanent incisors

permanent incisors
permanent canine

premolars
first permanent molar
second permanent molar

second permanent molar
first permanent molar
premolars

Teeth of a six-year-old child. The permanent teeth are coloured black.

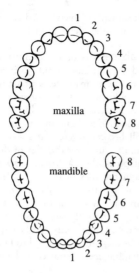

1 central incisor
2 lateral incisor
3 canine
4 1st premolar
5 2nd premolar
6 1st molar
7 2nd molar
8 3rd molar

The permanent teeth of the upper (top) and lower (bottom) jaws.

Teeth, Disorders of

Teething, or the process of eruption of the teeth in infants, may be accompanied by irritability, salivation and loss of sleep. The child will tend to rub or touch the painful area. Relief may be obtained in the child by allowing it to chew on a hard object such as a toy or rusk. Mild ANALGESICS may be given if the child is restless and wakens in the night. A serious pitfall is to assume that an infant's symptoms of ill-health are due to teething, as the cause may be more serious. Fever and fits (see SEIZURE) are not due to teething.

Toothache is the pain felt when there is inflammation of the pulp or periodontal membrane of a tooth (see TEETH – Structure). It can vary in intensity and may be recurring. The commonest cause is caries (see below) when the cavity is close to the pulp. Once the pulp has become infected, this is likely to spread from the apex of the tooth into the bone to form an abscess (gumboil – see below). A lesser but more long-lasting pain is felt when the dentine is unprotected. This can occur when the enamel is lost due to decay or trauma or because the gums have receded. This pain is often associated with temperature-change or sweet foods. Expert dental advice should be sought early, before the decay is extensive. If a large cavity is accessible, temporary relief may be obtained by inserting a small piece of cotton wool soaked, for example, in oil of cloves.

Alveolar abscess, dental abscess or gumboil This is an ABSCESS caused by an infected tooth. It may be present as a large swelling or cause trismus (inability to open the mouth). Treatment is drainage of the PUS, extraction of the tooth and/or ANTIBIOTICS.

Caries of the teeth or dental decay is very common in the more affluent countries and is most common in children and young adults. Increasing awareness of the causes has resulted in a considerable improvement in dental health, particularly in recent years; this has coincided with a rise in general health. Now more than half of five-year-old children are caries-free and of the others, 10 per cent have half of the remaining carious cavities. Since the start of the National Health Service, the emphasis has been on preventive dentistry, and now edentulous patients are mainly found among the elderly who had their teeth removed before 1948.

The cause of caries is probably acid produced by oral bacteria from dietary carbohydrates, particularly refined sugar, and this dissolves part of the enamel; the dentine is eroded more quickly as it is softer (see TEETH – Structure). The exposed smooth surfaces are usually protected as they are easily cleaned during normal eating and by brushing. Irregular and overcrowded teeth are more at risk from decay as they are difficult to clean. Primitive people who chew coarse foods rarely get caries. Fluoride in the drinking water at about one part per million is associated with a reduction in the caries rate.

Prolonged severe disease in infancy is associated with poor calcification of the teeth, making them more vulnerable to decay. As the teeth are formed and partly calcified by the time of birth, the diet and health of the mother are also important to the teeth of the child. Pregnant mothers and children should have a good balanced diet with sufficient calcium and vitamin D. A fibrous diet will also aid cleansing of the teeth and stimulate the circulation in the teeth and jaws. The caries rate can be reduced by regular brushing with a fluoride toothpaste two or three times per day and certainly before going to sleep. The provision of sweet or sugary juices in an infant's bottle should be avoided.

Irregularity of the permanent teeth may be due to an abnormality in the growth of the jaws or to the early or late loss of the deciduous set (see TEETH – Development). Most frequently it is due to an imbalance in the size of the teeth and the length of the jaws. Some improvement may take place with age, but many will require the help of an orthodontist (specialist dentist) who can correct many malocclusions by removing a few teeth to allow the others to be moved into a good position by means of springs and elastics on various appliances which are worn in the mouth.

Loosening of the teeth may be due to an accident or inflammation of the GUM. Teeth loosened by trauma may be replaced and splinted in the socket, even if knocked right out. If the loosening is due to periodontal disease, the prognosis is less favourable.

Discoloration of the teeth may be intrinsic or extrinsic: in other words, the stain may be in the calcified structure or stuck on to it. Intrinsic staining may be due to JAUNDICE or the antibiotic tetracycline. Extrinsic stain may be due to tea, coffee, tobacco, pan (a mixture of chuna and betel nuts wrapped in a leaf), iron-containing medicines or excess fluoride.

Gingivitis or inflammation of the gum may occur as an acute or chronic condition. In the acute form it is often part of a general infection of the mouth, and principally occurs in children or young adults – resolving after 10–14 days. The chronic form occurs later in life and tends to be progressive. Various micro-organisms may be found on the lesions, including anaerobes. Antiseptic mouthwashes may help, and once the painful stage is past, the gums should be thoroughly cleaned and any calculus removed. In severe conditions an antibiotic may be required.

Periodontal disease is the spread of gingivitis (see above) to involve the periodontal membrane of the tooth; in its florid form it used to be called pyorrhoea. In this, the membrane becomes damaged by the inflammatory process and a space or pocket is formed into which a probe can be easily passed. As the pocket becomes more extensive, the tooth loosens. The loss of the periodontal membrane also leads to the loss of supporting bone. Chronic inflammation soon occurs and is difficult to eradicate. Pain is not a feature of the disease but there is often an unpleasant odour (halitosis). The gums bleed easily and there may be DYS-PEPSIA. Treatment is largely aimed at stabilising the condition rather than curing it.

Dental abscess is an infection that arises in or around a tooth and spreads to involve the bone. It may occur many years after a blow has killed the pulp of the tooth, or more quickly after caries has reached the pulp. At first the pain may be mild and intermittent but eventually it will become severe and a swelling will develop in the gum over the apex of the tooth. A radiograph of the tooth will show a round clear area at the apex of the tooth. Treatment may be by painting the gum with a mild counter-irritant such as a tincture of aconite and iodine in the early stages, but later root-canal therapy or apicectomy may be required. If a swelling is present, it may need to be drained or the offending teeth extracted and antibiotics given.

Injuries to teeth are common. The more minor injuries include crazing and the loss of small chips of enamel, and the major ones include a broken root and avulsion of the entire tooth. A specialist dental opinion should be sought as soon as possible. A tooth that has been knocked out can be re-implanted if it is clean and replaced within a few hours. It will then require splinting in place for 4–6 weeks.

Prevention of dental disease As with other disorders, prevention is better than cure. Children should be taught at an early age to keep their teeth and gums clean and to avoid refined sugars between meals. It is better to finish a meal with a drink of water rather than a sweetened drink. Fluoride in some of its forms is useful in the reduction of dental caries; in some parts of the UK natural water contains fluoride, and in some areas where fluoride content is low, artificial fluoridation of the water supply is carried out. Overcrowding of the teeth, obvious maldevelopment of the jaw and persistent thumbsucking into the teens are all indications for seeking the advice of an orthodontist. Generally, adults have less trouble with decay but more with periodontal disease and, as its onset is insidious, regular dental inspections are desirable.

Teeth-Grinding

See also BRUXISM. Teeth-grinding occurs in children during sleep and is of no significance unless really persistent. During the day it may be an attention-seeking device. There is no treatment for it.

In adults it is usually associated with stress or

anxiety, but may be due to some local condition in the mouth such as an unsatisfactory filling. It may also be caused by certain drugs, including fenfluramine and LEVODOPA. If not controlled, it produces excessive wear of the enamel covering of the teeth. Treatment consists of alleviation of any condition in the mouth and any anxiety and stress.

Teething

See under TEETH, DISORDERS OF.

Teichopsia

This refers to zigzag lines that patients with MIGRAINE often experience as a visual AURA preceding an attack.

Teicoplanin

A glycopeptide antibiotic (see ANTIBIOTICS) which acts against aerobic and anaerobic gram-positive (see GRAM'S STAIN) bacteria. Like the similar drug, VANCOMYCIN, it is given in the prophylaxis and treatment of ENDOCARDITIS and other serious infections caused by gram-positive cocci, including STAPHYLOCOCCUS, which have developed resistance to other antibiotics. Its long duration of action means that it need be given only once a day. Teicoplanin can be given intramuscularly or intravenously. Its use should be carefully monitored as there is a range of adverse effects.

Telangiectasis

Abnormal dilatation of ARTERIOLES and venules (see VENULE). In the skin it is seen in spider NAEVUS and ROSACEA particularly.

Telemedicine

A broad term used to describe medicine at a distance through a communications link. Although distance education has been used successfully for some time, more recently distance diagnosis and treatment have been successfully piloted. In teleradiology, radiographic images are transmitted to a distant site for interpretation by a radiologist. A telepathologist can look down, and in some cases control, a microscope located several hundred miles away. In a teleconsultation, the doctor and patient are in different places, joined by a communications link such as medical videoconferencing. In its simplest form, this kind of telemedicine uses the telephone; more recently, full-colour two-way video and audio links have been used. Telesurgery, combining televisual and robotic techniques, is also under development.

Telemedicine is useful for remote locations, such as the Antartic, or on board ships, or aero-planes, where it may be difficult or impossible to get a doctor to the patient. It can also speed up the referral process, reduce unnecessary referrals and improve communication between professionals. It has potential value in pilot projects of 'hospital at home' care.

Temazepam

A benzodiazepine anxiolytic (see BENZO-DIAZEPINES; ANXIOLYTICS) derived from diazepam. To be used with care for short-term treatment of insomnia, generally associated with difficulty in falling asleep, frequent nocturnal awakening or early-morning awakening. Temazepam is a relatively quick-acting hypnotic of short duration, so – although there is little hangover the next morning compared with other hypnotics – there may still be some drowsiness and effect on skilled tasks such as driving. It should be avoided in elderly people who are at risk of becoming ataxic and so liable to falling and injuring themselves. Temazepam is often abused by drug addicts.

Temperature

Body temperature is the result of a balance of heat-generating forces, chiefly METABOLISM and muscular activity, and heat-loss, mainly from blood circulation through and evaporation from the skin and lungs. The physiological process of homeostasis – a neurological and hormonal feedback mechanism – maintains the healthy person's body at the correct temperature. Disturbance of temperature, as in disease, may be caused by impairment of any of these bodily functions, or by malfunction of the controlling centre in the brain.

In humans the 'normal' temperature is around 37 °C (98·4 °F). It may rise as high as 43 °C or fall to 32 °C in various conditions, but the risk to life is only serious above 41 °C or below 35 °C.

Fall in temperature may accompany major loss of blood, starvation, and the state of collapse (see SHOCK) which may occur in severe FEVER and other acute conditions. Certain chronic diseases, notably hypothyroidism (see THYROID GLAND, DISEASES OF), are generally accompanied by a subnormal temperature. Increased temperature is a characteristic of many acute diseases, particularly infections; indeed, many diseases have a characteristic pattern that enables a provisional diagnosis to be made or acts as a warning of possible complications. In most cases the temperature gradually abates as the patient recovers, but in others, such as PNEUMONIA and TYPHUS FEVER, the untreated disease ends rapidly by a CRISIS in which the temperature falls, perspiration breaks out, the pulse rate falls, and breathing becomes quieter. This crisis is often preceded by an increase in symptoms, including an epicritical rise in temperature.

Body temperature is usually measured on the Celsius scale, on a thermometer reading from 35 °C to 43·3 °C. Measurement may be taken in the mouth (under the tongue), in the armpit, the external ear canal or (occasionally in infants) in the rectum. (See also THERMOMETER.)

Treatment Abnormally low temperatures may be treated by application of external heat, or reduction of heat loss from the body surface. High temperature may be treated in various ways, apart from the primary treatment of the underlying condition. Treatment of hyperthermia or hypothermia should ensure a gradual return to normal temperature (see ANTIPYRETICS.

Temple

The side of the head above the line between the eye and ear. The term, temporal, is applied to the muscles, nerves, and artery of this region. The hair usually begins to turn grey first at the temples.

Temporal

Referring or relating to the temporal region (see TEMPLE).

Temporal Arteritis

Inflammation of the TEMPORAL ARTERY. Also known as giant cell arteritis, it often affects other arteries too, mainly in the head. It predominantly affects the elderly. The artery becomes tender with reddening of the overlying skin; headache and blindness may also occur. The diagnosis is confirmed by temporal artery BIOPSY, and treatment is with steroids (see STEROID).

Temporal Artery

A branch of the external carotid artery that is the main vessel supplying blood to the temple and scalp.

Temporal Lobe

Part of the cerebral cortex in each hemisphere of the BRAIN. Areas of the temporal lobe are involved in the understanding of sound and spoken language.

Temporal Lobe Epilepsy

More accurately called complex partial seizures, this is a type of EPILEPSY in which the abnormal cerebral activity originates in the temporal lobe of the BRAIN. It is characterised by hallucinations of smell and sometimes of taste, hearing, or sight. There may be disturbances of memory, including *déjà vu* phenomena. AUTOMATISM may occur, but consciousness is seldom lost.

Tenderness

Pain experienced when a diseased part is handled.

Tendinitis

Inflammation of a TENDON. Usually caused by unusual or excessive physical activity, it may also be infective in origin or secondary to a connective-tissue disorder. The pain and inflammation may be treated with NON-STEROIDAL ANTI-INFLAMMATORY DRUGS (NSAIDS), immobilisation splinting, and STEROID injections. Repetitive strain injury (RSI), caused by constant use of a keyboard (typewriter, word processor or computer), is tendinitis occurring in the hands and arms (see UPPER LIMB DISORDERS).

Tendon

A tendon – also known as sinew, or leader – is the cord of tissue that attaches the end of a muscle to the bone or other structure upon which the muscle acts when it contracts. Tendons are composed of bundles of white fibrous tissue arranged in a very dense manner, and are of great strength. Some are rounded, some flattened bands, whilst others are very short – the muscle-fibres being attached almost directly to the bone. Most tendons are surrounded by sheaths lined with membrane similar to the SYNOVIAL MEMBRANE lining joint-cavities: in this sheath the tendon glides smoothly over surrounding parts. The fibres of a tendon pass into the substance of the bone and blend with the fibres composing it. One of the largest tendons in the body is the Achilles tendon, or tendo calcaneus, which attaches the muscle of the calf to the calcaneus or heel-bone.

Tendon injuries are one of the hazards of sports (see SPORTS MEDICINE). They usually result from indirect violence, or overuse, rather than direct violence.

Rupture usually results from the sudden application of an unbalanced load. Thus, complete rupture of the Achilles tendon is common in taking an awkward step backwards playing squash. There is sudden pain; the victim is often under the impression that he or she has received a blow. This is accompanied by loss of function, and a gap may be felt in the tendon.

Partial Rupture is also accompanied by pain, but there is no breach of continuity or complete loss of function. Treatment of a complete rupture usually means surgical repair followed by immobilisation of the tendon in plaster of Paris for six weeks. Partial rupture usually responds to physiotherapy and immobilisation, but healing is slow.

Tendon Transfer
Reconstructive surgery in which the TENDON from an unimportant muscle is removed and used to repair or replace a damaged tendon of a major muscle.

Tendovaginitis
Also called tenovaginitis: inflammation of a TENDON and of the sheath enveloping it.

Tenesmus
A symptom of disease affecting the lower part of the large INTESTINE, such as DYSENTERY, piles (HAEMORRHOIDS) or tumour. It consists of a constant sense of heavy discomfort about the lower bowel and desire to defaecate, coupled with straining when doing so, with the passage of mucus and often blood.

Tennis Elbow
The medical name for this condition is epicondylitis. The condition is characterised by pain and tenderness on the outside of the elbow and is the result of inflammation in the TENDON that attaches the muscles which extend the elbow to the HUMERUS bone. Epicondylitis can be the result of playing a lot of tennis or other racquet sports, gardening, 'do it yourself' work, or any activity that constantly pulls the tendon at its point of attachment. Lifting heavy objects aggravates the condition. Treatment is resting the arm, ANALGESICS and/or NON-STEROIDAL ANTI-INFLAMMATORY DRUGS (NSAIDS). Sometimes ULTRASOUND therapy may promote healing, but persistent severe pain may necessitate the local injection of CORTICOSTEROIDS. Rarely, surgery may be recommended to release the tendon.

Teno-
A prefix denoting some relation to a TENDON.

Tenosynovitis
Also called tenositis: inflammation of a TENDON.

Tenotomy
An operation in which one or more tendons (see TENDON) are divided, usually with the object of remedying some deformity.

Tenovaginitis
See TENDOVAGINITIS.

TENS
See TRANSCUTANEOUS ELECTRICAL NERVE STIMULATION (TENS).

Tentorium
A wide flap of DURA MATER forming a partition between the cerebrum and cerebellum (see BRAIN) and supporting the former.

Teratogenesis
The production of physical defects in the FETUS. A drug may interfere with a mechanism that is essential for growth, and result in arrested or distorted development of the fetus – and yet cause no disturbance in adults, in whom these growth processes have ceased. Whether and how the EMBRYO is affected depends on what stage of development it has reached when the drug is given. The age of early differentiation – that is, from the beginning of the third week to the end of the tenth week of pregnancy – is the time of greatest susceptibility. After this time the likelihood of CONGENITAL malformation resulting from drug treatment is less, although the death of the fetus can occur at any time as a result of drugs crossing the PLACENTA or as a result of their effect on the placental circulation.

Although the risks are nil or very small with most drugs, no medication should be given to a pregnant woman, particularly during the first few months of pregnancy, unless it is absolutely essential for her health or that of her unborn child. Alcohol is regarded as 'medication' in this context.

Teratoma
A tumour that consists of partially developed embryonic tissues. The most common sites of this tumour are the ovary (see OVARIES) and the TESTICLE.

Terbinafine
An antifungal drug given systemically. Used in the treatment of dermatophyte infections of the nails and RINGWORM infections (tinea pedis, cruris and corporis) which have not responded to topical antifungal preparations.

Terbutaline

A beta$_2$ adrenoreceptor agonist that acts as a BRONCHODILATOR (see also BETA-ADRENOCEPTOR-BLOCKING DRUGS). As an aerosol (see INHALANTS), it is of particular value in the treatment of mild to moderate attacks of ASTHMA; it is also available in oral and parenteral forms, as well as subcutaneous, intramuscular, or slow intravenous injection.

Tertian Fever

The name applied to that type of MALARIA in which the fever reappears every other day.

Testicle

Every man has two testicles or testes which are the sexual glands. In the fetus, they develop in the abdomen, but before birth they descend into a fold or pouch of skin known as the SCROTUM. Each testicle consists of up to 1,000 minute tubes lined by cells from which the spermatozoa (see SPERMATOZOON) are formed. Around 4·5 million spermatozoa are produced per gram of testicle per day. These tubes communicate with one another near the centre of the testicle, and are connected by a much coiled tube, the EPIDIDYMIS, with the ductus, or VAS DEFERENS, which enters the abdomen and passes on to the base of the bladder. This duct, after joining a reservoir known as the seminal vesicle, opens, close to the duct from the other side of the body, into the URETHRA where it passes through the PROSTATE GLAND. Owing to the convolutions of these ducts leading from the testicles to the urethra, and their indirect route, the passage from testicle to urethra is over 6 metres (20 feet) in length. In addition to producing spermotozoa, the testicle also forms the hormone TESTOSTERONE which is responsible for the development of male characteristics.

Testicle, Diseases of

The SCROTUM may be affected by various skin diseases, particularly eczema (see DERMATITIS) or fungal infection. A HERNIA may pass into the scrotum. Defective development of the testicles may lead to their retention within the abdomen, a condition called undescended testicle.

Hydrocoele is a collection of fluid distending one or both sides of the scrotum with fluid. Treatment is by withdrawal of the fluid using a sterile syringe and aspiration needle.

Hypogonadism Reduced activity of the testes or ovaries (male and female gonads). The result is impaired development of the secondary sexual characteristics (growth of the genitals, breast and adult hair distribution). The cause may be hereditary or the result of a disorder of the PITUITARY GLAND which produces GONADOTROPHINS that stimulate development of the testes and ovaries.

Varicocoele is distension of the veins of the spermatic cord, especially on the left side, the causes being similar to varicose veins elsewhere (see VEINS, DISEASES OF). The chief symptom is a painful dragging sensation in the testicle, especially after exertion. Wearing a support provides relief; rarely, an operation may be advisable. Low sperm-count may accompany a varicocele, in which case surgical removal may be advisable.

Orchitis or acute inflammation may arise from CYSTITIS, stone in the bladder, and inflammation in the urinary organs, especially GONORRHOEA. It may also follow MUMPS. Intense pain, swelling and redness occur; treatment consists of rest, support of the scrotum, analgesics as appropriate, and the administration of antibiotics if a definitive microorganism can be identified. In some patients the condition may develop and form an ABSCESS.

Torsion or twisting of the spermatic cord is relatively common in adolescents. About half the cases occur in the early hours of the morning during sleep. Typically felt as pain of varying severity in the lower abdomen or scrotum, the testis becomes hard and swollen. Treatment consists of immediate undoing of the torsion by manipulation. If done within a few hours, no harm should ensue; however, this should be followed within six hours by surgical operation to ensure that the torsion has been relieved and to fix the testes. Late surgical attention may result in ATROPHY of the testis.

Tuberculosis may occur in the testicle, especially when the bladder is already affected. Causing little pain, the infection is often far advanced before attracting attention. The condition generally responds well to treatment with a combination of antituberculous drugs (see also main entry for TUBERCULOSIS).

Tumours of the testes occur in around 600 males annually in the United Kingdom, and are the second most common form of malignant growth in young males. There are two types: SEMINOMA and TERATOMA. When adequately treated the survival rate for the former is 95 per cent, while that for the latter is 50 per cent.

Injuries A severe blow may lead to SHOCK and symptoms of collapse, usually relieved by rest in bed; however, a HAEMATOMA may develop.

Testis
See TESTICLE.

Test Meal
(1) The name given to a gastric-function test, involving injection of HISTAMINE – a powerful stimulator of gastric juice, or pentagastin. After the stimulant has been injected, the digestive juices are withdrawn through a stomach tube (inserted through the nose and throat) and their volume and chemistry measured. A similar test is used to assess the working of the PANCREAS.

(2) The second meaning (also called test feed) applies to a diagnostic procedure for congenital PYLORIC STENOSIS, whereby a paediatrician feels over the baby's abdomen while he or she is feeding. The pyloric mass can be felt as a firm swelling with the consistency of a squash ball, which comes and goes under the examiner's fingers.

Testosterone
The principal male sex hormone secreted by the testes. It has also been prepared synthetically and has the formula $C_{19}H_{28}O_2$. In true male HYPOGONADISM it has the power of restoring male sexual characteristics. (See also ANDROGEN.)

Test-Tube
A tube of thin glass closed at one end, which is used for observing chemical reactions or for bacterial culture.

Test-Tube Baby
See EMBRYO TRANSFER.

Tetanus
Also called LOCKJAW, this is a bacterial infection of the nervous system. Increased excitability of the SPINAL CORD results in painful and prolonged spasms of the voluntary muscles throughout the body, rapidly leading to death unless treated.

Causes The disease is caused by the bacillus *Clostridium tetani*, found generally in earth and dust and especially in places where animal manure is collected. Infection usually follows a wound, especially a deeply punctured or gunshot wound, with the presence of some foreign body. It is a hazard in war and also among farmers, gardeners and those in the construction industry. The bacillus develops a toxin in the wound, which is absorbed through the motor nerves into the spinal cord where it renders the nerves excitable and acutely sensitive to mild stimuli.

Symptoms Most commonly appearing within four to five days of the wound, the patient's symptoms may be delayed for several weeks – by which time the wound may have healed. Initially there is muscle stiffness around the wound followed by stiffness around the jaw, leading to lockjaw, or trismus. This extends to the muscles of the neck, back, chest, abdomen, and limbs, leading to strange, often changing, contorted postures, accompanied by frequent seizures – often provoked by quite minor stimuli such as a sudden noise. The patient's breathing may be seriously affected, in severe cases leading to ASPHYXIA; the temperature may rise sharply, often with sweating; and severe pain is common. Mental clarity is characteristic adding to the patient's anxiety. In severe infections death may be from asphyxia, PNEUMONIA, or general exhaustion. More commonly, the disease takes a chronic course, leading to gradual recovery. Outcome depends on several factors, chiefly the patient's immune status and age, and early administration of appropriate treatment.

Tetanus may occur in newborn babies, particularly when birth takes place in an unhygienic environment. It is particularly common in the tropics and developing countries, with a high mortality rate. Local tetanus is a rare manifestation, in which only muscles around the wound are affected, though stiffness may last for several months. STRYCHNINE poisoning and RABIES, although similar in some respects to tetanus, may be easily distinguished by taking a good history.

Prevention and treatment The incidence of tetanus in the United Kingdom has been almost abolished by the introduction of tetanus vaccine (see IMMUNISATION). Children are routinely immunised at two, three and four months of age, and boosters are given later in life to at-risk workers, or those travelling to tropical parts.

Treatment should be started as soon as possible after sustaining a potentially dangerous wound. An intravenous injection of antitoxin should be given immediately, the wound thoroughly cleaned and PENICILLIN administered. Expert nursing is most important. Spasms may be minimised by reducing unexpected stimuli, and diazepam (see BENZODIAZEPINES; TRANQUILLISERS) is helpful. Intravenous feeding should be started immediately if the patient cannot swallow. Aspiration of bronchial secretions and antibiotic treatment of pneumonia may be necessary.

Tetany

A condition characterised by SPASM of muscle, usually caused by a fall in blood CALCIUM levels. This results in hyperexcitability of muscles which may go into spasm at the slightest stimulus. This is well demonstrated in two of the classical signs of the disease: Chvostek's sign, in which the muscles of the face contract when the cheek is tapped over the facial nerve as it emerges on the cheek; and Erb's sign, in which muscles go into spasm in response to an electrical stimulus which normally causes only a contraction of the muscle. Tetany occurs in newborn babies, especially if they are premature, and in infants; as a result of RICKETS, excessive vomiting, or certain forms of NEPHRITIS. It may also be due to lack of the active principle of the PARATHYROID glands. Overbreathing may also cause it. Treatment consists of the administration of calcium salts, and in severe cases this is done by giving calcium gluconate intravenously or intramuscularly. High doses of vitamin D are also required.

Tetrabenazine

A drug used mainly to control disorders of movement in HUNTINGTON'S CHOREA and similar disorders. It probably acts by reducing DOPAMINE at the NERVE endings, thus slowing neural transmissions.

Tetracyclines

A group of broad-spectrum ANTIBIOTICS which include oxytetracycline, tetracycline, doxycycline, lymecycline, minocycline, and demeclocycline.

All the preparations are virtually identical, being active against both gram-negative and gram-positive bacteria (see GRAM'S STAIN). Derived from cultures of streptomyces bacteria, their value has lessened owing to increasing resistance to the group among bacteria. However, they remain the treatment of choice for BRUCELLOSIS, LYME DISEASE, TRACHOMA, PSITTACOSIS, Q FEVER, SALPINGITIS, URETHRITIS and LYMPHOGRANULOMA INGUINALE, as well as for infections caused by MYCOPLASMA, certain rickettsiae (see RICKETTSIA) and CHLAMYDIA. Additionally they are used in the treatment of ACNE, but are not advised in children under 12 as they may produce permanent discoloration of the teeth. Tetracyclines must not be used if a woman is pregnant as the infant's deciduous teeth will be stained.

Tetralogy of Fallot

The most common form of cyanotic congenital heart disease. The tetralogy consists of stenosis of the pulmonary valve (see PULMONARY STENOSIS); a defect in the septum separating the two ventricles (see VENTRICLE); the AORTA over-riding both ventricles; marked HYPERTROPHY of the right ventricle. Surgery is required to remedy the defects.

Tetraplegia

PARALYSIS of the body's four limbs, also called quadriplegia.

Thalamus

(Plural: thalami.) One of two masses of grey matter lying on either side of the third ventricle of the BRAIN. It is an important relay and coordinating station for sensory impulses such as those for sight.

Thalassaemia

Also known as Cooley's anaemia, this is a condition characterised by severe ANAEMIA, due to an abnormal form of HAEMOGLOBIN in the blood. It is an inherited disease which is widely spread across the Mediterranean through the Middle East and into the Far East. It has a particularly high incidence in Greece and in Italy. The abnormal haemoglobin prevents the affected red cells from functioning properly. This results in the anaemia. The SPLEEN enlarges and abnormalities occur in the BONE MARROW. If someone inherits the disease from both parents, he or she is seriously affected but, if only one parent had the abnormal gene (see GENES), the person could well be free of symptoms. The severe form of the disorder is called thalassaemia major and affected individuals need repeated blood transfusions as well as treatment to remove excessive iron from their body. The disease can be diagnosed by prenatal investigation.

Thalidomide

A sedative and hypnotic drug long withdrawn from the market because it causes TERATOGENESIS. If taken during the first trimester of pregnancy it may cause an unusual limb deformity in the fetus known as phocomelia ('seal' or 'flipper' extremities).

Thallium

An element that is toxic to nerve and liver tissues. A poisoned victim's hair falls out and does not regrow. Treatment is the administration of CHELATING AGENTS. (See also POISONS.)

The radio-isotope (see ISOTOPE) thallium-201 is used as a tracer during special imaging studies of blood flow through the heart muscle in the diagnosis of myocardial ischaemia (see HEART, DISEASES OF.)

Theca
A sheath-like structure enclosing an organ or part.

Thenar Eminence
The projecting mass at the base of the thumb: what is popularly known as the ball of the thumb.

Theophylline
An alkaloid (see ALKALOIDS) structurally similar to CAFFEINE, and found in small amounts in tea. Its main use is for the relief of BRONCHOSPASM, where beta-2 adrenoceptor stimulants have failed. It is given intravenously in combination with the stabilising agent ethylenediamine (as aminophylline) for the treatment of severe ASTHMA or paroxysmal nocturnal DYSPNOEA. Formerly used in the treatment of left ventricular failure, it has been largely superseded by more effective DIURETICS. When indicated, aminophylline should be given by very slow intravenous injection; acute overdose may cause convulsions and cardiac ARRHYTHMIA.

Therapeutic Index
In anticancer therapy, this is the ratio of a dose of the treatment agent that damages normal cells to the dose necessary to produce a determined level of anticancer activity. The index shows the effectiveness of the treatment against the cancer.

Therapeutics
The general name applied to different methods of treatment and healing.

Therapy
The treatment of injury or disease.

Thermo-
A prefix implying some relation to heat.

Thermography
A method of detecting the amount of heat produced by different parts of the body. This is done with an infra-red sensitive photographic film. High blood flow in an area shows up as a heat zone and thus tumours such as breast cancer can be identified. The process records such

changes in temperature in a record known as a thermogram. Unfortunately, such hot areas of skin are caused by a number of other conditions; this is therefore a diagnostic method that can be used only as a rough screening procedure.

Thermoluminescent Dosimeter
A commonly used device for measuring people's exposure to RADIATION. It contains activated sodium fluoride which luminesces in proportion to the radiation dose to which it is exposed.

Thermometer
An instrument for measuring a person's body TEMPERATURE. A traditional clinical thermometer comprises a glass capillary tube sealed at one end with a MERCURY-filled bulb at the other. The mercury expands (rises) and contracts (falls) according to the temperature of the bulb, which may be placed under the tongue or arm or in the rectum. Calibration is in degrees Celsius or Fahrenheit. Modern thermometers use an electric probe linked to a digital read-out display, providing an instant reading. Hospitals now have electronic devices that maintain constant monitoring of patients' temperatures, pulse rates and blood pressure.

Thermometer Scales
See TEMPERATURE.

Thermoreceptor
The end of a sensory NERVE that reacts to changes in temperature. Such receptors are widely distributed in the SKIN as well as the mucous membranes of the mouth and throat.

Thiabendazole
The drug of choice for adults infected with the intestinal parasite *Strongyloides stercoralis* (see STRONGYLOIDIASIS). Its side-effects, including ANOREXIA, nausea, vomiting, diarrhoea, abdominal pain, itching and drowsiness, are more troublesome in elderly patients.

Thiamine
The *British Pharmacopoeia* name for vitamin B_1. Also known as ANEURINE, it is found in the husks of cereal grains. Its deficiency may be produced by too careful milling of rice, or by a diet of white bread to the exclusion of brown bread and other cereal sources of this vitamin. The resulting disease is a form of NEURITIS with muscular weakness and heart failure known as BERIBERI. The best sources of this vitamin are wholemeal flour, bacon, liver, egg-yolk, yeast

and the pulses. The daily requirement is dependent, among other things, upon the total food intake, and has been estimated to be in the region of 0·5 mg of thiamine per 1,000 calories, increased during pregnancy to 2 mg daily as a minimum. (See APPENDIX 5: VITAMINS.)

Thiazides

Thiazides are a group of moderately potent DIURETICS which are effective when taken by mouth. They act by inhibiting the reabsorption of sodium and chloride in the renal tubules. They also have a blood-pressure-lowering effect. Chlorothiazide was the first member of this group to be introduced. Their main use is to relieve OEDEMA in heart failure.

All thiazides are active by mouth with an onset of action within 1–2 hours, and a duration of 12–24 hours. Chlorthalidone is a thiazide-related compound that has a longer duration of action and only requires to be given on alternate days. The other thiazide drugs available include bendrofluazide, cyclopenthiazide, hydrochlorothiazide, hydroflumethiazide, indapamide, mefruside, methychlothiazide, metolazone, polythiazide and xipamide.

Thiazolidinedione Drugs

A group of drugs used to treat type-2 diabetes (see under DIABETES MELLITUS) which work by suppressing the activity of RESISTIN, a recently discovered hormone that acts against INSULIN. Resistin links obesity to type-2 diabetes which has long been known to be associated with overweight subjects.

Thiersch's Graft

The term given to a method of SKIN-GRAFTING (see also GRAFT) in which strips of skin are shaved from a normal area and placed on a burned, injured or scarred area to be grafted.

Thigh

The portion of the lower limb above the knee. The thigh is supported by the femur or thigh-bone, the longest and strongest bone in the body. A large four-headed muscle, the quadriceps, forms most of the fleshy mass on the front and sides of the thigh and serves to straighten the leg in walking as well as to maintain the erect posture of the body in standing. At the back of the thigh lie the hamstring muscles; on the inner side the adductor muscles, attached above to the pelvis and below to the femur, pull the lower limb inwards. The large femoral vessels emerge from the abdomen in the middle of the groin, the vein lying to the inner side of the artery. These pass downwards and inwards deeply placed between the muscles, and at the knee they lie behind the joint. The great saphenous vein lies near the surface and can be seen towards the inner side of the thigh passing up to the groin, where it joins the femoral vein. The femoral nerve accompanies the large vessels and controls the muscles on the front and inner side of the thigh; while the large sciatic nerve lies close to the back of the femur and supplies muscles at the back of the thigh and muscles below the knee.

Deep wounds on the inner side of the thigh are dangerous by reason of the risk of damage to the large vessels. Pain in the back of the thigh is often due to inflammation of the sciatic nerve (see SCIATICA). The veins on the inner side of the thigh are specially liable to become dilated.

Thiopentone Sodium

An intravenous barbiturate whose main use is for inducing ANAESTHESIA, which it does rapidly and painlessly.

Thioridazine

A tranquilliser that is a useful antipsychotic drug. (See NEUROLEPTICS.)

Thiotepa

One of a dozen or so ALKYLATING AGENTS used to treat malignant disease. It is especially effective for cancer of the bladder. (See also CYTOTOXIC.)

Thirst

The sensation of thirst is generally felt at the back of the throat, because, when there is a deficiency of water in the system, the throat and mouth especially become parched by evaporation of moisture from their surface. Thirst is increased by heat, and is a constant symptom of FEVER; it is also present in diseases which remove a considerable amount of fluid from the system, such as diarrhoea, DIABETES MELLITUS and DIABETES INSIPIDUS, and after great loss of blood by haemorrhage. A demand for water is also a feature of many conditions associated with prolonged exertion, severe exhaustion and DEHYDRATION.

Thoracic Duct

The large lymph vessel which collects the contents of the lymphatics proceeding from the lower limbs, the abdomen, the left arm, and left side of the chest, neck, and head. It is provided with numerous valves, and opens into the veins at the left side of the neck. (See GLAND; LYMPHATICS.)

Thoracocentesis

The withdrawal of fluid from the pleural cavity. (See ASPIRATION.)

Thoracoplasty

The operation of removing a varying number of ribs so that the underlying lung collapses. It was formerly done to treat pulmonary TUBERCULOSIS.

Thorax

Another name for the CHEST. Also the title of a medical journal read by chest physicians.

Thought Disorders

Thought is a mental activity by which people reason, solve problems, form judgements and communicate with each other by speech, writing and behaviour. Disturbances of thought are reflected in how a person communicates: the normal logic of thought is broken up and a person may randomly move from one subject to another. SCHIZOPHRENIA is a mental illness characterised by thought disorder. Confusion, DEMENTIA, DEPRESSION and MANIA are other conditions in which thought disorders may be a marked feature. (See also MENTAL ILLNESS.)

Threadworm

See ENTEROBIASIS.

Threonine

One of the essential or indispensable AMINO ACIDS.

Threshold

The degree of stimulation, or electrical depolarisation, necessary to produce an action potential in a nerve-fibre (see NEURON(E); NERVE). Stimulation below this level elicits no conducted impulse, and supramaximal stimulation will elicit the same response as a threshold stimulus.

Thrill

A tremor or vibration felt on applying the hand to the surface of the body. It is felt particularly over the region of the heart in conditions in which the valve openings are narrowed or an ANEURYSM is present.

Throat

In popular language, this is a vague term applied indifferently to the region in front of the neck, to the LARYNX or organ of voice, and to the cavity at the back of the mouth. The correct use of the word denotes the PHARYNX or cavity into which the nose, mouth, gullet, and larynx all open. (See also TONSILS; NOSE.)

Throbbing

See PULSATION.

Thrombin

See COAGULATION.

Thromboangiitis Obliterans

Also known as Buerger's disease, this is an inflammatory disease involving the blood vessels and nerves of the limbs, particularly the lower limbs. TOBACCO is an important cause. Pain is the outstanding symptom, accompanied by pallor of the affected part; intermittent CLAUDICATION caused by a reduction in blood supply is common. Sooner or later ulceration and GANGRENE tend to develop in the feet or hands when AMPUTATION of the affected part may be necessary. There is no specific treatment, but, if seen in the early stages, considerable relief may be given to the patient. Regular walking exercise is helpful and affected individuals should not smoke.

Thrombocyte

See PLATELETS.

Thrombocytopenia

A fall in the number of PLATELETS (thrombocytes) in the blood caused by failure of production or excessive destruction of platelets. The result is bleeding into the skin (PURPURA), serious bleeding after injury and spontaneous bruising. (See also IDIOPATHIC THROMBOCYTOPENIC PURPURA (ITP).)

Thrombocytopenic

See THROMBOCYTOPENIA.

Thromboembolism

The formation of a thrombus (BLOOD CLOT) in one part of the circulatory system from which a portion becomes detached and lodges in another blood vessel, partially or completely obstructing the blood flow (an EMBOLISM). Most commonly a thrombus is formed in the veins of the leg – DEEP VEIN THROMBOSIS (DVT) – and the embolism lodges in the pulmonary (lung) circulation. PULMONARY EMBOLISM is a potentially fatal condition and requires urgent anticoagulant treatment (see ANTICOAGULANTS) and sometimes surgery. Extended periods lying in bed or prolonged sitting in a confined position such as a car or aeroplane can cause DVT; venous thromboses in the legs may occur after surgery and preventive anticoagulant treatment with HEPARIN and warfarin is often used. Similar treatment is needed if a thrombus develops. STREPTOKINASE is also used to treat thromboembolism.

Thrombolysis

The breakdown of a BLOOD CLOT by enzymic activity (see ENZYME). Naturally occurring enzymes limit the enlargement of clots, and drugs – for example, STREPTOKINASE – may be given to 'dissolve' clots (e.g. following a coronary THROMBOSIS – see under HEART, DISEASES OF). The drug needs to be given within 6–12 hours to be effective in reducing the death rate, so prompt diagnosis and transfer to hospital is essential: a short 'door-to-needle' time. An unwanted effect may be increased risk of bleeding, especially in the elderly. It has been used in trials in patients with PULMONARY EMBOLISM and with peripheral arterial disease, but its value in these conditions is uncertain.

Thrombolytic Agents

These are compounds with the property of breaking up blood clots in the circulatory system (see BLOOD CLOT; THROMBUS; THROMBOSIS; FIBRINOLYTIC DRUGS).

Thrombophlebitis

Inflammation of the veins combined with clot formation. (See BLOOD CLOT; VEINS, DISEASES OF.)

Thromboplastin

Also known as thrombokinase, this is an ENZYME formed in the preliminary stages of the COAGULATION of blood. It converts the inactive PROTHROMBIN into the enzyme THROMBIN.

Thrombosis

The formation of a BLOOD CLOT within the vessels or heart during life. The process of clotting within the body depends upon the same factors as that of clotting of blood outside the body, involving the fibrinogen and calcium salts circulating in the blood, as well as blood PLATELETS. The indirect cause of thrombosis is usually some damage to the smooth lining of the blood vessels brought about by inflammation, or the result of ATHEROMA, a chronic disease of the vessel walls. The blood is also specially prone to clot in certain general conditions such as ANAEMIA, the ill-health of wasting diseases like cancer, and in consequence of the poor circulation of old age.

Thrombosis may occur in the vessels of the brain and thus causes STROKE in people whose arteries are much diseased.

Thrombosis of a coronary artery of the heart is a very serious condition which affects, as a rule, middle-aged or elderly people.

(See also ARTERIES, DISEASES OF; COAGULATION; HEART, DISEASES OF – Coronary thrombosis; VEINS, DISEASES OF.)

Thromboxane

A substance produced in the blood PLATELETS which induces aggregation of platelets and thereby THROMBOSIS. It is also a vasoconstrictor (a substance that causes the constriction of blood vessels).

Thrombus

A BLOOD CLOT. Usually describing the formation of a clot within a vessel obstructing the flow of blood, but it can also describe blood which has escaped from a damaged vessel and clotted in the surrounding tissue. (See also THROMBOSIS.)

Thrush

See CANDIDA.

Thumb-Sucking

Also called finger-sucking, this is a universal and harmless habit in infancy. It is usually given up gradually during the pre-school period, but quite often persists after school age – especially if the child is tired, lonely or unhappy. In these cases the remedy is to deal with the cause. It is cruel to use threats or punishment to try to stop the habit.

Thymocyte

A cell that develops in the THYMUS GLAND, probably from a stem cell of bone marrow. It is a precursor of T-lymphocytes originating in the gland (see LYMPHOCYTE).

Thymoma

A tumour of the THYMUS GLAND. Such tumours are rare and are classified according to the variety of thymus tissue from which they develop. Epithelial thymomas grow slowly and rarely spread. If the tumour arises from LYMPHOID TISSUE, it may progress to a generalised non-Hodgkin's LYMPHOMA. Another variety is a thymic TERATOMA which is normally benign in women but malignant in men. Thymomas may affect the working of the immune system (see IMMUNITY), increasing the likelihood of infection. They are also associated with MYASTHENIA GRAVIS – an autoimmune disorder; removal of the gland may cure the disorder.

Thymus Gland

The thymus gland was given its name by Galen in the second century AD because of its resemblance to a bunch of thyme flowers. It has two lobes and lies in the upper part of the chest. The centre (cortex) resembles LYMPHOID TISSUE and is made up of masses of small round cells called thymocytes (see THYMOCYTE; LYMPHOCYTE). The medulla is more loosely cellular and consists of a stroma which contains far fewer lymphocytes than are in the cortex.

The thymus gland is a vital part of the immunological system. Stem cells (see STEM CELL) from the BONE MARROW come to the thymus where they develop into immunologically competent cells. There are two distinct populations of lymphocytes. One is dependent on the presence of the thymus (T-lymphocytes); the other is independent of the thymus (B-lymphocytes). Both are concerned with immune responses (see IMMUNITY). The T-lymphocyte is a cell which in the absence of antigenic stimulation (see ANTIGEN) circulates through the blood, lymph nodes and back into the circulation again over a period of more than ten years. It performs a policing role, awaiting recognition of foreign material which it is able to identify as such. It reacts by multiplication and transformation and these are the ingredients of the immune response. B-lymphocytes are produced in the bone marrow and are concerned with the production of the circulating humoral ANTIBODIES.

The most common clinical disorder associated with abnormality of the thymus is MYASTHENIA GRAVIS. Ten per cent of patients with myasthenia gravis will have a tumour of the thymus, whilst the remainder will have inflammatory changes in the thymus called thymitis.

Thyroid Cancer

A rare disease that accounts for around 1 per cent of all cancers, cancer of the THYROID GLAND usually presents as an isolated hard nodule in the neck. The rate at which the nodule grows depends upon the patient's age and type of cancer cell. Pain is not usually a feature, but the increasing size may result in the tumour pressing on vital structures in the neck – for example, the nerves controlling the LARYNX (resulting in hoarseness) and the PHARYNX (causing difficulty in swallowing). If more than one nodule is present, they are likely to be benign, not malignant. Treatment is by surgical removal after which the patient will need to take THYROXINE for the rest of his or her life. Radioactive iodine is usually given after surgery

to destroy any residual cancerous cells. If treated early, the outlook is good.

Thyroid Cartilage

The largest cartilage in the LARYNX and forms the prominence of the Adam's apple in front of the neck.

Thyroid Gland

A highly vascular organ situated in front of the neck. It consists of a narrow isthmus crossing the windpipe close to its upper end, and joining together two lateral lobes which run upwards, one on each side of the LARYNX. The gland is therefore shaped somewhat like a horseshoe, each lateral lobe being about 5 cm (2 inches) long and the isthmus about 12 mm (½ inch) wide, and it is firmly bound to the larynx. The weight of the thyroid gland is about 28·5 grams (1 ounce), but it is larger in females than in males and in some women increases in size during MENSTRUATION. It often reaches an enormous size in the condition known as GOITRE (see also THYROID GLAND, DISEASES OF).

Function The chief function of the thyroid gland is to produce a hormone (see HORMONES) rich in iodine – THYROXINE, which controls the rate of body METABOLISM. Thus, if it is deficient in infants they fail to grow and suffer LEARNING DISABILITY, a condition formerly known as CRETINISM. If the deficiency develops in adult life, the individual becomes obese, lethargic, and develops a coarse skin, a condition known as hypothyroidism (see under THYROID GLAND, DISEASES OF). Overactivity of the thyroid, or hyperthyroidism, results in loss of weight, rapid heart action, anxiety, overactivity and increased appetite. (See THYROID GLAND, DISEASES OF – Thyrotoxicosis.)

The production of the thyroid hormone is controlled by a hormone of the PITUITARY GLAND – the thyrotrophic hormone.

Thyroid Gland, Diseases of

Goitre

SIMPLE GOITRE A benign enlargement of the THYROID GLAND with normal production of hormone. It is ENDEMIC in certain geographical areas where there is IODINE deficiency. Thus, if iodine intake is deficient, the production of thyroid hormone is threatened and the anterior PITUITARY GLAND secretes increased amounts of thyrotrophic hormone with consequent overgrowth of the thyroid gland. Simple goitres in non-endemic areas may occur at puberty, during pregnancy and at the menopause, which are times of increased demand for thyroid hormone. The only effective treament is thyroid replacement therapy to suppress the enhanced production of thyrotrophic hormone. The prevalence of endemic goitre can be, and has been, reduced by the iodinisation of domestic salt in many countries.

NODULAR GOITRES do not respond as well as the diffuse goitres to THYROXINE treatment. They are usually the result of alternating episodes of hyperplasia and involution which lead to permanent thyroid enlargement. The only effective way of curing a nodular goitre is to excise it, and THYROIDECTOMY should be recommended if the goitre is causing pressure symptoms or if there is a suspicion of malignancy.

LYMPHADENOID GOITRES are due to the production of ANTIBODIES against antigens (see ANTIGEN) in the thyroid gland. They are an example of an autoimmune disease. They tend to occur in the third and fourth decade and the gland is much firmer than the softer gland of a simple goitre. Lymphadenoid goitres respond to treatment with thyroxine.

TOXIC GOITRES may occur in thyrotoxicosis (see below), although much less frequently autonomous nodules of a nodular goitre may be responsible for the increased production of thyroxine and thus cause thyrotoxicosis. Thyrotoxicosis is also an autoimmune disease in which an antibody is produced that stimulates the thyroid to produce excessive amounts of hormone, making the patient thyrotoxic.

Rarely, an enlarged gland may be the result of cancer in the thyroid.

Treatment A symptomless goitre may gradually disappear or be so small as not to merit treatment. If the goitre is large or is causing the patient difficulty in swallowing or breathing, it may need surgical removal by partial or total thyroidectomy. If the patient is deficient in iodine, fish and iodised salt should be included in the diet.

Hyperthyroidism is a common disorder affecting 2–5 per cent of all females at some time in their lives. The most common cause – around 75 per cent of cases – is thyrotoxicosis (see below). An ADENOMA (or multiple adenomas) or nodules in the thyroid also cause hyperthyroidism. There are several other rare causes, including inflammation caused by a virus, autoimmune reactions and cancer. The symptoms of hyperthyroidism affect many of the body's systems as a consequence of the much-increased metabolic rate.

Thyrotoxicosis is a syndrome consisting of diffuse goitre (enlarged thyroid gland), overactivity of the gland and EXOPHTHALMOS (protruding eyes). Patients lose weight and develop an increased appetite, heat intolerance and sweating. They are anxious, irritable, hyperactive, suffer from TACHYCARDIA, breathlessness and muscle weakness and are sometimes depressed. The hyperthyroidism is due to the production of ANTIBODIES to the TSH receptor (see THYROTROPHIN-STIMULATING HORMONE (TSH)) which stimulate the receptor with resultant production of excess thyroid hormones. The goitre is due to antibodies that stimulate the growth of the thyroid gland. The exoph-

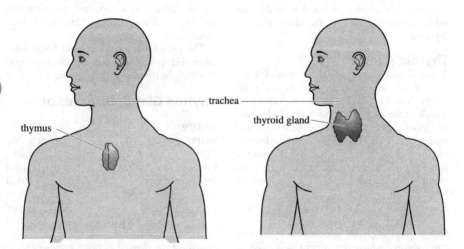

Anterior diagrammatic view showing positions of thymus (left) and thyroid (right) glands around the trachea between the lungs.

thalmos is due to another immunoglobulin called the ophthalmopathic immunoglobulin, which is an antibody to a retro-orbital antigen on the surface of the retro-orbital EYE muscles. This provokes inflammation in the retro-orbital tissues which is associated with the accumulation of water and mucopolysaccharide which fills the orbit and causes the eye to protrude forwards.

Although thyrotoxicosis may affect any age-group, the peak incidence is in the third decade. Females are affected ten times as often as males; the prevalence in females is one in 500. As with many other autoimmune diseases, there is an increased prevalence of autoimmune thyroid disease in the relatives of patients with thyrotoxicosis. Some of these patients may have hypothyroidism (see below) and others, thyrotoxicosis. Patients with thyrotoxicosis may present with a goitre or with the eye signs or, most commonly, with the symptoms of excess thyroid hormone production. Thyroid hormone controls the metabolic rate of the body so that the symptoms of hyperthyroidism are those of excess metabolism.

The diagnosis of thyrotoxicosis is confirmed by the measurement of the circulating levels of the two thyroid hormones, thyroxine and TRI-IODOTHYRONINE.

Treatment There are several effective treatments for thyrotoxicosis.

ANTITHYROID DRUGS These drugs inhibit the iodination of tyrosine and hence the formation of the thyroid hormones. The most commonly used drugs are carbimazole and propylthiouricil: these will control the excess production of thyroid hormones in virtually all cases. Once the patient's thyroid is functioning normally, the dose can be reduced to a maintenance level and is usually continued for two years. The disadvantage of antithyroid drugs is that after two years' treatment nearly half the patients will relapse and will then require more definitive therapy.

PARTIAL THYROIDECTOMY Removal of three-quarters of the thyroid gland is effective treatment of thyrotoxicosis. It is the treatment of choice in those patients with large goitres. The patient must however be treated with medication so that they are euthyroid (have a normally functioning thyroid) before surgery is undertaken, or thyroid crisis and cardiac arrhythmias may complicate the operation.

RADIOACTIVE IODINE THERAPY This has been in use for many years, and is an effective means of controlling hyperthyroidism. One of the disadvantages of radioactive iodine is that the inci-dence of hypothyroidism is much greater than with other forms of treatment. However, the management of hypothyroidism is simple and requires thyroxine tablets and regular monitoring for hypothyroidism. There is no evidence of any increased incidence of cancer of the thyroid or LEUKAEMIA following radio-iodine therapy. It has been the pattern in Britain to reserve radio-iodine treatment to those over the age of 35, or those whose prognosis is unlikely to be more than 30 years as a result of cardiac or respiratory disease. Radioactive iodine treatment should not be given to a seriously thyro-toxic patient.

BETA-ADRENOCEPTOR-BLOCKING DRUGS Usually PROPRANOLOL HYDROCHLORIDE: useful for symptomatic treatment during the first 4–8 weeks until the longer-term drugs have reduced thyroid activity.

Hypothyroidism A condition resulting from underactivity of the thyroid gland. One form, in which the skin and subcutaneous tissues thicken and result in a coarse appearance, is called myxoedema. The thyroid gland secretes two hormones – thyroxine and tri-iodothyronine – and these hormones are responsible for the metabolic activity of the body. Hypothyroidism may result from developmental abnormalities of the gland, or from a deficiency of the enzymes necessary for the synthesis of the hormones. It may be a feature of endemic goitre and retarded development, but the most common cause of hypothyroidism is the autoimmune destruction of the thyroid known as chronic thyroiditis. It may also occur as a result of radio-iodine treatment of thyroid overactivity (see above) and is occasionally secondary to pituitary disease in which inadequate TSH production occurs. It is a common disorder, occurring in 14 per 1,000 females and one per 1,000 males. Most patients present between the age of 30 and 60 years.

Symptoms As thyroid hormones are responsible for the metabolic rate of the body, hypothyroidism usually presents with a general sluggishness: this affects both physical and mental activities. The intellectual functions become slow, the speech deliberate and the formation of ideas and the answers to questions take longer than in healthy people. Physical energy is reduced and patients frequently complain of lethargy and generalised muscle aches and pains. Patients become intolerant of the cold and the skin becomes dry and swollen. The LARYNX also becomes swollen and gives rise to a hoarseness of the voice. Most patients gain weight and develop constipation. The skin becomes dry and yellow due to the presence of increased carotene. Hair becomes thinned and brittle and even baldness may develop. Swelling of the soft tissues may give rise to a CARPAL TUNNEL SYNDROME and middle-ear deafness. The diagnosis is confirmed by measuring the levels of thyroid hormones in the blood, which are low, and of the pituitary TSH which is raised in primary hypothyroidism.

Treatment consists of the administration of thyroxine. Although tri-iodothyronine is the metabolically active hormone, thyroxine is converted to tri-iodothyronine by the tissues of the body. Treatment should be started cautiously and slowly increased to 0·2 mg daily – the equivalent of the maximum output of the thyroid gland. If too large a dose is given initially, palpitations and tachycardia are likely to result; in the elderly, heart failure may be precipitated.

Congenital hypothyroidism Babies may be born hypothyroid as a result of having little or no functioning thyroid-gland tissue. In the developed world the condition is diagnosed by screening, all newborn babies having a blood test to analyse TSH levels. Those found positive have a repeat test and, if the diagnosis is confirmed, start on thyroid replacement therapy within a few weeks of birth. As a result most of the ill-effects of cretinism can be avoided and the children lead normal lives.

Thyroiditis Inflammation of the thyroid gland. The acute form is usually caused by a bacterial infection elsewhere in the body: treatment with antibiotics is needed. Occasionally a virus may be the infectious agent. Hashimoto's thyroiditis is an autoimmune disorder causing hypothyroidism (reduced activity of the gland). Subacute thyroiditis is inflammation of unknown cause in which the gland becomes painful and the patient suffers fever, weight loss and malaise. It sometimes lasts for several months but is usually self-limiting.

Thyrotoxic adenoma A variety of thyrotoxicosis (see hyperthyroidism above) in which one of the nodules of a multinodular goitre becomes autonomous and secretes excess thyroid hormone. The symptoms that result are similar to those of thyrotoxicosis, but there are minor differences.

Treatment The first line of treatment is to render the patient euthyroid by treatment with antithyroid drugs. Then the nodule should be removed surgically or destroyed using radioactive iodine.

Thyrotoxicosis A disorder of the thyroid gland in which excessive amounts of thyroid hormones are secreted into the bloodstream. Resultant symptoms are tachycardia, tremor, anxiety, sweating, increased appetite, weight loss and dislike of heat. (See hyperthyroidism above.)

Thyroidectomy
Surgical removal of the THYROID GLAND. Partial thyroidectomy – removal of part of the gland – is sometimes done in patients with hyperthyroidism (see under THYROID GLAND, DISEASES OF) when drug treatment has failed to control the disorder.

Thyroiditis
See under THYROID GLAND, DISEASES OF.

Thyrotoxicosis
See under THYROID GLAND, DISEASES OF.

Thyrotrophin-Releasing Hormone (TRH)
A hormone (see HORMONES) produced and released by the HYPOTHALAMUS which stimulates the release of THYROTROPHIN-STIMULATING HORMONE (TSH) by the PITUITARY GLAND.

Thyrotrophin-Stimulating Hormone (TSH)
A hormone (see HORMONES) manufactured and released by the anterior part of the PITUITARY GLAND which stimulates the THYROID GLAND to manufacture and release thyroid hormones (THYROXINE and TRI-IODOTHYRONINE).

Thyroxine
(T4) A crystalline substance, containing IODINE, isolated from the THYROID GLAND and possessing the properties of thyroid extract. It has also been synthesised. It is used in patients with defective function of the thyroid, such as myxoedema (see THYROID GLAND, DISEASES OF – Hypothyroidism).

TIA
See TRANSIENT ISCHAEMIC ATTACKS OR EPISODES (TIA, TIE).

Tibia
The larger of the two bones in the leg. One surface of the tibia lies immediately beneath the skin in front, forming the shin; fractures of this

bone are usually compound ones. The thigh bone abuts on the larger upper end of the tibia at the knee-joint, whilst below, the tibia and fibula together enter into the ankle-joint, the two bosses or malleoli at the ankle belonging, the inner to the tibia, the outer to the fibula.

Tic

A repetitive, usually involuntary SPASM that varies from being the simple twitch of a muscle – for example, affecting an eyelid – to complex coordinated actions. About 20 per cent of children suffer from tic which normally lasts several months. Emotional stress is a common cause (see GILLES DE LA TOURETTE'S SYNDROME).

Tic Douloureux

Another name for TRIGEMINAL NEURALGIA due to some affection of the fifth cranial nerve, and characterised by pain – situated somewhere about the temple, forehead, face, or jaw – and sometimes by SPASM in the muscles of the affected region.

Ticks

Ticks are blood-sucking arthropods which are responsible for transmitting a wide range of diseases to humans, including ROCKY MOUNTAIN SPOTTED FEVER, African tick typhus, LYME DISEASE and fièvre boutonneuse (see TYPHUS FEVER). Apart from being transmitters of disease, they cause intense itching and may cause quite severe lesions of the skin. The best repellents are dimethyl phthalate and diethyltoluamide. Once bitten, relief from the itching is obtained from the application of calamine lotion. Tick-bites are an occupational hazard of shepherds and gamekeepers. (See also BITES AND STINGS.)

Ticlopidine

A recently introduced antiplatelet drug, which decreases clumping of blood PLATELETS and thus inhibits the formation of clots (see BLOOD CLOT; THROMBUS). It is used to prevent episodes in patients with a history of symptomatic ischaemic disease such as STROKE and INTERMITTENT CLAUDICATION. The drug should be started under hospital supervision.

TIE

See TRANSIENT ISCHAEMIC ATTACKS OR EPISODES (TIA, TIE).

Timolol Maleate

A beta-adrenoceptor-blocking drug which is of value in the treatment of ANGINA PECTORIS, myocardial infarction (see HEART, DISEASES OF)

and HYPERTENSION. It is also used in the treatment of GLAUCOMA. (See also ADRENERGIC RECEPTORS.)

Tincture

An alcoholic solution used in PHARMACY, generally of some vegetable substance.

Tinea

See RINGWORM.

Tinnitus

A noise heard in the EAR without any external cause. It often accompanies DEAFNESS, and severely deaf patients find tinnitus as troubling as – if not more so than – the deafness. Tinnitus is described as 'objective' if it is produced by sound generated within the body by vascular tumours or abnormal blood flows. In patients with conductive hearing loss, tinnitus may be the consequence of the blocking of outside noises so that their own bodily activities become audible. Even normal people occasionally suffer from tinnitus, but rarely at a level which prompts them to seek medical advice. Present knowledge of the neurophysiological mechanisms is that the noise 'arises' high in the central nervous system in the subcortical regions of the BRAIN.

The resting level of spontaneous neuronal activity in the hearing system is only just below that at which sound enters a person's consciousness – a consequence of the fine-tuning of normal hearing; so it is not, perhaps, surprising that normally 'unheard' neuronal activity becomes audible. If a patient suffers sensorineural deafness, the body may 'reset' the awareness threshold of neural activity, with the brain attempting greater sensitivity in an effort to overcome the deafness. The condition has a strong emotional element and its management calls for a psychological approach to help sufferers cope with what are, in effect, physically untreatable symptoms. They should be reassured that tinnitus is not a signal of an impending stroke or of a disorder of the brain. COGNITIVE BEHAVIOUR THERAPY can be valuable in coping with the unwanted noise. Traditionally, masking sounds, generated by an electrical device in the ear, were used to help tinnitus sufferers by, in effect, making the tinnitus inaudible. Even with the introduction of psychological retraining treatment, these maskers may still be helpful; the masking-noise volume, however, should be kept as low as possible or it will interfere with the retraining process. For patients with very troublesome tinnitus, lengthy counselling and retraining courses may be required. Surgery is not recommended.

Under the auspices of the Royal National Institute for Deaf People, the RNID Tinnitus Helpline has been established. Calls are charged at local rates. (See also MENIÈRE'S DISEASE.)

Tissue Plasminogen Activator (TPA, tPA)

A natural PROTEIN that occurs in the body. It has the property of breaking down a THROMBUS in a blood vessel (see THROMBOLYSIS). It is effective only in the presence of FIBRIN and activates plasminogen, which occurs normally on the surface of the fibrin. TPA is an important thrombolytic treatment immediately after a myocardial infarction (see HEART, DISEASES OF).

Tissues of the Body

The simple elements from which the various parts and organs are found to be built. All the body originates from the union of a pair of CELLS, but as growth proceeds the new cells produced from these form tissues of varying character and complexity. It is customary to divide the tissues into five groups:

● Epithelial tissues, including the cells covering the skin, those lining the alimentary canal, those forming the secretions of internal organs. (See EPITHELIUM.)
● Connective tissues, including fibrous tissue, fat, bone, cartilage. (See under these headings.)
● Muscular tissues (see MUSCLE).
● Nervous tissues (see NERVE).
● Wandering corpuscles of the BLOOD and LYMPH.

Many of the organs are formed of a single one of these tissues, or of one with a very slight admixture of another, such as cartilage, or white fibrous tissue. Other parts of the body that are widely distributed are very simple in structure and consist of two or more simple tissues in varying proportion. Such are blood vessels (see ARTERIES; VEINS), lymphatic vessels (see LYMPHATICS), lymphatic glands (see GLAND), SEROUS MEMBRANES, synovial membranes (see JOINTS), mucous membranes (see MUCOUS MEMBRANE), secreting glands (see GLAND; SALIVARY GLANDS; THYROID GLAND) and SKIN.

The structure of the more complex organs of the body is dealt with under the heading of each organ.

Tissue Typing

The essential procedure for matching the tissue of a recipient in need of transplanted tissue or organ to that of a potential donor. Unless there is a reasonable match, the recipient's immune system (see IMMUNITY) will reject the donor's organ. The main factors that are relevant to an individual's reaction to donor tissue are called histocompatability antigens (see ANTIGEN). These are mostly human leucocyte antigens (HLAs – see HLA SYSTEM) present on the surface of cells. HLAs are inherited and, like fingerprints, unique to an individual, although identical twins have identical HLAs and hence are perfect matches for TRANSPLANTATION procedures.

Titration

A form of chemical analysis by standard solutions of known strength.

Titre

The strength of a solution as determined by TITRATION. In medicine it is used to describe the amount of antibody (see ANTIBODIES) present in a known volume of SERUM.

Titubation

A regular nodding movement of the head that sometimes involves the trunk. The term can also refer to a staggering or reeling condition, especially due to disease of the SPINAL CORD or cerebellum (see BRAIN).

Tizanidine

A recently introduced skeletal-muscle relaxant used in patients whose muscle spasticity is associated with MULTIPLE SCLEROSIS (MS) or injury to the SPINAL CORD. Its side-effects include drowsiness, tiredness, dizziness, dry mouth, nausea and lowered blood pressure.

T-Lymphocyte

See LYMPHOCYTE.

TNM Classification

A method of classifying cancers to determine how far they have spread. This helps doctors to determine the best course of treatment and the prognosis; it is also useful in research. Originally defined by the American Joint Committee on Cancer, the T applies to the primary tumour, the N to any lymph-node involvement, and the M to any metastatic spread. (See CANCER; METASTASIS; TUMOUR; LYMPH NODES.)

Tobacco

The leaf of several species of nicotiana, especially of the American plant *Nicotiana tabacum*.

The smoking of tobacco is the most serious public-health hazard in Britain today. It causes

100,000 premature deaths a year in the United Kingdom alone. In addition to the deaths caused by cigarette smoking, it is also a major cause of disability and illness in the form of myocardial infarction (see HEART, DISEASES OF), PERIPHERAL VASCULAR DISEASE, and EMPHYSEMA. Tobacco-smoking is also a serious hazard to the FETUS if the mother smokes. Furthermore, passive smoking – inhalation of other people's tobacco smoke – has been shown to be a health hazard to non-smokers.

Composition In addition to vegetable fibre, tobacco leaves contain a large quantity of ash, the nature of this depending predominantly upon the minerals present in the ground where the tobacco plant has been grown. Of the organic constituents, the brown fluid alkaloid known as NICOTINE is the most important. The nicotine content of different tobacco varies, and the amount absorbed depends upon whether or not the smoker inhales. Nicotine is the substance that causes a person to become addicted to tobacco smoking (see DEPENDENCE).

Tobacco smoke also contains some 16 substances capable of inducing cancer in experimental animals. One of the most important of these is benzpyrene, a strongly carcinogenic hydrocarbon. As this is present in coal tar pitch, it is commonly referred to in this context as tar. Other constituents of tobacco smoke include pyridine, ammonia and carbon monoxide.

Nicotine addiction is a life-threatening but treatable disorder, and nicotine-replacement treatment is available on NHS prescription. This includes the provision of bupropion – trade name Zyban®. The availability of this drug – which should be used with caution as it has unwelcome side-effects in some people – and the introduction of specialist smoking-cessation services to provide behavioural support to people who wish to stop smoking should result in a reduction in tobacco-related diseases. Given the critical position of nicotine in leading people to become addicted to smoking, it is anomalous that there are no effective government regulations covering the sales of tobacco. Because it is not a food, tobacco is not regulated by the Food Standards Agency; it is not classified as a drug so is not controlled by legislation on medicines. Furthermore, despite being a consumer product, tobacco is exempt from the Consumer Protection Act (1987) and other government safety regulations. So the NHS is left to try to ameliorate the serious health consequences – lung cancer, cardiovascular disease, peripheral vascular disease, chronic bronchitis, and emphysema – of a sub-

stance for which there are no effective preventive measures except the willpower of the individual smoker or non-smoker. (Escalating taxation of tobacco seems to have been circumvented as a deterrent by the rising incidence of smuggling cigarettes into Britain.)

Action on Smoking and Health (ASH) is a small charity founded by the Royal College of Physicians in 1971 that attempts to alert and inform the public to the dangers of smoking and to try to prevent the disability and death which it causes.

Tobramycin
An aminoglycoside antibiotic used to treat serious infections such as MENINGITIS and PERITONITIS as well as those affecting bones, joints and lungs. It is given by injection, sometimes in conjunction with penicillin. It has a range of side-effects including damage to the balance and hearing mechanisms as well as to the kidney.

Toes
See CORNS AND BUNIONS; SKIN – Nail.

Tolazomide
See SULPHONYLUREAS.

Tolbutamide
A sulphonamide derivative, or sulphonylurea (see SULPHONYLUREAS), which lowers the level of the blood sugar in DIABETES MELLITUS. As it is rapidly excreted from the body, it has to be taken twice daily. Like CHLORPROPAMIDE, it may induce undue sensitivity to alcohol.

Tolerance
This occurs when the response to a particular amount of a drug or physiological messenger decreases, so that a larger dose must be given to produce the same response as before. It is particularly common with certain drug dependencies (see DEPENDENCE): for example, with MORPHINE or HEROIN.

Toluene
Also called methylbenzene: a product of the distillation of coal tar widely used as a solvent in the manufacture of paint and rubber and plastic cements.

Tomography
A technique using X-RAYS or ULTRASOUND to build up a focused image of a 'slice' through the body at a given level. By producing a series of such slices at different depths, a three-dimensional image of the body structures can be built up.

-tomy

A suffix indicating an operation by cutting.

Tongue

The tongue is made up of several muscles, is richly supplied with blood vessels and nerves, and is covered by highly specialised MUCOUS MEMBRANE. It consists of a free part known as the tip, a body, and a hinder fixed part or root. The under-surface lies upon the floor of the mouth, whilst the upper surface is curved from side to side, and still more from before backwards so as to adapt it to the roof of the mouth. At its root, the tongue is in contact with, and firmly united to, the upper edge of the LARYNX; so that in some persons who can depress the tongue readily the tip of the EPIGLOTTIS may be seen projecting upwards at its hinder part.

Structure The substance of the tongue consists almost entirely of muscles running in various directions. The tongue also has numerous outside attachments: one muscle on each side unites it to the lower jaw-bone just behind the chin, and this muscle serves to protrude the tongue from the mouth; other muscles, which retract the tongue, attach it to the hyoid bone, the larynx, the PALATE, and the styloid process on the base of the SKULL.

The mucous membrane on the under-surface of the tongue is very thin. In the middle line, a fold of mucous membrane, the frenum, passes from the under-surface to the floor of the mouth; when this frenum is attached too far forwards towards the tip of the tongue, the movements of the organ are impeded – the condition being known as tongue-tie. On the upper surface or dorsum of the tongue, the mucous membrane is thicker, and in its front two-thirds is studded with projections or papillae, most of which are conical. Some of them end in long filaments, and are then known as filiform papillae. On the tip, and towards the edges of the tongue, small, red, rounded fungiform papillae are seen, which act as end-organs for the sense of taste – as do circumvallate papillae, each of which is surrounded by a trench along which open numerous taste-buds. These taste-buds are also found in the fungiform papillae, scattered over

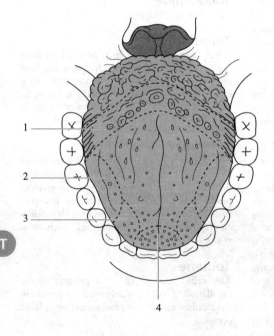

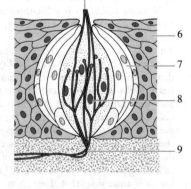

1 bitter	5 gustatory pore
2 sour	6 stratified epithelium
3 salt	7 sustentacular cell
4 sweet	8 gustatory cell with hairlet
	9 nerve

(Left) Tongue from above showing different areas of taste discrimination. (Right) Vertical section through surface of tongue showing taste-bud (x 400).

the throat, FAUCES, and palate. Five nerves, originating from the fifth, seventh, ninth, tenth and 12th cervical nerves supply the tongue.

Functions The chief uses of the tongue are:
- to push the food between the teeth for mastication, and then mould it into a bolus preparatory to swallowing;
- as the organ of the sense of taste, and as an organ provided with a delicate sense of touch; and
- to play a part in the production of speech. (See VOICE AND SPEECH.)

It is usual to classify any taste as: sweet, bitter, salt and acid, since finer distinctions are largely dependent upon the sense of smell. The loss of keenness in taste brought about by a cold in the head, or even by holding the nose while swallowing, is well known. Sweet tastes seem to be best appreciated by the tip of the tongue, acids on its edges, and bitters at the back. There are probably different nerve-fibres and end-organs for the different varieties of taste. Many tastes depend upon the ordinary sensations of the tongue.

Like other sensations, taste can be very highly educated for a time, as in tea-tasters and wine-tasters, but this special adaptation is lost after some years.

Tongue, Disorders of

Conditions of the tongue At rest, the TONGUE touches all the lower teeth and is slightly arched from side to side. It has a smooth surface with a groove in the middle and an even but definite edge. It is under voluntary control and the tip can be moved in all directions.

Ankyloglossia or tongue-tie is a rare disorder in which the frenum or band connecting the lower surface of the tongue to the floor of the mouth is so short or tight that the tongue cannot be protruded. Surgery can remedy the defect. It is easy to overdiagnose and is not a common cause of difficulty in feeding at birth or speech defects in infancy.

Gross enlargement of the tongue can make speech indistinct or make swallowing and even breathing difficult. This is known as macroglossia and may be such that the tongue is constantly protruded from the mouth. The cause may be CONGENITAL, as in severe cases of DOWN'S (DOWN) SYNDROME, or it may occur as a result of ACROMEGALY or be due to abnormal deposits as in AMYLOIDOSIS.

A marked tremor of the tongue when pro-truded may be seen in various neurological diseases, but may be caused by alcoholism.

After a STROKE involving the motor nerve centre, the control of one side of the tongue musculature will be lost. This will result in the protruded tongue pointing to the side of the body which is paralysed. The sense of taste on one side of the tongue may also be lost in some diseases of the brain and facial nerve.

The presence of fur on the tongue may be obvious and distressing. This is due to thickening of the superficial layers of the tongue which may appear like hairs which trap food debris and become discoloured. Furring is common during fever and as a result of mouth-breathing and smoking.

In some conditions the tongue may appear dry, red and raw (GLOSSITIS). An inflamed beefy tongue is characteristic of pellagra, a disease caused by deficiency of NICOTINIC ACID in the diet. A magenta-coloured tongue may be seen when there is a lack of RIBOFLAVIN.

Ulcers of the tongue are similar to those elsewhere in the mouth. The most common are aphthous ulcers which are small, red and painful and last for about ten days. They are associated with stress, mild trauma (such as from jagged teeth), and occasionally with folic acid and vitamin B_{12} deficiency. Ulcers of the tongue are sometimes found in patients with chronic bowel disease.

Tonics

These are placebos (see PLACEBO) and may be used in conditions for which there is no known remedy, to strengthen and support the patient. Available tonics range from rhubarb compound mixture to various mineral and vitamin supplements.

Tonsillitis

Tonsillitis is the inflammation of the TONSILS. The disorder may be the precurosor of a virus-induced infection of the upper respiratory tract such as the COMMON COLD, INFLUENZA or infectious MONONUCLEOSIS, in which case the inflammation usually subsides as other symptoms develop. Such virus-induced tonsillitis does not respond to treatment with antibiotics. This section describes tonsillitis caused by bacterial infection.

Acute tonsillitis The infection is never entirely confined to the tonsils; there is always some involvement of the surrounding throat or pharynx. The converse is true that in many cases of 'sore throat', the tonsils are involved in the generalised inflammation of the throat.

Causes Most commonly caused by the β-haemolytic STREPTOCOCCUS, its incidence is highest in the winter months. In the developing world it may be the presenting feature of DIPH-THERIA, a disease now virtually non-existant in the West since the introduction of IMMUNISATION.

Symptoms The onset is usually fairly sudden with pain on swallowing, fever and malaise. On examination, the tonsils are engorged and covered with a whitish discharge (PUS). This may occur at scattered areas over the tonsillar crypts (follicular tonsillitis), or it may be more extensive. The glands under the jaw are enlarged and tender, and there may be pain in the ear on the affected side: although usually referred pain, this may indicate spread of the infection up the Eustachian tube to the ear, particularly in children. Occasionally an ABSCESS, or quinsy, develops around the affected tonsil. Due to a collection of pus, it usually comes on four to five days after the onset of the disease, and requires specialist surgical treatment.

Treatment Most cases need no treatment. Therefore, it is advisable to take a throat swab to assess the nature of any bacterial treatment before starting treatment. Penicillin or erythromycin are the drugs of choice where beta-haemolytic streptococci are isolated, together with paracetamol or aspirin, and plenty of fluids. Removal of tonsils is indicated: when the tonsils and adenoids are permanently so enlarged as to interfere with breathing (in such cases the adenoids are removed as well as the tonsils); when the individual is subject to recurrent attacks of acute tonsillitis which are causing significant debility, absence from school or work on a regular basis (more than four times a year); when there is evidence of a tumour of the tonsil. Recurrent sore throat is not an indication for removing tonsils.

Tonsils

Two almond-shaped glands (see GLAND) situated one on each side of the narrow FAUCES where the mouth joins the throat. Each has a structure resembling that of a lymphatic gland, and consists of an elevation of the mucous membrane presenting 12–15 openings, which lead into pits or lacunae. The mucous covering is formed by the ordinary mucous membrane of the mouth, which also lines the pits; and the main substance of the gland is composed of loose connective tissue containing lymph corpuscles in its meshes, and packed here and there into denser nodules or follicles. The tonsils play an important role in the protective mechanism of the body against infection.

Tooth
See TEETH.

Tooth, Supernumerary
Malformed extra TEETH are frequently found, particularly in the upper incisor region. They often do not erupt, but prevent the eruption of the permanent teeth.

Toothache
See TEETH, DISORDERS OF.

Tophus
The name given to urate-based deposits which form in connection with joints or tendon sheaths as the result of attacks of GOUT. At first the tophus is a soft mass, but later becomes quite hard. It is composed of biurate of soda.

Topical
Pertaining to drugs or other treatment applied locally to the area being treated – e.g. the skin, eye, etc.

Torasemide
A loop diuretic (see DIURETICS) used in the treatment of OEDEMA and HYPERTENSION.

Torpor
A condition of bodily and mental inactivity, not amounting to sleep, but interfering greatly with the ordinary habits and pursuits. It is often found in people suffering from fever, and is a common symptom in aged people whose arteries are diseased.

Torsion
Twisting. The term is applied to the process in which organs, or tumours, which are attached to the rest of the body by a narrow neck or pedicle, become twisted so as to narrow the blood vessels or other structures in the pedicle. (See TESTICLE, DISEASES OF.)

Torsion is also the term applied to the twisting of the small arteries severed at an operation, by which bleeding from them is stopped.

Torticollis
This is shortness of the sternomastoid muscle on one side, resulting in asymmetry and limitation of movement of the neck. (See SPASMODIC TORTICOLLIS; WRY-NECK.)

Touch

The sense that enables an individual to assess the physical characteristics of objects – for example, their size, shape, temperature and texture. The sense of touch is considered here along with other senses associated with the skin and muscles. The cutaneous senses comprise:

Touch sense proper, by which we perceive a touch or stroke and estimate the size and shape of bodies with which we come into contact, but which we do not see.

Pressure sense, by which we judge the heaviness of weights laid upon the skin, or appreciate the hardness of objects by pressing against them.

Heat sense, by which we perceive that an object is warmer than the skin.

Cold sense, by which we perceive that an object touching the skin is cold.

Pain sense, by which we appreciate pricks, pinches and other painful impressions.

Muscular sensitiveness, by which the painfulness of a squeeze is perceived. It is produced probably by direct pressure upon the nerve-fibres in the muscles.

Muscular sense, by which we test the weight of an object held in the hand, or gauge the amount of energy expended on an effort.

Sense of locality, by which we can, without looking, tell the position and attitude of any part of the body.

Common sensation, which is a vague term used to mean composite sensations produced by several of the foregoing, like tickling, or creeping, and the vague sense of well-being or the reverse that the mind receives from internal organs. (See the entry on PAIN.)

The structure of the end-organs situated in the skin, which receive impressions from the outer world, and of the nerve-fibres which conduct these impressions to the central nervous system, have been described under NERVOUS SYSTEM. (See also SKIN.)

Touch affects the Meissner's or touch corpuscles placed beneath the epidermis; as these differ in closeness in different parts of the skin, the delicacy of the sense of touch varies greatly. Thus the points of a pair of compasses can be felt as two on the tip of the tongue when separated by only 1 mm; on the tips of the fingers they must be separated to twice that distance, whilst on the arm or leg they cannot be felt as two points unless separated by over 25 mm, and on the back they must be separated by more than 50 mm. On the parts covered by hair, the nerves ending around the roots of the hairs also take up impressions of touch.

Pressure is estimated probably through the same nerve-endings and nerves that have to do with touch, but it depends upon a difference in the sensations of parts pressed on and those of surrounding parts. Heat-sense, cold-sense and pain-sense all depend upon different nerve-endings in the skin; by using various tests, the skin may be mapped out into a mosaic of little areas where the different kinds of impressions are registered. Whilst the tongue and finger-tips are the parts most sensitive to touch, they are comparatively insensitive to heat, and can easily bear temperatures which the cheek or elbow could not tolerate. The muscular sense depends upon the sensory organs known as muscle-spindles, which are scattered through the substance of the muscles, and the sense of locality is dependent partly upon these and partly upon the nerves which end in tendons, ligaments and joints.

Disorders of the sense of touch occur in various diseases.

HYPERAESTHESIA is a condition in which there is excessive sensitiveness to any stimulus, such as touch. When this reaches the stage when a mere touch or gentle handling causes acute pain, it is known as hyperalgesia. It is found in various diseases of the SPINAL CORD immediately above the level of the disease, combined often with loss of sensation below the diseased part. It is also present in NEURALGIA, the skin of the neuralgic area becoming excessively tender to touch, heat or cold. Heightened sensibility to temperature is a common symptom of NEURITIS.

ANAESTHESIA, or diminution of the sense of touch, causing often a feeling of numbness, is present in many diseases affecting the nerves of sensation or their continuations up the posterior part of the spinal cord. The condition of dissociated analgesia, in which a touch is quite well felt, although there is complete insensibility to pain, is present in the disease of the spinal cord known as SYRINGOMYELIA, and affords a proof that the nerve-fibres for pain and those for touch are quite separate. In tabes dorsalis (see SYPHILIS) there is sometimes loss of the sense of touch on feet or arms; but in other cases of this disease there is no loss of the sense of touch, although there is a complete loss of the sense of locality in the lower limbs, thus proving that these two senses are quite distinct. PARAESTHESIAE are abnormal sensations such as creeping, tingling, pricking or hot flushes.

Tourette's Syndrome
See GILLES DE LA TOURETTE'S SYNDROME.

Tourniquet
A device – usually a rubber cord or tight bandage – that is bound around a limb to stop temporarily the arterial blood supply and so control severe bleeding. Tourniquets should be applied with caution; unless untied within 15 minutes, GANGRENE may result, necessitating AMPUTATION. Because of this serious hazard, they are rarely used nowadays; direct pressure on the bleeding points is simpler, safer and equally effective in emergencies. A temporary tourniquet to an arm to increase the distension of veins when taking a sample of blood does no harm.

Toxaemia
A term applied to forms of blood-poisoning due to the absorption of bacterial products (TOXINS) formed at some local site of infection, such as an ABSCESS. In other cases the toxaemia is due to defective action of some excretory organ, such as the kidney (see KIDNEYS). As regards treatment, the most important consideration is to remove the source of infection.

Toxaemia of pregnancy is a term sometimes used to describe the two complications of pregnancy known as PRE-ECLAMPSIA and ECLAMPSIA (see also PREGNANCY AND LABOUR).

Toxbase
This the main toxicology database of the National Poisons Information Service (see POISONS). It is available on the Internet (www.spib.axl.co.uk). Toxbase gives information about routine diagnosis, treatment and management of people exposed to drugs, household products and industrial and agricultural chemicals. Further information is available on 0131 536 2298.

Toxic
Poisonous or likely to be lethal.

Toxicology
The science dealing with POISONS.

Toxic Shock Syndrome
First described in 1978, this disorder is characterised by high fever, diarrhoea, SHOCK and a rash. It is frequently associated with the use of tampons (see TAMPON), but has occasionally been reported in men. The syndrome may also be linked to the use of contraceptives such as the diaphragm, cap and sponge (see under CONTRACEPTION), and skin wounds or infections may also be a cause. The disease is due to a staphylococcal toxin (see STAPHYLOCOCCUS; TOXINS). Treatment consists of supportive measures to combat shock and eradication of the staphylococcus by ANTIBIOTICS. The design of tampons has been improved. Recurrence of the disorder has been reported and women who have had an episode should stop using tampons and vaginal contraceptives.

Toxins
Poisons produced by BACTERIA. (See also IMMUNITY; IMMUNOLOGY; MICROBIOLOGY.) Toxins are usually soluble, easily destroyed by heat, sometimes of the nature of crystalline substances, and sometimes ALBUMINS. When injected into animals in carefully graduated doses, they bring about the formation of substances called antitoxins which neutralise the action of the toxin. These antitoxins are generally produced in excessive amount, and the SERUM of the animal when withdrawn can be used for conferring antitoxic powers upon other animals or human beings to neutralise the disease in question. The best known of these antitoxins are those of DIPHTHERIA and TETANUS. Toxins are also found in many plants and in snake venom.

Some toxins are not set free by bacteria, but remain in the substance of the latter. They are known as endotoxins and are not capable of producing antitoxins.

Toxocariasis
A disease acquired by swallowing the ova (eggs) of a roundworm which lives in the intestine of cats (*Toxocara cati*) or dogs (*Toxocara canis*). In humans, the small larval worms produced by these ova migrate to various parts of the body, including the retina of the EYE, where they then die, producing a small GRANULOMA which in turn may produce allergic reactions. In the eye it may cause choroidretinitis. It is said that 2 per cent of apparently healthy people in Britain have been infected in this way. A course of treatment with thiabendazole is recommended, though the drug has side-effects and should be used with caution in the elderly.

Toxoid
A toxin (see TOXINS) which has been rendered non-toxic by certain chemicals, or by heat, or

by being partly neutralised by antitoxin. The best-known example is DIPHTHERIA toxoid. (See also IMMUNITY.)

Toxoplasmosis

Toxoplasmosis is a disease due to infection with protozoa of the genus *Toxoplasma*. The infection may be acquired from eating raw or undercooked meat, from cats, or from gardening or playing in contaminated soil. It occurs in two forms: an acquired form, and a congenital form. The acquired form may run such a benign course that it is not recognised, the patient scarcely feeling ill. In the congenital form the unborn child is infected by the mother. The congenital form, the incidence of which in the United Kingdom is one in 5,000 pregnancies (one in 2,000 pregnancies in Scotland), may develop in one of two ways. The infant may either appear generally ill, or the brunt of the infection may fall on the nervous system causing HYDROCEPHALUS, mental retardation, or loss of sight. In some cases the infection may be so severe that it kills the fetus, resulting in a miscarriage or stillbirth. In other cases the infection is so mild that it is missed until, in later life, the child begins to show signs of eye trouble. As the congenital form of the disease, which is most serious, seems to develop only if the mother acquires the infection during pregnancy, it would appear to be a wise precaution that pregnant women should avoid contact with cats and eating raw or undercooked meat foods.

tPA/TPA

See TISSUE PLASMINOGEN ACTIVATOR (TPA, tPA).

Trabecula

(1) Thin strips of bony tissue occurring in cancellous BONE – sometimes called spongy bone. (2) A band of CONNECTIVE TISSUE passing from the outer part of an organ to the interior, separating the organ into discrete chambers.

Trace Elements

Chemical elements that are distributed throughout the tissues of the body in very small amounts and are essential for the nutrition of the body. Nine such elements are now recognised: cobalt, copper, fluorine, iodine, iron, manganese, molybdenum, selenium and zinc.

Tracer

A compound introduced into the body, the progress of which can subsequently be followed and information obtained about the body's metabolic activities. Radioactive tracers are compounds labelled with RADIONUCLIDE which give off radiation. This can be measured with a gamma camera or a scintigram. The information is used in the investigation of suspected tumours in the BRAIN or malfunctioning of the THYROID GLAND.

Trachea

Popularly known as the windpipe, this tube extends from the LARYNX above to the point in the upper part of the chest, where it divides into the two large bronchial tubes, one to each lung (see LUNGS). It is about 10 cm (4 inches) in length and consists of a fibrous tube kept permanently open by about 20 strong, horizontally placed hoops of cartilage, each of which forms about two-thirds of a circle, the two ends being joined behind by muscle-fibres. This fibrocartilaginous tube is lined by a smooth mucous membrane, richly supplied with mucous glands and covered by a single layer of ciliated epithelium. (See also AIR PASSAGES.)

Tracheitis

Inflammation of the TRACHEA. It may occur along with BRONCHITIS, or independently, due to similar causes. Usually a viral condition, treatment may be unnecessary (see CROUP). A rare condition, bacterial tracheitis, is more dangerous as the patient produces large amount of thick, sticky SPUTUM which may block the airway causing respiratory failure and collapse. Treatment is by insertion of an endotracheal tube under general anaesthesia (see ENDOTRACHEAL INTUBATION), removing the secretions and using high-dose antibiotics.

Tracheostomy

Also known as tracheotomy. The operation in which the TRACHEA or windpipe is opened from the front of the neck, so that air may be directly drawn or passed into the lower AIR PASSAGES. The opening is made through the second and third rings of the trachea.

Reasons for operation The cause of laryngeal obstruction should be treated but, if obstruction is acute and endangering the patient's life, urgent intervention is necessary. In most cases the insertion of an endotracheal tube either through the nose or mouth and down the pharynx through the larynx to bypass the obstruction is effective (see ENDOTRACHEAL INTUBATION). If not, tracheostomy is performed. The majority of tracheostomies performed nowadays are for patients in intensive-therapy-unit situations. These patients require airway intervention for prolonged periods to facilitate artificial ventilation which is performed by means of a mechanical ventilator. The presence of a tube passing through the larynx for a prolonged period of time is associated with long-term damage to the larynx, and therefore any patients requiring prolonged intubation usually undergo a tracheostomy to prevent further damage. Endotracheal intubation is also the preferred method of airway-intervention for acute inflammatory disorders of the upper airway (as opposed to tracheostomy); tracheostomy in these cases is performed only in the emergency situation if facilities for endotracheal intubation are not available or if they are unsuccessful. Tracheostomy may also be performed for large tumours which obstruct the larynx until some form of treatment is instituted. Similarly it may be needed in conditions whereby the nerve supply to the larynx has been jeopardised, impairing its protective function of the upper airway and its respiratory function.

Tracheostomy tubes When the trachea has been opened – by an incision through the skin between the Adam's apple and the clavicles; another through the THYROID GLAND followed by a small vertical incision in the trachea – a metal or plastic tube is inserted to maintain the opening. There is always an outer tube which is fixed in position by tapes passing round the neck, and an inner tube which slides freely out of and into the other, so that it may be removed at any time for cleansing, and is readily coughed-out should it happen to become blocked by mucus.

After-treatment When the operation has been performed for some permanent obstruction, the tube must be worn permanently; and the double metal tube is in such cases replaced after a short time by a soft plastic single one. When the operation has relieved some obstruction caused, say, by diphtheria, the tube is left out now and then for a few hours, and finally, at the end of a week or so, is removed altogether, after which the wound quickly heals up.

Trachoma

Trachoma is a severe type of conjunctivitis (see under EYE, DISORDERS OF). This chronic contagious condition is caused by *Chlamydia trachomatis*, a bacterium with virus-like characteristics. The disease affects 150 million people worldwide and is common in developing countries, where it is the leading cause of preventable blindness. It may be seen in immigrant populations in developed countries, although it is usually inactive. The bacterium is transmitted by flies and causes inflammation of the conjunctiva and cornea (see EYE) with consequent scarring. The active disease is treated with tetracycline tablets and eye drops; cure is usually satisfactory. In theory, trachoma should be easy to eliminate. The World Health Organisation, which aims to do this by 2020, is using a four-pronged strategy to tackle the disease. This comprises:

- surgery to correct deformed eyelids before blindness occurs.
- antibiotics to kill *Chlamydia*.
- regular face-washing to stop bacterial spread.
- environmental improvements – for example, better sanitation and rubbish disposal – to eliminate the bacteria.

Traction

The application of a pulling force to the distal part of a fracture in order to allow the fracture to heal with the bone in correct alignment. There are many different methods for applying traction, usually involving weights and pulleys.

Tractotomy

A neurological operation to relieve intractable PAIN. The thalamic tracts of the SPINAL CORD contain the nerve-fibres that signal pain. They travel from the source of the pain – in an organ or tissue such as skin or bone – via the cord to the brain stem and cortex (see BRAIN) where the individual becomes 'conscious' of the pain. The operation aims to sever these tracts within the medulla oblongata of the brain.

Training

See DIET; EXERCISE.

Trance

A profound SLEEP from which a person cannot for a time be aroused, but which is not due to organic disease. The power of voluntary movement is lost, although sensibility and even consciousness may remain. It is a disturbance in mental functions and may be associated with CATALEPSY, AUTOMATISM and petit mal EPILEPSY. A trance may be induced by HYPNOTISM. (See also ECSTASY).

Tranexamic Acid

A drug used in the control of bleeding. It inhibits the activation of PLASMINOGEN and FIBRINOLYSIS, and may be useful when bleeding cannot be stopped – for instance, dental extraction in HAEMOPHILIA. The drug is also useful in MENORRHAGIA.

Tranquillisers

A tranquilliser is a popular name for a drug which induces a mental state free from agitation and anxiety, and renders the patient calm. Tranquillisers are classified as major and minor. The former are used to treat psychotic illness such as SCHIZOPHRENIA; the latter are sedatives used to treat anxiety and emotional upsets (see NEUROSIS) and are called antianxiety drugs or ANXIOLYTICS. Major tranquillisers or antipsychotic drugs are given to patients with psychotic disorders which disrupt their normal lives (see PSYCHOSIS). They do not cure the patient, but do help to control his or her symptoms so that the person can live in the community and be admitted to hospital only for acute episodes. The drug chosen depends upon the type of illness and needs of a particular patient as well as the likely adverse effects. Antipsychotic drugs modify the transmission of nerve-signals by making brain cells less sensitive to the excitatory neurotransmitter chemical called DOPAMINE. Among the antipsychotic tranquillisers are CHLORPROMAZINE, HALOPERIDOL, CLOZAPINE and flupenthixol.

Anxiety is a consequence of too much STRESS and may occur without being serious enough to need treatment. Clinically it arises when the balance between certain chemicals in the brain is disturbed: this increases activity in the sympathetic system, thus provoking physical symptoms such as breathlessness, tachycardia, headaches and indigestion. Anxiolytics help to alleviate these symptoms but do not necessarily cure the underlying cause. Two main classes of drug relieve anxiety: BENZODIAZEPINES and beta blockers (see BETA-ADRENOCEPTOR-BLOCKING DRUGS). The latter, which include atenolol and propanolol, reduce the physical symptoms such as tachycardia and are useful in circumstances – for example, examinations – known to cause anxiety attacks. They block the action of NORADRENALINE, a key chemical of the sympathetic nervous system. Benzodiazepines depress activity in that part of the brain controlling emotion by stimulating the action of a chemical called gamma-aminobutyric acid (GABA). Among the benzodiazepines are chlordiazepoxide and diazepam. (See also MENTAL ILLNESS.)

Transcervical Resection of Endometrium (TCRE)

An operation, usually done under local anaesthetic, in which the lining membrane of the UTERUS (womb) is excised using a type of LASER or DIATHERMY surgery that utilises a hysterescope (a variety of ENDOSCOPE) through which the operator can visualise the inside of the uterus. The operation is done to treat MENORRHAGIA (heavy blood loss during MENSTRUATION) and its introduction has reduced the need to perform HYSTERECTOMY for the condition.

Transcutaneous Electrical Nerve Stimulation (TENS)

A method of electrical stimulation that is being used for the relief of PAIN, including that of MIGRAINE, NEURALGIA and phantom limbs (see AMPUTATION). Known as TENS, its mode of action appears to have some resemblance to that of ACUPUNCTURE. Several controlled trials suggest that it provides at least a modicum of relief of pain after operations, thereby reducing the amount of ANALGESICS that may be called for.

Transfusion

The administration of any fluid into a person's vein using a drip. This apparatus facilitates a continuous injection in which the fluid flows by force of gravity from a suspended bottle, via a tube that is fixed to a hollow needle inserted into a vein (usually in the front of the elbow). Saline solution, PLASMA and whole BLOOD (see below) are the most commonly administered fluids. Saline is used to restore fluid to a seriously dehydrated individual (see DEHYDRATION) and may be used as a temporary measure in SHOCK due to blood loss while the appropriate type of blood is being obtained for transfusion. Saline may also be useful as a way of administering a regular supply of a drug over a period of time. Plasma is normally used as a temporary measure in the treatment of shock until appropriately matched blood is available or if for any reason, such as for a patient with severe burns, plasma is preferable to blood.

Transfusion of blood is a technique that has been used since the 17th century – although, until the 20th century, with a subsequent high mortality rate. It was only when incompatibility of BLOOD GROUPS was considered as a potential cause of this high mortality that routine blood-testing became standard practice. Since the National Blood Transfusion Service was started in the United Kingdom (in 1946), blood for transfusion has been collected from voluntary, unpaid donors: this is screened for infections such as SYPHILIS, HIV, HEPATITIS and nvCJD (see CREUTZFELDT-JAKOB DISEASE (CJD)), sorted by group, and stored in blood-banks throughout the country.

In the UK in 2004, the National Blood Authority – today's transfusion service –

announced that it would no longer accept donations from anyone who had received a blood transfusion since 1980 – because of the remote possibility that they might have been infected with the PRION which causes nvCJD.

A standard transfusion bottle has been developed, and whole blood may be stored at 2–6 °C for three weeks before use. Transfusions may then be given of whole blood, plasma, blood cells, or PLATELETS, as appropriate. Stored in the dried form at 4–21 °C, away from direct sunlight, human plasma is stable for five years and is easily reconstituted by adding sterile distilled water.

The National Blood Authority prepares several components from each donated unit of blood: whole blood is rarely used in adults. This permits each product, whether plasma or various red-cell concentrates, to be stored under ideal conditions and used in appropriate clinical circumstances – say, to restore blood loss or to treat haemostatic disorders.

Transfusion of blood products can cause complications. Around 5 per cent of transfused patients suffer from a reaction; most are mild, but they can be severe and occasionally fatal. It can be difficult to distinguish a transfusion reaction from symptoms of the condition being treated, but the safe course is to stop the transfusion and start appropriate investigation.

In the developed world, clinicians can expect to have access to high-quality blood products, with the responsibility of providing blood resting with a specially organised transfusion service. The cause of most fatal haemolytic transfusion reactions is a clerical error due to faulty labelling and/or failure to identify the recipient correctly. Hospitals should have a strict protocol to prevent such errors.

Artificial blood Transfusion with blood from donors is facing increasing problems. Demand is rising; suitable blood donors are becoming harder to attract; the processes of taking, storing and cross-matching donor blood are time-consuming and expensive; the shelf-life is six weeks; and the risk of adverse reactions or infection from transfused blood, although small, is always present. Artificial blood would largely overcome these drawbacks. Several companies in North America are now preparing this: one product uses purified HAEMOGLOBIN from humans and another from cows. These provide oxygen-carrying capacity, are unlikely to be infectious and do not provoke immunological rejections. Yet another product, called Oxygene®, does not contain any animal or human blood products; it comprises salt water and a substance called perflubron, the molecules of which store oxygen and absorb carbon dioxide more effectively than does haemoglobin. Within 24 hours of being transfused into a person's bloodstream, perflubron evaporates and is harmlessly breathed out by the recipient. Artificial blood is especially valuable in that it contains no unwanted proteins that can provoke adverse immunological reactions. Furthermore, it is disease-free, lasts for up to three years and is no more expensive than donor blood. It could well take the place of donor blood within a few years.

Autologous transfusion is the use of an individual's own blood, provided in advance, for transfusion during or after a surgical operation. This is a valuable procedure for operations that may require large transfusions or where a person has a rare blood group. Its use has increased for several reasons:
● fear of infection such as HIV and hepatitis.
● shortages of donor blood and the rising cost of units of blood.
● substantial reduction of risk of incompatible transfusions.

In practice, blood transfusion in the UK is remarkably safe, but there is always room for improvement. So, in the 1990s, a UK inquiry on the Serious Hazards of Transfusion (SHOT) was launched. It established (1998) that of 169 recently reported serious hazards following blood transfusion, 81 had involved a blood component being given to the wrong patient, while only eight were the result of viral or bacterial infections.

There are three ways to use a patient's own blood in transfusion:
(1) predeposit autologous donation (PAD) – taking blood from a patient before operation and transfusing this blood back into the patient as required during and after operation.
(2) acute normovalaemic haemodilution (ANH) – diluting previously withdrawn blood and thus increasing the volume before transfusion.
(3) perioperative cell salvage (PCS) – the use of centrifugal cell separation on blood saved during an operation, particularly spinal surgery where blood loss may be considerable.

The government has urged NHS trusts to consider the introduction of PCS as a possible adjunct or alternative to banked-blood transfusion. In one centre (Nottingham), PCS has been used in the form of continuous autologous transfusion for several years with success.

Exchange transfusion is the method of treatment in severe cases of HAEMOLYTIC DISEASE OF THE NEWBORN. It consists of replacing the whole of the baby's blood with Rh-negative blood of the correct blood group for the baby.

Transient Ischaemic Attacks or Episodes (TIA, TIE)

Episodes of transient ISCHAEMIA of some part of the cerebral hemispheres or the brain stem (see BRAIN) lasting anything from a few minutes to several hours and followed by complete recovery. By definition, the ischaemic episode must be less than 24 hours. These episodes may be isolated or they may occur several times in a day. The cause is ATHEROMA of the carotid or vertebral arteries (see ARTERIES, DISEASES OF) and the embolisation (see EMBOLISM) of PLATELETS or CHOLESTEROL. These attacks present with strokes (see STROKE) that rapidly recover.

Translocation

The term used to describe an exchange of genetic material between CHROMOSOMES. It is an important factor in the etiology, or causation, of certain congenital abnormalities such as, for example, DOWN'S (DOWN) SYNDROME. It is one of the main abnormalities sought for in AMNIOSCOPY.

Transplantation

Transplantation of tissues or organs of the body are defined as an allotransplant, if from another person; an autotransplant, if from the patient him or herself – for example, a skin graft (see GRAFT; SKIN-GRAFTING); and a xenotransplant, if from an animal.

The pioneering success was achieved with transplantation of the kidney in the 1970s; this has been most successful when the transplanted kidney has come from an identical twin. Less successful have been live transplants from other blood relatives, while least successful have been transplants from other live donors and cadaver donors. The results, however, are steadily improving. Thus the one-year functional survival of kidneys transplanted from unrelated dead donors has risen from around 50 per cent to over 80 per cent, and survival rates of 80 per cent after three years are not uncommon. For a well-matched transplant from a live related donor, the survival rate after five years is around 90 per cent. And, of course, if a transplanted kidney fails to function, the patient can always be switched on to some form of DIALYSIS. In the United Kingdom the supply of cadaveric (dead) kidneys for transplantation is only about half that necessary to meet the demand.

Other organs that have been transplanted with increasing success are the heart, the lungs, the liver, bone marrow, and the cornea of the eye. Heart, lung, liver and pancreas transplantations are now carried out in specialist centres. It is estimated that in the United Kingdom, approximately 200 patients a year between the ages of 15 and 55 would benefit from a liver transplant if an adequate number of donors were available. More than 100 liver transplants are carried out annually in the United Kingdom and one-year-survival rates of up to 80 per cent have been achieved.

The major outstanding problem is how to prevent the recipient's body from rejecting and destroying the transplanted organ. Such rejection is part of the normal protective mechanism of the body (see IMMUNITY). Good progress has been made in techniques of tissue-typing and immunosuppression to overcome the problem. Drugs are now available that can suppress the immune reactions of the recipient, which are responsible for the rejection of the transplanted organ. Notable among these are CICLOSPORIN A, which revolutionised the success rate, and TACROLIMUS, a macrolide immunosuppressant.

Another promising development is anti-lymphocytic serum (ALS), which reduces the activity of the lymphocytes (see LYMPHOCYTE) cells which play an important part in maintaining the integrity of the body against foreign bodies.

Donor cards are now available in all general practitioners' surgeries and pharmacies but, of the millions of cards distributed since 1972, too few have been used. The reasons are complex but include the reluctance of the public and doctors to consider organ donation; poor organisation for recovery of donor kidneys; and worries about the diagnosis of death. A code of practice for procedures relating to the removal of organs for transplantation was produced in 1978, and this code has been revised in the light of further views expressed by the Conference of Medical Royal Colleges and Faculties of the United Kingdom on the Diagnosis of Brain Death. Under the Human Tissue Act 1961, only the person lawfully in possession of the body or his or her designate can authorise the removal of organs from a body. This authorisation may be given orally.

Patients who may become suitable donors after death are those who have suffered severe and irreversible brain damage – since such patients will be dependent upon artificial ventilation. Patients with malignant disease or systemic infection, and patients with renal disease, including chronic hypertension, are unsuitable.

If a patient carries a signed donor card or has otherwise recorded his or her wishes, there is no legal requirement to establish lack of objection on the part of relatives – although it is good practice to take account of the views of close relatives. If a relative objects, despite the known request by the patient, staff will need to judge, according to the circumstances of the case, whether it is wise to proceed with organ removal. If a patient who has died is not known to have requested that his or her organs be removed for transplantation after death, the designated person may only authorise the removal if, having made such reasonable enquiry as may be practical, he or she has no reason to believe (*a*) that the deceased had expressed an objection to his or her body being so dealt with after death, or (*b*) that the surviving spouse or any surviving relative of the deceased objects to the body being so dealt with. Staff will need to decide who is best qualified to approach the relatives. This should be someone with appropriate experience who is aware how much the relative already knows about the patient's condition. Relatives should not normally be approached before death has occurred, but sometimes a relative approaches the hospital staff and suggests some time in advance that the patient's organs might be used for transplantation after death. The staff of hospitals and organ exchange organisations must respect the wishes of the donor, the recipient and their families with respect to anonymity.

Relatives who enquire should be told that some post-mortem treatment of the donor's body will be necessary if the organs are to be removed in good condition. It is ethical (see ETHICS) to maintain artificial ventilation and heartbeat until removal of organs has been completed. This is essential in the case of heart and liver transplants, and many doctors think it is desirable when removing kidneys. Official criteria have been issued in Britain to recognise when BRAIN-STEM DEATH has occurred. This is an important protection for patients and relatives when someone with a terminal condition – usually as a result of an accident – is considered as a possible organ donor.

Transplant Support Services Authority

In the UK, this NHS authority (UKTSSA) provides a 24-hour service for matching, allocating and distributing organs. It is also responsible for keeping the records of all patients awaiting transplants. Established in 1991, the authority allocates donor organs without favour, following protocols set by advisory groups. It also administers the Human Organ Transplant Act on behalf of the Department of Health. (See TRANSPLANTATION.)

Trans-Sexualism

The psycho-sexual condition characterised by feelings of belonging to the gender opposite to that of the genitalia and the secondary sex characteristics. Subjects may be helped by counselling, drug therapy and in some circumstances an operation to change their physical sexual characteristics. Trans-sexuals or their families wanting help and guidance should contact the Gender Identity Consultancy.

Transudation

The passage of liquid – called the transudate – through a membrane: for example, the passage of blood through the wall of a capillary vessel.

Transurethral Resection

The use of a special CYSTOSCOPE (a resectoscope) inserted through the URETHRA to resect the PROSTATE GLAND or bladder tumours. (See also RESECTION.)

Transverse

An anatomical description of a line, plane or structure at right-angles to the long axis of an organ or the body.

Transvestitism

Also called transvestism. The term given to a psycho-sexual condition in which there is a repetitive compulsion to dress in the clothes of the opposite sex to achieve ORGASM.

Tranylcypromine

One of the monoamine oxidase inhibitor ANTIDEPRESSANT DRUGS.

Trapezium

A bone in the wrist, one of the carpal group (see HAND).

Trauma

A term used in a physical sense as a wound or injury – such as a severe blow, maybe leading to a fracture. Physical traumas such as events of birth, severe accidents and any form of childhood or sexual abuse are considered to be overwhelming stressful events and regarded as psychological traumas. Various scoring techniques have been formed for traumas; generally seen as numerical systems for assessing the severity and prognosis of severe injuries.

Traumatology

Branch of SURGERY specialising in the treatment of wounds and disabilities arising from injuries.

Travel Medicine

Many countries have reciprocal health arrangements with Britain under which British visitors may receive emergency treatment free or at reduced cost. Information about these arrangements is available from any local DSS office. General and specific advice for travellers on such matters as immunisations needed can be obtained from their general practitioner, through travel agents or one of the high street travel 'health shops'. Travellers are advised to consult a doctor if they develop an illness after an overseas visit: some tropical disorders may take days or even weeks to produce symptoms.

Travel Sickness

Sickness induced by any form of transport, whether by sea, air, motor-car or train. (See also MOTION (TRAVEL) SICKNESS.)

Traveller's diarrhoea is an all-too-common affliction of the traveller, which basks in a multiplicity of names: for example, Aden gut, Aztec two-step, Basra belly, Delhi belly, Gippy tummy, Hong Kong dog, Montezuma's revenge, Tokyo trots, turista. It is caused by a variety of micro-organisms, usually *E. coli*. Some people seem to be more prone to it than others, although for no good cause. Obvious preventive measures include the avoidance of salads, unpeeled fruit and ice cream, and never drinking unboiled or unbottled water. If diarrhoea occurs, co-phenotrope and loperamide are often used to reduce the frequency of bowel movements in adults. Prophylactic antibacterial drugs are not advisable.

Tremor

A fine involuntary movement. Tremors may be seen in projecting parts like the hands, head and tongue, or they may involve muscles. Coarse tremors, which prevent a person from drinking a glass of water without spilling it, are found in MULTIPLE SCLEROSIS (MS) and in CHOREA; somewhat finer tremors, which produce trembling of the hands or tongue when they are stretched out, are caused by alcoholism (see ALCOHOL) and other forms of poisoning, by PARKINSONISM, and by the weakness which follows some acute disease or characterises old age. A fine tremor of the outstretched fingers is a characteristic of thyrotoxicosis (see under THY-

ROID GLAND, DISEASES OF); very fine tremors, visible in the muscles of face or limbs and known as fibrillary tremors, are present in general paralysis of the insane (see SYPHILIS), and in progressive muscular atrophy or wasting palsy. Tremors may occur at rest and disappear on movement as in Parkinsonism, or they may occur only on movement (intention tremors) as in cerebellar disease.

Trench Fever

An infectious disease caused by *Rickettsia quintana* which is transmitted by the body louse. Large epidemics occurred among troops on active service during World War I. It recurred on a smaller scale in World War II, but is now rare.

Trench Foot

This is due to prolonged exposure of the feet to water – particularly cold water. Trench warfare is a common precipitating factor, and the condition was rampant during World War I. Cases also occurred during World War II and during the Falklands campaign. (The less common form, due to warm-water immersion, occurred with some frequency in the Vietnam war.) It is characterised by painful swelling of the feet accompanied in due course by blistering and ulceration which, in severe, untreated cases, may progress to GANGRENE. In mild cases recovery may be complete in a month, but severe cases may drag on for a year. (See also IMMERSION FOOT.)

Treatment Drying of the feet overnight, where practicable, is the best method of prevention, accompanied by avoidance of constrictive clothing and tight boots, and of prolonged immobility. Frequent rest periods and daily changing of socks also help. The application of silicone grease once a day is another useful preventive measure. In the early stages, treatment consists of rest in bed and warmth; in more severe cases treatment is as for infected tissues and ulceration. ANALGESICS are usually necessary to ease the pain. Technically, smoking should be forbidden, but the adverse psychological effects of this in troops on active service may outweigh its advantages.

Trendelenberg Position

This is a steep head-down tilt so that the patient's pelvis and legs lie above the heart. It is used to improve access, and to limit blood loss, during surgery to the pelvis. It has been used to treat shocked patients (see SHOCK), but, as the position increases pressure on the DIAPHRAGM and embarrasses breathing, raising the legs by themselves is better.

Trepanning

An operation in which a portion of the CRANIUM is removed. Originally the operation was performed with an instrument resembling a carpenter's brace and known as the trephine or trepan, which removes a small circle of bone; but now this instrument is only used, as a rule, for making small openings, whilst, for wider operations, gouge forceps, circular saws driven by electric motor, or wire saws are used.

Trepanning is used in cases of fracture, with splintering of the skull; the operation is performed to remove fragments of bone and any foreign bodies, like a bullet, which may have entered. In compression of the brain with unconsciousness following an injury, the skull is trephined and any blood clots removed, or torn vessels ligatured. The operation may also be done for an ABSCESS within the skull and for other conditions where operative access to the brain is required.

Trephining

See TREPANNING.

Treponema

The name of a genus of spirochaetal microorganisms which consist of slender spirals and which progress by means of bending movements. *Treponema pallidum* (formerly called *Spirochaeta pallida*) is the causative organism of SYPHILIS.

Triage

Derived from the French word for 'sorting', triage is a universal term applied to methods of allocating treatment prioritisations for casualties from disasters or in warfare. The procedure helps a medical team to treat casualties who, although badly injured, can be saved; to defer those whose treatment is less urgent; and to provide care and comfort for those with fatal injuries.

Triage is now operated in accident and emergency departments by a 'triage nurse' who allocates a degree of priority so that patients are seen in order of severity rather than according to their time of arrival.

Triamcinolone

One of the CORTICOSTEROIDS with a potency equivalent to that of PREDNISONE, but less likely to cause retention of sodium. It is used for the suppression of inflammatory and allergic disorders, and is used particularly for treating

the skin and joints by local injection.

Triceps

A muscle of the posterior upper arm which acts to extend the forearm. So-named because it originates from three heads.

Trichiasis

A condition in which the eyelashes become ingrown. (See EYE, DISORDERS OF.)

Trichiniasis

See TRICHINOSIS.

Trichinosis

Trichinosis, or trichiniasis, is a disease caused by eating meat infected with the parasitic nematode worm, *Trichinella spiralis*. Although it infects more than 100 animal species, this nematode usually infects humans via pig meat in which the immature spiralis is encysted. The full-grown female worm, which inhabits the intestine, is 3 mm in length, and the larvae, to whose movements the disease is due, are much smaller. The disease is acquired by eating raw or underdone pork from pigs that have been infected with the worm. When such a piece of meat is eaten, the embryos contained in it are set free and develop into full-grown trichinellae; from each pair of these, 1,000 or more new embryos may arise in a few weeks. These burrow through the walls of the gut, spread throughout the body and settle in voluntary muscle.

Prevention is based on thorough inspection of meat in slaughterhouses; even cooking, unless the meat is in slices, is not an efficient protection. Pigs should not be fed on unboiled garbage. Rats may be a source of sporadic outbreaks, as infected rats have been found near piggeries. The disease is widely distributed throughout the Americas, Asia, Africa and the Arctic. Sporadic cases and epidemics occur and outbreaks also appear in Europe, although rarely in Britain.

Treatment Thiabendazole or mebendazole are usually effective, while STEROID treatment helps patients with systemic illness and muscle tenderness.

Tricho-

Tricho- is a prefix denoting relation to hair.

Trichomonas Vaginalis

A protozoon normally present in the VAGINA of about 30–40 per cent of women. It sometimes becomes pathogenic and causes inflammation of the genital passages, with vaginal discharge. A man may become infected as a result of sexual intercourse with an infected woman and suffer from a urethral discharge; it may also cause prostatitis (see under PROSTATE GLAND, DISEASES OF). METRONIDAZOLE is usually an effective treatment, and to obtain a satisfactory result it may be necessary to treat both partners. Should metronidazole not work, then tinidazole may be tried.

Trichomoniasis
The disease caused by infection with TRICHOMONAS VAGINALIS.

Trichophyton
See DERMATOPHYTES.

Trichotillomania
An obsessional impulse to pull out one's own hair.

Trichuriasis
A worldwide infection, particularly common in the tropics. It is caused by *Trichuris trichiura*, or whipworm, so-called because of its shape – the rear end being stout and the front end hair-like, resembling the lash of a whip. The male measures 5 cm and the female 4 cm in length. Infection results from eating vegetables, or drinking water, polluted with the ova (eggs). These hatch out in the large INTESTINE and the diagnosis is made by finding the eggs in the stools (FAECES). The worms seldom cause any trouble unless they are present in large numbers when, especially in malnourished children, they may cause bleeding from the bowels, ANAEMIA and PROLAPSE of the RECTUM. The most effective drug is MEBENDAZOLE.

Tricuspid Incompetence
Failure of the TRICUSPID VALVE in the HEART to close fully, thus permitting blood to leak back into the right atrium during contractions of the right ventricle. This reduces the heart's pumping efficiency, and right-sided heart failure usually results. Treatment for heart failure (using DIURETICS and ACE inhibitor drugs) usually restores function, but sometimes heart surgery is required to repair or replace the defective valve.

Tricuspid Stenosis
The normal working of the TRICUSPID VALVE in the HEART is impeded by a narrowing of the opening, often as a sequel of RHEUMATIC FEVER. As with TRICUSPID INCOMPETENCE,

heart failure may result and treatment is similar, with surgery to repair or replace the faulty valve an option.

Tricuspid Valve
The valve, with three cusps or flaps, that guards the opening from the right atrium into the right ventricle of the HEART.

Tricyclic Antidepressant Drugs
This group of drugs is one of three main types of drugs used to treat DEPRESSION, and was the first to be introduced (in the 1950s). Tricyclic drugs work by blocking the re-uptake of the neurotransmitters SEROTONIN and NORADRENALINE (see NEUROTRANSMITTER), thus increasing the amount of the neurotransmitters at the nerve cell's receptors. In people with depression, fewer neurotransmitters than normal are released, resulting in a slowing of neural activities. The drugs have a sedative effect, which can be useful for depressives with sleep problems, and an antimuscarinic action which can cause dry mouth and constipation (see ANTIMUSCARINE). Overdosage can produce COMA, fits (see SEIZURE) and irregular heart rhythm (ARRHYTHMIA). They are sometimes used for treating bed-wetting. (See also ANTIDEPRESSANT DRUGS.)

Trifluoperazine
See NEUROLEPTICS.

Trigeminal Nerve
The fifth cranial nerve (arising from the BRAIN). It consists of three divisions: (1) the ophthalmic nerve, which is purely sensory in function, being distributed mainly over the forehead and front part of the scalp; (2) the maxillary nerve, which is also sensory and distributed to the skin of the cheek, the mucous membrane of the mouth and throat, and the upper teeth; and (3) the mandibular nerve, which is the nerve of sensation to the lower part of the face, the tongue and the lower teeth, as well as being the motor nerve to the muscles concerned in chewing. The trigeminal nerve is of special interest, owing to its liability to NEURALGIA – TRIGEMINAL NEURALGIA, or tic douloureux as it is also known, being the most painful form known.

Trigeminal Neuralgia
Also called tic douloureux, this is one of the most severe forms of NEURALGIA. It affects the main sensory nerve in the face (TRIGEMINAL NERVE), and may occur in one or more of the three divisions in which the nerve is distributed.

It is usually confined to one side. It is more common in women than in men, usually occurring over the age of 50. The attack is often precipitated by movements of the jaw, as in talking or eating, or by tactile stimuli such as a cold wind or washing the face. When the first or upper division of the nerve is involved, the pain is mostly felt in the forehead and side of the head. It is usually of an intensely sharp, cutting, or burning character, either constant or with exacerbations each day while the attack continues. There is also pain in the eyelid, redness of the eye and increased flow of tears. When the second division of the nerve is affected, the pain is chiefly in the cheek and upper jaw. When the third division of the nerve suffers, the pain affects the lower jaw. Attacks may recur for years; and, although interfering with sleeping and eating, they rarely appear to lead to any serious results. Nevertheless, the pain may become intolerable.

Treatment The outlook in trigeminal neuralgia was radically altered by the introduction of the drug CARBAMAZEPINE, which usually relieves the pain. If the side-effects – for example, dizziness, headache, nausea or drowsiness – are unacceptable or pain not relieved, PHENYTOIN SODIUM may help. Otherwise, surgery is needed in the shape of controlled, radiofrequency heat damage to the appropriate part of the trigeminal nerve.

Trigger Finger

Also called snapping finger. This is the condition in which, when the fingers are straightened on unclenching the fist, one finger – usually the ring or middle finger – remains bent. The cause is obscure. In severe cases treatment consists of opening up the sheath surrounding the tendon of the affected finger. When confined to the thumb, the condition is known as trigger thumb.

Trigger Thumb

See TRIGGER FINGER.

Triglyceride

A LIPID or neutral FAT comprising GLYCEROL and three fatty-acid molecules. Triglycerides are manufactured in the body from the digested products of fat in the diet. Fats are stored in the body as triglycerides.

Trigone

The base of the URINARY BLADDER between the openings of the two ureters (see URETER) and of the URETHRA.

Tri-Iodothyronine

(T3) The substance which exerts the physiological action of thyroid hormone (see THYROID GLAND). It is formed in the body cells by the de-iodination of THYROXINE (tetra-iodothyronine) which is the active principle secreted by the thyroid gland. It has also been synthesised, and is now available for the treatment of hypothyroidism (see THYROID GLAND, DISEASES OF). It is three times as potent as thyroxine.

Trimester

A period of three months. Normal human GESTATION is divided into three trimesters – see PREGNANCY AND LABOUR.

Trimethoprim

Trimethoprim is an antibacterial agent used in the treatment of infections of the URINARY TRACT. It is also a constituent of CO-TRIMOXAZOLE – a combination that should be used with caution as it can damage kidney function. Trimethoprim is also used to treat acute and chronic BRONCHITIS.

Trimipramine

One of the TRICYCLIC ANTIDEPRESSANT DRUGS which also acts as a sedative.

Trinitrin

See GLYCERYL TRINITRATE.

Trinitrophenol

See PICRIC ACID.

Triplets

See MULTIPLE BIRTHS.

Triple Vaccine

Also known as DPT vaccine, this is an injection that provides IMMUNITY against DIPHTHERIA, pertussis (whooping-cough) and TETANUS. It is given as a course of three injections at around the ages of two, three and four months. A booster dose of diphtheria and tetanus is given at primary-school age. Certain infants – those with a family history of EPILEPSY, or who have neurological disorders or who have reacted severely to the first dose – should not have the pertussis element of DPT. (See MMR VACCINE; IMMUNISATION.)

Trismus

Another name for TETANUS.

Trocar

An instrument provided with a sharp three-sided

point fitted inside a tube or cannula, and used for puncturing cavities of the body in which fluid has collected.

Trochanter

The name given to two bony prominences at the upper end of the thigh-bone (FEMUR). The greater trochanter can be felt on the outer side of the thigh; the lesser trochanter is a small prominence on the inner side of this bone.

Trochlear Nerve

The fourth cranial nerve (arising from the BRAIN), which acts upon the superior oblique muscle of the EYE.

Trophic

A term applied to the influence that nerves exert with regard to the healthiness and nourishment of the parts to which they run. When the nerves become diseased or injured, this influence is lost and the muscles waste, while the skin loses its healthy appearance and is liable to break down into ulcers (see ULCER).

Trophoblast

The outer layer of the fertilised OVUM which attaches the ovum to the wall of the UTERUS (or womb) and supplies nutrition to the EMBRYO.

Trophozoite

A stage in the life of the parasite *Plasmodium,* that is the cause of MALARIA. It has a ring-shaped body and single nucleus and grows in the blood cell, after which it divides to form a schizont.

Tropical Diseases

Technically, those diseases occurring in the area of the globe situated between the Tropic of Cancer and the Tropic of Capricorn: pertaining to the sun. They include many 'exotic' infections – many of them parasitic in origin – which fall under the umbrella of 'TROPICAL MEDICINE'. However, disease in the tropics is far broader than this and includes numerous other infections, many of them with a viral or bacterial basis: for example, the viral hepatidises, streptococcal and pneumococcal infections, and tuberculosis. The prevalence of other diseases, such as rheumatic cardiac disease, cirrhosis, heptocellular carcinoma ('hepatoma'), and various nutrition-related problems, is also much increased in most areas of the tropics. With people from developed countries increasingly travelling to worldwide destinations for business and holiday, the

'importation' of tropical diseases to temperate climates should be borne in mind when people fall ill.

The following diseases and conditions are treated under their separate dictionary entries: ANCYLOSTOMIASIS; BERIBERI; BLACKWATER FEVER; CHOLERA; DENGUE; DRACONTIASIS; DYSENTERY; ELEPHANTIASIS; FILARIASIS; HEAT STROKE; LEISHMANIASIS; LEPROSY; LIVER, DISEASES OF; MALARIA; ORIENTAL SORE; PLAGUE; PRICKLY HEAT; SCHISTOSOMIASIS; SLEEPING SICKNESS; STRONGYLOIDIASIS; SUNBURN; YAWS; YELLOW FEVER.

Tropical Medicine

The diagnosis and treatment of diseases that occur most commonly in tropical zones of the world. Examples are LEPROSY, MALARIA, SCHISTOSOMIASIS and TRYPANOSOMIASIS. With the great increase in international travel in the past 30 or so years, TROPICAL DISEASES are appearing more often in temperate climates. Global warming may also be enlarging the areas in which tropical disorders naturally occur.

Tropical Ulcer

Also called Nagra sore, this is a skin disease of unknown cause occurring in humid tropical areas. A simple wound or abrasion develops into an open sloughing sore that commonly occurs on the leg or foot. The ULCER is often infected with spirochaetes (see SPIROCHAETE) and BACTERIA and may be so deep as to destroy muscle and bone. Antiseptic dressing and an antibiotic, usually PENICILLIN (by intramuscular injection), is the best treatment. Sometimes a skin-graft is required to produce healing (see GRAFT; SKIN-GRAFTING).

Trunk

A major vessel or nerve from which lesser ones arise; or the main part of the body excluding the head, neck and limbs.

Truss

A device used to support a HERNIA; or to retain the protruding organ within the cavity from which it tends to pass. Every truss possesses a pad of some sort to cover the opening and a belt or spring to keep it in position.

Before applying a truss the wearer must make certain that the hernia has been reduced; this may mean lying down beforehand. A truss will rarely control a hernia satisfactorily, and it should be considered as a temporary measure only until surgical correction is possible. In the past, trusses have been supplied to patients considered too frail for surgery, but modern anaesthetic techniques mean that most people can have their hernias surgically repaired.

Trypanosoma

A genus of microscopic parasites, several of which are responsible for causing SLEEPING SICKNESS and some allied diseases.

Trypanosomiasis

See SLEEPING SICKNESS.

Trypsin

The chief protein ENZYME of the pancreatic secretion. Secreted by the PANCREAS as trypsinogen (an inactive form), it is converted in the duodenum by another enzyme, enteropeptidase. It changes proteins into peptones and forms the main constituent of pancreatic extracts used for digestion of food. (See PEPTONISED FOODS.)

Tryptophan

(1) One of the nine indispensable (essential) AMINO ACIDS. Like other amino acids, tryptophan is needed by the body to synthesise the proteins necessary for its growth and functioning. The description indispensable – previously the adjective used was essential – is applied because the body is unable to manufacture these amino acids, which have to be obtained from food or drink.

(2) A drug that has helped some patients with resistant DEPRESSION. Used as a supporting drug with other treatment, tryptophan was withdrawn because of side-effects; it has, however, been reintroduced for use in hospital for patients for whom no alternative treatment is suitable. (See also MENTAL ILLNESS.)

Tsetse Fly

An African fly of the genus *Glossina*. One or more of these is responsible for carrying the trypanosome which causes SLEEPING SICKNESS and thus spreads the disease among cattle and from cattle to humans.

Tsutsugamushi

Also called Japanese river fever, this is a disease of the typhus group. (See TYPHUS FEVER.)

Tubal Pregnancy

Also known as ECTOPIC PREGNANCY. Implantation of the EMBRYO in one of the FALLOPIAN TUBES, rather than in the lining of the UTERUS. The patient usually complains of pain between six and ten weeks' gestation and, if the Fallopian tube is not removed, there may be rupture with potentially life-threatening haemorrhage.

Tubercle

The term is used in two distinct senses. As a descriptive term in anatomy, a tubercle means a small elevation or roughness upon a BONE, such as the tubercles of the ribs. In the pathological sense, a tubercle is a small mass, barely visible to the naked eye, formed in some organ as the starting-point of TUBERCULOSIS. The name of tubercle bacillus was originally given to the micro-organism that causes this disease, but was subsequently changed to *Mycobacterium tuberculosis*. The term 'tubercular' should strictly be applied to anything connected with or resembling tubercles or nodules, and the term 'tuberculous' to anything pertaining to the disease tuberculosis.

Tuberculide

The term given to any skin lesion which is the result of infection with the tubercle bacillus, or *Mycobacterium tuberculosis* as it is now known.

Tuberculin

Tuberculin is the name originally given by Koch in 1890 to a preparation derived from the tubercle bacillus, or *Mycobacterium tuberculosis* as it is now known, and intended for the diagnosis or treatment of TUBERCULOSIS.

Varieties

OLD TUBERCULIN (OT) is the heat-concentrated filtrate from a fluid medium on which the human or bovine type of *Mycobacterium tuberculosis* has been grown for six weeks or more. TUBERCULIN PURIFIED PROTEIN DERIVATIVE (TUBERCULIN PPD) is the active principle of OT (see above), and is prepared from the fluid medium on which the *Mycobacterium tuberculosis* has been grown. It is supplied as a liquid, a powder, or as sterile tablets. The liquid contains 100,000 units per millilitre, and the dry powder contains 30,000 units per milligram. It is distributed in sterile containers sealed so as to exclude micro-organisms. It is more constant in composition and potency than OT.

Uses The basis of the tuberculin reaction is that any person who has been infected with the *Mycobacterium tuberculosis* gives a reaction when a small amount of tuberculin is injected into the skin. A negative reaction means either that the individual has never been infected with the tubercle bacillus, or that the infection has been too recent to have allowed of sensitivity developing.

There are various methods of carrying out the test, of which the following are the most commonly used. The Mantoux test is the most satisfactory of all, and has the advantage that the size of the reaction is a guide to the severity of the tuberculous infection: it is performed by injecting the tuberculin into the skin on the forearm. The Heaf multiple puncture test is reliable: it is carried out with the multiple puncture apparatus, or Heaf gun. The Vollmer patch test, using an impregnated filter paper, is useful in children because of the ease with which it can be carried out.

Tuberculosis

Tuberculosis results form infection with *Mycobacterium tuberculosis*. The lungs are the site most often affected, but most organs in the body can be involved in tuberculosis. The other common sites are LYMPH NODES, bones, gastrointestinal tract, kidneys, skin and MENINGES.

The weight loss and wasting associated with tuberculosis before treatment was available led to the disease's popular name of consumption. Enlargement of the glands in the neck, formerly called scrofula, was known also as the 'king's evil' from the supersition that a touch of the royal hand could cure the condition. Lupus vulgaris (see under LUPUS) is another of the skin manifestations of the disease.

The typical pathological change in tuberculosis involves the formation of clusters of cells called granulomas (see GRANULOMA) with death of the cells in the centre producing CASEATION.

It is estimated that there are 7–8 million new cases of tuberculosis worldwide each year, with 2–3 million deaths. The incidence of tuberculosis in developed countries has shown a steady decline throughout the 20th century, mainly as a result of improved nutrition and social conditions and accelerated by the development of antituberculous chemotherapy in the 1940s. Since the mid-1980s the decline has stopped, and incidence has even started to rise again in inner-city areas. In 2002, 7,239 cases of tuberculosis were notified in the UK compared with 6,442 a decade earlier; more than 390 deaths in 2003 were attributed to the disease. Factors involved in this rise are immigration from higher-prevalence areas, poorer social conditions and homelessness in some urban centres and the association with HIV infection and drug abuse. The incidence of tuberculosis is also rising in many developing countries because of the emergence of resistant strains of the tubercle bacillus (see below). In the UK recently there have been serious outbreaks in a handful of urban-based schools.

Nature of the disease Tuberculosis has been recognised from earliest times. Evidence of the condition has been found in Egyptian mummies; in the fourth century BC Hippocrates, the Greek physician, called it phthisis because of the lung involvement; and in 1882 Koch announced the discovery of the causative organism, the tubercle bacillus or *Mycobacterium tuberculosis*.

The symptoms depend upon the site of the infection. General symptoms such as fever, weight loss and night sweats are common. In the most common form of pulmonary tuberculosis, cough and blood-stained sputum (haemoptysis) are common symptoms.

The route of infection is most often by inhalation, although it can be by ingestion of products such as infected milk. The results of contact depend upon the extent of the exposure and the susceptibility of the individual. Around 30 per cent of those closely exposed to the organism will be infected, but most will contain the infection with no significant clinical illness and only a minority will go on to develop clinical disease. Around 5 per cent of those infected will develop post-primary disease over the next two or three years. The rest are at risk of reactivation of the disease later, particularly if their resistance is reduced by associated disease, poor nutrition or immunosuppression. In developed countries around 5 per cent of those infected will reactivate their healed tuberculosis into a clinical problem.

Immunosuppressed patients such as those infected with HIV are at much greater risk of developing clinical tuberculosis on primary contact or from reactivation. This is a particular problem in many developing countries, where there is a high incidence of both HIV and tuberculosis.

Diagnosis This depends upon identification of mycobacteria on direct staining of sputum or other secretions or tissue, and upon culture of the organism. Culture takes 4–6 weeks but is necessary for differentiation from other non-tuberculous mycobacteria and for drug-sensitivity testing. Newer techniques involving DNA amplification by polymerase chain reaction (PCR) can detect small numbers of organisms and help with earlier diagnosis.

Treatment This can be preventative or curative. Important elements of prevention are adequate nutrition and social conditions, BCG vaccination (see IMMUNISATION), an adequate public-health programme for contact tracing, and chemoprophylaxis. Radiological screening with mass miniature radiography is no longer used.

Vaccination with an attenuated organism (BCG – Bacillus Calmette Guerin) is used in the United Kingdom and some other countries at 12–13 years, or earlier in high-risk groups. Some studies show 80 per cent protection against tuberculosis for ten years after vaccination.

Cases of open tuberculosis need to be identified; their close contacts should be reviewed for evidence of disease. Adequate antibiotic chemotherapy removes the infective risk after around two weeks of treatment. Chemoprophylaxis – the use of antituberculous therapy in those without clinical disease – may be used in contacts who develop a strong reaction on tuberculin skin testing or those at high risk because of associated disease.

The major principles of antibiotic chemotherapy for tuberculosis are that a combination of drugs needs to be used, and that treatment needs to be continued for a prolonged period – usually six months. Use of single agents or interrupted courses leads to the development of drug resistance. Serious outbreaks of multiply resistant *Mycobacterium tuberculosis* have been seen mainly in AIDS units, where patients have greater susceptibility to the disease, but also in developing countries where maintenance of appropriate antibacterial therapy for six months or more can be difficult.

Streptomycin was the first useful agent identified in 1944. The four drugs used most often now are RIFAMPICIN, ISONIAZID, PYRAZINAMIDE and ETHAMBUTOL. Three to four agents are used for the first two months; then, when sensitivities are known and clinical response observed, two drugs, most often rifampicin and isoniazid, are continued for the rest of the course. Treatment is taken daily, although thrice-weekly, directly observed therapy is used when there is doubt about the patient's compliance. All the antituberculous agents have a range of adverse effects that need to be monitored during treatment. Provided that the treatment is prescribed and taken appropriately, response to treatment is very good with cure of disease and very low relapse rates.

Tuberous Sclerosis

Also called epiloia: a rare inherited disease transmitted as an autosomal dominant trait. EPILEPSY in childhood is often the first manifestation (see INFANTILE SPASMS), although ovoid hypopigmented macules ('ash leaf patches') in the skin may be detected in infancy. Later an ACNE-like eruption of the face (aden-oma sebaceum), fibrous outgrowths around the nails and fibrous plaques on the lower back (shagreen patch) can all occur. Half of those affected have learning difficulties and behaviour problems, and autistic symptoms may occur (see AUTISM).

Characteristic white streaks appear on the optic fundi (see EYE). Molecular genetic testing can identify up to 90 per cent of individuals with a tuberin gene. Genetic counselling of families is helpful. Relatives of those with this condition can obtain help and guidance from the Tuberous Sclerosis Association of Great Britain.

Tubocurarine

A voluntary-muscle relaxant given by intravenous injection before surgery under general ANAESTHESIA. The drug is also used to treat conditions such as TETANUS, ENCEPHALITIS and POLIOMYELITIS in which severe muscle spasms occur. Overdosage may result in respiratory failure because the muscles essential for breathing are paralysed.

Tubule

A small tube. There are several named tubules in the body: examples include convoluted tubules in the NEPHRON of the kidney (see KIDNEYS) and the seminiferous tubules in the testes (see TESTICLE).

Tularaemia

A disease of rodents such as rabbits and rats, caused by the bacillus, *Francisella tularense*, and spread either by flies or by direct inoculation – for example, into the hands of a person engaged in skinning rabbits. In humans the disease takes the form of a slow fever lasting several weeks, with much malaise and depression, followed by considerable emaciation. It was first described in the district of Tulare in California, and is found widely spread in North America and in Europe, but not in Great Britain. STREPTOMYCIN, the TETRACYCLINES and CHLORAMPHENICOL offer effective treatment.

Tulle Gras

A wound dressing of gauze impregnated with soft paraffin to prevent it from sticking to the wound.

Tumescence

A swelling usually caused by blood or other body fluids accumulating in the tissues, often as a consequence of injury. An erect PENIS, when blood fills the corpus cavernosa in the organ, is sometimes described as tumescent.

Tumour

This literally means any swelling, but the term does not usually include temporary swellings caused by acute inflammation. The consequences locally, however, of chronic inflammation – for example, TUBERCULOSIS, SYPHILIS and LEPROSY – are sometimes classed as tumours, according to their size and appearance.

Varieties Some are of an infective nature, as already stated; some arise as the result of injury, and several contributing factors are mentioned under the heading of CANCER.

Traditionally tumours have been divided into benign (simple) and malignant. Even benign tumours can be harmful, because their size or position may distort or damage nerves, blood vessels or organs. Usually, however, they are easily removed by surgery. Malignant tumours or cancers are harmful and potentially lethal, not just because they erode tissues locally but because many of them spread, either by direct growth or by 'seeding' to other parts – 'metastasising'. Malignant tumours arise because of an uncontrolled growth of previously normal cells. Heredity, environmental factors and lifestyle all play a part in malignancy (see also ONCOGENES). Symptoms are caused by local spread and as a result of metastases. These cause serious local damage, for example, in the brain or lungs, as well as disturbing the body's metabolism. Unless treated with CHEMO-THERAPY, RADIOTHERAPY or surgery or a combination of these, malignant tumours are ultimately fatal. Many, however, can now be cured. The original site and type of a malignant tumour usually determine the rate and extent of spread.

The type of cell and organ site determine the characteristics of a malignant tumour. The prognosis (outlook) for a patient with a malignant tumour depends largely upon how soon it is diagnosed. Staging criteria have been developed to assess the local and metastatic spread of a tumour, its size and also likely sensitivity to the types of available treatment. The ability to locate a tumour and its metastases accurately has vastly improved with the introduction of radionuclide and ULTRASOUND scanning, CT scanning and magnetic resonance imaging (MRI). Screening for cancers such as those in the breast, cervix, colorectal region and prostate help early diagnosis and usually improve treatment outcomes.

Tumours are now classed according to the tissues of which they are built, somewhat as follows:

- simple tumours of normal tissue.
- hollow tumours or cysts, generally of simple nature.
- malignant tumours: (*a*) of cellular structure, resembling the cells of skin, mucous membrane, or secreting glands; (*b*) of connective tissue.

Turgor

Being or becoming swollen or engorged.

Turner's Syndrome

This occurs in one in 2,500 live female births. It is caused by either the absence of or an abnormality in one of the two X CHROMO-SOMES. Classical Turner's syndrome is a complete deletion of one X so that the karyotype is 45XO. Half of the people with Turner's syndrome have MOSAICISM with a mixture of Turner cells and normal cells, or other abnormalities of the X chromosome such as partial deletions or a ring X. They are females, both in appearance and sexually; clinical features are variable and include short stature, with final height between 1·295 m and 1·575 m, and ovarian failure. Other clinical features may include a short neck, webbing of the neck, increased carrying angle at the elbow (cubitus valgus), widely spaced nipples, cardiovascular abnormalities (of which the commonest is coarctation of the aorta [about 10 per cent]), morphological abnormalities of the kidneys (including horseshoe kidney and abnormalities of the pelviureteric tracts), recurrent otitis media (see under EAR, DISEASES OF), squints, increased incidence of pigmented naevi (see NAEVUS), hypothyroidism (see under THYROID, DISEASES OF) and DIABETES MELLITUS. Intelligence is across the normal range, although there are specific learning defects which are related to hand-eye coordination and spatial awareness.

Patients with Turner's syndrome may require therapeutic help throughout their life. In early childhood this may revolve around surgical correction of cardiovascular disease and treatment to improve growth. Usually, PUBERTY will need to be induced with oestrogen therapy (see OES-TROGENS). In adult life, problems of oestrogen therapy, prevention of osteoporosis (see under BONE, DISORDERS OF), assessment and treatment of HYPERTENSION and assisted fertility predominate. For the address of the UK Turner Syndrome Society, see Appendix 2.

Twins

See MULTIPLE BIRTHS.

Tympanic Membrane

The ear-drum, which separates the external and middle ear. (See EAR.)

Tympanites

Also known as meteorism. Distension of the abdomen due to the presence of gas or air in the INTESTINE or in the peritoneal cavity (see PERITONEUM). The abdomen when struck with the fingers, gives under these conditions a drum-like (tympanitic) note.

Tympanum

Another name for the middle EAR.

Typhoid Fever

See ENTERIC FEVER.

Typhus Fever

An infective disease of worldwide distribution, the manifestations of which vary in different localities. The causative organisms of all forms of typhus fever belong to the genus RICKETTSIA. These are organisms which are intermediate between bacteria and viruses in their properties, and measure 0·5 micrometre or less in diameter.

Louse typhus, in which the infecting rickettsia is transmitted by the louse, is of worldwide distribution. More human deaths have been attributed to the louse via typhus, louse-borne RELAPSING FEVER and trench fever, than to any other insect with the exception of the MALARIA mosquito. Louse typhus includes epidemic typhus, Brill's disease – which is a recrudescent form of epidemic typhus – and TRENCH FEVER.

Epidemic typhus fever, also known as exanthematic typhus, classical typhus, and louse-borne typhus, is an acute infection of abrupt onset which, in the absence of treatment, persists for 14 days. It is of worldwide distribution, but is largely confined today to parts of Africa. The causative organism is the *Rickettsia prowazeki*, so-called after Ricketts and Prowazek, two brilliant investigators of typhus, both of whom died of the disease. It is transmitted by the human louse, *Pediculus humanus*. The rickettsiae can survive in the dried faeces of lice for 60 days, and these infected faeces are probably the main source of human infection.

Symptoms The incubation period is usually 10–14 days. The onset is preceded by headache, pain in the back and limbs and rigors. On the third day the temperature rises, the headache worsens, and the patient is drowsy or delirious. Subsequently a characteristic rash appears on the abdomen and inner aspect of the arms, to spread over the chest, back and trunk. Death may occur from SEPTICAEMIA, heart or kidney failure, or PNEUMONIA about the 14th day. In those who recover, the temperature falls by CRISIS at about this time. The death rate is variable, ranging from nearly 100 per cent in epidemics among debilitated refugees to about 10 per cent.

Murine typhus fever, also known as flea typhus, is worldwide in its distribution and is found wherever individuals are crowded together in insanitary, rat-infested areas (hence the old names of jail-fever and ship typhus). The causative organism, *Rickettsia mooseri*, which is closely related to *R. prowazeki*, is transmitted to humans by the rat-flea, *Xenopsylla cheopis*. The rat is the main reservoir of infection; once humans are infected, the human louse may act as a transmitter of the rickettsia from person to person. This explains how the disease may become epidemic under insanitary, crowded conditions. As a rule, however, the disease is only acquired when humans come into close contact with infected rats.

Symptoms These are similar to those of louse-borne typhus, but the disease is usually milder, and the mortality rate is very low (about 1·5 per cent).

Tick typhus, in which the infecting rickettsia is transmitted by ticks, occurs in various parts of the world. The three best-known conditions in this group are ROCKY MOUNTAIN SPOTTED FEVER, fièvre boutonneuse and tick-bite fever.

Mite typhus, in which the infecting rickettsia is transmitted by mites, includes scrub typhus, or tsutsugamushi disease, and rickettsialpox.

Rickettsialpox is a mild disease caused by *Rickettsia akari*, which is transmitted to humans from infected mice by the common mouse mite, *Allodermanyssus sanguineus*. It occurs in the United States, West and South Africa and the former Soviet Union.

Treatment The general principles of treatment are the same in all forms of typhus. PROPHYLAXIS consists of either avoidance or destruction of the vector. In the case of louse typhus and flea typhus, the outlook has been revolutionised by the introduction of efficient insecticides such as DICHLORODIPHENYL TRICHLOROETHANE (DDT) and GAMMEXANE.

The value of the former was well shown by its use after World War II: this resulted in almost complete freedom from the epidemics of typhus which ravaged Eastern Europe after World War I, being responsible for 30 million cases with a mortality of 10 per cent. Now only 10,000–20,000 cases occur a year, with around a few hundred deaths. Efficient rat control is another measure which reduces the risk of typhus very considerably. In areas such as Malaysia, where the mites are infected from a wide variety of rodents scattered over large areas, the wearing of protective clothing is the most practical method of prophylaxis.

CURATIVE TREATMENT was revolutionised by the introduction of CHLORAMPHENICOL and the TETRACYCLINES. These antibiotics altered the prognosis in typhus fever very considerably.

Tyramine

A variety of the chemical compound amine, which is derived from ammonia. A sympatho-mimetic agent with an action which resembles that of ADRENALINE, tyramine occurs in mistle-toe, mature cheese, beers, red wine and decaying animal matter. This adrenaline effect is potentially dangerous for patients taking MONOAMINE OXIDASE INHIBITORS (MAOIS) – ANTIDEPRESSANT DRUGS – because, when combined with tyramine, the blood pressure rises sharply. Such patients should avoid taking cheese, beers and red wine.

Tyrosine

One of the AMINO ACIDS. Tyrosine is important in the production of CATECHOLAMINES, MELANIN and THYROXINE.

UKCC

United Kingdom Central Council for Nursing, Midwifery and Health Visiting, now known as the Council for Nursing and Midwifery. (See APPENDIX 7: STATUTORY ORGANISATIONS.)

UKTSSA

United Kingdom Transplant Support Service Authority (see TRANSPLANT SUPPORT SERVICES AUTHORITY).

Ulcer

Destruction of the skin's surface tissues resulting in an open sore. A similar breach may occur in the surface of the mucous membrane lining body cavities – for example, the stomach, duodenum or colon (see COLITIS). Usually accompanied by pain and local inflammation, ulcers can be shallow or deep, with a crater-like shape. An ulcer may heal naturally, but on certain parts of the body – legs (venous ulcers, see below) or bony protuberances (decubitus ulcers, see below) – they can become chronic and difficult to treat. When an ulcer heals, granulations (well-vascularised connective tissue) form which become fibrous and draw the edges of the ulcer together. Any damage to the body surface may develop into an ulcer if the causative agent is allowed to persist – for example, contact with a noxious substance or constant pressure on an area of tissue with poor circulation. Treatment of skin ulcers is effected by cleaning the area, regular dry dressings and local or systemic ANTI-BIOTICS depending upon the severity of the ulcer.

Decubitus ulcer Also known as pressure or bed sore. Occurs when there is constant pressure on and inadequate oxygenation of an area of skin, usually overlying a bony protuberance. Elderly or infirm people, or individuals with debilitating, emaciating or neurological illnesses, are vulnerable to the condition. Long-term pressure from a bed, wheelchair, cast or splint is the usual cause. Loss of skin sensation is a contributory factor, and muscle and bone as well as skin may be affected.

Treatment The most important treatment is prevention, keeping the patient's back, but-tocks, heels and other pressure-points clean and dry, and regularly changing his or her position. If ulcers do develop, repeated local DEBRIDE-MENT, protective dressings and (in serious cases) surgical treatment are required, accompanied by an appropriate antibiotic if infection is persistent.

Venous ulcer This occurs on the lower leg or ankle and is caused by chronic HYPERTEN-SION in the deep leg VEINS, usually the consequences of previous deep vein thrombosis (DVT) – see THROMBOSIS; VEINS, DISEASES OF – which has destroyed the valvular system in the vein(s). The ulcer is usually preceded by chronic OEDEMA, often local eczema (see DERMATITIS), and bleeding into the skin that produces brown staining. Varicose veins may or may not be present. Control of the oedema by compression and encouragement to walk is central to management.

Ulcerative Colitis

Chronic inflammation of the lining of the COLON and RECTUM. The disease affects around 50 people per 100,000; it is predominantly a disease of young and middle-aged adults.

Symptoms The onset may be sudden or insidious. In the acute form there is severe diarrhoea and the patient may pass up to 20 stools a day. The stools, which may be small in quantity, are fluid and contain blood, pus and mucus. There is always fever, which runs an irregular course. In other cases the patient first notices some irregularity of the movement of the bowels, with the passage of blood. This becomes gradually more marked. There may be pain but usually a varying amount of abdominal discomfort. The constant diarrhoea leads to emaciation, weakness and ANAEMIA. As a rule the acute phase passes into a chronic stage. The chronic form is liable to run a prolonged course, and most patients suffer relapses for many years. SIGMOIDOSCOPY, BIOPSY and abdominal X-RAYS are essential diagnostic procedures.

Treatment Many patients may be under-nourished and need expert dietary assessment and appropriate calorie, protein, vitamin and mineral supplements. This is particularly important in children with the disorder. While specific nutritional treatment can initiate improvement in CROHN'S DISEASE, this is not the case with ulcerative colitis. CORTICO-STEROIDS, given by mouth or ENEMA, help to control the diarrhoea. Intravenous nutrition may be required. The anaemia is treated with iron supplements, and with blood infusions if necessary. Blood cultures should be taken, repeatedly if the fever persists. If SEPTICAEMIA is suspected, broad-spectrum antibiotics should be given. Surgery to remove part of the affected colon may be necessary and an ILEOSTOMY is sometimes required. After recovery, the patient should remain on a low-residue diet, with regular follow-up by the physician, Mesalazine and SULFASALAZINE are helpful in the prevention of recurrences.

Patients and their relatives can obtain help and advice from the National Association for Colitis and Crohn's Disease.

Ulcer Healing Drugs

A variety of drugs with differing actions are available for the treatment of peptic ulcer, the composite title covering gastric ulcer (see STOMACH, DISEASES OF) and DUODENAL ULCER. Peptic ulceration may also involve the lower OESOPHAGUS, and after stomach surgery the junction of the stomach and small intestine.

The drugs used in combination are:

- The receptor antagonists, which reduce the output of gastric acid by histamine H_2-receptor blockade; they include CIMETIDINE, FAMOTIDINE and RANITIDINE.
- ANTIBIOTICS to eradicate *Helicobacter pylori* infection, a major cause of peptic ulceration. They are usually used in combination with one of the PROTON-PUMP INHIBITORS and include clarithomycin, amoxacillin and metronidazole.
- BISMUTH chelates.
- The prostaglandin analogue misoprostol has antisecretory and protective properties.
- Proton-pump inhibitors omeprazole, lansoprazole, pantaprazole and rabeprazole, all of which inhibit gastric-acid secretion by blocking the proton pump enzyme system.

Ulna

The inner of the two bones in the forearm. It is wide at its upper end, and its olecranon process forms the point of the elbow. In its lower part it is more fragile and liable to be broken by a fall upon the forearm while something is grasped in the hand. Chipping-off of the olecranon process is a not uncommon result of falls upon the elbow. (See BONE, DISORDERS OF – Bone fractures.)

Ulnar Nerve

A major NERVE in the arm, it runs from the brachial plexus to the hand. The nerve controls the muscles that move the fingers and thumb and conveys sensation from the fifth and part of the fourth and from the adjacent palm. Muscle weakness and numbness in the areas supplied by the nerve is usually caused by pressure from an abnormal outgrowth from the epicondyle at the bottom of the humerus (upper-arm bone).

Ultrafiltration

Filtration carried out under pressure. Blood undergoes ultrafiltration in the KIDNEYS to remove the waste products, urea and surplus water that constitute URINE.

Ultrasonography

The use of ULTRASOUND to produce images of structures in the body that can be viewed on a television screen and transferred to photographic film.

Ultrasound

Ultrasound, or ultrasonic, waves comprise very-high-frequency sound waves above 20,000 Hz that the human ear cannot hear. Ultrasound is widely used for diagnosis and also for some treatments. In OBSTETRICS, ultrasound can assess the stage of pregnancy and detect abnormalities in the FETUS (see below). It is a valuable adjunct in the investigation of diseases in the bladder, kidneys, liver, ovaries, pancreas and brain (for more information on these organs and their diseases, see under separate entries); it also detects thromboses (clots) in blood vessels and enables their extent to be assessed. A non-invasive technique that does not need ionising radiation, ultrasound is quick, versatile and relatively inexpensive, with scans being done in any plane of the body. There is little danger to the patient or operator: unlike, for example, X-RAYS, ultrasound investigations can be repeated as needed. A contrast medium is not required. Its reliability is dependent upon the skill of the operator.

Ultrasound is replacing ISOTOPE scanning in many situations, and also RADIOGRAPHY. Ultrasound of the liver can separate medical from surgical JAUNDICE in approximately 97 per cent of patients; it is very accurate in detecting and defining cystic lesions of the liver, but is less accurate with solid lesions – and yet will detect 85 per cent of secondary deposits (this is less than COMPUTED TOMOGRAPHY [CT] scanning). It is very accurate in detecting gall-stones (see GALL-BLADDER, DISEASES OF) and more accurate than the oral cholecystogram. It is useful as a screening test for pancreatic disease and can differentiate carcinoma of the pancreas from chronic pancreatitis with 85 per cent accuracy.

Ultrasound is the first investigation indicated in patients presenting with renal failure, as it can quickly determine the size and shape of the kidney and whether there is any obstruction to the URETER. It is very sensitive to the presence of dilatation of the renal tract and will detect space-occupying lesions, differentiating cysts and tumours. It can detect also obstruction of the ureter due to renal stones by showing dilatations of the collecting system and the presence of the calculus. Adrenal (see ADRENAL GLANDS) tumours can be demonstrated by ultrasound, although it is less accurate than CT scanning.

The procedure is now the first test for suspected aortic ANEURYSM and it can also show the presence of clot and delineate the true and false lumen. It is good at demonstrating subphrenic and subhepatic abscesses (see ABSCESS) and will show most intra-abdominal abscesses; CT scanning is however better for the retroperitoneal region. It has a major application in thyroid nodules as it can differentiate cystic from solid lesions and show the multiple lesions characteristic of the nodular GOITRE (see also THYROID GLAND, DISEASES OF). It cannot differentiate between a follicular adenoma and a carcinoma, as both these tumours are solid; nor can it demonstrate normal parathyroid glands. However, it can identify adenomas provided that they are more than 6 mm in diameter. Finally, ultrasound can differentiate masses in the SCROTUM into testicular and appendicular, and it can demonstrate impalpable testicular tumours. This is important as 15 per cent of testicular tumours metastasise whilst they are still impalpable.

Ultrasonic waves are one of the constituents in the shock treatment of certain types of gallstones and CALCULI in the urinary tract (see LITHOTRIPSY). They are also being used in the treatment of MENIÈRE'S DISEASE and of bruises and strains. In this field of physiotherapy, ultrasonic therapy is proving of particular value in the treatment of acute injuries of soft tissue. If in such cases it is used immediately after the injury, or as soon as possible thereafter, prompt recovery is facilitated. For this reason it is being widely used in the treatment of sports injuries (see also SPORTS MEDICINE). The sound waves stimulate the healing process in damaged tissue.

Doppler ultrasound is a technique which shows the presence of vascular disease in the carotid and peripheral vessels, as it can detect the reduced blood flow through narrowed vessels.

Ultrasound in obstetrics Ultrasound has particular applications in obstetrics. A fetus can be seen with ultrasound from the seventh week of pregnancy, and the fetal heart can be demonstrated at this stage. Multiple pregnancy can also be diagnosed at this time by the demonstration of more than one gestation sac containing a viable fetus. A routine obstetric scan is usually performed between the 16th and 18th week of pregnancy when the fetus is easily demonstrated and most photogenic. The fetus can be measured to assess the gestational age, and the anatomy can also be checked. Intra-uterine growth retardation is much more reliably diagnosed by ultrasound than by clinical assessment. The site of the placenta can also be recorded and multiple pregnancies will be diagnosed at this stage. Fetal movements and even the heartbeat can be seen. A second scan is often done between the 32nd and 34th weeks to assess the position, size and growth rate of the baby. The resolution of equipment now available enables pre-natal diagnosis of a wide range of structural abnormalities to be diagnosed. SPINA BIFIDA, HYDROCEPHALUS and ANENCEPHALY are probably the most important, but other anomalies such as multicystic kidney, achondroplasia and certain congenital cardiac anomalies can also be identified. Fetal gender can be determined from 20 weeks of gestation. Ultrasound is also useful as guidance for AMNIOCENTESIS.

In gynaecology, POLYCYSTIC OVARY SYNDROME can readily be detected as well as FIBROID and ovarian cysts. Ultrasound can monitor follicular growth when patients are being treated with infertility drugs. It is also useful in detecting ECTOPIC PREGNANCY. (See also PREGNANCY AND LABOUR.)

Ultraviolet Rays (UVR)

Invisible light rays of very short wavelength beyond the violet end of the sun's spectrum. Ultraviolet-C (UVC) (wavelength <290 nm [nanometre – see APPENDIX 6: MEASUREMENTS IN MEDICINE]) is entirely absorbed by the earth's atmosphere and would otherwise be lethally damaging. Ultraviolet-B (UVB – 290–320 nm) intensity increases with altitude: it is greatest in midsummer and at midday and penetrates cirrhus cloud. UVB causes sunburn and also tanning. Ultraviolet-A (UVA – 320–400 nm) penetrates deeper into our skins but does not cause sunburn; it is implicated in many photochemical reactions and PHOTO-

DERMATOSES and in CARCINOGENESIS. UVR helps the skin to synthesise vitamin D.

Ultraviolet lamps produce UVR and are used to tan skin but, because of the risk of producing skin cancer (see SKIN, DISEASES OF), the lamps must be used with great caution.

Umbilical Cord

The fleshy tube containing two arteries and a vein through which the mother supplies the FETUS with oxygen and nutrients. The cord, which is up to 60 cm long, ceases to function after birth and is clamped and cut about 2·5 cm from the infant's abdominal wall. The stump shrivels and falls off within two weeks, leaving a scar which forms the UMBILICUS. (See also PREGNANCY AND LABOUR.)

Umbilicus

The scientific name for the navel, a circular depression in the ABDOMEN that marks the areas where the UMBILICAL CORD was attached when the fetus was in the uterus.

Uncinate Fit

A type of temporal lobe EPILEPSY in which a patient has a hallucination of smell or of taste; it may also be the result of a tumour pressing on that part of the BRAIN concerned with the appreciation of smell and taste.

Unconscious

A state of UNCONSCIOUSNESS or a description of mental activities of which an individual is unaware. The term is also used in PSYCHOANALYSIS to characterise that section of a person's mind in which memories and motives reside. They are normally inaccessible, protected by inbuilt mental resistance. This contrasts with the subconscious, where a person's memories and motives – while temporarily suppressed – can usually be recalled.

Unconsciousness

The BRAIN is the organ of the mind. Normal conscious alertness depends upon its continuous adequate supply with oxygen and glucose, both of which are essential for the brain cells to function normally. If either or both of these are interrupted, altered consciousness results. Interruption may be caused by three broad types of process affecting the brain stem: the reticular formation (a network of nerve pathways and nuclei-connecting sensory and motor nerves to and from the cerebrum, cerebellum, SPINAL CORD and cranial nerves) and the cerebral cortex. The three types are diffuse brain dysfunction – for example, generalised metabolic disorders such as URAEMIA or toxic disorders such as SEPTICAEMIA; direct effects on the brain stem as a result of infective, cancerous or traumatic lesions; and indirect effects on the brain stem such as a tumour or OEDEMA in the cerebrum creating pressure within the skull. Within these three divisions are a large number of specific causes of unconsciousness.

Unconsciousness may be temporary, prolonged or indefinite (see PERSISTENT VEGETATIVE STATE (PVS)), depending upon the severity of the initiating incident. The patient's recovery depends upon the cause and success of treatment, where given. MEMORY may be affected, as may motor and sensory functions; but short periods of unconsciousness as a result, say, of trauma have little obvious effect on brain function. Repeated bouts of unconsciousness (which can happen in boxing) may, however, have a cumulatively damaging effect, as can be seen on CT (COMPUTED TOMOGRAPHY) scans of the brain.

POISONS such as CARBON MONOXIDE (CO), drug overdose, a fall in the oxygen content of blood (HYPOXIA) in lung or heart disease, or liver or kidney failure harm the normal chemical working or metabolism of nerve cells. Severe blood loss will cause ANOXIA of the brain. Any of these can result in altered brain function in which impairment of consciousness is a vital sign.

Sudden altered consciousness will also result from fainting attacks (syncope) in which the blood pressure falls and the circulation of oxygen is thereby reduced. Similarly an epileptic fit causes partial or complete loss of consciousness by causing an abrupt but temporary disruption of the electrical activity in the nerve cells in the brain (see EPILEPSY).

In these events, as the brain's function progressively fails, drowsiness, stupor and finally COMA ensue. If the cause is removed (or when the patient spontaneously recovers from a fit or faint), normal consciousness is usually quickly regained. Strokes (see STROKE) are sometimes accompanied by a loss of consciousness; this may be immediate or come on slowly, depending upon the cause or site of the strokes.

Comatose patients are graded according to agreed test scales – for example, the GLASGOW COMA SCALE – in which the patient's response to a series of tests indicate numerically the level of coma.

Treatment of unconscious patients depends upon the cause, and range from first-aid care for someone who has fainted to hospital intensive-care treatment for a victim of a severe head injury or massive stroke.

U

Undescended Testis
See under TESTICLE, DISEASES OF.

Undulant Fever
Another name for BRUCELLOSIS.

Ungual
An adjective relating to the fingernails or toenails.

Unguentum
The Latin name for ointment.

Unit
The term applied to a quantity assumed as a standard for measurement. Thus, the unit of insulin is the specific activity contained in such an amount of the standard preparation as the Medical Research Council may from time to time indicate as the quantity exactly equivalent to the unit accepted for international use. The standard preparation consists of pure, dry, crystalline insulin. (See APPENDIX 6: MEASUREMENTS IN MEDICINE.)

Upper Limb Disorders
A group of injuries resulting from overuse of a part of the limb. One example is TENNIS ELBOW (epicondylitis) caused by inflammation of the tendon attaching the extensor muscles of the forearm to the humerus because of overuse of the muscles. Overuse of the shoulder muscles may cause inflammation and pain around the joint. Perhaps the best-known example is repetitive strain injury (RSI) affecting keyboard workers and musicians: the result is pain in and weakness of the wrists and fingers. This has affected thousands of people and been the subject of litigation by employees against their employers. Working practices have been improved and the complaint is now being recognised at an early stage. Treatment includes PHYSIOTHERAPY, but some sufferers have been obliged to give up their work.

Urachus
A corded structure which extends from the bladder up to the navel, and represents the remains of the canal which in the FETUS joins the bladder with the ALLANTOIS.

Uraemia
The clinical state which results from renal failure (see KIDNEYS, DISEASES OF). It may be due to disease of the KIDNEYS or it may be the result of pre-renal causes where a lack of circulating blood volume inadequately perfuses the kidneys. It may result from acute necrosis in the tubules of the kidney or it may result from obstruction to the outflow of URINE.

The word uraemia means excess UREA in the blood; however, the symptoms of renal failure are not due to the abnormal amounts of urea circulating, but rather to the electrolyte disturbances (see ELECTROLYTES) and ACIDOSIS which are associated with impaired renal function. The acidosis results from a decreased ability to filter hydrogen ions from blood into the glomerular fluid: the reduced production of ammonia and phosphate means fewer ions capable of combining with the hydrogen ions, so that the total acid elimination is diminished. The fall in glomerular filtration also leads to retention of SODIUM and water with resulting OEDEMA, and to retention of POTASSIUM resulting in HYPERKALAEMIA.

The most important causes of uraemia are the primary renal diseases of chronic glomerular nephritis (inflammation) and chronic PYELONEPHRITIS. It may also result from MALIGNANT HYPERTENSION damaging the kidneys and amyloid disease destroying them. Analgesic abuse can cause tubular necrosis. DIABETES MELLITUS may cause a nephropathy and lead to uraemia, as may MYELOMATOSIS and SYSTEMIC LUPUS ERYTHEMATOSUS (SLE). Polycystic kidneys and renal tuberculosis account for a small proportion of cases.

Symptoms Uraemia is sometimes classed as acute – that is, those cases in which the symptoms develop in a few hours or days – and chronic, including cases in which the symptoms are less marked and last over weeks, months, or years. There is, however, no dividing line between the two, for in the chronic variety, which may be said to consist of the symptoms of chronic glomerulonephritis, an acute attack is liable to come on at any time.

Headache in the front or back of the head, accompanied often by insomnia and daytime drowsiness, is one of the most common symptoms. UNCONSCIOUSNESS of a profound type, which may be accompanied by CONVULSIONS resembling those of EPILEPSY, is the most outstanding feature of an acute attack and is a very dangerous condition.

Still another symptom, which often precedes an acute attack, is severe vomiting without apparent cause. The appetite is always poor, and the onset of diarrhoea is a serious sign.

Treatment The treatment of the chronic type of uraemia includes all the measures which should be taken by a person suffering from chronic glomerulonephritis (see under KIDNEYS, DISEASES OF). An increasing number of these patients, especially the younger ones, are treated with DIALYSIS and/or renal TRANSPLANTATION.

Urates
See URIC ACID.

Urea
Urea, or carbomide, is a crystalline substance of the chemical formula $CO(NH_2)_2$, which is very soluble in water or alcohol. It is the chief waste product discharged from the body in the URINE, being formed in the liver and carried to the kidneys in the blood. The amount varies considerably with the quantity and nature of the food taken, rising greatly upon an animal (protein) dietary. It also rises during the continuance of a fever. The average amount excreted daily by a healthy adult on a mixed diet is about 33–35 grams. Kidney failure causes a rise in the concentration of urea in the blood (see URAEMIA; KIDNEYS, DISEASES OF).

Urea is usually administered for its diuretic action (see DIURETICS), and also as a test of kidney action, in doses of 5–15 grams. It is used, too, as a cream in the treatment of certain skin diseases, characterised by a dry skin.

Urea is rapidly changed, by a yeast-like micro-organism, into carbonate of ammonia – the cause of the ammoniacal smell associated with INCONTINENCE and inadequately cleaned toilets.

Ureaplasma
A group of micro-organisms which plays a larger part in the causation of disease than was at one time suspected. One of them, *Ureaplasma urealyticum*, is now recognised as a cause of chronic prostatitis (see under PROSTATE GLAND, DISEASES OF), NON-SPECIFIC URETHRITIS (NSU) – see also URETHRA, DISEASES OF AND INJURY TO – and INFERTILITY.

Ureter
The tube that carries URINE from the kidney (see KIDNEYS) to the URINARY BLADDER. There are two ureters, one for each kidney, and they originate from the kidney pelvis and track for 25–30 cm (10–12 inches) through the loins and pelvis. They open by a narrow slit into the base of the bladder. The lower end of the ureter pierces the wall of the bladder so obliquely (lying embedded in the wall for about 21 mm) that, although urine runs freely into the bladder, it is prevented from returning up the ureter as the bladder becomes distended.

Ureteroenterostomy
A surgically produced artificial channel between the URETER and the large bowel (see INTESTINE). A form of diversion of the URINE flow, the URINARY BLADDER is bypassed and the ureters drain into the sigmoid COLON. The operation is done when a bladder is removed, usually because of cancer.

Ureteroscope
A flexible or rigid endoscopic instrument (see ENDOSCOPE) that is inserted (via the URINARY BLADDER) into the URETER and up into the pelvis of the kidney (see KIDNEYS). The instrument is commonly used to identify a stone in the ureter and to remove it under vision with forceps or a stone basket. If the stone is large it is broken into fragments, using an ultrasound or electrohydraulic LITHOTRIPSY probe that is inserted through the instrument.

Urethra
The tube which leads from the URINARY BLADDER to the exterior, and by which the URINE is voided. It is about 20 cm (8 inches) long in the male and 3·5 cm (1½ inches) long in the female. In the male it passes along the PENIS; in the female the urethra opens to the exterior just in front of the VAGINA between the labial folds.

Urethra, Diseases of and Injury to

Trauma Injury to the urethra is often the result of severe trauma to the pelvis – for example, in a car accident or as the result of a fall. Trauma can also result from catheter insertion (see CATHETERS) or the insertion of foreign bodies into the urethra. The signs are the inability to pass urine, and blood at the exit of the urethra. The major complication of trauma is the development of a urethral stricture (see below).

Urethritis is inflammation of the urethra from infection.

Causes The sexually transmitted disease GONORRHOEA affects the urethra, mainly in men, and causes severe inflammation and urethritis. Non-specific urethritis (NSU) is an inflammation of the urethra caused by one of many different micro-organisms including BACTERIA, YEAST and CHLAMYDIA.

Symptoms The classic signs and symptoms are a urethral discharge associated with urethral pain, particularly on micturition (passing urine), and DYSURIA.

Treatment This involves taking urethral swabs, culturing the causative organism and treating it with the appropriate antibiotic. The complications of urethritis include stricture formation.

Stricture This is an abrupt narrowing of the urethra at one or more places. Strictures can be a result of trauma or infection or a congenital abnormality from birth. Rarely, tumours can cause strictures.

Symptoms The usual presenting complaint is one of a slow urinary stream. Other symptoms include hesitancy of micturition, variable stream and terminal dribbling. Measurement of the urine flow rate may help in the diagnosis, but often strictures are detected during cystoscopy (see CYSTOSCOPE).

Treatment The traditional treatment was the periodic dilation of the strictures with 'sounds' – solid metal rods passed into the urethra. However, a more permanent solution is achieved by cutting the stricture with an endoscopic knife (optical urethrotomy). For more complicated long or multiple strictures, an open operation (urethroplasty) is required.

Urethral Syndrome

A group of symptoms of unknown cause. It mainly affects women, and occasionally men, with pain and discomfort in the lower abdomen, a frequent urge to urinate and, in women, pain in the area of the VULVA. Investigation rarely results in any abnormal findings. Postmenopausal women (see MENOPAUSE), who are the most common sufferers, may have inflammation of the vulva due to thinning of the tissues in that area. Treatment is supportive, with the patient being advised to drink a lot of fluid and maintain a high standard of personal hygiene.

Urethritis

Urethritis means inflammation of the URETHRA (see NON-SPECIFIC URETHRITIS (NSU); URETHRA, DISEASES OF AND INJURY TO).

Urethrocele

PROLAPSE of the URETHRA into the wall of the VAGINA. The result is a bulbous swelling in the roof of the vagina which is worse when the woman strains to urinate or defaecate, or during childbirth. The condition is usually the consequence of a previous pregnancy. The condition is treated with surgical repair of the slack tissues to strengthen support for the urethra and vaginal wall.

Urethrography

Examination of the URETHRA using X-RAYS. A radio-opaque fluid is injected into the bladder and any abnormalities of the urethra can be observed on the X-ray films.

Urethroplasty

Surgical repair of the URETHRA, usually to relieve a stricture (see under URETHRA, DISEASES OF AND INJURY TO).

Uric Acid

A crystalline substance, very slightly soluble in water, of chemical formula, $C_5N_4H_4O_3$. The average daily quantity of uric acid passed by human beings is 0·5–1 gram. It is formed in the LIVER from the breakdown products of proteins and removed by the KIDNEYS from the blood. The amount is increased in the following conditions:

- Excessive consumption of meat, combined with sedentary habits.
- GOUT.
- Diseases in which the white corpuscles of the blood are increased: for example, LEUKAEMIA.
- The bi-urate of sodium and urate of ammonium occur in considerable amounts in the URINE during a feverish state or after great exertion, and produce, as the urine cools, a dense pink or yellow sediment. Owing to their insolubility, uric acid and the various urates often produce deposits in the urinary passages, which are known as urinary sand, gravel, or stones according to their size.

Uricosuric Drug

A drug that increases the amount of URIC ACID excreted in the URINE. Among the drugs used are PROBENECID or a sulfa derivative. Uricosurics are used to treat GOUT and other disorders which cause raised blood-uric-acid concentrations.

Urinalysis

Analysis of the physical and chemical composition of URINE to detect variations in the substances normally present, and to identify any abnormal constituents such as sugar, blood, drugs or alcohol. Sugar, protein and blood can be identified using chemically impregnated dipsticks which change colour in the presence of these substances. The presence of microscopic HAEMATURIA (blood in the urine) should be confirmed by microscopic examination of a fresh, midstream urine specimen. The specimen should also be sent for bacteriological culture to exclude or identify infection. If protein in the urine is suspected, a 24-hour collection of urine should be assessed. Cytological examination will identify abnormal or malignant cells in the urinary tract.

Urinary Bladder

The urinary bladder is a highly distensible organ for storing URINE. It consists of smooth muscle known as the detrusor muscle and is lined with urine-proof cells known as transitional cell epithelium.

The bladder lies in the anterior half of the PELVIS, bordered in front by the pubis bone and laterally by the side wall of the pelvis. Superiorly the bladder is covered by the peritoneal lining of the abdomen. The bottom or base of the bladder lies against the PROSTATE GLAND in the male and the UTERUS and VAGINA in the female.

Urinary Bladder, Diseases of

Diseases of the URINARY BLADDER are diagnosed by the patient's symptoms and signs, examination of the URINE, and using investigations such as X-RAYS and ULTRASOUND scans. The interior of the bladder can be examined using a cystoscope, which is a fibreoptic endoscope (see FIBREOPTIC ENDOSCOPY) that is passed into the bladder via the URETHRA.

Cystitis Most cases of cystitis are caused by bacteria which have spread from the bowel, especially *Escherichia coli*, and entered the bladder via the urethra. Females are more prone to cystitis than are males, owing to their shorter urethra which allows easier entry for bacteria. Chronic or recurrent cystitis may result in infection spreading up the ureter to the kidney (see KIDNEY, DISEASES OF).

Symptoms Typically there is frequency and urgency of MICTURITION, with stinging and burning on passing urine (dysuria), which is often smelly or bloodstained. In severe infection patients develop fever and rigors, or loin pain. Before starting treatment a urine sample should be obtained for laboratory testing, including identification of the invading bacteria.

Treatment This includes an increased fluid intake, ANALGESICS, doses of potassium citrate to make the urine alkaline to discourage

bacterial growth, and an appropriate course of ANTIBIOTICS once a urine sample has been analysed in the laboratory to confirm the diagnosis and determine what antibiotics the causative organism is likely to respond to.

Stone or calculus The usual reason for the formation of a bladder stone is an obstruction to the bladder outflow, which results in stagnant residual urine – ideal conditions for the crystallisation of the chemicals that form stones – or from long-term indwelling CATHETERS which weaken the natural mechanical protection against bacterial entry and, by bruising the lining tissues, encourage infection.

Symptoms The classic symptom is a stoppage in the flow of urine during urination, associated with severe pain and the passage of blood.

Treatment This involves surgical removal of the stone either endoscopically (litholapaxy); by passing a cystoscope into the bladder via the urethra and breaking the stone; or by LITHO-TRIPSY in which the stone (or stones) is destroyed by applying ultrasonic shock waves. If the stone cannot be destroyed by these methods, the bladder is opened and the stone removed (cystolithotomy).

Cancer Cancer of the bladder accounts for 7 per cent of all cancers in men and 2·5 per cent in women. The incidence increases with age, with smoking and with exposure to the industrial chemicals, beta-napththylamine and benzidine. In 2003, 2,884 men and 1,507 women died of bladder cancer in England and Wales.

Symptoms The classical presenting symptom of a bladder cancer is the painless passing of blood in the urine – haematuria. All patients with haematuria must be investigated with an X-ray of their kidneys, an INTRAVENOUS PYELOGRAM (UROGRAM) and a cystoscopy.

Treatment Superficial bladder tumours on the lining of the bladder can be treated by local removal via the cystoscope using DIATHERMY (cystodiathermy). Invasive cancers into the bladder muscle are usually treated with RADIO-THERAPY, systemic CHEMOTHERAPY or surgical removal of the bladder (cystectomy). Local chemotherapy may be useful in some patients with multiple small tumours.

Urinary Diversion

One of a variety of procedures for collecting and diverting URINE from its customary channel of excretion following surgical removal of the bladder for disease, usually cancer. The ureters (see URETER) may be implanted in the large bowel, or a reservoir or small pouch may be fashioned using a section of small or large INTESTINE. In the latter method the pouch is emptied through a small STOMA using a catheter (see CATHETERS), thus dispensing with the need for a urinary drainage bag.

Urinary Tract

A collective name for the KIDNEYS, ureters (see URETER), URINARY BLADDER and URETHRA, which between them produce, collect and void URINE.

Urination

The act of voiding URINE through the URETHRA. Abnormalities in urination such as difficulty in starting or stopping, greater than normal frequency, unusually small amounts of urine passed, a constant feeling of wanting to urinate or a sudden hard-to-control urge to urinate are all symptoms that suggest possible disorders of the urinary tract which merit investigation.

Urine

Waste substances resulting from the body's metabolic processes, selected by the KIDNEYS from the blood, dissolved in water, and excreted. Urine is around 96 per cent water, the chief waste substances being UREA (approximately 25 g/1), common salt (approximately 9 g/l), and phosphates and sulphates of potassium, sodium, calcium, and magnesium. There are also small amounts of URIC ACID, ammonia, creatinine, and various pigments. Poisons, such as MORPHINE, may be excreted in the urine; and in many infections, such as typhoid fever (see ENTERIC FEVER), the causative organism may be excreted.

The daily urine output varies, but averages around 1,500 ml in adults, less in children. The fluid intake and fluid output (urine and PERSPIRATION) are interdependent, so as to maintain a relatively constant fluid balance. Urine output is increased in certain diseases, notably DIABETES MELLITUS; it is diminished (or even temporarily stopped) in acute glomerulonephritis (see under KIDNEYS, DISEASES OF), heart failure, and fevers generally. Failure of the kidneys to secrete any urine is known as anuria, while stoppage due to obstruction of the ureters (see URETER) by stones, or of the URETHRA by a stricture, despite normal urinary secretion, is known as urinary retention.

Normal urine is described as straw- to amber-coloured, but may be changed by various diseases or drugs. Chronic glomerulonephritis or poorly controlled diabetes may lead to a watery appearance, as may drinking large amounts of water. Consumption of beetroot or rhubarb may lead to an orange or red colour, while passage of blood in the urine (haematuria) results in a pink or bright red appearance, or a smoky tint if just small amounts are passed. A greenish urine is usually due to BILE, or may be produced by taking QUININE.

Healthy urine has a faint aroma, but gives off an unpleasant ammoniacal smell when it begins to decompose, as may occur in urinary infections. Many foods and additives give urine a distinctive odour; garlic is particularly characteristic. The density or specific gravity of urine varies normally from 1,015 to 1,025: a low value suggests chronic glomerulonephritis, while a high value may occur in uncontrolled diabetes or during fevers. Urine is normally acidic, which has an important antiseptic action; it may at times become alkaline, however, and in vegetarians, owing to the large dietary consumption of alkaline salts, it is permanently alkaline.

Chemical or microscopical examination of the urine is necessary to reveal abnormal drugs, poisons, or micro-organisms. There are six substances which must be easily detectable for diagnostic purposes: these are ALBUMINS, blood, GLUCOSE, bile, ACETONE, and PUS and tube-casts (casts from the lining of the tubules in the kidneys). Easily used strip tests are available for all of these, except the last.

Excess of urine It is important to distinguish urinary frequency from increase in the total amount of urine passed. Frequency may be due to reduced bladder capacity, such as may be caused by an enlarged PROSTATE GLAND, or due to any irritation or infection of the kidneys or bladder, such as CYSTITIS or the formation of a stone. Increased total urinary output, on the other hand, is often a diagnostic feature of diabetes mellitus. Involuntary passage of urine at night may result, leading to bed wetting, or NOCTURNAL ENURESIS in children. Diagnosis of either condition, therefore, means that the urine should be tested for glucose, albumin, gravel (fragments of urinary calculi), and pus, with appropriate treatment.

Urine Retention

This occurs when URINE is produced by the kidneys but not voided by the bladder. It is generally less serious than ANURIA, in which urine is not produced.

Causes Neurological injury, such as trauma to the spinal cord, may cause bladder weakness, leading to retention, although this is rare. Obstruction to outflow is more common: this may be acute and temporary, for example after childbirth or following surgery for piles (HAEMORRHOIDS); or chronic, for example, with prostatic enlargement (see PROSTATE GLAND). Commonly seen in elderly men, this leads to reduced bladder capacity, with partial emptying every few hours. Total retention is rare, but may result from a stricture, or narrowing, of the URETHRA (see also URETHRA, DISEASES OF AND INJURY TO) – usually the result of infection or injury – or to pressure from a large neighbouring tumour.

Retention is generally treated by regular use of a urethral catether (see CATHETERS), various types of which are available. Tapping of the bladder with a needle passed above the pubis is rarely necessary, but may occasionally be required in cases of severe stricture.

Urinometer

A simple instrument designed for estimating the specific gravity of URINE – a test that can be helpful in diagnosing disorders of the URINARY TRACT.

Urobilinogen

A chemical compound formed when bacteria in the intestine act on BILIRUBIN. Some is reabsorbed and returns to the LIVER and some is eliminated in the faeces.

Urocele

A cystic swelling that develops in the SCROTUM when URINE escapes from the URETHRA, usually after injury. Prompt treatment is necessary and this is done by diverting the urine by inserting a suprapubic catheter (see CATHETERS) into the URINARY BLADDER, draining the cystocele and giving the patients antibiotics. The injured urethra can be surgically repaired later.

Urodynamics

The measurement of the pressures within the URINARY BLADDER as well as the pressures of the urethral sphincter. The technique is useful in the investigation of patients with urinary incontinence. Special equipment is needed to carry out the procedure.

Urogenital

An adjective relating to the organs and tissues involved in the anatomically closely related functions of excretion and reproduction.

Urography

Examination of the URINARY TRACT by means of contrast medium X-rays (see PYELOGRAPHY; URETHROGRAPHY).

Urokinase

Urokinase is an ENZYME obtained from URINE which dissolves blood clots. It is used to treat THROMBOLYSIS in the EYE, in arteriovenous shunts (see SHUNT) and deep-vein THROMBOSIS. It has the advantage over other fibrinolytic drugs of not causing immunological reactions.

Urology

The branch of medicine which treats disorders and diseases of the KIDNEYS, ureters (see URETER), URINARY BLADDER, PROSTATE GLAND, and URETHRA.

Ursodeoxycholic Acid

A preparation used in the treatment of cholesterol gall-stones when laparoscopic CHOLECYSTECTOMY and endoscopic biliary procedures cannot be used (see GALL-BLADDER, DISEASES OF).

URTI

An abbreviation for upper respiratory tract infection – that is colds (see COMMON COLD), otitis media (see EAR, DISEASES OF – Diseases of the middle ear), TONSILLITIS, PHARYNGITIS and laryngo-tracheo-bronchitis (see CROUP; LARYNX, DISORDERS OF).

Urticaria

The rash produced by the sudden release of HISTAMINE in the skin. It is characterised by acute itching, redness and wealing which subsides within a few minutes or may persist for a day or more. Depending upon the cause, it may be localised or widespread and transient or constantly recurrent over years. It has many causes.

External injuries to the skin such as the sting of a nettle ('nettle-rash') or an insect bite cause histamine release from MAST CELLS in the skin directly. Certain drugs, especially MORPHINE, CODEINE and ASPIRIN, can have the same effect. In other cases, histamine release is caused by an allergic mechanism, mediated by ANTIBODIES of the immunoglobulin E (IgE) class – see IMMUNOGLOBULINS. Thus many foods, food additives and drugs (such as PENICILLIN) can cause urticaria. Massive release of histamine may affect mucous membranes – namely the tongue or throat – and can cause HYPOTENSION and anaphylactic shock (see ANAPHYLAXIS) which can occasionally be fatal.

Physical factors can cause urticaria. Heat, exercise and emotional stress may induce a singular pattern with small pinhead weals, but widespread flares of ERYTHEMA, activated via the AUTONOMIC NERVOUS SYSTEM (CHOLINERGIC urticaria) may also occur.

Rarely, exposure to cold may have a smiilar effect ('cold urticaria') and anaphylactic shock following a dive into cold water in winter is occasionally fatal. The diagnosis of cold urticaria can be confirmed by applying a block of ice to the arm which quickly induces a local weal.

Transient urticaria due to rubbing or even stroking the skin is common in young adults (DERMOGRAPHISM or factitious urticaria). More prolonged deep pressure induces delayed urticaria in other subjects. IgE-mediated urticaria is part of the atopic spectrum (see ATOPY, and SKIN, DISEASES OF – Dermatitis and eczema). Allergy to peanuts is particularly dangerous in young atopic subjects. Notwithstanding the many known causes, chronic urticaria of unknown cause is common and may have an autoimmune basis (see AUTOIMMUNE DISORDERS).

Treatment Causative factors must be removed. Topical therapy is ineffective except for the use of calamine lotion, which reduces itching by cooling the skin. Oral ANTIHISTAMINES are the mainstay of treatment and are remarkably safe. Rarely, injection of ADRENALINE is needed as emergency treatment of massive urticaria, especially if the tongue and throat are involved, following by a short course of the oral steroid, prednisolone.

Angio-oedema is a variant of urticaria where massive OEDEMA involves subcutaneous tissues rather than the skin. It may have many causes but bee and wasp stings in sensitised subjects are particularly dangerous. There is also a rare hereditary form of angio-oedema. Acute airway obstruction due to submucosal oedema of the tongue or larynx is best treated with immediate intramuscular adrenaline and antihistamine. Rarely, TRACHEOSTOMY may be life-saving. Patients who have had two or more episodes can be taught self-injection with a preloaded adrenaline syringe.

Uterus

A hollow, triangular organ, flattened from front to back, the lower angle (or cervix) commincates through a narrow opening (the os uteri) with the VAGINA. The uterus or womb is where the fertilised ovum (egg) normally becomes embedded and in which the EMBRYO and FETUS develop. The normal uterus weighs 30–40 g; during pregnancy, however, enormous growth occurs together with muscular thickening (see MUSCLE – Development of muscle). The cavity is lined by a thick, soft, mucous membrane, and the wall is chiefly composed of muscle fibres arranged in three layers. The outer surface, like that of other abdominal organs, is covered by a layer of PERITONEUM. The uterus has a copious supply of blood derived from the uterine and ovarian arteries. It has also many lymphatic vessels, and its nerves establish wide connections with other organs (see PAIN). The position of the uterus is in the centre of the PELVIS, where it is suspended by several ligaments between the URINARY BLADDER in front and the RECTUM behind. On each side of the uterus are the broad ligaments passing outwards to the side of the pelvis, the utero-sacral ligament passing back to the sacral bone, the utero-vesical ligament passing forwards to the bladder, and the round ligament uniting the uterus to the front of the abdomen.

Uterus, Diseases of

Absence or defects of the uterus

Rarely, the UTERUS may be completely absent as a result of abnormal development. In such patients secondary sexual development is normal but MENSTRUATION is absent (primary amennorhoea). The chromosomal make-up of the patient must be checked (see CHROMOSOMES; GENES): in a few cases the genotype is male (testicular feminisation syndrome). No treatment is available, although the woman should be counselled.

The uterus develops as two halves which fuse together. If the fusion is incomplete, a uterine SEPTUM results. Such patients with a double uterus (uterus didelphys) may have fertility problems which can be corrected by surgical removal of the uterine septum. Very rarely there may be two uteri with a double vagina.

The uterus of most women points forwards (anteversion) and bends forwards (anteflexion). However, about 25 per cent of women have a uterus which is pointed backwards (retroversion) and bent backwards (retroflexion). This is a normal variant and very rarely gives rise to any problems. If it does, the attitude of the uterus can be corrected by an operation called a ventrosuspension.

Endometritis The lining of the uterine cavity is called the ENDOMETRIUM. It is this layer that is partially shed cyclically in women of

reproductive age giving rise to menstruation. Infection of the endometrium is called endometritis and usually occurs after a pregnancy or in association with the use of an intrauterine contraceptive device (IUCD – see CONTRACEPTION). The symptoms are usually of pain, bleeding and a fever. Treatment is with antibiotics. Unless the FALLOPIAN TUBES are involved and damaged, subsequent fertility is unaffected. Very rarely, the infection is caused by TUBERCULOSIS. Tuberculous endometritis may destroy the endometrium causing permanent amenorrhoea and sterility.

Menstrual disorders are common. Heavy periods (menorrhagia) are often caused by fibroids (see below) or adenomyosis (see below) or by anovulatory cycles. Anovulatory cycles result in the endometrium being subjected to unopposed oestrogen stimulation and occasionally undergoing hyperplasia. Treatment is with cyclical progestogens (see PROGESTOGEN) initially. If this form of treatment fails, endoscopic surgery to remove the endometrium may be successful. The endometrium may be removed using LASER (endometrial laser ablation) or electrocautery (transcervical resection of endometrium). Hysterectomy (see below) will cure the problem if endoscopic surgery fails. Adenomyosis is a condition in which endometrial tissue is found in the muscle layer (myometrium) of the uterus. It usually presents as heavy and painful periods, and occasionally pain during intercourse. Hysterectomy is usually required.

Oligomenorrhoea (scanty or infrequent periods) may be caused by a variety of conditions including thyroid disease (see THYROID GLAND, DISEASES OF). It is most commonly associated with usage of the combined oral contraceptive pill. Once serious causes have been eliminated, the patient should be reassured. No treatment is necessary unless conception is desired, in which case the patient may require induction of ovulation.

Primary amenorrhoea means that the patient has never had a period. She should be investigated, although usually it is only due to an inexplicable delay in the onset of periods (delayed menarche) and not to any serious condition. Secondary amenorrhoea is the cessation of periods after menstruation has started. The most common cause is pregnancy. It may be also caused by endocrinological or hormonal problems, tuberculous endometritis, emotional problems and severe weight loss. The treatment of amenorrhoea depends on the cause.

Dysmenorrhoea, or painful periods, is the most common disorder; in most cases the cause is unknown, although the disorder may be due to excessive production of PROSTAGLANDINS.

Irregular menstruation (variations from the woman's normal menstrual pattern or changes in the duration of bleeding or the amount) can be the result of a disturbance in the balance of OESTROGENS and PROGESTERONE hormone which between them regulate the cycle. For some time after the MENARCHE or before the MENOPAUSE, menstruation may be irregular. If irregularity occurs in a woman whose periods are normally regular, it may be due to unsuspected pregnancy, early miscarriage or to disorders in the uterus, OVARIES or pelvic cavity. The woman should seek medical advice.

Fibroids (leiomyomata) are benign tumours arising from the smooth muscle layer (myometrium) of the uterus. They are found in 80 per cent of women but only a small percentage give rise to any problems and may then require treatment. They may cause heavy periods and occasionally pain. Sometimes they present as a mass arising from the pelvis with pressure symptoms from the bladder or rectum. Although they can be shrunk medically using gonadorelin analogues, which raise the plasma concentrations of LUTEINISING HORMONE and FOLLICLE-STIMULATING HORMONE, this is not a long-term solution. In any case, fibroids only require treatment if they are large or enlarging, or if they cause symptoms. Treatment is either myomectomy (surgical removal) if fertility is to be retained, or a hysterectomy.

Uterine cancers tend to present after the age of 40 with abnormal bleeding (intermenstrual or postmenopausal bleeding). They are usually endometrial carcinomas. Eighty per cent present with early (Stage I) disease. Patients with operable cancers should be treated with total abdominal hysterectomy and bilateral excision of the ovaries and Fallopian tubes. Post-operative RADIOTHERAPY is usually given to those patients with adverse prognostic factors. Pre-operative radiotherapy is still given by some centres, although this practice is now regarded as outdated. PROGESTOGEN treatment may be extremely effective in cases of recurrence, but its value remains unproven when used as adjuvant treatment. In 2003 in England and Wales, more than 2,353 women died of uterine cancer.

Disorders of the cervix The cervix (neck of the womb) may produce an excessive

U

discharge due to the presence of a cervical ect-opy or ectropion. In both instances columnar epithelium – the layer of secreting cells – which usually lines the cervical canal is exposed on its surface. Asymptomatic patients do not require treatment. If treatment is required, cryocautery – local freezing of tissue – is usu-ally effective.

Cervical smears are taken and examined in the laboratory to detect abnormal cells shed from the cervix. Its main purpose is to detect cervical intraepithelial neoplasia (CIN) – the presence of malignant cells in the surface tissue lining the cervix – since up to 40 per cent of women with this condition will develop cervical cancer if the CIN is left untreated. Women with abnormal smears should undergo colposcopy, a painless investigation using a low-powered microscope to inspect the cervix. If CIN is found, treatment consists of simply removing the area of abnormal skin, either using a diathermy loop or laser instrument.

Unfortunately, cervical cancer remains the most common of gynaecological cancers. The most common type is squamous cell carcinoma and around 4,000 new cases (all types) are diagnosed in England and Wales every year. As many as 50 per cent of the women affected may die from the disease within five years. Cervical cancer is staged clinically in four bands accord-ing to how far it has extended, and treatment is determined by this staging. Stage I involves only the mucosal lining of the cervix and cone BIOPSY may be the best treatment in young women wanting children. In Stage IV the dis-ease has spread beyond the cervix, uterus and pelvis to the URINARY BLADDER or REC-TUM. For most women, radiotherapy or radical Wertheim's hysterectomy – the latter being preferable for younger women – is the treat-ment of choice if the cancer is diagnosed early, both resulting in survival rates of five years in 80 per cent of patients. Wertheim's hyster-ectomy is a major operation in which the uterus, cervix, upper third of vagina and the tissue surrounding the cervix are removed together with the LYMPH NODES draining the area. The ovaries may be retained if desired. Patients with cervical cancer are treated by radiotherapy, either because they present too late for surgery or because the surgical skill to perform a radical hysterectomy is not available. These operations are best performed by gynae-cological oncologists who are gynaecological surgeons specialising in the treatment of gynae-cological tumours. The role of CHEMOTHERAPY in cervical and uterine cancer is still being evaluated.

Prolapse of the uterus is a disorder in which the organ drops from its normal situ-ation down into the vagina. First-degree pro-lapse is a slight displacement of the uterus, second-degree a partial displacement and third-degree when the uterus can be seen outside the VULVA. It may be accompanied by a CYSTO-COELE (the bladder bulges into the front wall of the vagina), urethrocoele (the urethra bulges into the vagina) and rectocoele (the rectal wall bulges into the rear wall of the vagina). Prolapse most commonly occurs in middle-aged women who have had children, but the condition is much less common now than in the past when prenatal and obstetric care was poor, women had more pregnancies and their general health was poor. Treatment is with pelvic exercises, surgical repair of the vagina or hysterectomy. If the woman does not want or is not fit for

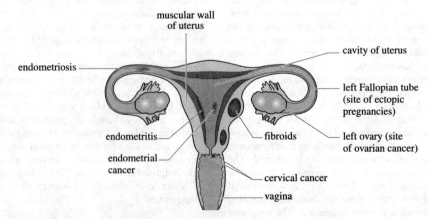

Vertical section of female reproductive tract (viewed from front) showing sites of common gynaecological disorders.

muscular wall of uterus

cavity of uterus

endometriosis

left Fallopian tube (site of ectopic pregnancies)

endometritis

fibroids

left ovary (site of ovarian cancer)

endometrial cancer

cervical cancer

vagina

surgery, an internal support called a pessary can be fitted – and changed periodically.

Hysterectomy Many serious conditions of the uterus have traditionally been treated by hysterectomy, or removal of the uterus. It remains a common surgical operation in the UK, but is being superseded in the treatment of some conditions, such as persistent MENOR-RHAGIA, with endometrial ablation – removal of the lining of the uterus using minimally invasive techniques, usually using an ENDOSCOPE and laser. Hysterectomy is done to treat fibroids, cancer of the uterus and cervix, menorrhagia, ENDOMETRIOSIS and sometimes for severely prolapsed uterus. Total hysterectomy is the usual type of operation: it involves the removal of the uterus and cervix and sometimes the ovaries. After hysterectomy a woman no longer menstruates and cannot become pregnant. If the ovaries have been removed as well and the woman had not reached the menopause, hormone replacement therapy (HRT – see MENOPAUSE) should be considered. Counselling helps the woman to recover from the operation which can be an emotionally challenging event for many.

Utricle

(1) Part of the membraneous labyrinth within the vestibule of the EAR.
(2) Prostatic utricle is a small sac extending out of the male URETHRA into the matrix of the PROSTATE GLAND.

Uvea

Uvea is a term applied to the middle coat of the EYE, including the iris, ciliary body and choroid.

Uveitis

An inflammation of the uveal tract (see EYE). Iritis is inflammation of the iris; cyclitis, inflammation of the ciliary body; and choroiditis, inflammation of the choroid. The symptoms and signs vary according to which part of the uveal tract is involved and tend to be recurrent. The patient may experience varying degrees of discomfort or pain, with or without blurring of vision. In many cases a cause is never found. Some known associations include various types of arthritis, some bowel diseases, virus illnesses, tuberculosis, syphilis, parasites and fungi. Treatment is with anti-inflammatory drops and occasionally steroid tablets, plus drops to dilate the pupil.

Uvula

The small mass of muscle covered by mucous membrane that hangs down from the middle of the soft PALATE on its posterior aspect. Its function is not certain and it seldom causes problems.

Uvulopalatopharyngoplasty

Surgery to excise the UVULA, part of the soft PALATE and the TONSILS. It is done to help people with severe SNORING problems but it does not always achieve a cure.

U

Vaccination

Named from vacca, Latin for cow, vaccination means inoculation with the material of cow-pox, performed to afford protection to the inoculated person against an attack of SMALL-POX, or to reduce seriousness of, and averting a fatal result from, any such attack. The term is often used, inaccurately, to refer to IMMUNISATION.

Vaccine

The name applied generally to dead or attenuated living infectious material introduced into the body, with the object of increasing its power to resist or to get rid of a disease. (See also IMMUNITY.)

Healthy people are inoculated with vaccine as a protection against a particular disease; this produces ANTIBODIES which will confer immunity against a subsequent attack of the disease. (See IMMUNISATION for programme of immunisation during childhood.)

Vaccines may be divided into two classes: stock vaccines, prepared from micro-organisms known to cause a particular disease and kept in readiness for use against that disease; and autogenous vaccines, prepared from micro-organisms which are already in the patient's body and to which the disease is due. Vaccines intended to protect against the onset of disease are of the former variety.

Autogenous vaccines are prepared by cultivating bacteria found in SPUTUM, URINE and FAECES, and in areas of inflammation such as BOILS (FURUNCULOSIS). This type of vaccine was introduced by Wright about 1903.

Anthrax vaccine was introduced in 1882 for the protection of sheep and cattle against this disease. A safe and effective vaccine for use in human beings has now been evolved. (See ANTHRAX.)

BCG vaccine is used to provide protection against TUBERCULOSIS. (See also separate entry on BCG VACCINE.)

Cholera vaccine was introduced in India about 1894. Two injections are given at an interval of at least a week; this gives a varying degree of immunity for six months. (See CHOLERA.)

Diphtheria vaccine is available in several forms. It is usually given along with tetanus and pertussis vaccine (see below) in what is known as TRIPLE VACCINE. This is given in three doses: the first at the age of two months; the second at three months; and the third at four months, with a booster dose at the age of five years. (See DIPHTHERIA.)

Hay fever vaccine is a vaccine prepared from the pollen of various grasses. It is used in gradually increasing doses for prevention of HAY FEVER in those susceptible to this condition.

Influenza vaccine A vaccine is now available for protection against INFLUENZA due to the influenza viruses A and B. Its use in Britain is customarily based on advice from the health departments according to the type of influenza expected in a particular year.

Measles, mumps and rubella (MMR) vaccines are given in combination early in the second year of life. A booster dose may prove necessary, as there is some interference between this vaccine and the most recent form of pertussis vaccine (see below) offered to children. Uptake has declined a little because of media reports suggesting a link with AUTISM – for which no reliable medical evidence (and much to the contrary) has been found by investigating epidemiologists. (See also separate entry for each disease, and for MMR VACCINE.)

Pertussis (whooping-cough) vaccine is prepared from Bordetella pertussis, and is usually given along with diphtheria and tetanus in what is known as triple vaccine. (See also WHOOPING-COUGH.)

Plague vaccine was introduced by Haffkine, and appears to give useful protection, but the duration of protection is relatively short: from two to 20 months. Two injections are given at an interval of four weeks. A reinforcing dose should be given annually to anyone exposed to PLAGUE.

Poliomyelitis vaccine gives a high degree of protection against the disease. This is given in the form of attenuated Sabin vaccine which is taken by mouth – a few drops on a lump of sugar. Reinforcing doses of polio vaccine are recommended on school entry, on leaving school, and on travel abroad to countries where POLIOMYELITIS is ENDEMIC.

Rabies vaccine was introduced by Pasteur in 1885 for administration, during the long incubation period, to people bitten by a mad dog, in order to prevent the disease from developing. (See RABIES.)

Rubella vaccine, usually given with mumps and measles vaccine in one dose – called MMR VACCINE, see also above – now provides protection against RUBELLA (German measles). It also provides immunity for adolescent girls who have not had the disease in childhood and so ensures that they will not acquire the disease during any subsequent pregnancy – thus reducing the number of congenitally abnormal children whose abnormality is the result of their being infected with rubella via their mothers before they were born.

Smallpox vaccine was the first introduced. As a result of the World Health Organisation's successful smallpox eradication campaign – it declared the disease eradicated in 1980 – there is now no medical justification for smallpox vaccination. Recently, however, there has been increased interest in the subject because of the potential threat from bioterrorism. (See also VACCINATION.)

Tetanus vaccine is given in two forms: (1) In the so-called triple vaccine, combined with diphtheria and pertussis (whooping-cough) vaccine for the routine immunisation of children (see above). (2) By itself to adults who have not been immunised in childhood and who are particularly exposed to the risk of TETANUS, such as soldiers and agricultural workers.

Typhoid vaccine was introduced by Wright and Semple for the protection of troops in the South African War and in India. TAB vaccine, containing *Salmonella typhi* (the causative organism of typhoid fever – see ENTERIC FEVER) and *Salmonella paratyphi* A and B (the organisms of paratyphoid fever – see ENTERIC FEVER) has now been replaced by typhoid monovalent vaccine, containing only *S. typhi*. The change has been made because the monovalent vaccine is less likely to produce painful arms and general malaise, and there is no evidence that the TAB vaccine gave any protection against paratyphoid fever. Two doses are given at an interval of 4–6 weeks, and give protection for 1–3 years.

Yellow fever vaccine is prepared from chick embryos injected with the living, attenuated strain (17D) of pantropic virus. Only one injection is required, and immunity persists for many years. Re-inoculation, however, is desirable every ten years. (See YELLOW FEVER.)

Haemophilus vaccine (HiB) This vaccine was introduced in the UK in 1994 to deal with the annual incidence of about 1,500 cases and 100 deaths from haemophilus MENINGITIS, SEPTICAEMIA and EPIGLOTTITIS, mostly in pre-school children. It has been remarkably successful when given as part of the primary vaccination programme at two, three and four months of age – reducing the incidence by over 95 per cent. A few cases still occur, either due to other subgroups of the organism for which the vaccine is not designed, or because of inadequate response by the child, possibly related to interference from the newer forms of pertussis vaccine (see above) given at the same time.

Meningococcal C vaccine Used in the UK from 1998, this has dramatically reduced the incidence of meningitis and septicaemia due to this organism. Used as part of the primary programme in early infancy, it does not protect against other types of meningococci.

Varicella vaccine This vaccine, used to protect against varicella (CHICKENPOX) is used in a number of countries including the United States and Japan. It has not been introduced into the UK, largely because of concerns that use in infancy would result in an upsurge in cases in adult life, when the disease may be more severe.

Pneumococcal vaccine The pneumococcus is responsible for severe and sometimes fatal childhood diseases including meningitis and septicaemia, as well as PNEUMONIA and other respiratory infections. Vaccines are available but do not protect against all strains and are reserved for special situations – such as for patients without a SPLEEN or those who are immunodeficient.

Vaccinia

Vaccinia is another term for cowpox, a disease in which vesicles form on the udders and teats of cows, due to the same virus as is responsible for SMALLPOX in humans. It is also the term used to describe the reaction to smallpox VACCINATION.

Vacuole

A space inside the cytoplasm of CELLS. It is

formed by a folding-in of the cellular membrane when the cell ingests material from the outside – for example, when white blood cells attack BACTERIA.

Vacuum Extractor

Also called a ventouse. The idea of the glass suction cup applied to the emerging head of the baby to assist in delivery was first considered by Younge in 1706, but it was not until 1954 that the modern (ventouse) vacuum extractor was introduced. The value of the ventouse as against the FORCEPS has been disputed in different clinics, the former being less popular in the UK. Indications are similar for the use of obstetric forceps. Even if the OCCIPUT is not in the anterior position, the extractor may still be applied; many obstetricians would choose forceps or perform manual rotation of the fetus in such cases.

In cases of prolongation of the first stage of labour, the ventouse may be used to accelerate dilatation of the cervix – provided that the cervix is already sufficiently dilated to allow application of the cup. The ventouse cannot be applied to the breech or face; in urgent cases of fetal distress the operation takes too long, and forceps delivery is preferred. There is some doubt about its safety when used on premature babies; many obstetricians feel that forceps delivery reduces the risk of intracranial haemorrhage. The vacuum extractor, while resulting in a slower delivery than when forceps are used, has a lower risk of damage to the mother's birth canal. (See PREGNANCY AND LABOUR – Some complications of labour.)

Vagina

The lower part of the female reproductive tract (see REPRODUCTIVE SYSTEM) through which a baby is delivered. It is a muscular passage leading from the labial entrance to the UTERUS. It is lined with mucous membrane and receives the erect PENIS during sexual intercourse. The semen is ejaculated into the upper part of the vagina; from there the sperms must pass through the cervix and uterus to fertilise the ovum in the Fallopian tube.

Vaginismus

Spasmodic painful, involuntary contraction of the opening of the VAGINA on attempted coitus (sexual intercourse). It is usually psychological in origin – due, for instance, to fear that penetration by the penis will be painful, or because of some previous traumatic incident of sexual intercourse such as rape or sexual abuse as a

child. It may also be due to some local, painful condition such as inflammation.

Vaginitis

Inflammation of the VAGINA. (See LEUCORRHOEA.)

Vagotomy

The operation of cutting the fibres of the VAGUS nerve to the stomach. It was once part of the routine surgical treatment of DUODENAL ULCER, the aim being to reduce the flow or acidity of the gastric juice. The operation is now performed on those patients who fail to respond to drug treatment. (See also STOMACH, DISEASES OF – Gastric ulcer).

Vagus

The tenth cranial nerve. Unlike the other cranial nerves, which are concerned with the special senses, or distributed to the skin and muscles of the head and neck, this nerve (as its name implies – Latin for 'wanderer'), passes downwards into the chest and abdomen, supplying branches to the throat, lungs, heart, stomach and other abdominal organs. It contains motor, secretory, sensory and vasodilator fibres.

Valgus

This term means literally knock-kneed, and is a bending inward at the knees (genu valgum), or at the ankle, as occurs in FLAT-FOOT (pes planus).

Validity

An indication of how much a clinical test or sign is an accurate indicator of the presence of disease. Reduced validity may occur because (1) identical tests repeated on the same person in similar circumstances produce variable results; (2) the same observer gets different results on successive occasions – intraobserver error; (3) different observers produce different results.

Valine

One of the essential (indispensable) AMINO ACIDS.

Valium

The proprietary name for diazepam, a widely used anxiolytic drug (see ANXIOLYTICS).

Valsalva's Manoeuvre

This is carried out by closing the mouth, holding the nose and attempting to blow hard. The manoeuvre raises pressure in the chest – and, indirectly, the abdomen – and forces air from

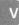

the back of the nose down the EUSTACHIAN TUBES to the middle ear. This latter effect can be used to clear the tube during descent in an aircraft, when it sometimes becomes blocked or partially blocked, producing differential pressures on the two sides of each eardrum, usually accompanied by temporary pain and deafness.

Valsalva's manoeuvre is involuntarily performed when a person strains to open his or her bowels: in these circumstances the passage of air to the lungs is blocked by instinctive closure of the vocal cords in the LARYNX. The resultant raised abdominal pressure helps to expel the bowel contents. The manoeuvre is also used in the study of cardiovascular physiology because the rise in pressure in the chest restricts the return of venous blood to the right atrium of the HEART. Pressure in the peripheral VEINS is raised and the amount of blood entering and leaving the heart falls. This drop in cardiac output may cause the subject to faint because the supply of oxygenated blood to the brain is reduced.

Valves
These cup-like structures are found in the HEART, VEINS, and lymphatic vessels (see LYMPH); they ensure that the circulation of the blood and lymph goes always in one direction.

Valvotomy
An operation that opens a stenosed heart valve (see STENOSIS; HEART, DISEASES OF) and allows it to function properly again. Various techniques are used, including a dilating instrument, a balloon or open-heart surgery.

Valvular Disease
See under HEART, DISEASES OF.

Valvuloplasty
An operation to repair or reconstruct a defective heart valve (see VALVES). It may be done as an open-heart procedure (with the patient temporarily connected to a HEART-LUNG MACHINE that maintains the circulation of oxygenated blood); alternatively, valvuloplasty can now be performed using a specially designed balloon-ended catheter (see CATHETERS) passed through the skin into a blood vessel and on to the heart. The balloon is inflated and the flaps of a narrowed (stenosed) valve are prised apart.

Vancomycin
An antibiotic derived from streptomyces, which is active against a wide range of gram-positive organisms (see BACTERIA; GRAM'S STAIN), including the STAPHYLOCOCCUS. The drug has a limited use by the intravenous route in the prophylaxis and treatment of ENDOCARDITIS and other serious infections caused by gram-positive cocci – in particular, METHICILLIN-RESISTANT STAPHYLOCOCCUS AUREUS (MRSA). It need be given only every 12 hours, although plasma concentrations should be monitored (especially in patients with renal impairment, when the dose may need marked reduction). It can both damage the middle ear and the kidney. A short course of vancomycin is effective in the treatment of antibiotic-associated COLITIS, for which it is given by mouth.

Van Den Bergh Test
A test done on SERUM from patients with JAUNDICE to discover whether the excess BILIRUBIN in the blood – which causes the jaundice – is conjugated or unconjugated. If conjugated, this indicates that HAEMOLYSIS is causing the jaundice; if unconjugated, disease of the LIVER or BILE DUCT is the likely diagnosis.

Vaporiser
A device that via a narrow nozzle turns water or a drug into a fine spray, thus enabling medicine to be taken by INHALATION. It is used, for example, in the treatment of ASTHMA.

Variance
See STANDARD DEVIATION.

Varicella
Another name for CHICKENPOX.

Varicocele
A condition in which the veins of the TESTICLE are distended. (See TESTICLE, DISEASES OF.)

Varicose Veins
VEINS that have become stretched and dilated. (See VEINS, DISEASES OF.)

Variola
Another name for SMALLPOX.

Varix
An enlarged and tortuous vein (see VEINS).

Varus
A term meaning inward displacement of a part of the body – for example, the knee (genu varum) or the ankle (talipes varus).

Vas
The Latin term for a vessel or duct, especially a blood vessel.

Vasa Efferentia
Efferent seminal ducts of the testis (see TESTICLE); these carry SEMEN from the testis to the head of the EPIDIDYMIS.

Vascular
Relating to the blood vessels.

Vasculitis
Inflammation of the blood vessels. This may damage the lining of the vessels and cause narrowing or blockage, thus restricting blood flow. This, in turn, may harm or destroy the tissues supplied by the affected blood vessels. Vasculitis is probably caused by small particles called immune complexes, circulating in the blood, that adhere to the vessel walls and provoke inflammation. Normally these complexes are consumed by the white blood cells. Vasculitis is the basic disease process in several disorders such as POLYARTERITIS NODOSA, ERYTHEMA nodosum, TEMPORAL ARTERITIS and SERUM SICKNESS.

Vas Deferens
A narrow tube that leads from each testis (see TESTICLE) through the PROSTATE GLAND to join a tube from the seminal vesicles to form the ejaculatory duct. Sperm (see SPERMATOZOON) and seminal fluid pass through this duct during ejaculation.

Vasectomy
The surgical operation performed to render men sterile, or infertile. It consists of ligating, or tying, and then cutting the ductus, or vas, deferens (see TESTICLE). It is quite a simple operation carried out under local anaesthesia, through a small incision or cut (or sometimes two) in the upper part of the SCROTUM. It has no effect on sexual drive or ejaculation, and does not cause impotency. It is not immediately effective, and several tests, spread over several months, must be carried out before it is safe to assume that sterility has been achieved. Fertility can sometimes be restored by a further operation, to restore the continuity of the vas; this cannot be guaranteed, and only seems to occur in about 20 per cent of those who have had the operation.

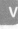

Vasoconstriction
Narrowing of blood vessels which results in the blood flow to a particular part of the body being reduced. Cold will cause vasoconstriction of the vessels under the skin, thus reducing heat loss. SHOCK due to injury or loss of blood will also provoke vasoconstriction.

Vasoconstrictors
Vasoconstrictor sympathomimetic drugs, such as EPHEDRINE and NORADRENALINE, raise the BLOOD PRESSURE temporarily by acting on receptors that constrict peripheral blood vessels. They are occasionally used as a quick way of raising blood pressure when other measures have failed, but they have potentially serious side-effects on the kidney. Vasoconstrictors are also used with local anaesthetics (see under ANAESTHESIA) to counteract the latter's vasodilator effect. Adrenaline will reduce local blood flow, slow the absorption of anaesthetic and prolong its effect.

Vasodilators
Substances that dilate blood vessels. Coronary vasodilators, such as NITRATES, CALCIUM-CHANNEL BLOCKERS and POTASSIUM-CHANNEL ACTIVATORS, are used in heart failure to improve blood supply to the heart. Peripheral vasodilators affect the blood vessels in the limbs and are used to treat conditions due to poor circulation such as CHILBLAIN and RAYNAUD'S DISEASE.

Vasomotor Centre
The description 'vasomotor' refers to control of the muscular walls of blood vessels, particularly ARTERIES, dilating or constricting their diameters. The vasomotor centre is a group of neurons (see NEURON(E)) in the MEDULLA OBLONGATA of the BRAIN; they receive messages from sensory receptors in the circulatory system, and engineer reflex alterations in the heart rate and blood-vessel diameters in order to adjust the blood pressure. The centre also receives transmission from other parts of the brain enabling emotions – fear or anger – to influence blood pressure. The vasomotor centre operates through the vasomotor nerves of the SYMPATHETIC NERVOUS SYSTEM and the PARASYMPATHETIC NERVOUS SYSTEM.

Vasomotor Nerves
Small nerve fibres that lie upon the walls of blood vessels and connect the muscle fibres of their middle coat with the NERVOUS SYSTEM. Through these nerves the blood vessels are retained in a state of moderate contraction. There are vasodilator nerves, through which are transmitted impulses that dilate the vessels, and, in the case of the skin vessels, produce the condition of blushing; there are also vasoconstrictor nerves which transmit impulses that constrict, or narrow, the blood vessels – as occurs on exposure to cold (see HYPOTHERMIA). Various drugs produce dilatation or contraction

of the blood vessels, and several of the substances produced by ENDOCRINE GLANDS in the body have these effects: for example, ADRENALINE.

Vasopressin

The fraction isolated from extract of the posterior PITUITARY GLAND lobe which stimulates intestinal activity, constricts blood vessels, and inhibits the secretion of URINE. It is also known as the antidiuretic hormone (ADH) because of this last effect, and its only use in medicine is in the treatment of DIABETES INSIPIDUS.

Vasovagal Attack

The temporary loss of consciousness caused by an abrupt slowing of the heartbeat. This may happen following SHOCK, acute pain, fear, or stress. A common cause of fainting in normal people, a vasovagal attack may be a consequence of overstimulation of the VAGUS nerve which is involved in the control of breathing and the circulation.

VD

The abbreviation for venereal disease (see SEXUALLY TRANSMITTED DISEASES (STDS)). The word 'venereal' is derived from Venus, the Roman goddess of love.

Vector

An animal that is the carrier of a particular infectious disease (see INFECTION). A vector picks up the infectious agent (bacterium – see BACTERIA; also RICKETTSIA; VIRUS) from an infected person's blood or faeces and carries it in or on its body before depositing the agent on or into a new host. Fleas, lice, mosquitoes and ticks are among common vectors of disease to humans. When a vector is used by the infectious agent to complete part of its life-cycle – for example, the malarial agent PLASMODIUM conducts part of its life-cycle in the mosquito – the vector is described as biological. If the vector simply carries the agent but is not a host for part of its life-cycle, the vector is described as mechanical. Flies, for example, may carry an infection such as bacterial dysentery from infected faeces to the fingers of another 'host'.

Veganism

A strict form of VEGETARIANISM. Vegans do not eat meat, dairy produce, eggs or fish.

Vegetarianism

Restriction of one's diet, for health, cultural or humanitarian reasons, to foods of fruit or vegetable origin. Most vegetarians, while excluding

meat and fish from their diets, include foods of animal origin, such as milk, cheese, eggs, and butter. Such a diet should supply an adequate balance of nutrients, although people with special dietary requirements – such as pregnant or feeding mothers, and very strict vegetarians – may require dietary supplements (see APPENDIX 5: VITAMINS).

Vegetations

Roughenings, comprising FIBRIN and blood cells, that appear upon the valves of the heart, usually as the result of acute RHEUMATISM. They lead in time to narrowing of the openings from the cavities of the heart, or to imcompetence of the valves that close these openings. (See HEART, DISEASES OF.)

Vehicle

A pharmaceutical term to describe the medium in which a drug is administered – for example, a fluid, gel, powder or aerosol.

Veins

The vessels which return the blood to the heart after it has circulated through the tissues; they are both more numerous and more capacious than the ARTERIES.

Structure While of similar structure to an artery, veins have much thinner walls, with much less muscular tissue. Furthermore, most veins have one-way VALVES to ensure that the blood flows in the right direction. These are most numerous in the legs, then the arms, with few in the internal organs.

Chief veins Four pulmonary veins open into the left atrium of the heart, two from each lung. The superior vena cava returns the blood from the head, neck, and arms; while the inferior vena cava returns blood from the legs and abdomen. The large basilic vein that runs up the inner side of the upper arm is the vein usually opened in blood-letting (see VENESECTION). The great saphenous vein is of special interest, because of its liability to become distended or varicose. Within the abdomen, the inferior vena cava receives branches corresponding to several branches of the aorta, its largest branches being the hepatic veins, which return not only the blood that has reached the liver in the hepatic arteries, but also blood which comes from the digestive organs in the PORTAL VEIN to undergo a second capillary circulation in the liver.

There are several connections between the superior and inferior cava, the most important

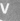

being three azygos veins that lie upon the sides of the spinal column, the veins on the front of the abdomen, and some veins that emerge from the abdomen at the navel and connect the portal system with those of the inferior and superior vena cava. (See also CIRCULATORY SYSTEM OF THE BLOOD.)

Veins, Diseases of

Veins are the blood vessels that convey blood back from the tissues towards the heart. Two common conditions that affect them are THROMBOSIS and varicosities (see below).

Varicose veins are dilated tortuous veins occurring in about 15 per cent of adults – women more than men. They most commonly occur in the legs but may also occur in the anal canal (HAEMORRHOIDS) and in the oesophagus (due to liver disease).

Normally blood flows from the subcutaneous tissues to the superficial veins which drain via perforating veins into the deep veins of the leg. This flow, back towards the heart, is aided by valves within the veins. When these valves fail, increased pressure is exerted on the blood vessels leading to dilatations known as varicose veins.

Treatment is needed to prevent complications such as ulceration and bleeding, or for

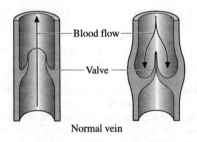

Normal vein

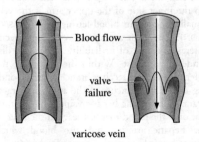

varicose vein

(Top) Normal vein showing how a closed valve prevents back flow of blood. (Bottom) Vein with faulty valve which allows some blood to leak back through the part-opened valve.

cosmetic purposes. Treatment alternatives include injection with sclerosing agents to obliterate the lumen of the veins (sclerotherapy), or surgery; in the elderly or unfit, an elastic stocking may suffice. One operation is the Trendelenburg operation in which the saphenous vein is disconnected from the femoral vein and individual varicose veins are avulsed. (See also VASCULITIS.)

Thrombosis Thrombosis occurs when blood, which is normally a liquid, clots within the vein to form a semisolid thrombus (clot). This occurs through a combination of reduced blood flow and hypercoagulability (a reduced threshold for clotting). The most common site for this to occur is in the deep veins of the leg, where it is known as a deep-vein thrombosis (DVT).

Predisposing factors include immobility (leading to reduced blood flow), such as during long journeys (e.g. plane flights) where there is little opportunity to stretch one's legs; surgery (leading to temporary post-operative immobility and hypercoagulability of blood); oestrogen administration (low-dose oestrogen oral contraceptives carry a very low relative risk); and several medical illnesses such as heart failure, stroke and malignancy.

Deep-vein thrombosis presents as a tender, warm, red swelling of the calf. Diagnosis may be confirmed by venogram (an X-ray taken following injection of contrast medium into the foot veins) or by ultrasound scanning looking for flow within the veins.

Prevention is important. This is why patients are mobilised and/or given leg exercises very soon after an operation, even major surgery. People should avoid sitting for long periods, particularly if the edge of the seat is hard, thus impeding venous return from the legs. Car drivers should stop regularly on a long journey and walk around; airline travellers should, where possible, walk round the aisle(s) and also exercise and massage their leg muscles, as well as drinking ample non-alcoholic fluids.

Diagnosis and treatment are important because there is a risk that the clotted blood within the vein becomes dislodged and travels up the venous system to become lodged in the pulmonary arteries. This is known as PULMONARY EMBOLISM.

Treatment is directed at thinning the blood with ANTICOAGULANTS, initially with heparin and subsequently with WARFARIN for a period of time while the clot resolves.

Blocked superficial veins are described as superficial thrombophlebitis, which produces inflammation over the vein. It responds to anti-inflammatory analgesics. Occasionally heparin and ANTIBIOTICS are required to treat associated thrombosis and infection.

Vena Cava

The name of either of the two large vessels that open into the right atrium of the HEART. (See VEINS.)

Venepuncture

The insertion of a needle into a vein (see VEINS), usually for the purpose of injecting a drug or withdrawing blood for haematological or bio-chemical analysis. The usual site for venepuncture in adults is the median cubital vein in the forearm.

Venereal Diseases

See SEXUALLY TRANSMITTED DISEASES (STDS).

Venesection

Venesection, or blood-letting, may be employed for two purposes. Most commonly, small quantities of blood may be required for analysis, as an aid to diagnosis or control of various diseases. For example, knowledge of the plasma glucose concentration is important in the diagnosis and management of DIABETES MELLITUS, or blood may be required in order to test for infections such as HIV or HEPATITIS. Blood may be obtained by pricking a fingertip, or inserting a needle into a vein, depending on the amount required. Controlled bleeding of larger amounts may rarely be used in certain cases of acute heart failure, as a rapid and temporary method of relieving the strain on the heart. It is also used in the treatment of POLYCYTHAEMIA.

Venography

The study of the VEINS, particularly by means of X-rays after the veins have been injected with a radio-opaque substance.

Venous Ulcer

See under ULCER.

Ventilation

(1) Passage of air into and out of the RESPIRATORY SYSTEM.

(2) The process by which air is purified and circulated in domestic, occupational, industrial, and other settings. Ideally, the air we breathe should be of the right temperature and humidity, and free of dust, smoke, pollen, and other contaminants. Ventilation aims to produce such an atmosphere. Air-conditioning is frequently used in hospitals, offices, and other public places. Special filters may be used to reduce the risk of airborne infections and allergies (see ALLERGY), but poorly maintained and contaminated systems may result in outbreaks of serious disorders, such as LEGIONNAIRE'S DISEASE. Sterilisation of air is rarely required, but ultraviolet light is sometimes used to kill pathogenic organisms. (See also ASTHMA; BRONCHITIS; HUMIDIFICATION.)

Ventilation, Artificial

The procedure, usually carried out in an operating theatre or intensive-care unit, in which a device called a VENTILATOR takes over a person's breathing. This is done for someone who is unable to breathe normally. Damage to the respiratory centre of the brain as a result of head injury, disease of the brain, or an overdose of sedative or narcotic drugs may affect the respiratory centre. Chest injuries, disease of the lungs, nerve or muscle disorders or surgery of the chest or abdomen can also affect breathing and require the use of a ventilator to maintain normal breathing. Artificial ventilation can also be carried out as an emergency by mouth-to-mouth resuscitation. (See also ANAESTHESIA; ARTIFICIAL VENTILATION OF THE LUNGS.)

Ventilator

Machinery used to provide artificial ventilation. Also called a respirator or life-support machine, it is an electric pump linked to a supply of air which it pumps into the patient through an endotracheal tube passed through the nose or mouth into the trachea (see ENDOTRACHEAL INTUBATION). Sometimes the air is pumped straight into the trachea through an artificial hole called a TRACHEOSTOMY. During ventilation the patient's blood gases are closely monitored and other bodily activities such as pulse and heart pressure are regularly measured. Some patients need to be kept on a ventilator for several days or even weeks if their medical condition is serious. (See also ARTIFICIAL VENTILATION OF THE LUNGS.)

Ventouse

See VACUUM EXTRACTOR.

Ventral

Positioned or relating to the front of a body or to the front part of an organ.

Ventricle

(1) The term applied to the two lower cavities of the HEART, and also to the four main cavities within the BRAIN.

Ventricular Fibrillation
A potentially life-threatening and rapid ARRHYTHMIA of the ventricle of the HEART.

Ventricular Hypertrophy
Enlargement of the ventricular chambers of the HEART, a common complication of HYPERTENSION and coronary artery disease (see HEART, DISEASES OF). Treatment is of the underlying conditions and cardiac drugs which facilitate the working of the heart.

Ventricular Septal Defect
An inherited defect of the HEART. The septum (partition) separating the two ventricles is pierced by a hole which, if large, results in blood being diverted to the LUNGS at a greater pressure than normal. This may lead to irreversible PULMONARY HYPERTENSION, which early surgical intervention (repair of the septal defect) should prevent. A quarter of patients with VSD have other cardiac defects. Half of the defects seal themselves spontaneously.

Ventriculography
The process of taking an X-ray photograph of the BRAIN after the fluid in the lateral ventricles of the brain has been replaced by air; in this way any alteration in the outline of the ventricles (e.g. from pressure by a tumour) can be detected.

Ventrosuspension
This is a surgical procedure to fixate a displaced UTERUS to the front wall of the abdomen. It is usually done by shortening the supporting round ligaments either where they are attached to the uterus, or to the abdominal wall.

Venule
A very small blood vessel that drains blood from CAPILLARIES. Several venules join up to form a vein (see VEINS).

Verapamil
Verapamil is a drug used in the treatment of HYPERTENSION, disordered rhythms of the heart, and ANGINA PECTORIS. The drug is one of the CALCIUM-CHANNEL BLOCKERS and acts by reducing cardiac output and slowing heart rate. It may, however, precipitate heart failure, cause HYPOTENSION and aggravate conduction problems in the heart, so should be prescribed with care. It should not be used with BETA-ADRENOCEPTOR-BLOCKING DRUGS.

Vermicides
Also called vermifuges, these are substances that kill, or expel, parasitic worms from the intestines.

Vernix
The white, cheese-like substance that covers the skin of a newborn infant. It consists of dead cells in a fatty secretion, protects the infant's skin, and helps lubricate its passage through the cervix and vagina during delivery.

Verruca
See WARTS.

Verrucose
This term means having a surface resembling verrucae (see WARTS). Certain skin diseases may become verrucose.

Version
The name given to an operation in OBSTETRICS which consists in turning the FETUS in the UTERUS where the fetus is lying in an abnormal position which may make eventual delivery difficult. In particular, version (which can take place spontaneously) may be done on a fetus between the 34th and 37th weeks of pregnancy when its buttocks rather than its head are positioned at the cervical end of the uterus. The procedure carries a small risk of precipitating premature labour, and it is not always successful, in which case a breech delivery is attempted or, in difficult cases, a CAESAREAN SECTION is performed. (See also PREGNANCY AND LABOUR.)

Vertebra
One of the irregularly shaped bones that together form the vertebral column. (See SPINAL COLUMN.)

Vertebrobasilar Insuffiency
Intermittent incidents of double vision, dizziness, weakness and speaking difficulties caused by a reduced blood supply to parts of the BRAIN. The cause is usually obstruction in the basilar, vertebral and other arteries at the base of the brain. The condition is sometimes the precursor of a STROKE.

Vertigo
A condition in which the affected person loses the power of balancing him or herself, and has a false sensation as to his or her own movements or those of surrounding objects. The power of balancing depends upon sensations derived partly through the sense of touch, partly from the eyes, but mainly from the semicircular canals of the internal EAR – the vestibular

mechanism. In general, vertigo is due to some interference with this vestibular ocular reflex mechanism or with the centres in the cerebellum and cerebrum (see BRAIN) with which it is connected. Giddiness is often associated with headache, nausea and vomiting.

Causes The simplest cause of vertigo is some mechanical disturbance of the body affecting the fluid in the internal ear; such as that produced by moving in a swing with the eyes shut, the motion of a boat causing sea-sickness, or a sudden fall. (See also MOTION (TRAVEL) SICKNESS.)

Another common positional variety is benign paroxysmal positional vertigo (BPPV) caused by sudden change in the position of the head; this causes small granular masses in the cupola of the posterior semicircular canal in the inner ear to be displaced. It may subside spontaneously within a few weeks but can recur. Sometimes altering the position of the head so as to facilitate return of the crystals to the cupola will stop the vertigo.

The cause which produces a severe and sudden giddiness is MENIÈRE'S DISEASE, a condition in which there is loss of function of the vestibular mechanism of the inner ear. An acute labyrinthitis – inflammation of the labyrinth of the ear – may result from viral infection and produce a severe vertigo lasting 2–5 days. Because it often occurs in epidemics it is often called epidemic vertigo. Vertigo is sometimes produced by the removal of wax from the ear, or even by syringing out the ear. (See EAR, DISEASES OF.)

A severe upset in the gastrointestinal tract may cause vertigo. Refractive errors in the eyes, an attack of MIGRAINE, a mild attack of EPILEPSY, and gross diseases of the brain, such as tumours, are other causes acting more directly upon the central nervous system. Finally, giddiness may be due to some disorder of the circulation, for example, reduced blood supply to the brain produced by fainting, or by disease of the heart.

Treatment While the attack lasts, this requires the sufferer to lie down in a darkened, quiet room. SEDATIVES have most influence in diminishing giddiness when it is distressing. After the attack is over, the individual should be examined to establish the cause and, if necessary, to be given appropriate treatment.

Vertigo and nausea linked to Menière's disease – or following surgery on the middle ear – can be hard to treat. HYOSCINE, ANTI-

HISTAMINE DRUGS and PHENOTHIAZINES – for example, prochlorperazine – are often effective in preventing and treating these disorders. Cinnarizine and betahistine have been marketed as effective drugs for Menière's disease; for acute attacks, cyclizine or prochlorperazine given by intramuscular injection or rectally can be of value. Research in America is exploring the use of virtual-reality technology to change subjects' visual perception of the outside world gradually during several 30-minute sessions, helping them to adjust to the abnormal sensations that occur during an attack. Early results are promising.

Vesical
The term applied to structures connected with, or diseases of, the URINARY BLADDER.

Vesicants
Vesicants are blistering agents.

Vesicle
A PAPULE containing fluid, for example as seen in CHICKENPOX.

Vesico-Ureteric Reflux
The back flow of URINE from the URINARY BLADDER into the ureters (see URETER). The cause is defects in the VALVES which normally prevent this reflux from occurring. If, in addition, the patient – usually a child – acquires bacteria in the bladder, the consequence may be one or more attacks of PYELONEPHRITIS caused by the infected urine gaining access to the kidney pelvis. Diagnosis is by imaging techniques. Treatment is by long-term antibiotics while awaiting spontaneous recovery. Occassionally, corrective surgery is required.

Vesicovaginal Fistula
A false communication between the URINARY BLADDER and the VAGINA. The result is urinary INCONTINENCE. Surgical damage to the bladder during operations for gynaecological disorders is one possible cause. Another is tissue damage following radiotherapy for cancer in the pelvis.

Vesicular Breathing
Normal breath sounds heard in the lung by means of a stethoscope. These are soft regular sounds which become altered by disease; the changed characteristics may help the physician to diagnose a disease in the lung.

Vestibule
An anatomical term for a cavity positioned at

the entrance to a hollow part in the body. An example is the nasal vestibule at the entrance of the NOSE.

Vestibulocochlear Nerve

The eighth cranial nerve. It consists of two sets of fibres, which constitute two separate nerves. One is known as the vestibular nerve, which connects the semicircular canals and inner ear to the BRAIN and conveys information on posture and movement of the body; it is the nerve of equilibration or balance. The other is known as the cochlear nerve, which links the COCHLEA (organ that responds to sounds) with the brain and is the nerve of hearing. Disturbance of the former causes giddiness (VERTIGO), whilst disturbance of the latter causes DEAFNESS.

Vestibulo-Ocular Reflex

Eye movement that occurs after or during the slow injection of 20 ml of ice-cold water into each external auditory meatus (see EAR) in turn.

Vestigial

An adjective referring to an organ which exists in a rudimentary form and whose function and structure have declined during the course of evolution. An example is the appendix.

Viable

The ability of an organism to survive on its own. In the United Kingdom, the legal age of the viability of a FETUS is 24 weeks.

Viagra

See SILDENAFIL CITRATE.

Vibrator

(1) An instrument used for vibratory massage to improve the tone of muscles and to relax them. It is of help in speeding the healing process after muscle or ligament strains.
(2) A penis-shaped, battery-driven device used by women to attain sexual stimulation and climax.

Vibrio

A bacterium with a curved shape, such as the vibrio of CHOLERA.

Villus

One of the minute processes thickly distributed upon the inner surface of the small INTESTINE, giving it, to the naked eye, a velvety appearance, and greatly assisting absorption of digested food. (See also DIGESTION; ABSORPTION; ASSIMILATION.)

Vinca Alkaloids

A group of powerful CYTOTOXIC (anticancer) drugs used to treat acute LEUKAEMIA, LYMPHOMA and some solid tumours such as breast and lung cancers. Originally derived from the periwinkle plant, the latest vinca alkaloid (VINORELBINE) is a semi-synthetic drug. These alkaloids, which are given intravenously, have potentially serious side-effects on the nervous system and also suppress the production of MYELOID cells in the bone marrow.

Vincent's Angina

An ulcerative inflammation of the throat, often foul-smelling, and caused by large, spindle-shaped bacilli (fusobacterium) and spirilla.

Vinorelbine

A semi-synthetic vinca alkaloid (see VINCA ALKALOIDS) CYTOTOXIC drug recently introduced for the treatment of advanced breast cancer, when anthracycline cytotoxic antibiotics such as DOXORUBICIN have failed. Vinorelbine is also used to treat advanced non-small-cell lung cancer (see LUNGS, DISEASES OF). As with all vinca alkaloids, the drug has neurotoxic effects, usually affecting the PERIPHERAL NERVOUS SYSTEM and AUTONOMIC NERVOUS SYSTEM. It may also cause (reversible) hair loss (ALOPECIA). The drug is given intravenously.

Vinyl Ether

An inhalational anaesthetic used in minor surgical procedures of short duration, and for the induction of ANAESTHESIA for longer surgical operations.

Viraemia

A condition occurring at various times in some viral infections in which the infecting VIRUS is present in large amounts in the blood. In other viral infections, the organisms are merely transported in the blood on their way to target tissues or organs.

Viral Haemorrhagic Fever

Also called EBOLA VIRUS DISEASE. A usually fatal infection caused by a virus related to that of MARBURG DISEASE. Two large outbreaks of it were recorded in 1976 (one in the Sudan and one in Zaïre), with a mortality, respectively, of 50 and 80 per cent, and the disease reappeared in the Sudan in 1979. After an incubation period of 7–14 days, the onset is with headache of increasing severity, and fever. This is followed by diarrhoea, extensive internal bleeding and vomiting. Death usually occurs on the eighth to ninth day. Infection is by person-to-person contact. Serum from patients convalescent from the disease is a useful source of ANTIBODIES to the virus.

Viral Pneumonia

Infection of the lung tissue by a VIRUS. Causes of this type of pneumonia include ADENOVI-RUSES, COXSACKIE VIRUSES and influenza virus. Viral infections do not respond to ANTIBIOTICS and treatment is symptomatic, with antibiotics used only if the patient develops secondary bacterial infection. In a previously healthy individual the viral infection is usually self-limiting, but in vulnerable patients – the elderly or those with pre-existing disease – it can be fatal.

Virilisation

The masculinisation of women suffering from excessive production of the male hormone ANDROGEN. The person develops temporal balding, a male body shape, increased muscular bulk, deepening of the voice, an enlarged CLIT-ORIS and HIRSUTISM. Virilisation may also occur in women who take synthetic androgens, a practice sometimes used (illegally) to increase physical strength and endurance in sport.

Virilism

The condition in which masculine character-istics develop in the female; it is commonly the result of an overactive suprarenal gland (see ADRENAL GLANDS), or of a tumour of its cortex. It may also result from an ANDROGEN-secreting ovarian tumour (see OVARIES, DISEASES OF) and also from the POLYCYSTIC OVARY SYNDROME. The overproduction of male-sex (androgen) hormones can produce excess growth of hair, male pattern hairline, stopping or disruption of MENSTRUATION, enlargement of the CLITORIS and conversion to a masculine body shape.

Virology

The scientific study of viruses (see VIRUS).

Virtual Hospital

See HOSPITAL.

Virulence

The power of a bacterium or virus to cause dis-ease. Virulence can be measured by how many people the micro-organism infects, how quickly it spreads through the body, and how many people die from it.

Virus

The term applied to a group of infective agents which are so small that they are able to pass through the pores of collodion filters. They are responsible for some of the most devastating diseases affecting humans: for example, INFLU-ENZA, POLIOMYELITIS, SMALLPOX and YELLOW FEVER. The virus of influenza measures 80 nanometres, whereas the STAPHYLOCOCCUS measures 1,000 nanometres (1 nanometre = one thousand-millionth of a metre).

A single virus particle, known as a virion, comprises an inner core of NUCLEIC ACID which is surrounded by one or two protective cover-ings (capsid) made of protein. Sometimes the capsid is enclosed by another layer called the viral envelope (also a protein structure). The envelope often disintegrates when the virus invades a cell. Viruses enter cells and then indulge in a complex and variable process of replication using some of the cells' own struc-ture. Viruses may stay in a host's nucleus, being reactivated months or years later. There are more than a score of large families of viruses, from papoviruses, which cause WARTS, through HERPES viruses (cold sores, CHICKENPOX, SHINGLES) and orthomyxoviruses (influenza), to corona viruses (common cold) and retro-viruses (AIDS/HIV). Viral diseases are more dif-ficult to treat than those caused by bacteria; ANTIBIOTICS are ineffective but INTERFERON, a group of natural substances, shows promise. IMMUNISATION is the most effective way of combating viral infections; smallpox, polio-myelitis, MUMPS, MEASLES and RUBELLA are examples of viral diseases which have been suc-cessfully combated. Research is progressing to find a vaccine against HIV.

Viscera

The general name given to the larger organs lying within the cavities of the chest and abdomen. The term 'viscus' is also applied individually to these organs.

Vision

Broadly speaking, vision is the ability to see.

Pathway of light from the eye to the brain
Light enters the EYE by passing through the transparent cornea, then through the aque-ous humour filling the anterior chamber. It then passes through the pupil, through the lens and the vitreous to reach the retina. In the ret-ina, the rod and cone photoreceptors detect light and relay messages in the form of electro-chemical impulses through the various layers of the retina to the nerve fibres. The nerve fibres carry messages via the optic nerve, optic chi-asma, optic tract, lateral geniculate body and finally the optic radiations to the visual cortex.

Here in the visual cortex these messages are interpreted. It is therefore the visual cortex of the BRAIN that 'sees'.

Visual acuity Two points will not be seen as two unless they are separated by a minimum distance. This distance is such that the objects are so far apart that the lines joining them to the eye enclose between them (subtend) an angle of at least one minute of a degree. This amount of separation allows the images of the two points to fall on two separate cones (if the light from two points falls on one cone, the two points would be seen as a single point). There are many tests of visual acuity. One of the more common is the Snellen test type. This is made up of many letters of different size. By conventions the chart is placed 6 metres away from the patient. Someone able to see the lowest line at this distance has a visual acuity of 6/4. If they are only able to see the top letter they have 6/60 vision. 'Normal' vision is 6/6.

Colour vision 'White light' is made up of component colours. These can be separated by a prism, thereby producing a spectrum. The three cardinal colours are red, green, and blue; all other colours can be produced by a varying mixture of these three. Colour vision is a complex subject. The trichromat theory of colour vision suggests that there are three types of cones, each type sensitive to one of the cardinal colours. Colour perception is based on differential stimulation of these cone types. The opponent colour theory suggests that each cone type can generate signals of the opposite kind. Output from some cones can collaborate with the output from others or can inhibit the action of other cones. Colour perception results from these various complex interactions.

Defective colour vision may be hereditary or acquired, and can occur in the presence of normal visual acuity.

HEREDITARY DEFECTIVE COLOUR VISION is more common in men (7 per cent of males) than women (0·5 per cent of females). Men are affected, but women convey the abnormal gene (see GENES) to their children. It occurs because one or more of the photopigments of the retina are abnormal, or the cones are damaged. Red-green colour defect is the most common.

ACQUIRED DEFECTIVE COLOUR VISION is the result of disease of the cones or their connections in the retina, optic nerve or brain – for example, macular disease, optic neuritis. Colour vision can be impaired but not lost as a result of corneal opacification or cataract formation (see under EYE, DISORDERS OF).

TESTS OF COLOUR VISION These use specially designed numbers made of coloured dots surrounded by dots of confusing colour (e.g. plates).

Vision, Disorders of

The list of disorders resulting in poor or dim vision is huge. Disturbance of vision can result from an uncorrected refractive error, disease or injury of the cornea, iris, lens, vitreous, retina, choroid or sclera of the EYE. It may also result from disease or injury to the structures comprising the visual pathway from the retina to the occipital cortex (see VISION – Pathway of light from the eye to the brain) and from lesions of the structures around the eye – for example, swollen lids, drooping eyelids. (See EYE, DISORDERS OF.)

Vision, Field of

When the eye looks at a specific point or object, that point is seen clearly. Other objects within a large area away from this fixation point can also be seen, but less clearly. The area that can be seen around the fixation point, without moving the eye, is known as the field of vision. The extent of the field is limited inwards by the nose, above by the brow and below by the cheek. The visual field thus has its greatest extent outwards from the side of the head. The field of vision of each eye overlaps to a large extent so that objects in the centre and towards the inner part of each field are viewed by both eyes together. Because the eyes are set slightly apart, each eye sees objects in this overlapping part of the field slightly differently. It is because of this slight difference that objects can be perceived as three-dimensional.

Defects in the visual field (scotomas) can be produced by a variety of disorders. Certain of these produce specific field defects. For example, GLAUCOMA, some types of brain damage and some TOXINS can produce specific defects in the visual field. This type of field defect may be very useful in diagnosing a particular disorder. The blind spot is that part of the visual field corresponding to the optic disc. There are no rods nor cones on the optic disc and therefore no light perception from this area. The blind spot can be found temporal (i.e. on the outer side) of the fixation point. (See also EYE.)

Vision Tests

Most vision tests examine a person's sharpness of VISION (visual acuity) and often of the field of vision (see VISION, FIELD OF). Refraction tests assess whether a person has an error that can be corrected with glasses such as ASTIGMATISM, HYPERMETROPIA or MYOPIA. Visual acuity is tested using a Snellen chart when the patient tries to read letters of differing standard sizes from 6 metres away. The optician will prescribe lenses to correct any defects detected by vision tests.

Visual Acuity
See VISION.

Visual Evoked Response
Stimulation of the retina of the EYE with light causes changes in the electrical activity of the cerebral cortex (see BRAIN). These changes can be measured from outside the skull and can give valuable information about the state of the visual pathway from the retinal ganglion cells to the occipital cortex. Not only can it determine that function is normal, it can also help to diagnose some causes of poor VISION.

Vital Capacity
The amount of air that can be forcibly exhaled from the lungs after a deep inspiration. (See RESPIRATION.)

Vital Centres
Groups of neurons (see NEURON(E)), usually sited in the HYPOTHALAMUS and the BRAIN stem, that are the control centres for various essential body functions. Examples are: blood pressure, breathing, heart rate and temperature control. The centres are part of the body's reflex adjustments to the outside world and its internal environment and are essential in maintaining HOMEOSTASIS.

Vitallium
A commercially trademarked alloy of cobalt and chromium used to make instruments, prostheses (see PROSTHESIS), surgical appliances and dentures. Its inert properties make it ideal for use in contact with live tissues such as bone and muscle.

Vital Sign
An indication that an individual is still alive. Chest movements (resulting from respiration), the existence of a pulse (showing that the heart is still beating) and constriction of the pupil of the eye in response to bright light are all vital signs. Other tests such as assessment of brain activity may also be needed in some circumstances: for example, when a patient is on a life-support machine. (See also GLASGOW COMA SCALE.)

Vitamin
A term applied to a group of substances which exist in minute quantities in natural foods, and which are necessary to normal nutrition, especially in connection with growth and development. Some – A, D, E and K – are fat-soluble and can be stored in the body. The remainder – C, B_{12} and other members of the B complex – are water-soluble and are quickly excreted. Most vitamins have now been synthesised. When they are absent from the food, defective growth takes place in young animals and children, and in adults various diseases arise; whilst short of the production of actual disease, persistent deprivation of one or other vitamin is apt to lead to a state of lowered general health. Certain deficiencies in DIET have long been known to be the cause of SCURVY, BERIBERI, and RICKETS. A diet containing foods such as milk, eggs, butter, cheese, fat, fish, wholemeal bread, fresh vegetables and fruit should contain sufficient vitamins. Details of the various vitamins are given in APPENDIX 5: VITAMINS.

Vitiligo
A disease in which small or large areas of skin lose their pigment and become white because of a reduction in the body's production of MELANIN. The hair may be similarly affected. Probably a consequence of an autoimmune mechanism, vitiligo is associated with other autoimmune diseases such as thyroiditis (see THYROID GLAND, DISEASES OF) and ADDISON'S DISEASE. There is no cure; the vitiliginous skin must be protected from sunburn.

Vitreous Body
A semi-fluid, transparent substance which fills most of the globe of the EYE behind the lens.

Viviparous
A term used to describe animal groups – including most mammals – in which the embryos (see EMBRYO) develop inside the mother's body with the young being born alive (in contrast to, say, birds and reptiles which hatch from eggs).

Vivisection
For more than a century the medical profession has aimed at maintaining as high a standard as possible for vivisection. It was the medical profession led by Dr James Paget that was responsible for the passing of the Cruelty to Animals Act 1876, which aimed to eliminate cruelty. The infliction of pain was reduced to a minimum by the use of anaesthetics (see ANAESTHESIA), and the licensing and surveillance of animal experiments was ensured.

Most experiments are carried out on specially bred mice and rats. Fewer than 1 per cent are done on cats, dogs, non-human primates, farm animals, frogs, fish and birds. Control on experiments has recently been strengthened.

The great majority of animal experiments are done without anaesthesia because feeding experiments, taking blood, or giving injections does not require anaesthetics in animals any more than in humans. Universities in Britain are responsible for fewer than one-fifth of animal experiments; commercial concerns and government institutions are responsible for most of the rest. Tests on cosmetics account for under 1 per cent of all animal work, but are necessary because such materials are often applied with great frequency – and for a long time – to the skin of adults and infants.

The use of tissue cultures and computer models instead of live animals are methods of research and investigation that are being increasingly used. There is, however, a limit to the extent to which infection, cancer, or drugs can be investigated on cultures of tissue cells. Computerised or mathematical modelling of experiments is probably the most promising line of development.

Vocal Cords
See LARYNGOSCOPE; LARYNX; VOICE AND SPEECH.

Vocal Resonance
The air carrying the voice produced in the LARYNX passes through the throat, mouth and nose. The shape and size of these structures will influence the timbre of the voice, or vocal resonance. This will vary from person to person and even within an individual; for example, with a cold.

Voice and Speech
Terms applied to the sounds produced in the upper AIR PASSAGES which form one of the means of communication between human beings. Air passes through the LARYNX to produce the fundamental notes and tones known as voice. This is then modified during its passage through the mouth so as to form speech or song.

Voice This has three varying characteristics: loudness, pitch, and quality or timbre. Loudness depends on the volume of air available and therefore on the size of the chest and the strength of its muscles. Pitch is determined by larynx size, the degree of tenseness at which the vocal cords are maintained, and whether the cords vibrate as a whole or merely at their edges.

In any given voice, the range of pitch seldom exceeds two and a half octaves. Typically, the small larynx of childhood produces a shrill or treble voice; the rapid growth of the larynx around PUBERTY causes the voice to 'break' in boys. Changes in the voice also occur at other ages as a result of the secondary action of the SEX HORMONES. Generally speaking, the adult voice is bass and tenor in men, contralto or soprano in women. Timbre is due to differences in the larynx, as well as to voluntary changes in the shape of the mouth.

Speech Rapid modifications of the voice, produced by movements of the PALATE, tongue and lips. Infants hear the sounds made by others and mimic them; hence the speech centres in the BRAIN are closely connected with those of hearing.

Defects of speech See below, and also SPEECH DISORDERS.

MUTISM, or absence of the power to speak, may be due to various causes. LEARNING DISABILITY that prevents the child from mimicking the actions of others is most common; in other cases the child has normal intelligence but some neurological disorder, or disorder of the speech organs, is responsible. Alternatively, complete DEAFNESS or early childhood ear disease may be the cause.

STAMMERING is a highly individual condition, but is basically a lack of coordination between the different parts of the speech mechanism. (See also main entry on STAMMERING.)

DYSPHASIA is the inability to speak or understand speech, most commonly following brain disease, such as STROKE.

APHONIA or loss of voice may be caused by LARYNGITIS or, rarely, a symptom of conversion and dissociative mental disorders – traditionally referred to as HYSTERIA. It is generally of short duration.

Volar
A term relating to the palm or sole.

Volkmann's Contracture
A rare condition in which, as a result of too great a pressure from splint or bandage in the treatment of a broken arm, the flexor muscles of the forearm contract and thus obstruct free flow of blood in the veins; the muscles then swell and ultimately become fibrosed.

Voluntary Admission
The term applied in the UK to the admission of a mentally ill person to a psychiatric unit with

his or her agreement. Patients with mental illnesses that may endanger their own safety or that of others can be compulsorily admitted using special legal powers – this is traditionally called 'sectioning'. (See MENTAL ILLNESS.)

Voluntary Muscle

Also known as skeletal muscle, this forms the muscles which are under a person's conscious control. Muscles that control walking, talking and swallowing are examples of those under such control (see INVOLUNTARY MUSCLE; MUSCLE; NERVOUS SYSTEM).

Volvulus

An obstruction of the bowels produced by the twisting of a loop of bowel round itself. (See also STRANGULATION; INTESTINE, DISEASES OF.)

Vomiting

Vomiting means the expulsion of the STOMACH contents through the mouth. When the effort of vomiting is made, but nothing is brought up, the process is known as retching. When vomiting occurs, the chief effort is made by the muscles of the abdominal wall and by the diaphragm contracting together and squeezing the stomach. The contraction of the stomach wall is no doubt also a factor, and an important step in the act consists in the opening at the right moment of the cardiac or upper orifice of the stomach. This concerted action of various muscles is brought about by a vomiting centre situated on the floor of the fourth ventricle in the BRAIN.

Causes Vomiting is brought about by stimulation of this nervous centre, and in most cases this is effected through sensations derived from the stomach itself. Thus, of the drugs which cause vomiting, some act only after being absorbed into the blood and carried to the brain, although most are irritants to the mucous membrane of the stomach (see EMETICS); various diseases of the stomach, such as cancer, ulcer and food poisoning act in a similar way. Stimulation – not only of the nerves of the stomach, but also of those supplying other abdominal organs – produces vomiting; thus in obstruction of the bowels, peritonitis, gall-stone colic, renal colic, and even in some women during pregnancy, vomiting is a prominent symptom.

Severe emotional shock may cause vomiting, as may acute anxiety and unpleasant experiences such as seeing an accident, suffering severe pain or travel sickness.

Direct disturbance of the brain itself is a cause: for example, a blow on the head, a cerebral tumour, a cerebral abscess, meningitis. Nausea and vomiting are common symptoms that may arise from local disease of the gastro-intestinal tract, but they are also associated with systemic illness – for example, DIABETES MELLITUS or kidney failure (see KIDNEYS, DISEASES OF) – and also with disturbances of labyrinthine function, such as motion sickness and acute labyrinthitis.

Treatment The cause of the vomiting must be sought and treatment directed towards this. Symptomatic treatment for vomiting can be dangerous since accurate diagnosis of the cause may be hindered. If antinauseant drug treatment is indicated, the choice of drug depends on the cause of the vomiting.

Granisetron and ondansetron are 5-hydroxytryptamine ($5HT_3$) antagonists valuable in the treatment of nausea and vomiting induced by cytotoxic CHEMOTHERAPY or RADIOTHERAPY and prevention and treatment of post-operative nausea and vomiting. Prochlorperazine is valuable in the treatment of severe nausea, vomiting, VERTIGO and disorders of the LABYRINTH of the EAR, although extrapyramidal symptoms may occur, particularly in children, elderly and debilitated patients.

Vomiting may occur after surgical operations and this is due to the combined effects of analgesics, anaesthetic agents and the psychological stress of operation. Various drugs can be used to prevent or stop post-operative vomiting.

Nausea and vomiting are common symptoms in pregnancy. Drugs are best avoided in this situation as they may damage the developing FETUS. Simple measures, such as the taking of food before getting up in the morning and reassurance, are often all that is necessary.

Von Recklinghausen's Disease

An inherited disease, now called neurofibromatosis. About one case occurs every 3,000 live births. The disease is characterised by tumours along the course of nerves which can be felt beneath the skin. Soft tumours may also develop beneath the skin. The condition may have other associated abnormalities such as SCOLIOSIS, decalcification of the bones due to overactivity of the PARATHYROID glands, and fibrosis in the lungs. Surgery may be needed for cosmetic reasons or to relieve pressure on the nervous system.

Von Willebrand's Disease

A genetically determined blood disorder in

which the affected person suffers episodes of spontaneous bleeding similar to that occurring in people with HAEMOPHILIA. It may be associated with a lack of FACTOR VIII (see COAGULATION) in the blood. The disorder is inherited as an autosomal dominant gene (see GENETIC DISORDERS).

Voyeurism

The regular viewing of people who are naked or part-naked or who are taking part in intimate sexual activities. The voyeur's subjects are unaware that they are being watched. The voyeur, nearly always a man, usually becomes sexually excited and may induce ORGASM by MASTURBATION.

Vulva

The external genitalia of the female. The LABIA majora and minora – comprising folds of flesh, the latter inside the former – surround the openings of the VAGINA and URETHRA. The folds extend upwards as an arch over the CLITORIS. The vulva also contains vestibular glands which provide profuse mucoid secretions during sexual activity.

Vulvectomy

Surgical excision of the external genitals (see VULVA). In simple vulvectomy the LABIA majora and minora and the CLITORIS are surgically removed, usually to treat a non-malignant growth. A more extensive operation is radical vulvectomy in which there is wide excision of the two labia and the clitoris along with complete removal of all regional LYMPH NODES on both sides and the covering skin. This procedure is carried out to treat cancer of the vulva.

Vulvo-Vaginitis

Inflammation of the VULVA and VAGINA. It may be due to infection, and may be a presenting feature of late onset DIABETES MELLITUS. Trauma may sometimes be the cause.

V

Waiting List

A term widely used in the NHS to show the number of people waiting for hospital admission, usually for non-acute surgery. The size of the waiting list has come to be perceived over the past 20 years– especially by politicians – as a measure of the Service's effectiveness. To the individual patient, however, what matters is the 'waiting time' – how long they have to wait before admission. This figure – along with the time a patient has to wait for an outpatient appointment to see a consultant – is increasingly being recognised as one important measurement of how well a hospital is serving its local communities.

Walk

See GAIT.

Warfarin

An anticoagulant (see ANTICOAGULANTS), usually given by mouth on a daily basis. The initial dose depends upon the PROTHROMBIN or coagulation time; this should be determined before starting treatment, and then at regular intervals during treatment. It is indicated for the prophylaxis of embolisation (see EMBOLISM) in rheumatic heart disease and atrial fibrillation (see HEART, DISEASES OF); after prosthetic heart-valve insertion; prophylaxis and treatment of venous thrombosis and PULMONARY EMBOLISM; and TRANSIENT ISCHAEMIC ATTACKS OR EPISODES (TIA, TIE). When given in tablet form, its maximum effect generally occurs within about 36 hours, wearing off within 48 hours. Special caution is appropriate in patients with disease of the liver or kidneys or who have had recent surgery. Warfarin is contra-indicated throughout pregnancy (especially the first and third trimesters), and in cases of PEPTIC ULCER, severe HYPERTENSION and bacterial ENDOCARDITIS. The most important adverse effect is HAEMORRHAGE. Other reported side-effects include HYPERSENSITIVITY, rash, ALOPECIA, diarrhoea, unexplained drop in HAEMATOCRIT readings, purple toes, skin NECROSIS, JAUNDICE, liver dysfunction, nausea, vomiting and pancreatitis (see PANCREAS, DISEASES OF). (See also COAGULATION.)

Warts

Warts (verrucae) are small, solid outgrowths from the SKIN arising from the epidermis and caused by various subtypes of 'human papilloma virus'. The causal viruses are ubiquitous and most people probably harbour them. Whether or not warts develop depends upon age, previous infection and natural resistance.

Common warts (verruca vulgaris) are seen mainly in children and young adults on the backs of the fingers and hands, and less often on the knees, face or scalp. They may be single or numerous and range from 1 mm to 10 mm or more in size. Untreated, they often resolve spontaneously after weeks or months. They may be occupationally contracted by butchers and meat-handlers.

Plane warts (verruca plana) are small, flat-topped, yellowish papules seen mainly on the backs of the hands, wrists and face in young people. They may persist for years.

Digitate warts (verruca digitata) are finger- or thread-like warts up to 5 mm in length with a dark rough tip. They tend to grow on the eyelids or neck.

Plantar warts (verruca plantaris) occur on the soles of the feet, most commonly in older children, adolescents and young adults. Spread by walking barefoot in swimming pools, changing rooms, etc., these warts may appear as minor epidemics in institutions, such as schools. They are flattened, yellow-white discrete lesions in the sole or heel, tender when squeezed. Multiple black points in the wart are thrombosed capillaries. Occasionally, aggregates of plantar warts form a mosaic-like plaque, especially in chronically warm, moist feet.

Genital warts are sexually transmitted. In the male they occur on the shaft of the PENIS and on the PREPUCE or around the anus. In women they occur around the entrance to the VAGINA and LABIA minora. Genital warts vary from 1–2 mm pink papules to florid, cauliflower-like masses. Pregnancy facilitates their development.

Mucosal warts may develop on the mucous membranes of the mouth.

Laryngeal warts may be found in children whose mothers had genital warts (see above) at the time of delivery. Some subtypes of genital wart can infect the uterine cervix (see UTERUS), causing changes which may lead eventually to cancer.

Treatment CRYOTHERAPY – freezing with liquid nitrogen – is the principal weapon against all types of warts, but curettage (scraping out the wart with a CURETTE) and cauterisation (see ELECTROCAUTERY) or LASER therapy may be required for resistant warts. Genital warts may respond to local application of PODOPHYLLIN preparations. Sexual partners should be examined and treated if necessary. Finally, treatment of warts should not be more onerous or painful than the disease itself, since spontaneous resolution is so common.

Washing
See DISINFECTION.

Washing Out of the Stomach
See GASTRIC LAVAGE.

Wassermann Reaction
A test introduced for the diagnosis of SYPHILIS by examination of the blood. It has now been largely supplanted by other, more specific tests.

Wasting
See ATROPHY.

Water Bed
A bed with a water-filled mattress can help prevent bed sores (see ULCER – Decubitus ulcer) in patients confined to bed for more than a few days. Its flexibility provides uniform support for the whole body. Air beds are now more often used: they are light and more comfortable and the modern version, called a ripple bed, has a little motor that fills and empties tubes in the mattress. The patient's circulation is stimulated and pressure is regularly changed on susceptible parts of the body – elbows, buttocks and heels – thus reducing the likelihood of pressure sores developing, particularly in the elderly.

Waterbrash
Also called pyrosis. A symptom of indigestion; during the course of DIGESTION, the mouth fills with tasteless or sour fluid, which is generally saliva, but is sometimes brought up from the stomach. This is accompanied by a burning pain often felt at the pit of the stomach or in the chest. The condition is a symptom of excessive acidity of the stomach contents, due sometimes to an injudicious diet, and often characteristic of a DUODENAL ULCER. (See also DYSPEPSIA.)

Water-Hammer Pulse
The peculiarly sudden PULSE that is associated with incompetence of the AORTIC VALVE of the heart.

Water Intoxication
A disorder resulting from excessive retention of water in the brain. Main symptoms are dizziness, headaches, confusion and nausea. In severe cases the patient may have fits (see SEIZURE) or lose consciousness. Several conditions can disturb the body's water balance causing accumulation of water in the tissues. Heart or kidney failure, CIRRHOSIS of the liver and disorders of the ADRENAL GLANDS can all result in water retention. Other causes are stress as a result of surgery, when increased secretion of antidiuretic hormone (VASOPRESSIN) by the adrenal gland may occur. Treatment is of the underlying condition and the judicious use of DIURETICS, with careful monitoring of the body's ELECTROLYTES.

Wax
This is used in medicine as an ingredient of ointments, plasters, and suppositories (see SUPPOSITORY). It is used either as yellow wax derived directly from honeycomb, or as white wax, which is the same substance bleached. It is also used in the form of paraffin wax to apply heat in the relief of rheumatic pains.

For wax in the ear, see under EAR, DISORDERS OF.

Weakness
See ATROPHY; CACHEXIA; PARALYSIS; TONICS.

Weals
Or wheals: raised white areas of OEDEMA in the skin with reddened margins, which may result from sharp blows, or accompanied by itching, may be a symptom of URTICARIA.

Weaning
The process by which a baby is introduced to solid foods after having only had breast milk or artificial milk to drink. The transfer usually starts at around 4–5 months of age but many parents prefer not to wait. (See INFANT FEEDING.)

Webbed Fingers
Or toes – see also SYNDACTYLY. A deformity sometimes present at birth, and which tends to run in families. The web may be quite a thin structure, or the fingers may be closely united by solid tissue. In any case, separation is a matter of considerable difficulty, because, if the web is simply divided, it heals up as before. A special operation is necessary, consisting in turning

back a flap of the web upon each of the united fingers, or some other device to produce healing in the new position.

Weber's Test
A test with a tuning fork that is used to assess a person's DEAFNESS.

Weight and Height
Charts relating height to age have been devised, and give an indication of the normal rate of growth. (See APPENDIX 6: MEASUREMENTS IN MEDICINE for more details.) The wide variation in normal children is immediately apparent on studying such charts. Deviations from the mean of this wide range are called percentiles. Centile or percentile charts describe the distribution of a characteristic in a population. They are obtained by measuring a specific characteristic in a large population of at least 1,000 of each sex at each age. For each age there will be a height, above and below which 50 per cent of the population lies: this is called the 50th centile. The 50th centile thus indicates the mean height at a particular age. Such tables are less reliable around the age of PUBERTY, because of variation in age of onset.

Minor variations from the mean do not warrant investigation, but if the height of an individual falls below the third centile (3 per cent of normal children have a height that falls below the third centile) or above the 97th centile, investigation is required. Changes in the rate of growth are also important, and skeletal proportions may provide useful information. There are many children who are normal but who are small in relation to their parents; the problem is merely growth delay. These children take longer to reach maturity and there is also a proportional delay in their skeletal maturation – so that the actual height must always be assessed in relation to maturity. The change in skeletal proportions is one manifestation of maturity, but other features include the maturing of facial features with the growth of nose and jaw, and dental development. Maturity of bone can readily be measured by the radiological bone age.

Failure to gain weight is of more significance. Whilst this may be due to some underlying disease, the most common cause is a diet containing inadequate calories (see CALORIE). Over the last six decades or so there has been quite a striking increase in the heights and weights of European children, with manufacturers of children's clothing, shoes and furniture having to increase the size of their products. Growth is now completed at 20–21 years, compared with 25 at the turn of the century. It has been suggested that this increase, and earlier maturation, have been due to a combination of genetic mixing as a result of population movements, with the whole range of improvement in environmental hygiene – and not merely to better nutrition.

In the case of adults, views have changed in recent years concerning 'ideal' weight. Life-insurance statistics have shown that maximal life expectancy is obtained if the average weight at 25–30 years is maintained throughout the rest of life. These insurance statistics also suggest that it is of advantage to be slightly over the average weight before the age of 30 years; to be of average weight after the age of 40; and to be underweight from ages 30–40. In the past it has been usual, in assessing the significance of an adult's weight, to allow a 10 per cent range on either side of normal for variations in body-build. A closer correlation has been found between thoracic and abdominal measurements and weight.

Weights and Measures
It is more than a hundred years since the metric system was legalised in Britain, but it was not until 1969 that it became illegal to use any system of weights and measures other than the metric system for dispensing prescriptions.

A rationalisation of the metric system is now used, known as the International System of Units (SI – see APPENDIX 6: MEASUREMENTS IN MEDICINE).

Weil's Disease
See LEPTOSPIROSIS.

Werner's Syndrome
A rare inherited condition in which the affected person suffers from premature ageing from adolescence onwards. His or her growth may be retarded, the skin become thin, and arterial disease, DIABETES MELLITUS and leg ulcers (see ULCER) develop. Treatment is symptomatic.

Wernicke's Encephalopathy
Also called the Wernicke-Korsakoff syndrome, this uncommon disorder is characterised by mental confusion or DELIRIUM that occurs in combination with an unsteady GAIT, nystagmus (see under EYE, DISORDERS OF) and paralysis of the eye muscles and eventually PSYCHOSIS. It is caused by a deficiency of vitamin B$_1$ (THIAMINE – see APPENDIX 5: VITAMINS) which affects the brain and nervous system. It occurs in alcoholic individuals and in patients with persistent vomiting. As soon as the condition is

W

diagnosed, it must be treated with large doses of thiamine. Unless the patient has developed symptoms of psychosis, the condition is usually reversible with treatment.

Werthheim's Hysterectomy
A major operation done to remove cancer of the UTERUS or ovary (see OVARIES). The ovaries, FALLOPIAN TUBES, the uterus and its ligaments, the upper VAGINA, and the regional LYMPH NODES are all excised.

West Nile Virus
A mosquito-borne viral infection that is normally harmless to healthy people who, if infected, develop a mild flu-like illness. However, if the elderly and those in poor health, particularly immunocompromised patients, are infected, they may develop fatal inflammation of the brain and spinal cord. In Israel in 2000, 12 people died and more than 155 survived an outbreak; and in New York in 1999, more than 60 people were infected, of whom six died. The disease was first reported in Uganda in 1937 and became ENDEMIC in the Middle East and Africa, recently spreading to Europe, central Asia, Oceania and America. Mosquitoes bearing the flaviviridae-family virus usually contract it by biting infected poultry, but the infection has been found in mammals, such as cats, dogs and horses.

Wheals
See WEALS.

Wheezing
A popular name applied to the various sounds produced in the chest when the bronchial tubes are narrowed. It is applied particularly to the long-drawn breathing of ASTHMA, and to the whistling or purring noises that accompany breathing in cases of BRONCHITIS.

Whiplash Injury
An injury to the neck region caused by the neck being forcibly bent backwards and forwards (or the other way around). Car accidents are a common cause, when a driver or passenger is suddenly decelerated. The injury usually affects the ligaments, spinal joints and soft tissues of the neck. Subluxation (partial dislocation) of a cervical joint sometimes occurs and cervical vertebra may occasionally be fractured if the forces are severe. Pain and stiffness of the neck result and these may worsen after a day or so. Treatment includes immobilisation of the neck in a collar, and analgesic and muscle-relaxing drugs. PHYSIOTHERAPY may be necessary. The patient usually recovers fully but may take several weeks to do so.

Whipworm
A popular name for *Trichuris trichiura*. (See also TRICHURIASIS.)

White Blood Cell
See LEUCOCYTES.

White Finger
Spasm of the blood vessels in the finger, resulting in a white appearance. The condition is common in RAYNAUD'S DISEASE but it can be caused by the long-term use of percussion implements such as mechanical road drills or hammers. It is a recognised industrial disease. Treatment is to remove or treat the underlying cause.

White Hair
The greying or whitening of hair which takes place with age is due to a loss of its pigment, MELANIN, and the collection of air bubbles in the shaft of the hair. There is no evidence that hair ever goes white overnight, whether in response to shock, strain or any other cause. Rapid whitening may occur patchily in a matter of days, but it is more often a matter of weeks or months. In the more rapid cases the cause is thought to be a form of ALOPECIA in which the dark hairs which fall out are replaced by white hairs. An alternative cause is VITILIGO. Certain drugs, including mephenesin and CHLOROQUINE, may also cause whitening of the hair.

Whitehead
A common benign blemish of the skin (see MILIA).

Whitlow
A popular term for PARONYCHIA.

Whooping-Cough
Whooping-cough, or pertussis, is a respiratory-tract infection caused by *Bordetella pertussis* and spread by droplets. It may occur at all ages, but around 90 per cent of cases are children aged under five. Most common during the winter months, it tends to occur in epidemics (see EPIDEMIC), with periods of increased prevalence occurring every three to four years. It is a notifiable disease (see NOTIFIABLE DISEASES). The routine vaccination of infants with TRIPLE VACCINE (see also VACCINE; IMMUNISATION), which includes the vaccine against whooping-cough, has drastically reduced the incidence of this potentially dangerous infection. In the 1990s

over 90 per cent of children in England had been vaccinated against whooping-cough by their second birthday. In an epidemic of whooping-cough, which extended from the last quarter of 1977 to mid-1979, 102,500 cases of whooping-cough were notified in the United Kingdom, with 36 deaths. This was the biggest outbreak since 1957 and its size was partly attributed to the fall in vaccination acceptance rates because of media reports suggesting that pertussis vaccination was potentially dangerous and ineffective. In 2002, 105 cases were notified in England.

Symptoms The first, or catarrhal, stage is characterised by mild, but non-specific, symptoms of sneezing, conjunctivitis (see under EYE, DISORDERS OF), sore throat, mild fever and cough. Lasting 10–14 days, this stage is the most infectious; unfortunately it is almost impossible to make a definite clinical diagnosis, although analysis of a nasal swab may confirm a suspected case. This is followed by the second, or paroxysmal, stage with irregular bouts of coughing, often prolonged, and typically more severe at night. Each paroxysm consists of a succession of short sharp coughs, increasing in speed and duration, and ending in a deep, crowing inspiration, often with a characteristic 'whoop'. Vomiting is common after the last paroxysm of a series. Lasting 2–4 weeks, this stage is the most dangerous, with the greatest risk of complications. These may include PNEUMONIA and partial collapse of the lungs, and fits may be induced by cerebral ANOXIA. Less severe complications caused by the stress of coughing include minor bleeding around the eyes, ulceration under the tongue, HERNIA and PROLAPSE of the rectum. Mortality is greatest in the first year of life, particularly among neonates – infants up to four weeks old. Nearly all patients with whooping-cough recover after a few weeks, with a lasting IMMUNITY. Very severe cases may leave structural changes in the lungs, such as EMPHY-SEMA, with a permanent shortness of breath or liability to ASTHMA.

Treatment Antibiotics, such as ERYTHROMY-CIN or TETRACYCLINES, may be helpful if given during the catarrhal stage – largely in preventing spread to brothers and sisters – but are of no use during the paroxysmal stage. Cough suppressants are not always helpful unless given in high (and therefore potentially narcotic) doses, and skilled nursing may be required to maintain nutrition, particularly if the disease is prolonged, with frequent vomiting.

Widal Reaction
See AGGLUTINATION.

Wilms' Tumour
Also called nephroblastoma. This is the commonest kidney tumour in infancy. It is a malignant tumour, which occurs in around one per 10,000 live births. The survival rate with modern treatment (removal of the kidney followed by radiotherapy and chemotherapy) is now around 80 per cent.

Wilson's Disease
Wilson's disease, or hepatolenticular degeneration, is a familial disease in which there is an increased accumulation of COPPER in the liver, brain, and other tissues including the kidneys. Its main manifestation is the development of tremor and rigidity, with difficulty in speech. In many cases there is improvement following the administration of dimercaprol, penicillamine, or trientine dihydrochloride; these substances cause an increased excretion of copper.

Windpipe
The popular name for the TRACHEA, which extends from the LARYNX above to the point in the upper part of the chest where it divides into the two large bronchial tubes, one to each lung. It is about 10 cm (4 inches) in length and consists of a fibrous tube kept permanently open by about 20 strong, horizontally placed hoops of cartilage, each of which forms about two-thirds of a circle, the two ends being joined behind by muscle fibres. This fibrocartilaginous tube is lined by a smooth mucous membrane, richly supplied with mucous glands and covered by a single layer of ciliated epithelium. (See also AIR PASSAGES.)

Winter Vomiting Disease
Winter vomiting disease, or epidemic nausea and vomiting, is a condition caused by subtypes of the genus Norwalk-like virus and is characterised by nausea, vomiting, diarrhoea and giddiness, which occurs during the winter. Outbreaks of it usually involve whole families or may affect communities like schools. The incubation period is 24–48 hours, and attacks seldom persist for more than 72 hours. In England and Wales in 2000, more than 1,600 infections were reported compared to more than 16,400 cases of salmonella infections and 56,420 of CAMPYLOBACTER. However, in England it is estimated that around 1,500 times more people are infected in the community than are reported. Humans are the only

W

known hosts of the virus and infection can be acquired via contaminated food or water or, more commonly, from an infected individual via the faeco-oral route, aerosol-spread and FOMITES.

Wisdom Tooth

A popular name for the last molar tooth on either side of each jaw (see TEETH). These teeth are the last to appear and should develop in early adult life, but often they do not cut the gum till the age of 20 or 25; indeed, they may sometimes remain permanently impacted in the jaw-bone. This occurs in up to 25 per cent of individuals. The lower third molar is often impacted against the second because of the direction in which it erupts.

Witch-Hazel

A preparation of the bark, twigs, and dried leaves from *Hamamelis virginiana*, a plant found in the United States. It has strong astringent properties and is used to check haemorrhages and excessive mucous discharges, and also for piles (see HAEMORRHOIDS).

Withdrawal Bleeding

Loss of blood from the UTERUS via the VAGINA occurring when the women's level of oestrogen hormones (OESTROGENS), PROGESTERONE hormone or PROGESTOGEN drugs falls quickly. The withdrawal bleeding that happens at the end of each month's cycle of combined oral contraceptive pills (see CONTRACEPTION) imitates the woman's menstrual period (see MENSTRUATION) but is normally briefer and less in amount.

Withdrawal Symptoms

Unpleasant physical and mental symptoms that occur when a person stops using a drug or substance on which he or she is dependent (see DEPENDENCE). The symptoms include tremors, sweating, and vomiting which are reversed if further doses are given. Alcohol and hard drugs, such as morphine, heroin, and cocaine, are among the substances that induce dependence, and therefore withdrawal symptoms, when stopped. Amphetamines and nicotine are other examples.

Womb

See UTERUS.

Womb Music

The name given to the playing to crying babies of sounds comparable to those by which the unborn babe is surrounded in the womb (UTERUS), such as the beating of the mother's heart, the bowel sounds of the baby and the like. The claim is that the replaying of these brings back the 'peaceful music of the womb', to which they have become conditioned, and thus 'sings' them to sleep.

Wool-Sorters' Disease

Another name for ANTHRAX.

Word Blindness

Alexia: a condition in which, as the result of disease in the brain, a person becomes unable to associate their proper meanings with words, although he or she may be quite able to spell the letters.

Word deafness is an associated condition in which, although hearing remains perfect, the patient has lost the power of referring the names heard to the articles they denote. (See also DYSPHASIA.)

World Medical Association

See ETHICS.

Worms

See ASCARIASIS; ENTEROBIASIS; TAENIASIS.

Wounds

A wound is any breach suddenly produced in the tissues of the body by direct violence. An extensive injury of the deeper parts without corresponding injury of the surface is known as a bruise or contusion.

Varieties These are classified according to the immediate effect produced:
INCISED WOUNDS are usually inflicted with some sharp instrument, and are clean cuts, in which the tissues are simply divided without any damage to surrounding parts. The bleeding from such a wound is apt to be very free, but can be readily controlled.
PUNCTURE WOUNDS, or stabs, are inflicted with a pointed instrument. These wounds are dangerous, partly because their depth involves the danger of wounding vital organs; partly because bleeding from a stab is hard to control; and partly because they are difficult to sterilise. The wound produced by the nickel-nosed bullet is a puncture, much less severe than the ugly lacerated wound caused by an expanding bullet, or by a ricochet, and, if no clothing has been carried in by the bullet, the wound is clean and usually heals at once.
LACERATED WOUNDS are those in which tissues are torn, such as injuries caused by machinery.

Little bleeding may occur and a limb can be torn completely away without great loss of blood. Such wounds are, however, especially liable to infection.

CONTUSED WOUNDS are those accompanied by much bruising of surrounding parts, as in the case of a blow from a cudgel or poker. There is little bleeding, but healing is slow on account of damage to the edges of the wound. Any of these varieties may become infected.

First-aid treatment The first aim is to check any bleeding. This may be done by pressure upon the edges of the wound with a clean handkerchief, or, if the bleeding is serious, by putting the finger in the wound and pressing it upon the spot from which the blood is coming.

If medical attention is available within a few hours, a wound should not be interfered with further than is necessary to stop the bleeding and to cover it with a clean dry handkerchief or bandage. When expert assistance is not soon obtainable, the wound should be cleaned with an antiseptic such as CHLORHEXIDINE or boiled water and the injured part fixed so that movement is prevented or minimised. A wounded hand or arm is fixed with a SLING, a wounded leg with a splint (see SPLINTS). If the victim is in SHOCK, he or she must be treated for that. (See also APPENDIX 1: BASIC FIRST AID.)

Wrinkle

A natural furrow in the skin commonly associated with AGEING. Wrinkles are most prominent on the face and other exposed body parts. Overexposure to sunlight causes premature wrinkling. Cosmetic preparations may temporarily improve excessive wrinkling, but a face lift, which stretches the skin using surgery, can improve a person's face for up to five years.

Wrist

The joint situated between the arm above and the hand below. The region of the wrist contains eight small carpal bones, arranged in two rows, each containing four bones. Those in the row nearest the forearm are – from the outside inwards when looking at the palm of the hand – the scaphoid, lunate, triquetrum, and pisiform.

Those in the row nearest the hand are the trapezium, trapezoid, capitate and hamate. These latter articulate with the metacarpal bones in the hand and are closely bound to one another by short, strong ligaments; and the wrist-joint is the union of the composite mass thus formed with the RADIUS and ULNA in the forearm. The wrist and the radius and ulna are united by strong outer and inner lateral ligaments, and by weaker ligaments before and behind, whilst the powerful tendons passing to the hand and fingers strengthen the wrist.

The joint can move in all directions, and its shape and many ligaments mean that it rarely dislocates – although stretching or tearing of some of these ligaments is a common accident, constituting a sprain. (See JOINTS, DISEASES OF.) Inflammation of the tendon-sheaths may occur as a result of injury or repetitive movement (see UPPER LIMB DISORDERS). A fairly common condition is the presence of a GANGLION, in which an elastic swelling full of fluid develops on the back or front of the wrist in connection with the sheaths of the tendons. (See also HAND.)

Wrist-Drop

See DROP WRIST.

Writer's Cramp

A SPASM which affects certain muscles when a person is writing, and which may not occur when the same muscles are employed in other acts. Similar symptoms are observed in the case of musicians (guitar, clarinet and piano in particular), typists, word-processor and computer operators and artists.

Wry-Neck

A condition in which the head is twisted to one side. It may be caused by the contraction of a scar, such as that resulting from a burn or by paralysis of some of the muscles; as a result of injury at birth; or trauma to the area later in life. Treatment is by an orthopaedic collar, heat or ULTRASOUND, or PHYSIOTHERAPY. Sometimes a local injection of BOTULISM toxin will produce temporary relief. Rarely, surgery is necessary. (See also MUSCLES, DISORDERS OF – Cramp; SPASMODIC TORTICOLLIS.)

W

Xanthelasma Palpebrarum
These yellow smooth nodules of LIPID-laden cells occur in and around the eyelids (see EYE). Blood lipids are usually normal, but there is an association with hypercholesterolaemia (see CHOLESTEROL; HYPERLIPIDAEMIA) in a minority of sufferers.

Xanthoma
(Plural: xanthomata.) A deposit of fatty material in the skin, subcutaneous fat and tendons. The presence of a xanthoma may be the first sign that a person has primary or secondary HYPERLIPIDAEMIA – a raised concentration of lipids (see LIPID) in the blood. This can lead to ATHEROMA, and appropriate clinical and laboratory examinations should be done to determine the diagnosis and treatment.

When fatty deposits occur in various parts of the body – skin, brain, cornea, internal organs and tendons – the condition is called xanthomatosis. Treatment is of the underlying conditions, an important aim being to lower the concentrations of fats in the body.

Xanthomata have a variety of manifestations which may point to the underlying cause. These include:

Eruptive Eruptive yellow papules on the buttocks.

Plane Yellow plaques or macules in the skin.

Tuberous Nodules on the elbows or knees.

Tendinous Subcutaneous nodules fixed to tendons, particularly those on the back of the fingers and the ACHILLES TENDON.

X Chromosome
One of two SEX CHROMOSOMES. Every normal female body cell has a pair of X chromosomes. Men have only one X chromosome and this is paired with a Y chromosome. The sex cells in men and women each have one X and one Y chromosome. Certain diseases are linked to the presence of an X chromosome: these include HAEMOPHILIA (see GENETIC DISORDERS). (See also GENES.)

Xenograft
A transplant (see TRANSPLANTATION) from one animal to another of a different species. It is also known as a heterograft.

Xenotransplantation
TRANSPLANTATION of organs from one species to another – for example, from pigs to humans. The use of organs from appropriately cloned animals was seen as a possible solution to the shortage of human organs for transplantation; however, research has shown that rejection remains a problem and there is also an unresolved possibility that diseases might be transmitted across the species barrier. It seems likely that STEM CELL research will provide a more realistic source of tissues for transplantation to replace diseased organs in humans.

Xeroderma
The term means dry skin. Normal skin may become dry when exposed to very low ambient humidity and is then vulnerable to irritation by soaps, detergents and other chemicals which cause 'chapping'. Dryness of the skin may also be a feature of skin disease, especially atopic eczema (see ATOPY; DERMATITIS). Genetically determined xeroderma is called ICHTHYOSIS.

Xeroderma Pigmentosum
A rare disease in which DNA repair mechanisms fail, rendering the skin especially vulnerable to damage from ultraviolet light (see ULTRAVIOLET RAYS (UVR)). Extreme photosensitivity begins in infancy; later, marked freckling occurs and premature CARCINOGENESIS in the skin usually leads to early death. There may also be neurological complications.

Xerosis
Abnormal dryness, especially of the eye.

Xerostomia
Dryness of the mouth due to lack of SALIVA. Its most extreme form occurs following radiotherapy of the mouth, and in the condition known as Sjögren's syndrome. No satisfactory substitute for natural saliva has been found though some find a methyl-cellulose substitute gives partial relief, as may a glycerin mouthwash.

Xiphisternum
See XIPHOID PROCESS.

Xiphoid Cartilage
See XIPHOID PROCESS.

Xiphoid Process

Also known as the xiphisternum or xiphoid cartilage, this is the small oval-shaped projection forming the lowest of the three parts of the STERNUM or breastbone.

X-Rays

Also known as Röntgen rays, these were discovered in 1895 by Wilhelm Conrad Röntgen. Their use for diagnostic imaging (radiology) and for cancer therapy (see RADIOTHERAPY) is now an integral part of medicine. Many other forms of diagnostic imaging have been developed in recent years, sometimes also loosely called 'radiology'. Similarly the use of chemotherapeutic agents in cancer has led to the term oncology which may be applied to the treatment of cancer by both drugs and X-rays.

The rays are part of the electro-magnetic spectrum; their wavelengths are between 10^{-9} and 10^{-13} metres; in behaviour and energy they are identical to the gamma rays emitted by radioactive isotopes. Diagnostic X-rays are generated in an evacuated tube containing an anode and cathode. Electrons striking the anode cause emission of X-rays of varying energy; the energy is largely dependent on the potential difference (kilovoltage) between anode and cathode. The altered tissue penetration at different kilovoltages is used in radiographing different regions, for example in breast radiography (25–40 kV) or chest radiography (120–150 kV). Most diagnostic examinations use kilovoltages between 60 and 120. The energy of X-rays enables them to pass through body tissues unless they make contact with the constituent atoms. Tissue attenuation varies with atomic structure, so that air-containing organs such as the lung offer little attenuation, while material such as bone, with abundant calcium, will absorb the majority of incident X-rays. This results in an emerging X-ray pattern which corresponds to the structures in the region examined.

Radiography The recording of the resulting images is achieved in several ways, mostly depending on the use of materials which fluoresce in response to X-rays.

CONTRAST X-RAYS Many body organs are not shown by simple X-ray studies. This led to the development of contrast materials which make particular organs or structures wholly or partly opaque to X-rays. Thus, barium-sulphate preparations are largely used for examining the gastrointestinal tract: for example, barium swallow, barium meal, barium follow-through (or enteroclysis) and barium enema. Water-soluble

iodine-containing contrast agents that ionise in solution have been developed for a range of other studies.

More recently a series of improved contrast molecules, chiefly non-ionising, has been developed, with fewer side-effects. They can, for example, safely be introduced into the spinal theca for myeloradiculography – contrast X-rays of the spinal cord. Using these agents, it is possible to show many organs and structures mostly by direct introduction, for example via a catheter (see CATHETERS). In urography, however, contrast medium injected intravenously is excreted by the kidneys which are outlined, together with ureters and bladder. A number of other more specialised contrast agents exist: for example, for cholecystography – radiological assessment of the gall-bladder. The use of contrast and the attendant techniques has greatly widened the range of radiology.

IMAGE INTENSIFICATION The relative insensitivity of fluorescent materials when used for observation of moving organs – for example, the oesophagus – has been overcome by the use of image intensification. A faint fluorographic image produced by X-rays leads to electron emission from a photo-cathode. By applying a high potential difference, the electrons are accelerated across an evacuated tube and are focused on to a small fluorescent screen, giving a bright image. This is viewed by a TV camera and the image shown on a monitor and sometimes recorded on videotape or cine.

TOMOGRAPHY X-ray images are two-dimensional representations of three-dimensional objects. Tomography (Greek *tomos* – a slice) began with X-ray imaging produced by the linked movement of the X-ray tube and the cassette pivoting about a selected plane in the body: over- and underlying structures are blurred out, giving a more detailed image of a particular plane.

In 1975 Godfrey Hounsfield introduced COMPUTED TOMOGRAPHY (CT). This involves (i) movement of an X-ray tube around the patient, with a narrow fan beam of X-rays; (ii) the corresponding use of sensitive detectors on the opposite side of the patient; (iii) computer analysis of the detector readings at each point on the rotation, with calculation of relative tissue attenuation at each point in the cross-sectional plant. This invention has enormously increased the ability to discriminate tissue composition, even without the use of contrast.

The tomographic effect – imaging of a particular plane – is achieved in many of the newer forms of imaging: ULTRASOUND, magnetic resonance imaging (see MRI) and some forms of nuclear medicine, in particular positron emission tomography (PET SCANNING). An alternative term for the production of images of a given plane is cross-sectional imaging.

While the production of X-ray and other images has been largely the responsibility of radiographers, the interpretation has been principally carried out by specialist doctors called radiologists. In addition they, and interested clinicians, have developed a number of procedures, such as arteriography (see ANGIOGRAPHY), which involve manipulative access for imaging – for example, selective coronary or renal arteriography.

The use of X-rays, ultrasound or computerised tomography to control the direction and position of needles has made possible guided biopsies (see BIOPSY) – for example, of pancreatic, pulmonary or bony lesions – and therapeutic procedures such as drainage of obstructed kidneys (percutaneous nephrostomy), or of abscesses. From these has grown a whole series of therapeutic procedures such as ANGIOPLASTY, STENT insertion and renal-stone track formation. This field of interventional radiology has close affinities with MINIMALLY INVASIVE SURGERY (MIS).

Radiotherapy, or treatment by X-rays The two chief sources of the ionising radiations used in radiotherapy are the gamma rays of RADIUM and the penetrating X-rays generated by apparatus working at various voltages. For superficial lesions, energies of around 40 kilovolts are used; but for deep-seated conditions, such as cancer of the internal organs, much higher voltages are required. X-ray machines are now in use which work at two million volts. Even higher voltages are now available through the development of the linear accelerator, which makes use of the frequency magnetron which is the basis of radar. The linear accelerator receives its name from the fact that it accelerates a beam of electrons down a straight tube, 3 metres in length, and in this process a voltage of eight million is attained. The use of these very high voltages has led to the development of a highly specialised technique which has been devised for the treatment of cancer and like diseases.

Protective measures are routinely taken to ensure that the patient's normal tissue is not damaged during radiotherapy. The operators too have to take special precautions, including limits on the time they can work with the equipment in any one period of time.

The greatest value of radiotherapy is in the treatment of malignant disease. In many patients it can be used for the treatment of malignant growths which are not accessible to surgery, whilst in others it is used in conjunction with surgery and chemotherapy.

Xylose

A sugar containing five carbon atoms involved in the metabolic conversion of carbohydrates (see CARBOHYDRATE) inside cells. Xylose is used in diagnostic tests on the functioning of the INTESTINE.

X

Yawning

An involuntary opening of the mouth, which is accompanied by marked dilatation of the pharynx, a characteristic distortion of the face and usually stretching of the limbs. The cause and function of yawning are quite obscure. It is classically regarded as a sign of drowsiness or boredom, but it it may be the result of raised concentrations of CARBON DIOXIDE (CO_2) in the blood – the physiological aim being to cut the amount of CO_2 and raise the level of oxygen in the blood.

Yaws

A non-venereal spirochaetal infection caused by *Treponema pertenue*; it was formerly widespread in most tropical and subtropical regions amongst the indigenous population, florid disease being more common in children than adults. The term is of Carib-Indian (native to north-eastern South America, the east coast of Central America, and the lesser Antilles) origin. It is directly contagious from person to person; infection is also transmitted by flies, clothing, and living in unclean huts. Clinically, the primary stage is characterised by a granulomatous lesion, or papule (framboesioma or 'mother yaw') at the site of infection – usually the lower leg or foot; this enlarges, crusts, and heals spontaneously. It appears some 2–8 weeks after infection, during which time fever, malaise, pains, and pruritus may be present. In the secondary stage, a granulomatous, papular, macular or squamous eruption occurs; periostitis may also be present. The late, or tertiary stage (which appears 5–10 years later), is characterised by skin plaques, nodules, ulcers, hyperkeratosis (thickening of the skin of the hands and feet) and gummatous lesions affecting bones. Recurrence of infection in individuals suffering from a concurrent infection (e.g. SYPHILIS or TUBERCULOSIS) renders the infection more serious. Diagnosis is by demonstration of *T. pertenue* in exudate from a suspected lesion. Treatment is with PENICILLIN, to which *T. pertenue* is highly sensitive. Extensive eradication campaigns (initiated by the WHO in 1949) have been carried out in endemic areas; therefore, the early stages of the infection are rarely counted; only tertiary stages come to the attention of a physician. Failure of surveillance can lead to dramatic local recurrences.

Y Chromosome

One of two SEX CHROMOSOMES that is present in every male body cell where it is paired with an X CHROMOSOME. The sex or germ cells in women as well as men contain one X and one Y chromosome (see also GENES).

Yeast

This consists of the cells and spores of unicellular fungi belonging to the family of *Saccharomycetaceae*. The main species of yeast used in medicine is *Saccharomyces cerevisiae*, which is used in the fermentation industries, such as brewing. It is a rich source of the vitamin B complex (see APPENDIX 5: VITAMINS), but its use has largely been given up since the various components of the vitamin B complex became available as separate entities.

Yellow Fever

An acute arbovirus (see ARBOVIRUSES) infection caused by a flavivirus of the togavirus family, transmitted from animals to humans by various species of forest mosquito (jungle/sylvan yellow fever), and from human to human by *Aëdes aegypti* (urban yellow fever). Mosquito transmission was shown by Walter Reed and his colleagues in 1900. It is ENDEMIC in much of tropical Africa and Central and South America but does not occur in Asia. In the urban cycle, humans constitute the reservoir of infection, and in the jungle/sylvan variety, mammals – especially subhuman primates – are involved in transmission. Historically, yellow fever was enormously important, causing devastating epidemics (see EPIDEMIC); it also carried a high mortality rate in travellers and explorers. Differentiation from other infections associated with JAUNDICE was often impossible.

Clinically, yellow fever is characterised by jaundice, fever, chills, headache, gastrointestinal haemorrhage(s), and ALBUMINURIA. The incubation period is 3–6 (up to 10) days. Differentiation from viral hepatitides, other viral haemorrhagic fevers, severe *Plasmodium falciparum* malaria, and several other infections is often impossible without sophisticated investigative techniques. Infection carries a high mortality rate. Liver histology (biopsy is contraindicated due to the haemorrhagic diathesis) shows characteristic changes; a fulminating hepatic infection is often present. Acute inflammation of the kidneys and an inflamed, congested gastric mucosa, often accompanied by haemorrhage, are also demonstrable;

myocardial involvement often occurs. Diagnosis is primarily based on virological techniques; serological tests are also of value. Yellow fever should be suspected in any travellers from an endemic area.

Management consists of instituting techniques for acute hepatocellular (liver-cell) failure. The affected individual should be kept in an isolation unit, away from mosquitoes which could transmit the disease to a healthy individual. Formerly, laboratory infections were occasionally acquired from infected blood samples. Prophylactically, a satisfactory attenuated VACCINE (17D) has been available for around 60 years; this is given subcutaneously and provides an individual with excellent protection for ten years; international certificates are valid for this length of time. Every traveller to an endemic area should be immunised; this is mandatory for entry to countries where the infection is endemic.

Yersinia

A genus of BACTERIA which includes the causative organism of PLAGUE, *Yersinia pestis.*

Yin and Yang

Basic concepts in traditional Chinese medicine and philosophy. Yang represents active, positive masculine qualities. Yin embodies passive, negative feminine qualities.

Yoga

A system of Hindu philosophy and physical discipline involving special breathing techniques and a series of prescribed physical poses. These are intended to relax the body and teach the individual mental and physical control. Yoga is best learned from experienced teachers, or those practising it may damage their backs.

Yoghurt

Sour milk curdled with one of the LACTIC ACID producing bacilli, such as *Lactobacillus acidophilus* or *Lactobacillus bulgaricus.* It contains all the protein, fat, calcium, and vitamins of the original milk, and is therefore a nutritious food, but there is no evidence that it has any unique beneficial properties of its own. In countries where standards of hygiene are low, it has the advantage of having been sterilised by boiling and is therefore unlikely to be contaminated with dangerous micro-organisms.

Yohimbine

This substance is derived from the bark of *Pausinystalia yohimbie,* a West African tree. Once widely used as an aphrodisiac – an action for which there is no good evidence, it is now being used in the treatment of certain cases of postural HYPOTENSION and for the treatment of IMPOTENCE.

Yttrium-90

An artificially produced ISOTOPE of the element Yttrium. The isotope is radioactive and emits beta rays which are utilised for the treatment of tumours.

Y

Zalcitabine

A nucleoside REVERSE TRANSCRIPTASE INHIBITOR used in the treatment of HIV, in combination with other antiretroviral drugs. Serious side-effects include the risk of peripheral NEUROPATHY and of pancreatitis (see PANCREAS, DISEASES OF).

Zanamivir

An antiviral drug (trade name Relenza©) which ameliorates the symptoms of INFLUENZA. It is licensed in the United Kingdom for treating the A or B varieties, 48 hours after the onset of symptoms. In otherwise healthy people it reduces the duration of symptoms by around 24 hours. It is not yet known to what extent zanamivir can prevent complications in high-risk patients such as the elderly.

Zidovudine

An antiviral drug used to treat AIDS (see AIDS/ HIV) and its related conditions, such as pneumocystis PNEUMONIA. The drug slows down the growth of human immunodeficiency virus (HIV) but does not cure the disease. It may be given intravenously or by mouth. Also called AZT, zidovudine has been in use since 1987, and it works by blocking the ENZYME that stimulates HIV to grow and multiply. It may cause ANAEMIA so regular blood tests are necessary.

Zinc

A metal, several salts of which are used in medicine for external application. It is essential for growth and development in animals and plants. The average human body contains a total of 1– 2 grams, and most human diets contain 10–15 mg. In human beings, deficiency of zinc results in lack of growth, slow sexual development and ANAEMIA. Deficiency is also associated with a skin disorder known as acrodermatitis enteropathica.

Uses Zinc chloride is a powerful caustic and astringent which, combined with zinc sulphate, is used as an astringent mouthwash. Zinc sulphate is also used in the form of eyedrops in the treatment of certain forms of conjunctivitis (see under EYE, DISORDERS OF).

Zinc oxide, zinc stearate, and zinc carbonate are made up in dusting powders, in ointments, in paste bandages or suspended in water as lotions for the astringent action they exert upon abraded surfaces of the skin. Zinc and castor oil ointment of the British Pharmacopoeia is a well-tried treatment for nappy rash.

Zinc undecenoate is used as an ointment and as a dusting-powder in the treatment of RINGWORM.

Zollinger-Ellison Syndrome

A rare disorder in which severe peptic ulcers recur in the stomach and duodenum (see DUODENAL ULCER; STOMACH, DISEASES OF). It is caused by a tumour in the PANCREAS that produces a hormone, GASTRIN, which stimulates the stomach and duodenum to produce excess acid: this causes ulceration. Treatment is by surgery.

Zona and Zoster

Two names for the eruption popularly known as shingles. (See HERPES ZOSTER.)

Zonulolysis

The process whereby the zonule (see EYE) is dissolved by an ENZYME (chymotrypsin) as part of intracapsular cataract surgery. Once the zonule has been dissolved the cataract can be lifted out of the eye. (See EYE, DISORDERS OF – Cataract.)

Zoonoses

Animal diseases which can be transmitted to humans. There are more than 150 infections of domestic and wild vertebrates which can be transmitted in this way, including BOVINE SPONGIFORM ENCEPHALOPATHY (BSE), bovine tuberculosis, BRUCELLOSIS, HYDATID cysts, RINGWORM, TOXOCARIASIS, TOXOPLASMOSIS, LEPTOSPIROSIS, LISTERIOSIS, and RABIES.

Zygoma

Or zygomatic bone. The name given to a bridge of bone formed by the union of a process from the temporal bone in the skull with one from the malar (cheek) bone. It lies in the region of the temple, gives attachment to the powerful masseter muscle which moves the lower jaw, and forms a protection to the side of the head.

Zygote

This is the cell produced when an OVUM is fertilised by a SPERMATOZOON. A zygote contains all the hereditary material for a new individual: half comes from the sperm and half from the

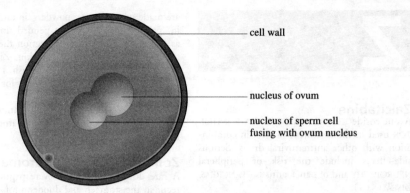

cell wall

nucleus of ovum

nucleus of sperm cell
fusing with ovum nucleus

Fertilisation of the female ovum by the male sperm cell to form the zygote.

ovum. After passing down the Fallopian tube, when the zygote starts dividing, it becomes implanted in the UTERUS and develops into an EMBRYO.

Zymolysis
The mechanism of fermentation initiated by an ENZYME during DIGESTION.

APPENDIX 1: BASIC FIRST AID

This appendix is designed to cover the basic principles involved in the immediate treatment of some common emergencies. It is not comprehensive, and anyone wishing to become proficient at first aid should attend a course run by a reputable organisation such as the British Red Cross, St John Ambulance, and the St Andrew's Ambulance Association. A knowledge of first aid can be of great practical value whether at home, at work or when travelling. On occasions its prompt application may save someone's life or lessen the potential harm of an accident.

First-aid treatment in an emergency is intended:
- to preserve life and stop the victim's condition from deteriorating.
- to help recovery and save the victim from further harm.
- to make the casualty as comfortable as possible and reassure him/her and the family.
- to assess the events surrounding the illness or accident so that relevant facts can be given to a doctor, nurse or paramedical staff.

No ill or badly injured person should be moved without skilled assistance – especially if a neck or spinal injury is suspected – unless the individual's life is in immediate danger from the surroundings (e.g. a fire). He or she should be kept warm; constricting clothing should be loosened; and a clear airway should be established, with any false teeth removed.

Bleeding This may occur from arteries, veins or capillary beds. The former is easily recognised as the blood tends to spurt from the wound at the same rate as the pulse; with the latter two types the blood tends to flow from the wound. Minor bleeding is usually treated in the home by the application of bandages, etc. However, the basic principles of treatment for major haemorrhages may be applied. Pressure should be applied to the bleeding point, via gauze or a clean piece of cloth if available, firmly enough to stop the flow of blood. With the pressure applied, the wound should be raised above the level of the heart. The patient should then be transferred to a place where medical care is available. If the loss of blood is severe enough for the victim to have become shocked (see SHOCK), he or she should be laid flat with the legs raised, if possible. (See also HAEMORRHAGE.)

Burns and scalds Burns can be caused by dry heat, severe cold, corrosive materials, radiation (including rays from the sun) and friction (such as results from a body sliding along a road surface after a motorcycle accident). Scalds are caused by hot fluids or steam. Burns and scalds may be associated with other injuries caused, say, by an escape from a burning building, a road traffic accident or an explosion: casualties should therefore be examined for other injuries. Most burns and scalds affect the skin, and the area(s) and site(s) of skin damaged are important in assessing a victim's condition. Muscles and other tissues may be damaged by burns, and inhalation of smoke or fumes may damage the linings of the mouth, throat and lungs. Shock, sometimes severe, is common – the result of pain and loss of body fluids. All but the most minor burns should be seen by a doctor, as it is difficult to assess the severity of the burn immediately after it occurs. If the person or his or her clothing is actually on fire, then the first move must be to smother the flames – by covering them with a blanket or coat, for example – and 'patting out' the flames without sustaining burns yourself. Many burns, however, are caused by hot liquids, hot gases, flashes from explosions or contact with a very hot object so that the person is not actually on fire. The treatment for all these burns is the same – to remove any clothing over the affected area, if possible, and to put the affected area under cold running water until the pain has stopped or the ambulance has arrived (the cold water should be applied for several minutes, as cooling of the tissues, particularly the deeper layers of the skin, will limit the extent of the burn). The burn should be left exposed or covered with a piece of clean wet linen (e.g. a pillowcase), for the transfer to hospital. No lotions or potions should be applied to the burn until it has been seen by a doctor or a nurse. (See also main dictionary entry for BURNS AND SCALDS.)

Choking Severe life-threatening CHOKING occurs when a piece of food or a foreign object becomes lodged in the LARYNX or TRACHEA causing obstruction. The person may cough, gag, or wheeze and will become cyanosed (blue) as he or she fights to take a breath. Infants or small children should be held along the arm, head down, and several gentle blows with the flat of the hand should be delivered to the back between the shoulder-blades: this will usually dislodge the foreign body. In older children or adults the Heimlich manoeuvre should be employed. Stand behind the victim with your arms wrapped around the waist. Make a fist with one hand, with the thumb placed at a point half-way between the victim's navel and the bottom of the breastbone. Grasp the fist with your other hand and give a quick inward and upward thrust. This may be repeated several times if necessary. Alternatively, if the person is unconscious, he or she should be placed on the back, face up, and the same thrust performed with the heel of the hand whilst kneeling astride the hips. If a choking person is alone, he or she can perform the manoeuvre by placing a fist in the correct position and delivering the thrust by pressing it against a firm surface.

Cardiac/respiratory arrest The measures described here are basic life-support procedures – they can be performed if necessary without any equipment. Before commencing cardiopulmonary resuscitation on a person who has collapsed, it is essential to establish that it is in fact required. Performing artificial ventilation and cardiac massage on a person who is breathing and whose heart is still beating can be dangerous. The person's chest and abdomen should be observed for respiratory movement and the PULSE should be checked either at the neck or groin or by feeling directly over the heart.

The technique for simple resuscitation may be remembered by means of the mnemonic 'ABC' (Airway, Breathing and Circulation). The aim of basic resuscitation is to maintain the flow of oxygenated blood to vital organs until the person's heartbeat and breathing can be restarted, if that is possible.

AIRWAY If the airway is obstructed, no air can enter the lungs; therefore the mouth should be checked for foreign bodies, which can be removed by hooking them out with an index finger. False teeth should be removed. To prevent the tongue from obstructing breathing, the jaw should be pulled forwards (using a finger behind the angle of the chin) and the head extended on the neck so that the person looks as if he or she is 'sniffing the morning air'.

Care must be taken if there is any suspicion of neck injury.

BREATHING If clearing the airway does not allow breathing to recommence, then artificial ventilation of the lungs must be started. Mouth-to-mouth ventilation, using the rescuer's expired air to inflate the victim's lungs, is probably the easiest and most satisfactory technique. The victim is positioned as described above. The rescuer uses one hand to obstruct

the nose and steady the head, and the other to pull the jaw forwards and open the mouth. The rescuer then places his or her mouth completely over that of the victim and blows out so as to inflate the victim's lungs, starting with two slow breaths to reinflate the lungs. It is important to observe the victim's chest rise and fall normally before commencing the next breath. If the chest does not rise, or if there is marked resistance to the inflating breath, then the airway is probably obstructed and the head should be repositioned.

CIRCULATION Ventilating the lungs without any blood circulating will not provide oxygenated blood to vital organs. Therefore, if there is no pulse or heartbeat, cardiac massage should be started to produce this circulation. The person performing cardiac massage – who should preferably have been trained in the technique – should kneel beside the victim with the heel of one hand over the lower two-thirds of the breastbone and the other hand placed on top. Downward pressure is applied, keeping the arms straight with the elbows locked, so as to depress the breastbone 4–5 cm. Pressure is released slowly so that it takes the same time as compression. The rate of compressions should be 80 per minute. If there are two rescuers, then the person performing cardiac massage should stop after every five compressions to allow the other to perform one cycle of artificial ventilation. A lone rescuer should perform two breaths after every 15 compressions.

Once spontaneous ventilation and cardiac output have returned, the patient should be placed in the recovery, or coma, position. This consists of rolling the person on to his or her side, with the lower arm and leg straight and in line with the body. The upper arm and leg are flexed and brought forwards to prevent the patient from rolling on to his or her front.

Drowning Around 500 people die from drowning each year in Britain, and an unknown number survive a near-drowning. About one-fifth of drownings occur in salt water. Wet drowning (when water is aspirated into the lungs) occurs in 85 per cent of cases; the remaining 15 per cent develop laryngospasm so that, although they also die of ASPHYXIA, no water enters the lungs.

There has been some controversy about what type of water carries the worst prognosis, but it is now thought that salt and fresh water are equally bad. The effect of salt water is to draw fluid into the alveoli (see ALVEOLUS) from the vascular compartment with concomitant damage to the lung. This results in PULMONARY

OEDEMA and HYPOXIA. Fresh water washes out pulmonary SURFACTANT (causing pulmonary atelectasis and leading to hypoxia) and is absorbed into the vascular compartment causing volume overload and electrolyte disturbances. Both types may result in ACIDOSIS and circulatory collapse, and may be complicated by HYPOTHERMIA and trauma (which may indeed have precipitated the drowning).

Treatment Cardiopulmonary resuscitation (see cardiac/respiratory arrest in this appendix) should be started as soon as possible and the patient transferred to hospital. This should include people who recover consciousness fairly quickly, as pulmonary oedema may develop over the next few hours. If the patient is hypothermic (see HYPOTHERMIA), resuscitation should continue until he or she has been warmed to normal body temperature. Patients may require admission to an intensive care unit for artificial ventilation, circulatory support, or correction of electrolyte imbalance or acidosis.

Electrocution People may be electrocuted when they touch an object which is live so that a current passes through them to earth. A lightning strike has a similar effect. The severity of the outcome depends upon the frequency and amplitude of the current which flows through them. Below 2mA there is only a feeling of strong PARAESTHESIA; 15–100mA will produce muscular contraction in the muscles near the point of contact, which makes letting go of the object impossible; and 50mA–2A is the threshold for producing VENTRICULAR FIBRILLATION. (These thresholds are for the mains electricity supply, which in Britain has a frequency of 50Hz – one that is particularly liable to induce ventricular fibrillation.) Thus electrocution can cause burns (see burns and scalds, above) to the tissues at the sites where the current enters and leaves the body, and may also induce ventricular fibrillation. If a person is seen being electrocuted, no attempt should be made to touch the victim until the power supply is turned off, as the helper may also be electrocuted. If the switch or mains supply cannot be found, then the victim should be knocked away from the power source using a non-conducting object such as wood. Burns should be treated as described above and, if the patient has developed ventricular fibrillation, then cardiopulmonary resuscitation should be started (see cardiac/respiratory arrest in this appendix). Any person experiencing significant electrocution should be seen by a doctor.

Foreign bodies Unwanted objects may enter the eyes, ears, nose, mouth and gullet (OESOPHAGUS), the lungs and wounds. Foreign bodies in wounds, the lungs, mouth, gullet and stomach should be treated by a doctor or nurse; unskilled attempts to remove them may harm the patient.

EYES Dust, eyelashes and displaced contact lenses that have not penetrated the tissue of the eye are usually easily removed by washing with clean water, preferably using an eyebath. If the foreign body is stuck to or has penetrated the surface of the eye, the eye should be covered with a clean pad and medical attention obtained.

EARS AND NOSE Do not attempt to remove the foreign body: obtain medical attention.

Heatstroke This occurs when the body becomes dangerously overheated because of a high fever or prolonged exposure to heat – for example, being out in the hot sun or working in a hot environment (e.g. near a furnace). Heatstroke may suddenly occur or manifest itself by the victim's feeling uncomfortable, ill or confused. Remove the casualty from the heat source and lower the body TEMPERATURE by removing clothing and wrapping the patient in a cold wet sheet or towel, fanning him or her and sponging with cold water. Obtain urgent medical attention.

Inhalation of fumes The inhalation of gases, smoke or toxic vapours can rapidly cause death. Victims need to be removed quickly from the source of the fumes, but the rescuer(s) may need protective equipment in order to do this. Attempts by inexperienced, unprotected persons may well result in further casualties, so emergency services should be called promptly. CARBON MONOXIDE (CO) is particularly dangerous because it has neither taste nor smell and can speedily overcome anyone exposed to the gas, especially in a confined space such as kitchen or garage. Victims need to be taken into the open air and their breathing quickly restored with artificial respiration (see cardiac/respiratory arrest, above) and oxygen, if available. (Remember that oxygen is very inflammable and is normally given by skilled staff using appropriate equipment.)

Poisoning The number of substances with which people are poisoned, either deliberately or accidentally, is too great to list individually. This section will merely cover some basic principles to follow on discovering a person who has been poisoned.

If the person is unconscious, he or she should be nursed in the coma position (see cardiac/respiratory arrest in this appendix). Vomiting should never be induced at home except under medical supervision. If corrosive substances have been ingested, then water or milk should be drunk to dilute the effects on the oesophagus and stomach, and any remaining on the skin should be washed away with copious volumes of water. The container from which the tablets or other substance came should be taken to hospital with the patient to help medical staff correctly identify the poison. Likewise if it is a plant, a leaf or a berry. (See also POISONS.)

Seizures A major SEIZURE or fit is known as a Grand Mal convulsion (see EPILEPSY) and consists of two phases: the tonic phase when the person may let out a cry, falls to the ground and is observed to be rigid; and the clonic phase when he or she shakes. At the end of the fit there is usually a period of unconsciousness. The most important task in looking after people undergoing a fit is to prevent them from doing any damage to themselves. Any objects which might cause harm, particularly hot food and liquids, should be moved out of their way, but there is no need to try to move the person themselves unless they are in danger (it may, however, be necessary to roll them on to their side to prevent asphyxiation). No attempt should be made to protect the tongue, and a finger should not be inserted in the mouth to straighten the tongue. Clothing around the patient's neck should be loosened and, if possible, a pillow placed under the neck. At the end of the fit, when the person is unconscious, he or she should be placed in the coma or recovery position (see cardiac/respiratory arrest, above).

APPENDIX 2: ADDRESSES: SOURCES OF INFORMATION, ADVICE, SUPPORT AND SELF-HELP

Addresses for other information and support groups can be found in the *Voluntary Agencies Directory* (published by NCVO Publications, National Council for Voluntary Organisations, Regent's Wharf, 8 All Saints Street, London N1 9RL [020 7713 6161, distribution: 01536 399016]). Telephone helpline numbers can be found in the *Telephone Helplines Directory* (published by the Telephone Helplines Association, 4th Floor, 9 Marshalsea Road, Borough, London SE1 1EP 020 7089 6321, fax: 020 7089 6320, website: www.helplines.org.uk]) and in the helpline sections of *Thomson Local* telephone directories. Information on many rare disorders may be found in *The CaF Directory* (see children, below). Helpline numbers beginning 0800 and 0808 are free; 0845 calls are charged at local rates; and 0870 calls at national rates.

ACCIDENT PREVENTION IN THE HOME Child Accident Prevention Trust, 4th floor, 18–20 Farringdon Lane, London EC1R 3HA (020 7608 3828, fax: 020 7608 3674, e-mail: safe@capt.demon).

Royal Society for the Prevention of Accidents, Edgbaston Park, 353 Bristol Road, Birmingham B5 7ST (0121 248 2000, fax: 0121 248 2001, website: www.rospa.com, e-mail: help@rospa.com).

ADOPTION See child adoption.

AGEING Age Concern England, Astral House, 1268 London Road, Norbury, London SW16 4ER (020 8765 7200, helpline: 0800 00 99 66 (7 days, 0700–1900), fax: 020 8765 7211, website: www.ageconcern.org.uk, e-mail: ace@ ace.org.uk).

Help the Aged, 207–221 Pentonville Road, London N1 9UZ (020 7278 1114, fax: 020 7278 1116, website: www.ageconcern.org.uk, e-mail: info@helptheaged.org.uk).

AGORAPHOBIA See phobias.

AIDS Terrence Higgins Trust Lighthouse (THTL), 52–54 Gray's Inn Road, London WC1X 8JU (020 7831 0330, helpline: 0845 1221 200 [M–F, 1000–2200, S–S, 1200–1800], fax: 020 7242 0121, website: www. tht.org.uk, e-mail: info@ tht.org.uk).

Communicable Diseases Surveillance Centre: see public health laboratory services, appendix 7: statutory organisations.

ALCOHOL ACCEPT: Alcohol and Substance Misuse, 724 Fulham Road, London SW6 5SE (administration: 020 7371 7555, clients: 020 7371 7477).

Alcoholics Anonymous, PO Box 1, Stonebow House, Stonebow, York YO1 7NJ (01904 644026, helpline: 0845 769 7555, fax: 01904 629091, website: www.alcoholics-anonymous.org.uk).

Al-Anon Family Groups UK and Eire (including Alateen), 61 Great Dover Street, London SE1 4YF (helpline: 020 7403 0888, fax: 020 7378 9910, website: www.al-anonuk.org.uk).

Alcohol Concern, Waterbridge House, 32–36 Loman Street, London SE1 0EE (020 7928 7377, fax: 020 7928 4644, website: www.alcoholconcern.org.uk, e-mail: contact@ alcoholconcern.org.uk).

Alcohol Focus Scotland, 2nd Floor, 166 Buchanan Street, Glasgow G1 2LW (0141 572 6700, fax: 0141 333 1606, website: www.alcohol-focus-scotland.org.uk, e-mail: enquiries@alcohol-focus-scotland.org.uk).

ALZHEIMER'S DISEASE Alzheimer's Society, 2nd Floor, Gordon House, 10 Greencoat Place, London SW1P 1PH (020 7306 0606, helpline: 0845 300 0336, fax: 020 7308 0808, website: www.alzheimers.org.uk, e-mail: enquiries@ alzheimers.org.uk).

ANKYLOSING SPONDYLITIS The National Ankylosing Spondylitis Society (NASS), PO Box 179, Mayfield, East Sussex TN20 6ZL (01435 873527, fax: 01435 873027, website: www.nass.co.uk, e-mail: nass@nass.co.uk).

ANOREXIA See eating disorders.

ARTHRITIS Arthritis Care, 18 Stephenson Way, London NW1 2HD (020 7380 6500, helpline: 0808 800 4050 [M–F, 1200–1600], or 020 7380 6555 (1000–1600), fax: 020 7380 6505, website: www. arthritiscare.org.uk).

ASTHMA Asthma UK, Providence House, Providence Place, London N1 0NT (020 7226 2260, helpline: 0845 701 0203, fax: 020 7704 0740, website: www.asthma.org.uk).

ATAXIA UK Room 10, Winchester House, Kennington Park, 11 Cranmer Road, London SW9 6EJ (020 7582 1444, helpline: 0845 644 0606, fax: 020 7582 9444, website: ataxia. org.uk, e-mail: enquiries@ataxia.org.uk).

AUTISM The National Autistic Society, 393 City Road, London EC1V 1NG (020 7833 2299, helpline: 0845 070 4004 [M–F, 1000-1600], fax: 020 7833 9666, website: www.nas.org.uk, e-mail: nas@nas.org.uk).

BACK PAIN Back Care, 16 Elmtree Road, Teddington, Middlesex TW11 8ST (020 8977 5474, fax: 020 8943 5318, website: www.backcare.org.uk, e-mail: website@ backcare.org.uk).

BLINDNESS Royal National Institute for the Blind (RNIB), 105 Judd Street, London WC1H 9NE (020 7388 1266, helpline: 0845 766 9999, fax: 020 7388 2034, website: www.rnib.org.uk, e-mail: helpline@ rnib.org.uk).

BLOOD TRANSFUSION National Blood Service, Oak House, Reeds Crescent, Watford, Herts. WD24 4QN, (0845 7 711 711, website: www.blood.co.uk). The authority is responsible for 15 regional centres in England.

BRAIN INJURIES Headway – the brain injury association, 4 King Edward Court, King Edward Street, Nottingham NG1 1EW (0115 924 0800, textphone: 0115 950 7825, fax: 0115 958 4446, website: www.headway.org.uk, e-mail: enquiries@headway.org.uk).

BREAST CANCER CARE Breast Cancer Care, Kiln House, 210 New Kings Road, London SW6 4NZ (020 7384 2984, helpline: 0808 800 6000, textphone: 0808 800 6001, fax: 020 7384 3387, website: www.breastcancercare. org.uk, e-mail: info@breastcancercare.org.uk).

Scottish office: 4th Floor, 40 St Enoch Square, Glasgow, G1 4DH, (0845 0771 892, fax: 0141 221 9499, e-mail: sco@breastcancercare.org.uk).

BREAST FEEDING National Childbirth Trust (see childbirth), Alexandra House, Oldham Terrace, London, W3 6NH (0870 4448 707, breastfeeding line: 0870 4448 708).

La Leche League of Great Britain (LLLGB), PO Box 29, West Bridgford, Nottingham, NG2 7NP (helpline 0845 120 2918 [24 hours], website: www.laleche.org.uk).

BRITTLE BONE DISEASE Brittle Bone Society, 30 Guthrie Street, Dundee DD1 5BS (01382 204446, helpline: 0800 028 2459, fax: 01382 206771, website: www.brittlebone.org, e-mail: bbs@brittlebone.org).

CANCER CARE Macmillan Cancer Relief, 89 Albert Embankment, London SE1 7UQ (020 7840 7840, helpline: 0808 808 2020, fax: 020 7840 7841, website: macmillan.org.uk).

Marie Curie Cancer Care, 89 Albert Embankment, London SE1 7TP (020 7599 7777, fax: 020 7599 7785, website: www. mariecurie. org.uk, e-mail: info@mariecurie.org.uk).

CANCER INFORMATION SERVICE Cancer BACUP, 3 Bath Place, Rivington Street, London EC2A 3DR (020 7696 9003, helpline: 0808 800 1234 or 0207 739 2280 standard rate [M–F 0900–1900], fax: 020 7696 9002, website: www.cancerbacup.org.uk).

CARERS Carers National Association, 20–25 Glasshouse Yard, London EC1A 4JT (020 7490 8818, helpline: 0845 573 369, fax: 020 7490 8824, e-mail: info@ukcarers.org, website: www. carersuk.org.

Women's Royal Voluntary Service, Garden House, Milton Hill, Steventon, Oxfordshire OX13 6AD (01235 442900, fax: 01235 861166, website: www.wrvs.org.uk).

CARE SERVICES Counsel and Care, Twyman House, 16 Bonny Street, London NW1 9PG (020 7241 8555, helpline: 0845 300 7585 [M–F 1000–1300], fax: 020 7267 6877, website: www.counselandcare.org.uk, e-mail: advice@counselandcare.org.uk).

CEREBRAL PALSY SCOPE, PO Box 833, Milton Keynes MK12 5NY (020 7619 7100, helpline: 0808 800 3333 [M–F, 0900–2100, S–S, 1400–1800], fax: 020 7619 7399, website: www.scope.org.uk).

Advice Service Capability Service Scotland (ASCS), 11 Ellersly Road, Edinburgh EH12 6HY (0131 313 5510, textphone: 0131 346 2529, fax: 0131 346 1681, website: www.capability-scotland.org.uk, e-mail: ascs@ capability-scotland.org.uk).

CHILD ADOPTION Adoption UK, 46 The Green, South Bar Street, Banbury OX16 9AB (helpline: 0870 7700 450, tel: 01295 752240, fax: 01295 752241, website: www.adoptionuk.org.uk, e-mail: helpdesk@ adoptionuk.org.uk).

Adoptions Section, Office for National Statistics, Smedley Hydro, Trafalgar Road, Birkdale, Southport PR8 2HH (0151 471 4313, fax: 0151 471 4755).

British Agencies for Adoption and Fostering (BAAF), Skyline House, 200 Union Street, London SE1 0LX (020 7593 2000, fax: 020 7593 2001, website: www.baaf.org.uk, e-mail: mail@baaf.org.uk).

National Organisation for Counselling Adoptees and Parents (NORCAP), 112 Church Road, Wheatley, Oxfordshire OX33 1LU (01865 875000 [M–Th 1000–1600], fax: 01865 875686, website: www.norcap.org.uk, e-mail: enquiries@norcap.org).

CHILDBIRTH National Childbirth Trust, Alexandra House, Oldham Terrace, Acton, London W3 6NH (enquiries: 0870 444 8707, breastfeeding line: 0870 444 8708, fax: 0870 770 3237, website: www.nctpregnancyandbabycare.com), e-mail: enquiries@national-childbirth-trust.co.uk).

CHILDREN Action for Sick Children, National Children's Bureau, 8 Wakley Street, London EC1V 7QE, (020 7843 6444, website: www. actionforsickchildren.org, e-mail: enquiries@ actionforsickchildren.org).

Contact a Family, 209–211 City Road, London EC1V 1JN (020 7608 8700, helpline: 0808 808 3555 [M–F, 1000–1600], fax: 020 7608 8701, website: www.cafamily.org.uk, e-mail: info@cafamily.org.uk). A charity which provides families who care for children with any disability or special need with authoritative, accessible, descriptive information. It is a main source of information about rare disorders and helps adults as well as children. *The CaF Directory* lists established UK support organisations and is available on the charity's website: www.cafamily.org.uk/dirworks.html.

National Society for the Prevention of Cruelty to Children (NSPCC), Weston House, 42 Curtain Road, London EC2A 3NH (020 7825 2500, helpline: 0808 800 5000, fax: 020 7825 2525, website: nspcc.org.uk).

NCH Action for Children, 85 Highbury Park, London N5 1UD (020 7704 7000, helpline: 0845 762 6579, fax: 020 7226 2537, website: nch.org.uk).

CHIROPODY See appendix 8: professional organisations.

CLEFT LIP AND PALATE See palate malformations.

COCHRANE COLLABORATION Update Software Ltd, Oxford OX2 7LG (01865 513902, website: www.cochrane.co.uk, e-mail: info@update.co.uk).

COELIAC DISEASE Coeliac Society of the United Kingdom, PO Box 220, High Wycombe, Buckinghamshire HP11 2HY (01494 437278, helpline 0870 444 8804, fax: 01494 474349, website: www.coeliac.co.uk, e-mail: helpline@ coeliac.co.uk).

COLITIS AND CROHN'S DISEASE National Association for Colitis and Crohn's Disease, 4 Beaumont House, Sutton Road, St Albans, Hertfordshire AL1 5HH (01727 830038, helpline: 0845 130 2233, fax: 01727 862550, website: www.nacc.org.uk, e-mail: nacc@nacc.org.uk).

COLOSTOMY British Colostomy Association, 15 Station Road, Reading, Berkshire RG1 1LG (0118 939 1537, helpline: 0800 328 4257, fax: 0118 956 9095, website: www.bcass. org.uk, e-mail: sue@bcass.org.uk).

CORONARY HEART DISEASE Coronary Prevention Group, 2 Taviton Street, London WC1H 0BT (020 7927 2125, fax: 020 7927 2127, website: www.healthnet.org.uk, e-mail: cpg@lshtm.ac.uk).

CYSTIC FIBROSIS Cystic Fibrosis Trust, 11 London Road, Bromley, Kent BR1 1BY (020 8464 7211, fax: 020 8313 0472, website: www.cftrust.org.uk, e-mail: enquiries@ cftrust.org.uk).

DEAFNESS Royal National Institute for Deaf People, 19–23 Featherstone Street, London EC1Y 8SL (020 7296 8000, info: 0808 808 0123, 0808 808 9000 (text), fax: 020 7296

8199, website: www.rnid.org.uk, e-mail: information@rnid.org.uk).

Defeating Deafness (Hearing Research Trust), 330–332 Gray's Inn Road, London WC1X 8EE (020 7833 1733, fax: 020 7278 0404, website: www.defeatingdeafness. org, e-mail: contact@defeatingdeafness.org).

National Deaf Children's Society, 15 Dufferin Street, London EC1Y 8UR (020 7490 8656, helpline: 0808 800 8880 [both voice and text], fax: 020 7251 5020, website: www.ndcs. org.uk, e-mail: ndcs@ndcs.org.uk).

Sense, 11–13 Clifton Terrace, Finsbury Park, London N4 3RS (020 7272 7774, fax: 020 7272 6012, website: www.sense.org.uk, e-mail: info@sense.org.uk).

Sense Scotland, 43 Middlesex Street, Kinning Park, Glasgow G41 1EE (0141 429 0294, 0141 418 7170 (text), fax: 0141 429 0295, website: www.sensescotland.org.uk, e-mail: info@sensescotland.org.uk).

DERMATITIS National Eczema Society, Hill House, Highgate Hill, London N19 5 NA (020 7281 3553, helpline: 0870 241 3604, fax: 020 7281 6395, website: www.eczema.org).

DIABETES Diabetes UK, 10 Parkway, London NW1 7AA (0207 424 1000, helpline: 0845 120 2960, fax: 0207 424 1001, website: www.diabetes.org.uk, e-mail: info@diabetes. org.uk).

DISABLED LIVING British Red Cross, British Red Cross UK Office, 44 Moorfields, London, EC2Y 9AL (0870 170 7000, fax: 020 7562 2000, website: www.redcross.org.uk, e-mail: information@ redcross.org.uk).

Disabled Living Foundation, 380–384 Harrow Road, London W9 2HU (020 7289 6111, helpline: 0845 130 9177, textphone: 020 7432 8009, fax: 020 7266 2922, website: www.dlf.org.uk, e-mail: dlf@dlf.org.uk).

Motability Operations, City Gate House, 22 Southwark Bridge Rd, London SE1 9HB (0845 456 4566, fax: 020 7928 1818, website: www.motability.co.uk).

Royal Association for Disability and Rehabilitation (RADAR), 12 City Forum, 250 City Road, London EC1V 8AF (020 7250 3222, textphone: 020 7250 4119, fax: 020 7250

0212, website: www.radar.org.uk, e-mail: radar@radar.org.uk).

Shaftesbury Society, 16 Kingston Road, London SW19 1JZ (0845 330 6033, fax: 020 8239 5580, website: www.shaftesburysoc.org.uk, e-mail: info@shaftesburysoc.org.uk).

DONORS BODY: British Organ Donor Society, Balsham, Cambridge CB1 6DL (telephone and fax: 01223 893636, website: www. argonet.co.uk/body, e-mail: body@argonet.co.uk).

HM Inspector of Anatomy, Department of Health, Wellington House, 133–155 Waterloo Road, London SE1 8UG (020 7972 4342, fax: 020 7972 4791, e-mail: karen.huscroft@doh.qsi.gov.uk).

National Blood Service: 0845 7 711 711.

NHS Organ Donor Register, FREEPOST (SWB1474), Patchway, Bristol BS34 8ZZ, 0845 60 60 400.

DOWN'S SYNDROME Down's Syndrome Association, Langdon Down Centre, 2a Langdon Park, Teddington TW11 9PS (0845 230 0372, fax: 0845 230 0373, website: www.downs-syndrome.org.uk, e-mail: info@downs-syndrome.org.uk).

DRUG DEPENDENCE National Drugs Helpline: 0800 776600, website: www.talktofrank.com.

DYSLEXIA British Dyslexia Association, 98 London Road, Reading, Berkshire RG1 5AU (0118 966 2677, fax: 0118 935 1927, helpline: 0118 966 8271, website: www.bda-dyslexia. org.uk, e-mail: helpline@bdadyslexia.org.uk).

DYSPHASIA Speakability, 1 Royal Street, London SE1 7LL (020 7261 9572, fax: 020 7928 9542, helpline: 080 8808 9572, website: www.speakability.org.uk, e-mail: speakability@speakability.org.uk).

The Stroke Association, 240 City Road, London EC1V 2PR (0845 3033 100, fax: 020 7490 2686, website: www.info.org.uk, e-mail: info@ stroke.org.uk).

DYSTONIA Dystonia Society, 46–47 Britton Street, London EC1M 5UJ (020 7490 5671, fax: 020 7490 5672, website: www.dystonia. org.uk, e-mail: info@dystonia.org.uk).

EATING DISORDERS Eating Disorders Association, 1st Floor, Wensum House, 103 Prince of Wales Road, Norwich NR1 1DW (01603 619090, helpline: 0870 770 3256, textphone: 01603 753322, fax: 01603 664915, website: www.edauk.com, e-mail: info@edauk.com).

ECLAMPSIA AND PRE-ECLAMPSIA Action on Pre-Eclampsia (APEC), 84–88 Pinner Road, Harrow, Middlesex HA1 4HZ (020 8863 3271, helpline: 020 8427 4217 [M–F, 1000–1300, recorded advice at other times], fax: 020 8424 0653, website: www.apec.org.uk, e-mail: enquiries@ apec.org.uk).

ECZEMA See dermatitis.

EPILEPSY British Epilepsy Association, New Anstey House, Gate Way Drive, Yeadon, Leeds LS19 7XY (0113 210 8000, fax: 0113 391 0300, website: www.epilepsy.org.uk, e-mail: epilepsy@epilepsy.org.uk).

Epilepsy Action Scotland, 48 Govan Road, Glasgow G51 1JL (0141 427 4911, helpline: 0808 800 2200, fax: 0141 419 1709, website: www.epilepsyscotland.org.uk, e-mail: enquiries@epilepsyscotland.org.uk).

FAMILY PLANNING fpa, 2–12 Pentonville Road, London N1 9FP (020 7837 5432, helpline: 0845 310 1334, fax: 020 7837 3042, website: www.fpa.org.uk).

FERTILITY Infertility Network UK, Charter House, 43 St Leonards Road, Bexhill on Sea, East Sussex TN40 1JA (08701 188 088, website: www.infertilitynetworkuk.com).

FIRST AID British Red Cross, 44 Moorfields, London EC2Y 9AL (0870 170 7000, fax: 0207 562 2000, website: www.redcross.org.uk, e-mail: information@redcross.org.uk).

St Andrew's Ambulance Association, Strachan House, 16 Torphichen Street, Edinburgh EH3 8JB (0131 229 5419, fax: 0131 228 2424).

St John Ambulance, 27 St John's Lane, Clerkenwell, London EC1M 4DA (0870 10 49 50, fax: 0870 10 40 65, website: www.sja.org.uk).

HAEMOPHILIA Haemophilia Society, First Floor, Petersham House, 57a Hatton Garden, London EC1N 8JG (020 7831 1020, fax: 020 7405 4824, website: www.haemophilia.org.uk, e-mail: info@haemophilia.org.uk).

HEAD INJURIES See brain injuries.

HEARING AIDS See deafness.

HOSPITAL FRIENDS National Assocation of Hospital and Community Friends, 11–13 Cavendish Square, London W1G 0AN (0845 450 0285, website: www.hc-friends.org.uk, e-mail: info@hc-friends.org.uk).

HUNTINGTON'S CHOREA Huntington's Disease Association, 108 Battersea High Street, London SW11 3HP (020 7223 7000, fax: 020 7223 9489, website: www.hda.org.uk, e-mail: info@hda.org.uk).

ILEITIS See colitis and crohn's disease.

ILEOSTOMY The Ileostomy and Internal Pouch Support Group (ia), Peverill House, 1–5 Mill Road, Ballyclare, Co. Antrim BT 39 9DR (0800 0184 724, 028 9334 4043, fax: 028 9332 4606, info@the-ia-org.uk, website: www.the-ia.org.uk).

LARYNGECTOMY The National Association of Laryngectomee Clubs, Ground Floor, 6 Rickett Street, Fulham, London SW6 1RU (020 7381 9993, fax: 020 7381 0025).

LEARNING DISABILITY British Institute of Learning Disabilities, Green Street, Kidderminster, Worcestershire DY10 1JL (01562 723010, fax: 01562 723029, website: www.bild.org.uk).

ENABLE (Scottish Society for the Mentally Handicapped), 7 Buchanan Street, Glasgow G1 3HL (0141 226 4541, fax: 0141 204 4398, website: www.enable.org.uk: e-mail: enable@enable.org.uk).

MENCAP (Royal Society for Mentally Handicapped Children and Adults), 123 Golden Lane, London EC1Y 0RT (020 7454 0454, fax: 020 7696 5540, website: www.mencap.co.uk, e-mail: information@ mencap.org.uk).

Mental Health Foundation, 20 Upper Ground, London SE1 9QB (0207 803 1100, fax: 020 7803 1111, website: www.mhf.org.uk, e-mail: mhf@mhf.org.uk).

LUPUS Lupus UK, St James House, Eastern Road, Romford, Essex RM1 3NH (01708 731251, fax: 01708 731252).

MARRIAGE GUIDANCE Relate (National Marriage Guidance), Herbert Gray College, Little Church Street, Rugby, Warwickshire CV21 3AP (01788 573241, fax: 01788 535007, website: www.relate.org.uk, e-mail: enquiries@relate.org.uk).

MASTECTOMY See breast cancer care.

MEDICAL ACCIDENTS Action for the Victims of Medical Accidents (AVMA), 44 High Street, Croydon, Surrey, CR0 1YB (0845 123 2352, fax: 020 8667 9065, website: www.avma.org.uk, e-mail: advice@avma.org.uk).

MENINGITIS Meningitis Trust, Fern House, Bath Road, Stroud, Gloucestershire GL5 3TJ (01453 768000, helpline: 080 8800 3344 [24 hours], fax: 01453 768001, website: www.meningitis-trust.org.uk, e-mail: info@meningitis-trust.org.uk).

Meningitis Research Foundation, Midland Way, Thornbury, Bristol BS35 2BS (01454 281811, fax: 01454 281094, website: www.meningitis.org, e-mail: info@meningitis.org).

MENTAL HEALTH Mental Aftercare Association (MACA), 1st Floor, Lincoln House, 296–302 High Holborn, London WC1V 7JH (020 7061 3400, fax: 020 7061 3401, website: www.maca.org.uk, e-mail: info@maca.org.uk).

Mental Health Act Commission See appendix 7: statutory organisations.

MIND (National Association for Mental Health), 15–19 Broadway, London E15 4BQ (020 8519 2122, fax: 020 8522 1725, website: www.mind.org.uk, e-mail: contact@mind.org.uk).

RETHINK, 30 Tabernacle Street, London EC2A 4DD (0845 456 0455, website: www.rethink.org, e-mail: info@rethink.org).

See also alzheimer's disease.

MIGRAINE Migraine Action Association (British Migraine Association), Unit 6, Oakley Hay Lodge Business Park, Great Folds Road, Great Oakley, Northamptonshire NN18 9AS (01536 461 333, fax: 01536 461 444, website: www.migraine.org.uk, e-mail: info@migraine.org.uk).

MOTOR NEURON DISEASE See paralysis.

MULTIPLE BIRTHS TAMBA (Twins and Multiple Births Association), 2 The Willows, Gardner Road, Guildford, Surrey GU1 4PG (0870 770 3305, fax: 0870 770 3303, website: www.tamba.org.uk, e-mail: enquiries@tamba.org.uk).

MULTIPLE SCLEROSIS Multiple Sclerosis Society of Great Britain and Northern Ireland, MS National Centre, 372 Edgeware Road, London NW2 6ND (020 8438 0700, helpline: 0808 800 8000, fax: 020 8438 0701, website: www.mssociety.org.uk, e-mail: info@mssociety.org.uk).

Multiple Sclerosis Resources Centre, 7 Peartree Business Centre, Peartree Road, Stanway, Colchester CO3 5JN (01206 505444, 0800 783 0518, fax: 01206 505 449, website: www.msrc.co.uk, e-mail: msrc@yahoo.com).

MUSCULAR DYSTROPHY Muscular Dystrophy Campaign, 7/11 Prescott Place, London SW4 6BS (020 7720 8055, fax: 020 7498 0670, website: www.muscular-dystrophy.org, e-mail: info@muscular-dystrophy.org).

MYALGIC ENCEPHALITIS The ME Association, 4 Top Angel, Buckingham Industrial Park, Buckinghamshire MK18 1TH (0870 444 8233, fax: 01280 821602, website: www.meassociation.org.uk, e-mail: meconnect@meassociation.org.uk).

MYASTHENIA GRAVIS Myasthenia Gravis Association, Keynes House, Chester Park, Alfreton Road, Derby DE21 4AS (01322 290219, fax: 01332 293641, website: www.mgauk.org, e-mail: mg@mgauk.org.uk).

MYOPATHY See muscular dystrophy.

NARCOLEPSY Narcolepsy Association (UK), UKAN, PO Box 13842, Penicuik EH25 8WX (0845 450 0394, fax: 0870 777 3039, website: www.narcolepsy.org.uk, e-mail: info@narcolepsy.org.uk).

NHS DIRECT HELPLINE (24 hours) 0845 4647.

NOTIFIABLE DISEASES See AIDS.

NURSING See appendix 8: professional organisations.

OSTEOARTHRITIS See arthritis.

OSTEOGENESIS IMPERFECTA See brittle bone disease.

OSTEOPATHY See appendix 10: complementary and alternative medicine.

OSTEOPOROSIS National Osteoporosis Society, Camerton, Bath BA2 0PJ (01761 471771, fax: 01761 471104, website: www.nos.org.uk, e-mail: info@nos.org.uk).

PAGET'S DISEASE National Association for the Relief of Paget's Disease, 323 Manchester Road, Walkden, Worsley, Manchester M28 3HH (0161 799 4646, fax: 0161 799 6511, website: www.paget.org.uk, e-mail: director@paget.org.uk).

PALATE MALFORMATIONS Cleft Lip and Palate Association (CLAPA), 1st Floor, Green Man Tower, 332 Goswell Road, London EC1V 7LQ (020 7833 4883, fax: 020 7833 5999, website: www.clapa.com, e-mail: info@clapa.com).

Maxillofacial and Dental Department, Great Ormond Street Hospital for Children, Great Ormond Street, London WC1N 3JH (020 7813 8439, e-mail: godbec@gosh.nhs.uk).

PARALYSIS Motor Neurone Disease Association, PO Box 246, Northampton NN1 2PR (01604 250505, helpline: 0845 762 6262, fax: 01604 624726, website: www.mndassociation.org, e-mail: enquiries@ mndassociation.org).

Spinal Injuries Association, Acorn House, 387–391 Midsummer Boulevard, Milton Keynes MK9 3HP (0845 678 6633, helpline: 0800 980 0501, fax: 01908 608 492, website: www.spinal.co.uk, e-mail: sia@spinal.co.uk).

Spinal Injuries Scotland, Festival Business Centre, 150 Brand Street, Glasgow G51 1DH (0141 314 0056, fax: 0141 314 0057, website: www.sisonline.org, e-mail: info@sisonline.org).

PARKINSONISM Parkinson's Disease Society of the United Kingdom, 215 Vauxhall Bridge Road, London SW1V 1EJ (020 7931 8080, fax: 020 7233 9908, website: parkinsons.org.uk, e-mail: enquiries@parkinsons.org.uk).

PHENYLKETONURIA National Society for Phenylketonuria (UK) Ltd (NSPKU), PO Box 26642, London N14 4ZF (helpline: 0845 603 9136, website: www.nspku.org, e-mail: info@nspku.org).

PHOBIAS National Phobics Society, Zion Community Resource Centre, 339 Stretford Road, Hulme, Manchester M15 4ZY (0870 7700 456, fax: 0161 227 9862, website: www.phobics-society.org.uk, e-mail: nationalphobic @btconnect.com).

PHYSIOTHERAPY See appendix 8: professional organisations.

PITUITARY-LINKED CONDITIONS The Pituitary Foundation, PO Box 1944, Bristol BS99 2UB (telephone and fax: 0845 450 0375, website: www.pituitary.org.uk, e-mail: helpline@pituitary.org.uk).

POISONS National Poisons Information Service: 0870 600 6266.

PSORIASIS Psoriasis Association, Milton House, 7 Milton Street, Northampton NN2 7JG (helpline: 01604 711129, fax: 01604 792894, e-mail: mail@psoriasis.demon.co.uk).

RABIES – PET TRAVEL SCHEME Department for Environment, Food and Rural Affairs (DEFRA), 1a Page Street, London SW1P 4PQ (020 7904 6000, helpline: 0870 241 1710, website: www.defra.gov.uk/animalh/quarantine/index.htm).

RESTRICTED GROWTH Restricted Growth Association (RGA), PO Box 4744, Dorchester DT2 9FA (telephone and fax: 01308 898445, website: www.restrictedgrowth.co.uk, e-mail: office@restrictedgrowth.co.uk).

SICKLE-CELL ANAEMIA Sickle Cell Society, 54 Station Road, Harlesden, London NW10 4UA (020 8961 7795, fax: 020 8961 8346, website: www.sicklecellsociety.org, e-mail: info@sicklecellsociety.org.uk).

SMOKING ASH (Action on Smoking and Health), 102 Clifton Street, London EC2A 4HW (020 7739 5902, fax: 020 7613 0531, website: www.ash.org.uk, e-mail: enquiries@ash.org.uk).

National Smoking Helpline: 0800 169 0 169 (0700–2300 daily).

SPEECH DISORDERS AFASIC (Unlocking Speech and Language), 2nd floor, 50–52 Great Sutton St, London EC1V 0DJ (020 7490 9410, helpline: 0845 355 5577, fax: 020 7251 2834, website: www.afasic.org.uk, e-mail: info@afasic.org.uk).

SPEECH THERAPY See appendix 8: professional organisations.

SPINA BIFIDA Association for Spina Bifida and Hydrocephalus, ASBAH House, 42 Park Road, Peterborough PE1 2UQ (01733 555988, fax: 01733 555985, website: www.asbah.org, e-mail: info@asbah.org).

Scottish Spina Bifida Association, 190 Queensferry Road, Edinburgh EH4 2BW (0131 332 0743, fax: 0131 343 3651, website: www.ssba.org.uk, e-mail: mail@ssba.org.uk).

STAMMERING BSA (British Stammering Association), 15 Old Ford Road, London E2 9PJ (020 8983 1003, fax: 020 8983 3591, website: www.stammering.org, e-mail: mail@stammering.org).

STOMA See colostomy and ileostomy.

STROKE See dysphasia.

SUDDEN INFANT DEATH SYNDROME Foundation for the Study of Sudden Infant Deaths, Artillery House, 11–19 Artillery Row, London SW1P 1RT (0870 787 0885, 24-hour helpline: 0870 787 0554, fax: 0870 787 0725, website: www.sids.org.uk, e-mail: fsid@sids.org.uk).

TALKING BOOKS Calibre, New Road, Weston Turville, Aylesbury, Buckinghamshire HP22 5XQ (01296 432339, fax: 01296 392599, website: www.calibre.org.uk, e-mail: enquiries@calibre.org.uk).

Listening Books, 12 Lant Street, London SE1 1QH (020 7407 9417, fax: 020 7403 1377, website: www.listening-books.org.uk, e-mail: info@listening-books.org.uk).

TINNITUS See deafness.

TOY LIBRARIES The National Association of Toy and Leisure Libraries/Playmatters, 68 Churchway, London NW1 1LT (020 7255 4600, fax: 020 7255 4602, website: www.natll.org.uk, e-mail: admin@playmatters.co.uk).

TRANS-SEXUALISM Gender Identity Consultancy (GICS), BM Box 5434, London WC1N 3XX (telephone and fax: 020 7828 9575, website: www.members.aol.com/gic).

TRAVEL See appendix 3: travel and health.

TUBEROUS SCLEROSIS Tuberous Sclerosis Association, PO Box 9644, Bromsgrove, Worcestershire B61 0FP (01527 871898, fax: 01527 579452, website: www.tuberoussclerosis.org, e-mail: support@tuberoussclerosis.org).

TURNER'S SYNDROME The Turner's Syndrome Support Society (UK), 12 Irving Quadrant, Hardgate, Clydebank G81 6AZ (01389 380 385, fax: 01389 380 384, website: www.tss.org.uk, e-mail: turner.syndrome@tss.org.uk).

VOLUNTARY ORGANISATIONS National Council for Voluntary Organisations, Regent's Wharf, 8 All Saints Street, London N1 9RL (020 7713 6161, helpdesk: 0800 2798 798, fax: 020 7713 6300, website: www.ncvo-vol.org.uk, e-mail: helpdesk@ncvo-vol.org.uk).

INTRODUCTION

Whether a person is travelling abroad for business or pleasure or is going to live in another country, he or she should obtain information about the climate, environment and health risks at their destination (including any stopovers that involve personal contacts with local people). Certain risks to health in another country may always be present; sometimes hazards to health may be temporary because of a local epidemic or sudden adverse environmental circumstance, such as a drought, earthquake or volcanic eruption, any of which can cause problems in obtaining supplies of food, clean water and medicine.

Any intending travellers with an existing illness should find out from their doctors whether they are fit to travel; whether the country of destination will admit them; whether they will be able to obtain appropriate treatment; and if so, how it will be paid for.

Healthy travellers are also advised to enquire about health-care arrangements (including payments) in their destination country in case they fall ill while away. Some countries have reciprocal arrangements with the UK. Travellers should take sensible precautions about drinking water and food, as hygiene standards vary widely throughout the world. Pharmacists are usually helpful with advice on over-the-counter remedies for travel sickness and traveller's tummy.

Recent media publicity has alerted air travellers, especially those flying long distances, about the risks of developing deep vein thrombosis (DVT), sometimes called 'economy-class syndrome'. Sitting in a relatively confined position for several hours can cause blood clots to form in the deep veins of the legs: ocasionally small clots break away and are carried in the bloodstream to the lungs where they form clots in the circulation called pulmonary emboli (see PULMONARY EMBOLISM) – a potentially fatal disorder. The risk of developing DVT is greatly reduced by exercising the feet and knees while sitting, by walking around the aircraft when possible, drinking plenty of water but little or no alcohol, and wearing (properly fitting) elastic stockings on the legs. Anyone who has already had a DVT should seek medical advice before travelling by air.

Travel agents have a responsibility to advise their clients about health risks, and the travel trade has access to directories giving up-to-date information on visa requirements, recommended immunisations (see VACCINE; IMMUNISATION), climate, current health hazards and currency allowances. They cannot, however, be expected to give detailed individual advice, especially if the traveller has an existing medical condition.

There are many publications of help to travellers, and authoritative advice is available from organisations listed in this appendix.

Travellers returning home who fall ill – even several months later – should always tell their doctor where they have visited and when, in case their illness originated in another country.

USEFUL ADDRESSES

Tropical medical advice can be obtained by *those advising travellers* from PHLS Communicable Disease Surveillance Centre, 61 Colindale Avenue, London NW9 5EQ (020 8200 6868); London School of Hygiene and Tropical Medicine, Keppel Street, London WC1E 7HT (020 7636 8636); Medical Advisory Services for Travellers (MASTA) (www.masta.org); Communicable Diseases (Scotland) Unit, and Department of Tropical Medicine, Ruchill Hospital, Glasgow G20 9NB (0141 946 7120); Department of Infectious and Tropical Diseases, Birmingham Heartlands Hospital, Bordesley Green East, Birmingham B9 5ST (0121 766 6611 – enquiries from doctors and pharmacists only); Department of Infectious Diseases and Tropical Medicine, North Manchester General Hospital, Delaunays Road, Manchester M8 6RB (0161 795 4567); and Liverpool School of Tropical Medicine, Pembroke Place, Liverpool L3 5QA (0151 708 9393).

SOURCES OF 'OFFICIAL' ADVICE

The Department of Health produces annually the T4 booklet *Health Advice for Travellers,* and this is available free from post offices or by telephoning an order to 0800 555777. It contains information on what compulsory and recommended immunisations apply to countries. Advice is given on reducing health risks and on entitlement to medical treatment at reduced cost. Certificate E111 entitles nationals of European Community countries to care in other member states and the leaflet explains how to get this. Advice can be obtained from UK Department of Health Public Enquiries Office, Richmond House, 79 Whitehall, London SW1A 2NS (020 7210 4850); a free booklet can be ordered from 0800 555777.

Another source of advice is Foreign &

Commonwealth Office Travel Advice (website: www.fco. gov. uk/travel/countryadvice. gov/).

The health departments in Scotland, Wales and Northern Ireland also produce information on immunisation against infectious diseases; this is published by HMSO and referred to as the 'green book'.

The World Health Organisation in Geneva issues annually *International Travel and Health Vaccination Requirements and Health Advice*, also available from HMSO. It is written primarily for a medical readership. Designated yellow-fever vaccination centres are distributed throughout the UK and details of these can be obtained from local departments of public health, and in Scotland and Northern Ireland from health boards.

Most good bookshops contain a range of travel books and specific travel-health guides that contain information relating to health. Books may, however, become quickly out of date because of changing circumstances and health regulations in different countries. *The Traveller's Handbook*, published by Wexas Ltd, is a good and comprehensive guide. Among several specialist organisations giving travel advice, for instance, to handicapped people, and publishing books and leaflets, are the following: International Association for Medical Assistance to Travellers (www.iamat.org –

membership free but voluntary contributions welcome; publishes a directory of English-speaking doctors and leaflets on climate, acclimatisation, immunisation, etc.); Air Transport Users Council, Room K705, CAA House, 45-59 Kingsway, London WC2B 6TE (020 7240 6061 – *Care in the Air*, advice for handicapped travellers); Intermedic, 77 Third Avenue, New York, United States of America NY 10017 (members may obtain a list of recommended English-speaking doctors in many countries); US State Department website: www.travel.state.gov; British Airways Medical Service, Queens Building (N121), Heathrow Airport, Hounslow, Middlesex (020 8562 7070, website: www.british-airways.com; *Your Patient and Air Travel* is useful for medical practitioners); Diabetes UK, 10 Parkway, London NW1 7AA (020 7424 1000 – leaflets including travel guides concerning the more popular destinations); Royal Association for Disability and Rehabilitation (RADAR), 12 City Forum, 250 City Road, London EC1V 8AF (020 7250 3222 – leaflets available to help the handicapped arrange their travels); National Association for Maternal and Child Welfare Ltd, 1st Floor, 40–42 Osnaburgh Street, London NW1 3ND (020 7383 4117 – also *The Care of Babies and Young Children in the Tropics* by D. Morley, *Travelling with Children*).

APPENDIX 4: COMMON MEDICAL TESTS AND PROCEDURES

ACETONE (URINE)
Aim: Detection of diabetic ketoacidosis.
Method: Using Acetest tablets, Chemstrip or Multistix.
Normal: Negative. Positive result can be provoked by starvation and/or vomiting as well as various metabolic diseases including diabetes mellitus.

ACID PHOSPHATASE
Aim: Aid in diagnosis of prostatic cancer.
Increased concentrations of this enzyme, which is present in the kidney, semen, serum and the prostate gland, may occur in this condition.
Normal: 1–5 international units per litre.

ADRENOCORTICOTROPHIC HORMONE (ACTH) (PLASMA)
Aim: Diagnosis of Addison's disease, Cushing's syndrome and other disturbances of the hypothalamo-pituitary-adrenal axis.
Normal: Sleep–wake cycle of ACTH production, with highest levels at 06.00–08.00 (soon after getting up) and lowest levels at 21.00–22.00 (after going to bed). Secretion is increased by pregnancy and stress.

ALKALINE PHOSPHATASE
Aim: Evaluation of liver or bone disease.
This enzyme may be present in greater than normal amounts in several disorders including bone metastases, Paget's disease, rickets, liver disease, pulmonary infarction and heart failure.
Normal: 30–300 international units per litre.

AMNIOCENTESIS
Aim: Assessment of fetal maturity and diagnosis of fetal abnormalities.
Method/hazards: With ultrasound guidance, a needle is inserted through the mother's abdominal wall and uterus, and a specimen of amniotic fluid withdrawn. There is a small risk to the fetus and the test should only be performed when essential.

AMYLASE (SERUM)
Aim: Investigation of pancreatic and hepatic disease.
Normal: 25–125 U/1 (units per litre).

APGAR SCORE
Aim: Assessment of neonate's need for resuscitation.
Method: Evaluation at 1 minute and 5 minutes after delivery of skin colour, muscle tone, respiratory effort, heart rate, and response to stimulus. Points are awarded and resuscitation started if needed. An Apgar score still low at 10 or even 15 minutes represents a high risk for developing cerebral palsy.

BICARBONATE (WHOLE ARTERIAL BLOOD)
Aim: Investigation of acidosis and alkalosis.
An important investigation when managing patients with respiratory or renal disease or anyone whose metabolism is profoundly disturbed, for example in any intensive care situation.
Normal: 18–23 mmol/l.

BILIRUBIN
Aim: To help assess liver function (and sometimes degree of breakdown of blood cells – haemolysis)
A breakdown product of the blood pigment haemoglobin that is excreted in the bile, its concentration is raised in liver disease, obstructive jaundice, haemolytic anaemia and pulmonary infarction.
Normal: 2–17 m mol.1.

BIOPSY OF TUMOURS
Aim: Histological diagnosis of type of tumour and malignancy.
Methods: Fine-needle and large-needle aspiration biopsy – excision biopsy.

CALCIUM (SERUM)
Aim: Diagnosis of hyperparathyroidism, hypoparathyroidism, etc.
Normal: See table B1 (page 804). Range may be affected by other drugs.

CARDIAC STRESS TEST
Aim: Assessment of cardiac efficiency.
Method: Heart rate, blood pressure, and electrocardiograph are recorded continuously while the patient performs an incremental work test. The test is stopped whenever requested, e.g. in the presence of excessive dyspnoea, chest pain.
Contraindications include acute infection, recent myocardial infarction, unstable angina, congestive heart failure, uncontrolled dysrhythmia, etc.

CERVICAL CANCER SCREENING
Aim: Early detection of changes in cervical cells, allowing earlier treatment.
Method: Starting 6 months after first inter-

course, then at 3-yearly intervals for rest of life. The test involves a cervical smear with a spatula, the cells then being examined histologically.

CHOLECYSTOGRAM

An X-ray of the gall-bladder after the patient has taken a contrast medium by mouth; it is concentrated in the gall-bladder, thus enabling identification of abnormalities such as gallstones, tumours and restricted patency of the cystic duct (which carries the bile from the gallbladder to the duodenum).

CHOLESTEROL

Aim: A fatty substance present in several forms in tissues and blood where its concentration ranges from 3.6–7.8 mmol/l. Raised concentrations (hypercholesterolaemia) are often associated with atheroma, which can cause cardiovascular or cerebral vascular disease, and are linked with a high intake of saturated fats and cholesterol, though damage to blood vessels may be caused by one form of cholesterol called low-density lipoprotein (LDL) at a concentration above 4.4 mmol/l.

CHORIONIC GONADOTROPHIN

(URINE, FIRST MORNING SPECIMEN)
Aim: Diagnosis of pregnancy.
Methods: Agglutination inhibition assay: positive in pregnancy 8–14 days after first missed period. Monoclonal antibody test: positive in pregnancy 14–18 days from conception.

CHORIONIC VILLUS SAMPLING

Aim: Ascertainment of fetal chromosome pattern.
Method: A small sample of trophoblastic tissue is obtained from the placenta, by ultrasound guidance either transvaginally or transabdominally, taken between the 9th and 11th weeks of pregnancy. There is a small risk of abortion.

CORDOCENTESIS

Aim: Investigation of the chromosome pattern and haemoglobinopathies in mid-pregnancy.
Method: Blood is withdrawn from the umbilical cord at about the 18th week of pregnancy and extensively analysed.

ENZYME-LINKED IMMUNOSORBENT ASSAY (ELISA) (URINE)

Aim: Diagnosis of presence of antibodies, for example to infective agents.

ERYTHROCYTE COUNT (WHOLE BLOOD)

Aim: Investigation of anaemia.

Normal: See table B1 (pages 804–805).

ERYTHROCYTE SEDIMENTATION RATE (ESR)

Aim: Investigation and monitoring of fever, inflammatory, malignant, or autoimmune disease.
Method: Anticoagulated whole blood is used. The result obtained may be influenced by numerous factors, notably various disorders and different drugs.
Normal:

male	<50	<15 mm/h
	>50	<20 mm/h
female	<50	<20 mm/h
	>50	<30 mm/h

GLASGOW COMA SCALE (MODIFIED)

Aim: To test the depth of coma, particularly following head injury, as a guide to the need for neurosurgical intervention.
Method: Opening of the eyes, best verbal response, and best motor response are scored separately, giving a total quantitative index of the level of cerebral dysfunction.

GLOMERULAR FILTRATION RATE (GFR)

Aim: Investigation of renal function.
Method: Plasma and urinary creatinine levels are measured and the creatinine clearance rate calculated. This corresponds closely to the GFR, normally 120 ml/min in adults.

GLUCOSE (BLOOD, URINE)

Aim: Diagnosis and monitoring of diabetes mellitus.
Method: Stick tests available for urine and blood samples.
Normal: See tables B1 and B4 (pages 804, 805).

GLUCOSE TOLERANCE TEST (ORAL)

Aim: Diagnosis of diabetes mellitus/impaired glucose tolerance.
Method: Pre-test patient, ensure no recent illness, accident, or surgery. Discontinue nonessential drugs. Patient fasts for 10–16 hours, then takes 75 g glucose over 5 minutes. Serum glucose level is measured at 0, 30, 60, 90 and 120 minutes. The test should be performed in the morning.
Normal:

fasting	3.9–5.8 mmol/l
30 minutes	6.1–9.4 mmol/l
60 minutes	6.7–9.4 mmol/l
90 minutes	5.6–7.8 mmol/l
120 minutes	3.9–6.7 mmol/l

GLYCATED HAEMOGLOBIN (WHOLE BLOOD)
Aim: Monitoring of diabetes mellitus.
Method: The test reflects the mean blood-glucose concentration over the previous 4–8 weeks. It is a measure of long-term control and should be repeated at around 3-monthly intervals.
Normal: (In insulin-dependent diabetic) 7–9 per cent.

HAEMATOCRIT (PACKED RED CELL VOLUME) (WHOLE BLOOD)
Aim: Investigation of anaemia and polycythaemia.
Normal: See table B1 (page 804).

HEPATITIS A ANTIGEN (SERUM)
Aim: Diagnosis of hepatitis A infection.
Normal: Negative.
Anti-HAV IgG appears about four weeks after infection and persists indefinitely.

HEPATITIS B SURFACE ANTIGEN (SERUM)
Aim: Diagnosis of active or chronic hepatitis B virus infection.
Normal: Negative.

HUMAN IMMUNODEFICIENCY VIRUS (HIV) ANTIBODY (SERUM)
Aim: Diagnosis of HIV infection.
Method: HIV antibodies are usually detectable from 4 weeks to 4 months after infection, and persist indefinitely. The test is by enzyme-linked immunosorbent assay (ELISA).
Normal: Negative.

IRON (SERUM)
Aim: Investigation of anaemia.
Normal: See table B1 (page 804).

LIVER FUNCTION TESTS
The liver is a complex organ with metabolic, excretory and protective functions that are interdependent, so there is no single test to assess overall function. Liver biopsy, done under local anaesthetic with entry through the skin, gives helpful diagnostic information with little risk or discomfort to the patient. The procedure enables liver tissue to be examined in the laboratory for structural changes and the presence of abnormal cells.

Several tests of blood chemistry detect changes in the various functions, as well as assessing the healthiness of liver cells. These include tests on blood serum for the amounts of bilirubin (yellow breakdown products of red blood cells), albumin (a key body protein made in the liver) and alkaline phosphatase (an enzyme in bile) and aminotransferases or transaminases (enzymes entering the blood following liver-cell damage). Prothrombin time (see below) tests how well the blood clots: the process depends on the presence in the blood of vitamin K (see APPENDIX 5: VITAMINS) which is produced by the normal liver; damage to liver cells lengthens the time blood takes to clot. X-ray and ultrasound assessment of liver and gall-bladder structure are valuable, as are radio-nuclide scanning and computed tomography.

LUMBAR PUNCTURE
Aim: To obtain samples of cerebrospinal fluid (CSF) for investigation of central nervous system diseases, especially meningitis.
Method: With the patient lying on his or her side, and under local anaesthesia, a long needle is inserted between the third and fourth lumbar vertebrae. When performed correctly, a small volume of fluid should flow out spontaneously; this is collected and analysed (see table B2 [page 805] for normal values).

The test should never be carried out in the presence of a raised CSF pressure, since it may precipitate transtentorial or tonsillar herniation in the brain.

MYOGLOBIN (SERUM)
Aim: Diagnosis of myocardial infarction.
Normal:
men   19–92 mg/l
women   12–76 mg/l
The increase in value begins 30–60 minutes after onset of myocardial infarction and continues for 2–3 days.

POTASSIUM
Aim: To test for raised or lowered concentrations of this essential element present as an electrolyte in the blood. Abnormally low or high levels are found in a wide range of disorders. Low: cirrhosis of liver, malnutrition, vomiting, diarrhoea, diuresis, hyperadrenalism. High: diabetic acidosis, hypoadrenalism, haemolysis, renal tubular defect, thrombocytosis.
Normal: 3.5–5.0 m mol/l.

PROSTATE SCREENING TESTS
These tests for prostate cancer are still being evaluated. One test is for the protein, prostate-specific antigen (PSA); its drawback is that it detects small areas of cancerous cells which might not necessarily go on to develop and cause symptoms. Raised concentrations of acid phosphatase occur in prostate cancer and in

certain other conditions such as liver and bone disease.

Normal: 0–4 ng/ml.

Ultrasound scanning and biopsy of the gland are useful tests.

PROTHROMBIN TEST

Aim: To test quantitatively the amount of prothrombin in the blood based on the time it takes blood plasma to clot in the presence of thromboplastin and calcium chloride. It measures the integrity of the blood-clotting function.

Normal: 10–14 seconds.

The time is extended in haemophilia, serious liver disorders and when the diet is deficient in vitamin K.

SKIN BIOPSY

Aim: Histological or immunofluorescent examination of skin lesions, especially if there is any suspicion of malignancy.

Method: Various techniques are used, depending on the amount of skin required and the degree of doubt of the diagnosis.

SODIUM

Aim: To test for raised or lowered concentrations of this essential element present as an electrolyte (sodium chloride) in the blood. Abnormally low or high levels are found in several disorders. Low: nephrosis, myxoedema, heart failure, diarrhoea and vomiting, diabetic acidosis, diuresis, adrenocortical insufficiency. High: dehydration, diabetes insipidus, excessive salt intake, diabetes mellitus.

Normal: 135–145 mmol/l.

THYROXINE, FREE (FT4) (SERUM)

Aim: Measurement of thyroid function.

Method: Various methods are used. The normal value is 10–31 pmol/l, but varies with the technique used.

TROPONIN

Aim: Diagnosis of myocardial infarction.

A raised level of this enzyme is now part of the definition of myocardial infarction. False positives can occur, for example after strenuous exercise such as marathon running.

TUBERCULIN SKIN TESTS

Aim: Diagnosis of tuberculosis.

Method: Antigens of *Mycobacterium tuberculosis* are injected intradermally. In the Heaf test, six skin punctures are then made through the antigen. The test is read at 3–7 days and a positive result is the appearance of four or more papules. It means that the patient has encountered the tubercle bacillus at some time in their life but not necessarily that they are currently infected.

APPENDIX 5: VITAMINS

Introduction A general description of vitamins is in the main text. Vitamins are divided into those that are fat-soluble and those that are water-soluble. Fat-soluble vitamins are A, D, E and K; the water-soluble ones, B group and C.

The water-soluble vitamin B group is complex. Although often found together in similar types of food – cereals, milk, liver, etc. – they are not related chemically. These vitamins are all coenzymes – organic (non-protein) compounds which, when the appropriate ENZYME is present, have an essential function in the chemical reaction catalysed by the enzyme. The vitamin B group comprises B_1 (thiamine, aneurine), B_2 (riboflavin), B_3 (niacin, nicotinic acid), B_6 (pyridoxine), B_{12} (cobalamin, cyanocobalamin), biotin, folacin (folic acid) and pantothenic acid.

Unlike fat-soluble vitamins, the water-soluble ones are not stored in large amounts in the body so deficiency of these is more likely.

Fat-soluble vitamins

VITAMIN A (Preformed specific compounds: RETINOL, retinal, RETINOIC ACID. Precursor: CAROTENE)
Functions Maintenance of epithelial cells and mucous membranes. Constituent of visual purple (for night vision). Necessary for normal growth, development and reproduction. Maintenance of immune system.
Symptoms of deficiency Keratinised skin, dry mucous membranes, xerophthalmia. Night blindness. Susceptibility to disease.
Symptoms of toxicity Dry skin. Loss of appetite and hair, enlarged spleen and liver, abnormal pigmentation of skin. Fetal malformations.
Food sources *Preformed vitamin A* Liver, especially cod and halibut liver oil; egg yolk; milk and butter. *Carotene* Dark-green, leafy vegetables, especially spinach, broccoli, kale. Deep orange vegetables and fruits, especially carrots, tomatoes, apricots.
Recommended daily amounts (IUs*)
Babies and children   1,875–3,500
Boys (>11 years) and men   5,000
Girls (>11 years) and women   4,000
Lactating women   6,000–6,500
*International Units

VITAMIN D (ERGOCALCIFEROL or CALCIFEROL [vitamin D_2]; cholecalciferol [vitamin D_3]; 25-hydroxycholecalciferol [main circulating form

of vitamin D]; 1,25-dihydroxy-cholecalciferol [main active form of vitamin D]; precursor of vitamin D_2: ergosterol [plants]; of vitamin D_3: 7-dehydrocholesterol [in skin])
Functions Helps in absorption of calcium and phosphorus. Regulates blood concentrations of calcium. Promotes mineralisation of teeth and bones.
Symptoms of deficiency Rickets in children. Osteomalacia in adults.
Symptoms of toxicity Calcification of soft tissues, hypercalcaemia, renal stones, loss of weight and appetite, nausea and fatigue, failure of growth.
Sources Cod and halibut liver oils, bony fish, egg yolk, fortified milk, butter and polyunsaturated margarine. Sunlight acts on ergosterol in plants to produce vitamin D2 and on the skin to produce vitamin D3.
Recommended daily amounts (IUs)
Babies and children   300–400
Subjects aged11–25   400
Subjects over 25   200
Pregnant and lactating women   400

VITAMIN E
Functions Prevents oxidation of vitamin A in gut. Protects red blood cells from haemolysis. Maintains cell membranes by reducing the oxidation of polyunsaturated fats.
Symptoms of deficiency Breakdown of red blood cells.
Symptoms of toxicity Headache, nausea, longer blood-clotting times.
Food sources Wheat germ, vegetable oils, legumes, nuts, whole grains, fish, green, leafy vegetables.
Recommended daily allowances (mg)
Babies and children   3–7
Boys (>11 years) and men   10
Girls (>11 years) and non-pregnant women   8
Pregnant and lactating women   10–12

VITAMIN K
(PHYTOMENADIONE, phylloquinone)
Functions Necessary for the formation of prothrombin and other factors necessary for blood clotting.
Symptoms of deficiency Haemorrhage.
Symptoms of toxicity Haemolytic anaemia, liver damage.
Sources Dark-green leafy vegetables, especially alfalfa, spinach, cabbage. Cauliflower. Egg yolk. Soybean oil. From synthesis by intestinal bacteria.

Recommended daily amounts (µg)

Babies and children	5–20
Boys (>11 years) and men (increasing with age)	45–80
Girls (>11 years) and women (increasing with age)	45–65
Pregnant and lactating women	65

CHOLINE The basic compound participates in the synthesis of LECITHIN and other phospholipids as well as of acetylcholine. Choline, which helps to transport fat in the body, and is essential to life, is sometimes classed as a vitamin, but the body is able to produce the compound.

Water-soluble vitamins

VITAMIN B₁ (THIAMINE, ANEURINE)

Functions Has role in carbohydrate metabolism. Helps nervous system, heart and muscles to function properly. Promotes appetite and functioning of digestive tract.

Symptoms of deficiency Polyneuritis, beriberi, fatigue, depression, poor appetite and functioning of digestive tract.

Symptoms of toxicity Anaphylactic shock, lethargy, ataxia, nausea, hypotension.

Sources Whole grains, wheat germ, enriched white-flour products, legumes. Brewer's yeast. Heart, liver, kidney; pork.

Recommended daily amounts (mg)

Babies and children	0.3–1.0
Boys (>11 years) and men	1.2–1.5
Girls (>11 years) and women	1.0–1.1
Pregnant women	1.5
Lactating women	1.6

VITAMIN B₂ (RIBOFLAVIN [formerly vitamin G])

Functions Essential for certain enzyme systems important in the metabolism of food (carbohydrate, protein and fat).

Symptoms of deficiency Inflamed tongue, scaling and burning skin, sensitive eyes, angular stomatitis and cheilosis, cataracts.

Symptoms of toxicity None recorded.

Sources Green, leafy vegetables, peanuts, whole grains. Milk and its products, eggs, liver, kidney, heart.

Recommended daily amounts (mg)

Babies and children	0.4–1.2
Boys (>11 years) and men	1.4–1.8
Girls (>11 years) and women	1.2–1.3
Pregnant women	1.6
Lactating women	1.7–1.8

VITAMIN B₃ (niacin, NICOTINIC ACID [a derivative of pyridine])

Functions Part of two important enzymes regulating energy metabolism. Promotes good physical and mental health and helps maintain the health of the skin, tongue and digestive system.

Symptoms of deficiency Pellagra, gastrointestinal disturbances, photosensitive dermatitis, depression.

Symptoms of toxicity Flushing, loss of appetite, nausea and vomiting, abnormal energy metabolism, anaphylaxis, circulatory collapse.

Sources Whole grain flour, enriched white flour, legumes. Brewer's yeast. Meat; heart, liver, kidney.

Recommended daily amounts (mg)

Babies and children	5–13
Boys (>11 years) and men	15–20
Girls (>11 years) and women	13–15
Pregnant women	17
Lactating women	20

VITAMIN B₆ (PYRIDOXINE [pyridoxal is a coenzyme of pyridoxine])

Functions Important in metabolism of proteins, amino acids, carbohydrate and fat. Essential for growth and health.

Symptoms of deficiency Not fully known but possibly convulsions, peripheral neuropathy, secondary pellagra, depression and oral symptoms.

Symptoms of toxicity Reduces prolactin secretion, which is important for milk pro-duction. Damage to sensory nerves. Liver damage.

Sources Whole grains, potatoes, green vegetables, maize. Liver; red meat.

Recommended daily amounts (mg)

Babies and children	0.3–1.4
Boys (>11 years) and men	1.7–2.0
Girls (>11 years) and women	1.4–1.6
Pregnant women	2.2
Lactating women	2.1

VITAMIN B₁₂ (cobalamin, CYANOCOBALAMIN)

Functions Important for haemoglobin synthesis. Essential for normal functioning of all cells, especially of the nervous system, bone marrow, and gastrointestinal tract.

Symptoms of deficiency Pernicious anaemia, subacute degeneration of the spinal cord, various psychological disorders, possibly loss of appetite (anorexia).

Symptoms of toxicity Not known.

Sources Not found in significant amounts in plant foods. Eggs, dry milk and milk products. Meat; liver, kidney, heart.

Recommended daily amounts (µg)

Babies and children	0.3–1.4
Subjects over 11 years	2.0
Pregnant women	2.2
Lactating women	2.6

VITAMIN B COMPLEX (folate, FOLIC ACID)
Functions Formation of red blood cells. Normal function of gastrointestinal tract. Helps in metabolism of protein.
Symptoms of deficiency Possible neural tube defect in fetuses, anaemia.
Symptoms of toxicity Possible hypersensitivity reactions.
Sources Dark-green, leafy vegetables, legumes, whole grains. Yeast. Kidneys, heart and pancreas.

Recommended daily amounts (µg)

Babies and children	25–100
Boys (>11 years) and men	150–200
Girls (>11 years) and women	150–180
Pregnant women	400
Lactating women	260–280

VITAMIN B COMPLEX (BIOTIN)
Functions Takes part in amino-acid and fatty-acid metabolism.
Symptoms of deficiency Rare: dermatitis, soreness of the tongue, dependency.
Symptoms of toxicity Not known.
Sources Egg yolk, cauliflower, kidney, legumes, liver, nuts, yeasts.
Recommended daily amounts 150–300 µg.

VITAMIN B COMPLEX (PANTOTHENIC ACID)
Functions An essential component of coenzyme A, which is a key factor in many of the body's metabolic activities.
Symptoms of deficiency Rare, but in a trial on volunteers malaise, abdominal discomfort and sensory disturbances occurred.
Symptoms of toxicity Not known.
Sources Widely distributed in foodstuffs.
Recommended daily amounts Adults probably need about 4 to 7 mg/day.

VITAMIN C (ASCORBIC ACID, dehydroascorbic acid)
Functions Protects against infection and helps in wound healing. Important for tooth dentine, bones, cartilage, connective tissue and blood vessels.
Symptoms of deficiency Scurvy, anaemia, swollen and bleeding gums, loose teeth, bruising (from rupture of small blood vessels).
Symptoms of toxicity Kidney stones.
Sources Citrus fruits, tomatoes, strawberries, currants, green, leafy vegetables, broccoli, cabbage, potatoes.

Recommended daily amounts (mg)

Babies and children	30–45
Subjects over 11 years	50–60
Pregnant women	70
Lactating women	90–95

Introduction This appendix gives a brief description of the System of International Units (SI UNITS) and tables of 'normal' values for the composition of body fluids and body wastes. In addition there are tables of desirable body weights according to age (infants) and height and body build (adults).

Readers should bear in mind that 'normal' values may vary, sometimes quite widely, in healthy individuals. Furthermore, the relationships between height, build and weight are flexible and should not be treated as absolute targets.

A: SI units and multiples The International System of Units (Système International) usually referred to as SI units, was introduced in the 1970s and has been expanded and developed since. Now the SI units and symbols and certain units derived from the system are used for measurements in most scientific disciplines and are an integral part of scientific language. The units comprise three classes: base units, supplementary units and derived units. The seven base units are the metre (length), kilogram (weight), second (time), ampere (electric current), kelvin (temperature), mole (amount of substance: one mole of a compound has a mass equal to its molecular weight in grams) and candela (luminous intensity). The SI units used commonly in medicine are shown below. Some traditional measurements are still used, one example being millimetres of mercury (Hg) which is the unit for blood pressure.

SI UNITS COMMONLY USED IN MEDICINE

Quantity	SI unit (abbreviation)
Length	metre (m)
Area	square metre (m²)
Volume	cubic metre (m³) = 100 litre (l or L)
Mass	kilogram (kg)
Amount of substance at molecular level	mole (mol)
Energy	joule (J)
Pressure	pascal (Pa)
Force	newton (N)
Time	second (s)
Frequency	hertz (Hz)
Power	watt (w)
Temperature	degree Celsius (°C)

MULTIPLES AND SUBMULTIPLES

Factor	Prefix	Abbreviation
10^6	mega	m
10^3	kilo	k
10^{-1}	deci	d
10^{-2}	centi	c
10^{-3}	milli	m
10^{-6}	micro	μ
10^{-9}	nano	n
10^{-12}	pico	p

B: 'Normal' body values
1 BLOOD (PLASMA, SERUM)
Biochemical values

Substance	Approximate adult range
Ammonium	24–48 μmol/l
Ascorbate	45–80 μmol/l
Base excess	0±2 mmol/l
Bicarbonate (serum)	23–29 mmol/l
Bilirubin, total (plasma)	5–17 μmol/l
Caeruloplasmin (serum)	1.5–2.9 μmol/l
Calcium (serum)	2.1–2.6 mmol/l
Carbon dioxide tension (Pco2)	4.5–6.1 kPa
β-carotene	0.9–5.6 mmol/l
Chloride (serum)	95–105 mmol/l
Cholesterol (serum)	3.9–6.5 mmol/l
Copper (serum)	13–24 mmol/l
Cortisol (plasma)	280–700 nmol/l
Creatine (serum)	15–61 μmol/l
Creatinine (serum)	62–133 μmol/l
Fibrinogen (plasma)	5.9–11.7 μmol/l
Folate (serum)	11–48 nmol/l
Glucose, fasting (serum)	3.9–6.4 mmol/l
Iron (serum)	13–31 μmol/l
Iron binding capacity, total (serum)	45–73 μmol/l
Lactate	0.6–1.8 mmol/l
Lipids, total (plasma)	4.0–10.0 g/l
Osmolality (serum)	280–295 mmol/kg
Oxygen tension (Po2)	11–14 kPa
pH	7.35–7.45
Potassium (serum)	3.5–5.0 mmol/l
Prostate specific antigens	0–4 ng/l
Protein (serum)	
total	62–82 g/l
albumin	35–55 g/l
globulin	25–35 g/l
Pyruvate	45–80 μmol/l
Sodium (serum)	135–145 mmol/l
Triglycerides (serum)	0.3–1.7 mmol/l
Urate (serum)	0.1–0.4 mmol/l
Urea (serum)	4.0–8.0 mmol/l

Haematological values

Measurement	Adult daily range
Bleeding time (Ivy)	5 minutes
Cell counts	
Erythrocytes, men	4.6–6.2 × 10 12/l
women	4.2–5.8 × 10 12/l
Leucocytes, total	4.5–11.0 × 10 9/l
Differential:	
Neutrophils	3.0–6.5 × 10 9/l
Lymphocytes	1.5–3.0 × 10 9/l
Monocytes	0.3–0.6 × 10 9/l
Eosinophils	50–300 × 10 6/l
Basophils	15–60 × 10 6/l
Platelets	150–350 × 10 9/l
Reticulocytes	25–75 × 10 9/l
Haemoglobin, men	2.2–2.8 mmol/l
	(13.5–18.0 g/dl)
women	1.9–2.5 mmol/l
	(11.5–16.0 g/dl)
Haematocrit, men	0.40–0.54
women	0.37–0.47
Mean corpuscular haemoglobin (MCH)	0.42–0.48 fmol
Mean corpuscular volume (MCV)	80–105 fl
Mean corpuscular haemoglobin concentration (MCHC)	0.32–0.36
Red cell life span (mean)	120 days

2 CEREBROSPINAL FLUID

Measurement	Approximate adult range
Cells	5 μl; all mononuclear
Chloride	120–130 mmol/l
Glucose	2.8–4.2 mmol/l
Pressure	70–180 mm water
Protein, total	0.2–0.5 g/l
IgG	0.14 of total protein

3 FAECES

Measurement	Approximate adult range
Bulk	100–200 g/24 hours
Dry matter	23–32 g/24 hours
Fat, total	6.0 g/24 hours
Nitrogen, total	2.0 g/24 hours
Urobilinogen	40–280 mg/24 hours
Water	0.65 g/24 hours

4 URINE

Measurement	Approximate adult range
Albumin	0.2–1.5 μmol/24 hours
Calcium	2.5–7.5 mmol/24 hours
Catecholamines (adrenalin)	55 nmol/24 hours
Chloride	110–250 mmol/24 hours
Copper	0.8 μmol/24 hours
Creatine, men	300 μmol/24 hours
women	700 μmol/24 hours
Creatinine	9–17 mmol/24 hours
Glucose	11 mmol/l
Magnesium	3.0–4.5 mmol/24 hours
Osmolality	38–1400 mmol/kg water
pH	4.6–8.0
Phosphorus (inorganic)	20–45 mmol/24 hours
Porphyrins:	
Coproporphyrin	77–380 nmol/24 hours
Uroporphyrin	12–36 nmol/24 hours
Potassium	25–100 mmol/24 hours
Protein	10–150 mg/24 hours
Sodium	130–260 mmol/24 hours
Urate	1.2–3.0 mmol/24 hours

5 TEMPERATURE

Normal, adults	36.6–37.2 °C
children	36.5–37.5 °C
infants	37.5–38.5 °C
Hyperpyrexia (q.v.)	41.6 °C
Hypothermia (q.v.)	35.0 °C

NB The temperature in the axilla or groin is about 0.5 °C lower, and in the rectum about 0.5 °C higher, than the oral temperature.

C: Desirable body weights and heights

1 CHILDREN, BIRTH TO 5 YEARS, SEXES COMBINED

Age	Standard weight (kg)	Standard height (cm)
0 (birth)	3.4	55
1 month	4.3	
2 months	5.0	
3 months	5.7	60
4 months	6.3	
5 months	6.9	
6 months	7.4	65
8 months	8.4	
10 months	9.3	
12 months	9.9	75
18 months	11.3	80
2 years	12.4	85
3 years	14.5	95
4 years	16.5	100
5 years	18.4	105

2 ADULTS, ACCORDING TO HEIGHT AND BUILD

Men				Women			
Height	Build (weight in kg)			Height	Build (weight in kg)		
(m)	Small	Medium	Large	(m)	Small	Medium	Large
1.550	50.8–54.4	53.5–58.5	57.2–64.0	1.425	41.7–44.5	43.5–48.5	47.2–54.0
1.575	52.2–55.8	54.9–60.3	58.5–65.3	1.450	42.6–45.8	44.5–49.9	48.1–55.3
1.600	53.5–57.2	56.2–61.7	59.9–67.1	1.475	43.5–47.2	45.8–51.3	49.4–56.7
1.625	54.9–58.5	57.6–63.0	61.2–68.9	1.500	44.9–48.5	47.2–52.6	50.8–58.1
1.650	56.2–60.3	59.0–64.9	62.6–70.8	1.525	46.3–49.9	48.5–54.0	52.2–59.4
1.675	58.1–62.1	60.8–66.7	64.4–73.0	1.550	47.6–51.3	49.9–55.3	53.5–60.8
1.700	59.9–64.0	62.6–68.9	66.7–75.3	1.575	49.0–52.6	51.3–57.2	54.9–62.6
1.725	61.7–65.8	64.4–70.8	68.5–77.1	1.600	50.3–54.0	52.6–59.0	56.7–64.4
1.750	63.5–68.0	66.2–72.6	70.3–78.9	1.625	51.7–55.8	54.4–61.2	58.5–66.2
1.775	65.3–69.9	68.0–74.8	72.1–81.2	1.650	53.5–57.7	56.2–63.0	60.3–68.0
1.800	67.1–71.7	69.9–77.1	74.4–83.5	1.675	55.3–59.4	58.1–64.9	62.1–69.9
1.825	68.9–73.5	71.7–79.4	76.2–85.7	1.700	57.2–61.2	59.9–66.7	64.0–71.7
1.850	70.8–75.7	73.5–81.6	78.5–88.0	1.725	59.0–63.5	61.7–68.5	65.8–73.9
1.875	72.6–77.6	75.7–83.9	80.7–90.3	1.750	60.8–65.3	63.5–70.3	67.6–76.2
1.900	74.4–79.4	78.0–86.2	82.6–92.5	1.775	62.6–67.1	65.3–72.1	69.4–78.5

An individual assessment of a person's size can be made by using the BODY MASS INDEX (BMI). (See also OBESITY.)

APPENDIX 7: STATUTORY ORGANISATIONS

Names, addresses and functions of a selection of government-funded bodies whose activities are related to the provision of health care in the United Kingdom.

AUDIT COMMISSION, 1 Vincent Square, London SW1P 2PN (020 7828 1212, website: www.auditcommission.gov.uk). Appoints auditors to local authorities, health authorities and NHS trusts and promotes studies to encourage economy, efficiency and effectiveness in the NHS and local government.

CLINICAL STANDARDS ADVISORY GROUP, Room 19, Wellington House, 133–155 Waterloo Road, London SE1 8UG (020 7972 4918). Advises health ministers and the NHS on standards of clinical care for, access to and availability of services to NHS patients

COMMITTEE ON SAFETY OF MEDICINES See MEDICINES CONTROL AGENCY.

COMMON SERVICES AGENCY FOR THE SCOTTISH HEALTH SERVICE, Trinity Park House, South Trinity Road, Edinburgh EH5 3SE (0131 552 6255, website: www.show.scot.nhs.uk). Provides the NHS in Scotland with a range of services and products as directed and ensures they are delivered to customer requirements and to defined standards of quality.

COUNCIL FOR NURSING AND MIDWIFERY (formerly UNITED KINGDOM CENTRAL COUNCIL FOR NURSING, MIDWIFERY AND HEALTH VISITING), 23 Portland Place, London W1N 4JT (020 7637 7181). A regulatory body which sets standards for education and conduct of the nursing, midwifery and health-visiting professions and maintains the professional registers.

GENERAL DENTAL COUNCIL, 37 Wimpole Street, London W1G 8DQ (020 7887 3800, e-mail: information@gdc-uk.org). Maintains a register of dentists; promotes high standards of dental education at all stages and of professional conduct among dentists. The council has disciplinary powers in respect of dentists' professional conduct.

GENERAL MEDICAL COUNCIL (GMC), Regents Place, 350 Euston Rd, London NW1 3JN (0845 357 8001, website: www.gmc-uk.org).

The GMC is the medical profession's regulatory body and also has responsibility for setting educational and ethical standards. The council is a statutory body, set up in 1858, which is responsible to the Privy Council. It has powers under the Medical (Professional Performance) Act 1995 to act in respect of doctors whose professional performance is seriously deficient. The GMC has the authority to investigate and, where appropriate, discipline doctors for professional misconduct. The council has proposed a revalidation procedure to monitor doctors' continuing professional competence during their careers.

GENERAL OPTICAL COUNCIL, 41 Harley Street, London W1N 2DJ (020 7580 3898, website: www.optical.org). Registers and regulates the professions of ophthalmic opticians and dispensing opticians.

HEALTH AND SAFETY COMMISSION AND HEALTH AND SAFETY EXECUTIVE (HSE), Rose Court, 2 Southwark Bridge, London SE1 9HS (020 7717 6000, information line: 08701 545500, fax: 020 717 6717, website: www.hse.gov.uk, e-mail: hseinformationservices@ natbrit.com). Both these bodies are dedicated to securing the health, safety and welfare of persons at work and to protect the public generally against risks to health or safety arising from work activities. The HSE has powers to inspect the health and safety arrangements of organisations and, where these fail to meet statutory requirements or where accidents have occurred, it can investigate and prosecute offenders.

HEALTHCARE COMMISSION, Finsbury Tower 103–5 Bunhill Row, London EC1Y 8TG (020 7448 9200, website: www.healthcarecommission.org.uk). A statutory body set up in 1999 and accountable to the Secretary of State for Health. It provides an independent guarantee that systems are in place to monitor and improve clinical standards in general practice, community services and hospitals. The commission provides national leadership to develop and disseminate clinical governance principles and to monitor local arrangements. It comprises 14 members (including a chairman) and these include health professionals and academics, along with eight lay members. The commission's activities cover England and Wales; Scotland's equivalent to the HCC is the Clinical Standards Board.

HEALTH DEVELOPMENT AGENCY (HDA), Trevelyan House, 30 Great Peter Street, London SW1P 2HW (020 7222 5300, fax: 020 7413 8900, website: www.hda-online.org.uk, e-mail: hda.enquirydesk@hda-online.org.uk).

HEALTH PROFESSIONS COUNCIL (FORMERLY COUNCIL FOR PROFESSIONS SUPPLEMENTARY TO MEDICINE), Park House, 184 Kennington Park Road, London SE11 4BU (020 7582 0866, website: www.hpc-uk.org.com). Supervises the professional education and discipline in chiropody, dietetics, medical laboratory sciences, occupational therapy, orthoptics, physiotherapy and radiography.

HEALTH SERVICE COMMISSIONER FOR ENGLAND (OMBUDSMAN), 11th Floor, Millbank Tower, Millbank, London SW1P 4QP (020 7217 4051, fax: 020 7217 4000, website: www.ombudsman.org.uk, e-mail: OHSC.Enquiries@ombudsman.gsi.gov.uk). Appointed by the government, the Commissioner investigates complaints about services provided under the NHS and presents regular reports to Parliament.

HUMAN FERTILISATION AND EMBRYOLOGY AUTHORITY, Paxton House, 30 Artillery Lane, London E1 7LS (020 7377 5077, website: www.hfea.gov.uk). A government licensing body concerned with storage of human gametes (sperm and eggs) and embryos, research on human embryos, and any infertility treatment which involves the use of donated gametes or embryos created outside the body.

MEDICAL RESEARCH COUNCIL (MRC), 20 Park Crescent, London W1N 4AL (020 7636 5422, website: www.mrc.ac.uk). The MRC's main objectives are to promote the balanced development of medical and related biological research so as to improve health care. It employs its own research staff in more than 40 research establishments, and also provides grants to individual scientists.

MEDICINES COMMISSION   See MEDICINES CONTROL AGENCY.

MEDICINES CONTROL AGENCY (MCA), Market Towers, Nine Elms Lane, London SW8 5NQ (020 7273 0393, website: www.mca.gov.uk). The MCA is an executive agency of the Department of Health. Its main function is to safeguard public health by ensuring that branded and non-branded human medicines in the UK meet appropriate criteria of safety, quality and efficiency. It applies standards laid down in the Medicines Act of 1968 and by European Community legislation. The agency seeks advice from expert professional committees such as the Committee on Safety of Medicines and the Medicines Commission, both statutory committees based at the same address as the MCA. The MCA operates the Yellow Card reporting scheme for adverse reactions to drugs.

MENTAL HEALTH ACT COMMISSION, Maid Marian House, 56 Houndsgate, Nottingham NG1 6BG (0115 943 7100, fax: 0115 943 7001, website: www.mhac.trent.nhs.uk, e-mail: chief.exec@mhac.trent.nhs.uk). Set up in 1983 as a special health authority, the commission is responsible for protecting the interests of patients detained in England and Wales under the Act. Scotland and Northern Ireland have separate legislation.

MENTAL WELFARE COMMISSION FOR SCOTLAND, Argyle House, 3 Lady Lawson Street, Edinburgh EH3 9SH (0131 222 6111, website: www.mwcscots.org.uk). This body has similar responsibilities in Scotland to those of the Mental Health Act Commission in England and Wales (see above).

NATIONAL AUDIT OFFICE (NAO), 157–197 Buckingham Palace Road, Victoria, London SW1W 9SP (020 7798 7000, website: www.nao.gov.uk). The NAO audits public expenditure and is accountable to Parliament that money is spent for the purpose intended by Parliament and is properly accounted for.

NATIONAL BLOOD AUTHORITY (NBA), Oak House, Reeds Crescent, Watford, Herts. WD1 1QH (01923 486800, fax: 01923 486801, website: www.blood.co.uk). Created in 1993 to manage all NHS blood services, the NBA manages 15 regional transfusion services. Its objectives are to maintain blood and blood-product supply, based on a system of two million voluntary donors; and to ensure a safe, high-quality, cost-effective supply of blood and blood products for national needs.

NATIONAL INFECTION CONTROL AND HEALTH PROTECTION AGENCY   See entry in main dictionary.

NATIONAL INSTITUTE FOR CLINICAL EXCELLENCE (NICE), 90 Long Acre, Covent Garden,

London WC2E 9RZ (020 7849 3444, website: www.nice.org.uk). A special NHS health authority which produces guidelines for clinical treatments in hospitals and general practice based on scientific evidence. It appraises new and existing technologies and promotes clinical audit and confidential inquiries into clinical practices in the NHS. As well as a chairman, seven non-executive directors and four executives, NICE has a partners' council comprising representatives from patient and care groups, the health professions, NHS interests and health-care industries.

NATIONAL RADIOLOGICAL PROTECTION BOARD, Chilton, Didcot, Oxfordshire OX11 0RQ (01235 831600, website: www.nrpb.org.uk). An independent government body which acts as the national point of authoritative reference for radiological protection.

NORTHERN IRELAND CENTRAL SERVICES AGENCY FOR THE HEALTH AND SOCIAL SERVICES, 25–27 Adelaide Street, Belfast BT2 8FH (02890 324431). Offers a range of services to GPs and the four health and social-services boards.

PRESCRIPTION PRICING AUTHORITY, Bridge House, 152 Pilgrim Street, Newcastle upon Tyne NE1 2SN (0191 232 5371, website: www.ppa.org.uk). The authority's main functions are to calculate and make payments to dispensing pharmacists and doctors in England for NHS prescriptions, and to provide information on prescribing and dispensing to NHS GPs and NHS authorities.

PUBLIC HEALTH LABORATORY SERVICE (PHLS), Headquarters Office, 61 Colindale Avenue, London NW9 5DF (020 8200 1295, website: www.phls.co.uk). The PHLS co-operates with the NHS to provide national facilities for the diagnosis, prevention and control of infectious and communicable diseases. The network of 50

laboratories in England and Wales is led by the headquarters complex at Colindale, where the Central Public Health Laboratory and Communicable Disease Surveillance Centre is sited.

STANDING MEDICAL ADVISORY COMMITTEE, Department of Health, Room 919, Wellington House, 135–155 Waterloo Road, London SE1 8UG (020 7972 4919); STANDING NURSING AND MIDWIFERY ADVISORY COMMITTEE, Department of Health, Room 919, Wellington House, 135–155 Waterloo Road, London SE1 8UG (020 7972 4919); and STANDING PHARMACEUTICAL ADVISORY COMMITTEE, Department of Health, Room 301, Richmond House, 79 Whitehall, London SW1A 2NS (020 7210 5117). The three standing advisory committees advise health ministers in England and Wales on matters relating to medicine, nursing, midwifery and pharmaceutical services.

STANDING COMMITTEE ON POSTGRADUATE MEDICAL AND DENTAL EDUCATION (SCOPME), One Park Square West, London NW1 4IJ (020 7935 3916). There are separate councils for Scotland, Wales and Northern Ireland. Advises the secretary of state on the delivery of postgraduate and continuing medical and dental education.

UNITED KINGDOM CENTRAL COUNCIL FOR NURSING, MIDWIFERY AND HEALTH VISITING See COUNCIL FOR NURSING AND MIDWIFERY.

UNITED KINGDOM TRANSPLANT SUPPORT SERVICE AUTHORITY, Fox Den Road, Stoke Gifford, Bristol BS12 6RR (0117 975 7575, website: www.uktransplant.org.uk). A special health authority providing a support service for the matching, allocating and distribution of donor organs for transplant.

YELLOW CARD SCHEME See MEDICINES CONTROL AGENCY.

APPENDIX 8: PROFESSIONAL ORGANISATIONS

A selection of health-related non-statutory professional organisations.

Specialist organisations of the medical profession

The royal colleges and faculties in the list that follows represent the range of recognised specialties in medicine in the United Kingdom. They are responsible for setting the criteria for specialist training; for approving and monitoring training posts in the NHS; for organising appropriate specialist examinations; and for admitting successful candidates to membership or fellowship of the relevant institution. This enables doctors to be registered with the General Medical Council as specialists. Representatives of the colleges and faculties join with representatives of hospital doctors in the British Medical Association and the British Dental Association to form the Joint Consultants Committee. This Committee meets regularly with ministers and officials from the UK's health departments and NHS management to discuss the provision and standards of NHS specialist care along with the postgraduate educational requirements of NHS doctors.

The royal colleges and faculties also have an umbrella organisation called the Academy of Medical Colleges (1 Wimpole Street, London W1M 8AE [020 7290 3913]). The academy protects and preserves health and the relief of sickness by supporting, promoting and coordinating the work of the medical royal colleges, offering a forum for discussion and collaboration.

ACADEMY OF MEDICAL COLLEGES (see above).

ROYAL COLLEGE OF ANAESTHETISTS, 48–49 Russell Square, London WC1B 4JP (020 7813 1900, website: www.rcoa.ac.uk).

ROYAL COLLEGE OF GENERAL PRACTITIONERS, 14 Prince's Gate, London SW7 1PU (020 7581 3232, website: www.rcgp.org.uk, e-mail: info@rcgp.org.uk).

ROYAL COLLEGE OF OBSTETRICIANS AND GYNAE-COLOGISTS, 27 Sussex Place, Regent's Park, London NW1 4RG (020 7772 6200, website: www.rcog.org.uk, e-mail: coll.sec@rcog.org.uk).

ROYAL COLLEGE OF OPHTHALMOLOGISTS, 17 Cornwall Terrace, London NW1 4QW (020 7935 0702, website: www.rcopth.ac.uk).

ROYAL COLLEGE OF PAEDIATRICS AND CHILD HEALTH, 50 Hallam Street, London W1W 6DE (020 7307 5600, website: www.rcpch.ac.uk).

ROYAL COLLEGE OF PATHOLOGISTS, 2 Carlton House Terrace, London SW1Y 5AF (020 7451 6700, website: www.rcpath.org, e-mail: info@rcpath.org).

ROYAL COLLEGE OF PHYSICIANS, 11 St Andrews Place, London NW1 4LE (020 7935 1174, website: www.rcplondon.ac.uk).

ROYAL COLLEGE OF PHYSICIANS OF EDINBURGH, 9 Queen Street, Edinburgh EH2 1JQ (0131 225 7324, website: www.rcpe.ac.uk).

ROYAL COLLEGE OF PHYSICIANS AND SURGEONS OF GLASGOW, 234–242 St Vincent Street, Glasgow G2 5RJ (0141 221 6072, website: www.rcpsglasg.ac.uk).

ROYAL COLLEGE OF PHYSICIANS OF IRELAND, 6 Kildare Street, Dublin 2 (00353 1 6616677, website: www.rcpi.ie).

ROYAL COLLEGE OF PSYCHIATRISTS, 17 Belgrave Square, London SW1X 8PG (020 7235 2351, website: www.rcpsych.ac.uk, e-mail: awoolf@rcpsych.ac.uk).

ROYAL COLLEGE OF RADIOLOGISTS, 38 Portland Place, London W1N 3DG (020 7636 4432, website: www.rcr.ac.uk/enquiries, e-mail: enquiries@rcr.ac.uk).

ROYAL COLLEGE OF SURGEONS OF EDINBURGH, 18 Nicolson Street, Edinburgh EH8 9DW (0131 556 6206, website: www.rcsed.ac.uk, e-mail: information@rcsed.ac.uk).

ROYAL COLLEGE OF SURGEONS OF ENGLAND, 35–43 Lincoln's Inn Fields, London WC2A 3PN (020 7405 3474, website: www.rcseng.ac.uk).

ROYAL COLLEGE OF SURGEONS OF IRELAND, 123 St Stephen's Green, Dublin 2 (00353 1 4022100, website: www.rcsi.ie).

FACULTY OF OCCUPATIONAL MEDICINE, 6 St Andrews Place, Regent's Park, London NW1 4LE (020 7487 3414).

FACULTY OF PHARMACEUTICAL MEDICINE, 1 St Andrews Place, Regent's Park, London NW1 4LB (020 7224 0343, website: www.fpm. org.uk, e-mail: fpm@f-pharm.med.org.uk).

FACULTY OF PUBLIC HEALTH MEDICINE, 4 St Andrews Place, London NW1 4LB (020 7935 0243, website: www.fester.his.path.cam. ac.uk/ health/fphm.htm, e-mail: enquiries@fphm. ac.uk).

Voluntary organisations BRITISH MEDICAL ASSOCIATION, BMA House, Tavistock Square, London WC1H 9JP (020 7387 4499, website: www.bma.org.uk). The BMA is a voluntary professional association of doctors from all branches of medicine, with more than 80 per cent of practising doctors in the UK in membership. It is a scientific and educational body, an independent trade union and a publishing house.

BRITISH DENTAL ASSOCIATION, 64 Wimpole Street, London W1M 8AL (020 7935 0875, website: www.bda-dentistry.org.uk, e-mail: enquiries@bda-dentistry.org.uk). A voluntary professional body representing the dental profession; it also has scientific and educational responsibilities.

CHARTERED SOCIETY OF PHYSIOTHERAPY, 14 Bedford Row, London WC1R 4ED (020 7306 6666, fax: 020 7306 6611, website: www.csp.org.uk, e-mail: pr@csphysio.org.uk). The professional and educational body and trade union for chartered physiotherapists.

COLLEGE OF HEALTH-CARE CHAPLAINS, Registrar: Mr C. Webber, 49 Chesterton Park, Cirencester, Gloucestershire GL7 1XS (01285 643660, e-mail: cjw@dialin.net). Provides educational opportunities for health-care chaplains, sets and maintains high standards of chaplaincy and provides support through a regional branch structure.

THE COLLEGE OF OPTOMETRISTS, 42 Craven Street, London WC2N 5NG (020 7839 6000, website: www.college-optometrists.org, e-mail: optometry@college-optometrists.org). Members of the college have passed its qualifying examination and met its training requirements. The college's aims are to improve and conserve human vision, to study and research ophthalmic optics and to maintain high professional standards and competence.

MEDICAL WOMEN'S FEDERATION, Tavistock House North, Tavistock Square, London WC1H 9HX (020 7387 7765). The federation promotes equal opportunities for women doctors and patients through a network of local associations in the UK. Membership is open to women doctors and medical students, and the federation organises local and national seminars and conferences.

NHS CONFEDERATION, 1 Warwick Row, London SW1E 5ER (020 7959 7272, website: www.nhsconfed.net). The NHS Confederation is a representative organisation with more than 500 trusts, health authorities and health boards as members.

ROYAL COLLEGE OF MIDWIVES, 15 Mansfield Street, London W1M 0BE (020 7872 5100, website: www.rcm.org.uk). A professional organisation, educational trust and trade union for midwives.

ROYAL COLLEGE OF NURSING OF THE UNITED KINGDOM (RCN), 20 Cavendish Square, London W1M 9AE (020 7409 3333, website: www.rcn.org.uk). The RCN is the voluntary professional association for registered, student and pupil nurses, midwives and health visitors. It has a worldwide membership of over 300,000. The college promotes the science and art of nursing, the training of nurses and the professional standing and interests of members and the profession. It represents nurses and negotiates on their behalf with the government and other employers.

ROYAL COLLEGE OF SPEECH AND LANGUAGE THERAPISTS, 2 White Hart Yard, London SE1 1NX (020 7378 1200, fax: 020 7403 7254, website: www.rcslt.org, e-mail: postmaster-@rcslt.org). Responsible for the accreditation of courses and examinations leading to qualification to practise as a speech and language therapist and the maintenance of a register.

ROYAL PHARMACEUTICAL SOCIETY OF GREAT BRITAIN, 1 Lambeth High Street, London SE1 7JN (020 7735 9141, website: www.rpsgb. org.uk). A professional body, promoting pharmaceutical education and science and the interests of its members.

ROYAL SOCIETY OF MEDICINE (RSM), 1 Wimpole Street, London W1M 8AE (020 7290 2900, website: www.rsm.ac.uk). An independent, apolitical society of mainly medical members which provides a neutral forum for the exchange of views on medical, educational and other health-care issues. It also provides continuing medical education and possesses one of the most comprehensive medical libraries in the world.

THE SOCIETY OF CHIROPODISTS AND PODIATRISTS, 1 Fellmongers Path, Tower Bridge Road, London SE1 3LY (020 7234 8620, fax: 929 7234 8621, website: www.feetforlife.org, e-mail: enq@scp.org).

Medical defence bodies The three commercial institutions listed below assist doctors, dentists and other health-care professionals with complaints and negligence claims arising from clinical practice and payments of legal costs and damages. They also provide advice on medicolegal and professional problems associated with clinical practice.

MEDICAL DEFENCE UNION, 230 Blackfriars Road, SE1 8PJ (020 7202 1500, fax: 020 7202 1666, website: www.the-mdu.com, e-mail: mdu@the-mdu.com).

MEDICAL PROTECTION SOCIETY, 33 Cavendish Square, London W1G 0PS (020 7399 1300, 020 7399 1301, website: www.mps.org.uk, e-mail: info@mps.org.uk).

MEDICAL AND DENTAL DEFENCE UNION OF SCOTLAND, Mackintosh House, 120 Blythwood Street, Glasgow G2 4EA (0141 221 5858, fax: 0141 228 1208, website: www.mddus.com).

APPENDIX 9: HEALTH-POLICY RESEARCH ORGANISATIONS

This is a list of some of the bodies involved in health-policy research and consultancy; it is not exhaustive but includes those bodies that publish regularly for a national audience.

CENTRE FOR HEALTH ECONOMICS, University of York, Heslington, York YO10 5DD (01904 321401, website: www.york.ac.uk/inst/che). Director: Professor Michael Drummond. The centre specialises in health-economics research. Principal areas of research activity include economic evaluation of health technologies, outcome measurement, primary care, community care, and the determinants of health.

CENTRE FOR HEALTH SERVICES RESEARCH, University of Newcastle upon Tyne, 21 Claremont Place, Newcastle upon Tyne NE2 4AA (0191 222 7045). A multidisciplinary organisation that mainly does research aimed at improving the health status of people in Europe, the United Kingdom and North-East England. Among its research interests are health-technology assessment and effective practice and organisation of care.

CENTRE FOR POLICY ON AGEING, 25/31 Ironmonger Row, London EC1V 3QP (020 7553 6500). Director: Dr Gillian Dalley. Using research and analysis, this organisation aims to formulate better policies for older people.

HEALTH ECONOMICS RESEARCH UNIT, University of Aberdeen, Polworth Building, Foresterhill, Aberdeen AB25 2ZD (01224 553480, website: www.abdn.ac.uk/heru). The unit receives core funding from the Chief Scientist's Office of the Scottish Office Departments of Health and from competitive research grants and funding. It has two underlying aims: to develop methods within health economics; and to encourage use of the techniques of economic appraisal by clinicians and managers in the NHS. Produces regular discussion papers and undertakes consultancy in the NHS in Scotland.

HEALTH POLICY AND ECONOMIC RESEARCH UNIT, British Medical Association, BMA House, Tavistock Square, London WC1H 9JP (020 7387 4499, e-mail: hperu@bma.org.uk). Director: Jon Ford. Established in January 1994 to help the BMA make contribution to wider debates about health policy by producing briefing and discussion documents and conducting original research. The documents it produces are not BMA policy as such, and are intended to provoke debate inside and outside the association. Some work is 'commissioned' internally; otherwise it is free to determine the topics it studies.

HEALTH SERVICES MANAGEMENT CENTRE, University of Birmingham, Park House, 40 Edgbaston Road, Birmingham, B15 2RT (0121 414 7050, website: www.hmsc.bham.ac.uk). The aim of the centre is to strengthen the management of health services and so promote better health. Current areas of activity include primary-care provision and management; quality management and clinical effectiveness; priority setting and rationing, involving users and the public in health-service decision making. The centre conducts research, postgraduate programmes, courses and seminars and undertakes consultancy.

INSTITUTE FOR PUBLIC POLICY RESEARCH, 30–32 Southampton Street, London WC2E 7RA (020 7470 6100, website: www.ippr.org.uk). Independent charity whose purpose is to contribute to public understanding of social, economic and political questions through research, discussion and publications. Established to provide an alternative to the free-market think tanks.

KING'S FUND, 11–13 Cavendish Square, London W1G 0AN (020 7307 2400, website: www.kingsfund.org.uk). Chief executive: Niall Dickson. Independent charity, the original aim of which was to improve the health and health care of Londoners. It now carries out research and development, audit and education across the UK. Undertakes health-policy research and analysis, promotes good practice in health and social care, supports leadership development and offers grants to London projects. Also runs King's Fund organisational audit for hospitals. Comprehensive health-policy library open to researchers.

LSE HEALTH, London School of Economics and Political Science, Houghton Street, London WC2A 2AE (020 7955 6840, website: www.lse.ac.uk/collections/LSEHealthand SocialCare). Co-directors: Professor Elias Mossialos and Professor Martin Knapp.

Multidisciplinary research centre which brings together members of LSE academic staff from different departments working on health-policy issues. Its fundamental mission is to undertake research consultancy and training in the area of international health policy and to influence thereby international health policies.

NATIONAL PRIMARY CARE RESEARCH AND DEVELOPMENT CENTRE, University of Manchester, Williamson Building, Oxford Road, Manchester M13 9PL (0161 275 7601, website: www.npcrdc.man.ac.uk). Multidisciplinary centre which brings together academic disciplines, clinical professions and health-service managers to engage in a broad programme of policy-relevant research and to promote research-based service development in primary care.

NUFFIELD INSTITUTE FOR HEALTH, University of Leeds, 71–75 Clarendon Road, Leeds LS2 9PL (0113 343 6633, website: www.nuffield.leeds.ac.uk). Interests include health and social policy and management practice, public health, health services, research and community-care research with particular attention to needs assessment and health and social-care outcomes. Offers courses and undertakes research and consultancy.

NUFFIELD TRUST, 59 New Cavendish Street, London W1G 7LP (020 7631 8450, website: www.nuffieldtrust.org.uk). Secretary: John Wyn Owen, CB. Describes itself as an independent observer of the UK health scene and the NHS. Main areas of activity are invited meetings, workshops and seminars, publications, a grant programme and fellowships. Activities currently include an investigation of policy futures for UK health and work on globalisation and devolution.

OFFICE OF HEALTH ECONOMICS, 12 Whitehall, London SW1A 2DY (020 7930 9203, website: www.ohe.org). Director: Adrian Towse. Supported from an annual grant from the Association of the British Pharmaceutical Industry. Its terms of reference are to commission and undertake research on the economics of health and health care; to collect and analyse health and health-care data from the UK and other countries; and to disseminate the results of this work and stimulate discussion of them and their policy implications. Publishes on a regular basis a comprehensive compendium of UK health statistics.

POLICY STUDIES INSTITUTE, 100 Park Village East, London NW1 3SR (020 7468 0468, website: www.psi.org.uk). Director: Malcolm Rigg. Independent research organisation undertaking studies of social and economic policy. A registered charity and, since January 1998, a wholly owned subsidiary company of the University of Westminster. Among areas of interest in health-related research are doctors' careers.